Activity intolerance
Activity intolerance, high risk for
Adjustment, impaired
Airway clearance, ineffective
Anxiety
Aspiration, high risk for
Body image disturbance
Body temperature, altered, high risk for
Breastfeeding, effective
Breastfeeding, ineffective
Breastfeeding, interrupted
Breathing pattern, ineffective
Cardiac output, decreased
Caregiver role strain
Caregiver role strain, high risk for
Communication, impaired verbal
Constipation
Constipation, colonic
Constipation, perceived
Coping, defensive
Coping, family: potential for growth
Coping, ineffective family: compromised
Coping, ineffective family, disabling
Coping, ineffective individual
Decisional conflict (specify)
Denial, ineffective
Diarrhea
Disuse syndrome, high risk for
Diversional activity deficit
Dysreflexia
Family processes, altered
Fatigue
Fear
Fluid volume deficit (1)
Fluid volume deficit (2)
Fluid volume deficit, high risk for
Fluid volume excess
Gas exchange, impaired
Grieving, anticipatory
Grieving, dysfunctional
Growth and development, altered
Health maintenance, altered
Health-seeking behaviors (specify)
Home maintenance management, impaired
Hopelessness
Hyperthermia
Hypothermia
Incontinence, bowel
Incontinence, functional
Incontinence, reflex
Incontinence, stress
Incontinence, total
Incontinence, urge
Infant feeding pattern, ineffective
Infection, high risk for
Injury, high risk for
Knowledge deficit (specify)

Mobility, impaired phy
Noncompliance (specify)
Nutrition, altered: less than body requirements
Nutrition, altered: more than body requirements
Nutrition, altered: high risk for more than body
   requirements
Oral mucous membrane, altered
Pain
Pain, chronic
Parental role conflict
Parenting, altered
Parenting, altered, high risk for
Peripheral neurovascular dysfunction, high risk for
Personal identity disturbance
Poisoning, high risk for
Post-trauma response
Powerlessness
Protection, altered
Rape-trauma syndrome
Rape-trauma syndrome, compound reaction
Rape-trauma syndrome, silent reaction
Role performance, altered
Self-care deficit, bathing/hygiene
Self-care deficit, dressing/grooming
Self-care deficit, feeding
Self-care deficit, toileting
Self-esteem disturbance
Self-esteem, chronic low
Self-esteem, situational low
Self-mutilation, high risk for
Sensory/perceptual alterations (specify) (visual, auditory,
   kinesthetic, gustatory, tactile, olfactory)
Sexual dysfunction
Sexuality patterns, altered
Skin integrity, impaired
Skin integrity, impaired, high risk for
Sleep pattern disturbance
Social interaction, impaired
Social isolation
Spiritual distress (distress of the human spirit)
Stress syndrome, relocation
Suffocation, high risk for
Swallowing, impaired
Therapeutic regimen (individual), ineffective
   management of
Thermoregulation, ineffective
Thought processes, altered
Tissue integrity, impaired
Tissue perfusion, altered (specify type) (renal, cerebral,
   cardiopulmonary, gastrointestinal, peripheral)
Trauma, high risk for
Unilateral neglect
Urinary elimination, altered patterns
Urinary retention
Ventilation, inability to sustain spontaneous
Ventilatory weaning response, dysfunctional (DVWR)
Violence, high risk for: self-directed or directed at others

MENTAL HEALTH—
PSYCHIATRIC NURS

A Holistic Life-Cycle Approach

MENTAL HEALTH– PSYCHIATRIC NURSING
A Holistic Life-Cycle Approach

THIRD EDITION

EDITED BY

Ruth Parmelee Rawlins, RN, DSN, CS
Associate Professor, School of Nursing,
University of Central Arkansas,
Conway, Arkansas

Sophronia R Williams, RN MSN
Associate Professor, College of Nursing,
University of Arkansas for Medical Sciences,
Little Rock, Arkansas

Cornelia Kelly Beck, RN, PhD
Professor and Associate Dean for Research and Evaluation, College of Nursing;
Assistant Professor, Department of Psychiatry and Behavioral Sciences,
College of Medicine,
University of Arkansas for Medical Sciences,
Little Rock, Arkansas

illustrated

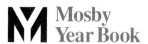

Mosby
Year Book

St. Louis Baltimore Boston Chicago London Philadelphia Sydney Toronto

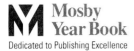

Mosby
Year Book
Dedicated to Publishing Excellence

Executive Editor: Linda L Duncan
Developmental Editor: Teri Merchant
Project Manager: Karen Edwards
Production Editor: Amy Adams Squire Strongheart
Designer: Jeanne Wolfgeher

Cover Photograph: © David Bishop/PHOTOTAKE, NYC

Third Edition
Copyright © 1993 by Mosby–Year Book, Inc.
A Mosby imprint of Mosby–Year Book, Inc.

Previous editions copyrighted 1984, 1988

Printed in the United States of America

Mosby–Year Book, Inc.
11830 Westline Industrial Drive
St. Louis, Missouri 63146

Library of Congress Cataloging in Publication Data

Mental health–pyschiatric nursing : a holistic life-cycle approach /
    edited by Ruth Parmelee Rawlins, Sophronia R. Williams, Cornelia
    Kelly Beck.—3rd ed.

        p.   cm.
        Includes bibliographical references and index.
        ISBN 0-8016-6331-8
        1. Psychiatric nursing.   2.   Holistic nursing.   I.   Rawlins, Ruth
    Parmelee.   II.   Williams, Sophronia R.   III.   Beck, Cornelia Kelly.
        [DNLM: 1.   Holistic Health—nurses' instruction.   2.   Mental
    Disorders—nursing.   3.   Psychiatric Nursing.   WY 160 M549]
    RC440.M355   1992
    610.73'68—dc20
    DNLM/DLC
    for Library of Congress   92-49347
                                               CIP

93   94   95   96   97   GW/VH/VH   9   8   7   6   5   4   3   2   1

To Hildegard E Peplau

- A PIONEER in psychiatric nursing who prepared the way for others in the field

- A SCHOLAR who significantly contributed to the theoretical bases for the practice of psychiatric nursing

- A MENTOR who generously shared her knowledge so that others might benefit from her wisdom

- An INSPIRATION as she influences future directions in psychiatric nursing education and practice

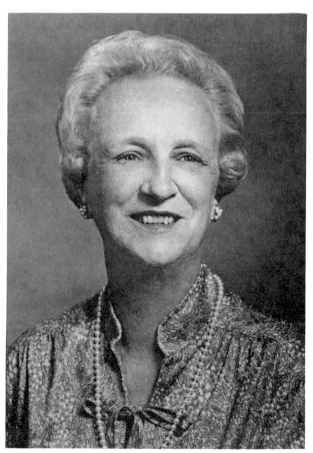

Hildegard E. Peplau

Contributors

Ann Adams, RN, MNSc
Private Practice
Eureka Springs, Arkansas
Clinical Specialist, St. John's Adolescent Treatment Center
Springfield, Missouri

Bertram Bandman, PhD
Professor of Philosophy,
Long Island University, Brooklyn Campus
Brooklyn, New York

Elsie L Bandman, RN, EdD, FAAN
Professor Emeritus and Adjunct Professor,
Hunter-Bellevue School of Nursing,
Hunter College of the City University of New York,
New York, New York

Margaret T Beard, BA, MS, PhD
Professor, College of Nursing,
Texas Woman's University
Denton, Texas

Cornelia Kelly Beck, RN, PhD
Professor and Associate Dean for Research and Evaluation, College
    of Nursing;
Assistant Professor, Department of Psychiatry and Behavioral
    Sciences, College of Medicine,
University of Arkansas for Medical Sciences
Little Rock, Arkansas

Doris E Bell, RN, PhD
Professor of Nursing, School of Nursing,
Southern Illinois University at Edwardsville,
Edwardsville, Illinois

Virginia Trotter Betts, MSN, JD
Senior Research Associate and Research Associate Professor of
    Human Resources,
Vanderbilt Institute for Public Policy Studies;
President, HealthFutures, Inc.
Nashville, Tennessee

Elizabeth B Brophy, RN, PhD
Associate Professor, Niehoff School of Nursing,
Loyola University of Chicago,
Chicago, Illinois

Margery Menges Chisholm, RN, EdD, CS
Associate Professor, Northeastern University;
Lecturer in Psychiatry, Harvard University;
Professor Emeritus, Boston University,
Boston, Massachusetts

Patricia Ann Clunn, EdD, ARNP, CS
Professor, University of Miami School of Nursing,
Miami, Florida

Jackie Coombe-Moore, RN, MNSc, MD
University of Arkansas for Medical Sciences,
Little Rock, Arkansas

Virginia K Drake, RN, DNSc, CS
Psychotherapist in Private Practice,
Vienna, Virginia

Nancy Kowal Ellis, RN, MS
Worcester, Massachusetts

Rauda Salkauskas Gelazis, RN, PhC
Doctoral Candidate, Wayne State University,
Detroit, Michigan;
Associate Professor, Ursuline College,
Pepper Pike, Ohio

Laina M Gerace, RN, PhD
Assistant Professor, Psychiatric Nursing,
University of Illinois at Chicago,
Chicago, Illinois

Lynne Goodykoontz, RN, PhD, CNAA
Dean and Professor, School of Nursing,
The University of North Carolina at Greensboro,
Greensboro, North Carolina

James L Harris, RN, DSN, CS
Associate Chief, Nursing Service for Education,
Veterans Administration Medical Center,
Durham, North Carolina

Diane M Hedler, RN, MS
Consultant, Regional Accreditation and Regulation,
Kaiser Permanente, Northern California,
Oakland, California

Nancy L Hedlund, RN, PhD
Associate Researcher, Cancer Research Center of Hawaii;
Associate Professor, School of Nursing
University of Hawaii,
Honolulu, Hawaii

Sharon K Holmberg, RN, MSN
Doctoral Student, University of Rochester School of Nursing;
Nurse Clinical Specialist, St. John's Home,
Rochester, New York

Ann P Hutton, RN, MS
Assistant Professor, College of Nursing,
University of Utah,
Salt Lake City, Utah

Finis Breckenridge Jeffrey, MA
Instructor of History, Chaminade University,
Research Analyst, United States Pacific Command,
Honolulu, Hawaii

Margie N Johnson, RN, PhD
Dean, School of Nursing and Allied Health,
Tuskegee University,
Tuskegee, Alabama

Virginia Burke Karb, RN, PhD
Assistant Dean and Associate Professor, School of Nursing,
University of North Carolina at Greensboro
Greensboro, North Carolina

Norman L Keltner, RN, EdD
Associate Professor, School of Nursing,
University of Alabama at Birmingham,
Birmingham, Alabama

Alice R Kempe, MEd, MSN
Doctoral Candidate, Wayne State University,
Detroit, Michigan;
Associate Professor, Ursuline College,
Pepper Pike, Ohio

Sydney D Krampitz, RN, PhD
Partner, Krampitz, Berry and Associates;
Director, Shift Operations, Truman Medical Center,
Kansas City, Missouri

Peggy A Landrum, RN, PhD, CS
Psychotherapist, Private Practice;
Corporate Consultant;
Adjunct Professor, Texas Woman's University,
Houston, Texas

Judith R Lentz, RN, MSN, MA
Doctoral Candidate, Rice University,
Houston, Texas;
Adjunct Instructor, St. Louis University School of Nursing
St. Louis, Missouri

Joyce Levy, RN, MS, CS
Psychiatric Clinical Nurse Specialist, Brigham and Women's
    Hospital;
Adjunct Assistant Professor, College of Nursing,
Northeastern University,
Boston, Massachusetts

Anita Lewis, RN, MS, CS
Psychiatric Liaison Nurse, Department of Nursing;
Assistant Clinical Professor, Department of Psychiatry,
Tufts University School of Medicine,
New England Medical Center Hospitals, Inc.,
Boston, Massachusetts

Eva Hester Lin, RN, MS
Psychiatric Liaison Nurse, The Cambridge Hospital,
Cambridge, Massachusetts;
Lecturer, Psychiatry, Harvard Medical School,
Boston, Massachusetts

Sonja H Lively, RN, MS
Assistant Professor, College of Nursing,
University of Iowa,
Iowa City, Iowa

Elizabeth G Maguire, RN, MSN, CS
Clinical Nurse Specialist, Acute Care and Evaluation Unit,
Central State Hospital,
Peterburg, Virginia

Susan H McCrone, RN, PhD
Assistant Professor, School of Nursing,
University of Maryland at Baltimore,
Baltimore, Maryland

Tomye J Modlin, RN, MNSc
Psychiatric Clinical Nurse Specialist,
University Hospital,
Little Rock, Arkansas

Eleanor Gilliam Moon, RN, MSN, C
Clinical Nurse Specialist/Community Liaison,
Behavioral Medicine, Alamance Health Services,
Burlington, North Carolina

Ann Mabe Newman, RNC, DSN
Assistant Professor of Nursing;
Adjunct Assistant Professor of Women's Studies,
University of North Carolina at Charlotte,
Charlotte, North Carolina

Benni S Ogden, RN, MSE
Director of Student Affairs;
Assistant Professor, College of Nursing,
University of Arkansas for Medical Sciences,
Little Rock, Arkansas

Alice R Parkinson, RN, MS
Assistant Professor, Clinical, College of Nursing,
University of Utah,
Salt Lake City, Utah

Sarah M Powell, RN, MS
Clinical Specialist/Consultant, Private Practice,
Hattiesburg, Mississippi

Ruth Parmelee Rawlins, RN, DSN, CS
Associate Professor, School of Nursing,
University of Central Arkansas,
Conway, Arkansas

Lenora Richardson, RN, DSN
Assistant Professor, School of Nursing,
University of North Carolina at Greensboro,
Greensboro, North Carolina

Ethel Rosenfeld, RN, MSE, C
Associate Professor of Nursing (Retired)
University of Central Arkansas,
Conway, Arkansas;
President, Arkansas Alliance for the Mentally Ill

Judith A Saifnia, RN, MNSc
Psychiatric Clinical Nurse Specialist;
Biofeedback Coordinator,
St. Vincent's Infirmary Medical Center,
Little Rock, Arkansas

Anne H Shealy, RN, DNS, CS
Assistant Professor, School of Nursing,
University of Alabama at Birmingham,
Birmingham, Alabama

Cathleen M Shultz, RN, PhD
Professor and Dean, School of Nursing,
Harding University,
Searcy, Arkansas

Louise Bradford Suit, RN, EdD
Professor, Harding University,
Searcy, Arkansas

Toni Tripp-Reimer, RN, PhD, FAAN
Professor and Director, Office of Nursing Research,
College of Nursing, University of Iowa,
Iowa City, Iowa

Christine Gorman Walton, RN, MNSc
Clinical Nurse Specialist, Austin State Hospital,
Austin, Texas

Sophronia R Williams, RN, MSN
Associate Professor, College of Nursing,
University of Arkansas for Medical Sciences,
Little Rock, Arkansas

Preface

The intent of the third edition of *Mental Health–Psychiatric Nursing: A Holistic Life-Cycle Approach* is to provide a basic, comprehensive nursing text that presents current content for the beginning student in mental health–psychiatric nursing. Since the basic concepts are defined behaviorally, this text is appropriate for use in either an integrated or nonintegrated curriculum. The textbook will be most meaningful for students who have a general knowledge base in anatomy, physiology, psychology, sociology, and chemistry. In addition, an understanding of the nursing process and the relationship of a philosophy and conceptual framework to nursing practice will enhance the reader's use of the text. Chapters about issues, current treatment methods, and mental health–psychiatric nursing across the life cycle may be of special interest to graduate students in mental health–psychiatric nursing and practical mental health–psychiatric nurses.

In the first and second editions of *Mental Health–Psychiatric Nursing* we integrated content essential to the practice of mental health–psychiatric nursing into a holistic approach that addressed the five dimensions of the person as an organizing framework for the nursing process. The individual's responsibility in maintaining and promoting his or her health and in participating in restoration of his or her mental health was emphasized in these earlier editions. In both editions NANDA diagnoses pertinent to mental health–psychiatric nursing, the latest research, and content on DSM-III-R classifications were integrated throughout the text.

CONTENT

This third edition retains the strengths of the previous editions, and the content has been reordered, expanded, and added to to enhance the usefulness of the text for the student. This edition is based on the same philosophy about nursing and the individual as the previous ones. To introduce the conceptual framework early in the text, The Person as a Client is now Chapter 2. We clarified the conceptual model of holistic nursing care and related philosophical positions by expanding the discussion. In keeping with the current emphasis on the biological basis for psychiatric problems, content has been added on the biological theoretical approaches.

To meet the student's need for detailed information on medical diagnoses, we expanded the discussion of the DSM-III-R classifications. The Standards of Psychiatric Mental Nursing Practice are included in the discussion of the nursing process. The 1993 NANDA diagnoses pertinent to mental health–psychiatric nursing and the latest research continue to be integrated throughout the text.

Loss and Addictive Behavior are two new chapters that have been added. In keeping with a current trend in psychiatry, content previously discussed as psychophysiological disorders has been revised and discussed behaviorally in Chapter 19, entitled Somatization.

ORGANIZATION

Mental Health–Psychiatric Nursing continues to be divided into five parts. Part I is concerned with the foundations for the practice of mental health–psychiatric nursing. Included in this focus is an examination of (1) the historical evolution of psychiatric nursing and (2) the conceptual base for practice and selected philosophical positions about the nature of the person and the relationship of these positions to an understanding of mental health and illness. Theoretical approaches that contribute to the development of frameworks for mental health–psychiatric nursing are explored, including the work of nursing theorists. The organizing theme of Part I is a holistic approach to the individual within the five dimensions.

Part I also views the nursing process in mental health–psychiatric nursing as focusing on (1) basic communication, (2) the establishment of a therapeutic relationship, and (3) cultural diversity in therapy. Skills and attitudes basic to this process are interwoven throughout the discussion. The five dimensions of the person are viewed as a basis for the effective use of self in developing a therapeutic relationship characterized by self-responsibility and advocacy. A detailed discussion of communication is included.

Part II focuses on the concepts that are basic to human functioning in health and illness throughout the life cycle. The concepts presented are anxiety, anger, guilt, loss, hope-hopelessness, flexibility-rigidity, dependence-independence, trust-mistrust, addictive behaviors, somatization, pain, loneliness, boredom, and manipulation. We have added a box highlighting medical and nursing diagnoses characteristic of the behavioral concept. Selected medication monographs have been added to the pharmacological therapy sections. Each chapter begins with a discussion of the dynamics of these behaviors within the five dimensions of the individual. Based on an organizing framework of the five dimensions, the steps in the nursing process are discussed, with specific nursing interventions strengthened. Key interventions highlighted, and guidelines for primary/tertiary prevention listed. Each chapter includes a therapeutic interaction that exemplifies the concept. Current research related to each concept and instruments for measuring related behaviors are included.

Part III presents a description of specific treatment methods designed for health promotion, maintenance, and restoration. Chapter 24, Psychotropic Medications, has been updated to include the new antidepressants. Chapter 26, Community Mental Health Nursing, has been completely revised, with new sections on AIDS, homelessness, rural populations, the elderly, and the abused. Milieu therapy; crisis intervention; and group, family, and couples therapy are also discussed. Part III concludes with chapters on therapy with clients with eating disorders and with clients who are chronically mentally ill, who have dementia, and who are victims of abuse.

In Part IV concepts and principles of mental health–psychiatric nursing are applied to the care of clients across the life cycle. The various periods of life discussed are infancy; childhood; adolescence; and the young, middle, and aged adult years. For each life period, content essential to using the nursing process is presented. In addition, specific nursing interventions for mental health–psychiatric nursing are discussed for each stage of life.

An exploration of issues that are basic to the practice of mental health–psychiatric nursing in today's society is the focus of Part V. Value clarification and ethical principles are provided as bases for making decisions about professional practice issues. The chapter on legal issues includes a discussion of laws that have relevance for mental health–psychiatric nursing, the role of the nurse as a client advocate, and the responsibility of the nurse in effecting mental health care legislation. Issues and suggestions regarding research and various aspects of quality assurance, including credentialing, are also presented. The book concludes with a chapter on consultation liaison nursing.

FEATURES

The manner in which content is structured is a study aid to reinforce the student's orientation to a holistic, conceptual approach to mental health–psychiatric nursing.

As in the first and second editions, we have begun each chapter with a list of student **learning objectives.** Within each chapter we have continued to highlight important concepts and information in tabular, boxed, or illustrative form. These include nursing diagnoses, DSM-III-R classifications, and psychopharmacological considerations. Many new **case examples** and **research highlights** have been included to facilitate understanding of clinical application. **Nursing care plans** for common problems are also featured.

The text is also extensively cross-referenced for easy location of selected topics. The inside covers contain separate listings of where specific **nursing diagnoses, DSM-III-R diagnoses,** and discussions of **personality disorders** can be found in text. We have retained the glossary to familiarize students with key terms, which are italicized in text.

Because a thorough understanding of mental health–psychiatric nursing in its current state is facilitated by viewing its substance and issues within a historical perspective, each chapter contains a **historical overview.**

TERMINOLOGY AND LANGUAGE

The term *client* instead of *patient,* the traditional term used in medicine, is used in this text in keeping with the current thinking that health care consumers have rights, responsibilities, and a participatory role in their care. "Patient" denotes a subservient or dependent position in relation to the caregiver and may imply that the consumer is passive, without responsibility, and subordinate to the caregiver. The term *client* suggests a reciprocal relationship between consumer and caregiver.

We have attempted to delete evidence of sexism in the language of this textbook. However, this has not always been possible. Therefore for clarity the client is referred to as "he," and the nurse is referred to as "she." No slight is intended to the growing numbers of men in nursing.

ACKNOWLEDGMENTS

We greatly appreciate the expertise of the authors contributing chapters to this text. Without their continued efforts, a project of this magnitude would have been many years in the making. We also wish to thank the instructors, students, and clinicians who reviewed the third edition or who offered valuable comments and suggestions for the revision. Many thanks to our supportive friends and colleagues who are too many to mention by name.

Ruth Parmelee Rawlins
Sophronia R Williams
Cornelia Kelly Beck

Contents

MENTAL HEALTH—
PSYCHIATRIC NURSING

A Holistic Life-Cycle Approach

PART I

Foundations for Practice

An important element in understanding the contemporary practice of mental health–psychiatric nursing is an awareness of its history. Thus Chapter 1 gives an overview of mental health–psychiatric nursing. Both societal trends and changes in health care delivery have had an impact on the development of mental health–psychiatric nursing.

Chapters 2 and 3 provide a behavioral and philosophical approach to the individual. The foundation for the holistic approach to the client, which is developed throughout the text, is delineated in Chapter 2. Major philosophical positions are discussed in Chapter 3, with holism presented as the philosophical base for this text's ideas and approaches.

Arising from various philosophical positions are the many theoretical approaches that form the basis for practice. Chapter 4 is an exposition of a variety of approaches from which a nurse may choose.

Chapter 5, Nursing Theorists' Approaches, describes the attempts of several theorists to explain the phenomenon of nursing practice. The concepts and relationships that have emerged are applied to the holistic approach of mental health–psychiatric nursing practice.

Chapter 6 examines basic communication, emphasizing factors that facilitate or impede the development of therapeutic communication. Therapeutic communication and behavior change through communication are also discussed. Chapter 7 addresses the development of a therapeutic relationship with clients. Applying the nursing process within the therapeutic relationship to mental health–psychiatric nursing is the focus of Chapter 8. The way psychotherapy differs among various cultures is the focus of Chapter 9.

Armed with a sense of the past and a set of beliefs about the individual and mental health and mental illness, nurses select theories from other disciplines as well as nursing theorists to guide their practice with individuals, families, and communities.

CHAPTER 1

Overview of Psychiatric Nursing

Nancy L Hedlund
Finis Breckenridge Jeffrey

After studying this chapter, the student will be able to:

- Define mental health and mental illness
- Describe major trends in the development of treatment methods for mental illness
- Discuss the processes by which mental health–psychiatric nursing developed in the United States
- State the importance of the National Mental Health Act of 1946 and the Community Mental Health Centers Act of 1963 in moving mental health–psychiatric nursing into the community
- Describe present and future challenges for mental health–psychiatric nursing

Mental health implies that individuals function comfortably within society and are generally satisfied with themselves and their achievements. A mentally healthy person's behavior demonstrates a balance among the body, mind, and environment. However, states of mental health or illness are defined by the values of the society in which a person lives. A person whose behavior is consistent with the values of the society in which he or she lives is generally considered mentally healthy. A person whose behavior is not consistent with those values is generally considered maladaptive, or mentally ill. Based on behavior then, the presence or absence of mental health is inferred. Behavior that is acceptable in one cultural group may not be tolerated in another.

Mental health implies mastery in the areas of life involving love, work, and play. Evidence of mental health is usually manifested by physical health; meaningful work; enjoyment of life; satisfying relationships with others; and the ability to make sound judgments and decisions, to accept responsibility for one's actions, to give and receive, and to express feelings appropriately.

Mental illness is conceptualized as the mind expressing its discomfort or pain in feelings, thoughts, or behavior. For example, the person may feel anxious or depressed, may think obsessively or in a psychotic manner, or may behave impulsively so as to endanger himself or others.

Mental illness is defined in numerous ways with little consensus. For the purpose of this text, *mental illness* is defined as a substantial disorder in one's thoughts or mood that significantly impairs judgment, behavior, the capacity to recognize reality, or the ability to cope with the ordinary demands of life.

Psychiatric nursing as defined by the ANA Division on Psychiatric and Mental Health Nursing is a specialized area of nursing practice employing theories of human behavior as its science and the purposeful use of self as an art. It is directed toward both preventive and corrective impacts on mental disorders and their sequelae and is concerned with the promotion of optimal mental health for the individual, the community, and society. Psychiatric nursing is recognized as one of the four core mental health disciplines that include psychiatry, psychology, and social work. This chapter traces the origins of mental health care and psychiatric nursing and describes future challenges for mental health–psychiatric nursing.

ORIGINS OF MENTAL HEALTH CARE

Societies have always had to deal with the actions of those considered to be deviant, or "crazy." Throughout history, the mentally ill have primarily been cared for by their family and friends. Those without such support were banished from society or executed. Treating unproductive members has been an unaffordable luxury for most societies. However, some societies such as certain Native American tribes have held the insane in high regard and have treated them as prophets or oracles. Similarly, other tolerant societies have permitted the insane the freedom to move about with little restraint. Only in recent decades have methods of treatment been developed and applied to a large segment of the population.

The practice of taking care of the sick has been a part of most societies. However, the specific role of nurses and nursing is relatively recent. As an organized profession, nursing originated in the middle nineteenth century with the work of Florence Nightingale. However, nursing at that time focused on the care of the physically sick and those wounded in war. As nursing developed into the care of the sick and injured in hospital settings, the practice of psychiatric nursing emerged quite separately within the distinct settings where care of the mentally ill was gradually becoming a part of the social order. Psychiatric nurses considered themselves distinct in training from their general hospital counterparts until well into the twentieth century. This distinction was removed when the nursing profession agreed that its members should receive one standard education, which occurred some years ahead of the development of advanced clinical nursing specialties.

Mental health–psychiatric nursing is a relatively recent development in care of the mentally ill and exists primarily in the United States. The addition of mental health to psychiatric nursing, resulting in the term *psychiatric–mental health nursing,* dates back to the early 1900s. At that time, state public health departments employed mental health consultants who taught their staff, including public health nurses, mental health principles. This movement led nurse educators to believe that psychiatric nurses had an important community health role to play. The term *psychiatric–mental health* was created as the designation for what had been graduate psychiatric nursing programs. They accepted the dual hospital-community challenges after the passage of the 1946 NMH act by developing large numbers of graduate psychiatric mental health nursing programs.[31]

Psychiatric nursing as it is today is the result of combining knowledge from psychiatry (medicine), psychology, physiology, pharmacology, and philosophy with the basic concept of caring that is fundamental to nursing practice. Originally, psychiatric nursing consisted of little more than physical restraint and physical care. However, as more sophisticated treatment methods evolved, and the public came to demand more effective care, nurses began to develop therapeutic systems of care that focused on methods of improving communication with clients. These nursing approaches were designed to help clients learn to communicate more effectively and thereby learn ways to function more effectively in everyday life.

The rapidly expanding complexity of psychiatric treatment motivated many nurses in this field to continue their education. This interest in learning and increased availability of federal funding resulted in a relatively high percentage of psychiatric nurses pursuing advanced college degrees compared with nurses in other clinical specialties. For example, although psychiatric nurses constitute only a comparatively small percentage of all nurses, during the 1970s they accounted for 30% of the doctoral degrees held among nurses as a whole.

Psychiatric nursing in the United States is unique in comparison to the field in other countries. Outside of Europe, psychiatry as a profession is little known; thus it is not surprising that the overall number of psychiatric nurses in the world is low. Even in Europe, nurses primarily provide supportive care to clients and play a small role in treatment. In Western Europe nurses remain substantially subordinate to physicians, a pattern U.S. psychiatric nurses actively challenged so they could participate equally in therapeutic services based on multidisciplinary, team-based care.

Primitive Times Through Early Christianity

Psychology is the study of human behavior and the mind. As human beings began to contemplate what they thought about and what made them think and act, they realized that people could suffer from disorders of the mind as well as the body. Medicine evolved as the discipline treating disease, with psychiatry emerging as the special field of medicine that treated disease of the mind. The disciplines of psychology and psychiatry (medicine) have long paralleled each other's efforts to understand human behavior in mental health and mental illness.

Philosophy embraces the human search to understand the basic truths and principles of the universe, life, morals, and human perception. Philosophy applies logical reasoning to such questions as What is life? Who are we? Why are we here? Where do we come from? Three basic philosophical concepts of mental health and illness include organic; cerebral, or mental; and magical thinking.[1] The organic approach explains the cause of mental or behavioral disorders in physical terms. Cerebral explanations identify mental or psychological factors as causing these disorders. Magical thinking attributes these disorders to magic forces or powers.

Five different belief models shaped the reactions to mental illness of early humans and their primitive descendants[12]:

1. The person's soul had fled the body; the wandering soul needed to be convinced to return.
2. A foreign body with magical powers entered the body; the cure required that it be extracted and neutralized.
3. Evil spirits had entered the body; these had to be exorcised before the victim could have relief.
4. The person had infringed on a taboo; the person and situation required ritualistic purification.
5. The person had sinned (Hebraic and other traditions attributed mental illness to sin), requiring confession in the hope that the sins would be expiated.

Early people confronted irrational behavior with fantastic or unreasonable responses. Regardless of whether the disease was physical or mental or whether or not some form of treatment was involved, the effectiveness of the healing was often attributed to magic. Primitive medicine or psychiatry was believed to cure if the client accepted and believed in the treatment. Ellenberger[12] identifies five key elements in the success of primitive medicine's healing:

1. The healer occupied a central role in society.
2. Confidence was in the healer, not the medication.
3. Healers were learned people, as defined by the culture.
4. Psychological methods of healing were most important.
5. The healing was almost always a public affair.

Jaynes[22] provides explanation for this early approach to healing, arguing that people originally were under the influence of the right, or nonverbal, side of the brain. They responded to what he calls the "inner voices" from the brain that in time came to be attributed to gods or superhuman forces. Jaynes argues, however, that many centuries ago, the left side of the brain became dominant, and the perceived healing potential of these inner voices lost prominence as a method of care.

Jaynes' ideas are still open to debate, since evidence also

supports the theory that 2500 years ago certain imaginative individuals developed concepts that laid the foundation for modern thought. These concepts included the idea that physical and mental afflictions can rationally be explained through cause and effect. Individual effort was also believed to play a role in cure. This "psychology without demons" developed over a long period and is one of the many significant contributions by the Greeks to Western culture.[1]

The kinds of care practiced by the Greeks did not reveal the depth and quality of the philosophical concepts they developed. They believed that humans were not subject to impersonal forces or demons but instead possessed within themselves the knowledge of their ills and the appropriate cure for them. The Greek aristocracy, however, lacked concern for the fate or lower classes. Afflicted members of the upper classes fared reasonably well, but the less fortunate received little or no care.

The Roman Empire followed a similar pattern, producing a remarkable legacy of ideas and culture. Their success can be traced to an emphasis on the virtues that produced victory in war and tight control of citizens in peace. This emphasis on military virtues, however, was reflected in their ideas about dealing with mentally ill people. The majority of the mentally ill were probably eliminated in some way as an unnecessary disturbance to the public order. Individuals from wealthy families probably fared better, being confined and treated in a kindly manner. Persons whose mental illness appeared "magical" were seen either as oracles or healers and were often honored for their special view of reality.

Different approaches to care of the mentally ill appear throughout the Middle East and Asia. The records are scant but suggest that many of the mentally ill were sent away or hidden by their families. However, some of these societies believed such people were empowered with special gifts, and they were protected as sources of power; they occupied important positions in society for religious and political purposes.

The Middle Ages

After the fall of the Roman Empire in 476 AD, concern for the less fortunate members of society became the responsibility of the religious orders of the Roman Catholic church; it was not unusual, however, for lay workers to provide care in places where the church did not.

St. Benedict of Nursia (480-547 AD) laid the foundation for monastic medicine.[1] Small centers staffed by religious orders offered sanctuary and care to the sick. The Greek tradition of rational medicine declined during the Middle Ages but was preserved to some extent in monastic libraries and even more so by the Arabs. These monastic orders accepted the responsibility of ministering to the ill. They provided what physical comfort they could and trusted simple medicine and divine intervention to achieve a cure.

At the beginning of the Middle Ages the mentally ill were not treated as outcasts but rather as persons to be helped. A few places, such as Gheel in Belgium, became famous for its care of psychotic individuals. This tolerance seems to have lasted until the fourteenth century, when a wave of general unrest swept through Europe. As a result, the insane were persecuted as witches and would not receive humane

care on a consistent basis until the nineteenth century.[1]

St. Augustine was one of the great figures of the early Middle Ages. Although not directly involved with care, he developed through his *Confessions* ideas about introspection and self-awareness that would provide a model for later developments in psychotherapy.[1] As a Christian he believed that God acted directly in human affairs but that persons were responsible for their own actions. God was a necessary participant in the struggle with evil but was not viewed as acting alone.

In the East the Byzantine Empire ruled half of the original Roman Empire until it fell in 1453. Perhaps its most important contribution was the preservation of Greek culture and medicine until the Renaissance.

Beginning in the seventh century, the Byzantines faced the growing power of the Arab world, unified under the banner of Islam. The Arabs considered their mentally ill to be in some way divinely inspired and treated them with great kindness. A number of their philosophers also continued the Greek tradition of rational investigation, some of it dealing with irrational or disturbed behavior.[24]

Throughout the Middle Ages, the insane received care ranging from good to poor. Despite a harsh environment, concern for their well-being persisted in communities and families. This response would in time be replaced by the conviction that unacceptable behavior could be cured through the powers of the intellect. This belief in reason became the foundation for modern theories of mental health and treatment.

The Renaissance in Europe

In fifteenth-century Europe, the Renaissance led to increasing secularization and a weakening of religious influence on intellectual life and moral conduct. Greek and Roman culture, with its frank and questioning attitude toward life was rediscovered. The religious Reformation, which accompanied the Renaissance, represented a powerful demand for fundamental change in the religious and political activities of the Roman Catholic church. As a result, the rational approach to the study of people and their place in the universe was resurrected, emphasizing internal and logical forces that acted on the person in an orderly and predictable manner.

This view forced individuals to consider themselves responsible for their own actions, not victims of dark and demonic forces. One consequence of this view was the idea that nonrational individuals are affected by factors that can be alleviated or cured by rational methods. Rather than appealing for divine intervention, the healer could use human methods.[16]

The transition to a more rational view of mental illness was not instantaneous. For the most part, the mentally ill were still considered to be afflicted by evil spirits. They were often neglected and were even confined, beaten, and starved. Therefore the new spirit of rational treatment was paradoxically accompanied by a violent reaction by some people against the insane.[1] With the decline in the authority of the Church, increased power was assigned to the devil, whose followers were thought to be witches and sorcerers. Fear of those not viewed as normal led to such extremes as burning at the stake for those accused of witchcraft, driving the insane outside the city walls, or paying sailors to carry them away on the "Ship of Fools."

Views of traditional European care for the mentally ill have probably been negatively influenced by highly publicized scenes of London's Hospital of St. Mary of Bethlehem, which was popularly named "bedlam." Although these descriptions paint a dark picture, they actually occurred well after the significant reforms of the nineteenth century. In general, European society probably dealt with its sick much more humanely than these popular images suggest.

THE AMERICAN EXPERIENCE

Responses to the mentally ill in the United States reflected many of the European attitudes and treatments. The New World demanded a great deal of its inhabitants, and few resources remained for humane care of the mentally ill. During the colonial period, the insane were left in the care of their families, who were judged the ones most responsible and most able to perform this task. Local government demonstrated no social obligation to erect special buildings to meet unrecognized need. The few eighteenth-century institutions that existed for the mentally ill were clearly places of last resort, designed for the custody of those with no family or friends.

Yet the picture is again one of contrasts and so is probably not as grim as suggested. The famous example of American barbarity, the Salem witch trials (involving some mentally ill defendants), was an aberration. With this one exception, the execution of so-called witches was a rare occurrence in American history.[10]

In the Jacksonian era (after 1820), Americans began to erect asylums for the insane at an increased rate[36] (Figure 1-1). Although some might argue that this reflected a growing awareness of the problem and a more humane approach to its solution, it was more likely a much needed attempt to promote the stability of a new society. Before 1820 the insane had been an expected part of life and an unfortunate problem to be taken care of within the family. The new society of the Jacksonian era saw this deviant behavior as a reflection of faulty community to be corrected by organized care and treatment. The most effective solution lay in bringing healers and clients together at a centrally located site, an institution incorporating the latest ideas in architecture and treatment. In such a setting, the chances for significant cure or improvement were enhanced.

The new asylums emphasized treatment of individuals with recent or milder symptoms of mental distress. Through rational and humane methods of treatment, the client could quickly be helped and returned to society. Such treatment included clean, well-ventilated surroundings and periods of discussion and reading when the client's condition permitted. A strict schedule that included appropriate levels of work and reading therapy was followed from 5 AM until 9:30 PM. The reformers, as administrators considered themselves, were adamant that these institutions not become dumping grounds for the chronically ill but rather be short-term hospitals for persons with a good chance of being cured.

This optimistic concept broke down soon after the new asylums were occupied. Reformers such as Dorothea Dix had been tireless in their efforts to promote humane care

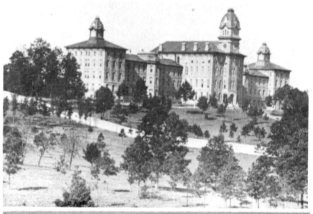

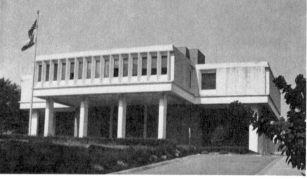

FIGURE 1-1 A, This photograph of the Arkansas Lunatic Asylum was taken in 1883 by I.W. Banks. **B,** Arkansas State Hospital in 1991. (**A** *courtesy the Heiskell Library Collection at the Arkansas Gazette.*)

and treatment for the mentally ill. However, these efforts were hampered by the reality of increasing numbers of admissions for long-term care and the deterioration of facilities caused by inadequate funds.[40] By the end of the Civil War, the facilities had become custodial rather than short term. The promise of reform built the asylums, but the functionalism of custody perpetuated them. By 1870 custody was definitely the norm, with increased use of *mechanical restraints* and harsh punishments. The asylum lost its place as a symbol of hope and instead became a forbidding place of last resort, the home of the incurable. Society in turn replaced its vision of cure and recovery with one of isolation from a disease that was now considered contagious. The America of the late nineteenth century grew fearful of mental illness and demanded protection from those who would spread the "contagion."[36]

PSYCHIATRIC NURSING IN AMERICA
Origins of Modern Psychiatric Nursing

Complex forces interacted to produce the psychiatric–mental health nursing practice of modern times. Developments in hospital organization and services, as well as in the medical profession, significantly affected the early course of nursing in general and the progress of psychiatric nursing in particular. World Wars I and II radically changed ideas about mental health care, particularly with respect to knowledge about the effectiveness of short-term care and treatment of clients in their home communities. The Community Mental Health Centers legislation consolidated knowledge with public policy to revolutionize the entire scope of national public mental health services. Finally, scholars in psychiatric nursing and other professions provided considerable direction for the advancement of this developing nursing specialty.

Hospitals and the medical profession

Psychiatric nursing and nursing in general developed from the need for hospitals to provide socially acceptable levels of care for clients. Although many nurses found employment in private duty roles, the major impetus for establishing nursing as an organized profession can be traced to the demands of nineteenth century reformers for social services, such as hospital treatment of both physical and mental diseases. Hospitals differed in types of care and recruited suitably trained people to staff them.

General and mental hospitals differed little in the way they attracted nurses. As hospitals sought to meet increasing demands for services, the ideas of Florence Nightingale and the traditional role of women as caregivers of the sick prompted hospital administrators to recruit women to provide the continuous care known as *nursing*. Although ideas of care have existed for as long as there have been people, the specifics of nursing were new. Thus hospitals created nursing education as they began to train nurses to meet the unique standards for general and psychiatric care.

The first training school for mental health nurses started at McLean Hospital, Waverly, Massachusetts, in 1882. This school, and those that followed, ostensibly trained nurses for later employment. However, student nurses performed basically the same tasks as graduate nurses but at far less cost to the hospital. As a result, hospital training schools typically furnished the majority of nursing personnel for institutions but replaced them as they graduated with new enrollees. In general and mental hospitals the young profession had to face the fact that graduates of educational programs could not readily find jobs.[3]

The American Psychiatric Association (APA) played a directive role in shaping the course of psychiatric nursing in the early part of the twentieth century, illustrating not only the influence of the medical profession on nursing but also on the social status and image of both nursing and women. For example, in 1906 the APA began a program to standardize the training of nurses practicing in mental institutions. Although this predominantly male professional group sought to improve client care through improved education of nurses, the APA also assumed it was appropriate that they should implement and oversee educational preparation for the predominantly female nursing profession. Not until the mid-1930s did organized nursing actively define psychiatric nurses as a separate group with unique educational requirements.[35]

Influence of the two world wars

The two world wars provided important clinical understandings about short-term treatment as a result of treating soldiers who were experiencing *battle fatigue* or acute stress reactions, as well as post-traumatic stress disorder (PTSD). Before both wars combat reactions were erroneously assumed to be continuations of preexisting neuroses. An alternative view, supported by empirical evidence, explained war neuroses as syndromes precipitated by combat experience, without preexisting emotional difficulty. Treatment in the stressful environment relatively near the front lines minimized the soldier's sense of guilt and shame and prevented his identifying himself as a failure. Withdrawal from the situation was rarely needed, and soldiers seemed to fare better in overcoming stress-related symptoms than if they were shipped to "the rear" or to the States.

Salmon[37] pioneered the World War I treatment of battle reactions with short-term, intensive approaches provided in close proximity to the combat situation. Classic descriptions of similar but seemingly unrelated work during World War II are provided by Ferenczi and others,[15] Kardiner,[25,26] and Grinker and Spiegel.[18,19]

The two world wars provided at least two lessons significant to mental health–psychiatric nursing: (1) the effective short-term treatments for stress-related syndromes developed for combat situations should be refined and made available to the population at large, with appropriate research and evaluation; and (2) more psychiatric nurses with training in these short-term, crisis-oriented methods were needed to meet the demand for professional staff.

After World War II, the need for more psychiatric nurses and more educational programs became increasingly clear; war casualties turned out to be more than physical wounds and battle fatigue, which was described as an equally disabling condition. At the same time, short-term intensive treatment of any person with mental problems was increasingly thought to be superior. As a result, public awareness of the problems faced by soldiers and civilians was translated into a demand for legislative action. The National Mental Health Act of 1946 changed nursing practice to include more direct involvement of the nurse in communication with mentally ill clients and other therapies. In addition, the legislation encouraged nursing education to incorporate mental health content in basic nursing education. The addition of this content improved the quality of care given to clients and promoted research in mental health aspects of client care.

Community mental health centers legislation

Significantly more progressive attitudes and practices have come to characterize much of the care provided to the mentally ill as the twentieth century has advanced. As nursing knowledge has taken shape, ideas about teamwork in treating clients have generated more therapeutic treatment environments. The Community Mental Health Centers Act of 1963 dramatically transferred the psychiatric nurse's efforts out of the institution and into the community. This program focused on mental health and the prevention of severe mental illness by early intervention, short-term treatment approaches, and outpatient care.

This 1963 act was a visionary approach to widespread mental health problems that had long been ignored and neglected. As with any such movement, however, it produced its own problems as nurses and other health professionals struggled to establish their own limits. Significant questions for nursing became the focus of debate: How should nurses prepare for this new role—in traditional hospital settings or in the community? Should their preparation be united with that of social workers and other mental health workers, or should it be independent? Finally, once prepared, how should psychiatric nurses deal with public health nurses within their own profession and social workers, psychiatrists, and psychologists from without? To understand the factors that led to the community mental health movement and subsequent controversy, one needs to consider the development of more progressive psychiatric treatments.

Scholars in nursing and other professions

Hildegard Peplau's[33] concise history of psychiatric nursing was published in 1959, shortly before the passage of the Community Mental Health Centers Act of 1963. She defined *psychiatric nursing* as both (1) a vital skill of general nursing practice to be acquired and used by all nurses, and (2) an area of clinical specialization to be practiced by those with a graduate education. Over the years the education required for specialization in psychiatric nursing included a certificate, diploma, or degree, but increasingly it meant the baccalaureate degree. Today, the term refers to nurses wth postbaccalaureate training. Peplau divided her history of psychiatric nursing into five periods, as shown in Table 1-1.

Peplau[33] concluded her optimistic view of the future of psychiatric nursing by raising some important questions and suggesting possible answers. She believed that the historical division of psychiatric and general nursing had been resolved and that psychiatric nursing had been recognized as an aspect of all nursing and a specialized field of advanced nursing practice. She advocated that the basic education of all nurses be unified and that those choosing to work in psychiatric hospitals receive an introduction to psychiatric concepts in the general curriculum, followed by basic experience with psychiatric clients. The question of who would provide the basic psychiatric nursing experience—the psychiatric hospital or the school of nursing—was still unresolved.

Peplau[33] argued that a philosophy of psychiatric nursing had not yet been explicitly defined. She was critical of the fact that organized symposia and papers by nurses about actual nursing practice were not available. She concluded that much remained to be achieved to improve standards and increase the impact of nurses on the client care environment.

Sills[38] discussed the history of psychiatric nursing in 1973, drawing largely from an unpublished paper by Peplau.[34] She took the story past 1959 into the period following the Community Mental Health Centers Act of 1963. She pointed out that two issues confronting the field in 1882 still remained: (1) dominance of untrained or poorly educated service personnel, and (2) uncertainty about where nurses should receive training for the care of emotionally troubled people.

The first issue has yet to be resolved. Strong support for the continued use of custodial types of staff in mental health facilities has been provided by (1) reduced public spending in mental health care, (2) increased demands by nurses for better salaries, and (3) the continuing and pervasive custodial care mentality about mental health care in the United States. This philosophy ranges from extensive employment of psychiatric aides who have little or no training to retention and promotion of nurses who have only completed beginning levels of education in nursing. Not uncommonly, only a few if any nurses with graduate or even undergraduate degrees in nursing will be found on the staff of an inpatient psychiatric facility. The second concern about education of psychiatric nurses has been resolved, as noted by Peplau, in favor of the general nursing school over the single-focus school.

Sills described how the nursing profession required undergraduate programs to incorporate psychiatric nursing into their curricula after 1955. During the 1930s and 1940s, the seeds of the community mental health movement were sown; eventually, the Community Mental Health Centers Act was passed in 1963. During this transition in philosophy about mental health and the treatment of mental illness, nursing increasingly considered the role mental factors play in all matters of health and illness. Basic nursing education of the time included knowledge of psychiatric concepts.

▼ **TABLE 1-1** Peplau's History of Psychiatric Nursing

Period	Events
1773-1881	Psychiatric nursing did not exist as such.
	Psychiatric care was generally custodial and harsh.
1882-1914	Mental health nurses were trained and introduced into mental health facilities.
	New methods of treatment that avoided the use of restraints were used.
	The mental hygiene movement began and emphasized prevention and more humane treatment.
	Nurses played a subordinate and custodial role as managers of the ward and keepers of the keys; their primary function was to implement treatment programs devised by others.
	Psychiatric nurse's training did not include much psychology or psychiatry.
1915-1935	The number of undergraduate programs, including courses in psychiatric nursing, increased to half of the existing programs by 1935.
	The first psychiatric nursing textbook was published.
	Some training at the postgraduate level for psychiatric nurses was given in psychiatric hospitals.
1936-1945	Three universities offered courses in postgraduate psychiatric nursing education.
	The establishment of the Mental Health and Psychiatric Nursing Project within the National League for Nursing Education brought psychiatric nursing into the mainstream of nursing.
1946-1959	Postgraduate education in psychiatric nursing was firmly established.
	The National League for Nursing assumed responsibility for the accreditation of psychiatric nursing curricula.

The changes produced by the two world wars and the community mental health centers legislation required creative responses from dedicated psychiatric nursing leaders. Sills' classic analysis[38] singles out Theresa Muller and Hildegard Peplau as providing the field with a comprehensive framework for understanding psychiatric nursing. Muller[30] studied coping mechanisms for dealing with stress in everyday life. Peplau[32] defined the therapeutic roles that nurses have in the mental health setting. Among her specific contributions to clinical practice is the conceptualization of the nature of anxiety and how increasing levels of anxiety affect thought, feeling, and action. She defined how nursing care could be specifically tailored to respond to the client's particular degree of functional impairment from anxiety.

Peplau's 1952 clinical analysis of anxiety,[32] Gwen Tudor Will's 1952 conceptualization of the process of nurse-patient withdrawal in the psychiatric ward milieu,[39] June Mellow's 1964 consideration of nursing therapy,[27] and the results of clinical studies contributed by other nurse clinicians helped create a substantial body of psychiatric nursing knowledge. This knowledge has helped to develop a professional climate in which the nurse is a coordinator of care, assembling a variety of treatment methods and helping determine which are most effective. Simultaneously, opportunities have increased for psychiatric nurses to have direct involvement in client treatment.

Esther Lucile Brown, an anthropologist who directed the Russell Sage Foundation for many years, studied nursing as one of the foundation's studies of professions in the 1940s. She reported her findings in 1948 in *Nursing for the Future,* otherwise known as the "Brown Report."[7] In general, she effectively argued in support of college education for nurses, and in particular she recommended increases in our society's emphasis on mental health nursing. She stressed the importance of integrating mental health nursing into a general curriculum and ending single-focus training schools in mental hospitals.

Contemporary Social and Cultural Influences

Modern day psychiatric nursing began with the inception of comprehensive community mental health centers in the 1960s and continues into the present decade. These years have been characterized by innovation, study, growth, and the consolidation of skills, as nurses have moved into new roles emerging from the community mental health movement. Many forces have shaped the course of psychiatric nursing. The following review of the social and cultural factors affecting this developmental process provides a basis for understanding advances in the profession during this contemporary period. Major influences on psychiatric—mental health nursing include (1) developments in the organized profession; (2) society's use and misuse of mind-altering chemicals; (3) societal changes in mental health treatment needs and services; (4) holistic health and the self-help revolution; and (5) increased consciousness about sex, class, and color barriers to social equality.

Developments in the profession

The 1946 National Mental Health Act stimulated development of graduate training programs and psychiatric nursing content in baccalaureate nursing programs. These baccalaureate programs increasingly integrated mental health concepts into the total curriculum. Strong graduate programs in psychiatric nursing have increasingly offered specializations in education, administration, and advanced practice in both psychiatric settings as well as general nursing care settings.

Major events affecting contemporary psychiatric nursing include (1) delineation of levels of nursing through standards defined by the ANA, (2) formation of specialty subgroups with the ANA, and (3) *certification* of advanced practitioners in psychiatric nursing. The overall effect of these events is clarity in role definition and assurance of quality in practice.

The ANA standards established two levels of mental health—psychiatric nursing practice. The first level requires at least baccalaureate level preparation in nursing; the second requires graduate education, supervised clinical experience, and knowledge and skill as evidenced in testing. ANA certification recognizes excellence in practice through examination, clinical competence, and achievement of appropriate education credentials. These ANA procedures and achievements are described in Chapter 44.

Society's use and misuse of mind-altering chemicals

The contemporary era, described by some as "better living through chemistry," has significantly challenged psychiatric nursing. The explosion of knowledge about the biochemistry of mind and behavior and the nation's everworsening problem with drug and alcohol abuse has created this complex challenge. Entire new biochemical explanations have been proposed for such serious diseases as depression, schizophrenia, and addiction, as well as certain so-called neurotic disorders such as panic reactions and eating disorders.

As a result, just as nursing was approaching success in establishing its role as a full participant in the mental health team, a new wave of physicians and biomedical researchers moved into the treatment arena to argue that only time and medication were required for the successful return of the client to the community. Consequently, treatment approaches in many settings dramatically shifted from reliance on the "therapeutic community" to a renewed reliance on antidepressants and major antipsychotic drugs in inpatient and outpatient services.

Increasing visibility of the diseases of addiction and alcoholism and the simultaneous recognition of the co-occurrence of addiction with other psychiatric disorders such as schizophrenia and depression have presented mental health nurses with entirely new treatment challenges. The new wave of so-called recreational drugs, popularized in the 1960s, eventually progressed to the widespread abuse of crack cocaine and "ice" (crystal methamphetamine) and other serious stimulants, hallucinogens, and narcotics. Publicity about the use of these drugs and the homicides and suicides associated with these drugs has forced our society to face painful realities about the addictive and destructive potential of both drug and alcohol abuse. Treatment efforts with this little understood disease of addiction to alcohol or drugs have had limited value, given the steadily increasing availability of drugs, the number of users, and the social encouragement to use drugs. Clients with a dual-diagnosis of addiction with schizophrenia or a depressive disorder suffer from two diseases, each of which compounds the severity of the other even when actively treated. For some people simultaneous remission of these two chronic diseases has been extremely difficult to achieve.

Societal changes in mental health treatment needs

Two treatment challenges have assumed major proportions during the last decade: chronic, severe mental illness (schizophrenia and depression) and alcohol and drug addiction. In addition, a wide variety of other mental health problems in adults, children, and families, including family violence, child abuse, and neurotic disorders, present opportunities for psychiatric nursing involvement. Widespread homelessness in both urban and rural areas has greatly intensified the impact of these mental health disorders.

A major shift in the care of the chronically mentally ill called *deinstitutionalization* brought clients out of mental hospitals and into the community. Care and services were adapted to the community mental health center model, including significant attention to the rehabilitation needs of this population. For many clients, years of confinement in mental institutions resulted in significant deficits in education, social skills, and occupational capabilities. Although inventive, this broad-based approach to integrating the chronically mentally ill into the community has required intensive application of staff and resources to the long-standing problems of this population. In reality, this effort has failed in many instances to achieve its goal of significantly improving the day-to-day experiences and opportunities of the chronically mentally ill.

One major complicating force in the care of the chronically mentally ill has been the high rate of alcohol and drug addiction that has emerged in this population. Thrust into the community without adequate social supports, many clients responded to their new freedom by entering into dysfunctional social patterns that included easy access to alcohol and drugs. For those with severe mental disorders and/or the genetic predisposition to addiction, this social pattern has had devastating consequences. Typical residential treatment programs of 1 to 3 months frequently have been inadequate to meet the complex challenges presented by these severely and chronically ill clients.

Widespread problems of homelessness have increasingly compounded the problems of the severely disabled mentally ill, as these troubled people continue to flow back into the community. Factors contributing to homelessness, in addition to deinstitutionalization, have included economic recession, unemployment, alcohol and drug abuse, cutbacks in federal programs, and shortages in low-income housing resulting from the redevelopment of inner-city areas.

Holistic health and the self-help revolution

The philosophy of holistic health will be discussed in Chapter 2. Its importance for psychiatric nursing comes from its focus on the interrelationship of mind, body, and spirit. The holistic health movement has functioned much like the consumer movement in that individuals seek and demand the rights and responsibilities associated with being informed participants in decisions about their health and health care. Self-help groups aid individuals in con-fronting a wide range of health issues, from illness prevention to recovery during chronic and/or terminal disease.

A parallel influence has been increased knowledge and increased public awareness of the interrelationship between body, mind, and spirit. Accordingly, many self-help groups place particular emphasis on the power of spiritual faith and prescribe various affirmations to influence the outcome of disease. Such groups now bring hope and recovery to clients and families facing diseases that were once erroneously believed to be either entirely physical in nature, such as cancer, or entirely the result of the sick person's moral weakness and inner evil, such as alcohol and drug addiction.

Obvious obstacles limit the application of self-help group principles to diseases commonly known as mental illness. For one thing, many persons suffering from mental illness have limitations in social skills, which can alter their willingness or ability to "join" a group focused on health or recovery. In addition, the various forms of mental illness typically affect cognitive and emotional functioning, so that it may be difficult to understand how to utilize the group or difficult to handle feelings associated with being in the group, or both.

Another challenge is the strength of many clients' social support systems. While some clients have strong support from family or friends, others meet with indifference or even rejection from their family. These difficulties arise because mental illness in a family member affects everyone in the family. Progress in recovery requires difficult changes in communication and relationships for everyone, and each family member progresses at his or her own pace. As a result, the support network of family and friends frequently fails to function as a consistent and cohesive helping force. Instead one or more members may be actively engaged in recovery and change, while others cling to the old ideas and defenses associated with the person's mental illness.

Finally, mental illnesses produce various human responses and behaviors, many of which are the object of social stigma. For example, a person who talks out loud to herself, urinates in public, or acts in other inappropriate ways is often stigmatized or ostracized. This sense of being a social disgrace contributes to the client's shame and hopelessness about having a mental illness. Society applauds the efforts of the physically ill or handicapped to carve out meaningful lives; but even the most compassionate citizens often become suspicious and retaliatory in response to the plight of the severely mentally ill, addicted, or homeless in their midst. In fact a major challenge for holistic and self-help movements is to confront negative community attitudes about the mentally ill so as to create a greater sense of community support and caring.

A unique "turning point" for clients suffering from chronic mental illness, alcoholism, or drug abuse often comes through involvement in self-help and recovery groups. This turning point is achieved when they begin to view the illness as their *responsibility* instead of their *fault*. This acceptance of responsibility creates the opportunity to learn to act on one's own behalf, which in turn produces hope. Reduction of shame and resistance to future experiences with social stigma are often direct consequences of accepting personal responsibility for recovering.

Groups based on a spiritual approach to recovery help

new members learn to trust in the spiritual force or higher power that they understand as "ruling the universe." For those clients who have no faith, group members often say, "Believe in us until you can believe in something more." As a result, clients are encouraged to accept ideas and suggestions from members who have more experience, based on the idea that spiritual enlightenment usually comes through relatedness to other people rather than through visions or large-scale miracles.

New members in self-help groups are urged to try to live life a day at a time by ceasing to worry endlessly about all the possible catastrophes of the future and instead addressing the problems or tasks that can be worked on that day. These basic problem-solving approaches and the social support of group members can quite dramatically contribute to the client's recovery process. Various theories propose explanations for why or how these self-help groups affect people and succeed in improving health and well-being. However, further mental health research is needed to determine the extent to which the beneficial effects result from (1) increased hope; (2) rebalancing emotional responses and physiological processes associated with anxiety, arousal, and emotion; (3) restoring relationships, when possible, that might be supportive to the client; (4) fuller participation in self-care, including compliance with treatments such as medication or therapy; (5) potential strengthening of the immune system; and/or (6) greater involvement in work and play.

Social consciousness of barriers to opportunity

A wide range of social movements has emerged over the past 20 to 30 years, characterized by shared concern about perceived experiences of stigma or disadvantage. The individuals in many of these movements have sought to increase each other's awareness of their common experiences with race, sex, social class, or other identity barriers to equal access to society's opportunities. This spirit of social action based on solidarity has had major influences on both mentally ill clients and psychiatric nursing.

For mentally ill clients, changes were sought that included major improvements in services and social opportunities. Action groups of family members and other concerned citizens found considerable political influence, as they lobbied to affect local, state, and national policies and priorities. Their efforts have brought about changes affecting budget decisions, adequacy of services, access to housing, and availability of community services. As these groups have worked to increase public awareness of the problems and needs of the mentally ill, the severe social stigma that has always been associated with the mentally ill has been somewhat reduced.

The evolution of nursing in general, and psychiatric nursing in particular, over the past 30 years has paralleled an important era of activity in the women's movement. Nursing is still primarily a profession of women. Rich detail about the mutual influence of nursing and the women's movement is provided by contemporary authors who have sought to address the nursing profession's obstacles to economic security and social status.[3,29]

At the turn of the century, nurses advancing the cause of nursing were often the same women who were advancing women's rights, such as the right to vote and later the right to use birth control. Today, however, these are two fairly distinct movements. No leading feminist theorist and few public feminist activists are nurses, even though many nurses actively promote the concerns of women through feminist groups and political activities. Some contemporary nurse leaders are concerned that the social changes promoted by feminist thought have only "trickled down" to nursing rather than originating in nursing as they did in the past.

Major issues of the contemporary women's movement have become critical issues for nursing as well. For example, professional issues involving collaboration and autonomy in the workplace have emerged as central to nursing's definition of its place in health care and in society. Increased competition has brought status concerns and economic goals to the forefront as nurses seek higher and more powerful organizational positions and greater economic rewards. A few nurses have found their way into public office, in addition to those who have sought political influence through professional roles within nursing.

Nurses also confront the same personal issues about career and family life as other women, as they seek to integrate family, parenthood, and career roles in a society that still rewards the more "male" career orientation of full-time work with no disruptions for childbirth and child care. Recent court rulings may help society to become more flexible in this regard. Legal and other organized challenges have achieved acceptance of such workplace opportunities as sharing professional positions; parental leave for men and women, including adoptions; and leave associated with care of a sick child, parent, or other family member.

American Psychiatric Nursing Today

Modern day psychiatric nursing is best characterized by describing ways that clinical practice has evolved across a wide variety of settings and the theoretical developments that have most importantly shaped the course of this clinical specialty.

Developments in clinical practice

Contemporary mental health–psychiatric nursing methods and practice settings create diverse opportunities for nurses practicing in the mental health arena. Figure 1-2 presents a simple three-by-four matrix showing twelve different combinations of practice methods and settings, including varying individual, family, and group methods across inpatient, day-care, outpatient, and community settings. In reality these combinations probably do not each occur separately. Rather, the matrix is just a way of thinking about how practice and setting combine to create various types of mental health services. The following discussion briefly reviews selected typical mental health services to illustrate their diversity as well as certain improvements in care during this contemporary period.

Inpatient facilities vary in the length of time the client typically stays in the hospital and the type of institution. Inpatient stay can vary from a few days to a few years. Most comprehensive community mental health centers have short-stay inpatient units; those that do not have such units make arrangements with a nearby institution to provide this care.[1] State mental hospitals also provide inpatient care.

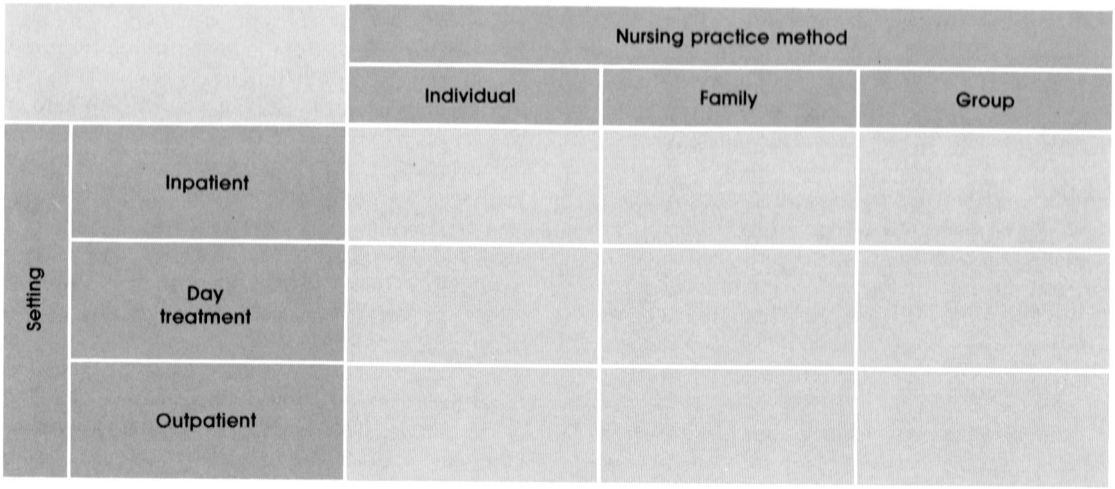

		Nursing practice method		
		Individual	Family	Group
Setting	Inpatient			
	Day treatment			
	Outpatient			

FIGURE 1-2 Two-way matrix. Nursing practice opportunities are created by variations in practice method and setting.

Inpatient units are also located in general hospitals and private psychiatric institutions.

Although one kind of inpatient unit cannot be defined as always better than another, comparisons are made because people naturally try to decide whether or when one option for care is a better choice than another. Factors that particularly influence the quality of care on inpatient units include the ratio of staff to clients, the philosophy of nursing care, and the attitudes of family and friends in the client's support system.

The first factor, staff-client ratio, suggests the extent to which clients are under a nurse's direct observation and care as well as the degree of opportunity for the client to learn from nurse-client interaction. This ratio varies greatly; some units are staffed with a nurse for every 4 to 6 clients, while others only have a nurse for one or even several wards. Ideally, the nurse needs time with a client to develop a relationship that will help him work through his resistance to treatment, manage fears about illness and treatment, and learn new skills for living life in the outside world. Conversely, the stereotypical picture of an old state hospital "back ward" is one in which psychiatric aides or technicians staff the unit and a nurse supervises an entire building containing a number of wards.

In the past most inpatient units were locked, and nurses carried keys. This was necessitated in part by the low ratio of nurses to clients and was a way of ensuring that clients would remain in the hospital, even when there were not enough nurses to provide direct care. Many psychiatric nursing leaders today call this type of ward outmoded. Across the United States many back ward units still exist. Nurses in some settings are still very much the keepers of the keys, and some inpatients still spend very little of their hospital stay with a nurse. However, one is more likely to find nurses on inpatient units actively involved in the treatment team's decision making process and in direct client care.

A second factor is the underlying philosophy of the setting, which determines the treatment offered. For example, some inpatient treatment settings strongly emphasize the therapeutic potential of the client's social milieu.[17] Nurses in these settings work with other members of the team to develop therapeutic relationships with clients and environmental situations that help clients develop skills to cope with the feelings and events of everyday living.

In other settings a strong medical model prevails with an emphasis on one or both of the following methods of treatment: intensive psychotherapy between the client and a psychiatrist (a physician who is often a resident) and/or use of psychotropic drugs. In these treatment settings, it is not unusual for the nurse's role to be that of a "social chairperson," in which the client's nursing care is limited to superficial conversation, playing games, and being escorted on recreational outings. The ability of the nurse to establish therapeutic communication with the client often has little value in these settings and may even be discouraged or prohibited.

On some inpatient units that have been strongly influenced by the medical model, the client is under the care of a private psychiatrist who makes brief rounds each day and leaves the remainder of the client's care to the hospital staff. These clients often receive large doses of psychotropic medications and/or electroconvulsive therapy (ECT), either of which may cause side effects that limit their capacity for therapeutic communication. Despite various medical "justifications" for these treatments based on their outcomes over time, many nurses agree there are too many disadvantages associated with the frequent side effects of drowsiness, memory loss, and confusion. Nurses in these settings typically do little more than monitor clients' vital signs, orientation, and safety in performing activities of daily living; this supportive care represents limited attention to developing social or therapeutic relationships.

A third factor concerns the willingness of treatment staff to work with family members in planning the client's care during and after hospitalization. Attitudes of family members toward the client, as well as toward the treatment staff and setting, can vary widely and are influenced by such variables as previous knowledge and experience, culture, and social class. What matters is whether family members support the client or withdraw, whether they offer understanding or condemnation, whether the client will return to a supportive family system or hostility and rejection, and whether they are willing to learn new ways of relating to the client and to each other or whether they choose to withdraw.

Evaluating the quality of care in mental health services in any setting begins with an open mind. It is best to refrain from premature judgment and, instead, to seek accurate information and direct contact with the staff as a way of becoming familiar with the care and treatment. For example, traditional stereotypes about quality of health care often imply that private care is superior to that provided by public facilities.

Mental health services provided by public facilities, however, frequently offer higher ratios of nurses to clients and/or more progressive team approaches to client care with less reliance on psychotropic drugs. Alternatively, private facilities may discourage or restrict nurses from developing therapeutic, problem-solving oriented relationships with clients and may rely essentially on brief physician contact with clients and treatments such as psychotropic drugs and ECT. This means a client in a public facility might receive better care than a client in a private psychiatric setting. Quality of care cannot be predicted by the name of an institution, by whether it is public or private, or by the neighborhood in which is it located.

Outpatient care has developed over the past 20 to 30 years, primarily influenced by the community mental health movement, whose services can be found in mental health clinics, schools, churches, prisons, storefronts, and hospital emergency departments. Every type of care except inpatient hospitalization is available in these settings; sometimes even a short stay of a few hours or a day is the treatment of choice.

Community practice settings offer nurses positions in private practice, consultation, and community organizations, as well as in schools, industry, and child care. Psychiatric nurses are increasingly turning to community settings because these roles typically offer increased autonomy and substantially better utilization of the nurse's knowledge and skills. Many states have enacted legislation empowering advanced practice nurses (master's degree in nursing) to prescribe medication within defined legal limits. As a result, psychiatric nurses in community settings are increasingly moving into roles in which they are responsible for "total patient care," including the monitoring of responses to ongoing treatment with psychotropic medications.

A major difficulty for nurses establishing a private practice is being paid for services. In many instances nurses are not reimbursed through *third-party payment* for psychiatric nursing services, even when the nurse has become certified in this specialty. Psychiatric nurses in private clinical practice utilize a variety of approaches for setting fees; for example, the fair market price in their community can range from $50 to $150 per hour. An alternative approach is the "value received" method, in which the nurse and client discuss the value of the service received and reach an agreement as to what is fair payment. Fair payment can be money, services, or other types of bartered goods.

Psychiatric nurse consultants charge anywhere from $100 to $500 (or more) per day, depending on the client, the work to be performed, and the typical rate in a given setting. For example, some nurse consultants charge lower fees when consulting or speaking to a nursing student organization or honor society. Also, consultant fees paid by federal grants tend to be lower than the typical rate paid by other organizations. The considerable variance in private practice earnings is probably caused by problems associated with third-party reimbursement as well as the reluctance of nurses to share facts with each other about their fees. This certainly differs from the pattern observed in psychiatrists, psychoanalysts, and clinical psychologists, who typically charge the same fee in their respective communities.

Psychiatric nursing roles in schools, industry, and child care vary widely. These systems have increasingly recognized the applicability of psychiatric–mental health nursing in such areas as counseling, teaching, group services, and home visits. Both specialized and generic roles are available because of their consistent success in providing prevention services.

Psychiatric nurses are increasingly involved in studying and attempting to treat social problems that have mental health implications. For example, many psychiatric nurses now work in the areas of child abuse and other forms of family violence, abortion and family planning, single parenting, and crisis hot lines. This trend can be partially explained by the influence of the community mental health movement, with its strong emphasis on prevention. In addition, this trend logically follows the increased reliance on biomedical models of treatment. There is also the increasingly obvious concern of professional women about social problems affecting women and children. And finally, nursing is a profession substantially composed of women, and women have traditionally been prime movers in motivating societal concern about human problems, particularly problems affecting women and children. As a result of this trend, nursing may well be on its way to reestablishing its position among other female social activists who seek to eradicate hunger, poverty, child abuse, family violence, homelessness, alcohol and drug addiction, and discrimination.

Developments in psychiatric nursing theory

The development of psychiatric nursing over the past 20 to 30 years should be contemplated as this book is studied. Some psychiatric nurses are troubled by the fact that no dramatically new ideas or thinkers seem to have emerged—at least not in significant numbers—since the outstanding contributions of Peplau, Mellow, Orlando, and others in the 1950s and early 1960s. Are we falling behind or failing to progress? Perhaps the full impact of the community mental health movement, especially such roles as the nurse as therapist or the nurse as community organizer, is still unfolding.

Alternatively, perhaps we are observing the natural consequence of the holistic health movement in which the integrating forces and synergistic processes of the system or organization become superior to the uniqueness and separateness of its component parts. Psychiatric nursing had to become somewhat "separate" in order to find its place in the mental health arena. Now, perhaps, it must join other forces moving in such diverse new directions as (1) biomedical knowledge about the cause and treatment of mental illness; (2) political and social action to effectively confront such problems as homelessness, family violence, poverty, and addiction; and (3) psychological and spiritual healing for cancer, AIDS, and other chronic and often fatal diseases.

Looking Forward to the Twenty-First Century

As the 1990s bring the world to the turn of the century, how will ideas about mental health and mental illness change? How will mental health problems be prioritized? In other words, how will the United States address its problems of alcohol and drug addiction; homelessness; poverty; family violence; and severe, disabling mental illness? And how will psychiatric nursing participate fully in society's decisions about these serious problems as we move into the next century?

Public support of mental health services—at federal, state, and local levels—will probably continue to decline. This trend has adversely affected nursing in recent decades and will continue to present a challenge to the growth and development of the profession. Expecting to solve problems by simply adding more resources is neither realistic nor justifiable, given the scope of our nation's limited resources and the extent of our federal debt. The population of the United States continues to increase in size and diversity, and unemployment and educational deficits continue to present a powerful challenge to the national economy and social well-being.

The decline of government support poses a dilemma if social problems continue to rise in seriousness and frequency. Increased tension between government as provider and government as controller has produced a society divided over issues relating to government support for social programs, extent of government controls needed to ensure quality, and protection of individual rights and freedom. An alternative and more hopeful prediction for the 1990s is that in the face of worsening problems, reduced resources, and increased consciousness about individual rights, Americans will be inspired to renew their commitment to volunteer service, charitable giving, and educational programs to promote self-reliance.

How, then, will psychiatric nursing change? The profession already has increased its involvement in social problems, in both clinical practice and political and social action. Practice, research, and education all reveal this shift in emphasis. Nevertheless, as a group of professionals, mental health–psychiatric nurses are at risk of being spread too thin. Because of limited expansions in public services, "more is better" solutions are not being applied. Development of alternative clinical activities within the private and public sector is clearly needed to bring creative responses to America's social and mental health problems.

For example, self-care and emphasis on responsibility for self are now accepted concepts in mental health, among both professionals and lay persons. Self-help groups and activities permeate most areas of health and illness, suggesting that the human instinct to seek and offer support during difficult times is alive and well. These activities will play an increasingly critical role with people experiencing emotional and social distress. Some examples of such groups include contemporary spiritual recovery fellowships for people with addictions, support groups for cancer clients and their families, and rehabilitation-support groups for clients and families coping with severe, disabling mental illness. Nurses will continue to increase their involvement in these groups, filling such key roles as consultants, health educators, counselors, community organizers, and advocates.

Scientific advances will continue to challenge accepted practices in mental health care. Already, dramatic inroads have been made regarding the physiological processes associated with affective disorders, schizophrenia, borderline personality disorder, violence, and other important mental health problems. Many professionals believe we have moved solidly into an era in which biological and physiological factors in mental illness are the leading topics of research and critical thought.

As a result, scientific advances will continue to alter the nature of treatment and will also shape the course—and even the future—of psychiatric–mental health nursing. Despite the achievement of interpersonal "answers" to many questions and issues in client care, mental health professionals have failed to show that these interpersonal treatment methods can effectively prevent or treat severe mental illnesses. Other solutions are needed. These trends in science and social policy confront psychiatric nursing with certain painful realities and challenges that will affect mental health nursing roles in practice, research, and social action.

Research

Psychiatric nurses have not generally been the researchers inquiring into the origins or processes of severe mental disorders, especially the study of biological and physiological functions at the cellular level of the brain and nervous system. Professional identity and practice issues have inspired nurses to pursue their own research ideas and interests, producing certain areas of knowledge about interpersonal aspects of care, therapeutic intervention in social problems such as family violence, and application of mental health concepts to other health issues such as stress management.

However, this focus has left the profession substantially out of the mainstream of contemporary scientific inquiry addressing the relationship between psychobiological factors and mental health. As we move toward the next century, new research roles will be defined because more psychiatric nurses pursuing doctoral study will specialize in the study of mind and behavior from a neuropsychobiological frame of reference. These nurse researchers will assume leadership and collaborative roles in scientific pursuits, exploring as yet unknown frontiers of the mind. These research endeavors will embrace the traditional concerns of nursing for the caring and "humanistic" dimensions of behavior, producing a new era of holistic inquiry in the mental health arena.

Nursing research will also broaden our scientific knowledge about a wider range of mental health phenomena. For example, nurse researchers are studying the effectiveness of treatments designed to prevent or reduce the severity of social problems such as family violence. Interventions will be designed to prevent and treat stress-related disease, such as cardiovascular disease and psychosomatic disorders. Nurse researchers can also be found investigating the effect of the mind on the immune system, as might apply to nursing care of people with AIDS or cancer.

Clinical practice

The interpersonal techniques at which psychiatric nurses have worked so hard to become proficient will be given progressively less credence in the mental health treatment arena, if biochemical theories continue to promote the use of medications and deinstitutionalization. For example, when medications effectively eliminate seizures or hallucinations in a severely mentally ill person, then reliance on medications to return people to "normal" life becomes a compelling possibility. As these approaches increasingly leave the severely disabled mentally ill out in the community, the interpersonal talents and skills of psychiatric nurses will be in greater demand in new and alternative community settings instead of in institutional treatment environments.

If the United States is inspired during this decade to find ways to solve such problems as family violence, poverty, homelessness, and severe disabling mental illness, then treatment and needed social services will increasingly evolve through private and not-for-profit organizations. Psychiatric nursing practice will expand, and nurses' sources of income will probably change as well. New combinations of practice (including private practice) and work site will evolve as nurses develop alternative roles incorporating skills in interpersonal relationships, case management, and monitoring clients receiving psychotropic medications (including practice with prescription privileges where state laws permit).

Psychiatric nurses will increasingly become involved in facilitative roles with self-help approaches of all kinds, for individuals, families, and groups. These roles will include consultation and education in many contexts, ranging from crisis intervention to social rehabilitation, for example. Community organization will gain importance as a component of these nurses' roles, as clients become more capable of using help to function collectively within their communities.

Social-political action

In the social-political arena, possibilities for psychiatric nurses will be limitless. Many roles will be apparent, resulting from increasing numbers of psychiatric nurses seeking forms of influence as citizens, as professionals in strategic positions in health care systems, as nurses within their profession, as participants in political campaigns, and as candidates themselves who campaign successfully and are elected to public office.

One major challenge to be confronted is advocacy of public support for mental health treatment, training, and research. Broader definitions of mental health issues will be reinforced, to embrace the problems of family violence, child abuse, poverty, and homelessness, as well as the needs of the mentally ill. Encouragement of continuing development of our nation's resources in the private sector will complement advocacy of public support; this will include encouragement of both charitable giving as well as volunteer service.

A second major challenge, or focus, for social-political action is the nursing profession, particularly psychiatric–mental health nursing, as a specialty group. Increasing involvement in substantive research is needed, especially research that follows a line of inquiry with multiple studies and approaches. More nurse researchers who have expertise in the study of psychobiological processes and who are willing to join with other researchers in large-scale investigations will be needed.

Action within organized psychiatric nursing is needed to stimulate serious research rather than the myriad of small studies that often characterize the field in nursing journals. Action is also needed to establish clearer standards for research and scholarly work, including increased valuing of large-scale substantive studies in mental health over small studies that at best suggest "implications" for nursing and lack generalizability. Dissemination and integration of knowledge into the mainstream of day-to-day psychiatric nursing practice will require widespread commitment and increased valuing of scientific inquiry as a basis for improving psychiatric nursing practice.

In conclusion, significant political, economic, scientific, and social realities will affect the future of mental health–psychiatric nursing. Strongly conservative political party forces continue to work in opposition to the liberal ideas that shaped the community mental health movement of the late 1950s and early 1960s. Major cutbacks in public spending for social services, accompanied by increased defense spending, characterize recent so-called attempts to restore economic stability. Some observers note that social responses reveal greater unrest and disorder in certain sectors; others point out that improvements in social conditions that heighten expectations have also resulted in disappointment and increased dissatisfaction.

Opportunity more than risk characterizes the immediate future. Choices range from embarking on independent practice roles to undertaking the academic study necessary to become clinical researchers. Psychiatric nurses can work and develop collectively with other nurses and collaborate with other health professionals. Opportunities to become advocates in the community and to devote energy to creating alternative forms of care are currently challenging old ways of thinking and former practices in psychiatric nursing. Achievement of better third-party reimbursement of mental health nursing services and better compensation for nurses in institutional roles will ensure clients more opportunity to experience the holistic form of care that characterizes modern day mental health–psychiatric nursing.

BRIEF REVIEW

The psychiatric nurse's treatment of mental health problems is a relatively recent response to an age-old human dilemma: What is the best way to care for the mentally ill? Through the ages, care has been the product of two different traditions, one stressing a need to appease magical or supernatural forces and the other attempting to understand, through rational methods, the causes and cure of the disease.

Training of psychiatric nurses has changed from experience acquired solely in mental hospitals to enrollment in colleges and universities to study nursing. Concepts of psychiatric care have been added to the curriculum for all nursing students. Nurses specialize today by means of postgraduate training. Psychiatric nursing has received extensive federal support in this endeavor, primarily as a result of the National Mental Health Act of 1946.

The Community Mental Health Centers Act of 1963 has been a powerful force in moving care out of the mental hospital into the community. This was a natural development in mental health policy, after innovations in psychiatric care during the two world wars crystallized the nation's recognition of the power and possibility of prevention. Some of the consequences of this expansion of services have brought nurses into conflict with other mental health professionals. The ongoing progress of this conflict process promises to be a determinant of the future course of psychiatric nursing.

Advances in scientific knowledge are among the factors affecting psychiatric nursing over the past few decades. For example, new knowledge about the fundamental psychobiological bases of mental illness increased reliance on psychotropic medications, moving away from the therapeutic milieu and communication-based interventions. Reduced public spending for mental health resulted in fewer hospital beds and a treatment approach called *deinstitutionalization*; this was said to be in the client's best interest for both therapeutic and ethical reasons. However, overall reductions in public spending and a shrinking economy combined with deinstitutionalization to produce large numbers of homeless mentally ill.

The holistic and self-help movements incorporated many attributes of consumerism by stressing the importance of the individual being responsible for and knowledgeable about the creation and maintenance of a healthy existence. These movements were compatible with psychiatric nursing's trend toward development of roles outside institutional settings in more varied and autonomous community activities. With this increased participation in community settings has come greater involvement in mental health problems more typically called *social problems*, such as family violence, child abuse, and rape. As a result, psychiatric nursing has once again moved closer to the women's movement and joined forces with feminist and other social action groups committed to improving health for people disadvantaged by our society.

The psychiatric nurse today faces a present and future of both risk and opportunity. Practicing in a wide range of settings, the psychiatric nurse integrates conflicting values of tradition and progress, of humanism and science, and of caring and "curing." The future challenges psychiatric nursing to find creative responses to decreasing public support, increasing emphasis on biological theories of mental disorder, and the perception that mental problems and social disorder are on the rise. The importance of nursing care in treating the mentally ill and the socially deviant will be confirmed through continued progress in research, practice, and education.

REFERENCES AND SUGGESTED READINGS

1. Alexander F, Selesnick S: *The history of psychiatry*, New York, 1966, Harper & Row.
2. American Nurses Association Council on Psychiatric and Mental Health Nursing: guidelines for private practice, *Pacesetter*, p 3, Spring 1985.
3. Ashley J: *Hospitals, paternalism and the role of the nurse*, New York, 1976, Teachers College Press.
4. Bailey H: *Nursing mental diseases*, New York, 1920, Macmillan.
5. Beers C: *A mind that found itself*, ed 7, Garden City, NY, 1948, Doubleday.
6. Block S, Reddaway P: *Psychiatric terror: how Soviet psychiatry is used to suppress dissent*, New York, 1977, Basic Books.
7. Brown EL: *Nursing for the future*, New York, 1948, Russell Sage Foundation.
8. Chamberlain J: The role of the federal government in development of psychiatric nursing, *Journal of Psychosocial Nursing and Mental Health Services* 21(4):11, 1983.
9. Church OM: Emergence of training programs for asylum nursing at the turn of the century, *Advances in Nursing Science* 7(2):35, 1985.
10. Davidson J, Lytle M: *After the fact: the art of historical detection*, vol 1, New York, 1982, Alfred A. Knopf.
11. Donahue MP: *Nursing: the finest art—an illustrated history*, St Louis, 1985, Mosby–Year Book.
12. Ellenberger F: *The discovery of the unconscious*, New York, 1970, Basic Books.
13. Fagin CM: Psychiatric nursing at the crossroads: quo vadis, *Perspectives in Psychiatric Care* 19(3-4):99, 1981.
14. Fagin CM: Concepts for the future: competition and substitution, *Journal of Psychosocial Nursing and Mental Health Services* 21(3):36, 1983.
15. Ferenczi S and others: Psychoanalysis and the war neuroses, New York, 1921, International Psychoanalytic Press.
16. Foucalt M: *Madness and civilization*, New York, 1965, Pantheon Books.
17. Greenblatt M, York R, Brown EL: *From custodial to therapeutic patient care in mental hospitals*, New York, 1955, Russell Sage Foundation.
18. Grinker R, Spiegel J: *War neurosis in North Africa*, New York, 1943, Josiah Macy, Jr. Foundation.
19. Grinker R, Spiegel J: *Men under stress*, New York, 1945, Blakiston.
20. Hardin S, Durham J: First rate: structure, process and effectiveness of nurse psychotherapy, *Journal of Psychosocial Nursing and Mental Health Services* 23(5):8, 1985.
21. Hume TB: General principles of community psychiatry. In Arieti S, editor: *American handbook of psychiatry*, vol 3, New York, 1966, Basic Books.
22. Jaynes J: *The origin of consciousness in the breakdown of the bicameral mind*, Boston, 1977, Houghton Mifflin.
23. Joint Commission on Mental Illness and Health: *Action for mental health*, New York, 1961, Basic Books.
24. Kaplan HI, Freedman AM, Sadock BJ: *Comprehensive textbook of psychiatry/IV*, ed 4, Baltimore, 1985, Williams & Wilkins.
25. Kardiner A: *Traumatic neuroses of war*, New York, 1941, Paul B. Hoeber.
26. Kardiner A: Traumatic neuroses of war. In Arieti S, editor: *American handbook of psychiatry*, New York, 1959, Basic Books.
27. Mellow J: The evolution of nursing therapy and its implications for education, doctoral dissertation, Boston, 1964, Boston University.
28. Mitsunaga BK: Designing psychiatric/mental health nursing for the future: problems and prospects, *Journal of Psychosocial Nursing and Mental Health Services* 20(12):15, 1982.

29. Muff J, editor: *Socialization, sexism, and stereotyping: women's issues in nursing*, St Louis, 1982, Mosby–Year Book.

30. Muller T: *Fundamentals of psychiatric nursing*, Totowa, NJ, 1962, Littlefield, Adams & Co.

31. Osborn O, Thomas M: On public sector psychosocial nursing: a conceptual framework, *Journal of Psychosocial Nursing and Mental Health Services* 29(8):13, 1991.

32. Peplau H: *Interpersonal relations in nursing*, New York, 1952, GP Putman's Sons.

33. Peplau H: Principles of psychiatric nursing. In Arieti S, editor: *American handbook of psychiatry*, vol 2, New York, 1959, Basic Books.

34. Peplau H: Historical development of psychiatric nursing: a preliminary statement of some facts and trends, Paper presented at working conference on graduate education in psychiatric nursing, Williamsburg, Va, November, 1956. Reprinted in Smoyak SA, Rouslin S, editors: *A collection of classics in psychiatric nursing literature*, Thorofare, NJ, 1982, Charles B. Slack.

35. Roberts M: *American nursing: history and interpretation*, New York, 1954, Macmillan.

36. Rothman D: *The discovery of the asylum*, Boston, 1971, Little, Brown, & Co.

37. Salmon TW: War neuroses: shell shock, *Military Surgery* 41:674, 1917.

38. Sills G: Historical developments and issues in psychiatric mental health nursing. In Leininger M, editor: *Contemporary issues in mental health nursing*, Boston, 1973, Little, Brown & Co.

39. Tudor G: Sociopsychiatric nursing approach to intervention in a problem of mutual withdrawal on a mental hospital ward, *Psychiatry* 15:193, 1952.

40. Wilson D: *Stranger and traveler: the story of Dorothea Dix, American reformer*, Boston, 1975, Little, Brown & Co.

ANNOTATED BIBLIOGRAPHY

Ashley J: *Hospitals, paternalism and the role of the nurse*, New York, 1976, Teachers College Press.

This important study traces the development of nursing in hospitals, exploring questions about why nurses have had so little influence on hospital management and health care delivery. Ashley argues that the problem is rooted in sexism and the exploitation of nurses over the years by hospital administrators and physicians. By illuminating the historical basis for contemporary problems, the author convincingly argues that nurses need to become more politically active in both health care and general social policy arenas.

Church O: From custody to community in psychiatric nursing, *Nursing Research* 36(1):48, 1987.

This article presents a review of psychiatric nursing that adds perspective and insight to current nursing practice issues.

McBride A: Psychiatric nursing in the 1990's, *Archives of Psychiatric Nursing* 4(1):21, 1990.

The author reviews nursing's accomplishments over the past years. She describes limitations and makes recommendations for the future of nursing, including the approaching "Decade of the Brain."

Peplau H: Future directions in psychiatric nursing from the perspective of history, *Journal of Psychosocial Nursing and Mental Health Services* 27(2):18, 1989.

Peplau, an early leader in nursing, reviews historical influences that have been integrated into the present perspective of psychiatric nursing.

Roberts MM: *American nursing: history and interpretation*, New York, 1954, Macmillan.

This is the "grand" book of nursing history, a work that provides a standard that regrettably is rarely equaled in later works. Roberts writes in a sympathetic yet unsparing style that clearly identifies the issues surrounding the development of nursing in the United States. Her work is meticulously documented and even today, 30 years later, is the best discussion of American nursing up to 1950. Unfortunately, throughout most of the period covered she does not deal with psychiatric nursing as it relates to nursing in general.

Smoyak S, Rouslin S: *A collection of classics in psychiatric nursing literature*, Thorofare, NJ, 1982, Charles B. Slack.

A collection of articles written by early nurse leaders in psychiatric nursing. This book provides the foundation for psychiatric nursing as it is today.

The Person as a Client

Peggy A Landrum
Cornelia Kelly Beck
Ruth Parmelee Rawlins
Sophronia R Williams

After studying this chapter, the student will be able to:

- Discuss the historical development of the holistic approach to the person
- Describe the qualities of each dimension of the person
- Describe the person-environment relationship

- Describe the nature of stress and adaptation within each dimension of the person
- Discuss the impact of self-responsibility on health status

The primary goal of nursing care is to help clients develop strategies to achieve harmony within themselves and with others, nature, and the world. Integrative functioning of the client's physical, emotional, intellectual, social, and spiritual dimensions is emphasized. Each person is considered as a whole with many factors contributing to health and illness.

This chapter presents an overview of the person within the framework of holistic philosophy. The following general concepts of the holistic approach to health care are explored: (1) human dimensions, (2) relationship of the person with the environment, (3) stress and adaptation, and (4) self-responsibility. The chapter is intended to challenge the student to consider the highly interactive nature of human functioning in relation to both health and illness.

HOLISTIC HEALTH CARE CONCEPTS

Several concepts are generally accepted as premises of a holistic orientation to health care. The general concepts discussed in this chapter are shown in Table 2-1.

Dimensions of the Person

Recognizing all human dimensions encourages a balanced and whole view of a person. Each facet of an individual is important and contributes to the quality of life experience. If any facets are ignored, the person has diffi-

culty living in a balanced state, resulting in fewer available options to the individual. For instance, people who ignore their physical aspect probably do not view exercise as an outlet for emotional stress. If intellectual capacities are not developed, people may lack the knowledge and cognitive skills necessary for problem solving. If their spiritual component is ignored, they may be unable to construct meaningful life goals. Individuals create options for themselves by respecting their needs in each dimension and by fully developing each dimension. To the extent that they are willing to do this, they increase available alternatives regarding any life situation.

The dimensions are separated here for exploration purposes, but this is an artificial separation that can occur only in an analysis. In reality they are intricately interwoven, and the person as a whole functioning organism is more than the simple combination of dimensions.

Physical dimension The physical aspect involves everything associated with one's body, both internal and external. Inputs to the body (such as food, water, and air), transformation of these inputs within the body, and outputs from the body (such as waste products, energy for exercise, and energy for healing) are included in the physical dimension.[9] Some issues related to this dimension are genetics, nutrition, breathing, touching, rest, body weight, the sleep-wake cycle, autoimmunological functioning, energy, fitness, movement, body image, healing capacity of the body, stress reduction through physical activity and relaxation, and the physical environment. In this section, ge-

HISTORICAL OVERVIEW

DATES	EVENTS
Ancient Times	Primitive people perceived their bodies as the dwelling place of the soul, and illness was seen as the result of malevolent spirits projecting some noxious object into the body.
	Indian and Chinese philosophers saw all of life as a whole, and the spirit was unseparated from the rest of the person.
400-300 BC	Plato contended that human beings possess a spirit with direct access to the realm of the nonphysical, seen in prophesy and healing.
	Aristotle distinguished between experiences that involved physical activities (sensations, appetites, passions) and those that involved activity of the soul (thinking).
1600s-1700s	Descartes' suggestion that the body and mind were two different entities encouraged the establishment of medical systems in which physical problems were solved by dealing exclusively with the body and mental problems were approached by dealing with the mind.
	Repressive measures by the Church of England led a small religious group to separate from the main church to seek religious freedom. This group of separatists, known as Puritans, believed that an austere life released their soul from bondage to the body and permitted union with a divine being.
1800s	William James proposed relationships between experiences that involved emotional stimulus, emotional behavior (visceral reactions and overt actions), and emotional experience.
1960s	The emergence of mass society identified by such factors as depersonalization, mechanization, and loss of individuality and privacy has promoted the view that people are a mass target of influence rather than individual human beings.
1970s	The women's movement contributed to altering sex role differentiation particularly in areas of work and education.
	Dramatic changes were seen in childrearing practices, male and female roles, and concerns about the environment and the structure of society.
1980s	Research indicated that intellectual capacity is not predetermined, that individuals use less than half of their brains and that the decline in intellectual functioning can be prevented.
1990s	Current health care models recognize the interrelationships of the mind, body, and environment.
Future	As the elderly population increases, nurses will need to provide holistic care to this population in an era of decreased funding.

netics, physiological processes, and body image are selected for discussion because of the relevance of these concepts to mental health–psychiatric nursing.

Genetics involves a complex process through which individuals inherit particular characteristics, potentials, predispositions, and limitations. Hereditary factors in mental illness are typically investigated by twin studies, genetic marker studies, and adoption studies. Evidence of genetic influence on psychiatric dysfunction is continually increasing. The contribution of heredity to the development of alcoholism, the major affective disorders, and schizophrenia have most often been studied, with some attention to the role of genetics in the development of antisocial personality disorder. All of these disorders show tendencies to cluster in biological relatives, even when the related individuals do not grow and develop in the same family environments. Studies on familial clustering of various disorders support genetic theory.[56]

Currently, evidence shows that heredity contributes to the potential for such disorders. However, the manifestation of symptoms and specific behaviors is then triggered by physiological, social, and environmental forces. Mental health–psychiatric nurses recognize that genetic influence is not absolute. Such risk can be modified or counteracted by other forces.

Sleep is necessary for good health, and sleep alterations can be one of the earliest indicators of behavioral and somatic disturbance. Two types of sleep occur. Non-rapid eye movement (NREM) is a quiet sleep that encompasses the first four stages of sleep; rapid eye movement (REM) is the active final stage of sleep, characterized by extremely rapid eye movement (see the box on p. 19).

REM sleep is necessary for mental restorative processes, including learning, memory, and psychological adaptation. Emotional and mental stress increases the need for REM sleep. Decreased sleep time results in loss of REM sleep,

▼ **TABLE 2-1**   Holistic Health Care Concepts

Concept	Assumptions
Multidimen-sionality	Interaction and balance of the physical, emotional, intellectual, social, and spiritual dimensions is evident.
	Emphasis is on respect of needs and development of potential in each dimension.
Relationship with the environment	The person-to-environment interaction is a crucial factor in determining the quality of life experiences in both health and illness.
Self-responsibility	Each person is an active participant in the maintenance of optimal health status. The health care system cannot "make" people healthy; individuals choose their own life-styles and directions.
Life-cycle development	Each person progresses through the stages of life with particular needs, issues, feelings, and behaviors affecting that person at different times. Growth and development at any one stage affects later stages.
Stress and adaptation	An individual's ability to cope with stressful events is a primary factor in each person's experience of health and illness. Stressful conditions are unique to each person, are experienced throughout the life cycle, and affect the whole person.

▼ **THE STAGES OF SLEEP**

Stage 1	Twilight phase: person is easily aroused; lasts up to 30 minutes
Stage 2	Sound sleep, but person is aroused with ease
Stage 3	Deep level of sleep; strong stimulus is needed to wake person
Stage 4	Deepest phase of sleep, reached approximately 30 to 40 minutes after beginning Stage 1
REM	Final stage of sleep cycle; person is difficult to arouse; dreaming and nightmares occur

for which the body tries to compensate by increasing REM sleep during the next sleep period. Chronic disruption of REM sleep interferes with healthy psychological functioning. Lack of sleep for prolonged periods can produce psychosis. Disruption of sleep-rest activity can exhaust individuals and contribute to the experience of illusions and hallucinations.

Stage 4 sleep is necessary for physical restorative processes; thus strenuous physical activity creates additional need for Stage 4 sleep. Integumentary cellular renewal occurs during the deepest sleep period, usually midnight to 4 AM; constant disruption can significantly extend healing time.[28] Mental health–psychiatric nurses recognize the important role of adequate sleep cycles in overall functioning of their clients.

Body image is a significant aspect of the physical dimension. Body image is determined by how one views oneself. This view of self is fairly well established by the end of toddlerhood and relatively fixed by the end of adolescence. Messages received by children as they are maturing lay the foundation for the development of body image. Words such as "cute," "ugly," "strong," "weak," "awkward," "good," and "bad" are incorporated into the body image. *Ideal* body image and *perceived* body image constitute the physical aspect of the total self-concept. The body is considered by some to be the most significant avenue for expression of the total self.[45] It is the body that others see, that acts and demonstrates competencies, and that in these acts reveals emotions.

The way people perceive their physical bodies may also have important emotional consequences. A realistic body image may significantly enhance one's potential for successful achievement throughout life. When one's body image is not distorted, a correlation exists between self-perception and perception by others. Individuals who have a consistent, realistic, and stable body image are demonstrating their ability to appropriately assess reality.

One's body image—shape, size, mass, structure, function, and significance of the body and its parts—is dynamic and open to change. Body image may change as alterations occur in the individual's anatomy or personality. For example, an adolescent girl may gain extra pounds if she constantly snacks on high-calorie foods to relieve anxious feelings. As she becomes aware of tight clothing, she may also become acutely aware of her excess body bulk and withdraw from selected social contacts until she returns to her original weight and shape.

The idea that personality is correlated with body build was introduced in the 1920s and further refined in the 1940s. Three basic body types were described: endomorph (pyknic), mesomorph (athletic), and ectomorph (esthetic).[64] The term *endomorph* denoted a round, soft body, frequently associated with an affectionate, sociable personality, subject to mood swings. Traits attributable to the endomorph included love of comfort and eating, sociability, politeness, tolerance, and complacency. The athletic *mesomorph* was a person of average size with a muscular build who preferred physical activity and displayed traits of assertiveness, adventurousness, courage, callousness, ruthlessness, and indifference to pain. Finally, the *ectomorph* was a tall, thin, fragile person who tended to possess a withdrawn temperament and demonstrated traits of restraint, privacy, secretiveness, and introversion. This system of correlating personality and body build is not universally accepted. However, social reactions to different body builds vary. The components of a person's body structure set up expectations about the person's abilities and greatly influence what the person can do.

The various aspects of the physical dimension interact constantly with each other. For instance, a person's nutritional status directly affects other areas such as energy, weight, and physiological processes. Eating excessive amounts of sugar is known to decrease energy levels and cause fatigue and shakiness. Heredity establishes certain parameters for physical growth and development. Exercise leads to better eating habits, better ability to sleep, weight control, improved cardiovascular and pulmonary functioning, joint flexibility, fewer injuries, faster healing response, fat reduction, increased energy, and stamina.

A person's physical dimension affects emotions, intellectual functioning, social experiences, and even spirituality. Physical fitness is associated with an improved body image, positive attitudes, self-confidence, fewer periods of depression, greater ability to relate to other people, increased assertiveness, and an increased number of spiritual experiences. Physical activity is an effective way of counteracting emotional stress and tension. Factors such as body image, physical energy, and sexuality affect social interactions. When people neglect themselves physically, they limit their potential in other areas as well; for example, it is difficult to be sociable or to think clearly when one is fatigued or sick.

The degree to which people experience physical well-being is an indicator of how effectively they are taking care of their total selves, as well as how effectively they are integrating the healthy aspects of their other four dimensions—emotional, intellectual, social, and spiritual.

Emotional dimension Terms such as mood, emotion, and affect are used interchangeably by professionals and lay persons. Dozens of instruments are designed to measure emotional states, and a multitude of descriptive terms are used to describe moods and emotions. The richness of language reflects the importance of this dimension to our culture. In this book, the term "emotional" rather than "psychological" is used to describe this dimension. "Psychological" implies a combination of emotional and intellectual components, whereas "emotional" refers to affective states and feelings. In general, *emotion* refers to a fleeting feeling, *mood* refers to a prolonged feeling, and *affect* represents the observable manifestation of a person's feelings. Some terms commonly used to describe mood include those in the accompanying box.

The various theories of emotion attempt to integrate the following three components: the motor behavior associated with emotion (what is expressed), the experienced aspect (what is felt), and the physiological mechanisms that underlie emotions (what happens inside the body). Although emphasis varies, each of the components receives attention in most existing theories of emotion.

In all theories of emotion, the activation of the physiological systems (the parasympathetic and sympathetic nervous systems, the limbic system, and the reticular formation) is related to emotional experiences, and cognitive processes mediate emotional experiences. Secondly, most theories of emotion accept the concept of adaptation level, which is a physiological or cognitive state that assists the individual in maintaining homeostasis. A third common element suggests that a related social event can elicit and define the nature of a particular emotional experience, such as fear in response to a loss of power. No theory of emotion views individuals as passive receptacles of emotional experiences.

Emotional experiences are actively constructed by *appraisal processes*; some emotional experiences are actively sought, and others are avoided. These appraisal processes are determined partially by learned patterns of reponse. One person may react to a particular situation with fear, whereas another reacts with anger. A final persistent theme in theories of emotion is that control helps determine emotional experiences. Individuals can maximize positive feelings and minimize negative feelings by exercising control (for example, over social events or their degree of involvement).

For the purposes of this book emotion is defined in the following manner: (1) emotion is affective and includes a feeling element or awareness; (2) the central nervous system and the autonomic nervous system are involved in emotion by producing motor, glandular, and visceral activities; and (3) emotion is related to motivation as an energizer of behavior.[35]

The first component of emotion is the affective property. Affect is the observable manifestation of an individual's feelings. Observation of behavior, including posture, facial expressions (Figure 2-1), tone of voice, gestures, crying, sweating, and clenched fists, provides objective data about one's affect.

The feeling element is perhaps the most commonly recognized aspect of the emotional dimension. Feelings are harder to conceptualize than aspects of the physical realm because they are less tangible, but they are still a vital part of each person. Feelings such as joy, anger, sadness, and fear occur most naturally in young children, who are not yet restricted by many *should's* and *should not's* regarding the experience and expression of feelings. Adults, however, often attach judgments to their feelings, and consequently ignore uncomfortable ones. Certain cultures are more likely to label particular feelings as good or bad, but all feelings are subject to being ignored at one time or another. For example, a person may not feel joy if it seems "undeserved." Anger may be ignored because it is considered "impolite." Sadness, or grief, may not be acknowledged when it "makes someone else uncomfortable." Fear may be suppressed because of a need to "be strong." Feelings in themselves are neither good nor bad; they are simply a part of human experience. Each individual has the capacity to experience the entire realm of feelings, which are meant to be experienced, not ignored. By ignoring or suppressing

▼ ···
TERMS USED TO DESCRIBE MOOD

Angry	Lonely
Anxious	Mad
Bored	Mean
Calm	Miserable
Cheerful	Outraged
Confused	Pained
Despairing	Pleasant
Distraught	Relaxed
Enraged	Remorseful
Exasperated	Sad
Fearful	Scared
Frightened	Solemn
Furious	Stunned
Grieving	Terrified
Happy	Worried
Infuriated	

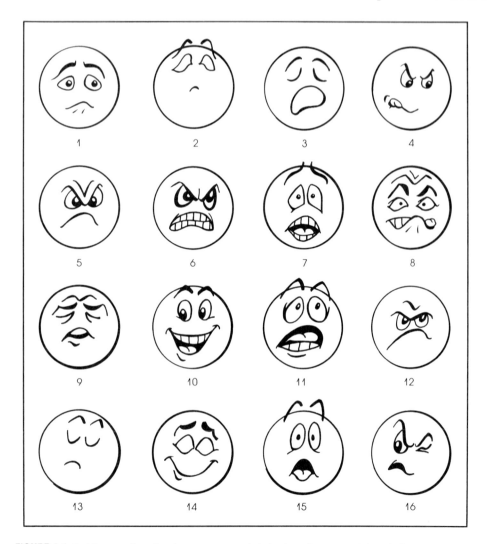

FIGURE 2-1 Facial expressions that demonstrate mood. *1,* Anxious; *2,* arrogant; *3,* bored, *4,* concentrating; *5,* disapproving; *6,* enraged; *7,* frightened; *8,* frustrated; *9,* grieving; *10,* happy; *11,* horrified; *12,* negative; *13,* prudish; *14,* satisfied; *15,* surprised; *16,* suspicious.

feelings, people limit their opportunities to function as whole persons.[54]

Feelings assist people to stay in touch with themselves, with what pleases them and what does not. Often they may be one's first source of information about what is going on and about how one is responding or wants to respond to a situation. The emotionally aroused person generally is aware of feelings, for example, excitement, fear, anger, or joy.

Individuals learn at an early age how to express feelings. Words, voice tone and volume, body posture and movements, and facial expressions are among the behaviors people use to communicate their feelings. The way that an individual expresses a particular feeling is influenced greatly by the culture in which the person lives. Studies have found that American women receive emotional cues more accurately than do American men. One explanation is that during socialization girls are encouraged to express their emotions openly and to pay close attention to the emotions of others, whereas boys are actively discouraged from engaging in these behaviors.[1]

The second component of the definition of emotion is motor, glandular, and visceral activities, produced by the central and autonomic nervous systems. During stimulation, the reticular system and the hypothalamus send simultaneous impulses to the cortex of the brain and to the viscera; these impulses result in physiological changes (Table 2-2).

Physiological changes that occur with emotional arousal are referred to as the "emergency" function of emotions. The physical aspects of emotions such as fear and anger seem to help individuals survive in case of danger. Stress responses such as increased heart rate, blood pressure, and rate of breathing make available an increased supply of oxygen for strenuous muscle activity. Changes in blood composition make more sugar available for quick energy and cause clotting in case of injury. Blood is taken from digestive organs and distributed where it is needed most. Pupil response produces greater visual acuity. Increased perspiration carries away waste products of intense muscle action.

The final component of emotion is motivation as an en-

▼ **TABLE 2-2   Summary of Physiological Changes that May Occur with Emotional Arousal**

Change	Description
Increase in heart rate	The increased epinephrine released from the pituitary gland accelerates heart rate.
Increase in blood pressure	The increased heart rate may cause a rise in blood pressure. Other changes take place in the distribution of blood. A greater volume is made available to the lungs and muscles, and internal organs receive less. Flushing of the face and neck during anger or embarrassment result from these changes in blood pressure and circulation.
Muscle tension tremor	Muscle tone is increased. Tremor ("knocking of the knees") often occurs when opposing groups of muscles are contracted simultaneously.
Changes in blood composition	The amount of blood sugar, the acid-base balance, and the epinephrine (adrenalin) content of the blood are significantly increased.
Increase in perspiration	Shaking hands with a person provides a quick and fairly reliable indication of the degree of emotional tension the person is experiencing by the presence or absence of perspiration.
Increase in respiration	Both rate and depth of breathing accelerate.
Gastrointestinal changes	Peristaltic movements of the stomach and intestines may cease. The flow of digestive juices, including saliva, decrease, producing feelings of dry mouth, being "sick to the stomach" and a lack of appetite.
Galvanic skin response (GSR)	Minute but detectable changes occur in the electric properties of the skin. These can be recorded and measured by means of an instrument called a galvanometer. An electrode is attached to the skin, usually the palms of the hands. A swing of the instrument's needle indicates a GSR. GSR is a sensitive indicator of changes in emotional state and is used as one component of the lie detector test. Blood pressure and rate of respiration also are monitored in persons taking a lie detector test.
Pilomotor response	This is the technical term for "goose pimples." The small hairs on the skin rise.
Pupil response	The pupils of the eye tend to dilate.

ergizer of behavior. The Latin word *emovere* means to stir up, agitate, excite, and move. To be moved in an emotional sense means to "stir up oneself" or to be "pushed." At times, emotion not only stirs one up, but also causes one to push (motivate) oneself.[50] When a person experiences emotions such as fear and anger, body resources are mobilized to meet emergencies. Mobilization of resources as described in the preceding paragraph enables the threatened person to either fight or flee more effectively.

Emotional states are significantly determined by cognitive factors. When individuals are physiologically aroused, they label, interpret, and identify their stirred-up state according to the precipitating situation. What is perceived in the immediate situation is interpreted through past experience, allowing the feeling to be labeled and understood. The same increase in heart rate, rapid breathing, and trembling can be experienced as "joy" or "anger," depending on how the immediate situation is perceived. For example, parents send their estranged adolescent a letter. The boy is aware of his trembling hands and pounding heart while holding the envelope. When he opens the envelope, he finds that it contains an airplane ticket to return home. The adolescent may feel anger or joy, depending on whether the gesture is interpreted as manipulative or caring.

Mild emotions may be constructive in their overall effect by motivating one toward worthwhile goals. Once an emotion has become attached to an object or situation, one's behavior is directed toward reaching the goal. Mild anxiety sharpens a student's cognitive abilities and facilitates the achievement of educational goals. For example, college students who love the color and excitement of football games are not likely to stay home when invited to go.

As emotions reach the intermediate range of intensity, they may prompt a person to take action, such as leaving an unhealthy situation; conversely, the intensity of the emotion may be detrimental to problem solving and task performance. When people do not cope adequately with a highly intense emotion, it becomes increasingly disruptive to organized behavior. Severe emotional upheavals actually defeat their emergency function, and prolonged emotional mobilization produces physiological changes that are only not useless but also are actually harmful to the person.[63] For example, when fear is aroused in situations requiring struggle or escape, the accompanying physiological conditions may provide incredible energy and lend "wings to our feet." However, if emotional activation is too intense, the fear may paralyze our action, "rooting us to the spot" or "freezing us in our tracks."

The way a person expresses or ignores feelings and copes with emotional stress has implications for the whole person. When emotionally aroused, the person undergoes changes that affect every activity. Emotional reactions are altered, thoughts and actions are affected, and overall adjustment may be disturbed. Physical manifestations of feelings are constantly present. Consider, for example, the tingling and expansive sensation of joy, the tight muscles and clenched body posture of anger, the gut level sickness of grief, and the rapid heart rate and breathing associated with fear. Although these reactions vary from one person to another and from one situation to another, every person's body and emotions are always interacting in some way. Receptors, muscles, internal organs, and nervous mechanisms interact, resulting in changes in brain waves, physiological reactions, and behaviors. When not coped with adequately, emotional stress can contribute to physical discomfort and illness, ranging from muscle tension, general fatigue, and mild aches to cardiovascular disorders, cancer, rheumatoid arthritis, and migraine headache.[55] The emotional dimension also affects intellectual functioning; the ability to evaluate new ideas and to make effective decisions is influenced by feelings. When emotionally aroused, one may say or do something one would not normally say or do, such as threaten or attempt suicide. Feelings and emotional stress influence how individuals fulfill social roles and relate to other people, both personally and professionally.

Intellectual dimension A variety of definitions of the intellectual dimension have been developed. The one chosen for this discussion divides intellectual functions into the following four main classes: (1) *receptive functions*, which involve the ability to acquire, process, classify, and integrate information; (2) *memory and learning*, by which information is stored and recalled; (3) *cognition*, or thinking, which concerns the mental organization and reorganization of information; and (4) *expressive functions*, through which information is communicated or acted on.[42] Although each function represents a distinct set of behaviors, they normally operate cooperatively.

The two main receptive functions are sensation and perception. Although sensory reception is classified as an intellectual function, it is actually a physiological arousal process that triggers the central registering and integrating activities. The individual receives sensation passively and shuts it out only by voluntary actions, such as holding the nose to avoid an unpleasant odor.[42] The sensory processes include vision, hearing, smell, taste, and touch.

Perception involves an active awareness and interpretation of stimuli. For example, as sound waves cause movement of the tympanic membrane, auditory sensation occurs. As the impulses transmitted by the tympanic membrane are organized, a sound is heard. The same sound, such as thunder, ocean waves, or a slamming door, can be perceived in many different ways with a variety of meanings attached to it. Thus perception provides a bridge between the reception of stimuli by all of the senses and the integration of these sensations into meaningful data; these data are then organized within the context of the person's experience and used for adaptive functioning.

Memory and learning comprise the second main class of intellectual functions. Preceding any memory or learning is the process of registration, in which perceptions are selected, recorded, and programmed in the memorizing centers of the brain. The attention focusing components of perception and the individual's emotional state play an important role in the registration process. For example, two people experiencing the same sensory event may register completely different information depending on their selective attention and their emotional state.

Three types of memory are clinically distinguished by the length of time information is retained: two types of short-term memory (immediate and recent) and long-term, or remote, memory.

Immediate memory involves the fixation of information that is selected for retention during the registration process. It lasts from about 30 seconds to several minutes, unless sustained by rehearsal. With repetition or rehearsal, a memory trace of registered information can be maintained for hours.[42] *Recent memory* involves the retention of infor-

mation from about an hour to 1 or 2 days; this is longer than information could be maintained by conscientious repetition, but the information is not yet fixed in long-term storage as learned material. *Long-term memory*, or learning, is the individual's ability to store information. The process of storage begins as early as ½ second after information enters short-term storage and lasts as long as the information remains in long-term memory. Information that was recently learned can be disrupted or dissipated more easily than older memories because traces become progressively strengthened with time. Evidence exists that information in short-term storage is organized on the basis of contiguity and sensory properties, such as similar shapes, colors, and sounds, whereas information in long-term storage is organized on the basis of meaning.[42]

The third class of intellectual functions is thinking, or cognition, which is any mental operation that relates two or more bits of information. Cognitive operations may be defined by the nature of the information being manipulated (numbers, words, designs, concepts) and the actual operation (comparing, compounding, abstracting, ordering, judging). For example, the operations of "distance judgment" involve abstracting and comparing ideas about space, whereas "computation" may involve the operations of ordering and compounding numbers.

Thinking processes also can be hierarchically arranged according to the degree to which the concept being considered is concrete or abstract.[42] *Concrete thinking* involves focus on a particular aspect of an object or situation, such as the idea of "a round table." Although useful in focusing on particulars, concrete thinking binds the person to immediate experience. *Abstract thinking* involves making generalizations about a category of objects or drawing relationships between situations, such as the idea that "knowledge is power." Abstract thinking considers the past and the future in responding to situations. In essence, it frees the person to think and act based on the construction of possibilities.

The nature of one's thoughts, positive or negative, influences the quality of one's experience by affecting the judgments one makes about the experience. Individuals create their own experience of reality through thoughts and beliefs. They "program" themselves with the information that they acquire and by the way that they process and organize it.[58] When people give themselves positive messages, they are more likely to succeed. When they harbor thoughts of failure, they increase the probability of failure.

The fourth case of intellectual functions is expression, which includes activities such as speaking, drawing, writing, facial expressions, and physical gestures and movements. These activities comprise the observable behavior from which all other mental activity is inferred. Language is particularly important because it influences the way people perceive, interpret, and respond to their world.

The intellectual dimension makes possible such processes as acquiring information through the senses; filtering and integrating incoming stimuli; sorting and recalling information; organizing information; and communicating information through words, gestures, facial expressions, and movements.[42] Using these intellectual processes, one can engage in such activities as goal setting, problem solving, and decision making.

The intellectual dimension interacts with and influences the other human dimensions. Any thought or message one communicates to oneself can induce physical changes. Thoughts of stressful or relaxing conditions affect heart rate, respiration rate, skin temperature, and other physiological functions. Mental images affect one's body in much the same way that equivalent events in the external world affect it; for example, visualization of running creates muscle contraction, and images of danger elicit autonomic nervous system responses such as increased pulse rate and sweating.[59] Many civilizations throughout history have used visualization techniques to affect physical healing. Today mental imagery is being incorporated successfully in the treatment of conditions ranging from headaches to cancer.[65]

The effect of intellectual functioning on the emotional dimension is evident when one judges one's feelings as right or wrong, expects that one should or should not feel certain emotions, and is either able or not able to communicate emotional experiences to oneself and others. The intellectual dimension also influences one's relationships with other people. For instance, positive or negative thoughts about a relationship contribute to the actual evolution of that relationship. If people think that they have no friends or that they have lost intimacy with someone, they tend to selectively gather and organize information from the environment to support that thought. Ultimately, individuals communicate based on this selected information, resulting in the exact situation that they believe has occurred. Intellectual functioning also contributes to the nature of one's spiritual dimension through such processes as visualization, meditation, creative thinking, ability to communicate, and ability to develop meaning in one's life. Finally, one's thoughts are influenced by environmental factors, such as people and places; conversely, people influence their surroundings by what they think and communicate.

Social dimension The aspects of individuals that enable them to function in society are what comprise the social dimension. Intrinsic to the social dimension are interactions and relationships with others. People constantly interact with the social system (society) in which they live. Through socialization, people acquire the knowledge, skills, and dispositions that allow them to function within their society. As individuals are socialized, they experience dependence, independence, and interdependence in their interactions. Their relationships with others contribute to the development of self-concept and varying degrees of trust and mistrust. The interrelationship of society, the environment, culture, and the individual evolves from continuous social interaction.

Social interaction is action that mutually affects two or more individuals. A *social relationship* is a continuing pattern of social interaction. Basic human needs can be satisfied only by interaction with other people. Through these interactions, social relationships are established in the family and in the larger community. Individuals who have had satisfying social interactions in early life are usually comfortable with both social interaction and being alone in the adult years. When an individual's needs for social interaction have not been met during early development, it may be difficult to successfully interact in the adult years.

A group of people who interact and maintain relationships over time is referred to as a *society*. A link exists between the health of the individual and the health of the society, each affecting the other. The society encompasses several generations of individuals at any given time. Because of varying views and perceptions, a generation gap may lead to stress as these different generations engage in social interaction.

Two mechanisms hold society together.[13] The first is mutual interdependence, or reciprocal interaction between individuals to promote survival. In mutual interdependence, members of society adapt to the needs and interests of others. At certain times, individuals depend on others for survival; at other times, independence is an essential aspect of survival. Dependence and independence constitute the extremes on either end of the continuum of interdependence. Throughout life, individuals progress through various stages of dependence and independence, with the ideal being a balance between the two.

The second mechanism in a cohesive society is the internalization of common norms. *Norms* are rules that govern social behavior in a wide variety of situations. Without norms as a guide to behavior, every situation would be problematic, and individuals would spend much time deciding how to behave in a given situation. Individuals are unaware of the norms that govern a great deal of their behavior; they simply have learned appropriate responses in given situations and automatically behave according to the norms.

The process by which norms are internalized is *socialization*. Socialization is the basic process by which a person becomes a functioning member of society. Persons are continually integrated into groups by acquiring as their own the norms, values, and perspectives of such groups.[46] Socialization affects people in such areas as beliefs, attitudes, values, habits, customs, motives, and behaviors. Individuals learn through socialization how to interact with others, and how to behave in interpersonal relationships. The process of socialization, which begins at birth and ends only at death, consists of deliberate as well as unconscious activities.

The family is one of the primary mechanisms of socialization. The family provides the setting for an individual's initial experiences of social interaction and relationships, as well as exposure to social norms, values, and perspectives. Within the family framework, individual members learn socially acceptable attitudes, values, behaviors, and expectations. Healthy families facilitate the growth and development of their members throughout the life cycle, whereas maladaptive families may restrict individual functioning in one or more dimensions.

The community also represents a major socializing force. Each community adopts variations of the prevalent norms in its society. Community attitudes and values, as well as physical restrictions and resources, influence the individual. (Chapters 26 and 29 of this text provide in-depth discussions of the community and the family, respectively.)

Socialization prepares individuals for the roles they will assume in society. *Social roles* are patterns of attitudes, values, goals, and behaviors that are expected of individuals by virtue of the position they occupy in society. Society defines a number of social roles that influence the individual's relationship with others. A concept related to role is status. A *status* is a position in society, and a *role* is the behavioral counterpart of a position. For example, nurse is a status, and provision of care for clients is the role. Statuses and role characteristics may be achieved, ascribed, or assumed. Individuals occupy achieved statuses, such as educational and occupational statuses, as a result of their own motivation, efforts, and competence. Ascribed statuses, such as family of origin, sex, age, and ethnicity, are socially assigned.

Throughout the life cycle people assume many social roles with corresponding expectations. Each person occupies several roles at any given time in the life cycle, such as parent, child, student, friend, and spouse. *Role transitions* occur when statuses are acquired or discarded. The student status, for example, is discarded once the individual graduates.

Role change refers to situations in which status is retained while role expectations change. Occupation of any particular role entitles a person to certain privileges and imposes certain limitations. The ability to enter into and enjoy a variety of roles increases one's options and allows optimal development of one's capabilities.

During socialization the individual develops a *self-concept*. The self-concept consists of one's ideas, feelings, values, and beliefs about oneself that result from social interactions with others. Cooley[14] coined the phrase "looking-glass self" to describe people's perceptions of themselves as reflective of how they think others perceive and evaluate them. Thus children learn to think of themselves as good because they perceive that others evaluate them as good. Many factors influence the development of self-concept, including expectations of and evaluation by significant others, genetic and environmental factors, and development tasks and crises. Redefining oneself in response to developmental and situational crises occurs throughout the life cycle.

Self-concept may be positive or negative. A positive self-concept implies acceptance of one's own strengths and weaknesses, and it enhances self-confidence in one's social interactions. A negative self-concept is reflected in feelings of worthlessness and lack of respect for oneself and one's abilities.

Self-esteem is a major component of self-concept. Self-esteem is judging or evaluating one's own worth in relation to one's ideal self and to the performance of others. Self-esteem may be high or low. Individuals with a positive self-concept and high self-esteem tend to be autonomous and to display a basic trust of themselves and other people. Mistrust of oneself and others is manifested by persons with a negative self-concept and low self-esteem. Self-concept and self-esteem influence how one relates to others.

Personal identity is the component of self-concept that allows individuals to maintain a consistent sense of themselves, and thus enables them to occupy a stable position in the environment. Personal identity is based on one's overall pattern of qualities. These patterns are considered to be personal and distinctive. It provides a reference point from which to monitor and evaluate one's own thoughts, feelings, and behavior in relation to the surrounding environmental reality. Personal identity regulates and coordinates one's view both of outside reality and of oneself within that reality. Information is available from oneself and from the environment at any given time; personal identity

is a primary factor in a person's determination of what information is relevant. For example, an individual whose personal identity includes self-competence may view a potentially difficult situation as easily manageable; however, someone with a personal identity of inadequacy could view the same situation as threatening or impossible to resolve. People tend to interpret information so that it confirms their own theories of reality based on their own personal identities. One person may interpret benign comments as critical, whereas another may not perceive intended criticism. Although personal identity forms the basis for a sense of continuity, feedback from ongoing self-perception, self-evaluation, and interaction with the environment allows continuous development over time.[27]

Human *sexuality*, an important aspect of all dimensions, is influenced significantly by the social dimension. Sexuality refers to qualities associated with one's expression of oneself as either male or female. Thus, sexuality encompasses a broad spectrum, ranging from attitudes, beliefs, and feelings to social roles and actual behaviors. People learn to identify and value their masculinity or feminity through interacting with others. Sexuality is interdependent with one's self-concept, self-esteem, and personal identity. People with a positive self-concept and high self-esteem are likely to feel comfortable with their sexuality. A positive attitude toward and acceptance of one's sexuality can also enhance self-esteem and strengthen personal identity.

Social norms that govern the expression of sexuality are learned primarily through socialization and differ greatly among societies. Social norms determine the acceptable sexual roles in any society. The norms are used to establish the attitudes, values, and behaviors that are expected of people by virtue of their sexual identity. Sexual role behavior includes all behaviors that express or disclose a person as being male or female. As with deviation from other social norms, individuals who choose nontraditional sexual roles may be considered aberrant. In recent years sexual roles have become less restrictive in this society.[33]

The social dimension interacts with and influences each of the other human dimensions. Social interaction enables one to meet physical needs such as nourishment, touch, clothing, shelter, and health care. The social and emotional dimensions are intertwined, as witnessed by the feelings elicited and experienced in any kind of relationship. Social roles also assist people in meeting their emotional needs: a maternal role may allow the expression of tenderness; a child role may encourage playfulness. The interrelatedness of the social and intellectual dimensions is evident in communication. Socialization allows a person to develop communication skills, and communication is a primary factor that makes socialization possible.

Both verbal and nonverbal communication are primary factors in interpersonal relationships. In addition, social interaction is the primary framework in which communication skills are learned. Through communication individuals share experiences, thoughts, feelings, and information; express and meet their needs; make teaching and learning possible; and develop social support systems.[58] Through social contact people learn either positive or negative thought patterns. Social roles influence attitudes toward learning and thus educational and career choices. Society influences the particular way in which spirituality is expressed and consequently affects a person's individual spiritual experience.

Spiritual dimension *Spirituality* is at the core of the individual's existence, integrating and transcending the physical, emotional, intellectual, and social dimensions. Frequently, spirituality is defined as sensitivity or attachment to religious values. Religion refers to an organized system of faith, worship, and prescribed rituals and observances that allows the expression of one's spiritual needs. Organized traditional religions tend to adhere to the revelations of one or more persons that are passed along to those who follow.[20] A person's spiritual dimension encompasses much more than these revelations, more than established doctrine introduced by others. This dimension allows one to experience and understand the reality of existence in unique and direct ways that go beyond one's usual limits. Hence spirituality is not synonymous with religious beliefs.

The spiritual dimension is the most elusive for many people because of the individual nature of spirituality and because of a tendency, particularly in Western culture, to emphasize what is tangible. The spiritual dimension deals with a reality that is more than tangible. Spirituality permeates an individual's life principles and incorporate one's total being. When spiritual needs are met, an individual can function with a meaningful identity and purpose and can relate to reality with hope and confidence. Needs related to the spiritual dimension are experienced throughout the life cycle. These needs are basic to the individual's inner strivings toward goals in life that hold the deepest values for the individual. The extent to which spiritual needs are met directly affects feelings of hope.

Some needs that are related to the spiritual dimension include[12]:

1. A meaningful philosophy of life
2. A sense of the numinous and transcendent
3. A deep experience of trustful relatedness to God, a supreme being, or a universal power or force
4. A relatedness to people and nature
5. Self-actualization

All individuals have a philosophy of life, or a set of standards and ideals, that guides them in decision making about their goals and that largely determines the meaning they attribute to their lives. Beliefs, values, morals, and ethics are essential components of an individual's philosophy of life. A belief is a conviction in the truth or existence of something or someone, a state of mind in which confidence or trust is placed in some person or thing. An individual's beliefs are influenced by social and cultural belief systems. Through the socialization process, beliefs are internalized and modified throughout the life cycle.

Values are beliefs shared by the members of a society that determine what is desirable or what ought to be. Values are positive and negative; positive values indicate what is desirable, and negative values demonstrate what is undesirable. Through socialization, individuals learn the dominant values of a society; however, individuals also develop personal values.

Morals relate to the individual's conception of what behavior is right and wrong. Kohlberg[39] formulated and validated stages of moral development that begin in childhood and continue into adulthood. The stages are defined by ways of thinking about moral issues and by choices. He believed that morality represents a set of rational principles of judgment and justice that are valid for every culture. An individual's value judgment system and philosophy determine the level of moral development attained. Moral development is also influenced by reasoning abilities, problem-solving experiences, and the type of knowledge used in thinking. Individuals who receive little or no information regarding cultural and personal morality develop uncertainty because they have to work out so many answers for themselves. While morals relate to the concept of what is right and wrong, *ethics* is the set of values, moral codes, and rules of conduct by which an individual's morals are implemented.

One's values, beliefs, and goals are based largely on the meaning, or purpose, that one attributes to one's life. People play an active role in the choice and development of giving their life meaning and purpose.

A sense of the numinous and transcendent is the second spiritual need. *Numinous* refers to an appeal to the higher emotions, such as awe or reverence. *Transcendence* involves the ability to go beyond one's ordinary everyday limits to experience more than one's usual existence. Transcendence involves moments of enlightenment: "Oh, I see!" "Aha! That is it!" "Now it all fits!" These moments may be as simple as viewing another person, a flower, or a mountain in new ways and as mysterious as psychic healing or a strong feeling of oneness with the universe.[58] While searching for a meaning in life, individuals may attempt to transcend the limitations of their human condition or try to forget unpleasant experiences such as loneliness, restlessness, dissatisfaction, and aloneness. The stamina that enables individuals to persist until they arrive at a purpose to which they can commit themselves is determined by hope and faith. Hope, which is discussed in Chapter 14, is basic to survival in health and illness. Faith is a firm belief in something and always involves certainty, even without evidence or proof. The difference between life and death may be the presence or absence of hope and faith. For example, nurses encounter critically ill clients who recover against all expectations because they have hope and faith. Hope and faith are evident in the specific, personal meaning that motivates individuals to continue life and survive in the most unfavorable conditions.

One way of describing the third spiritual need—a deep experience of trustful relatedness to God, a supreme being, or a universal power or force—is in terms of the individual's religion. The concept of a deity refers to the meanings, ideas, thoughts, and expressions individuals have for a supreme being or universal power or force; these are determined primarily through culture. Several human behavior patterns are related to the concept of a deity. These behaviors are the tendency to congregate, the tendency to imitate, and the desire to appeal to a higher force when one's own resources fail. The need for trustful relatedness to the object of worship can be met through the belief that the object is loving and active in one's life. With this belief, there is reassurance that life has meaning and that one can appeal to a power outside one's personal realm.

The concept of a deity is closely related to worship, which is the reverent love and allegiance accorded a deity, idol, or sacred object. Each religious group subscribes to a particular form of worship within an institution such as a church, temple, synagogue, or other designated space. Worship involves a connectedness with a deity or power that may result in a spiritual relationship with others in the group. This spiritual relationship is expressed in love and care for other persons. Love is defined in this sense as intense concern for another person. Care is compassion as opposed to tolerance, tenderness as opposed to a sense of duty, and respect as opposed to obligation.

Attitudes of peace, dignity, and belonging are often communicated through an individual's own sense of accountability to a higher spiritual authority or deep sense of commitment to others. The presence of God, the integration of the universe, and the meaning of life are often evoked through continued participation in familiar religious rituals and ceremonies.

A relatedness to people and nature is a fourth spiritual need. Some individuals may not experience a trustful relatedness to a deity; however, they may have a meaningful relatedness to other people and to nature that enables them to grow spiritually.

Nurses can facilitate a client's spiritual, physical, and social well being through their role as an "advocate." (See the accompanying research highlight.) True advocacy involves more than speaking up for or speaking in behalf of another. An often neglected or forgotten meaning of the term advocate is the notion of walking along with or ac-

companying another on his or her journey through life.[12] Such sharing is not an easy or objective task because it opens the advocate to more anxiety and pain as well as more satisfaction and joy. Through such relationships, individuals often have the opportunity to experience another's core, or centeredness. It is then impossible to treat that person as an object that one needs to manipulate.

Spirit has been viewed throughout history as the force by which humans are related to the universe, to nature, and to other people. The spiritual dimension enables people to connect with a positive universal energy that makes it possible to "more fully develop our courage, our ability to genuinely love, our wisdom, and our compassion."[1] This sense of relatedness, or connectedness, is an important aspect of the spiritual dimension. A relationship with nature may evoke humility, respect, courtesy, and sometimes fear. Events that seem coincidental or accidental, such as psychic healing, encountering an old friend who recently appeared in a dream, or suddenly "knowing" that a family member is in danger, may exemplify a universal relatedness. This seems feasible in view of the thesis that the universe is one energy.[58] Without this sense of connectedness, an individual may experience isolation, hopelessness, and purposelessness.

Self-actualization, the fifth spiritual need, is the epitome of spiritual experience but is a need that is met less often than the others. Individuals who achieve self-actualization

RESEARCH HIGHLIGHT

Preferences for Spiritually Related Nursing Interventions Among Terminally Ill and Nonterminally Ill Hospitalized Adults and Well Adults

• P Reed

PURPOSE

This study focused on identification of specific nursing interventions regarded by adults as facilitative of their spirituality during hospitalization.

SAMPLE

The convenience sample consisted of 300 adults: 100 adults with incurable cancer, 100 hospitalized adults who did not have a serious illness, and 100 nonhospitalized well adults. The groups were comparable on four key variables known to influence spirituality: age, sex, years of education, and religious background.

METHODOLOGY

After securing consent the question was asked, "In what ways could hospital nurses help you in your spiritual needs?" The question was followed by seven response categories, six of which represented intervention approaches. The seventh possible response was open-ended and invited participants to describe approaches not listed.

FINDINGS

The category referring to arranging a visit with clergy obtained the highest frequency of responses within and across the three groups (n = 116, 27%). The next two most frequent categories focused on providing time for personal reflection (n = 74, 17%) and for family participation in spiritual activities (n = 64, 15%).

Terminally ill patients identified "read to you or with you" and "provide time for family involvement in spiritual activities" significantly more than nonterminally ill patients. The category "help you attend chapel" was selected significantly more often among the nonterminally ill patients than the terminally ill patients.

IMPLICATIONS

The participants identified several key interventions that fall within the domain of nursing practice. The difference found between terminally ill and nonterminally ill adults has implications for individualizing nursing care among clients who are dying versus those for whom the prognosis is less serious but who require hospitalization. Those differences translated into more one-to-one interactions with clients who were not seriously ill and more creative management of the environment for the terminally ill clients.

From *Applied Nursing Research* 4(3):122, 1991.

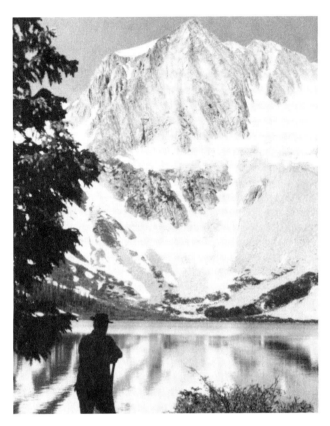

FIGURE 2-2 An individual's spirituality is enhanced by viewing the wonders of nature.

have transcended their limitations and realized their highest potentials. According to Maslow, the self-actualized person has experiences that are described as "limitless horizons opening up to the vision, the feeling of being simultaneously more powerful and also more helpless than one ever was before, the feeling of great ecstasy and wonder and awe, the loss of placing in time and space with, finally, the conviction that something extremely important and valuable has happened, so that the person is to some extent transformed and strengthened even in his daily life by such experience."[45] Maslow believes that to attain self-actualization, individuals need to be free of mundane worries, especially those related to survival. Once individuals experience self-actualization, they may develop an aesthetic sense that enables them to create and appreciate beauty in painting, sculpture, music, and nature (Figure 2-2).

Figure 2-3 shows the interrelationships of the five dimensions of the person and the components within each dimension. The components within each dimension form the basic framework for the five dimensions throughout this text.

Relationship with the Environment

The environment is an irrevocable aspect of human existence. As indicated in the discussion of systems theory (see Chapter 4), every living organism is interdependent with its environment. In addition, each individual organism constitutes an environment for the smaller systems within

itself. Just as a person is multidimensional, each individual's environment is composed of many factors that are influential in the person's life—people, places, things, events. At any moment and in any situation, one is in dynamic relationship both with one's immediate surroundings and with more distant environmental factors. An ongoing pattern of adapting occurs as person and environment contribute to the nature of each other.

Continual energy exchanges between people and their environment occur on many levels. In all exchanges between the person and environment, one takes in energy from outside sources, processes and uses it, and then returns some form of energy to the environment. Thus individuals are simultaneously affected by input from their surroundings and through their output, contribute to environmental characteristics. As a person's outputs are processed by and incorporated into the environment, they become new inputs that affect the person. Because of this ongoing relationship between people and their environment, one cannot fully understand individuals in isolation from their surroundings. People feel, think, and behave differently in various environmental settings.

Regardless of the actual content of the environment, one's interaction with it contributes significantly to who one is, how one lives, what one does, and certainly to one's state of health or illness.

A person relates to the environment through all human dimensions, often simultaneously, satisfying personal needs and helping satisfy the needs of the environment. As a result of the interdependent nature of the person-environment relationship, people must deal with their surroundings in ways that promote coordination and synchrony rather than conflict and chaos. Mutual adaption is necessary. Environmental factors may act as both resources and stressors; they can provide security and excitement or they can contribute to hardship and obstacles.

The physical environment may contain elements that help meet one's needs in all dimensions, needs such as adequate living quarters, a safe neighborhood, availability of cultural events, and opportunities for spiritual growth. Conversely, the physical environment can inhibit a person's development through crowded living conditions, excessive crime, and lack of various resources.

Emotional needs frequently are met through environmental interaction. One's environment is conducive to health when emotional support is readily available and when one has numerous avenues for expressing feelings. Such an environment encourages development in all dimensions.

Intellectual development is closely related to environmental situations. A healthy environment provides opportunities for intellectual growth and development as well as adequate stimulation and encouragement to learn. In turn such an environment facilitates the ability to meet one's needs in other areas.

By definition the social dimension is closely linked to the environment. People are simultaneously dependent parts of society and independent wholes within society. Through environmental resources, people can meet their physical needs such as food, shelter, and health care. One can create caring relationships primarily through the social dimension, fulfilling many basic needs. Thus one's environ-

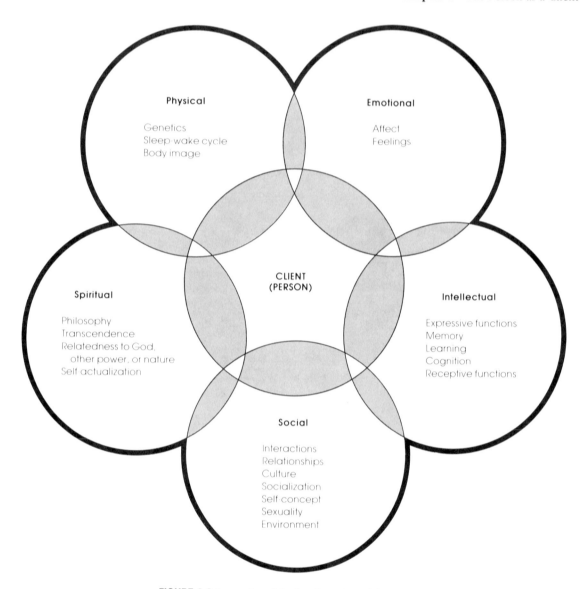

FIGURE 2-3 Integration of the five dimensions of the person.

ment is a crucial aspect of healthy development. When possibilities for social contact are limited or when the contacts are primarily negative, people find it more difficult to function optimally in all dimensions.

Spiritual beliefs and experiences are greatly affected by the beliefs of the society in which a person lives. A rich environment offers many opportunities for personal exploration and expansion, which enhances one's ability to cope effectively with stressors in all other dimensions as well.

Community resources play a large role in the support that can be offered by the environment. There are many health-related resources available, although a given community may have an abundance or a scarcity. Community health centers and community mental health centers often can provide information to individuals and families about available support, education, or intervention services.

Some health-related community resources are managed by health professionals. Examples of common educational topics offered by community agencies include parenting

and family relationships, stress management, health promotion and fitness, and addiction. Examples of other professional community services include halfway houses, community homes, alcohol and drug treatment programs, therapy groups, crisis management, crisis hotlines, various information hotlines, and smoking cessation clinics.

Self-help groups, generally led by lay people, have become an increasing source of support in recent years. Many self-help groups use the 12-step model originated by Alcoholics Anonymous, which offers a safe setting for members to challenge their old beliefs and behaviors and to explore new more constructive ones. There is a common bond among members, who have shared many similar experiences, feelings, and ways of thinking about their problems. Other examples of 12-step groups are Al-Anon, Narcotics Anonymous, Overeaters Anonymous, Emotions Anonymous, and Gamblers Anonymous. Other self-help groups offer support and encouragement to their members, who share some common problem or trauma, using approaches of discussion, ventilation of feelings, problem solving, and journaling. Examples of these are self-help groups for rape victims, adult survivors of incest, codependency, cancer clients, stroke victims, parents, and individuals who are grieving the death of a family member. Although self-help groups usually accept donations, they do not typically charge a fee.

When one considers the person-environment interrelationship, it is crucial to remember that each individual interacts with the environment based on subjective experience as well as actual external stimuli. One's perceptions of and responses to the environment are largely determined by one's attitudes, values, feelings, and beliefs. Past experience, attributed meanings, and expectations of the future contribute to an inner reality; from this reality, one interacts with and adapts to the environment.[8]

Self-Responsibility

Holistic health philosophy maintains that people are ultimately responsible for their own lives. They continually make choices and decisions that determine who they are, what they experience, and how they live. Although many factors contribute to these choices and decisions, individuals are responsible for those that they make. Even when options seem limited or nonexistent, people still choose among alternatives.

Self-awareness is a prerequisite to the genuine acceptance of responsibility for oneself. Awareness implies that one can focus attention on a particular experience and promote individual "knowing" of that experience. Awareness is a kind of "turning in to" and willingness to recognize what is currently significant. Experiences that have occurred in the past or that are anticipated in the future are meaningful only as they relate to the present and as they influence current choices and decisions.

To be a whole person, one must develop an awareness of oneself, including strengths and weaknesses, feelings and behaviors, attitudes and beliefs, social patterns, and meaning; one's environment, including people, places, objects, and energy; and one's connections with the environment, including expectations, energy exchange, interactions, and boundaries. As people develop this awareness, they can recognize the reality of their life situations. Only then can they identify their contributions to life events, acknowledge the choices they make, and fully assume responsibility for themselves.

Locus of control indicates how individuals perceive personal responsibility in life, and whether or not they believe they have power over events that affect them. Internal locus of control, or internality, means that an outcome is a consequence of the individual's own actions and is thus under personal control. External locus of control, or externality, refers to the belief that an outcome is determined by fate, chance, or powerful others and is thus beyond personal control.[3] If people can develop a locus of control that is more internal than external, they may learn to acquire more responsibility for their own health.[62]

The concept of locus of control, or self-responsibility, affects each person in all dimensions. For example, physically, people believe either that they can control their actions and general nutritional and fitness status or that outside circumstances make it impossible for them to change

their patterns. Emotionally, some people assume responsibility for their own feelings, whereas others believe that something or someone else can cause them to feel a particular way. Intellectually, individuals believe either that they choose their thoughts or that they learned them long ago and cannot change them. Socially, people may see how the contribute to the success and failure of interactions and relationships, or they may attribute outcome to the other person or persons involved. Spiritually, people believe either that they create meaning for themselves or that meaning is revealed to them by outside forces.

A holistic approach to living assumes that the individual exerts primary influence in all these areas. People are in fact responsible for the sum of their life experiences. In contrast to a sense of responsibility for oneself and control over one's own life, people may believe and act as if other people, circumstances, or fate exert more influence over their life situations than they do. Phrases such as "I have to . . . ," "I should . . . ," "I can't . . . ," and "I couldn't help it" indicate a sense of helplessness or a belief that one is not in control of oneself. People who feel responsible for themselves generally use more powerful phrases, such as "I choose to . . . ," "I want to . . . ," "I won't . . . ," and "I contributed by. . . ." The difference in the two sets of phrases reflects two distinct approaches to living. The former represents feeling at the mercy of outside forces (external locus of control); the latter allows people to assume both the power and the responsibility of directing their own lives (internal locus of control).

Historically, the health care system has encouraged specific and restricted roles for both health care professionals and clients. Those who represent the system often are expected to behave "professionally" rather than authentically, to act in a kind but detached manner rather than with true caring, and to view themselves as authorities rather than as coparticipants in the healing process. In contrast, consumers of health care services are expected to comply with instructions rather than to understand the rationale behind them, to allow others to make health care decisions for them rather than to participate in decision making, and to view health care professionals as authorities rather than consultants.

When accepting responsibility for personal health, individuals view themselves as active participants in their health status, including the occurrence of illness and accidents. They are not victims or passive recipients of any outside force, including the health care system; they maintain their sense of personal power rather than believing that others exert control over them.

Self-responsibility includes the recognition that people participate in or contribute to their illness and accidents, and need to seek information and evaluate the choices they make. For example, if people determine that they have contributed to the development of a cold by insufficient rest, an ulcer by inadequate relaxation, or a state of depression by lack of assertiveness, they may want to make different choices that are more likely to contribute to a healthier status. Individuals who assume responsibility for their health status actively strive to cope with stressors, reach their own potentials, and maintain balance within their lives.

As one develops a greater sense of responsibility, one is less able to accept the "fix-it" attitude that many people learn as children; that is, if something goes wrong, someone else will fix it. Although the health care system often can effectively treat illness or injury, it cannot be responsible for how people contribute to their state of health, to illness, or to an accident. Only the individual can, for instance, maintain fitness levels, wear seat belts, or deal effectively with stressors. As one assumes greater responsibility for one's health, one chooses healthier behaviors. In this way, each person retains personal power and integrity rather than relinquishing control to someone else.

For most people, the prospect of being responsible for their own health and illness is exciting and powerful. However, responsibility also contains an awesome and at times frightening element. People can no longer blame other persons or things for "making them" ill, "leading" them in a certain direction, or "running" their lives. An attitude of helplessness is replaced by resoluteness. These transitions are not always easy.

In considering self-responsibility for participation in illness or accident, it is important that the concept of responsibility not be confused with guilt, self-blame, or self-criticism. When people accept responsibility for illness, they are able to view their current situation as a starting point, explore how they have contributed to the present situation, determine the message or meaning, and choose a new direction. However, when individuals distort responsibility into guilt, they inhibit personal growth. Self-blaming and self-critical attitudes limit people. Self-responsibility does not mean that a person becomes paralyzed with guilt and self-blame but that the person learns from the illness and continually strives to make healthier choices.

Life-Cycle Development

Holistic concepts are applicable to all stages of the life cycle. (Part IV of this text provides an in-depth discussion of life-cycle development.) The dimensions of the person and the environment are interdependent at every age. Each stage of life is typically accompanied by particular kinds of stressors that require different kinds of coping mechanisms. Self-responsibility, recognizing one's needs and making choices to obtain what one wants, is an important component at every stage of life.

Stress and Adaptation

Holistic health philosophy recognizes stress as a primary factor in all states of health and illness. *Stress* is the body's arousal response to any demand, change, or perceived threat, and a *stressor* is the circumstance or event that elicits this response. Selye[63] has described a generalized reponse to stressors that involves the autonomic nervous system and the endocrine system. This general adaptation syndrome (GAS) has three states: (1) an alarm reaction, (2) resistance, and (3) exhaustion. The purpose of GAS is to assist the individual in resisting the stressor as efficiently as possible and in maintaining equilibrium. When stressors (real or perceived) are chronic, and there is no opportunity to regain equilibrium, the exhaustion state may lead to illness or death. (See Chapter 4.)

Stress is neither inherently good nor bad; it produces positive and negative effects. Stress is healthy when it fa-

cilitates stimulation and alertness, contributes to personal growth and development, or assists individuals in meeting their needs. Life is not very challenging, and people accomplish little if demands are not made on them. However, stress is not healthy when it creates a sense of helplessness, leaves one feeling tired and apathetic, inhibits optimal functioning, or predisposes one to illness. These conditions occur when a person does not create opportunities to regain equilibrium.

A stressor can be anything that elicits the stress response of physiological and biochemical change. Like the effects of stress, stressors may be positive or negative. On a physiological and biochemical level, positive and negative stressors elicit the same responses, and both can have positive or negative consequences. Although negative stressors often are more intense and of greater concern, events such as marriage, job promotion, moving to a new home, vacation, and graduation are demanding and require change. Positive life changes elicit the same stress response as situations such as divorce, loss of job, or academic failure. A negative stressor can be more harmful when a person prolongs arousal by continuing to worry or maintain other strong feelings long after the actual stressor is gone, as in the case of prolonged concern following an examination or reliving an argument a month after it has happened.

The range of events or circumstances that can act as stressors is wide and varied, affecting all human dimensions. Examples of negative stressors are physical deprivation or injury, emotional strain or loss, self-defeating thoughts and beliefs, social isolation or over-extension, and spiritual conflicts. Examples of positive stressors are athletic contests, emotional commitments such as marriage or parenthood, intellectual stimulation or accomplishment, expansion of social involvement, and spiritual enlightenment. Examples of negative environmental stressors include pollution, difficult weather conditions, lack of personal space or poor physical surroundings, and occupational settings.

An event or circumstance is a stressor when an individual consciously or unconsciously perceives it as such. What is stressful for one person may not be for another. For example, someone who enjoys the sun and water may perceive an ocean beach as a relaxing place; the same setting can be stressful for someone who is afraid of the water and is hypersensitive to the sun. A new assignment at work or graduation from school may be perceived as exciting by one person but frightening by another. An individual also perceives potential stressors differently according to particular life situations. For instance, divorce may be experienced primarily as relief at age 30 but overwhelming to the same person at age 60. The role of parenthood can be perceived as a welcome challenge at one point in life but an unwelcome obstacle at another. Many variables determine a person's perception and experience of stressors including age, sex, physical condition, personality, learned attitudes and beliefs, family situation, cultural background, social support system, spiritual beliefs, and environment.

Every individual develops coping patterns, or behaviors, used to maintain equilibrium when faced with stressful situations. Coping behaviors are numerous and may be adaptive or maladaptive. Adaptive coping behaviors enable an individual to change or reinterpret a stressful situation, or to control stress resulting from a situation, without adverse effects in other aspects of life. Examples include hobbies, conflict resolution, building relationships, time management, relaxation strategies, and exercise. Maladaptive coping occurs when the behaviors used to respond to stressors produce negative side effects and may be harmful or produce additional stress when used often or over a long period of time. Examples of maladaptive coping are drug abuse, overeating, tantrums, and social isolation. People tend to use coping behaviors that have worked in the past. If adaptive, the person can become stronger with each stressful situation; when maladaptive, the person may become more vulnerable to the effects of stress over time.

Approaches to *stress management* are numerous and varied. The first step of stress management is the identification of stressors in one's life. These stressors may be major events, such as marriage or moving to a new city, or daily occurrences, such as traffic or constant worry about a particular issue. They may originate outside oneself (the cranky boss, the alcoholic spouse, or depressed economic conditions) or within the individual (self-critical thoughts, poor nutritional habits, lack of assertiveness, or anxiety about the future). The stressors can affect any dimension of the individual.

To identify personal stressors, individuals examine how they react to what occurs in their particular situation. The following reactions indicate at least some degree of stress: feelings of helplessness or hopelessness, perceived loss of control, chronic anxiety and worry, a "knot" in the stomach, continual frustration, increased heart and respiration rates, cold hands and feet, neck and shoulder muscle tension, clenched jaw, feeling overwhelmed, excessive or constant fatigue, and nervous laughter. Once aware of one's physical and emotional reactions, one often can locate the stimulus of the reaction, that is, the stressor.

The second step of stress management is to determine which stressors to eliminate, if any, those with which one simply wants to reduce contact, and those to which one would like to diminish one's response. A person who is retaining beliefs and attitudes from the past that are now acting as stressors may wish to replace these with constructive, reinforcing thoughts. One may be able to make relatively simple changes in a home or work environment to make it less stressful; for example, furniture arrangement, new color scheme, sharing chores, or creating a private space. If one determines that a particular person is acting as a stressor, one may choose to become less involved or to detach completely.

When considering which stressors to eliminate, remember that it is neither possible nor desirable to completely empty one's life of stressors. Removing certain stressors may be impractical, and removing others simultaneously deprives the person of challenge and personal growth opportunities. Positive attitudes and the willingness to cope in healthy ways with stressors are much more critical to health than is the quantity of stressors that people encounter.

The third and crucial step of stress management then is to develop effective coping mechanisms so that one is able either to counteract one's own stress response when it occurs or to use the response constructively. Stress is a problem only when the body initiates physiological and biochemical activity in preparation to deal with the stressor

and then does not experience any release. This can easily occur as a person faces one stressor after another without any recovery time; the person's body stays in a constant state of readiness, which is destructive. Ultimately, individuals are in charge of whether they choose to counteract or use the stress response.

Physical dimension Stressors related to genetic factors, physiological processes, and body image are listed in the accompanying box. The reader is referred to other texts on physical health and illness for a further discussion of physical stressors and the individual's responses to them. Stressors affecting body image are discussed briefly in this section because of their impact on a person's mental or emotional health.

Stressors threatening one's body image are those that are perceived to alter or that actually do alter the person's physical structure. A person's perception determines his or her reality. Thus a perceived alteration in body image can be as stressful as an actual one. For example, adolescents may perceive themselves as "fat" if they exceed their personally defined ideal weight, regardless of how others perceive them. Personal definitions of "ideal weight" are partially determined by cultural standards; staying thin may be a desirable goal if the adolescent's culture places a premium on this characteristic. Threats to body image are stressful because the ability to relate in meaningful ways to others or develop a satisfactory sexual identity are related to the concept of self and body image. Major stressors to body image fall into six categories: (1) normal maturation, (2) elective surgical procedures, (3) disease or other disorders, (4) surgery or trauma, (5) drugs, and (6) social influences.

Norris[51] identified four factors that influence an individual's adjustment to alterations in body size, function, or structure: (1) the meaning the stressor has for the individual; (2) the extent to which the individual's pattern of adaptation is interrupted; (3) the support system and patterns of adaptation available to the individual; and (4) the nature of the threat, degree of change, and rate at which

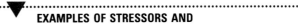

EXAMPLES OF STRESSORS AND MALADAPTIVE RESPONSES

Physical Dimension

Stressors	Maladaptive Responses
Genetic dysfunctions	Congenital abnormalities
Nutritional deficiencies	Physical defects
Drug use	Physical diseases
Disease, illness, injury, pain	Withdrawal symptoms
Aging process	Negative body image
Sensory deprivation	Sleeplessness
Environmental factors	Restlessness
Inadequate or excessive physical activity	Decreased energy
	Fatigue
Body image alterations	Impaired growth
Sleep disorders	Hyperalertness
	Metabolic disturbances
	Gastrointestinal disturbances
	Sexual dysfunction
	Cardiovascular deterioration
	Self-destruction

it occurs. The person's level of growth and development influences the significance of the loss.

Reactions to body image changes vary greatly as individuals attempt to handle threats to loss of self-control or control of their immediate space. Such threats occur when clients are faced with potentially threatening nursing procedures, such as enemas, catheterizations, and other restrictions that immobilize them so that they are dependent on others to care for intimate needs. Denial can lead to restlessness, fatigue, vulnerability, intractable pain, nervousness, insomnia, and phobias. Adaptation occurs more readily when the person is encouraged to express feelings, allowed time to develop healthy coping mechanisms, supported by meaningful others, and assisted in lowering the anxiety level.

Emotional dimension Any situation that elicits an emotion from the individual and generates a physiological response has the potential for producing stress. Stressors in every dimension may elicit strong emotions and place demands on one's emotional coping capacity.

Emotional health and illness occur along a continuum on which one's health status at any given time can be reflected. Intensity and duration of an emotion determine where one is placed on the continuum.

One's ability to satisfy needs and to fully experience and deal with feelings determines one's position on the continuum. Some healthy emotional responses include laughing, crying, loving, anger, trust, fear, hopefulness, and powerfulness. Unhealthy emotional responses may include excessive guilt, hurt, long-term resentment, and helplessness. Researchers are beginning to explore the interactive effects of various expressions of emotion; examples include biochemical changes that may occur in the brain during laughter, and the differing content of tears shed because of emotion and those caused by physical irritation.

One's position on the emotional continuum changes as one responds to stressors in healthy or unhealthy ways. No state of absolute emotional health or illness exists. Emotional health evolves as people meet their needs, recognize and accept their feelings, and choose to use their emotional energy to enhance their life situations. A sense of emotional health is maintained when harmony exists within oneself, with others, and in interactions with the environment. Emotional distress results when basic needs are not met, causing disruption, disorganization, and dysfunction in one's emotional equilibrium. See the accompanying box for examples of stressors and responses in the emotional dimension.

Intellectual dimension Stressors in the intellectual dimension are of either internal or external origin and interfere with receptive functions, memory and learning, cognitive functions, or expressive functions.

The complex processes of sensation and perception involve many aspects of the central nervous system; consequently, proper functioning is largely dependent on good physical health.

The healthy person has good recall for immediate, recent, or remote events and learns what is meaningful. Internal and external strategies to enhance memory can be used, such as increasing study time or tying a string around a finger. Although moderate levels of anxiety can enhance memory and learning, high anxiety levels often lead to forgetfulness or the inability to learn.

▼ **EXAMPLES OF STRESSORS AND MALADAPTIVE RESPONSES**

Emotional Dimension

Stressors	Maladaptive Responses
Anxiety	Crying
Anger	Restlessness
Depression	Substance abuse
Hopelessness	Isolation
Guilt	Aggression
Elation	Suicide
Fear	Homicide
Grief	Helplessness
	Hopelessness
	Feelings of worthlessness
	Hostility
	Addiction

The inability to recall specific information such as a friend's name or a significant historical date is an indication of memory loss. Memory defects can differentially affect motor skills, conceptual relationships, or speech patterns. For example, the motor speech ability to organize sounds into words may be retained but the ability to organize words into meaningful speech lost. Sensory modalities and output mechanisms involved in stored memories are also affected differentially. For example, a person may retain the ability to recognize a picture but not be able to recognize numbers or letters.[9]

Long-term memory is impaired in some types of brain disease. Time of onset of memory loss is estimated by eliciting the most recent of the remote memories, since all events preceding the disease onset may be poorly remembered or not remembered at all. In other types of brain injury or disease, only specific bits of remote memory are lost. An alteration in level of consciousness usually accompanies a global loss of long-term memory.[41]

Persons who have adapted well to stressors have attained Piaget's cognitive developmental level of formal operations[55]; they are realistic, rational, and logical; consider a range of differing viewpoints; and use their imagination to creatively solve problems. They also maintain positive thoughts that enhance growth. Poor adaptation to stressors results in a disintegration of cognition, occurring in form, content, or flow of thought.

In response to stressors, the form of thought may become unrealistic, irrational, or illogical, as in dereistic and autistic thinking. In *dereistic thought,* the laws of logic, experience, and reality are not followed. An extreme example is the person who jumps off a 12-story building, not "knowing" that death will occur. Autistic thinking focuses on internal processes; fantasy life becomes reality. *Symbolic associations* and *concrete associations* are other types of disintegrations of the form of thought. In symbolic associations, words or other symbols that have a common meaning take on specific meanings known only to the individual. In concrete associations, the individual is unable to generalize or to make abstract associations.

The thoughts of a person who has adapted to stressors are oriented to reality and under the person's control. Unhealthy adaptation to stressors may be reflected in chronically negative and self-defeating thoughts or even in a person's inability to maintain a realistic orientation or control the content of thought. This lack of control is reflected in delusions—false beliefs that are seen as reality by the individual. These beliefs may be classified as bodily delusions or delusions of persecution, control, influence, infidelity, or grandeur. A characteristic of delusions is their inability to be corrected by reason, argument, or logic.

The flow of thoughts in a person who has adapted well to stressors is regular and even. Unhealthy adaptation to stressors may result in an inability to regulate the flow of thoughts, including flight of ideas, thought retardation, and blocking. With flight of ideas, the person's thoughts rapidly digress from one idea to another, although some connecting train of thought is usually apparent. In thought retardation, thoughts form very slowly, and blocking is the spontaneous loss of a train of thought.

Healthy individuals possess the physical capabilities to use their expressive functions to express their ideas and feelings. Their verbal and nonverbal communication is organized, consistent, and a true expression of themselves. They have a variety of channels for self-expression, including speech, dance, and other artistic forms. An unhealthy response to stressors can be manifested in pressured speech, tangential speech, circumstantial speech, or muteness.

Like other disturbances in the intellectual dimension, expressive and receptive disabilities are associated with particular anatomical lesions. Specific sensory impairments can result in disturbances called *agnosia, apraxia,* and *aphasia* (Table 2-3). Language disturbances usually appear in clusters of related dysfunctions. Impaired intellectual function needed for language is usually reflected in more than one language modality. For example, *agraphia* (literally, no writing) and *alexia* (literally, no reading) rarely occur alone; they usually occur together, often with other language disturbances.[41] See the accompanying box for examples of stressors and responses in the intellectual dimension.

Social dimension Meaningful relationships that provide nurturance and support increase a person's ability to cope with all types of stressors. Social stressors arise from such sources as the family, the workplace, and social class. Potential stressors include family conflict, a hostile environment, poverty, unemployment, and social isolation. Because people often depend on families as a primary source of nurturance and support, familial conflict can be particularly stressful. The effects are compounded when the individual has not developed a social support system outside the family, such as close friends or trusted associates. When families cannot adapt to the normal growth and development of individual members, crises occur that are stressful to both the family member and the family unit.

Social isolation is an interpersonal stressor because it denies satisfaction of social needs and distorts social processes. Social interaction, the basis of social relationships, becomes a stressor when there is too much or too little.

▼ **TABLE 2-3** **Common Expressive and Receptive Disturbances**

Category of Deficit	Specific Deficits
AGNOSIA Sensory interpretation deficits characterized by an inability to recognize objects through the use of a particular sense	Spatial agnosia: disorder of spatial orientation; inability to recognize spatial relationships Autopagnosia: inability to locate and name parts of own body Finger agnosia: inability to recognize own fingers Tactile agnosia: inability to recognize objects by touch Auditory agnosia: inability to identify common environmental sounds without looking; inability to recognize sounds Visual agnosia (very rare): inability to recognize objects by sight or their pictoral representation
APRAXIA Loss of previous ability to perform skilled acts	Motor or kinetic apraxia: usually affects finer movements of the upper extremities and is believed to be caused by loss of kinesthetic memory traces Audiomotor apraxia: difficulty carrying out an action on verbal command Ideational apraxia: inability to formulate a plan of action successfully Constructional apraxia: inability to put parts together to make a whole Dressing apraxia: inability to dress properly
APHASIA Impairment in the reception, manipulation, or expression of the symbolic content of language	Expressive aphasia: trouble initiating speech Auditory receptive aphasia: trouble understanding speech Visual receptive aphasia: impaired ability to understand written language (dyslexia, alexia) Expressive writing aphasia (dysgraphic): inability to initiate written communication Amnestic or nominal aphasia: inability to identify people and things by their proper names

▼ EXAMPLES OF STRESSORS AND
MALADAPTIVE RESPONSES

Intellectual Dimension

Stressors	Maladaptive Responses
Brain dysfunction	Perceptual disturbances
Limited intelligence	Thought disintegration
Inability to express self	Disorientation
Altered level of consciousness	Loss of contact with reality
Brain lesions	Decreased cognitive functioning:
	Loss of memory
	Impaired judgment
	Impaired concentration
	Impaired decision making
	Delusion
	Illusions
	Hallucinations
	Forgetfulness
	Inability to learn
	Negative thinking
	Irrational thinking
	Illogical thinking
	Inability to speak (mute)
	Pressured speech
	Tangential/circumstantial speech
	Blocking
	Language disturbances

▼ EXAMPLES OF STRESSORS AND
MALADAPTIVE RESPONSES

Social Dimension

Stressors	Maladaptive Responses
Family conflict	Withdrawn behavior
Hostile environment	Alienation
Poverty	Criminal behavior
Unemployment	Impaired relationships
Social isolation	Sexual acting out
Threat to self-concept	Addiction (alcohol and drugs)
Threat to sexual role	Aggressive behavior
Role dysfunction	Low self-esteem
	Identity confusion
	Dependence
	Abusive behavior

Too much social interaction infringes on the individual's life space, whereas too little may be experienced as social isolation or deprivation.[40]

Circumstances adversely affecting one's self-concept are stressful. Chronic criticism and devaluation contribute to low self-esteem and a sense of worthlessness. Behavior that is incongruent with one's personal identity causes conflict and anxiety. Any event that necessitates a sudden change in self-concept is especially stressful because of minimal time for adaptation; examples may include an accident that results in disfigurement, death of a significant other, loss of a job, and a natural disaster.

Disturbances in social roles, such as conflicting pressures and strains, are stressors. An individual may feel role stress when a social structure creates very difficult, conflicting, or impossible demands for that position within the structure. The following are various types of role stress:

Role conflict—enactment of roles that conflict with one's value system or multiple roles that conflict with each other

Role ambiguity—enactment of roles that are not clearly defined in terms of expected behavior

Role incongruity—transition to a role that requires a significant modification in attitudes and values (for example, conflict between personal and professional values)

Role overload—enactment of roles in which excessive demands are made and insufficient time is available to fulfill obligations (for example, student, worker, parent, spouse); most likely in highly industrialized societies and in higher level positions[29]

Role incompetence—inability to fulfill role obligations associated with any given role (for example, inadequate occupational knowledge or expertise)

Role overqualification—enactment of a role which does not require full use of a person's resources (for example, experienced professional working in position designed for new graduate)

Many roles are temporary, existing only for a given age or status. The roles of children are replaced by a different set when they reach young adulthood and by still another when they reach their later years. The transition from old to new roles may create difficulty as one leaves the familiarity of settled positions and faces the uncertainty of new ones. Such stress accompanies developmental changes, such as the transitions from childhood to adolescence, high school to college, being single to being married, and going from working to being retired.

Experiences that threaten an individual's sexual identity or interfere with sexual role behaviors may be stressors. When one's attitudes, beliefs, or preferences regarding sexual behavior differ greatly from one's peer group, social isolation and self-doubt may occur. The inability to meet one's sexual needs because of internal or external obstacles can act as a stressor; examples include illness or injury that affects sexuality, value conflicts, guilt regarding sexual expression, and perceived sexual inadequacy. Stressors that affect sexuality can also limit a person's capacity to develop intimacy within significant relationships.

Responses to social stress are determined by the individual's cultural values, past experiences with similar conditions, adequacy of coping mechanisms, and attribution of meaning. The failure to master social stress may lead to mental illness, physical illness, addiction, and criminal behavior.

Complex urban life, crowded living arrangements, and disruptions in social relationships are possible determinants of physical illness. Such conditions require excessive adaptation and create chronic frustration, thus eliciting prolonged physiological arousal. Studies concerning diseases such as tuberculosis and other respiratory disorders concluded that individuals deprived of meaningful social contact are more likely than others to develop these conditions. Social factors have also been shown to be important determinants in rheumatoid arthritis, hypertension, and coronary heart disease. These latter diseases may indicate the individual's lack of preparedness for new and unfamiliar situations. (See the box above for examples of stressors and responses in the social dimension.)

▼ **TABLE 2-4   Social Readjustment Rating Scale**

Life Event	Mean Value
1. Death of spouse	100
2. Divorce	73
3. Marital separation from mate	65
4. Detention in jail or other institution	63
5. Death of a close family member	63
6. Major personal injury or illness	53
7. Marriage	50
8. Being fired at work	47
9. Marital reconciliation with mate	45
10. Retirement from work	45
11. Major change in the health or behavior of a family member	44
12. Pregnancy	40
13. Sexual difficulties	39
14. Gaining a new family member (e.g., through birth, adoption, older person moving in)	39
15. Major business readjustment (e.g., merger, reorganization, bankruptcy)	39
16. Major change in financial state (e.g., a lot worse off or a lot better off than usual)	38
17. Death of a close friend	37
18. Changing to a different line of work	36
19. Major change in the number of arguments with spouse (e.g., either a lot more or a lot less than usual regarding child rearing, personal habits)	35
20. Taking out a mortgage or loan for a major purchase (e.g., home, business)	31
21. Foreclosure on a mortgage or loan	30
22. Major change in responsibilities at work (e.g., promotion, demotion, lateral transfer)	29
23. Son or daughter leaving home (e.g., marriage, attending college)	29
24. Trouble with in-laws	29
25. Outstanding personal achievement	28

Reprinted with permission from Holmes TH, Rahe RH: The social readjustment rating scale, *Journal of Psychosomatic Research* 11:213, 1967.

Many events in a person's life contribute to social stress. Some of the life events cited in the Social Readjustment Rating Scale developed by Holmes and Rahe[35] are social stressors that may result in mental or physical illness (Table 2-4). These events require a high level of adaptation and elicit a stress response.

Spiritual dimension Stressors to the spiritual dimension interfere with one's ability to meet spiritual needs. Challenges to an individual's beliefs and actions that transgress a person's values or moral code are stressors. For instance, a woman who firmly believes that it is wrong to interfere with her body in any way but finds it necessary to have a hysterectomy may experience stress. A less severe stressor is a contradiction between a person's values and life-style. When people spend much time and energy on activities opposed to their values and beliefs, conflict arises and stress increases. Stress also occurs when an individual must choose between two conflicting values, such as clients' rights to know their diagnoses versus the need to protect their fragile emotional conditions. When two such values are in conflict, the person experiences stress until one value is affirmed as a priority and the other is surrendered, at least temporarily.[69]

Spiritually healthy persons who have adapted well to stressors have clarified their goals and values, are decisive, spend their time and energy in achieving their goals, and can make moral and ethical judgments based on these beliefs and values. Persons who have not adapted well to stressors may respond by wishing to undo, redo, or relive the past. They may express shame, regret, or guilt; relate their illness to their guilt for failing to meet some standard of conduct; be unable to forgive themselves or receive forgiveness from others; project blame onto others; or engage in self-destructive behavior.[9]

Events that precipitate a struggle with the meaning of life can serve as stressors. Such events may involve an anticipated role change, the loss of a meaningful relationship, personal illness, illness or death of a family member or close friend, or any kind of intense suffering. During such crises people are brought face-to-face with the ultimate issues of life, such as immortality, personal limitations, loss of control, and suffering in relation to the purpose of their lives.[66]

Spiritually healthy persons have found a reason for being that gives meaning to their existence. This meaning can be found in an organized religion involving the worship of a deity, in relationships with other persons, in a relationship with nature or the surrounding world, or in nonspiritual goals such as acquiring money. These persons have a sense of hope, believing that things can work out and difficulties, including illness, can be overcome.

In contrast, spiritually unhealthy persons feel a sense of meaninglessness or purposelessness that may be characterized by questioning the meaning of their own existence, by hopelessness or despair, feelings of uselessness, or a sense of abandonment. In a situation of intense suffering, these persons may question the meaning of their suffering; doubt their ability to endure it; question the credibility of their belief system; express that suffering is a necessary reparation; or become withdrawn, irritable, restless, self-pitying, or fatigued. Unresolved feelings about death can

▼
EXAMPLES OF STRESSORS AND MALADAPTIVE RESPONSES

Spiritual Dimension

Stressors	Maladaptive Responses
Challenge to personal beliefs or morals	Hopelessness
	Despair
Value conflicts	Decreased self-value
Loss of health, general well-being	No pleasure
	Decreased quality of life
Struggle with meaning, purpose in life	Meaninglessness
	Fragmentation or loss of sense of continuity
Fear of death or dying	
Lack of faith	Alienation
Abandonment	Isolation

be manifested in fears of darkness, being alone, or going to sleep; disturbing dreams; demanding behavior; or avoidance of, preoccupation with, or jokes about death. Chronic feelings such as these act as stressors and decrease an individual's ability to adapt.

Disruptions in relationships, including a sense of isolation from others, can elicit a chronic stress reaction. A sense of relatedness to or connectedness with others contributes to feelings of courage and hope, which help one continue even when the "odds" seem unfavorable.

Individuals require private time and space in which they can develop their own sense of meaning and relatedness and recharge themselves. When this time is unavailable because of external obligations or choice, people experience stress. The need for self-actualization with its accompanying aesthetic sensitivity cannot be met when people are constantly entrenched in the external world.

Spiritually healthy persons are keenly aware of the world about them and allow a variety of experiences to enter their consciousness. They have a sense of freedom and harmony and have developed their potential for creativity. Spiritually unhealthy persons block out events or distort them before they are allowed to enter consciousness. These persons feel little control over what happens to them or over their own response to events. (See the accompanying box for examples of stressors and responses in the spiritual dimension.)

BRIEF REVIEW

Five major concepts are generally accepted as premises of holistic health care philosophy. First, each person is multidimensional; one's physical, emotional, intellectual, social, and spiritual dimensions are in constant interaction with each other. Historically, interest has been shown in all five dimensions; however, Eastern views of human dimensions have typically been more holistic than Western views. The physical dimension involves everything associated with one's body, both internal and external. The emotional dimension consists of affective states and feelings, including motor behavior associated with emotion, the experienced aspect of emotion, and the physiological mechanisms that underlie emotion. The intellectual dimension includes the receptive functions, memory and learning, cognition, and

the expressive functions. The social dimension is based on social interaction and relationships as well as the more global concept of culture. The spiritual dimension is that aspect of a person from which meaning in life is determined and through which transcendence over the ordinary is possible.

The second premise of holistic health care philosophy is that the environment makes significant contributions to the nature of one's existence. Each person's environment consists of many factors that are influential in that person's quality of life. Consequently, people cannot be fully understood without consideration of environmental factors such as family relationships, culture, and physical surroundings. Individuals interact with their unique environments through all dimensions, based on subjective experience as well as external stimuli.

The third premise is that each person experiences development across his or her life cycle; in each stage of life, the individual experiences and confronts different issues or similar issues in different ways. One's experience of each stage of life forms the basis for further development as one moves through the life cycle.

Fourth, the holistic health care provider maintains that stress is a primary factor in health and illness. Any event or circumstance can act as a stressor. Regardless of the source, stress has an impact on the whole person. Stressors directly affecting the physical dimension are numerous; examples include stressors associated with genetic factors, physiological processes, and body image. Emotional stress may result from any experience or situation, related to any dimension that elicits an emotion from the individual and generates the physiological stress response. Examples include poor physical conditions, perceived social inequities, a significant loss, intellectual incompetence, and a sense of meaninglessness. Stressors affecting the intellectual dimension may be any factors that interfere with receptive functions, memory and learning, cognitive functions, or expressive functions. Social stressors may arise from interactions and relationships with other people, as well as from more general societal and cultural factors. Stressors affecting the spiritual dimension may be any factors that interfere with one's ability to meet spiritual needs. Value conflicts, perceived loss of meaning, and a sense of isolation are examples of stressors to the spiritual dimension.

Fifth, people are ultimately responsible for the directions their lives take and the life-styles they choose. Locus of control is a concept that indicates the extent to which individuals perceive a sense of personal responsibility in life. Within a holistic framework, people are viewed as active participants in and contributors to their health status; they are willing to learn from illness and to strive toward healthier choices.

REFERENCES AND SUGGESTED READINGS

1. Baron RA and others: *Psychology: understanding behavior,* ed 2, New York, 1980, Holt, Rinehart and Winston.
2. Bendich S: Appreciating bodily phenomena in verbally oriented psychotherapy sessions, *Issues in Mental Health Nursing* 9:1, 1988.
3. Blankstein K, Egner K: Relationship of the locus of control construct to the control of heart rate, *Journal of General Psychology* 97:291, 1977.
4. Brallier LW: Stress management as a path toward wholeness.

In Krieger D: *Foundations for holistic health nursing practices: the Renaissance nurse*, Philadelphia, 1981, JB Lippincott.

5. Brallier LW: The nurse as holistic health practitioner, *Nursing Clinics of North America* 13:643, 1978.

6. Brodsky C: *A study of norms for body form-behavior relationships,* Washington, DC, 1954, The Catholic University of America Press.

7. Burkhardt M: Dealing with spiritual concerns of clients in the community, *Journal of Community Health Nursing* 2(4):191, 1985.

8. Capra F: *The turning point: science, society, and the rising culture*, New York, 1982, Simon & Schuster.

9. Clark CC: *Enhancing wellness: a guide for self-care*, New York, 1981, Springer.

10. Clemmens E: Some psychological functions of language, *American Journal of Psychoanalysis* 43(4):294, 1988.

11. Clinebell H: *Basic types of pastoral counseling: new resources for ministering to the troubled*, New York, 1966, Abingdon Press.

12. Colston L: The handicapped. In Wicks R, Parson R, Capps D, editors: *Clinical handbook of pastoral counseling*, New York, 1985, Integration Books.

13. Cole S: *The sociological orientation: an introduction to sociology*, Chicago, 1975, Rand McNally & Co.

14. Cooley C: *Human nature and the social order*, New York, 1902, Charles Scribner's Sons.

15. Craig WJ: Caffeine update, *Adventist Review* 158(35):3, 1981.

16. Davis G: The hands of the healer: has faith a place? *Journal of Medical Ethics* 6:185, 1980.

17. Denver GEA: *Community health analysis: a holistic approach*, Germantown, Md, 1980, Aspen Systems.

18. Dunn HL: *High level wellness*, Thorofare, NJ, 1961, Slack.

19. Ellwood R: *Many peoples, many faiths*, ed 3, Englewood Cliffs, NJ, 1987, Prentice Hall.

20. Ferguson M: *The aquarian conspiracy: personal and social transformation in the 1980's*, Los Angeles, 1980, Jeremy P Tarcher.

21. Flynn PAR, editor: *The healing continuum: journeys in the philosophy of holistic health*, Bowie, Md, 1980, Robert J Brady.

22. Garsee J: The development of an ideology. In Schuster, CS, Ashburn SS: *The process of human development: a holistic approach*, Boston, 1980, Little, Brown & Co.

23. Giger J, Davidhizer R: Crosscultural nursing and implications for nursing care, *International Nursing Review* 37(1):199, 1990.

24. Girdano D, Everly G: *Controlling stress and tension: a holistic approach*, Englewood Cliffs, NJ, 1979, Prentice Hall.

25. Gordon JS: The paradigm of holistic medicine. In Hastings AC, Fadiman J, Gordon JS, editors: *Health for the whole person*, Boulder, Colo, 1980, Westview Press.

26. Greenspan S: *Intelligence and adaptation*, Madison, Conn, 1979, International Universities Press.

27. Guidano VF, Liotti G: *Cognitive processes and emotional disorders: a structural approach to psychotherapy*, New York, 1983, The Guilford Press.

28. Guyton AC: *Textbook of medical physiology*, ed 6, Philadelphia, 1981, WB Saunders.

29. Hardy M: Role strain and role stress. In Hardy M, Conway M, editors: *Role theory: perspectives for health professionals*, New York, 1978, Appleton-Century-Crofts.

30. Hayter J: The rhythm of sleep, *American Journal of Nursing* 80(3):457, 1980.

31. Heiniger MC, Randolph SL: *Neurophysiological concepts in human behavior: the learning tree*, St Louis, 1981, Mosby–Year Book.

32. Highfield MF: *Oncology nurses' awareness of their patients' spiritual needs and problems*, master's thesis, 1981, University of Arkansas for Medical Sciences.

33. Hogan RM: *Human sexuality: a nursing perspective*, Norwalk, Conn, 1985, Appleton-Century-Crofts.

34. Hollen P: A holistic model of individual and family health based on a continuum of choice, *Advances in Nursing Science* 3(4):27, 1981.

35. Holmes TH, Rahe RH: The social readjustment rating scale, *Journal of Psychosomatic Research* 11:213, 1967.

36. Jenny J: Classifying nursing diagnoses: self-care approach, *Nursing Health Care* 10(2):83, 1988.

37. Johnstone R: *Religion in society*, ed 3, Englewood Cliffs, NJ, 1988, Prentice Hall.

38. Kaluger G, Kaluger MF: *Human development: the span of life*, ed 3, St Louis, 1984, Mosby–Year Book.

39. Kohlberg L: Development of moral character and moral ideology. In Hoffman ML, Hoffman LW, editors: *Review of child development research*, vol 1, New York, 1964, Russell Sage Foundation.

40. Leininger M: *Transcultural nursing: concepts, theory, and practice*, New York, 1978, John Wiley & Sons.

41. Levine S, Scotch N: *Social stress*, Chicago, 1970, Aldine Publishing Co.

42. Lezak M: *Neuropsychological assessment*, New York, 1976, Oxford University Press.

43. Lugo J, Hershey G: *Human development: a multidisciplinary approach to the psychology of individual growth*, New York, 1974, Macmillan.

44. Maslow AH: *Motivation and personality*, ed 2, New York, 1970, Harper & Row.

45. Maslow AH: *Toward a psychology of being*, ed 2, New York, 1968, Van Nostrand Reinhold.

46. McKee J: Introduction to sociology, ed 2, New York, 1974, Holt, Rinehart and Winston.

47. Menninger W: *A psychiatrist for a troubled world*, New York, 1967, The Viking Press. (Edited by B. Hall.)

48. Molzahn A, Northcott H: The social basis of discrepancies in health/illness perceptions, *Journal of Advanced Nursing* 14(2):132, 1989.

49. Moore L and others: *The biocultural basis of health,* Prospect Heights, Ill, 1987, Waveland Press.

50. Munn N: *The fundamentals of human adjustment*, Boston, 1961, Houghton Mifflin.

51. Norris C: The professional nurse and body image. In Carlson C, coordinator: *Behavioral concepts and nursing intervention*, Philadelphia, 1970, JB Lippincott.

52. Nowakowski L: Health promotion/self-care programs for the community, *Topics in Clinical Nursing* 2(2):21, 1980.

53. Pelletier KR: *Mind as healer, mind as slayer: a holistic approach to preventing disorders*, New York, 1977, Dell Publishing.

54. Perls F, Hefferline RF, Goodman P: *Gestalt therapy*, New York, 1951, Bantam Books.

55. Piaget J: *The growth of logical thinking from childhood to adolescence*, New York, 1958, Basic Books.

56. Rainer J: Contributions of the biological sciences. In Kaplan H, Sadock B: *Comprehensive textbook of psychiatry*, ed 4, Baltimore, 1985, Williams & Wilkins.

57. Rew L: Exercises for spiritual growth, *Journal of Holistic Nursing* 4(1):20, 1986.

58. Ryan RS, Travis JW: *The wellness workbook*, Berkeley, Calif, 1981, Ten Speed Press.

59. Samuels M, Bennett H: *The well body book*, New York, 1973, Random House.

60. Schuster CS, Ashburn SS: *The process of human development: a holistic approach*, Boston, 1980, Little, Brown & Co.

61. Scott A: Human interaction and personal boundries, *Journal of Psychosocial Nursing and Mental Health Services* 26(8):23, 1988.

62. Segal J: Biofeedback as medical treatment, *Journal of the American Medical Association*, 2232:179, 1975.

63. Selye H: *The stress of life*, ed 2, New York, 1978, McGraw-Hill.

64. Sheldon W, Stevens S, Tucker W: *The varieties of human physique: and introduction to constitutional psychology*, New York, 1941, Harper & Brothers.

65. Simonton O, Mathews-Simonton S, Creighton J: *Getting well again*, New York, 1978, Bantam Books.

66. Stoll RI: Guidelines for spiritual assessment, *American Journal of Nursing* 79:1574, 1979.

67. Sun M: FDA caffeine decision too early, some say, *Science* 209:1500, 1980.

68. Topf M: Verbal interpersonal responsiveness, *Journal of Psychosocial Nursing and Mental Health Services* 26(7):8, 1988.

69. Tubesing DA: *Stress skills*, Oakland, Ill, 1979, Whole Person Associates.

70. White House Conference on Aging: *Spiritual well-being*, Washington, DC, 1971, Department of Health, Education, and Welfare, US Government Printing Office.

ANNOTATED BIBLIOGRAPHY

Baron RA and others: *Psychology: understanding behavior*, ed 2, New York, 1980, Holt, Rinehart & Winston General Book.

This comprehensive book includes a framework for understanding maladaptive behavior, details causes and treatment of maladaptive behavior, and discusses areas of assessment and prevention. Emphasis is given to the latest research findings on biological factors in the cause of disorders.

Belsky J: *Here tomorrow: making the most of life after fifty*, Baltimore, 1988, Johns Hopkins University Press.

This book reviews the healthy aspects of aging. A discussion of growing old as another stage of human growth and development is presented in a positive perspective.

Kaluger G, Kaluger MF: *Human development: the span of life*, ed 3, St Louis, 1984, Mosby—Year Book.

This books presents the basic universal principles of growth and development, while emphasizing the significance of individual differences and recognizing the environmental influences in creating differences.

Kreiger D: *Foundations of holistic health nursing practice: the Renaissance nurse*, Philadelphia, 1981, JB Lippincott.

This book focuses on the healing of the whole person and discusses human embryological development on a continuum through death. From prehistoric time to the present, it lays the foundations for modern holistic health nursing. The content includes articles covering therapeutic touch, imagery, stress management theories, and the holistic conceptual framework as it is used in the nursing process. Emphasis is placed on revitalizing humanism in nursing within the philosophy of holism.

CHAPTER

3 Philosophical Positions

Peggy A Landrum

After studying this chapter, the student will be able to:

- Discuss ways in which philosophy has influenced human life
- Examine contributions of philosophy to the Western health care system
- Describe the impact of philosophy on mental health–psychiatric nursing

- Identify components of various philosophical positions that have affected the nature of mental health–psychiatric nursing practice
- Identify the general view of human nature within the philosophical framework of holism
- Discuss the principles of holistic health care

Philosophy plays an important role in all aspects of human life. Any conceptual base for mental health–psychiatric nursing has a foundation in philosophy. Personal and professional philosophies influence the nature and quality of mental health–psychiatric nursing care, thus affecting both practitioner and client. The purposes of this chapter are (1) to introduce philosophy as a primary influence in human life, health care, and mental health–psychiatric nursing; (2) to briefly discuss several philosophical positions that are relevant to understanding health care in general and mental health–psychiatric nursing in particular; (3) to discuss the philosophical position of holism; and (4) to introduce basic principles of holistic health practice that may be used as guidelines in any setting to enhance the quality of the nurse-client relationship.

SIGNIFICANCE OF PHILOSOPHY

Philosophy and Human Nature

Philosophy has influenced every aspect of human life throughout recorded history. Philosophical thought probably occurred as soon as people began to question the nature of their own lives and surroundings. Beliefs, expectations about life, and the meaning of human existence have been profoundly affected by philosophical thinking. People have fought wars, explored new lands, and developed technology based on their philosophical positions. Cultural attitudes and beliefs have made it possible for various political systems to evolve—from those flourishing on freedom of human thought and behavior to those thriving on slavery and persecution. The meanings that people ascribe to life have also caused major changes in the course of history,

because those things that people value determine the direction of human development. Religions have been influenced by philosophy, as have ideals, goals, and standards of behavior. Throughout history, solutions to human problems and the acquisition of new knowledge have been interrelated with philosophy.

Individuals have their own personal philosophy, which consciously or unconsciously influences their lives. This philosophy and its accompanying behaviors are partially determined by culture. Personal philosophy determines how people view themselves, others, and the world in which they live. For instance, if one views the nature of people as essentially good, one is likely to approach people with positive expectations; if one believes that basic human nature is evil, one probably will have negative expectations. If one's personal philosophy asserts that people can exert some degree of control over their destiny, one is more likely to assume responsibility for oneself than if the belief is that outside or random forces control destiny. Personal philosophy regarding the environment will determine a person's interaction with physical surroundings, and the result may be respectful or destructive.

A person's philosophy is reflected in values, attitudes, beliefs, goals, and activities that are developed by that individual. Unique life circumstances—including familial, social, cultural, and environmental factors—contribute to developing personal values. Many values and attitudes are learned from parents and families, from educational and religious institutions, and from personal and professional peer groups. Some are adopted through exposure to the media or literature. Each person needs to actively develop a personal philosophy, otherwise one's directions and goals may be determined more by others than by oneself.

Philosophy is not static. It constantly evolves and may be influenced by any aspect of one's life situation. As children, people incorporate certain values into their lives without question. This is necessary for socialization and survival. However, throughout life values are reevaluated to determine which are still relevant and which are no longer conducive to growth and development. Frequently, the *should*'s and *should not*'s that we learn as children need to be modified to serve us more appropriately as adults. For instance, a child of an abusive family may need an attitude of strong skepticism to survive emotionally. But for an adult this attitude may be maladaptive. As individuals move among different peer groups throughout their lives, they adopt some of the values and attitudes of each group. Personal philosophy influences receptiveness to new knowledge and beliefs. Conversely, acquiring new knowledge and beliefs may affect overall personal philosophy.

Philosophy is an active partner of science; both are necessary and contribute to the quality of life. Science and technology provide necessary problem-solving tools. Philosophy guides people in their use of these tools. Science analyzes the process and examines the facts, whereas philosophy seeks the meaning and value of the process and attempts to interpret the facts. Science reduces the whole into parts, and philosophy reconstructs the parts in new and more meaningful ways.

Philosophy and Health Care

The general philosophy of a society affects the nature of health care in that society. For example, if people are viewed as primarily in charge of their own destiny, health care providers are likely to encourage personal responsibility for disease prevention and for health promotion. If people believe that everything in the universe is interrelated, the focus of health care is likely to be the many factors in a person's life contributing to health and illness. However, when cultural beliefs separate mind and matter, physical and emotional problems are probably approached as separate, unrelated disturbances.

In health care, as in other areas of life, philosophy and science fulfill complementary roles. Both are necessary for the health care system to operate at its optimal level. Science provides knowledge and technology that profoundly affect the quality of life and that often can make the difference between life and death. However, scientific expertise is most effective when used discriminately within guidelines. Philosophy creates a framework in which the health care system can apply its knowledge and technology to client care in meaningful and ethical ways.

Any particular health care system develops its own philosophy, which is reflected in the values, attitudes, beliefs, goals, and activities of its practitioners and of the system as a whole. The philosophy of a health care system determines the framework for applying knowledge and technology, thus greatly affecting the nature and quality of health care delivery. Consideration of many facets is necessary when exploring the philosophy of a particular health care system. Because health care affects the quality and even the existence of individual human lives, the system's basic assumptions about the value of human life are primary. The focus of the system is an important factor; it may be

on the person or the disease, aimed toward prevention or cure, and oriented toward health or illness. The system's view of the practitioner-client relationship as well as responsibility for health status influence the nature of health care. The practitioner-client relationship can range from authoritarian to coparticipatory and may or may not be considered relevant to the healing process. Clients may be encouraged to assume much responsibility or discouraged from assuming any. In general, the philosophy of a health care system determines how practitioners define and approach health and illness.

Philosophy and Mental Health–Psychiatric Nursing

Mental health and illness have been recognized throughout history, but beliefs have changed as human culture and philosophy have changed. Each culture holds its own beliefs about mental illness. The definition of mental health and illness is based on the current philosophy and value systems of the society and culture. Certain standards are used at any given time in the development of society. Deviance from these standards has often been labeled as mental illness.

The philosophy of mental health–psychiatric nursing in this text holds that people are multidimensional and in constant interaction with their environments. Nursing action focuses on people as they adapt to their environments, cope with illness, and pursue health.

Each nurse approaches mental health–psychiatric nursing in an individual way. To a large extent this approach is determined by the nurse's personal philosophy of life and concept of human nature. Each nurse has a philosophy that provides a framework for relationships with clients. A nurse's values, attitudes, and beliefs about people and about mental health and illness dictate many aspects of nursing care. For example, nurses may either value clients for who they are or show concern primarily with the illness or disease. Client perspectives may or may not influence the development of nursing care plans; primary emphasis may be on client needs or nurse-physician-institution needs. In addition, the nurse's philosophy determines whether authoritarian or coparticipatory relationships are formed with clients and whether mental health and physical health are viewed as separate or interrelated entities. Tendencies to label, judge, or fear clients also affect nursing care. In general, personal philosophy affects how individuals fulfill the nursing role, which in turn affects the well-being of their clients.

Because personal philosophies have a great impact on mental health–psychiatric nursing, nurses need to develop their own philosophical positions. This process provides useful information about how nurses and clients may influence each other, and begins with awareness of the self, the environment, and the interaction of the two. *Awareness of self* is developed as nurses clarify their values and beliefs, acknowledge their attitudes and opinions, and become consciously aware of the many choices and decisions that they constantly make. *Awareness of environment* includes recognizing client needs, belief systems, and behaviors; identifying factors that contribute to health and illness in the client; and assessing resources available to the client. *Awareness of interactions with the environment*—specif-

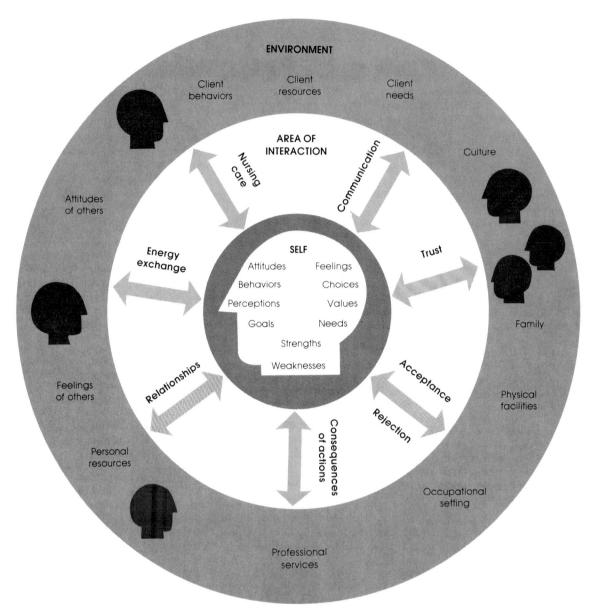

FIGURE 3-1 Awareness of self, of environment, and of interaction.

ically with clients—is enhanced when nurses identify their specific feelings and thoughts about clients (including feelings of acceptance or rejection), evaluate the consequences of their actions toward clients, and differentiate between their own needs and client needs (Figure 3-1).

Awareness of self and others helps nurses effectively promote self-awareness in their clients. Nurses who are aware of self can interact authentically with clients rather than reciting preprogramed instructions or standard notions about how things are or should be. Those who can evaluate their own strengths and weaknesses and determine personal needs and goals are in a much stronger position to facilitate the same processes in clients. Awareness is the foundation of change; the more clients understand about themselves and their situations, the more likely they are to accurately identify their needs and to choose healthier ways of meeting them.

OVERVIEW OF PHILOSOPHIES

Preliterate Ideologies

In humanity's earliest days most energy was necessarily devoted to survival. Humans were aware of their mortality and concerned about their uncertain and unknown future. Religious and magical concepts evolved to help cope with the uncertainty. Over tens of thousands of years humans adapted to environmental conditions by inventing tools, developing art forms, and creating social groups. They learned to cultivate food rather than simply gather it. Value and belief systems emerged that added order to human existence.

Complicated magic and symbolic rituals were intended to ensure safety and to help preliterate groups of people obtain what they needed and wanted. Visions such as dreams and sensing the invisible were considered legitimate ways to acquire information and formed the basis for certain decisions. Misfortune was believed to be sent by evil spirits; good fortune, such as successful hunts or good crops, was often attributed to good spirits.

Magic and symbolic rituals were also used to ensure the prevention of disease and injury. Outcomes of disease and injury were predicted by using extrasensory powers and dream interpretations. What is considered mental illness today was thought to be caused by violation of taboos, refusal to participate in rituals, loss of the soul from the body, possession by evil spirits, and witchcraft. In some cultures trephination, or surgical opening of the skull, was performed to release evil spirits or to allow the entrance of good spirits.

Shamanism evolved as a common practice in many preliterate cultures and is still practiced in some parts of the world. A *shaman* is a person with a special relationship to the spirit world that results in unique healing powers. Healing most often occurs when the shaman is in an altered state of consciousness. Public confessions by the afflicted individual and family, chants, symbolic rituals, and medicinal herbs are among the shaman's healing techniques.

Chinese Perspective

Although the early Chinese believed that human destiny initially depended on the gods, they also recognized the value of human virtue. As their civilization evolved, the Chinese considered destiny as primarily dependent on human actions and merit. Because human nature is considered essentially good, a strong sense of optimism exists in Chinese culture, and developing moral character is very important. Mencius (Chinese philosopher, c. 372-289 BC) asserted four basic human qualities—love, righteousness, propriety, and wisdom. When nourished through moral training and social education, these develop; when neglected, they are lost.

Chinese doctrine supports the concept of universal order; individuals, societies, and the physical universe are composed of the same elements and reflect universal principles. Love of both people and things is important, and harmony with nature is a primary goal of human life. Within the social order, the individual and society are equally significant and interdependent.[9]

Additionally, the natural cycles of the universe and of human life are intricately interrelated and respected. In Chinese philosophy *ch'i* is fundamental life energy that flows in orderly ways through the body along meridians. *Yin* and *yang* are polarized aspects of ch'i; yin is passive, or negative energy, and yang is active, or positive energy. An individual is healthy when yin and yang energies are in balance; illness is a disturbance in this energy flow.

A primary focus of Chinese health care is teaching people to prevent illness and to maintain and promote their own health. Responsibility for oneself is emphasized. When health problems occur, attention is given to the whole person by assessing the flow of life energy, physical and emotional states, natural cycles, environmental influences, behavior, dreams, and current life situation. Change between health and illness develops gradually and includes many contributing factors rather than a single cause and effect. Balance within the person and harmony with the environ-

ment are critical for health.[7] Because everything in the universe is related, mind and body are not considered separate entities; mental functions are not specific to or located in any single part of an individual.

Chinese history acknowledges mental illness; ancient writings refer to insanity, dementia, violent behavior, and convulsions. Acute psychosis may be attributed to loss of face or failure to fulfill family and social obligations, which can lead to suicide. An aspect of Chinese life that may have a positive influence on mental health is that people are encouraged to make primary emotional and social attachments to groups as a whole rather than to specific individuals. This arrangement offers a broader support system than most societies, and a person may feel less isolated and alone.

East Indian Perspective

The most pervasive notion in Indian thought is value of the subjective nature of humans. The highest value is to know one's true self, or *atman*. The atman is the most inward reality and the highest controlling power of a person. Because humans are the link between the supreme inward reality of spirit and the outward reality of matter, they are the center of the universe. A successful life depends on the degree of inwardness that a person deliberately pursues and attains, accounting for the Indian ideals of peace and quietism. This focus on the subjective nature of humans is not a general retreat from the external world or a passive approach to life. The universe is in meaningful and constant motion that provides order, and one must act if one wants life.[35]

The natural and moral laws of the universe govern life conditions that complicate human efforts to pursue the inward search. The laws relate to action, work, destiny, product, and effect, according to Buddhist tradition. Adhering to these laws allows individuals to satisfy their duty. To ignore them is to work against universal energy and create further suffering and additional limitations in one's life.[15]

Yoga, a system designed to facilitate physical, mental, and spiritual development, is the primary method for enhancing the pursuit of inward consciousness. Yoga hastens one's movement through the distressful conditions of life toward *samadhi,* a state of total enlightenment in which the body, mind, and spirit function as a harmonious whole.[12]

The *prana* is the life energy that unites the physical body into a whole and organizes the life process. Pranic energy currents give vitality to the physical body and convey the psyche's activities throughout the body; they relate to the natural cycles of the universe and to the state of the individual. *Chakras* are centers of swirling pranic energy that act as centers of consciousness. The practice of yoga activates these chakras so that human energies are more balanced.

Ancient Indian writings indicated that health depended on cooperating with nature's laws. People with disease were believed to have violated moral laws or to be out of balance. The client and the disease process were evaluated as a whole unit. Primary concerns, in addition to curing illness, were health promotion and longevity. Healers in ancient India had profound understanding of herbs and roots, an accurate knowledge of anatomy and physiology, and an awareness of the principles of some contagious diseases.[26]

In the *Atharuveda*, dated 700 BC, magic formulas were mentioned that counteracted demons and their human representatives. Early in their history the Indians differentiated between the brain and the mind, and the heart was considered to be the center of sensation and consciousness. Insanity was an imbalance within the person. At least four treatments for mental diseases were recognized: psychotherapy in the form of chanting, sacrifices, fasting, and purification rituals; drugs derived from plants or animals; divine agents such as sun, air, and water; and occasional physical or mental shocks.[17]

Ancient Greek Perspective

In early Greek history the primary philosophical interest was the order of nature as a whole; people were not objects of specific concern. Rather than having personal motivations, individuals received feelings and ideas from external sources. In the fifth century BC, the Sophists believed that the true nature of the universe was changeable. Community action was valued because of the belief that the individual could not effect change without help.

Socrates (c. 469-399 BC), following the Sophists, thought that nature was an ordered array of interactions rather than accidental chaos and that humans were a product of this ordered array. The soul allowed understanding and conscious direction of one's life, and diseases of the soul, such as ignorance and vice, were considered much worse than physical diseases. Socrates viewed the person as a physical body united with a nonphysical soul. The belief that mind and body are two separate, though interrelated, entities has occurred in many Western philosophies since the time of Socrates.

Plato (c. 429-347 BC), a student of Socrates, believed that mental health and justice were related. He contended that reason, spirit, and appetite are separate components of the psyche. Each part performs its unique task to enhance the person's ability to function in useful and healthy ways. Such functioning was viewed as justice.

Plato viewed reason as the dominant and logical part of the psyche, in charge of coordinating information and feedback, making decisions and plans, and instructing the other parts to carry out their own tasks. For reason to function at its peak level, its primary requirement is truth. The spiritual element of the psyche responds to human and social matters. Spirit provides energy to fulfill the conclusions of reason and to control the energy of appetite. Courage is the spirit's primary requirement. Appetite is the part of the psyche that is the source of one's desires and cravings, and in excess is a liability. Manageable degrees of desire are necessary for things that are really important. The primary requirement of appetite is temperance. So truth, courage, and temperance—within the general context of justice—were needed to qualify a person as mentally healthy. Plato explained irrational events in behavior as an unavoidable aspect of human life. He expected people to deal with these events through reason.

Aristotle (384-322 BC), Plato's student for 20 years, believed that the mind is clearly distinguished, but is not separate, from the body. Aristotle believed that regular catharsis would purge passion and thus avoid violence. He viewed music, wine, and aphrodisiacs as therapeutic because they aroused passion and helped release repressed emotions.

Hippocrates (c. 469-379 BC) believed that mental disease is not supernatural or sacred but that it has certain characteristics and specific causes.[17] He believed that health depended on interaction of the basic qualities in nature and the body humors. During ill health, a person's habits and irregularities that preceded illness were noted. Therapeutic interventions were also based on natural cycles. Dreams were used to gather information and to heal physical ills. A particular treatment induced states of consciousness in which the unconscious mind was instructed to heal body ills; this is evidence of an early belief in Western culture that mind and body influence each other.[26]

The popular concept in the early Greek days was that mental illness was caused by supernatural forces and possession by evil spirits sent by angry gods. Aimless wandering and violent behavior indicated mental disease. The personality functioned best when the appropriate interaction of internal and external forces had been achieved.

Asceticism

The philosophy of *asceticism* (from the Greek *asketos*, meaning "one who practices virtue") is basically a discipline of self-denial, renunciation, and detachment. The primary premise is that human purpose is to know, love, and be united with a spiritual force, and this purpose is more important than love of humans and earthly things. Enlightened spiritual states and salvation can be attained only through self-discipline and self-denial.

Asceticism was practiced in some Eastern religions and by proponents of some schools of Greek philosophy, particularly by the Stoics and the Cynics. In the Roman Empire, ascetic practices were characteristic of certain Gnostic sects who based their practices on the doctrine that matter is evil and only spirit is good. Judeo-Christian tradition asserts that humans are created in God's image. The purpose then of asceticism is to achieve peace with God through discipline of the body. Characteristics of early Christian asceticism were detachment from the world, practice of celibacy, renunciation of personal property, and martyrdom.

Asceticism's highest value is dedicating oneself to a mission, goal, purpose, or service that is divinely assigned. In the early history of nursing, both society—and nurses—viewed nursing as a mission that required self-denial, dedication to duty, self-discipline, and the refusal of rewards. Asceticism was a primary component of nursing philosophy and characterized nursing practice from the mid-nineteenth century through 1920. It then became less dominant.

The ascetic influence affected both clients and nurses. Redemption of the client's soul was the primary goal of nursing care during the ascetic phase. This duty took priority over any other nursing goal. A client's own personal beliefs about the world and his particular situations were not relevant, and the client was not viewed as a whole person with many kinds of needs.

During this period, institutions for mentally ill clients provided primarily custodial care. Because of large client populations and the severity of psychotic behavior, nursing care also was custodial, and nurses did not deal with interpersonal or psychodynamic issues.[11] Early psychiatric nursing texts written by both psychiatric nurses and psychiatrists[3,37] advocated personal qualities such as patience, self-sacrifice, cheerfulness, courage, and strong will for the psychiatric nurse to contend successfully with these clients. As in other areas, nurses in mental institutions worked long hours, functioned in poor conditions, and collected low wages. Service to clients and physicians took precedence over the nurse's own needs.

Romanticism

In the late eighteenth and early nineteenth centuries, a popular attitude of revolt against society and social institutions developed that included protest against rules governing language, artistic form, and subjective matter. *Romanticism* was a social and aesthetic movement, characterized in art, literature, and music by freedom of form, spontaneity of feeling, and a strong emphasis on imagination. The individual was glorified for personal merit rather than status; emotions, imagination, and creative powers determined personal merit. Self-fulfillment, emotionalism, freedom, and pursuit of the ideal were valued and often found expression in unrealistic and impractical ways. Delight in the mysterious, adventurous, and sentimental was evident; goals and aims were high but impractical.

Romanticism exerted a strong influence on nursing from the early 1920s through the early 1940s, perhaps as a reaction against the rigidity of nursing's earlier ascetic nature. Personal glory, emotionalism, and adventure characterized the common view of nursing; service and loyalty to others were often the ideal; and nurses allowed physicians and hospitals to set the standards of practice. Romanticism encouraged and idealized the dependence and subservience of women, and that ideal in nursing was for nurses to be dependent on physicians and hospitals. Nursing care was not primarily based on rationality or on practical consequences for clients or nurses. Instead, nursing practice followed the needs of the medical model and of hospitals. Due largely to ascetic and romantic influences, nursing did not value or reward autonomy, assertiveness, or independent thinking. In return for subservience, nurses did not have to accept responsibility for themselves; physicians and hospitals accepted responsibility for them.

Pragmatism

The focus of *pragmatism* is practical consequences; ideas are valued only for their consequences. Intellectual concepts and theories are not significant if they make no practical difference; they must be applied in some way to everyday human existence and problem solving. Pragmatists are active rather than thoughtful and deal with facts rather than abstractions; they examine issues to determine if they serve a specific purpose.

Pragmatism was a useful philosophy for nursing during and following World War II, primarily to cope with the nurse shortage that ensued. Many nursing care problems demanded practical and expedient solutions. Lack of sufficient nursing personnel and the increases in client pop-ulations of psychiatric hospitals made it necessary to delegate many duties to ancillary personnel; thus nurses became, to a large degree, teachers and supervisors. Nursing care was primarily directed toward the specific problem or disease alone; other needs of the client often were not considered.

Responding to physician and institution needs remained a nursing priority early in this era. Health care institutions specialized according to diseases and to stages of illness. Psychiatric units became more dynamic than custodial, and psychiatric nurses became more aware of interpersonal influences on behavior. The importance of therapeutic social interaction was recognized. The emergence of community psychiatry also created changes in the nursing role, and mental illness was viewed as more than an isolated internal psychological problem.[11]

Pragmatism emphasized realistic application of ideas, and psychiatric nurses began to realize that nursing care could make a real difference in client welfare. Thus psychiatric nurses began to explore new, more effective ways to view clients. Focus on the client's perspective encouraged responsiveness to client needs. Consequently, there was less emphasis on physician and hospital needs, and loyalties toward clients arose. When clients became the focus of nursing actions, nurses became accountable to them. Nurses could no longer allow physicians to assume responsibility for nursing care.[5]

Humanism

The basic tenets of *humanism* stress the importance of human abilities, aspirations, and achievements in the earthly life. Human nature is distinct from, though related to, the concrete physical universe and the metaphysical abstractions beyond it. Humanism was first expressed in the philosophy, literature, and art of ancient Greece and Rome but was submerged during the Middle Ages. It was revived when ancient culture was rediscovered during the Renaissance.

Renaissance humanism protested against the dogma of otherworldliness and the church. Humanists of the eighteenth century attacked political oppression, and those of the nineteenth century resisted attempts to interpret human nature through the categories and methods of the natural sciences.

Humanism today is a philosophical movement in which people and their interests, development, fulfillment, and creativity are central and dominant. This ethical doctrine supports the right to human freedom. Humanists emphasize self-understanding, self-determination, and human responsibility. Humanists advocate that people develop individual goals based on their personal life experience.

Within nursing, humanism emphasizes the value and importance of being human, and encourages caring for client dignity and welfare. When humanistic philosophy guides mental health–psychiatric nursing practice, nurses are aware of themselves and of clients in nursing interactions, and they assume responsibility for nursing decisions. The person is the focus of nursing care, and the client's well-being guides all nursing activities. The whole person, rather than only the specific disease or problem, receives attention in an accepting and nonjudgmental manner.

Clients are recognized as having the basic ability to make their own decisions concerning health care. The concern of nursing is to deal with each client's quality of life and to help people as they strive toward fulfilling their human potential.

Existentialism

The word *existentialism* was coined after World War I to designate the philosophical thinking of Karl Jaspers and Martin Heidegger. Both were indebted to the philosophy of Sören Kierkegaard (1813-1855), a nineteenth-century Danish theologian and philosopher. The writings of Jean-Paul Sartre brought existentialism to the attention of the English speaking world after World War II. Existential philosophy is concerned with the essence of human existence rather than logic or science and developed out of a conviction that most academic philosophy is too remote from human life and death. Existentialists are especially concerned with the most extreme human experiences, such as anguish, despair, and confrontation with death, because they enable a person to realize the true nature of existence.

The following three ideas and concerns are central to existentialism[40]:

1. The idea that individual existence is more important than theories regarding general human nature, since such theories often neglect the quality of uniqueness
2. Concern with the meaning and purpose of human lives on earth; inner experience is more important that objective truth
3. Concern with individual freedom, the most important and distinctively human property. People are free to choose their own attitudes, purposes, values, and way of life, and they must accept personal responsibility for these choices

The most radical division of existential thought is between the religious and the atheistic. Kierkegaard rejected abstract philosophies and advocated the prime importance of the individual and the individual's choices. He described three main ways of life (aesthetic, ethical, and religious) from which each person must choose. He believed the religious way—Christianity in particular—was the most desirable, but it could be reached only after struggling through the other two ways.

The views of Friedrich Nietzsche (1844-1900), the other main source of existential thought in the nineteenth century, were atheistic. He asserted that because religion and God are illusions people must find meaning and purpose for their lives in human terms alone. Nietzsche proposed that morality is individual and must come from within each person. If there were an absolute morality and all people had knowledge of it, they would be stranded in a static and frozen position. To seek an absolute morality is to avoid the kind of consciousness that actually characterizes human existence itself, one consisting of change, process, and decision making.

Consciousness is the focus of twentieth-century existentialism, which asserts that individuals must take responsibility for making their own choices and consequently for the direction of their lives. This process can be lonely and frightening, but it can also be a gratifying experience of change and growth and of fully appreciating one's potentials.

Existentialism in conjunction with humanism has influenced mental health–psychiatric nursing since the early 1960s. Together they imply that nurses can neither understand clients through science or metaphysical systems alone, nor adequately relate to clients in terms of only their disease or problem. An isolated aspect of a client neither explains how that client functions as a whole person nor indicates what the client needs. Only authentic, honest relationships with clients can help mental health–psychiatric nurses respond to the client as a whole person. Scientific principles and attempts to predict human responses are not excluded from nursing practice, but nurses with an existentialist viewpoint must accept the client's right to make choices about health care as well as life-style.

Existentialism supports accountability in nursing. Nurses are free to make choices regarding nursing care and are responsible for the consequences of their choices, which are best made after recognizing possibilities and alternatives. Mental health–psychiatric nurses have established themselves as self-directed peers of other mental health practitioners and have exerted a major influence on nursing as a profession. Thus they have many opportunities to practice responsibility and accountability. Nurses need to become more aware of their own experience, striving for authenticity and honesty with themselves. The nurse-client relationship is an opportunity for nurse and client to increase awareness, to experience freedom and growth, and to learn to make responsible choices.

HOLISTIC PHILOSOPHY AND HEALTH CARE

The philosophical position of holism is useful for examining human nature and health care philosophy. Holism and holistic health have been described and defined from several perspectives. A basic premise inherent in all definitions is that living and nonliving entities are viewed in terms of "wholeness, relationships, processes, interactions, freedom and creativity."[7] The patterns of interrelationship within and among entities determine reality; thus it is inaccurate to consider individuals, societies, or things in isolation.

A holistic philosophy of health care simultaneously grows out of and integrates all of these concepts of human nature. It incorporates ideas and principles from several philosophical positions, such as the Eastern beliefs of China and India, humanism, and existentialism. Holistic health philosophy accepts the Chinese concept of universal order, that everything in the universe is composed of the same elements. Therefore human nature is an intricate part of universal order, and harmony with nature is a primary value. A person's body is composed of active and passive energy forces, and health exists when these energies are balanced; illness occurs when they are disturbed. As in Chinese belief, holistic health care emphasizes prevention, personal responsibility, and mind-body unity.

A primary concept in holistic health, as in Indian philosophy, is the subjective nature of a person. To understand outward reality, individuals must know and understand themselves. Health is viewed within the context of the importance of inward reality and of the natural laws of the universe; the two must be balanced. Person and disease are evaluated as one unit, and health promotion and longevity are valued.[26]

Humanism emphasizes the value and importance of being human. In health care, a humanistic approach means that attention is paid to the whole person rather than only the specific problem, and the basic ability and right of clients to choose a personal life path is recognized.

Existentialism, the concern for individual existence rather than theories regarding human nature, the premise that inner experience provides people with meaning and purpose, and the view that individuals make choices throughout life for which they are personally responsible has also influenced health care philosophy. Only through authentic, honest relationships with clients can health care providers value them as whole persons. A crucial obligation

of health care providers is to encourage freedom, growth, and personal responsibility in relationships with clients.

A holistic orientation to health care then recognizes all aspects of a person as significant and considers how these interact to affect the whole person. Each individual is a whole person with physical, emotional, intellectual, social, and spiritual dimensions who is in constant interaction with other people and with the environment. What happens in one human dimension affects the others and, consequently, the whole person. All factors contribute to health and illness. The balance of all dimensions of a person is valued. Thus no one human dimension, either within the person or in that person's interactions with others, can be consid-

▼ **TABLE 3-1** Summary of Influence of Philosophical Positions on Views of Human Nature, Health Care, and Nursing

Position	View of Human Nature	View of Health Care	View of Nursing
Preliterate ideologies	Ruled by nonhuman forces Health and illness caused by good and evil spirits	Use of magic to appease spirits Trephination; transfer of disease to animals	
Chinese perspective	Importance of morality and harmony with nature Interdependence of person and society	Emphasis on prevention Health based on balanced flow of life energy; illness caused by disruption of that flow	
East Indian perspective	Inward reality most important In constant process with universe	Health based on cooperation with natural and moral laws of universe Concern for health promotion and longevity	
Ancient Greek perspective	Nature as ordered rather than accidental Mind and body separate but interrelated	Importance of natural cycles Use of mind to heal physical ills	
Asceticism	Primary purpose to serve spiritual force Insignificance of physical needs Self-denial and self-discipline	Focus on redemption of client's soul	Primarily service and duty Tolerance of poor working conditions Dedication to a mission
Romanticism	Glorification of the individual Encouraged subservience of women Personal merit determined by superiority, not status Value of mystery, adventure, and sentiment	Idealization of service and loyalty to others	Lack of rational foundation or consideration of practical consequences Dependence on physicians and hospitals
Pragmatism	Focus on practical consequences Value of facts, not abstractions	Specialization according to disease and stage of illness	Focus on client perspectives Realization of impact of nursing care on client welfare
Humanism	Value of human abilities and aspirations; rejection of supernatural Resistance to methods of science	Emphasis on individual freedom in health choices	Attention to whole person rather than only disease process Acceptance of responsibility for nursing actions
Existentialism	Concern for essence of human existence, especially extreme experience Value of individual freedom and personal responsibility	Importance of accountability and responsibility by both clients and practitioners	Focus on authentic, honest relationships Importance of learning to make responsible choices
Holism	Reality in terms of relationships and processes Multidimensionality	Focus on context of health and illness Illness as opportunity for growth	Active partnership of client and nurse Emphasis on stress management and health promotion

ered in isolation. For example, any attempt to consider only the social aspect or only the physical aspect gives an incomplete view of the whole person. If people are viewed in a fragmented way, the tendency is to interact with them in a fragmented manner.

Each individual actively participates in developing conditions that either enhance health or encourage illness; thus personal responsibility is valued as a crucial component of a holistic orientation to health care. See Table 3-1 for a summary of philosophical positions.

HOLISTIC HEALTH PRINCIPLES OF PRACTICE

Holistic health principles of practice constitute a framework that can be used in any nursing care setting and that will enhance the quality of the nurse-client relationship. They are intended as guidelines to stimulate self-exploration and to improve the effectiveness of nursing care. These principles are summarized in Table 3-2 and are discussed in the following sections.

Human Uniqueness

Within a holistic health framework, each individual is considered unique. Complex factors, including human dimensions, determine how people view themselves, the world, health, and illness. One individual's response in a given situation cannot be equated with that of another person. For any person, the interaction of different dimensions and the interaction of the person with the environment are unique.

This uniqueness requires individualized approaches to health and illness. What is healthy for one person may be detrimental to another; what contributes to illness in one individual may not affect another. People meet their needs in each dimension in different ways. For example, one person may consider jogging an excellent form of exercise, while another may consider aerobic dancing with a group of people best. Group therapy may help one person who is depressed, whereas individual therapy may help another. One person may cope with social isolation through group participation, another through individual friendships, and still another through school or work involvement. Some individuals need many details to process, incorporate, and make decisions regarding new information; others are comfortable with very few details. One person may develop and express spirituality through meditation, another through organized religion.

In addition, to stay balanced, individuals must meet different needs within themselves and in their particular life situations. Recognizing these needs helps the person to attain health. For instance, the person who is physically fit but is unaware of feelings needs help in developing the emotional dimension. One who is able to express feelings well but is not able to solve problems may need to attend to the intellectual dimension. Another person who has well-developed problem-solving skills but cannot maintain a support system may need help in developing the social dimension. Someone who has a well-developed social support system but experiences a loss of purpose in life may need to consider what is lacking in the spiritual dimension. The person who is attuned spiritually but neglectful of exercise

Concept	Principle
Human uniqueness	The individual's uniqueness requires an individual approach to health care
Context of health and illness	The various settings within which the individuals function influence their health care
Illness as opportunity	Discovering some personal meaning in illness may provide an opportunity for growth
Client-nurse partnership	The client and nurse are active in the relationship and both may experience growth and change
Self-care	Individuals, families, and communities have a responsibility for self-care
Health	Health focuses on health promotion and involves working toward optimum functioning in all areas

TABLE 3-2   Summary of Holistic Health Principles of Practice

or nutrition may need to direct some attention toward the physical dimension.

When a client's uniqueness is ignored, health care that has been effective with other clients may not help with this one. This happens when health care professionals consider only the disease process, the symptoms, or a label. When nurses categorize clients, they limit their ability to identify individual needs and innovative solutions. Labels encourage identical interventions for similar sets of conditions in different individuals. This approach is sometimes useful and at other times is not. Sole reliance on labels makes it difficult to view the needs of the individual as a priority; instead, the application of standard interventions and the expectation of standard results become the priorities.

Context of Health and Illness

People, with their states of health and illness, do not exist in isolation. They function within many settings, such as familial, occupational, communal, social, and cultural. The beliefs and behaviors developed in these settings influence health and illness, and a holistic perspective considers these factors significant. A family may be a safe place to express feelings, or it may interact on superficial levels only. A person's workplace may be a source of creative challenge or of chronic, unrelieved stress. A community may provide areas for physical exercise and activities that encourage social interaction; a different community may be physically unsafe and socially hostile. One individual may have a social network that supports self-development and growth, and another may have friends who are unreliable and unresponsive to the individual's needs. Some cultures value verbal and nonverbal expressions of affection, whereas others view displays of affection with distaste.

When nurses view health and illness within the context of the client's life, they can understand how the person experiences health and illness. They can see that people with similar symptoms react in different ways, individuals with similar diseases do not necessarily respond to identical interventions, and people differ in how they perceive health and illness.

A person's life context largely determines the options that are available at a given time. In any situation, people have access to various resources and not to others. The availability of financial, social, familial, and community resources will all influence health and illness. A holistic perspective helps identify and develop individual options and resources rather than assuming that what worked in one case will work in another.

Illness as Opportunity

Just as stressors are not inherently positive or negative, illness is not intrinsically good or bad. The impact of an illness is determined by one's attitudes toward it, what one is able to learn from it, and what growth results from the illness. Some people may view illness as a catastrophe that simply "happened" to them over which they had no control. They see themselves as victims being persecuted by the illness (and often by other factors in their life situation). They view themselves as helpless and are tempted to give up. In contrast, other people see illness as an opportunity to evaluate their current life situation, including the role of stressors. They view themselves as maintaining control of their lives and seek to discover the ways in which they may have contributed to the illness. Acknowledging that pertinent information is available in the illness, they use this information to set new goals and move in new directions. This approach is consistent with holistic health philosophy, which asserts that there is personal meaning, or a message, in any illness. Discovering what that is provides an opportunity for growth.

Illness may often be related to needs that a person has but is not meeting. People ideally strive to meet needs in the best available ways, such as asking for what they want, taking the time and space they need, or, in general, creating life to be what they want. However, when they are not conscious of or ignore certain needs, they may develop an illness or particular symptoms to meet their needs. This is usually an unconscious process and occurs when people do not have better coping mechanisms available to them.

The use of illness to meet one's needs may at first be a difficult issue to explore in one's own life. An initial and automatic response often is "but I don't want to be sick!" and this is certainly true. However, sometimes the person may not perceive any alternative. Possibly an individual is not even consciously aware of the need. A look at how one's situation changes as a result of illness, or what one gains from being ill or injured, will offer clues to needs that are not being met otherwise. These needs may be as simple as more time alone, less responsibility, or a few days' rest or as major as restructuring a relationship, changing jobs, or setting new priorities. If a person is forced to rest for a few days or to be dependent when he or she is normally independent, dependence may be a need that person is attempting to meet through illness. If illness or injury allows an individual to say "no" to certain demands without feeling guilty or provides permission to slow one's pace, perhaps one can learn to meet these needs in healthy ways.

At the very least, illness signals people to examine the stressors in their lives, the meaning that they ascribe to them, and their ways of coping with them. Their personal belief system and what various events and circumstances mean to them determine their range of possible coping responses. Illness and injury indicate that people need to reconsider these meanings and the ways they respond to life events. When individuals label an event as disastrous, they are likely to respond in harmful ways (such as by feeling helpless, hopeless, anxious, or panic-stricken). When they relabel the event as an opportunity for growth, they are able to respond in constructive ways (such as by feeling powerful, assertive, calm, and in charge of their lives). Illness can be an opportunity to the extent that people are willing to create various healthy meanings to illness, and thus broaden the scope of their responses.

Client-Nurse Partnership

A holistic health framework supports the relationship between client and nurse as an active partnership, and responsibility for healing and growth is shared. Because an energy exchange occurs between the two, the relationship itself has a healing effect. Teaching and learning operate in both directions, so the practitioner and the client both experience growth and change.

The nurse in a holistic health care setting attempts to create conditions that are conducive to healing and optimal health. The client's current belief system is the beginning framework, and from this point the nurse provides support and helps the client find healthy ways to meet individual needs. This process will include, but not be limited to, expanding self-awareness, evaluating life-style factors, identifying stressors and coping mechanisms, exploring meanings of illness, considering alternative beliefs and response patterns, and implementing health habits that are acceptable and appropriate for the client. Nurses are willing and able to share information and experience with clients rather than using their expertise to appear more powerful or more "professional." Actually nurses consider clients as the ultimate experts regarding their own health and illness and respect the client's subjective experience as highly relevant to the healing process.

Clients in a holistic setting are coparticipants in healing and health promotion, working closely with the nurse to determine necessary and appropriate interventions. To the greatest extent possible, clients maintain active roles in any treatment or decision making process and actively seek relevant information. They do not consider themselves passive recipients of health care but learn to consider themselves the experts regarding their own needs and health status. In this way they are able to retain their sense of personal power rather than conceding it to the health care system and assuming the role of helpless victim. Clients learn to recognize that health and illness or injury are multidimensional, with many contributing factors and possible outcomes. As whole persons with unique valid needs, they realize that many alternatives are available for meeting these needs. Rather than assuming that the nurse is able to decide for them, clients examine alternatives and choose from among them.

As practitioners, nurses' most powerful healing capacities come from who they are and how they relate to others. Holistic nurses who pursue their own personal growth and strive toward optimal health for themselves are better able to facilitate healing and optimal health in others. Incorporating such qualities as self-awareness, personal responsibility, and balance into their own lives is a first step in enhancing these qualities in clients. The nurse's own willingness to examine stressors and choose healthier response patterns demonstrates what clients can do for themselves.

The client-nurse relationship will have some effect on both individuals. To a large extent, the nurse assumes the responsibility of making this a positive effect. Practitioners have the opportunity to influence clients so that they are better able to strive toward optimal health and get what they want out of life. At the same time, practitioners have the opportunity to learn from each client and allow their own boundaries and experience of life to expand.

Self-Care

As implied in preceding sections, holistic health philosophy supports self-care as a valid and necessary component of the larger health care system. The formal health care system cannot provide all services associated with health and illness; it has no control over the choices that people make that contribute to health or illness, their responses to stressors, or their life-styles. Self-care proponents encourage individuals, families, and communities to assume more responsibility for health status improvement. Because people are, or can be, experts regarding themselves and their health, they can learn how to safely depend less on health professionals and more on themselves.

Self-care is based on the premise of personal responsibility and may range from health promotion behaviors to treatment of some illnesses, injuries, and chronic health conditions. A large portion of health care actually is self-care. Examples are coping effectively with stress, using vitamins and over-the-counter medications, increasing fluid intake, applying heat or cold, using elastic bandages, resting, and managing chronic conditions such as diabetes or asthma. Many common health problems can be prevented, alleviated, or eased by consumers, in many cases more efficiently and effectively than by the health care system.

Many factors, including cultural influence, familial patterns, personal value systems, and prior learning, affect the individual's capacity for self-care. Appropriate self-care implies knowledge; thus a crucial element of self-care is health education. Because people engage in some form of self-care with or without adequate knowledge, health care practitioners have a responsibility to create every possible opportunity to disseminate accurate information about self-care concepts and skills. Such information can be made available through schools, churches, clinical settings, community centers, study groups, and formal classes. Self-care education based on the needs and current level of knowledge of the individual or community is likely to be the most acceptable and useful. A variety of approaches can be used

to reach such diverse groups as children, adolescents, the elderly population, and minority groups.

Self-care is not an exclusive alternative to treatment by the health care system. However, with adequate knowledge about self-care, individuals are likely both to assume responsibility for their health and to recognize the importance of relationships with the health care system. The system operates in a consultant role, assisting and supplementing consumer skills. People who pursue self-care learn how and when to best use professional assistance.

Health

Holistic health philosophy also focuses on health promotion, or health as a positive process, rather than limiting itself to the elimination of illness. Health is more than the absence of disease; it is a dynamic, active process of continually striving to reach one's own balance and highest potentials. Health involves working toward optimal functioning in all areas. This process varies among people and even within individuals as they move from one situation or stage of life to another, and it depends on personal needs, imbalances, and individual perceptions of reality.

Health is a life-style that leads to optimal functioning, and therefore can be pursued only by the person, family, or community. Individuals create their own life-styles through life choices. Because everything in life has an impact on health, each choice leads toward or away from health. The goal is to improve one's ability and willingness to assess the effect of one's choices on health and to make healthy choices. A major assumption of a healthy life-style is that each person is responsible for creating a life situation that promotes health.

In addition to personal responsibility, a positive adaptation to stress is an important aspect of health. People must learn to recognize stressors in all dimensions of life, eliminate those that are harmful, and choose healthy responses for those that they keep. This includes recognizing needs, strengths and weaknesses, and internal and external factors that affect all dimensions: physical, emotional, intellectual, social, and spiritual. Each person needs to determine whether activities, feelings, attitudes, beliefs, expectations, and interactions with others contribute to or detract from the quality of health. Being able to deal effectively with change and maintain a sense of control over one's life, even while responding to change, greatly contributes to health.

Illness or injury also stimulates the pursuit of health by providing information that the individual needs to restore balance and optimal functioning. Often through such circumstances people become aware of the changes that are necessary to get more of what they want out of life. Individual and family health remains a goal and is possible even in acute or chronic illness or injury. Even the chronically ill or disabled have optimal functioning levels. The focus is on maintaining optimal energy levels and striving toward one's health potential.

The meaning of health and genuinely healthy life-styles varies among individuals and are determined by both objective and subjective factors. Some objective components, such as nutrition, exercise, meditation, psychotherapy, visualization, development of healthy relationships, and positive belief patterns, are generally agreed on as conducive to positive states of health. The relevance and usefulness of these objective factors, when applied to any particular individual, are determined by subjective factors such as cultural and familial belief systems, work and home environments, individual attitudes and values, the nature of the social network, past experiences, expectations for the future, and genetic predisposition. Holistic health practitioners consider objective and subjective factors while facilitating health in themselves and others.

BRIEF REVIEW

Philosophy has been a crucial factor in the evolution of human life, determining how people view themselves, others, and the universe in which they live. Individuals each have unique philosophies that are reflected in their values, attitudes, beliefs, goals, and activities. These influence their everyday lives through their choices and their behaviors. The relationship between philosophy and science is complementary in that both contribute to the human quest for knowledge and understanding.

Each society's health care system is affected by that society's philosophy. Both philosophy and science are necessary for health care to reach its highest potential. The philosophies of the health care system, the individual practitioner, and the client influence the quality of health care services.

Philosophy is an integral part of mental health–psychiatric nursing. Nurses' personal and professional philosophies affect the care they provide and the relationships they form with clients. For this reason nurses need to recognize and develop their own philosophical positions; the foundation of this process is awareness of self and others.

Numerous philosophies have developed throughout the history of human existence, including asceticism, romanticism, pragmatism, humanism, existentialism, and holism. These have affected the quality of life, nature of health care, and, more specifically, approaches to mental health and mental illness. Nursing has evolved through various philosophies, all of which have influenced the nature of nursing practice. Several principles that evolve from these philosophical concepts may be used as guidelines for improving the quality of mental health–psychiatric nursing care.

Holistic health philosophy has been influenced by Chinese and Indian thought and by the more recent philosophical positions of humanism and existentialism. The person is viewed as a complex whole affected by many factors at any given time. Even though these variables each exert a particular influence, every factor alters the person's relationships with other influential forces. Thus it is most meaningful to view people in terms of their relationships rather than to analyze their various aspects in isolation.

REFERENCES AND SUGGESTED READINGS

1. Ackermann RJ: *Beliefs and knowledge,* New York, 1972, Anchor Books.
2. Allen CE: Analysis of the pragmatic consequences of holism for nursing, *Western Journal of Nursing Research* 13(2):256, 1991.
3. Bailey H: *Nursing mental diseases,* New York, 1920, Macmillan.
4. Barker P: Philosophy of psychiatric nursing, *Nursing Standards* 5(12):28, 1990.
5. Bevis EO: Framework for nursing practice. In Bower FL, Bevis EO, coeditors: *Fundamentals of nursing practice: concepts, roles, and functions,* St Louis, 1979, Mosby–Year Book.
6. Black KM: An existential model for psychiatric nursing, *Perspectives in Psychiatric Care* 6:178, 1968.
7. Blattner B: *Holistic nursing,* Englewood Cliffs, NJ, 1981, Prentice Hall.
8. Bresler DE: Chinese medicine and holistic health. In Hastings AC, Fadiman J, Gordon JS, editors: *Health for the whole person,* Boulder, Colo, 1980, Westview Press.
9. Cadwallader EH: The main features of values experience, *Journal of Value Inquiry* 14:229, 1980.
10. Chan WT: The concept of man in Chinese thought. In Radhakrishnan S, Raju PT, editors: *The concept of man,* London, 1966, Allen & Unwin.
11. Critchley DL: Evolution of the role. In Critchley DL, Maurin JT, editors: *The psychiatric mental health clinical specialist: theory, research and practice,* New York, 1985, John Wiley & Sons.
12. Devi I: *Renew your life through yoga: the Indra Devi method for relaxation through rhythmic breathing.* Englewood Cliffs, NJ, 1963, Prentice Hall.
13. Dixon J and others: Psychometric and descriptive perspective of illness impact over the life span, *Nursing Research* 40(1):51, 1991.
14. Dossey B and others: *Holistic nursing: a handbook for practice,* Rockville, Md, 1988, Aspen Publishers.
15. Eliade M: *Yoga: immortality and freedom,* Princeton, NJ, 1969, Princeton University Press.
16. Farrell F: Western versus Chinese philosophy: cultural roots, *Journal of Chinese Philosophy* 8:59, 1981.
17. Freedman AM, Kaplan HI, and Sadock BJ: *Modern synopsis of comprehensive textbook of psychiatry/II,* ed 2, Baltimore, 1976, Williams & Wilkins.
18. Fuller SS: Holistic man and the science and practice of nursing, *Nursing Outlook* 26:700, 1978.
19. Gott M and others: Attitudes and beliefs in health promotion, *Nursing Standards* 5(2):30, 1990.
20. Graham B: Bridging the gap . . . conventional and alternative medicine, *Health* 23(1):62, 1991.
21. Kelly G and others: Zen in the art of occupational therapy. II, *British Journal of Occupational Therapy* 54(4):130, 1991.
22. Kershaw B: Nursing models as philosophies of care, *Nurse Practitioner* 4(1):25, 1990.
23. Keyes CD: *Four types of value destruction,* Washington, DC, 1978, University Press of America.
24. King M: Health as the goal for nursing, *Nursing Science Quarterly* 3(3):123, 1990.
25. Kollemorten I and others: Ethical aspects of clinical decision making, *Journal of Medical Ethics* 7:67, 1981.
26. Krieger D: *Foundations for holistic health nursing practices: the Renaissance nurse,* Philadelphia, 1981, JB Lippincott.
27. Kurtz P, editor: *The humanist alternative: some definitions of humanism,* Buffalo, 1973, Prometheus Books.
28. Lang NM and others: Standards and holism: a reframing, *Holistic Nurse Practitioner* 5(3):14, 1991.
29. Laszlo E, Wilbur JB: *Value theory in philosophy and social science,* New York, 1973, Gordon & Breach, Science Publishers.
30. Macklin R: Mental health and mental illness: some problems of definition and concept formation, *Philosophy of Science* 39:341, 1979.
31. Miller T: Advances in understanding the impact of stressful life events on health, *Hospital and Community Psychiatry* 39(6):615, 1988.
32. Paterson JG, Zderad LT: *Humanistic nursing,* New York,

1988, National League for Nursing (a reissue of the 1976 edition).

33. Pender NJ: Expressing health through lifestyle patterns, *Nursing Science Quarterly* 3(3):115, 1990.

34. Price JI, Drake RE, Hine LN: Value assumptions in humanistic psychiatric nursing education, *Perspectives in Psychiatric Care* 12:64, 1974.

35. Raju PT: The concept of man in Indian thought. In RadhakKrishnan S, and Raju, PT: *The concept of man*, London, 1966, Allen & Unwin.

36. Riccardo EP: *Introduction to humanistic philosophy*, Dubuque, Iowa, 1979, Kendall/Hunt Publishing Co.

37. Sadler WS: *Psychiatric nursing*, St Louis, 1937, Mosby—Year Book.

38. Smith MC: Nursing's unique focus on health promotion, *Nursing Science Quarterly* 3(3):105, 1990.

39. Smith MC: Existential-phenomenological foundations in nursing: a discussion of the differences, *Nursing Science Quarterly* 4(1):5, 1991.

40. Stevenson L: *Seven theories of human nature*, Oxford, England, 1974, Clarendon Press.

41. von Bertalanffy L: *General system theory: foundations, development, applications*, New York, 1968, George Braziller.

42. Weir M: Towards a holistic understanding of health and illness, *Health Visit* 64(3):77, 1991.

ANNOTATED BIBLIOGRAPHY

Bevis EO: Framework for nursing practice. In Bower FL, Bevis EO: *Fundamentals of nursing practice: concepts, roles, and functions*, St Louis, 1979, Mosby—Year Book.

Bevis discusses the influence of the following philosophical positions on the evolution of the nursing role: asceticism, romanticism, humanism, and existentialism. Examples of each of these philosophies' contribution to nurses' view of themselves and their clients throughout the history of professional nursing are given.

Critchley DL: Evolution of the role. In Critchley DL, Maurin JT, editors: *The psychiatric mental health specialist: theory, research and practice*, New York, 1985, John Wiley & Sons.

Critchley offers a historical overview of the development of psychiatric nursing and the major forces in society, nursing, and medicine that have contributed to the development. Previous trends as well as current issues are discussed and related to the role of psychiatric mental health clinical specialist.

CHAPTER 4

Theoretical Approaches

Tomye J Modlin
Ann Adams

After studying this chapter, the student will be able to:

- Discuss the historical development of major theoretical approaches
- Identify key concepts associated with each selected theory
- Identify basic assumptions of each theoretical approach
- Discuss the application of selected theories to the therapeutic process

A common theme in nursing is the importance of theory-based practice. Using theory as a basis for practice distinguishes professional nursing from technical nursing. The nurse practices in highly complex settings, and few theories deal with all the complex variables affecting clinical problems. Providing care based on a holistic approach greatly compounds the challenge.

The theories presented in this chapter bring significant understanding to clinical practice by providing frameworks for organizing and labeling perceptions of behavior. These theories also explain what behaviors mean with respect to the individual in a specifically defined context.

The mental health–psychiatric nurse's basic beliefs about human nature and the meaning of mental health and illness provide the basis for selecting theoretical approaches to psychiatric nursing. Other considerations in selecting a theoretical approach or combination of approaches to mental health–psychiatric nursing include the client's behavior, belief system, and resources; the treatment setting; and societal and political influences. Each nurse's *eclectic approach* demonstrates how theoretical approaches have influenced her.

PSYCHOANALYTICAL THEORY

A basic premise of psychoanalytical theory is that some knowledge of a person's thoughts, feelings, and motives is necessary to understand overt behaviors. Although focuses may differ in general, the psychoanalytical approach emphasizes the unconscious and the *psychodynamics* of behavior. Two basic theoretical assumptions of psychodynamics are that present behavior is influenced by past experiences and that mental forces influence development and motivate behavior.

Intrapsychic

Sigmund Freud[19,20] developed the ideas that became the foundation for psychoanalytical theory. He was the first theorist to develop a comprehensive theory of personality. One of his basic assumptions was that all behavior is meaningful. Each behavior that seems insignificant, such as slips of the tongue and forgetfulness, reveals significant information. Related to this assumption is the important role of the unconscious in influencing behavior. Anxiety (see Chapter 10) is viewed as a motivator for behavior.

The personality consists of three major systems: the *id,* the *ego,* and the *superego.* Each system has specific characteristics and functions and interacts with the others causing behavior. When the three systems function in harmony, individuals show relative stability. Discordant interaction among the three systems can lead to maladjusted behavior.

The id is the basic system of the personality structure, and consists of all psychological processes that are present at birth. The id functions on a primitive level and is characterized by irrationality, and a lack of sense of time and logic. The id is amoral, or lacking moral sensibility. It is in contact with body processes, experiences the world subjectively, and houses instinctual drives and *psychic energy (libido).*

The primary aim of the id is to experience pleasure and avoid pain. This tendency is referred to as the *pleasure principle.* Persons functioning according to the pleasure principle seek immediate gratification of needs, impulses, and wishes. Avoiding pain and seeking pleasure involves *primary process thinking,* which enables the individual to discharge tension by forming an image of the object that will remove the tension. For example, an infant has a hallucinatory experience (mental image) involving a symbol for milk. This experience is referred to as *wish fulfillment.*

53

	DATES	EVENTS
HISTORICAL OVERVIEW	Before 1800s	Approaches to the study of human behavior were nonscientific and almost exclusively in the domain of philosophy and theology. Scholars emphasized the biological foundation of behavior and believed the mind and body functioned independently of each other. Philosophers and theologians focused on the conscious actions of the individual's free will, reason, and memory.
		These scholars studied the soul and attended to supernatural forces, which they believed governed behavior.
	1800s	There was a transition from philosophy and theology to psychology and a scientific approach to the study of behavior.
		Experimental psychologists believed the field of psychology was the study of consciousness (mind) and that states of consciousness can be analyzed in terms of sensations, images, and feelings.
		A lasting contribution made by experimental psychologists is a framework for the measurement and study of individual differences.
		Psychologists associated with the functionalism school of thought also studied the conscious processes that affect behavior but were mainly interested in consciousness in relation to people's adaptation to the environment.
	Early 1900s	Kraepelin and colleagues, proponents of the biological views of psychiatry, influenced research related to the biological bases of behavior.
	Mid-1900s	Psychoanalytical and behavioral schools of thought dominated the study of human behavior.
		Psychoanalytical theory emphasized unconscious mental processes. Psychoanalytical theorists also agreed that the early years of development are important.
		The behaviorists focused on mechanistic thinking and emphasized conscious control of behavior. The behaviorists used physiological concepts such as receptors, effectors, and conditioning as a basis for studying behavior and conducted experiments under controlled laboratory conditions.
		The learning theorists focused on learning in response to stimulus and reinforcement (reward) as the major basis for explaining behavior.
		The humanists were a dominant force that influenced the study of behavior. A goal of this group was to develop a multidisciplinary approach to the study of behavior that was broader than the behavioral and psychoanalytical approaches. The humanists emphasized the ability of individuals to assume responsibility for their own behavior, basing their theory on the premise that the whole represents more than the sum of its parts.
	1960s	American psychiatry shifted the focus of attention to the biological bases of behavior.
		General systems theory made its appearance and has since been continuously expanded.
		Symbolic interactionism became important to psychiatrists.
	1970s	Flexibility of theoretical approaches was more apparent.
	1980s	Increased interest in the biological explanation of mental health and mental illness.
		Discovery of altered brain chemistry among persons with mental illness.
	1990s	Increased interest in clients with Alzheimer's disease and associated anatomical changes in the brain.
	Future	Psychiatric nurses will conduct research on biological factors related to mental illness to delineate the nurse's role in treatment.

With maturation and the growing recognition that mental images do not satisfy needs, reality intervenes and the ego becomes differentiated from the id. Along with maturation, interactions with the environment and heredity influence the ego's development. The ego is the aspect of the personality that is in contact with reality.

The primary function of the ego is to mediate between the instinctual impulses and the environment to satisfy needs. The ego is the executive of the personality, maintaining harmony between the id, the superego, and the external world. The ego is the aspect of the personality that experiences anxiety and uses defense mechanisms to control the level of anxiety. The psychological functions of perception, memory, thinking, and action are also functions of the ego.

The *reality principle* and *secondary process thinking* govern ego functions. The aim of the reality principle is to postpone immediate gratification until an appropriate object for satisfying the needs is available. This principle then functions in accord with the demands of reality. Secondary process thinking is logical, involving organized thought processes characterized by a causal relationship between events. This type of thinking is based on reality testing and consists of developing a plan of action as a result of problem solving.

The superego evolves from the ego in response to rewards and punishments from significant others. The superego begins its functions when the person has the capacity to identify with and internalize the prohibitions and demands of parental figures. This system is made up of two subsystems: the *conscience* and the *ego ideal.* The conscience is the prohibiting aspect of the superego that corresponds to the individual's conception of what parents consider morally wrong. The ego ideal is based on what parents consider morally good, and the individual strives to adhere to these ideals. The child learns what the parents perceive as morally good and bad through rewards and punishments. In addition to an emphasis on moral behavior are the ideals of beauty, strength, and success. To the extent that individuals are able to live up to the superego's ideal standards, they experience inner satisfaction and increased self-esteem. When persons fail to fulfill ego ideals, they feel shame and low self-esteem. Failure to live up to moral standards leads to feelings of guilt. The superego may be in conflict with the id and ego as it fulfills its functions of (1) inhibiting the expression of id impulses, (2) persuading the ego to substitute moralistic goals for realistic ones, and (3) striving for perfection.

The id, ego, and superego need energy to fulfill their functions. Psychic energy (libido) is the form of energy used for the id, ego, and superego interactions. Psychic energy is body energy used for psychological tasks such as thinking, perceiving, and remembering. Freud believed that each person has a specified amount of energy. The psychic energy used by the ego and superego is obtained from the id during the process of psychological development.

The psychic energy used by the three systems to perform their tasks is obtained from *instincts.* An instinct is an inborn psychological representation of a need. Body needs are the *source* of instincts. The instinct's *aim* is to remove a body need. For example, the aim of the instinct of a hungry person is to remove hunger. The *object* of the instinct is the means by which the aim is achieved. The *impetus,* or force, of the instinct is determined by the amount of energy used to achieve the aim. Freud believed that the source and aim of instincts remain constant throughout life unless the source is changed or eliminated by physical maturation. As new body needs emerge during development, new instincts may appear. The object varies throughout life.

There are two categories of instincts: *life* instincts and *death* instincts. The aim of the life instinct is survival and propagation of the species. Hunger, sex, and thirst are examples of life instincts. Death instincts are also called destructive and aggressive instincts.

Freud described three levels of consciousness that are closely related to structure of the personality. The levels of consciousness are *unconscious, preconscious,* and *conscious.* The unconscious level is the largest and consists of repressed memories, thoughts, and feelings. Instinctual impulses are in the unconscious and actively seek expression. Preconscious perception and memories are outside conscious awareness, but are immediately available to consciousness when the need arises. These experiences require only recall to be brought into full awareness. Conscious experiences are those within conscious awareness at the moment. When attention is directed away from the experiences, they become preconscious.

Freud believed that the individual passes through a series of predetermined stages of psychosexual development. During these stages, sexual instincts develop and psychic energy becomes concentrated at specified *erogenous zones* of the body: the mouth, the anus, and the genitals. Tension becomes concentrated in these zones and can be relieved by manipulation of the region. The relief of tension is experienced as pleasure.

Freud referred to the first 5 years of development as pregenital; the individual's life is characterized by infantile sexuality. He believed that the basic personality is formed by the end of the fifth year of life and that subsequent development builds on this basic structure. The stages of psychosexual development are summarized in Table 4-1. Failure to successfully achieve the tasks of each stage may lead to maladaptive traits (Table 4-2).

Carl Jung's analytical theory[34] is classified as psychoanalytical because of the emphasis placed on the role of the unconscious as a behavior determinant. Jung described the structure of the personality, or *psyche,* as a composite of partial personalities that interact as a system. He believed that the psyche is the only thing people experience directly and know immediately. The *collective unconscious* is the personality's most influential system. This inherited, racial foundation of the personality is a residue of evolutionary development, an accumulation of experiences passed down to the person from ancestors. Jung believed that the personality's racial origin gives direction to the individual's behavior and determines, in part, what will become conscious and how the person will respond to experiences. That is, people are predisposed to certain experiences, and these predispositions are universal. Jung viewed fear of the dark and snakes and easily formed ideas about a supreme being as examples of predispositions.

The *ego,* which is the conscious mind, develops from the collective unconscious. The ego is the aspect of the personality that relates to the individual's feelings of identity and continuity. Perceptions, thoughts, memories, and feelings comprise the ego. In close contact with the ego is the individual's *personal unconscious,* which consists of experiences that were once conscious but that have been transformed by defense mechanisms such as repression and suppression.

Archetypes are symbols derived from the collective experiences of the race. As structural components of the collective unconscious, archetypes relate to ideas and modes of thought, and provide clues to the hidden potentials and qualities of the person. The aim of archetypical symbols is the fulfillment of the individual personality as a whole. Jung

▼ **TABLE 4-1**   Freud's Stages of Psychosexual Growth and Development

Stage of Development	Critical Experiences	Developmental Task	Major Characteristics	Emergent Defense Mechanisms
Oral (birth to 18 months)	Weaning	Establishing trusting dependence	Autoeroticism, narcissism, omnipotence, pleasure principle, frustration, dependence	Denial, introjection, projection
Anal (18 months to 3 years)	Toilet training	Developing sphincter control, self-control, feeling of autonomy	Reality principle, fear of loss of object love, approval and disapproval, beginning superego development	Sublimation, displacement
Phallic (3 to 5 years)	Oedipal conflict, castration anxiety	Establishing sexual identity, beginning socialization	Differentiation between the sexes, superego more internalized	Identification, sublimation, reaction formation, undoing
Latency* (6 to 12 years)	Peer group experience, intellectual growth	Group identification	Superego influence in erotic interests, immense intellectual development	No new defense mechanisms; major operating defense mechanisms are partial sublimations and reaction formation
Prepuberty and adolescence* (12 to 15 years)	Establishing heterosexual relationships	Developing social control over instincts	Identity, turmoil, needs of others	Intellectualization and asceticism
Genital (15 years to adult)	Sexual maturity	Resolving dependence-independence conflict	Heterosexual relations	Use of all preceding defense mechanisms

*The latency and prepuberty and adolescence stages of psychosexual development were not included in Freud's original description of development. Anna Freud (1946) extended Freud's works when she described developments in these periods of life.

believed that archetypes are the source of the person's strength of will and inner resources that serve as motivators to self-discovery.

Other systems of the personality, the persona, the anima and animus, and the shadow, develop from archetypes. Jung's conception of the *persona* is basically the same as other theorists' views of social role. The persona is a mask worn in social situations. This mask is determined by the role which society has assigned to the individual. The per-

sona becomes a problem when the ego either identifies too closely with it or becomes too distant from it. A related problem is difficulty in differentiating between one's public self (persona) and one's private self.

Anima and *animus* relate to the essentially bisexual nature of people. The anima is the feminine archetype in the man, and the animus the masculine archetype in the woman. Anima and animus develop from the unconscious racial experiences of man with woman and woman with

▼ **TABLE 4-2**   Manifestations of Failure to Achieve Developmental Tasks

Stage of Development	Behavioral Manifestations
Oral	Behaviors centered around oral experiences, for example, smoking, obesity, substance (drug and alcohol) abuse; difficulty with trust; disturbed physiological (particularly gastrointestinal) reactions; pessimism; and excessive dependence, envy, and jealousy
Anal	Defiant behavior, bowel and bladder disorders; rage, diarrhea, constipation; obsessive-compulsive personality; perfectionism, stubbornness; and inability to control impulses and emotions
Phallic	Faulty sexual identity; problems with authority; sexual deviations; erotic attachment of male child to mother and of female child to father; phobic reactions; and conversion reactions
Latency	Lack of self-motivation in job; school problems, including lack of self-motivation; inability to accept proper social role; problems with relationships with persons of own sex; and behavior disorders such as stealing, lying, and sociopathic behaviors
Genital	Sexual acting out; excessively hostile attitudes toward authority; excessive dependence; unsatisfactory relationships with the opposite sex; serial marriages; and difficulty with sexual functioning such as frigidity and impotence

man. These elements of the personality also evolve from the person's experiences with the parent of the opposite sex. Jung believed that people of each sex need to accept their bisexual archetype as reality, try to understand it, and integrate the archetype into the personality. The archetype will then serve a creative and constructive purpose.

The *shadow* archetype represents unacceptable aspects and components of behavior. The shadow may operate within and outside consciousness; that is, the shadow archetype may account for an individual's lack of awareness of certain personal faults. To the extent that persons can accept the tendencies of the shadow as a part of self, they are able to work toward wholeness of personality. Jung believed the shadow becomes more positive in the later half of life.

Jung's investigations led to theories about personality in middle and later years. Some of these views are presented in Chapters 39 and 40.

Erik Erikson[16] used Freud's psychoanalytical theory as a framework for his theory of personality. Erikson's primary goal was to build a bridge between psychosexual and psychosocial development. Thus he emphasized the importance of social and environmental factors within the home and community that influence development of the personality. He also extended Freud's theory by focusing on human development throughout the life cycle. Some of his theoretical ideas are based on maladaptive behavior. However, unlike Freud, he derived the major portion of his theory from studying the play activities of normal children and the functioning of young adolescents.

Erikson accepted many of Freud's ideas regarding the structure of the personality. Erikson used the terms *id, ego,* and *superego* and emphasized the ego's psychosocial development. He viewed the id and superego as horizontal polarities. The goal of the id is to meet its excessive and undisciplined wishes, whereas the superego strives to adhere to the internalized wishes of parents and society.

Erikson believed the superego is as barbaric as the id. As the executive of the personality, the ego assumes the functions of organizing external experiences, testing perceptual experiences, and governing action. These ego functions are considered positive and lead to control of the id's and superego's strivings and to a sense of oneself in a state of well-being.

Erikson accepted Freud's theory that instincts and psychic energy (libido) motivate behavior. Erikson believed that the libido is characterized by two dynamically opposed strivings: a drive to live and an opposing drive to return to the earlier state before infancy. These drives are similar to Freud's life and death instincts and create a polarity. Erikson believed that drives stimulate growth through the developmental stages.

Erikson's theory includes the three levels of awareness described by Freud: the *conscious,* the *preconscious,* and the *unconscious.* Erikson views the last two as most influential in motivating behavior.

Erikson described eight stages of development that are based on biological, psychological, and social events. The first five stages roughly parallel Freud's psychosexual developmental stages, with the last three occurring within adulthood. Each stage is characterized by a positive and a negative experience and an emotional crisis. Development involves a struggle between two poles, with experiences of the two essential for healthy growth. For example, the task of developing a sense of basic trust versus mistrust necessitates that the infant experience trust as well as mistrust to learn to differentiate between the two. Ultimately, the infant needs to have more positive than negative experiences in order to grow psychologically. Erikson was optimistic in his views about continuous development throughout the life cycle and the possibility of new solutions to problems at each stage. The eight stages and their related tasks are summarized in Table 4-3 and are discussed in relation to each phase of the life cycle in Part IV.

▼ **TABLE 4-3** Erikson's Stages of Psychosocial Development

Stage of Development	Developmental Task	Major Characteristics
Oral-sensory (birth to 12 months)	Trust versus mistrust	Mothering person viewed as significant
Anal-muscular (1 to 3 years)	Autonomy versus shame and doubt	Ego skills; parallel play, negativism; ambivalence; self-control and will power; initial development of superego
Genital-locomotor (3 to 6 years)	Initiative versus guilt	Cooperative play; fantasy; imitation of adults; development of Conscience; directed and purposeful activities
Latency (6 to 12 years)	Industry versus inferiority	Intellectual curiosity; government of behavior by rules and regulations; acculturation
Puberty and adolescence (12 to 18 years)	Identity versus identity diffusion	Heterosexual relationships; establishment of identity
Young adult (18 to 25 years)	Intimacy and solidarity versus isolation	Close personal relationships with adults of both sexes
Adulthood (25 to 45 years)	Generativity versus stagnation	Creativity and productivity; parental sense; adjustment to life; lasting relationships
Maturity (older than 45 years)	Ego integrity versus despair	Adjustment to changes; acceptance of culture; sense of continuity of past, present, and future; acceptance of death

Interpersonal

Harry Stack Sullivan,[58] credited with developing the most comprehensive theory of interpersonal relations, believed that the essence of being human is the capacity to live effectively in relationships with others. Freud's theory, as well as social psychology and anthropology greatly influenced Sullivan's thinking about development. Sullivan believed the individual is a social being and that personality development is determined within the context of interactions with other humans. He recognized the influence of the person's biological system on development to the extent that the body is necessary for life. However, he believed society influences the individual's biological functions.

A central theme of Sullivan's theory is *anxiety* and its relationship to the formation of personality. He viewed anxiety as (1) a prime motivator of behavior, (2) a builder of self-esteem, and (3) the great educator in life. His ideas about anxiety are discussed in Chapter 10.

In keeping with his basic beliefs about the individual, Sullivan viewed the personality as consisting of interpersonal experiences rather than intrapsychic ones. The *self-system* is a significant aspect of the personality that develops in response to anxiety. Disapproving and forbidding gestures during interactions with significant others help develop the self-system. In response to these gestures, *security operations* become a part of the self-system to help the individual avoid or minimize anxiety. The security operations include *sublimation, selective inattention,* and *dissociation.* Sublimation is an unconscious process of substituting a socially acceptable activity pattern to partially satisfy a need for an activity that would give rise to anxiety. Selective inattention is an unconscious substitutive process that allows many meaningful details of one's life that are associated with anxiety to go unnoticed. Sullivan believed selective inattention causes individuals to fail to profit from experiences related to problem areas. Dissociation is a system of processes that minimizes or avoids anxiety by keeping parts of the individual's experiences called "not me" out of consciousness. The self-system becomes unable to objectively evaluate the individual's behavior, and, because of this, Sullivan believed the self-system to be the "principal stumbling block to favorable changes in personality."[58]

Sullivan believed that at an early age individuals develop *personifications* that influence their perceptions of people throughout life. A personification is an image that individuals have of themselves and other people resulting from experiences with anxiety and satisfaction of needs. Personifications of self and others develop in the infant's early need-satisfaction experiences with the mothering one. Depending on the infant's experience, the mother is personified as a good mother or a bad mother. For example, because the infant experiences discomfort, an anxious mother is personified as a bad mother. During development, the either/or personifications become fused and complex. When this fusion is not achieved, the individual goes through life with a polarized view of self, other people, and situations. Everything is viewed in dichotomous terms such as *black or white* and *good or bad.*

Sullivan believed that during infancy (through sensations of the body and the caregiving of significant others in response to body needs) three personifications of "me" gradually evolve: *"good me," "bad me,"* and *"not me."* The "good me" results from experiences of approval and tenderness and leads to good feelings about oneself. Experiences related to increased anxiety states result in the "bad me." The "not me" evolves in response to overwhelming anxiety and results from poorly understood experiences that retain an uncanny quality like horror, dread, and awe. These personifications belong to the self-system.

Sullivan described the cognitive processes in terms of the following three modes of experience: *prototaxic, parataxic,* and *syntaxic.* The prototaxic mode of experience is the initial type and is characterized by sensations, feeling, and fragmented images of short duration. These experiences occur at random, are not connected logically, and leave memory traces as a basis for the next level of experience. This primitive type of experience is found during the early months of infancy and may be observed in deep psychotic states.

With the parataxic mode of experience, events that occur at the same time but are not logically connected are viewed as being causally related. A child stated that every time he saw a police car, there was an accident, so he thought that police cars caused accidents. This type of thinking is characteristic of development and is normally evident throughout childhood. However, Sullivan believed that much of the individual's experience may not progress beyond this level. The parataxic mode of experience is frequently the foundation for adult prejudices and superstitious beliefs. The term *parataxic distortion* is used to label adult experiences in the parataxic mode.

The highest level of experience, which begins in the juvenile era, occurs in the syntaxic mode. Experiences that occur in this mode are logically interrelated and contribute to logical thinking. The syntaxic mode is characterized by consensually validated symbols—symbols accepted by enough people to have a universal meaning. Sullivan believed that individuals can have meaningful relationships with others only when they learn the syntaxic mode of experience.

Sullivan described six stages of personality development from birth to maturity, which he divides according to the capacity for communication and integration of new interpersonal experiences. Experiences during each stage are influenced by those of the previous one. The personality achieves some degree of stability at the end of the juvenile era, but continues to develop beyond this time and has the potential for corrective experiences. Sullivan believed that the juvenile and preadolescent eras contain the greatest opportunity for corrective experiences. The stages of personality development are summarized in Table 4-4.

Transactional

Eric Berne, the founder of transactional analysis, was trained in classic psychoanalysis. He departed from orthodox psychoanalysis when he developed his theory of transactional development; however, because of the influence of his psychoanalytical thinking, his theory can be grouped with the psychoanalytical theories of personality development.

Berne[5] assumed that the personality's structure consists of *ego states.* An ego state is a coherent system of feelings

▼ **TABLE 4-4** **Sullivan's Stages of Interpersonal Growth and Development**

Stage of Development	Developmental Tools*	Developmental Task	Interpersonal Needs	Cognitive Mode of Experience
Infancy (birth to 1½ years)	Cry, mouth, satisfaction response, empathic communication, emergency reactions, autistic invention	Learning to count on others to meet needs	Need for contact	Prototaxic
Childhood (19 months to 6 years)	Language, anus, self, identification, anxiety, autistic invention, emergency reaction; anger, shame, guilt, and doubt	Learning to accept, in relative comfort, interferences with wishes	Need for adult participation in activities	Largely parataxic
Juvenile (7 to 9 years)	Competition, compromise, cooperation	Learning to form satisfactory relationships with peers	Need for peers Need for acceptance	Mostly syntaxic
Preadolescence (10 to 12 years)	Capacity to love, collaboration, consensual validation	Learning to relate to chum of same sex	Need for chum, friend, or loved one	Syntaxic
Early adolescence (13 to 14 years)	Lust, anxiety	Learning to become independent; learning to establish satisfactory relationships with members of the opposite sex	Need for intimacy	Syntaxic
Late adolescence (15 to 21 years)	Genital organs	Learning to become interdependent; learning to form durable sexual relationship with selected member of opposite sex	Need for heterosexual relationship	Fully syntaxic

*Experimentation, exploration, and manipulation are tools used during each stage of development.

and related behavior patterns. Ego states are psychological realities because they represent real people. Each person has three ego states—the Parent, Adult, and Child.

The Parent ego state is a collection of recordings of external events experienced during the first 5 years of life. Everything the person saw the parental figures do and heard them say is recorded in the Parent. This ego state includes all of the rules and parental admonitions (the *should*'s and *should not*'s) as well as some pleasant experiences. The Parent has two forms—the direct and indirect. When the Parent is directly active, the message is "Do as I do." Indirect influence of the Parent is evident when the individual adapts to the parents' requirements. The message in this situation is "Don't do as I do; do as I *say.*"

The Child ego state represents archaic fears and expectations. It is characterized by autistic thinking, comparable to what Freud called primary process thinking. The Child state records the child's response to internal events that the child sees, hears, feels, and understands. Most stored information relates to feelings, because at the time the child had no words to give meaning to the experiences. The Child ego state consists of negative and positive information. The negative information is a by-product of the demands of socialization. For example, toilet training places demands on the child and causes frustration of desires. On the basis of these early, negative experiences the individual concludes, "I'm not OK." Some positive aspects are curiosity, creativity, and a desire to explore and have fun. Because of these positive attributes, Berne believed the Child ego

state is the most valuable part of the personality. This ego state allows access to childhood pleasures.

The Adult is characterized by reality testing and rational thinking, comparable to Freud's secondary process thinking. This ego state processes incoming information in accord with reality. The Adult state examines and regulates the activities of the Parent and Child. This ego state also decides what the individual will and will not do. These functions are essential for dealing with the outside world.

The ego states shift from one state of mind or one behavior pattern to another. Each ego state has its place and function and contributes to a healthy balance of the personality. When one or the other disturbs the balance, psychopathology may result.

Berne[7] identified four life positions that underlie behavior:

1. "I'm not OK; you're OK." This is the depressive, despair position.
2. "I'm not OK; you're not OK." This is the futility, giving up position.
3. "I'm OK; you're not OK." This is the destructive, arrogant position.
4. "I'm OK; you're OK." This is the healthy, mature position.

The first three positions are based on feelings. The fourth is based on thought. Individuals can move to new positions. These four positions are universal and learned during early development as the child has transactions with the parental figure. The positions are complex and contradictions may exist; however, each person usually has one basic position that governs life and from which games and scripts are played out.

Berne[6] defined a psychological *game* as a type of human behavior that is predictable, stereotyped, usually destructive, and directed by hidden motives. During childhood, the individual is taught what games to play and how to play them. These games are then played throughout life with change in external events such as place, person, and time. People tend to have a small collection of games that they use as a basis for social relationships, and they find people with whom they can share these games. The games determine how each individual will use opportunities in life. Games also determine the person's ultimate destiny, such as "payoffs" in marriage, career, and circumstances surrounding death.

A *script* is the person's unconscious life plan.[5] The script is based on questions that involve a person's identity and destiny. An individual begins developing a script at birth when he picks up messages about himself and his worth through transactions with the parental figures. The scripting messages are verbal and nonverbal. For example, the cuddling, hugging, and touching an infant receives gives him a nonverbal message about his worth. At the same time the infant may be given verbal messages such as "I love you. You are all boy." These scripting verbal messages give information about the person's worth as well the sexual identity he is expected to assume. As the person grows, script instructions are programmed into the Child Ego. The script has directions with expectations of how the person will live his life. Each person's script is influenced by family and cultural scripts. Examples of a family script are: "There has always been a doctor in our family" or "The women in our family have never worked outside the home." These messages contain an expectation that may be programmed into the person's script. A script is maintained by basic life positions, by games, and through strokes.

A *stroke* is any act that implies recognition of the presence of another person.[6] Strokes are given in the form of physical intimacy (actual physical contact), nonverbal acts such as a nod or a smile, and by words. Strokes are basic motivators of behavior[5] in that everyone needs strokes and normally behaves in ways to receive strokes. Stroking is basic to survival. Infants who do not experience enough stroking in the form of physical contact fail to thrive physically and mentally.

Strokes are positive and negative. Positive strokes contribute to healthy emotional development and convey to the person an "OK-ness" about himself. The person feels alive, secure, and significant. Positive strokes involve transactions that are complementary, direct, appropriate, and relevant to the situation. Positive strokes are expressed through compliments, a warm smile or hello, a direct answer to a question, affectionate feelings, and verbal expression of appreciation. Spontaneous expression of love to a spouse and a direct, aboveboard answer to a question from a supervisor are examples of positive strokes.

Since everyone needs strokes, a person who does not get sufficient positive strokes will provoke negative strokes. Negative strokes discount the person's feelings and needs and convey that the person is Not-OK. The person who receives negative recognition feels insignificant and experiences pain. However, negative strokes may be perceived as better than none at all and are important for survival. A child who does not receive positive strokes from parental figures may violate a family rule so that the parents will scold him. A husband who feels left out because of his wife's attention to the children may invite negative strokes by provoking a verbal confrontation with her.

The infant's earliest need for stroking is met through intimate physical contact, such as feeding, diapering, and hugging. As the person develops, he continues to have a desire to meet the need for stroking through infantile physical means. However, the person learns to compromise and get the need met through nonphysical acts. Also, each person develops an individualized way of expressing the need for stroking.

An exchange of strokes constitutes a *transaction.*[6] A transaction is a unit of social intercourse. It is a stimulus from the ego state of another person. Transactions begin at birth and continue throughout development. When any two or more people are in close proximity, eventually a transaction takes place. The simplest transactions are those in which stimulus and response arise from the Adult state of each person. The Child and Parent are the next, simplest transactions. Transactions may be (1) *complimentary,* when the response is what is appropriate and expected; (2) *crossed,* when communication is broken off; (3) *ulterior,* those transactions involving the activity of more than two ego states; or (4) *angular,* those transactions involving all three ego states.

The first transaction in the infant's life centers on getting nourishment during nursing. The rudiments of games are formed during these earliest transactions with the mother. As the child comprehends separateness from the mother and has some degree of independent existence, Adult functioning begins. The infant begins to learn some control of self when finding the nipple and releasing it at will.

A new set of transactions develops as the child realizes control over the body in ways acceptable to others. Bowel training involves a long, complicated series of transactions that have the potential for developing maneuvers and games by the child and the mother.

The child next discovers sharing the mother with other, more powerful people, such as the father, or a person the mother seems to prefer, such as a newborn sibling. The child, now 2 or 3 years old, develops games in an attempt to deal with these rivalries. At 4 to 7 years of age the child begins to make decisions, to take positions that justify the decisions, and to ward off influences that threaten a position. The actions taken determine the child's script (life plan) and affect social relationships in later life.

As the child has transactions with other children and teachers at school, he tries out games learned at home. The child may sharpen some, tone down others, abandon some, and pick up new ones. The child also tests decisions and positions. The influence of the family experiences is still evident in all transactions.

Adolescence is the first time the individual makes autonomous choices; however, these are still influenced by decisions made in early life. The adolescent reevaluates basic decisions and positions in light of new experiences with peers and may fluctuate between using actions learned early in life and trying out new ones. By the early twenties, the individual makes a decision to adhere to positions acquired earlier or to modify these positions. This decision remains relatively constant until the forties, when the individual must again struggle with new experiences that require a reevaluation of basic position. The remainder of life follows a similar pattern.

BEHAVIORAL THEORY

Behavioral theory is based on the premise that all behavior, adaptive and maladaptive, is a product of learning. Learning is a change in behavior resulting from reinforcement. A related assumption is that, since behavior is learned, it can be unlearned and adaptive behavior can be substituted.

Conditioning is a type of learning. The classic work of Pavlov—the evoking of salivation in dogs with the ringing of a bell—is an example of a conditioned reflex and response. With training, the dogs associated the bell (stimulus) with food (reinforcement).

Behavioral therapists and theorists such as Albert Bandura[3] have emphasized the reciprocal interactive relationship between individuals and their environments. Individuals are active in influencing the environment, which in turn influences their behavior. In the newer approach, called *social learning theory,* clients are encouraged to actively participate in therapy by defining problems, selecting objectives, and evaluating outcomes.

Behaviorist *BF Skinner*[56] avoided focusing on the inner mental functioning of repression and emphasized observable data when analyzing human behavior. He was interested in learning why a specific behavior starts and what in the current situation makes it rewarding for the person to continue the behavior. His theory is based on *operant conditioning* techniques. Operant responses are emitted by the person rather than elicited by a stimulus. In operant conditioning, the subject actively manipulates the environment. This characteristic distinguishes Skinner's approach from the more passive Pavlovian conditioning.

A key concept in Skinner's theory of operant conditioning is *reinforcement,* which is "any event, contingent upon the response of the organism, that alters the future likelihood of that response."[56] *Positive reinforcement* is a reward for selected behavior, and *negative reinforcement* brings anxiety producing sanctions against whatever behavior is in progress. Thus continued rewards tend strongly to enforce desired behaviors, whereas negative reinforcement tends to extinguish undesirable behaviors.

Another significant concept is *response frequency,* which refers to how often a response is given. In a treatment situation, the client's task is to adapt personal activities to behaviors approved by society and to abandon behaviors with negative sanctions. Guiding the individual in achieving the desired behavioral response is referred to as *shaping,* and the overall approach is called operant conditioning.

Joseph Wolpe[64] based many of his ideas on the concept that all behavior is learned; that is, individuals are conditioned to respond to a stimulus. Behavior then is a series of habitual responses to a familiar series of stimuli. Wolpe described neurosis as using maladaptive ways to respond to anxiety producing situations.

Wolpe began developing his conditioning theory by producing experimental neuroses in animals in the mid-1940s. Using this initial work, he developed a theory that considers anxiety a behavior generator. The individual with a neurosis crystallizes the behavior as a way of coping. Wolpe hypothesized the *principle of reciprocal inhibition;* that is, if a pleasant or anxiety reducing state is experienced at the same time the anxiety provoking stimulus is introduced, this new experience diminishes the anxiety response to the stimulus.

A related concept that is basic to Wolpe's theory is *anxiety hierarchy.* Hierarchical relationships are established among anxiety producing stimuli. With this approach, a more acceptable behavior is substituted for the symptom by learning another way of coping with the underlying anxiety. One such way developed by Wolpe is *systematic desensitization,* a counterconditioning technique for extinguishing maladaptive responses and replacing them with more acceptable (adaptive) responses. The details of this and related techniques are discussed later in the chapter.

John Dollard and *Neal Miller's stimulus-response theory*[13] emphasizes reinforcement or reward as the essential ingredient for forming a new stimulus response. They explored the determination of the conditions under which habits are formed and broken. A *habit* is a link of association between a stimulus and a response. Four concepts related to the learning process are basic to Dollard and Miller's theory: drive, cue, response, and reinforcement (reward).

A *drive* is a stimulus with sufficient strength to impel the person into the activity. *Primary drives,* essential for survival, are innate and in close contact with physiological processes such as hunger, pain, and sex. These drives are important determinants of behavior to the extent that the means for reducing the drive stimuli are available. The hunger drive of a person without sufficient food is strong and is an important determinant of the person's behavior. *Secondary drives* evolve during growth and incite and direct behavior. The stimuli of these drives generally replace primary drive stimuli. The person learns to respond to secondary drive stimulation with appropriate adaptive activity, such as eating before hunger pangs (primary drive stimuli) are experienced.

A *cue* is a stimulus that determines the nature of the person's *response.* The time, place, and type of response are related to the cue. The response relates to a given cue in the environment; during the growth process, individuals learn a hierarchy of responses. *Reinforcements (rewards)* strengthen the connection between a given response and a particular cue and lead to a repetition of the response. When the response is not reinforced, *extinction* of the behavior occurs.

Dollard and Miller[13] believed that in the process of growth a person experiences *conflict,* opposition between two drives experienced simultaneously in response to the same situation. This concept is discussed in Chapter 10. The frustration-aggression hypothesis, basic to their theory of human behavior, is discussed in Chapter 11.

COGNITIVE THEORY

Jean Piaget's theory of cognition[52] is based on the assumption that human personality evolves from a composite of interrelated intellectual and affective functions. He be-

▼ **TABLE 4-5** Piaget's Stages of Cognitive Development

Stage of Development	Critical Experience	Major Characteristics
Sensorimotor (birth to 2 years)	Learning to recognize the permanence of objects	Goal-directed behavior; imitation in terms of make believe
Preoperational		
Preconceptual (3 to 4 years)	Symbolic mental activity; learning to think in terms of past, present, and future	Egocentrism; use of language as major tool
Intuitive (5 to 7 years)	Learning to integrate concepts based on relationship	Comprehension of basic rules; increased exactness in imitation of reality
Stage of concrete operations (8 to 11 years)	Learning to use logic and objectivity in concrete thoughts	Classification of events; reversibility
Stage of formal operations (12 to 15 years)	Learning to think abstractly and logically	Use of scientific approach to problem solving

lieved that consciousness, judgment, and reasoning depend primarily on the individual's evolving intellectual capacity to organize experiences. A related view holds that the total experiences of individuals shape interests and the specific experiences they tend to pursue.

Piaget's theory of personality development says the developing child passes through four main, discrete stages: the sensorimotor stage, the preoperational stage, the stage of concrete operations, and the stage of formal operations (Table 4-5). Each stage reflects a range of organizational patterns that occur in definite sequence and within an approximate age span.

Development is influenced by biological maturation, social experiences, and experiences with the physical environment. During cognitive development, the individual strives to find equilibrium between self and environment. This striving, or *adaptation,* depends on the interrelated processes of *assimilation* and *accommodation.* During assimilation the child develops the ability to handle new situations and problems with existing mechanisms. Accommodation enables individuals to manage situations previously beyond their ability. *Schema,* another concept related to the child's development, is an innate knowledge structure that allows the child to organize ways to behave in the environment. Interaction between the child and the environment is directed by changes in cognitive processes that allow the child to adapt, accommodate, and assimilate in order to adjust to the environment.

Albert Ellis' rational emotive theory (RET) of personality[15] was developed as a therapeutic approach and consists of four basic premises:

1. All people start with a basic set of values and assumptions that govern much of their lives. Once these assumptions are made, subsequent rational and irrational thinking and behaving can be accurately specified, worked with, and understood.
2. All humans want to survive and be relatively happy while surviving. Ellis defines happiness as being satisfied and free from unnecessary pain.
3. Usually, individuals want to live in and get along with members of a social group or community.
4. Individuals want to relate intimately with a few selected members of this group.

Ellis believed that behaviors that support these basic values are rational while those that interfere with attaining values are irrational.

Ellis considered the ABC theory of personality in health and illness central to RET theory. A is the activating event; B is the person's belief system about A; and C is the emotional consequence. A person's appropriate or inappropriate emotional response to an experience is determined by the person's belief system about the experience and not by the experience itself. For example, if a person feels depressed (point C) after being rejected for a job (point A), the rejection does not cause the feeling of depression. Rather, it is the person's beliefs (point B) about the rejection. Rational beliefs and appropriate feelings related to the experience motivate the person to work harder to achieve the goal. A person with irrational beliefs and inappropriate feelings tends to resign to defeat.

Aron T. Beck[4] focused on the cognitive distortions characteristically seen in depression. Much depression, according to Beck, is the result of irrational, distorted thinking. The types of cognitive distortions are *arbitrary inference,* in which a negative conclusion is drawn from insufficient evidence ("My boss didn't smile at me this morning; therefore I have done something terrible"); *overgeneralization,* in which what is true for one event is assumed to be true for all others ("I botched dinner last night; I am a stupid wife, a failure as a mother, and a rotten person"); *selective abstraction,* in which focus on one aspect of an event negates all other aspects ("My marriage is failing because of my self-centered demands"); and *magnification* and *minimization,* in which marked distortions occur in evaluating oneself ("My anger at my friend for being late has destroyed our friendship").

Distorted thinking develops from a set of rules one holds about oneself, others, and the world. These rules are called *underlying assumptions,* and the individual regards them as unquestionably true. Because they are so basic to one's belief system, they are rarely critically examined, except in therapy. In cognitive theory, the underlying assumptions are the basis of conflict because they rigidly limit one's alternatives for solving ambiguous or new life situations. Some of these rules are assumptions of *entitlement* ("The world owes me a living"; "Things always work out for the best"; "I deserve better than this"), *perfection* ("Unless I do everything 100%, I am useless"; "Unless I am perfect, no one will love me"; "A mistake is shameful"), and *expectations* ("A good father never gets angry at his children"; "If he loves me, he'd understand me"; "I'm nothing without love"). Underlying assumptions generally divide the world into black-and-white alternatives. Therefore each time an ambiguous situation is encountered, an underlying assumption triggers the distorted thinking pattern, producing *automatic thoughts*, a kind of habitual shorthand conclusion about the situation not subject to critical evaluation. For example, the boss passes by the secretary without smiling, and the secretary *automatically* thinks, "The boss is going to fire me because I'm a terrible secretary." These thoughts arouse feelings of anger, helplessness, depression, or worthlessness, the hallmarks of a depressive episode.

SOCIOCULTURAL THEORY

Sociocultural theories introduce a change in emphasis from the intrapsychic, individualistic approach to an action-oriented, community-based theory that links a sociocultural system to mental health.[39] This approach emphasizes social processes and their roles in mental illness.

George Mead's formulations[45] on *symbolic interactionism* are influenced by sociocultural theory. This theory's major tenet is the concept of self that develops through interaction between the child and significant others. The self comes into being through trying out or testing behaviors, retaining those that result in social approval and rejecting those that are not acceptable. This approach is an extremely complex action-interaction network that falls under the term *socialization*. Significant others teach the child the *rules* by which to live. These rules acknowledge explicit or implicit norms defined by a particular culture. Deviation from these rules to any significant degree creates social or interpersonal pressures. In tandem with the rules is a set of *roles*. Deviation from the norms also may coincide with role rejection. As an example, failure to be a mother in the commonly accepted sense of the word depends on definitions of the mothering role in a given group or social setting. However, each definition has a recognizable core. To violate the core definition, to transgress the outer limits of the social definition may well lead to a *label*. The label may encompass a legal term (child abuse, for example) or a social definition ("poor mother").

Labels arise from norm deviations and are a powerful force in deciding the fate of people who are labeled "eccentric," "drunk," or "gambler." The label "crazy" is a familiar one. A pseudopsychiatric label like this may be a lifelong liability. In every society and every cultural group within each society, there are acceptable behaviors, unacceptable behaviors, and behaviors that receive a temporary label because of unusual circumstances perceived in the specific situation. Most of our everyday transactions are well within the "acceptable range." Those that exceed the usual expectations are labeled as deviant.

Thus social meaning, the consensus within a particular group, is at the heart of symbolic interactionism. Social meaning depends on *consensual validation*, a sometimes imperceptible but constant checking on what a given situation means to one's reference group. *Consensus* is the device that is used to establish social meaning.

Thomas Szasz,[59] a sociocultural theorist, also studied the effects of sociocultural variables on labeling behavior not conforming to social norms as deviant behavior. He recognized certain dangers in labeling other people's behavior but believed that getting rid of the label is almost impossible, despite social pressures to do so. He made an impact with his characterization of mental illness as "myth." Szasz viewed mental illness as a label assigned to a group of persons unable or unwilling to conform to societal norms. These individuals are institutionalized in mental hospitals, which is society's way of controlling disruptions of social life. His views served as a catalyst for reexamining many legal, moral, and ethical factors in the confinement and treatment of clients with psychiatric problems.

Erving Goffman made lasting contributions to the study of behavior in the culture at large. His work, *Asylums,*[26] has been used extensively in the psychiatric world to assess social factors that have an impact on client residence in large public hospitals. Also derived from *Asylums* is the concept of *total institution*. A total institution is "a place of residence and work where a large number of like-situated individuals, cut off from the wider society for an appreciable period of time, together lead an enclosed, formally administered round of life."[26] The traditional state hospital is an example of a total institution. For one thing, it is possible for both "inmates" and staff members to remain at the hospital for long periods without leaving the grounds. Food and other goods can be purchased in on-site stores, walks can be taken on the extensive grounds, gymnasiums are often available, movies are shown, and other forms of recreation are available. There is a barrier to social interaction with the outside world. The institution, not the person's illness, is the most important factor in forming a mental hospital client.

The concept of *stigma*[27] is also important for caring for the mentally ill. Goffman uses the term stigma to describe any attribute that makes one different or is discrediting in the categorization scheme employed by all societies, large and small. The mentally ill, as well as many others who do not meet selected norms of a social group, are prominent in the discredited group.

Another movement pioneered by *Maxwell Jones*[30] is the concept of the therapeutic community. The term *therapeutic community* originated with TF Main[42] in 1946 when he was working with a group of demobilized, psychoneurotic former soldiers. The institution (hospital) was seen as a community aimed at enhancing full participation in its daily life, resocialization, and return to society. The goal is met by full participation in the microcosm that the ward or hospital represents. The concept of therapeutic community encompasses use of the community's resources in a system of open and democratic communication.

GENERAL SYSTEMS THEORY

General systems theory is a science of "wholeness" characterized by dynamic interaction among components of the system and between the system and the environment. A basic premise of systems theory is that a phenomenon cannot be understood independent of the system of which it is a part. General systems theory assumes that an impact made on one component of a system affects the functioning of the total system. Instead of looking at parts of a person (for example, dealing only with the mind), general systems theory deals with both mind and body as they exist in a given environment. Systems can be persons, families, wards, or care units in hospitals, educational centers, or shopping centers.

Ludwig von Bertalanffy[61] viewed a person as an active system in the larger system of the world. He considered the world a complex but well-organized system. *Kurt Lewin*[40] suggested that each person or object exists in a particular field or environment. Within this person-field unit are two opposing forces. One set of forces produces change, and the other halts change, thus upsetting the state of equilibrium. Lewin calls the direction that these forces take a *vector.* The psychobiological forces are made up of mind, body, and societal factors.

A *system* is a set of parts meshing within a *boundary.* There are inputs, outputs, and throughputs across the boundary. Boundary lines delineating the shape of a system are an integral part of the systems concept.

Equilibrium, another important concept in systems theory, refers to a balance among parts of the system. The various parts inside the boundary have the following two possibilities: they can reach an even level, much as a scale can be balanced, or they can reach a steady state, in which they move dynamically through a process of exchange and rearrangement, maintaining a balanced relationship among all components. All systems tend to maintain a steady state, or balance, among subsystems.

Feedback is another key feature of systems theory. Systems maintain function and balance through communication, and feedback is necessary to communication. Since transmitting a message requires a sender and a receiver, the reply to the sender is feedback. The nature of the message sent determines the structure of the return message and how long the interchange will last. A pleasant message usually will be received in a pleasant manner, whereas a curt, negative message can end the feedback loop at that point. Chapter 6 includes a more complete description of the process.

Certain premises are related to the major terms just described. The first one suggests that all living systems are open, with contacts across boundaries with input, output, and a functioning feedback system. A person is an open system in a state of constant exchange with other people as well as with the physical world of components such as water, air, and food. According to the strict definition, no systems are truly closed, but a system may have minimal inputs and outputs for awhile.

EXISTENTIAL THEORY

Existentialism emphasizes the totality of an individual's existence. The individual is responsible for existence on a personal level, and recognition is given to the individual's values, mode of being in the world, and religious qualities. Individuals are in a state of "becoming," which they control.

Each individual is forced to confront the ultimate existential dilemmas of isolation, meaninglessness, and death. Suffering can result as the individual experiences anxiety, despair, and dread. The individual uses maladaptive defenses to deny the inevitability of death, fails to accept freedom and therefore responsibility, fails to come to terms with individual isolation, and unsuccessfully struggles to develop individual meaning in life.

Erich Fromm,[21] generally allied with the interpersonal group that focused on the social and cultural aspects of human behavior, was primarily an existentialist. Fromm identified positive and negative needs that must be met in a helpful, constructive way and saw the ideal individual as one free to live at maximum capacity. Fromm clearly stated that this is the ideal but that often, as a result of family and cultural pressures, other patterns emerge.

Fromm is credited with developing the idea that *sadomasochism* is a "mechanism" used to escape from situations that interfere with expansion of the true self. Sadistic and masochistic traits coexist in the person; they are opposite sides of the same coin and necessary for each other. A *sadist,* one who gains a feeling of power by inflicting pain on others, needs someone who is willing to incur the pain, the *masochist.* Both of these behaviors meet basic needs to relieve anxiety and to escape loneliness and powerlessness. In short, behaviors are mechanisms of escape from what are otherwise intolerable situations.

Fromm developed several character types of general, observable kinds of personalities molded in the family and in the culture. A culture is influential in developing a set of characteristics common to most people in that group or society. Fromm has called this set of characteristics a *social character.* On top of this social character, a unique pattern of interaction is developed. Among the types that develop are the following four unproductive orientations: (1) *marketing character,* (2) *receptive character,* (3) *exploitative character,* and (4) *hoarding character.* A *productive character* also develops. The types of character used determines the person's adjustment to life.

HUMANISTIC THEORY

Because humanistic theory draws heavily from existential theory, it is often referred to as existential-humanism.

Humanistic psychology identifies the person as the most reliable source of knowledge about personal capabilities, resources, and characteristics. This psychology values all dimensions of the human condition—physical, emotional, intellectual, social, and spiritual—from a holistic perspective (see Chapter 2).

Humanists are similar to ego psychologists in their emphasis on the conscious aspects of personality. According to the humanists, each person is an understanding, conscious, experiencing individual whose subjective impressions are as valid as the "hard data" of science. The total person responds with personal growth or self-actualization, which, from the humanistic perspective, is among the most highly valued goals. The current popularity of humanistic psychology is undoubtedly related to changing modern values such as personal freedom, individual responsibility, equal opportunity, and protection of the natural human environment. Humanists hold an optimistic view of human potential.

Among the diverse groups of theorists who are essentially humanistic are Frederick (Fritz) Perls, Abraham Maslow, Sidney Jourard, and RD Laing.

Perls[50,51] developed gestalt theory. This theory focuses on the here and now, encouraging people to become aware of psychological and physical functioning, since one affects and interacts with the other. Together they form a whole picture, or *gestalt*. Perls saw the individual as embedded or grounded in a situation that he or she deals with in terms of an open or closed gestalt. The open gestalt is unformed, incomplete, or contains parts of a situation that remain as "unfinished business." When needs in the situation are met, the person can move on to another situation with renewed energy. Once this occurs, the gestalt is closed. The individual is encouraged to become aware of open gestalts, that is, to be genuine in all facets of a situation and to devote energy to closing open gestalts. Open gestalts are anxiety producing psychological states standing in the way of productive living and must be removed so that an objective and subjective view of current reality is possible.

Maslow[43] viewed the personality as self-actualizing. This means that the ideal individual is at the peak capacity of fulfilling personal human potential. Before peak fulfillment of an individual's capacity can occur, more basic needs such as hunger, thirst, security, and physical safety must be met. Maslow devised a hierarchy of needs in the order of necessity for fulfillment (Figure 4-1). Once needs in the lower part of the hierarchy are met, those of a higher order can be met, such as the need to belong to a group, to be loved, to be looked on with esteem, and to be respected. As the lower group of needs are met, the self is freed, or actualized, to create in whatever mode suits that person. Individuals can then proceed to express themselves in personally creative ways—music, art, or, as Maslow puts it, "by baking a superlative cake."

Jourard[51,52] discussed self-actualizing and creative components of the personality in his book, *The Transparent Self.* His basic premise is that people who work with others in need must be in touch with their inner selves so that they are genuinely relating as one person to another. There must be honesty in the relationship, not manipulative control or irrational use of interpersonal power. Jourard believed that the ability to disclose oneself to others is a sign of health and a distinct advantage in attempting to help others. Persons who perceive themselves as capable and who have adequate self-esteem will act in ways that indicate interpersonal capacity. Those who see themselves as nonfunctional, weak, and unable to relate to others will have too much anxiety to experience freedom in self-disclosure.

Laing,[56,57] a British psychiatrist, is perhaps best known for his work with schizophrenic clients and the publication of a book entitled *Knots,* which expresses a series of communicative snarls in verse. Laing relates schizophrenia to lack of a core self; that is, the person tries to assume roles that others have imposed from the outside, usually through family rules and metarules. *Metarules* are rules about rules, often unspoken. The environment, the individual's perception of the environment, and the family who pass along what their ancestors handed down to them all affect the individual. The individual then superimposes perceptions or imaginings on the total picture. Laing called the process of handing down a set of patterns from one generation to another *mapping*. Each new generation has projections and inducements from the preceding generation. The preceding generation goes through the same process, and each generation develops its own response. Laing believed that at least three generations could be mapped.

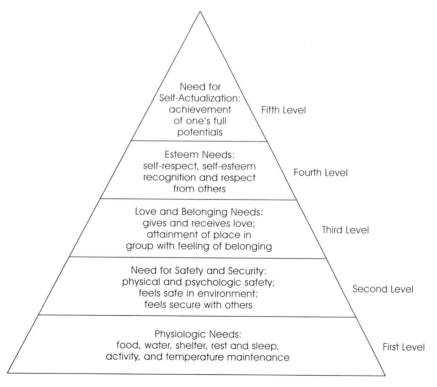

FIGURE 4-1 Maslow's hierarchy of needs. *(Based on data from Maslow A: Motivation and personality, ed 2, New York, 1970, Harper & Row.)*

BIOLOGICAL THEORY

Biological theory, sometimes referred to as the *medical model,* is based on the belief that mental illness is a disease in the same sense as diabetes or high blood pressure. Mental illness results from abnormalities in brain structure and chemistry.[2,60] The mental diseases of the brain manifest themselves primarily by abnormalities in behavior, emotion, and thinking. Presently these abnormalities cannot be traced to distinct areas of damage in the brain. According to biological psychiatrists, the biological model of mental illness derives from the work of Emil Kraepelin, who was the first psychiatrist to view mental illness as a disease.

Neurochemistry influenced the biological theory of mental illness.[2,28] Emphasis is given to the biochemical abnormalities of the brain that underlie mental illness. This focus is based on the belief that serious mental illnesses are due to problems in the regulation of specific neurotransmitter systems. "Neurotransmitters are chemicals that are stored in the boutons of the nerves and that are released, by depolarization of boutons, to stimulate other neurons."[28] Data support an association between catecholamine neuron dysfunction and several psychiatric disorders, including Parkinson's disease, depression, panic disorders, and schizophrenia. The catecholamines that have been given the most attention are dopamine, norepinephrine, epinephrine, and serotonin. Biological psychiatrists believe that certain medications normalize catecholamine activity and control the symptoms of the mental disorder. Thus if researchers can determine which neurotransmitter dysfunctions are associated with a certain mental illness, specific medication can be used to treat the illness.

According to biological psychiatrists, genetics provide support for consideration of biological and biochemical factors in mental illness since genes express themselves through chemical processes.[60] Support for the genetic explanation of some mental illnesses has been found through research of adopted persons and twins. It is believed that if genetic factors contribute to the cause of major psychoses then these disorders are illnesses rather than ways of life and the biological (medical) model is an appropriate model. Along with genetic factors, these psychiatrists support the importance of environmental factors in the development of mental illness. They believe that what is transmitted by the genes is a predisposition to the mental disorder. Everyone who has the genetic vulnerability does not necessarily develop the illness unless certain crucial environmental factors are present. The specific environmental factors are not known; they may be family interactions or psychosocial factors.

Psychiatrists who subscribe to the biological model of mental illness emphasize diagnosing each specific illness based on the symptoms the client presents.[2] Instead of a "50-minute hour," the biological psychiatrist believes a detailed medical history, family illness history, and physical examination are necessary to determine the type of mental illness the client has and the medication regimen to prescribe. Biological psychiatrists further believe that laboratory tests are valuable with the biological model.[2] The tests help to better understand the physical processes that underlie the client's symptoms. Tests that have been useful include various types of techniques for brain imaging, the use of blood and urine measures of neuroendocrine and neurotransmitter function, and electroencephalogram (EEG), especially during sleep, to evaluate the electrical activity of the brain. Theoretical approaches are summarized in Table 4-6.

Stress

Theories of stress as a cause of biological and psychological abnormalities are another area of interest within biological theory. *Walter Cannon, Harold Wolff,* and *Hans Selye* made significant contributions to the development of stress theories and the impact of stress on the human mind and body.

Cannon[10,11] was the first physician to mention stress as a causative factor of disease. In developing his ideas about *homeostasis,* he described the strains and stresses resulting from pressure placed on specific body mechanisms necessary to maintain a steady state, or homeostasis. Fluid and electrolyte balance, body temperature control, nervous system control, and immune system response are homeostatic mechanisms that help maintain equilibrium.

Cannon applied the body's fight-flight alert to stress. He viewed disease as a fight to maintain homeostasis in the body's tissues.

Wolff and Selye were the first to apply the term *stress* scientifically to medicine. Wolff[63] described stress as a dynamic state within the organism rather than an aspect of the external environment. He defined stress as an internal force produced by external forces and therefore viewed stress as the interaction between the external environment and the individual. Past experiences are a major factor in determining a person's response to stress.

Wolff[62,63] used a "protective reaction pattern" as a principle concept in developing his ideas about stress. According to this pattern, threats to the physical integrity of the body cause a complex reaction to rid the body of the threat. Symbolic as well as physical threats initiate similar reactions, which involve alterations in feeling, body processes, and behavior.

Selye's[54] biochemical model of stress focuses on an analysis of stress at the physiological and biochemical levels. Selye[54] viewed stress as the body's nonspecific response to any demand made on it. The response is considered nonspecific because no selectivity occurs, and all or most parts of the body must try to adjust to any specific agent of stress. Selye related stress to homeostasis when he described the body's adaptive response to cold, shivering. The goal of shivering is to return the body to its previous steady state.

A stressor produces stress. Any demands on the body, including those necessary to maintain life, are stessors. The body responds to both positive and negative stressors. Individuals experience multiple and constant stressors; these constitute the wear and tear on the body.

Selye[54] believed that people must adapt to stressors throughout life. Hereditary factors influence how an individual adapts to stress. However, Selye calls the process by which all people adapt to stress the *General Adaptation Syndrome* (GAS). GAS is the process by which the body's nonspecific responses to stress evolve through three stages of adaptation: (1) the *alarm reaction* (AR), (2) the *stage of resistance* (SR), and (3) the *stage of exhaustion* (SE).

The alarm reaction, the initial response to stress, is characterized by a generalized expression of the body's defense system. Selye found that maintaining the alarm reaction

▼ **TABLE 4-6**   **Summary of Theoretical Approaches**

Theory	Theorist	Emphasis	Key Concepts
Psychoanalytical	Freud	The study of unconscious mental processes and the psychodynamics of behavior	Personality structure: id, ego, superego; libido, pleasure principle, reality principle, instincts; stages of psychosexual development
	Jung	The role of the unconscious as a determinant of behavior; the inherited racial foundation of personality structure	Collective unconscious, archetypes, persona, anima and animus, shadow
	Erikson	Psychosocial factors that influence development throughout the life cycle	Id, ego, superego; conscious, preconscious, unconscious, developmental tasks; eight stages of biopsychosocial development
	Berne	Transactional development of the individual	Ego states, transactions; games, strokes, scripts
	Sullivan	Interpersonal experiences that influence development	Self-system, anxiety, security operations, personifications, modes of experience; stages of interpersonal growth and development
Behavioral	Pavlov	Mechanistic principles: individual's behavior is under the control of past learned experiences and current environmental circumstances	Conditioning; stimulus, reinforcement
	Skinner	Analysis of human behavior observed in the current situation	Operant conditioning; positive and negative reinforcement, response frequency, shaping
	Wolpe	Behavior is a series of habitual responses to a familiar series of stimuli	Principle of reciprocal inhibition, anxiety hierarchy, systematic desensitization
	Dollard and Miller	Reinforcement or reward as the essential ingredient for forming a new stimulus response	Drive: primary and secondary; habit, cue, response, reinforcement (rewards), extinction, conflict, frustration-aggression hypothesis
Cognitive	Piaget	The interrelationship of intellectual and affective functions in human development	Four discrete states in the stages of cognitive development; adaptation, assimilation, accommodation, schema
	Ellis	The values and assumptions that govern much of people's lives	ABC theory of rational emotive theory
	Beck	Cognitive distortions	Arbitrary inference, overgeneralization, selective abstraction, magnification and minimization, underlying assumptions, entitlement, perfection, automatic thoughts
Sociocultural	Mead	The development of self through the child's interaction with significant others	Socialization, rules, roles, labels, consensual validation
	Szasz	The effects of sociocultural variables on labeling behavior that does not conform to social norms as *deviant*	Labels; mental illness as a "myth"
	Goffman	Social factors that have an impact on client residence in large public hospitals	Total institution, stigma
	Jones	The hospital as a microcosm of the larger community	Therapeutic community
General Systems	Lewin	The interaction of the person-field as two opposing forces	System, boundary, equilibrium, feedback, vector
Existential Humanism	Fromm	Achievement of essence	Sadomasochism, social character
	Perls	The individual's awareness of his physical and psychological functioning	Gestalt
	Maslow	Fulfilling human potential	Hierarchy of needs, self-actualization
	Jourard	Self-actualizing creative components of personality	Self-disclosure
	Laing	Schizophrenia and lack of a core self	Family rules, metarules, mapping
Biological	Andreason	The influence of genetics and organic factors on the person's development of a psychiatric illness	Defective genes, environmental stresses
Stress	Cannon	The effect of strains and stresses of life on mechanisms of the body	Homeostasis, fight-flight, protective reaction pattern
	Wolff	Stress as a dynamic state within the organism	Protective reaction pattern
	Selye	Analysis of stress at the physiological and biochemical levels of functioning	Stressor, general adaptation syndrome: alarm reaction, stage of resistance, stage of exhaustion
	Lazarus	Cognitive model of stress	Appraisal, coping, outcome

stage for an extended period causes death. This led him to identify and describe the stage of resistance. Resisting changes in body organs leads to homeostasis and survival. The stage of exhaustion results from prolonged stress. The wear and tear on the body that accompanies this stage leads to premature aging. Selye believed that with most short-lived stressors, such as mental or physical exertion, only the first and second stages of GAS are manifested. People learn to adapt to the demands of their environment through repeated experiences with stages 1 and 2. Because stage 3 is initiated by severe stress that may lead to death, it is not experienced as often as the other stages.

Selye believed that a person's adaptability is probably life's most unique characteristic. The ability to adapt allows for the complexities of life, homeostasis, and resistance to stress.

Lazarus' theory,[38] though not a biological one, is pertinent to this discussion because of its focus on stress. Lazarus proposed that the degree of reaction produced by a stressor is related to the subjective appraisal each individual makes of the event as threatening or nonthreatening. The Lazarus cognitive model of stress involves the following three phases: (1) *appraisal,* (2) *coping,* and (3) *outcome.*

Primary appraisal occurs as the person evaluates the stressor and the perceived degree of danger. Secondary appraisal involves assessing the availability of adequate coping devices. Coping mechanisms can be palliative, or they can involve direct action. Palliative mechanisms alter the distress the individual experiences in response to the event. Direct action meets or avoids the approaching threat. The results of these actions lead to the overall outcome the event has on the person.

ECLECTIC APPROACH

An eclectic approach as a therapeutic modality includes selecting the most appropriate theories and approaches from various orientations. If diverse theories are viewed as complementary perspectives of the truth rather than competing or exclusive, one can readily acknowledge the usefulness of all of these theories in a variety of nurse-client situations.

Nurse-client interaction is affected by many variables such as respective philosophies of life, values, motivations, time restrictions, and emotional and intellectual capabilities. With a broad spectrum of theoretical approaches from which to select, the nurse is able to tailor interventions to the individual's needs or capabilities of the moment.

The following case example exemplifies an eclectic approach employed by a psychiatric nurse working with an adult woman who had survived severe long-term incestuous abuse as a child. Only those approaches that seemed most useful at different stages were applied.

▼ Case Example

Laura is a 30-year-old woman who initially responded to a flier advertising a support group for women who were sexually abused as children. The nurse of a local community mental health center facilitated this group. After a preliminary interview and assessment, Laura and the nurse decided that individual sessions would be initiated and the group experience would be an adjunct at a mutually agreed upon point. Laura and the nurse contracted to enter this process together. Weekly sessions lasted 1½ years.

After several sessions the nurse and Laura determined that, similar to other survivors of long-term incestuous abuse, Laura was experiencing difficulties with the life issues of trust and self-worth. Specifically, Laura's long-term response to the sexual abuse was severely affecting her ability to establish and maintain intimate interpersonal relationships and to develop her potentials. Laura also exhibited an immobilizing reaction to rain storms.

Approaches
Psychoanalytical

Because long-term traumas existed during Laura's ego-formative years, the nurse selected an approach that used principles of psychoanalytical theory. This modified approach provided Laura with an opportunity to examine the abuse within the context of life review, while developing insights into the psychogenic origins of her current problems. Interpretation and explanations were used as insight developed. During the process, the nurse became a surrogate nonabusive parent and, through support and acceptance, the therapeutic relationship provided opportunity for some degree of ego-restructuring and affirmation. Transferences, positive and negative, were discussed at appropriate times. For example, during one session the nurse reached up to scratch her head and Laura exhibited fear by wincing as if she were about to be struck. Laura acknowledged fear that the nurse was going to strike her, as her father had. This transference was discussed, providing an opportunity for Laura to relate to the nurse in the here and now. Laura was able to move past the assumption that she had to be hurt to be cared about.

Behavioral

Several episodes of Laura's abuse occurred during thunderstorms. Laura developed a phobic response to adverse weather conditions. A desensitization tape was constructed that introduced sound recordings of water splashing, light rain, heavy rain, and finally thunderstorms with rain. These were gradually introduced following relaxation exercises in the session. These relaxation exercises and storm recordings were also practiced at home between sessions. Toward the end of the densensitization process, Laura and the nurse went out into the rain together. Laura slowly became reconditioned to the rain through relaxation and pleasurable events.

Cognitive

After approximately 6 months of sessions, the nurse suggested that Laura read *Feeling Good,*[9] a self-help book that employs cognitive therapy techniques in identifying and modifying irrational thought assumptions and patterns. Laura did the suggested homework readings and, together in session, she and the nurse analyzed these readings. Laura was able to identify and diminish many of her automatic negative thought patterns and significantly reduce her tendency toward a depressive, low self-esteem state.

Existential

Using the gestalt technique of "empty chair" to facilitate dialogue, Laura expressed long withheld anger at her perpetrator father as well as grief and frustration about her unknowing, unprotective mother. The "empty chair" technique uses two chairs placed facing each other. One chair represents the client or an aspect of the client's personality, and the other represents another person or the opposing part of the personality. As the client alternates roles, she sits in one or the other chairs. This exercise provided Laura with a chance to express her feelings in a therapeutic way. In addition, she was able to do so within a safe and supportive environment.

During one difficult session, Laura was evasive, noncooperative, and antagonistic. After several traditional attempts at exploration and interpretation, the nurse stopped the process, admitting that she was confused and not quite certain what was happening. She then asked Laura if she was comfortable or satisfied with the way the session was going, or would she like to work with the nurse to begin again on a more authentic level. Laura responded that she was also confused. She immediately proceeded to deal with what was distressing her.

This demonstrates the existential use of the nurse as an authentic person, eliciting authentic behavior in the client. This new behavior in turn changes the nature of existence of the client—in this case from a shame-filled, secretive, and angry woman to one beginning to communicate more openly and responsibly.

Sociocultural

Understanding the nature of incestuous experiences and the tendency of the victim to maintain a sense of shame and secrecy, the nurse, after several individual sessions, encouraged Laura's participation in a support group for women survivors of childhood sexual abuse. This group provided social support with deep empathy among group members who shared similar childhood experiences. Consensual validation was shared as emotions and reactions were expressed. In addition, the group provided an excellent opportunity for the development of trust, intimacy, and communication skills.

In the group, sociocultural conditions were examined that currently contribute to the abuse of children. Several group members, including Laura, became involved in sexual abuse prevention programs. These empowering activities greatly enhanced self-esteem.

This case example is representative of a nurse's use of a variety of client-appropriate paths to healing. Use of an eclectic method allows variability and expression of the nurses' and clients' creative potentials. This process operates within the light of different theoretical orientations that examine the truth of human beings and how they live their lives and relate interpersonally as they share existence.

BRIEF REVIEW

Interest in the study of human behavior has existed for centuries, with theology and philosophy providing the earliest focus on behavior. Experimental psychologists introduced a scientific approach to the study of behavior. They continued to focus on conscious aspects of the mind.

The psychoanalytical school of thought, pioneered by Freud, initiated a change in the focus of behavior motivators from conscious to unconscious processes. Therapists strive to develop insights, uncover basic conflicts, and restructure the personality.

Sullivan emphasized interpersonal relations in his theory of personality. Anxiety in human relations is central to his theory. In interpersonal therapy, both therapist and client actively participate in the therapeutic process. Emphasis is on current issues and problems.

According to behaviorists, the basis for behavior is learning in response to a stimulus response and reinforcement. Skinner, Wolpe, Dollard, and Miller focus on behavioral change. Therapeutic techniques are used to promote relearning experiences that in turn change behavior. Piaget, Ellis, and Beck focused on cognitive development and processes, and alteration in patterns of thinking is the goal of therapy.

Sociocultural theorists address the effects of social processes, conditions, and attitudes on individuals. Therapy involves manipulating these conditions, such as in a therapeutic community or group. The focus is on developing harmony in human relations.

General systems theory emphasizes wholeness. An impact on one component of the system affects the functioning of the total system.

The existentialists give consideration to personal responsibility and the here and now. Humanism emphasizes health and human potential. The therapist participates in intense dialogue with the client, who assumes responsibility for establishing and achieving goals.

Biological theories contribute to our present knowledge of the human psychic condition and mental illness. Attention is given to genetic and organic factors that contribute to mental illness.

Cannon, Selye, Wolff, and Lazarus made major contributions to the theory of stress, thus increasing our understanding of the effects of stress on the body and mind as well as how to diminish or alleviate deleterious effects.

Theories of human behavior serve as a framework for the mental health–psychiatric nurse. None of the various approaches covers all the aspects of human functioning. Thus the nurse is able to select from several major theories and develop an eclectic approach to the study of behavior and application in practice.

REFERENCES AND SUGGESTED READINGS

1. Andreasen NC: *Can schizophrenia be localized in the brain?*, Washington, DC, 1984, American Psychiatric Press.
2. Andreasen NC: *The broken brain: the biological revolution in psychiatry,* New York, 1984, Harper & Row.
3. Bandura A: *Principles of behavior modification,* New York, 1969, Holt, Rinehart and Winston.
4. Beck AT: *Cognitive therapy and the emotional disorders,* New York, 1976, International Universities Press.
5. Berne E: *Transactional analysis in psychotherapy,* New York, 1961, Grove Press.
6. Berne E: *Games people play: the psychology of human relationships,* New York, 1964, Grove Press.
7. Berne E: *What do you say after you say hello: the psychology of human destiny,* New York, 1972, Grove Press.
8. Buckwalter KC: The decade of the brain and psychiatric nursing, *Archives of Psychiatric Nursing* 4(5):283, 1990.
9. Burns D: *Feeling good,* New York, 1980, Signet.
10. Cannon WB: *The wisdom of the body,* New York, 1932, WW Norton.
11. Cannon WB: Stresses and strain of homeostasis, *American Journal of Medical Sciences* 189(1):1, 1935.
12. Caudill W: *The psychiatric hospital as a small society,* Cambridge, Mass, 1958, Harvard University Press.
13. Dollard J, Miller NE: *Personality and psychotherapy: an analysis in terms of learning, thinking, and culture,* New York, 1950, McGraw-Hill.

14. Drew BJ: Devaluation of biological knowledge, *Image: Journal of Nursing Scholarship* 20(1):25, 1988.

15. Ellis A: The basic clinical theory of rational-emotive therapy. In Ellis A, Grieger R: *Handbook of rational-emotive therapy,* New York, 1978, Springer.

16. Erikson EH: *Childhood and society,* ed 2, New York, 1964, WW Norton.

17. Erikson EH: *Identity, youth and crisis,* New York, 1968, WW Norton.

18. Freud A: *The ego and mechanisms of defense,* New York, 1946, International Universities Press (Translated by C Baines).

19. Freud S: *The ego and the id,* New York, 1962, WW Norton & Co (Edited by J Strachey).

20. Freud S: *A general introduction to psychoanalysis,* New York, 1972, Pocket Books.

21. Fromm E: *Escape from freedom,* New York, 1941, Irvington Publishers.

22. Fromm E: *Man for himself,* New York, 1947, Rinehart & Winston.

23. Fromm E: *Psychoanalysis and religion,* New Haven, 1950, Yale University Press.

24. Fromm E: *The art of loving,* New York, 1956, Harper & Row.

25. Giannini JA, editor: *The biological foundations of clinical psychiatry,* New York, 1986, Elsevier Science Publishing Company.

26. Goffman E: *Asylums: essays on the social situation of mental patients and other inmates,* New York, 1961, Doubleday.

27. Goffman E: *Stigma: notes on the management of spoiled identity,* Englewood Cliffs, NJ, 1963, Prentice Hall.

28. Gold MS, Hamlin CL: Neurotransmitters and mental disorders. In Giannini AJ, editor: *The biological basis of clinical psychiatry,* New York, 1986, Elsevier Science Publishing Company.

29. Grinker RR Sr: *Toward a unified theory of human behavior,* New York, 1956, Basic Books.

30. Jones M: *The therapeutic community,* New York, 1953, Basic Books.

31. Jourard S: *Disclosing man to himself,* Princeton, NJ, 1968, D Van Nostrand.

32. Jourard S: *The transparent self,* New York, 1971, Van Nostrand Reinhold.

33. Jung CG: *The psychogenesis of mental disease,* New York, 1960, Pantheon Books.

34. Jung CG: *Two essays on analytical psychology,* Princeton, NJ, 1966, Princeton University Press.

35. Laing RD: *The politics of experience,* New York, 1967, Ballantine Books.

36. Laing RD: *Knots,* New York, 1972, Random House.

37. Laing RD: *Self and others,* Baltimore, 1975, Penguin Books.

38. Lazarus R: *Psychological stress and the coping process,* New York, 1966, McGraw-Hill Book Co.

39. Leighton A: *My name is legion: foundations for a theory of man in relation to culture,* vol 1, The Stirling County study of psychiatric disorders and sociocultural environment, New York, 1959, Basic Books.

40. Lewin K: *A dynamic theory of personality: selected papers,* New York, 1935, McGraw-Hill Book Co.

41. Liaschenko J: Changing paradigms with psychiatry: implications for nursing research, *Archives of Psychiatric Nursing* 3(3):153, 1989.

42. Main TF: *The hospital as a therapeutic institution, Bulletin of the Menninger Clinic* 10:66, January 1946.

43. Maslow A: *Toward a psychology of being,* Princeton, NJ, 1962, D Van Nostrand.

44. Maslow A: *Motivation and personality,* ed 2, New York, 1970, Harper & Row.

45. Mead GJ: *Mind, self, and society,* Chicago, 1934, University of Chicago Press.

46. McEnany GW: Psychobiological indices of bipolar mood disorder: future trends in nursing care, *Archives of Psychiatric Nursing* 4(1):29, 1990.

47. McGue M, Gottesman II: Genetic linkage in schizophrenia: perspective from genetic epidemiology, *Schizophrenia Bulletin* 15:453, 1989.

48. McKeon KL: Introduction: a future on psychiatric mental health nursing, *Archives of Psychiatric Nursing* 3(3):153, 1989.

49. Owen F and others: Neurotransmitter receptors in brain in schizophrenia, *Acta Psychiatrica Scandinavica* 291:20, 1981.

50. Perls F: *The gestalt approach,* Palo Alto, Calif, 1970, Science & Behavior Books.

51. Perls F: *The gestalt therapy book,* New York, 1973, Julian Press.

52. Piaget J: *The origin of intelligence in children,* New York, 1952, International Universities Press.

53. Piaget J: *The child's conception of the world,* Ames, Ia, 1963, Littlefield, Adams & Co.

54. Selye H: *The stress of life,* rev ed, New York, 1976, McGraw-Hill Book Co.

55. Sidman M: *Tactics of scientific research,* New York, 1960, Basic Books.

56. Skinner BF: *Science and human behavior,* New York, 1953, The Macmillan Co.

57. Skinner BF: *Beyond freedom and dignity,* New York, 1971, Alfred A Knopf.

58. Sullivan HS: *Interpersonal theory of psychiatry,* New York, 1953, WW Norton & Co.

59. Szasz T: *The myth of mental illness,* New York, 1974, Harper & Row.

60. Usdin E, Mandell AJ, editors: *Biochemistry of mental disorders,* New York, 1978, Marcel Dekker.

61. von Bertalanffy L: *General systems theory: foundations, development, applications,* New York, 1968, George Braziller.

62. Wolff HG: *Life stress and bodily diseases,* Baltimore, 1950, Williams & Wilkins.

63. Wolff HG: *Stress and disease,* Springfield, Ill, 1953, Charles C Thomas.

64. Wolpe J: *The practice of behavior therapy,* ed 2, New York, 1973, Pergamon Press.

65. Yalom I: *Existential psychotherapy,* New York, 1980, Basic Books.

ANNOTATED BIBLIOGRAPHY

Andreasen NC: *The broken brain: the biological revolution in psychiatry,* New York, 1984, Harper & Row.

This easy to read text includes content that is still relevant to the current focus on the relationship between the brain and psychiatry. The text presents a collection of articles that address various aspects of the biological basis of mental illness that have implications for the practice of psychiatric nursing. The author also intends to educate the reader about and increase sensitivity to mental illness.

Burton A, editor: *Operational theories of personality,* New York, 1974, Brunner/Mazel, Inc.

This book provides a discussion of personality theories that deal with change in the personality and that conceive personality as a growing entity. Each theory is described by its founder or a major apostle. The concepts and techniques of the theory are applied, using a case study.

McBride AB: Psychiatric nursing in the 1990s, *Archives of Psychiatric Nursing,* 4(11):21, 1990.

This article highlights the current biological focus on mental illness. The author emphasizes the need for psychiatric nurses to integrate biological knowledge with the psychological, social, and cultural factors that also influence human behavior.

Margaret T Beard
Margie N Johnson

After studying this chapter, the student will be able to:

- Discuss key factors in the historical development of mental health–psychiatric nursing theory
- Describe the philosophical foundations and major concepts characterizing each nursing theory
- Analyze the usefulness of theoretical frameworks in providing a holistic approach to mental health–psychiatric nursing concepts

- Assess relative strengths and weaknesses of the nursing theories in guiding nursing practice
- Identify research problems to test the applicability of selected theories to mental health–psychiatric nursing practice

Grand theories emerged as nurses began to focus on the content of their profession. A grand theory consists of broad concepts from which more specific theoretical frameworks are derived. Early theoretical writings depicted nursing as a process centered around the relationship between the client and nurse. Peplau's focus on interpersonal relationships,[47] Roger's formulation of person-environment interaction,[49] and King's view of nurse-client transaction[28] are examples of grand theories.

In the mid- to late 1970s several theorists and their followers began to develop middle range theories through the testing of grand theories. A middle range theory consists of a conceptual scheme from which working hypotheses can be derived and tested. The client's perspective forms middle range theory. Thus Orem's view of the client as a self-care agent,[43] Johnson's view of the client as a behavioral system,[25] and Roy's view of the client as a holistic adaptive person[51] are specific examples of attempts to develop middle range theory.

In the past decade many writers have stressed that nursing theories should be practice oriented. A theory of practice consists of a set of interrelated theories of action that specify, according to the situation, the action that will, under the relevant circumstances, yield the intended consequences.[38] Practice theory is needed to direct nursing therapeutics and to evaluate outcomes of nursing interventions.

The six major theoretical nursing approaches described in this chapter are in various stages of development, but each gives some direction to practice. The work of each theorist helps explain the holistic perspective of persons in a psychiatric–mental health context.

PEPLAU'S INTERPERSONAL THEORY

Hildegard Peplau's book *Interpersonal Relations in Nursing*[47] made a major contribution to theory-based practice. Her approach, which evolved from problems in clinical situations, is process oriented and focuses on interpersonal theory as applied to the nurse-client relationship.

Major Concepts

The core of Peplau's approach is interpersonal relations. The theory includes concepts such as communication, roles, and growth and development. All are used in expanding her conceptualization of the therapeutic nurse-client relationship. Communication is a problem-solving process whereby the nurse and client collaborate to meet the client's needs. The position assumed by the nurse during various phases of the relationship is know as a *role*. The nurse may assume the roles of counselor, leader, resource, surrogate, teacher, or technical expert to address the client's needs. In the therapeutic interaction, these roles are designed to lead to growth and development.

A diagram of the major concepts of Peplau's theory is provided in Figure 5-1. Peplau views the therapeutic relationship as being divided into four sequential phases: orientation, identification, exploitation, and resolution. The

HISTORICAL OVERVIEW

DATES	EVENTS
Before 1860	Atheoretical
1860-1951	Florence Nightingale: *Notes on nursing: what it is and what it is not* (environmental theory)
1952-1959	Grand theories formulations (for example, Hildegard E. Peplau)
1960-1964	Metatheoretical writings regarding the necessity of theory for nursing Grand theories Nursing science emphasized the need for a theoretical base for practice predicated on holism and the interconnectedness of person and environment
1965-1970	Nursing theory development conferences (Norris—1969, 1970, and 1971) WICHE Conferences
1971-1975	Conceptual frameworks for curriculua required by NLN Grand theories continue Middle range theories begin Nurse educator conferences Nursing theory conferences Theory construction writings
1978	Advances in Nursing Science (ANS) begun as a forum for testing and developing nursing theory and nursing science
1980	Postdoctoral theory conferences—Clemson University Practice theory
1984	Nursing Science Colloquia—Boston University theory
1990	Symposium on Knowledge Development—University of Rhode Island
1991	Biennial Nurse Theorist Conference. Nursing worldwide: a futuristic view, Tokyo, Japan
Future	Testing nursing theories in mental health—psychiatric nursing will contribute to their usefulness in practice

activities involved in each of these phases are described in Table 5-1.

Holistic Perspective

The holistic approach to the person, family, and community is inherent in Peplau's theory. The nurse's approach mobilizes the person's innate capacity for self-healing and growth. Individual therapy in the interpersonal process allows the client to discover and resolve potentially chronic intrapsychic and relationship patterns. Other holistic threads emphasize interpersonal relations, illness as an opportunity for discovery, and an appreciation for the quality of life and an interest in improving it. The interpersonal process affects both nurse and client because both experience growth.

Physical dimension The physical dimension is reflected in the client's somatic responses to life experiences. For example, the emotional and physical dimensions are interrelated in insomnia caused by emotional trauma. Insomnia may be brought on by anxiety generated by an emotional experience such as separation from a loved one, as an expression of hostile feelings toward certain family members, or as a result of physical illness. Extra attention given a client keeps the anxiety within tolerable limits.

The physical dimension is reflected in the following principles of Peplau's approach:

1. Instinctual drives are imperative individual needs that lead to tension and demand tension reduction.
2. Tension can be discharged in active or passive behavior, or it may become bound within the person.
3. When the energy of tension is bound, as in a symptom, relief is felt when the tension is reduced through constructive action.

The nurse and client discuss and agree on the value of the client's responses to various experiences.

Emotional dimension The emotional dimension of the person is inherent in Peplau's belief that nurses help individuals develop ways to convert tension and anxiety into purposeful action. Energy derived from needs, frustra-

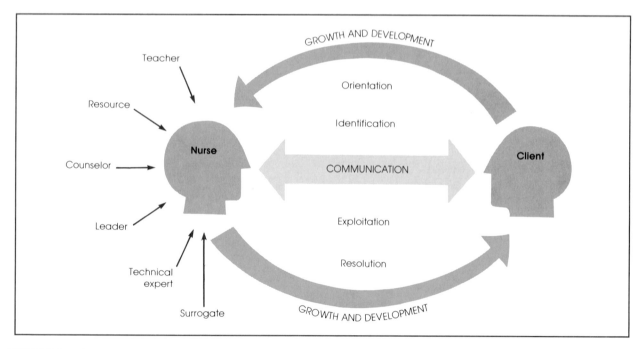

FIGURE 5-1 Peplau's nurse-client interpersonal framework.

tion, conflict, and anxiety is transformed into action. Because of the subjectivity of the client's emotional responses, the nurse must have a high level of self-awareness and be able to recognize the various types of overt and covert actions and reactions that the client may display through the various phases of the relationship.

Intellectual dimension The intellectual dimension is apparent in Peplau's emphasis on the individual's capacity and responsibility for development. The person has the ability to acquire, process, and integrate information obtained in the nurse-client relationship. Learning and memory allow the individual to store and recall information for problem solving in future situations. Information is organized and reorganized as the nurse works with the client through the various stages of the relationship.

Social dimension This dimension emphasizes the importance of socialization during growth and development. Nurse-client interactions can be a micromodel of general social interactions between the client and people from past and present relationships. Ways of functioning in society are learned over time as social exchange, values, perceptions, and behaviors are adopted. Disruptions in significant social relationships vary according to the amount of instability the individual experiences. Peplau contends that understanding the sociocultural context in which the client functions provides valuable information for assisting the client's return to healthy, spontaneous interactions in the social environment.

Spiritual dimension The spiritual dimension develops as a result of cultural forces. Children acquire the beliefs, values, and ethics of a given culture from caretaking adults who express and exemplify them. Peplau states that clients may question their faith in others and their social and ethical beliefs. She suggests using a method that explores doubts and feelings and discovers convictions. Pe-

TABLE 5-1   **Activities in Phases of the Therapeutic Relationship**

Phases	Activities
Orientation	Establish need to seek professional help
	Establish working relationship
	Listen for themes that may help define problem areas more clearly
	Determine whether to continue the relationship or whether referral needs to be made
Identification	Clarify perceptions and expectations
	Identify problems more clearly
	Discuss preliminary solutions to problems
Exploitation	Work out conscious and unconscious conflicts that may not be well understood by either client or nurse
	Create a nonthreatening atmosphere
	Demonstrate confidence in client's ability to become involved in problem solving
	Clarify, listen, accept, and interpret
Resolution	Determine whether client's needs have been met
	Work through difficulties in terminating the relationship
	Use the bond that has developed as a positive force for moving the client into other meaningful relationships
	Assist client in setting new goals

plau emphasizes the role of interprofessional relations with clergy.

Clinical Application

The following case example will be referred to in subsequent discussions about the clinical applications of each theorist's approach.

▼ Case Example

Susan, age 14, was admitted to the psychiatric unit from the emergency room after inflicting two cuts on her left arm in a suicide attempt. She stated that she had thought of killing herself by cutting her wrist but decided she did not want to die.

Two days earlier, Susan had run away with a 20-year-old female friend who was unhappy with her family situation. During the episode, Susan lost her bags that contained all her clothes when she left them unattended in a restaurant. On her return home, her mother gave her money to buy more clothes. However, Susan stated, "I threw the money away also."

At the time of admission her mother reported that Susan had suffered from depression 2 years earlier. On the unit Susan was fearful and wanted her mother to remain with her; however, her mother had to return to work and could spend only a short time with Susan. After the mother returned to work, Susan telephoned her several times, "just to talk."

Susan has a 22-year-old brother and a 19-year-old sister. Her father is an ex-military man who is beginning his own business as a television repairman. Her mother attends school full-time in the mornings and works in the evenings. Susan's family traveled a lot and moved frequently from one location to another because of her father's military career. The family has been in its present residence for about 5 months.

Using Peplau's theory, the nurse establishes a therapeutic relationship with Susan. The five dimensions are explored as the nurse proceeds through the orientation, identification, exploitation, and resolution phases of the relationship. In assessing the emotional dimension, for example, the nurse may focus on the tension and anxiety Susan is experiencing. The nurse seeks ways to assist Susan's release of the tension through constructive channels. Through the therapeutic nurse-client relationship Susan is allowed to discover the most effective ways to release tension. Basic physical and safety needs are met in response to Susan's self-destructive behavior. In the intellectual dimension, the nurse judges Susan as capable of self-control and responsibility. Susan integrates and processes information obtained from the relationship to recall old problem-solving techniques and to learn new ones. The nurse vigilantly evaluates Susan's behavior until she can use her skills for responsible self-control.

There is considerable evidence in this case that Susan has some doubts about her social relationships with her family and friends. Past and present disappointments have perhaps eroded her faith (spiritual dimension) in herself and others, significantly diminishing her hope for recovery and for a meaningful existence.

As the work with Susan progresses through the phases of relationship, the nurse is alert for indications of Susan's recovery. In some instances, however, a lessening of anxiety may actually reflect Susan's decision to repeat self-destructive behavior, but if open communcation is continually en-

couraged, trust between Susan and the nurse may motivate Susan to move toward health rather than toward illness.

As described in Table 5-5, a weakness of Peplau's approach is that little attention is given to the various dimensions. In particular, the spiritual dimension can only be assumed to be present within the nurse-client interpersonal framework.

OREM'S SELF-CARE MODEL

The self-care concept of nursing as perceived by Dorothea Orem was first published in 1959.[13] Orem, like other theorists, views nursing as an interpersonal process, with nurses given direct, necessary assistance to individuals who, because of health conditions, cannot provide self-care. Self-care is defined as the continuous contribution adults give to personal health and well-being.[44]

Major Concepts

The major concepts of Orem's theory are *self-care* and *nursing systems* (Figure 5-2). The word *self* in the term self-care is used in the sense of one's whole being. Self-care connotes "for oneself" and "given by oneself." Self-care agency is the ability to engage in self-care. The development of this ability is aided by intellectual curiosity, instruction, supervision from others, and experience performing self-care measures. Self-care deficits occur when health-related problems require nursing care. Self-care requisites are universal and include health deviations and developmental processes.

Universal self-care requisites, common to persons during all stages of life, are associated with life processes and with maintaining the integrity of human structure and functioning. Universal self-care includes sufficient intake of air, water, and foods; care related to excrements; balance of activity and rest; balance of solitude and social interactions; and prevention of hazards to one's well-being.[45]

Self-care requisites for healthy deviation are concerned with genetic and constitutional defects and structural and functional aberrations. The focus is on diagnosis and treatment. Health deviation self-care requisites include seeking and securing appropriate health assistance, carrying out prescribed measures effectively, and learning to live with the residual effects of illness and treatment.

Developmental self-care requisites are specialized expressions of the universal self-care requisites. They are associated with human developmental processes and with conditions and events occurring during the life cycle.

The nurse is concerned with the client's self-care deficit. When helping the client address self-care deficits, the nurse considers the orientation, skills, knowledge, and motivation of the client for overcoming deficits and improving self-care agency.

The second major concept, nursing systems, includes the approaches nurses use to assist clients with self-care deficits caused by health conditions. Nursing systems include all actions and interactions of nurses and clients in nursing practice situations. Compensatory processes are actions performed by nurses, clients, or both to meet client's self-care requisites. These compensatory processes may be partly or wholly educational.

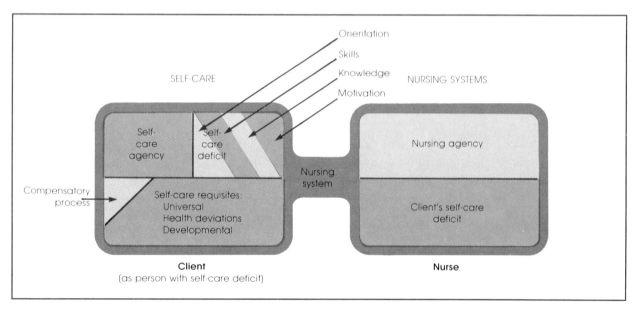

FIGURE 5-2 Orem's self-care framework.

Nursing agency is the special ability of nurses to provide total care as a unit. Nursing agency, analogous to self-care agency, constitutes ability for specialized types of deliberate nursing actions. Nursing agency is developed and exercised for the benefit and well-being of others, whereas self-care agency is for oneself.

Holistic Perspective

According to Orem, individuals are responsible for sustaining their own health. Therefore therapeutic techniques rely on the client rather than on the nurse. The emphasis on self-care encourages approaches that mobilize the individual's innate capacity for self-healing.

Physical dimension A person's physical dimension, according to Orem's theory, is addressed by the following categories of universal self-care demands: air, water, food, excretion, activity and rest, and physical hazards. Assessment of subjective and objective data for each of these self-care demands assists the nurse in helping the client develop an optimal level of self-care agency. The nurse then helps the client to meet self-care demands regarding respiration, fluids and electrolytes, metabolism, excretory processes, activity and rest, and protection against hazards.

Emotional dimension After determining the client's need, the nurse designs activities to foster self-care. The emotional dimension may be indicated by a need to foster bonds of affection, love, friendship and closeness, and managing impulses.

Intellectual dimension Developing the intellectual dimension of self-care agency involves learning in the course of day-to-day living. The nurse intervenes to prevent disturbances in cognition, memory, and learning. Optimal functioning is encouraged by activities that stimulate, engage, and balance intellectual efforts. Orem's framework emphasizes preventive health care. The primary prevention of self-care demands includes universal and developmental self-care requisites. Secondary and tertiary prevention self-

care demands include health deviation, universal, and developmental self-care requisites.

Social dimension Socialization is required in the nursing situation because both nurse and client are strangers entering a helping relationship. The client may need role preparation.[45] The client's ability to accept the role may be influenced by temperament, self-image, and life-style. The nurse may also be affected by those factors, in addition to the clients' age, sex, race, culture, social status, or disease.

Spiritual dimension The spiritual dimension in Orem's framework is the search for a meaningful philosophy of life. The goal of health care is to enable persons to understand the illness. A meaningful philosophy teaches the client to live with the effects of pathological conditions and to develop a life-style that promotes continued personal development. Orem advocates that nurses, in gathering personal information about clients, determine clients' religious orientations. This information helps nurses understand how such affiliations limit or qualify the values of the nursing system variables and the operation of nursing practice.

Clinical Application

Using Orem's theory within the holistic perspective, the nurse assists Susan in optimizing the development of self-care agency (see the case example on p. 74). The five dimensions are explored in an analysis of self-care agency and therapeutic self-care demand. Following this analysis, Susan's self-care deficits in orientation, skills, knowledge, and motivation are identified.

The self-care agency can be understood from the description of Susan as a client, a 14-year-old, and a daughter. Universal and health deviation self-care require that Susan develops self-care agency. Susan's self-care agency deficit requires intervention in terms of coping patterns.

Suicidal behavior is a deviation from health. The necessary interventions are focused on assessing Susan's self-care demands. These demands include guidance and teaching coping strategies to deal with destructive tendencies. The nurse gathers information about how Susan perceives and reacts in family or social situations. The nurse may use guided imagery as a technique for teaching Susan to improve her coping patterns. The nurse may also teach Susan to tense and relax muscle groups as a method of improving coping patterns and enhancing Susan's ability to meet her self-care demands. Susan's depressed feelings, suicidal thoughts, and self-injury represent health deviations within the emotional dimension. Developmentally, Susan is experiencing a time of emotional turmoil with mood swings.

Based on the limited case example data, it is assumed that no skills or orientation deficits exist. However, Susan may have deficits in knowledge and motivation. The goal is to overcome the deficits through self-care.

To overcome deficits in knowledge, the nurse helps Susan to identify stress as a precipitating factor for her hospitalization. The goal for Susan's self-care is to identify stressful situations. The health hazard consists of injurious behaviors as a function of stress. Intellectually, Susan is capable of understanding and learning to cope with stressful situations.

Socially, there are requisites to assist Susan in functioning optimally. Susan wants and needs guidance from a responsible adult, although she may resist these efforts from time to time. She can learn to be responsible for her health-related care.

The nurse determines and assesses deficits in motivation and implements self-care by encouraging Susan to talk about her long-term and short-term life goals. The nurse identifies and explores sources of support for Susan that are helpful to Susan spiritually as she regains faith in herself and in others.

The strengths and weaknesses of Orem's theory are presented in Table 5-5.

KING'S GOAL ATTAINMENT THEORY

The early works of Imogene King appeared in the literature in the mid-1960s. King's approach emphasizes the nursing process as a dynamic interpersonal process between the nurse and individuals in various social systems. Through reciprocal interactions, mutual nursing activities are defined to assist individuals to function in society. For King[28,29] health is the outcome of behaviors directed toward goal attainment.

Major Concepts

King's theory of goal attainment encompasses three broad, interlocking, open systems: the personal, interpersonal, and social systems. The personal systems (self) and the social systems (self and society) influence the quality of care, but the major elements in the goal attainment theory are contained in the interpersonal systems. In these systems two or more persons come together under the guidance of a health care organization to promote an optimal state of health. The major concepts within the interpersonal systems are interaction, perception, communication, transaction, role, stress, growth and development, and time and space (Figure 5-3).

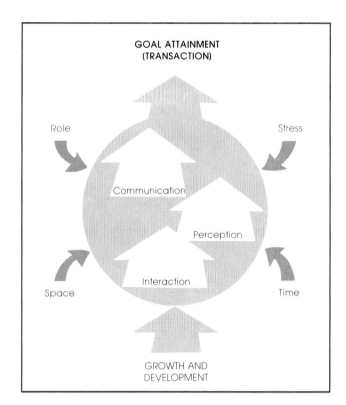

FIGURE 5-3 King's goal attainment theory.

Interactions are defined as actions and reactions between persons or between persons and the environment. Purposeful interactions establish a frame of reference, and mutually agreed upon goals are developed. Interactions become increasingly complex as more individuals become involved. As diversity (for example, in background, experience, and motivation) among individuals increases, so does the complexity of the interactions. However, if the diversity is too extreme, interactions may not occur at all. When interpersonal interactions are not successful, disruptive factors can usually be identified and resolved or alleviated.

King defines perception as "a process of organizing, interpreting and transforming information from sense data and memory. . . . [Perception] gives meaning to one's experience, represents one's image of reality and influences one's behavior."[28] A person's perceptual and intellectual tools are related to past experiences, concept of self, biological inheritance, educational background, and socioeconomic group. A nursing assessment takes into account the potential or actual differences between the perceptions held by the nurse and those held by the client. Accurate perception, by which both nurse and client interpret sensory data, is a primary step toward identifying mutual goals and determining strategies for goal attainment. A conflict between the nurse and client as they perceive problems and their resolution may delay the client's return to a healthy state. For example, a nurse assesses a client's pain and determines that medication is needed to decrease suffering. However, the nurse may actually do more harm than good if the client perceives the pain level as discomforting but within a personal range of tolerance. Each individual needs to be seen as unique with different needs, values, resources, and expectations.

The concept of communication is basic in King's framework. She defines communication as the exchange of feelings, perceptions, and values between and among individuals. Communication is the information portion of interaction and may be direct (verbal) or indirect (nonverbal). Although communication is universal, the verbal and nonverbal symbols vary from one culture to another and from one person to another. Communication is further influenced by an individual's stress level, development level, prior experience, and the current context of the interaction. Communication, whether verbal or nonverbal, is a function of the total person; the self cannot be separated from what is communicated. Any message that is conveyed has significance for the overall well-being of the individual. What an individual does not say or do is just as important as what the person does say or do. Effective communication assists individuals to gain a sense of understanding about themselves and helps meaningful relationships with others emerge.

Transaction is the contractual agreement resulting from a number of interactions. This product of communication is influenced by individual viewpoints. Transaction is the goal of the interpersonal process between the nurse and the client.

King emphasizes the importance of transaction in a therapeutic relationship. The implication is that individuals entering the relationship take active roles in defining goals and resolving problems. Continuous give-and-take occurs as the nurse and client progress toward a transaction. Ideas, beliefs, and values are communicated between the individuals as the process evolves. The social exchange between nurse and client should always be open, honest, and mutual. Any transaction between different individuals, or between the same individuals at different times, is unique; thus transactions have temporal and spatial dimensions. The data gathered through interactions provide the nurse with the tools for implementing the nursing process.

Role and stress continuously influence interaction, perception, communication, and transactions. Role, as defined by King, is a set of observable behaviors expected of individuals in the interpersonal system. The client and the nurse have expectations of each other based on accurate or inaccurate information. When roles are misinterpreted, conflict arises, and conflict decreases the effectiveness of the interpersonal relationship. Correct information about role behaviors and functions is communicated through ongoing interactions. To King, the purpose of nursing is mutual transaction between persons to assess health status and promote an optimal state of health. The roles of the nurse and client are defined within this context.

Stress involves an exchange of energy for the purpose of maintaining balance and promoting growth. Stress is dynamic and continuously influences interactions. Nurses are expected to assist clients and their families in reducing the stress that interferes with optimal functioning. Just as stress affects the health status of the client, it also affects the health status of the nurse. When noxious environmental stressors influence the nurse and the client, a narrowing of perception and a decrease in interactions occur. The result is that mutual goal setting for effective nursing care is diminished, and the opportunity for growth on the part of both individuals is limited. An outside source may be necessary to help the nurse regain equilibrium and increase the effectiveness of coping skills. When equilibrium is reestablished, the nurse can help the client examine the negative factors that were present in the situation. The process used by the nurse in coping with stress serves as a model for clients.

Holistic Perspective

Implicit in King's theory is a holistic orientation. Although her major focus is on the individual as a social being, she implies that persons use energy to react as whole organisms to experiences and events. Aspects of holism can also be found in King's definition of health as continuous adjustment to environmental stressors through optimal use of one's resources. King maintains that health is the way individuals deal with the stressors of growth and development while functioning in various roles and cultural environments. An analysis of the dimensions reflects King's emphasis on the social dimension of the person.

Physical dimension The physical dimension can be inferred from King's broad concept of growth and development. These two life processes represent continuous changes in individuals at the cellular and behavioral activity levels. Growth and development help persons move from a potential achievement level to self-actualization, a critical variable.

King's concept of time may also be included in the physical dimension. Time is a continuous flow of successive events, implying change, a past, and a future. It is related to rhythmicity and is observed in body temperature, elimination, sleep-wake cycles, metabolism, and fluid and electrolyte balance. Time and space perceptions are important in nurse-client interaction. Interactions in hospitals may occur in places that restrict space, such as a client's room. The client's territory is defined by behavior as well as the boundaries of actual space.

Emotional dimension King also addresses the emotional dimension in her discussion of growth and development. The developing individual has the potential for achievement and self-satisfaction. Nurses and clients share information as transactions are made to meet goals. This helps individuals achieve their greatest potential for a meaningful life.

Intellectual dimension For King the intellectual dimension may be inferred from the concept of perception. Perception leads the person to recall and attribute meaning based on past experience. In assessing the intellectual dimension, the nurse can ascertain disturbances in perception such as illusions, hallucinations, and autistic thinking.

Social dimension King addresses the social dimension more fully than the other dimensions. King's goal of nursing is assisting the individual, a social being, to function effectively within the following three dynamically interacting social systems: (1) the personal system, (2) the interpersonal system, and (3) the social system. To these systems the nurse may focus on such questions as What stress factors interfere with the individual's functioning in certain roles in society? What factors interfere with the development of meaningful relationships with others?

Spiritual dimension The person's spiritual dimension is implied in King's concept of health. Health relates to the way persons deal with the stress of personal, interpersonal, and social growth. One of the stressors is maintaining a level of health that enables a person to live a relatively useful, satisfying, productive, and happy life each day. In this way an assessment of personal, interpersonal, and social relationships as they contribute to the sense of well-being and fulfillment is an assessment of spiritual health.

Clinical Application

Using King's theory to assist the nurse in the clinical case of Susan (refer to the case example on p. 74) involves several concepts. Within the context of the interpersonal system, the nurse strives to develop a relationship in which both nurse and client are involved in identifying health problems and the changes needed to attain goals. Interpersonal interactions between the nurse and Susan involve perceiving and communicating to derive a transaction, or contractual agreement, for achieving goals. The assessment identifies stressors, primarily in the emotional and social realms. Interactions between the nurse and Susan are influenced by the needs and past experiences that each brings to the situation. Both nurse and client have values, goals, and expectations that affect the interaction. The nurse refrains from making a value judgment about Susan's suicidal behavior and about the family's apparent neglect of Susan's needs; however, the nurse may assume that Susan has difficulties in personal, interpersonal, and social relationships.

As described in Table 5-5, King's approach, perhaps more than the other approaches discussed in this chapter, emphasizes the social dimension almost to the exclusion of the other four dimensions. The specific directions for nurse-client interaction are a major strength of this approach.

JOHNSON'S BEHAVIORAL SYSTEMS THEORY

Dorothy Johnson presented her framework for nursing in 1968. Johnson's behavioral systems approach emphasizes the nurse's role in promoting optimal health for the individual. Health is maintained when the system's units (or subsystems) are kept in balance. The aim of the approach is to integrate the subsystem's functions for overall system stability and growth.[18,26]

Major Concepts

Johnson's theory is based on the broad concepts of system and behavior. Individuals, as systems, respond to environmental input and produce behavioral output. System units include the affiliative, dependence, achievement, ingestive, eliminative, sexual, and aggressive-protective subsystems. Behavior is linked with each subsystem in response to the subsystem's components: goal, set, choices, and action. Figure 5-4 depicts the feedback operation responsible for integrating environmental input and behavioral output. Behavior is the visible feature of the system and the nurse's most important concern.

These seven subsystems contribute to the functioning

▼ **TABLE 5-2** Subsystem Goals

Subsystems	Goals
Affiliative	Security
Dependence	Self-dependence and interdependence
Achievement	Mastery of self and environment according to an internalized standard of excellence
Ingestive	Taking in nourishment in socially and culturally acceptable ways
Eliminative	Ridding system of waste in socially and culturally acceptable ways
Sexual	Procreation and gratification
Aggressive-protective	Survival

of the overall behavioral system. The goals of each of the subsystems are described in Table 5-2.

The components of each subsystem (goal, set, choices, and action) provide its structure. The goal is the drive or motivational aspect of the system. The set is the predisposition to act with reference to the goal. Choices are the repertoire of available alternatives. Action leads to the system's behavioral output. Each subsystem is further guided by variables such as age, sex, motives, values, and rewards. These structural components of each subsystem give direction for nursing assessment, analysis, planning, intervention, and evaluation.

Holistic Perspective

Johnson sees the person as an open system with seven broadly defined subsystems, interacting with the environment by receiving input and displaying behavioral output. Each subsystem has a motivational component and a reservoir of potential behaviors, choices, and actions. The systems, which are interrelated, reflect the total person as a behavioral being. Although Johnson does not specifically address the following dimensions these aspects can be inferred from the subsystems.

Physical dimension The physical dimension encompasses the ingestive, eliminative, and sexual subsystems. Subsystem responses are affected by when, how much, and under what conditions subsystem behaviors occur. For example, in the sexual subsystem, the dual functions of procreation and gratification are considered. If a deficit exists in this subsystem, some type of sexual dysfunction may occur. Each subsystem can be assessed in terms of its behavioral response to stress within the various dimensions.

Intellectual dimension The intellectual dimension may be assessed through an evaluation of the achievement subsystem. The achievement subsystem's results include a sense of mastery over one's environment. Mastery implies memory, learning, and growth are elements of the intellectual dimension. Stress impinging on this subsystem may thwart the achievement of life goals. For example, an im-

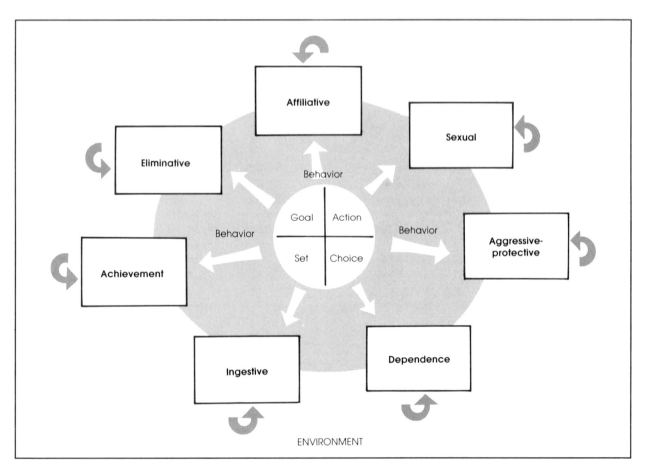

FIGURE 5-4 Basic structures of Johnson's behavioral subsystems.

prisoned individual may become intellectually dull and consequently unable to develop into a productive person. The nurse employing Johnson's theory to provide holistic mental health nursing care may find this dimension particularly useful in working with individuals in isolated situations. Helping the isolated person find creative and innovative ways to achieve optimal environmental control is a challenge to the nurse.

Social dimension Because the affiliative and dependence subsystems result in social inclusion and forming social bonds, both can be included in the social dimension. The nurse's goal in working with a recently widowed elderly woman, for example, may be to assist her in joining community groups in which other aged persons have regular, well-established recreational activities.

Spiritual dimension The client's relationship with himself and with another person in attaining personal inclusion and developing a meaningful existence are important to the spiritual dimension. The affiliative subsystem again gives the nurse the information necessary for assessment within this dimension.

Clinical Application

Johnson's theory directs the nurse to establish a data base regarding Susan's nursing care (see the case example on p. 74) by observing the subsystems and their structural components. The general goal of this nursing intervention is to help Susan achieve balance in all systems so she can function effectively.

Susan's aggressive and dependence subsystems seem most affected. The set in the aggressive-protective subsystem, as reflected by Susan's behavior, is a predisposition to act in a self-destructive manner by cutting her arm. The choice confronting Susan is to harm or not to harm herself. Susan chose to inflict only minor injury on herself. Finally, the goal of Susan's behavior in the aggressive subsystem is to seek protection from self-destructive impulses. Susan's ability to seek protection depends on internally and externally available resources. Thus the nurse's assessment and intervention in this subsystem takes into account the goal of protection. Active suicide precautions may be indicated initially, in conjunction with an opportunity to help Susan talk about her feelings of anger and hostility.

Regarding disruption in the dependence subsystem, the set exemplified by Susan is attention-seeking behavior, which has probably been present for some time. Susan's frequent telephone calls from the hospital to her mother exemplify her attention-seeking alliance with friends or family. Susan seems to have some ambivalence regarding this choice. Observable behavior, or action, is reflected in Susan's self-destructive behavior and running away from home and school. These are responses to frustration in meeting dependence needs. The goal in the dependence subsystem is seen in Susan's seeking reassurance from her mother. The nurse's focusing primarily on the dependence subsystem will assist Susan in reestablishing appropriate trusting relationships with significant others. Family therapy, as well as individual therapy, may be indicated.

The nurse using Johnson's theoretical approach needs to remember that disruption in one subsystem may cause disruption in one or several other subsystems. Therefore all subsystems need to be assessed for possible changes in system stability.

The strengths and weaknesses of Johnson's approach are highlighted in Table 5-5.

ROGERS' THEORY OF THE UNITARY PERSON

Because Martha Rogers' theory addresses the science of nursing, the terms and concepts are somewhat different from those used in the other theories discussed here. Pulling from fields such as anthropology, sociology, philosophy, and history, Rogers[49,50] has postulated a view of the person as a continuously evolving unitary person.

Major Concepts

Two broad concepts capture the essence of Rogers' theoretical framework of the unitary person—life process and homeodynamics (Figure 5-5). Life process encompasses energy fields embedded in a four-dimensional space-time matrix that becomes increasingly complex as it evolves rhyth-mically along life's longitudinal axis. Life process is continuous, dynamic, and changing. It evolves irreversibly and unidirectionally along a space-time continuum. Thus a living system (a person) is an evolving process that emerges and moves continually forward from birth through death. The system is characterized by identifiable patterns and rhythms.

The energy fields of the life process are the human field and the environmental field. The human and environmental fields are open systems. The environment, external to the individual, interacts and exchanges matter and energy with the person so that a pattern of wholeness emerges.

Homeodynamics includes principles of complementarity, helicy, and resonancy. Complementarity recognizes life as a continuously changing process, influenced by the interaction of person and environment. Helicy refers to the direction of change-forward, nonrepeatable, irreversible, and increasing in complexity and diversity. Resonancy suggests change that increases in rate and intensity over time. Thus principles of homeodynamics are a way of viewing persons in their complex wholeness.

Holistic Perspective

The holistic perspective of persons assumes that characteristics of wholeness and unity exists. A person's total response is the focus of concern.

Self-responsibility stems from self-regulation, a dynamic quality directed toward orderly innovation and fulfillment

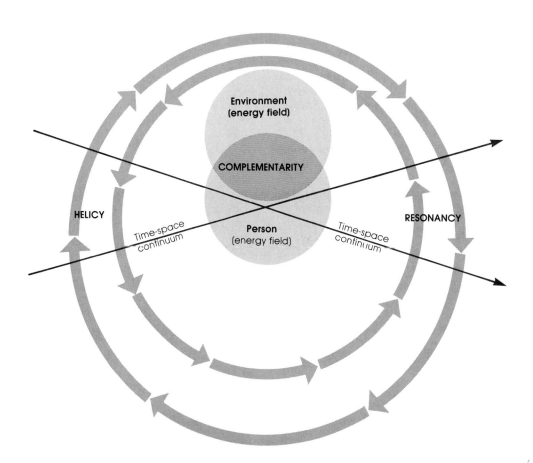

FIGURE 5-5 Rogers' unitary person framework.

of life's potential. Persons interacting with the environment have the capacity to arrange the environment and to exercise choice in fulfilling their potential.

Physical dimension Rogers' theory of a unitary wholeness of persons negates viewing people in a compartmental manner. Wholeness with regard to the individual's physical dimension may be observed in sleep-wake cycles, elimination, and respiratory processes. Rogers suggests that some physiological functions are subject to conscious control.

Emotional dimension An individual's emotional dimension is reflected in the unique nature of persons as feeling and sensing beings. People evolve through interaction with the environment. For example, pain thresholds vary greatly from one individual to another primarily as a result of the individual's emotional makeup and perception. Other feelings in this dimension involve expressions of joy, sorrow, affection, and sadness. Within the emotional realm, communication is the tool for transmitting feelings.

Intellectual dimension The intellectual dimension is based on the person as a thinking, rational being. An individual's capacity for abstraction, imagery, language, and thought are tools of the intellectual sphere. With these tools the individual seeks to organize and understand experiences and the environment. An emerging understanding surpasses an accumulation of facts and events.

Social dimension Rogers addresses the social dimension by assessing a person's history of such social behaviors as smoking, drinking, and employment. Cultural attitudes toward health and illness and the use of health resources are important determinants of an individual's behavior.

The social nature of the individual is implicit in the person-environment interaction. As an open system, the individual is continually affected by environmental forces that influence values and attitudes. The person tries to develop patterns of living that are in harmony with environmental forces. Factors such as social inequities, economic and educational deprivation, technological advances, and ecological disturbances cause disruptions in the individual's relationship with the environment. The individual is expected to participate in evaluating disruptive events and in reestablishment of patterns congruent with forward movement, growth, and health. Nursing's responsibility to the individual and society is to seek means to promote the person-environment interaction to attain maximal health potential.

Spiritual dimension In the spiritual dimension perception and thought are the basis for functioning. A person who can perceive and transcend his present state of consciousness and find expression in reasoning and creativity may alter his perception and attitude toward his health potential.

Clinical Application

The nurse applying Rogers' framework uses the principles of homeodynamics in the assessment process with Susan (refer to the case example on p. 74). The nurse understands that through person-environment interactions positive or negative patterns many emerge. The nurse, as a component of the environment, recognizes her behavior's influence on Susan's behavior and the importance of both the nurse's and Susan's cooperation in identifying problem areas.

Implicit in Rogers' approach are some questions that may generate useful information. First, information about the environment and the client is collected. The nurse attempts to discover the nature of the interaction between Susan, her family, and her friends. What patterns in these interactions reflect a breakdown in perception and communication? Are the home and school environments in which Susan interacts contributing to her behavior?

Second, information about life process (historical elements) is collected. For example, what has been the nature of Susan's interaction with family, friends, and environment in the past? What factors, over time, have contributed to pattern formation?

Finally, questions such as the following are asked: Have new relationships evolved in an attempt to cope with dysfunction in the rhythms and patterns? To what extent have these relationships influenced Susan's present behavior? What are the environmental factors that support or retard Susan's stability?

Working closely, both Susan and the nurse assess problems, establish diagnoses, and set goals. They establish strategies of intervention to assist Susan in repatterning her behavior. Adhering to the unitary person framework makes a simultaneous assessment of all dimensions necessary. The nurse working with Susan is likely to discover that factors in the home environment are contributing to Susan's present difficulties. Susan's patterns of coping are likely to become increasingly ineffective over time. Susan's suicidal gestures are viewed not as static behavior but rather as an evolving way of responding to her environment. Rogers' focus is on health and health potential rather than disease. Thus the goal is to use Susan's own resources and abilities to channel energy in a positive direction.

Congruence of Rogers' approach with the holistic perspective is a major strength. A significant area of weakness is a lack of direction for assessment and intervention. Other strengths and weaknesses of this approach are listed in Table 5-5.

ROY'S ADAPTATION THEORY

Sister Callista Roy placed her perspective of nursing in a systems model framework. In this model the person is viewed as an adaptive system; nursing intervention is needed when there is a deficit between the adaptation level and environmental demands.[51,52]

Major Concepts

The major concepts of Roy's theoretical approach are regulator, cognator, and adaptive modes (Figure 5-6). Adaptation is the process of coping with internal and external stimuli. It is determined by the effects of three classes of stimuli: focal, contextual, and residual. Focal stimuli immediately confront the person and an adaptive response is made. Contextual, or background, stimuli contribute to the behavior as a result of focal stimuli. Residual stimuli arise from the person's beliefs, attitudes, and past experiences.

The adaptive system has two main subsystems, the reg-

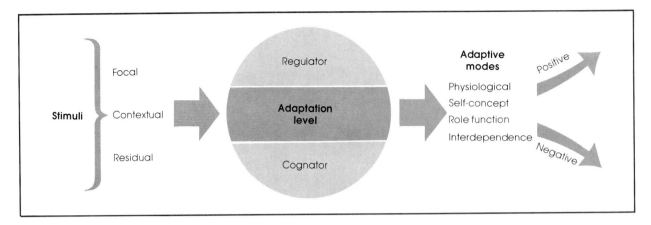

FIGURE 5-6 Roy's adaptation framework.

ulator and the cognator. Neural and endocrine body responses to stimuli are handled by the regulator subsystem. The cognator subsystem handles information processing, learning, and decision making in response to stimuli. When adaptation problems arise, the nursing process is used to assist the individual in one or several of the adaptive modes (physiological, self-concept, role function, and interdependence). The physiological mode encompasses needs such as circulation, temperature, activity, sleep, and nutrition. The self-concept mode is a composite of beliefs and feelings one holds about oneself at a given time that is formed from the perceptions and reactions of others. The role function mode regulates the performance of duties according to the expected behaviors to maintain a particular status in society. The interdependence mode achieves harmony and balance with others through a mutual exchange of recognition, praise, and approval. The adaptive modes are patterns of responses that make up the person's coping mechanisms, which parallel the kinds of demands the person encounters.

Holistic Perspective

According to Roy, individuals have biological, psychological, and social components as well as adaptive abilities. The person is viewed from this perspective as a unified whole.

Physical dimension The physical dimension is reflected in Roy's concept of a person's physiological needs in regard to exercise and rest, nutrition, elimination, fluid and electrolytes, and oxygen and circulation. These are handled by the regulator subsystem. Changes in mental activity (cognator subsystem) may influence physiological functions.

Emotional dimension The emotional dimension is inherent in the self-concept mode, which involves feelings and perception. Experiences enter the self-concept through perception of past and present events. Perceiving the adequacy of various experiences influences emotional adaptation. Roy emphasizes that emotional reactions may allow verbalization of fears, concerns, or anxiety. The self-concept mode also includes aspects of the intellectual and social dimensions.

Intellectual dimension The person's intellectual dimension is addressed in Roy's discussion of memory, information processing, and integrity. Sensory overload or deprivation can influence intellectual functioning. Maladaptive sensory responses can lead an individual to a level of disequilibrium and disorganization. Judgment is an intellectual function and is one of the psychosocial pathways of the cognator subsystem.

Social dimension The social dimension is emphasized in the interdependence and role function modes. Social experience reflects the external stimuli that surround the individual. Roy proposes social integrity, individual adaptation, and group adaptation as system functions. Interactions and relationships develop in the social dimension as the individual adapts within the culture.

Spiritual dimension Although not explicitly stated as a component of the theory, the spiritual dimension is among the person's innate needs. For successful adaptation, personal, social, and cultural aspects of life need to be fulfilled.

Clinical Application

In accordance with Roy's approach, the nurse establishes a data base regarding Susan's care by observing behavior in each of the adaptive modes. (See the case example on p. 74.) The nurse then describes the focal, contextual, and residual stimuli affecting Susan's behavior. The focal stimuli requiring immediate attention are Susan's self-destructive tendencies. The contextual stimuli are Susan's relationships with her mother and possibly with other members of her family. The residual stimuli for Susan may be repressed anger and frustration in response to unmet needs.

Further, the nurse assists Susan's move toward health by promoting and supporting her adaptive abilities in the social and interdependence modes. From a holistic perspective, the emotional and social dimensions are the primary ones affected in Susan's care. The adaptive modes of self-concept and interdependence are patterns of behavior or responses that constitute Susan's coping mechanisms for demands made on her. The nurse helps Susan meet the demands to develop a positive self-concept and to achieve a balance between dependence and independence.

The assessment of focal (for example, self-destructive tendencies), contextual, and residual stimuli determines the needed intervention. The intervention, directed at stimuli, constitutes the nursing action within the adaptive mode. The nurse supports and promotes Susan's adaptation. Following assessment, analysis, planning, and intervention, an evaluation is made to determine Susan's progress in adapting.

A major weakness of Roy's approach (Table 5-5) is the lack of direction given for a meaningful, reality-based assessment.

The philosophical foundations and assumptions of each theorist are illustrated in Table 5-3. Research using each of the theoretical approaches and the phenomena studied are listed in Table 5-4.

A brief summary of the major strengths and weaknesses of the theoretical approaches discussed is given in Table 5-5.

BRIEF REVIEW

The development of a theoretical base for the practice of nursing is still in its infancy. The importance of this scientific activity, however, is reflected in the serious effort put forth by nurses in research, education, and practice. A sound basis for the discipline of nursing depends on a critical examination of existing theories and conceptual models proposed for nursing practice.

In general, the six nursing theorists' approachs in their present level of development offer some degree of direction for the practice of mental health–psychiatric nursing from a holistic perspective. The applications in some instances are minimal, but they demonstrate the theory's potential for use in the practice of this nursing specialty.

Although the theories vary in strengths and weaknesses, appropriate research questions will, ideally, validate the usefulness of the theories in practice.

▼ **TABLE 5-3** Philosophical Foundations and Assumptions of the Theoretical Approaches

Theorist	Philosophical Foundations	Assumptions
Peplau	Individuals are organisms that strive to reduce tension generated by needs. Need is an internal requirement that creates tension. Individuals are unique beings, capable of new learning and positive change. Nursing is a therapeutic process. Society is culture.	The individual has the ability to adapt to tensions created by needs. Both nurse and client participate in determining what each will contribute and learn in the relationship.
Orem	An individual is an integrated whole biologically, symbolically, and socially. Health is a state of wholeness. Nursing's concern is self-care.	Needs are adapted to the environment. Functioning can be altered within flexible limits. Societal influence is reflected in the person-environment interaction.
King	Individuals are biopsychosocial organisms with continually evolving needs. Nursing's goal is the attainment of health.	Behavior is understood in terms of personal, interpersonal, and social systems. Health is adaptation to stress.
Johnson	Individuals are an aggregate of behavioral subsystems. Nursing assists individuals to develop a range of behavioral alternatives.	An individual is a system of interrelated physiological, psychosociocultural, and mental structures and functions. Persons interact with others within a group, family, and community by expressing behaviors that are intended to foster personal equilibrium and stability.
Rogers	The individual is a four-dimensional energy field evolving simultaneously with the environment. Individuals have the capacity for abstraction and imagery, language and thought, sensation and emotions. Individuals have self-regulating ability. Nursing's responsibility is to identify evolutionary patterns.	A continuous exchange of energy and matter between a person and his or her environmental field results in visible behavior. Individuals are capable of attaining integrity, unity, and growth.
Roy	An individual is a biopsychosocial adaptive being. The level of adaptation is influenced by external and internal stimuli.	Innate and acquired mechanisms are used to cope with a changing world. Adaptation is initiated by a stressor or focal stimulus.

▼ **TABLE 5-4** **Selected Research Studies Based on Theoretical Approaches**

Theorist	Researcher	Year	Phenomena
Peplau	Burd	1963	Anxiety
	Clack	1963	Aggression
	Oden	1963	Panic
	Morris	1967	Approach-avoidance
	Wrin	1968	Aspiration
	Werner	1973	Trust
	Walt, O'Toole	1989	Observation
Orem	Underwood	1978	Self-care behavior in psychiatric patients
	Spangler, Spangler	1983	Self-care in the aged
	Harper	1984	Self-care and behavior modification
	Chang and others	1985	Self-care and adherence to health care regimen in the aged
	Denyes	1988	Health promotion and self-care agency
	McBride	1991	Self-care agency
King	Given, Given, Simoni	1979	Process and outcome variables
	King	1981	Transaction predictive variables
	Michigan State Nurses Association (CURN project)	1982	Goal setting variables
Johnson	Holaday, Majesky	1974	Achievement behavior
	Brester, Nishio	1978	Client indicators of nursing care
	Damus	1980	Posttransfusion hepatitis
	Lovejoy	1981	Validation research
			Roy
	Roy	1967	Role adequacy
	Idle	1977	Self-perceived adaptation level
	Roy, Lewis	1977	Decision making and adaptation level
	Firsich, Parsell	1978	Health outcomes
	Roy	1978	Focal stimuli and distress
	Roy	1979	Powerlessness and decision-making activities
	Mitchell, Pilkington	1990	Totality
Rogers	Goldberg, Fitzpatrick	1980	Movement group therapy in the aged
	Engle	1981	Movement tempo and time perception
	Johnston, Fitzpatrick, Donovan	1982	Temporal orientation and depression
	Reed and others	1982	Temporal orientation and suicide
	Floyd	1983	Rhythmicity (sleep-wake cycle)
	Magan, Gibbon, Mrozek	1990	Value, movement, and creative patterns

REFERENCES AND SUGGESTED READINGS

1. Barrett EAM: Theory: of or for nursing? *Nursing Science Quarterly* 4(2):48, 1991.
2. Boykin A, Shoenhofer S: Caring in nursing: analysis of extant theory, *Nursing Science Quarterly* 3(4):146, 1990.
3. Burd SF, Marshall MA: *Some clinical approaches to psychiatric nursing,* New York, 1963, Macmillan.
4. Chalmers H and others: Nursing models: enhancing or inhibiting practice? *Nurse Standard* 5(11):34, 1990.
5. Clack J: *Some clinical approaches to psychiatric nursing,* New York, 1973, Macmillan Publishing.
6. Chang BL and others: Adherence to health care regimen among elderly women, *Nursing Research* 34(1):27, 1985.
7. Damus K: An application of the Johnson behavioral system model for nursing practice. In Riehl JP, Roy C, editors: *Conceptual models for nursing practice,* New York, 1980, Appleton-Century-Crofts.
8. Denyes M: Orem's model used for health promotion: directions for research, *Advances in Nursing Science* 11: 13, 1988.
9. Dickoff J, James P: Symposium on theory development in nursing. A theory of theories: a position paper, *Nursing Research* 17:197, 1968.
10. Engle V: *Movement and time as correlates of health.* Paper presented at the American Nurses' Association Council of Nurse Researchers Annual Meeting, Washington, DC, 1981 (abstract).
11. Fitch M and others: Developing a plan to evaluate the use of nursing conceptual frameworks, *Canadian Journal of Nursing Administration* 4(1):22, 1991.
12. Fitzpatrick JJ, Whall A: *Conceptual models of nursing: analysis* and application, ed 2, Norwalk, Conn., 1989, Appleton & Lange.
13. Forchuk C: Peplau's theory: concepts and their relevance, *Nursing Science Quarterly* 4(2):54, 1991.
14. Floyd JA: Research using Rogers' conceptual system: development of a testable theorem, *Advances in Nursing Science* 5(2):37, 1983.
15. Frey A, Denyes M: Health and illness self-care in adolescents with IDDM: a test of Orem's theory, *Advances in Nursing Science* 12(1):67, 1989.
16. Given B, Given CW, Simoni LF: Relationships of processes of care to patient outcomes, *Nursing Research* 28(2):85, 1979.
17. Goldberg WG, Fitzpatrick JJ: Movement therapy with the aged, *Nursing Research* 29(6):339, 1980.

▼ **TABLE 5-5** **Major Strengths and Weaknesses of the Theoretical Approaches**

Theorist	Strengths	Weaknesses
Peplau	Emphasis on interpersonal relationship	Dimensions of persons not in sufficient detail, particularly the spiritual dimension
	Exploration of client problems in a safe, trusting relationship	
	Guidelines for therapeutic interaction	Difficulty comparing phases of nurse-client relationship and the nursing process
Orem	Individual responsibility for self-care	Frequent reference to the medical perspective diminishes the independent responsibility of the nurse
	Inclusion of the nursing process helpful in organizing nursing care	
King	Process delineated for nurse-client interaction	Greater emphasis on social dimension than on other dimensions
	Similarity of the nurse-client interaction process to the nursing process useful to the nurse	
Johnson	Articulation of elements constituting human behavior	Person-environment interaction not well described
	Potential for growth when system stability is achieved	Empirical indexes for system stability and instability inadequately delineated
Rogers	Congruence with nursing's holistic view of persons	Rudimentary direction for assessment
	Broad conceptualization of ideas and relationships	Abstract guidelines for intervention strategies
Roy	Focus on the biopsychosocial nature of persons	Reciprocal influences of subsystems are not explicit
	Emphasis on physiological needs	

18. Grubbs J: An interpretation of the Johnson behavioral system model for nursing practice. In Riehl JP, Roy C, editors: *Conceptual models for nursing practice,* ed 2, New York, 1980, Appleton-Century-Crofts.
19. Harper DC: Application of Orem's theoretical constructs to self-care medication behavior in the elderly, *Advances in Nursing Science* 6(3):19, 1984.
20. Holaday BJ: Achievement behavior in chronically ill children, *Nursing Research* 23:25, 1974.
21. Huckaboy LMD: Nursing models and theories: do they work in practice? *Nursing Administration Quarterly* 15(3):80, 1991.
22. Idle BA: SPAL: a tool for measuring self-perceived adaptation level for an elderly population. In Bauwens EE, editor: *Clinical nursing research: its strategies and findings,* Monograph Series, Indianapolis, 1978, Sigma Theta Tau.
23. Ingram R: Why does nursing need theory? *Journal of Advances in Nursing* 16(3):350, 1991.
24. Jenny J: Self-care deficit theory and nursing diagnosis: a test of conceptual fit, *Journal of Nursing Education* 30(5):227, 1991.
25. Johnson DE: *One conceptual model of nursing.* Paper presented at Vanderbilt University, Nashville, Tenn, April 25, 1968.
26. Johnson DE: The Johnson behavioral system model for nursing. In Riehl JP, Roy C, editors: *Conceptual models for nursing practice,* ed 2, New York, 1980, Appleton-Century-Crofts.
27. Johnson RL, Fitzpatrick JJ, Donovan MJ: Developmental stage: relationship to temporal dimensions, *Nursing Research* 31:120, 1982 (abstract).
28. King IM: *A theory for nursing: systems, concepts, process,* ed 2, New York, 1981, John Wiley & Sons.
29. King IM: *Toward a theory for nursing,* New York, 1971, John Wiley & Sons.
30. Laben JK, Dodd D, Sneed L: King's theory of goal attainment applied in group therapy for inpatient juvenile offenders and community parolees, using visual aids, *Issues in Mental Health Nursing* 12(1):51, 1991.
31. Laschinger HK, Duff V: Attitudes of practicing nurses toward theory based nursing practice, *Canadian Journal of Nursing Administration* 4(1):6, 1991.
32. Lewis FM, Firsich SC, Parsell S: Development of reliable measures of patient health outcomes related to quality nursing care for chemotherapy patients. In Krueger JC, Nelson AH, Walanin MO, editors: *Nursing research development, collaboration, and utilization,* Rockville, Md, 1978, Aspen.
33. Lister P: Approaching models of nursing from a postmodernist perspective, *Journal of Advances in Nursing* 16(2):206, 1991.
34. Lovejoy NC: *An empirical verification of the Johnson behavioral system model for nursing,* doctoral dissertation, Birmingham, 1981, University of Alabama.
35. Magan SJ, Gibbon EJ, Mrozek R: 1990 Nursing theory applications: a practice model, *Issues in Mental Health Nursing* 11:297, 1990.
36. Majesky SJ, Brester MJ, Nishio K: Development of a research tool: patient indicators of nursing care, *Nursing Research* 27:6, 365, 1978.
37. McBride SH: Comparative analysis of three instruments to measure self-care agency, *Nursing Research* 40(1):12, 1991.
38. Meleis AJ: *Theoretical nursing: development and progress,* Philadelphia, 1985, JB Lippincott.
39. Michigan State Nurses Association: *CURN project: mutual goal setting in patient care,* New York, 1982, Grune & Stratton.
40. Mitchell GJ, Pilkington B: Theoretical approaches in nursing practice: a comparison of Roy and Parse, *Nursing Science Quarterly* 3(2):81-87, 1991.
41. Morris K: *Approach-avoidance conflict in the orientation phase of therapy,* ANA Regional Clinical Conference, New York, 1967, Appleton-Century-Crofts.
42. Oden G: Individual panic: elements and patterns. In Burd S, Marshall MA, editors: *Some clinical approaches to psychiatric nursing,* New York, 1963, Macmillan Publishing Co.
43. Orem DE: *Guides for developing curricula for the education of practical nurses,* Washington, DC, 1959, US Government Printing Office.

44. Orem DE: *Nursing concepts of practice,* New York, 1971, McGraw-Hill Book Co.

45. Orem DE: *Nursing concepts of practice,* ed 2, New York, 1980, McGraw-Hill Book Co.

46. Parker ME, editor: *Nursing theories in practice,* New York, 1990, National League for Nursing.

47. Peplau HE: *Interpersonal relations in nursing,* New York, 1952, GP Putnam's Sons.

48. Reed PG and others: Suicidal crisis: relationship to the experience, *Nursing Research* 31:2, 1982.

49. Rogers ME: *An introduction to the theoretical basis of nursing,* Philadelphia, 1970, FA Davis.

50. Rogers ME: Science of unitary man: a paradigm for nursing. In Laskar GE, editor: *Applied systems and cybernetics,* vol 4, Elmsford, NY, 1981, Pergamon Press.

51. Roy C: A conceptual framework for nursing, *Nursing Outlook* 18(3):42, 1970.

52. Roy C, Roberts SL: *Theory construction in nursing: an adaptation model,* Englewood Cliffs, NJ, 1981, Prentice Hall.

53. Roy C: Role cues and mothers of hospitalized children, *Nursing Research* 16(2):178, 1967.

54. Roy C: *Decision-making by the physically ill and adaptation during illness,* doctoral dissertation, Los Angeles, 1977, University of California.

55. Roy C: The stress of hospital events: measuring changes in level of stress (abstract). In Communicating nursing research, vol 11, *New approaches to communicating nursing research,* Boulder, Colo, 1978, Western Interstate Commission for Higher Education.

56. Roy C: Health-illness (powerlessness) questionnaire and hospitalized patient decision-making. In Ward MJ, Lindeman CA, editors: *Instruments for measuring nursing practice and other health variables,* vol 1, Hyattsville, Md, 1979, Department of Health, Education and Welfare.

57. Selanders L, Dietz-Omar M: Making nursing models relevant for the practising nurse, *Nurse Practitioner* 4(2):23, 1991.

58. Spangler FS, Spangler WD: Self-care: a testable model. In Chinn PL, editor: *Advances in nursing theory development,* Rockville, Md, 1983, Aspen Publishers.

59. Welt SR, O'Toole AW: Hildegard E. Peplau: observations in brief, *Archives of Psychiatric Nursing* 3(5):254, 1989.

60. Werner AM: Learning to trust. In Burd S, Marshall MD, editors: *Some clinical approaches to psychiatric nursing,* New York, 1963, Macmillan.

61. Wrin JT: *Nurse-patient interaction: nurse's level of aspiration.* In ANA Clinical Session, New York, 1968, Appleton-Century-Crofts.

ANNOTATED BIBLIOGRAPHY

Andrews AJ, Roy C: *Essentials of the Roy adaptation model,* Norwalk, Conn, 1986, Appleton-Century-Crofts.

The principles of Roy's conceptualization of adaptation theory for nursing practice are presented, emphasizing the nursing process. The concepts are depicted in diagrams. Individual and nursing activities are emphasized, including discussion of the person, environment, health, and nursing. The concepts are applied to common life situations with exercise for application.

Barrett EAM: *Visions of Rogers' science-based nursing,* New York, 1990, National League for Nursing

This book is a collection of scholarly papers that relate to Rogerian science-based nursing. The text is a useful resource for conceptual and practical activities. Attention is given to application of the conceptual model in education, research, and service. Rogers' postulates and principles of homeodynamic are addressed.

Johnson DE: The Johnson behavioral system model for nursing. In Riehl JI, Roy C, editors: *Conceptual models for nursing practice,* ed 2, New York, 1980, Appleton-Century-Crofts.

The author discusses the basis tenets of her behavioral system framework. She includes general assumptions regarding systems theory, which form the foundation of her framework, and describes the structural and functional components of the concepts. The author emphasizes the responsibility of the user to seek a foundation in the natural and social sciences.

King IM: *A theory for nursing: systems, concepts, process,* ed 2, New York, 1981, John Wiley & Sons.

The author describes and analyzes her framework. She expands concepts of the goal attainment theory as relevant to nursing. The focus is the promotion of health practices. Of particular interest are the author's presentation and illustration of a goal-oriented nursing record that can be used to document nursing care.

Orem DE: *Nursing concepts of practice,* New York, 1971, McGraw-Hill.

Nursing as a service to persons to promote self-reliance and responsibility is the theme of this text. The author acknowledges the absence in her book of specific solutions for health needs. Instead she describes a broad framework for the identification and search for resolution strategies.

Parker ME, editor: *Nursing theories in practice,* New York, 1991, National League for Nursing.

This book presents a discussion of major nursing theories by eminent theorists. Each theorist's contribution includes practical examples of how the theory is effectively implemented in a variety of settings.

Peplau HE: *Interpersonal relations in nursing,* New York, 1952, GP Putnam's Sons.

Considered the reference source for the application of interpersonal theory to nursing. This text contains a thorough interpretation of elements of the interpersonal process and nursing's responsibility in providing a therapeutic context for meeting the needs of individuals seeking health care. Peplau consistently emphasized the use of self in promoting mutual learning and growth.

Rogers ME: Science of unitary human beings. In Malinski VM, editor: *Explorations on Martha Rogers science of unitary human beings,* Norwalk, Conn, 1986, Appleton-Century-Crofts.

Rogers has further developed her conceptual system, advocating a new world view specific to phenomena of interest to nursing. Principles and theories derived from the system are validated in the real world. The three principles derived from the system are validated in the real world. The three principles derived from the concept of homeodynamics are helicy, resonancy, and integrality. Roger's theory suggests a world view different from the prevailing one. Seeing the world from this view requires a creative leap with new attitudes and values.

CHAPTER

6   Therapeutic Communication

Nancy L Hedlund
Finis Breckenridge Jeffrey

After studying this chapter, the student will be able to:

- Differentiate between verbal and nonverbal communication and metacommunication
- Give examples of the structural distinctions in communication
- Give examples of functions of communication
- Discuss theoretical approaches to communication

- Discuss techniques that facilitate therapeutic communication
- Discuss issues in therapeutic nurse-client communication
- Explain approaches to changing behavior through communication

Therapeutic communication in mental health–psychiatric nursing modifies ordinary communication to create client interactions that promote healing or improved mental health in two important ways. First, the nurse creates helpful client-nurse communication that addresses client difficulties with self-respect, problem solving, autonomy, and sense of purpose in life. Second, the nurse helps the client to heal through achieving more healthy internal communication between his various dimensions.

Learning effective communication in mental health–psychiatric nursing challenges the nurse to become a highly skilled listener who can plan and carry out interactions specifically designed to achieve client outcomes. Skill development includes using emotional and cognitive abilities in a variety of nursing interventions that include support, confrontation, trust, and affection.

DEFINITIONS OF COMMUNICATION

Verbal and Nonverbal Communication

Verbal communication refers to written and spoken messages exchanged in the form of words as the elements of language. An example of verbal communication is provided by the words "I am anxious." These written or spoken words convey an idea about the speaker's experience.

Nonverbal communication refers to messages that do not involve the spoken or written word but are conveyed by behavior, such as the presence or absence of body language or through any of the five senses. For example, the client's hands may tremble, accompanied by rapid breath-

ing, gesturing, and profuse sweating. This behavior may represent the message "I am anxious." However, the person may be conveying anger or respiratory distress. The correct meaning of the message can be achieved by verbal validation with the other person.

It is possible to further distinguish between (1) *communication,* which is the actual content of the message, and (2) *metacommunication,* which is how the message is to be understood, or the intended meaning. The actual message may be a compliment, such as "You look lovely," but the metacommunication of a frown may imply the actual message is not sincere. The metacommunication tells the receiver of the message how to interpret what the sender means.

Structure of Communication

The structure of communication includes the form of language and the use of words and behaviors to construct messages. Knowledge about the structure of language provides an important way to analyze communication. Assessing the client's communication includes analysis of how verbal and nonverbal modes are used to structure communication. You might ask: What messages are conveyed by each? Are the messages congruent? Are the messages consistent with the client's culturally defined and taken-for-granted rules? To what extent are stereotypes about the self or others conveyed by the structure of the client's communication? How does the client's communication structure contribute to the problem for which help is sought?

HISTORICAL OVERVIEW

DATES	EVENTS
Late 1800s to Mid-twentieth Century	With the exception of Florence Nightingale's *Notes on Nursing,* early nursing textbooks did not emphasize how to communicate effectively.
1950s	Acceptance of nurse-client communication as the core of clinical practice emerged with the publications of the mental health–psychiatric nursing theorists.
1960s	Theories of communication formulated by nonnurses were incorporated into nursing's knowledge base. Hays and Larson published first text on specific interpersonal techniques used in verbal communication with clients. Recognition of need for research on understanding communication between nurse and client and the consequences of communication for the client.
1970s	Increased publications by nurses on communicating with clients. The significance of communication as an aspect of the nurse's role and the role of the nurse as a therapist became well established.
1980s	The need for rapid assessment of the client's health status in response to short-term hospitalization increased the significance of therapeutic communication.
1990s	Nurses continued to use technological and theoretical advances in communication to enhance its expertise in therapeutic communication.
Future	Nurses will conduct research on communication behaviors as affected by such factors as diagnosis of client, phase of the nurse-client relationship, and length of the relationship.

Analysis of the structure of nurse-client communication also includes assessing whether the client's communication appears to be consciously intended or an unconsciously motivated message. The nurse also analyzes the degree of clarity in the message in conveying the intended information. For example, consider the following four actions:

1. Painting a picture
2. Saying, "It's good to wake up feeling ready for the day!"
3. Giving the instruction, "The normal temperature of the human being is 37° C."
4. Jaywalking

Each of the four examples of behaviors can be seen as containing an intention to create interaction. Painting a picture may be a request to another person: "Please buy my painting." Remarking on how good it feels to awaken feeling ready for the day may imply "Don't you agree?" Instructing another about the normal temperature of human beings may imply "Do you understand?" Jaywalking may imply a desire to be injured or a test of the alertness of the driver of an oncoming vehicle. Examining the intention of a client to interact and communicate a message is best accomplished by talking about the behavior, the possible messages that may be conveyed, and the kind of response being requested.

Functions of Communication

Consideration of the *functions of communication* refers to examining what the verbal or nonverbal communication messages accomplish rather than examining how the message is structured. The two are related because structuring the message affects the function, as in structuring a statement instead of a question.

Question: *Don't you think teenagers disobey parental rules a lot?*
Statement: *In my opinion, teenagers disobey parental rules a lot.*

One function of the question is specifically to request a response, which is not necessarily part of a declarative statement.

Another function of communication is to disclose information or create a specific message about the self, others, or objects. These messages can be sent with no expectation of a response. For example, consider the four behaviors cited earlier: (1) painting a picture, (2) saying, "It's good to wake up feeling ready for the day!" (3) instructing, "The normal temperature of the human being is 37° C," and (4) jaywalking. Each behavior involves disclosing information about an act that requests no response or interaction with others.

One important communication function is *self-disclosure,* which is communicating information or perceptions about the self. This includes intended and unintended acts that describe and evaluate the self. Through communication individuals convey what kind of person they perceive themselves to be and their level of self-esteem.

In the four examples of behavior previously listed, creating a painting may be a way of expressing a strong image of the self. Remarking on how good it feels to awaken feeling ready for the day may be a way of describing the self as a person who happily faces each day. The instruction about normal human body temperature may be a correct response to a student's question that simultaneously conveys the speaker's sense of worth in knowing the correct information. Jaywalking may be a way of describing the self as a risk-taking person. However, an alternative analysis of the meaning of these acts could suggest a negative self-view.

A variation on the idea of self-disclosure as a function of communication is the idea that behavior can also communicate a symptom or mental health difficulty. Behavior that appears to communicate such symptoms is sometimes interpreted as a request for help.

Using the four previously cited illustrations of behavior, a client may paint a picture depicting impending disaster to convey a concern about his own safety. Remarks about how good it feels to awaken feeling ready for the day may express a severely depressed person's temporary optimism just before a suicidal attempt. Instruction about normal human temperature may occur in a context in which fears of being cold and alone were being expressed. Finally, the act of jaywalking may be an expression of rebellion, lack of concern about self, or even suicidal intention. In each of these examples, the context significantly shapes the meaning of the event, which is then further clarified by validating the meaning of the behavior with the client.

Analysis of the known and unknown aspects of self as they relate to self-awareness and awareness of others can be described in a two-way matrix (Figure 6-1) known as *Johari's window.*[22] Four categories of self-awareness are shown: (1) aspects known to self and others, (2) aspects not known to self but known to others, (3) aspects known to self but not known to others, and (4) aspects not known to self or others.

Johari's window can be used to organize information that the nurse acquires in the assessment process. As the nurse develops greater intimacy with the client, more information can be added to categories 1 and 2. As the client's self-awareness increases, more information can be added to category 3 and, it is hoped, to category 1. In other words, as the nurse's relationship with the client deepens, the client will be able to share more about himself with the nurse, which is information transferred from category 3 to category 1. The developing relationship with the client permits the nurse to learn more about the client through observation and discussion with others; this process makes it possible to add information from category 2 to category 1 as the nurse's understanding of the client grows.

THEORIES FOR ANALYZING COMMUNICATION IN NURSING

Ruesch's Theory

Ruesch applied knowledge of people and cultures to the analysis of communication as the social matrix of psychiatry.[26,29] Ruesch proposed a general theory of communication that broadly defined communication as the full range of mechanisms or operations by which people affect one another. Communication includes written and oral speech as well as drama, dance, and the arts. The theory aims to provide a unified construct of human behavior, an understanding of psychopathological conditions such as disturbed communication, and a view of communication as a therapeutic tool.

Communication is defined as a circular process, as illustrated in Figure 6-2. A statement is the expression of internal events intended to convey information to other persons; it becomes a message when it has been perceived and interpreted by another. In other words, the message travels in a circle beginning with the internal events within one person, which are transmitted to another, and, after being affected by the internal events in the other person, result in a response message back to the original sender.

Language is a collection of signs or symbols of which two or more communicators or interpreters understand the significance. Statements in the communication process contain both content and instruction. Instruction refers to the process of communication itself, including references as to how a statement is to be interpreted. This instruction is also called metacommunication; it is, in effect, communication about the communication. Feedback is an essential element of the system because it exerts a control or corrective effect by feeding back information about the effects of the communication activity.

Communication is described as being successful when agreement of meaning, or concordance, is established. Alternatively, the lack of agreement, or discordance, results in unsuccessful communication (Figure 6-3).

Therapeutic communication is distinguished from ordinary communication by the intent of one or more of the

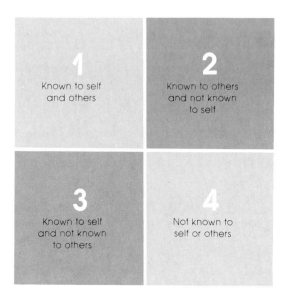

FIGURE 6-1 The Johari window.

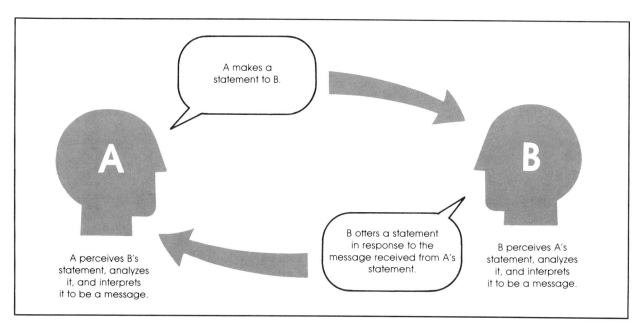

FIGURE 6-2 Ruesch's feedback loop of communication.

participants to bring about a change in the communication pattern in the system. Ruesch[27] defines a *therapist* as a person in charge of directing the change by steering communication in such a way that the client is exposed to situations and message exchanges that eventually will bring about more gratifying social relations. The nurse assumes this role in many different health care settings, in addition to traditional mental health care situations. As theories about therapeutic communication have evolved, a variety of practice approaches have become available to nurses seeking to assume therapeutic roles.

Disturbed communication can originate within the individual, as well as between individuals. Nursing assessment includes looking for any of the following occurrences of disturbed communication:

1. Interference with sending or receiving messages, as may be caused by disease, trauma, or malformation of communication organs; having a speech impediment; or being deaf.
2. Insufficient mastery of the language resulting from a poor-quality education or not speaking the same language as others in the environment.

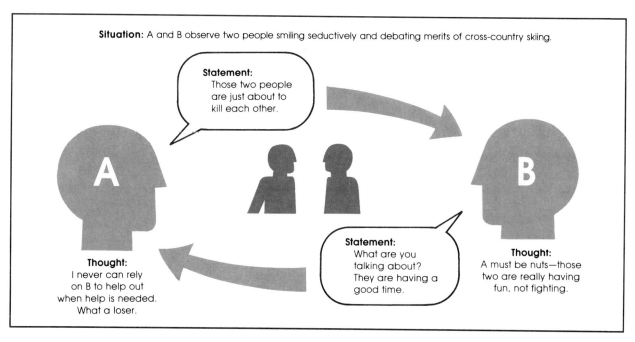

FIGURE 6-3 Unsuccessful communication produced by discordant information.

3. Incorrect or insufficient information about the self or others, as may be caused by misinterpreting a situation or having only partial information, for example, being adopted and not knowing facts about one's background or not knowing there is a familial history of diabetes.

4. Insufficient use of metacommunication devices, as may be caused by lack of understanding or lack of skill in interpreting one's messages to others or interpreting other's messages, for example, misinterpreting a slight smile to mean humor when it really is a sneer.

5. Inability to correct information through feedback circuits, as in being unskilled in correcting information or in having obstacles in the feedback loop within a person or between persons, for example, being unable to telephone a person or being told that the other person is not willing to talk.

Figure 6-4 illustrates how these disturbances impede communication between two persons seated next to one another at a workshop. Disturbances in communication can also result from circumstances in group dynamics.

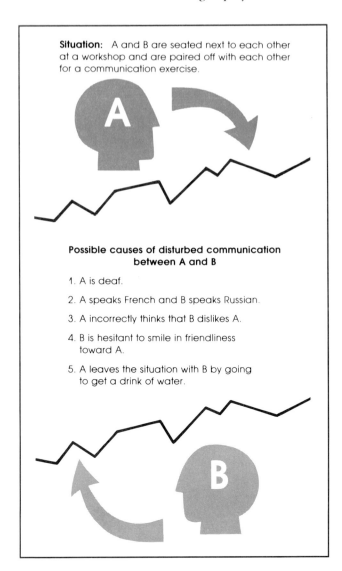

Situation: A and B are seated next to each other at a workshop and are paired off with each other for a communication exercise.

Possible causes of disturbed communication between A and B

1. A is deaf.

2. A speaks French and B speaks Russian.

3. A incorrectly thinks that B dislikes A.

4. B is hesitant to smile in friendliness toward A.

5. A leaves the situation with B by going to get a drink of water.

FIGURE 6-4 Sources of disturbed communication within the person.

Disturbed communications can also occur in large networks of people in which feedback devices are not effective. For example, when nurses work with large groups of clients as in some inpatient or day-care settings, disturbed communications can arise when the setting lacks adequate mechanisms for keeping the nurse informed about client concerns.

Subgroups of clients may form to express concern to the head nurse; however, different rules of communication concerning feedback may apply in such groups. Although the norm in the institution may be that people need to express concerns openly and communicate through proper channels when they are attempting to solve a problem, a suspicious member in a newly created subgroup may lead the group to resort to extreme secrecy. As a result, a disturbed communication pattern develops that is characterized by overlooking appropriate levels of communication and going directly to the medical director of the setting.

Needs for therapeutic communication can be created by acute or long-term disturbances, such as unexpected loss of a job or a long-standing marital conflict. Crises and environmental stresses also can create situations in which participants want to initiate changes in communication behavior. Human experience is the subject of study or concern in assessing and treating communication disturbances. In such disturbances and the distressing events in human experience that cause them, anticipatory adaptation and momentary adaptation are a person's most powerful survival tools.

Anticipatory adaptation means that a person can begin adapting in advance of a potentially distressing situation, such as when a person tries to relax before calling to receive the results of a laboratory test. Anticipatory adaptation is one human capacity that makes therapeutic communication possible; the client needs to have the capacity to imagine events in advance and analyze how to communicate more effectively in potentially distressing situations. In other words, people need to be able to conceptualize the future, or else they will be severely limited in their ability to solve problems that may occur in the future. *Momentary adaptation* is the ability to be effective at the moment the distressing situation actually occurs. The success of therapeutic communication also depends on the client's developing this ability.

However, the therapist has an advantage because she possesses a certain kind of *leverage* with the client. This leverage is developed in the process of the therapeutic relationship, and it occurs in many nurse-client communication situations. The leverage is the influence of the helping person on the client that adds to, but is different from, the motivation of the client to acquire or enter a state of well-being. This leverage is a kind of power or influence and is produced by the helper's efforts on the client's behalf. It refers to influence over the thoughts, feelings, and behaviors of another and is created through the processes of understanding communication, acceptance, and agreement. Figure 6-5 illustrates the three steps in developing this leverage.

In the first step, through communication with the client, the nurse seeks to gain an understanding of the nature of the client's distress. The nurse perceives the client's statements about himself and what needs to be changed. This

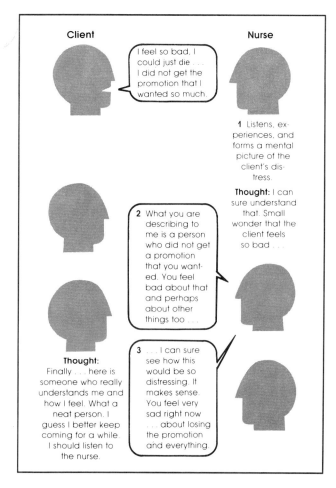

FIGURE 6-5 Steps in the therapeutic leverage the nurse develops with the client.

first step in developing leverage—understanding—is a process that occurs within the nurse, during which the client's distress becomes comprehensible. The nurse has a mental description or image of the client's distress and a cognitive acceptance of it as being the best picture of the client's reality that can be achieved at that moment.

The second step involves the nurse's engaging the client in communication in which information is shared between the client and the nurse about the nurse's observations and analysis of the client's behavior. Later in this chapter, a variety of communication approaches are described to assist the nurse in developing skills in sharing information with clients, conveying acceptance, and promoting greater self-understanding.

The third step is agreement. To whatever degree is possible, the nurse agrees with the client as a form of support that is relayed through communication. The agreement represents consensual validation of the client's distress and the need for improvement through change. That is, the nurse and client reach agreements about what the client is experiencing, what needs to change, and what may bring about those changes. Agreements reached through consensual validation represent a kind of negotiation, in that the nurse and client bring their respective viewpoints to some form of similar picture of what is happening and what is to be done.

It is important for nurses to understand that for a variety of possible reasons the nurse can influence the client in some nurse-client interactions. While many approaches, such as Ruesch's, perceive the therapist's leverage to have great therapeutic importance, an alternative view involved in a holistic approach encourages a balance of power in which the client perceives the power of healing to reside within himself. The resolution of this balance of power in the nurse-client relationship is a function of the nurse's beliefs about practice and the specific needs of each client.

The nurse's influence, or leverage, can persuade the client to listen to and consider new ideas and new ways of

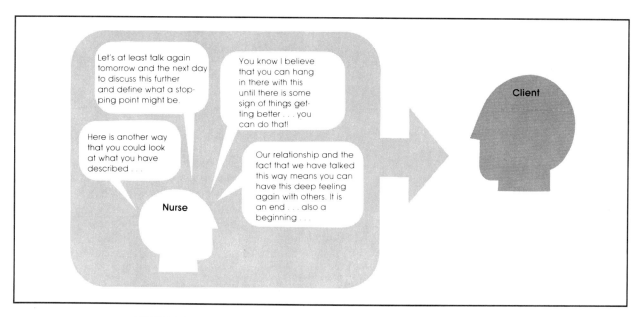

FIGURE 6-6 Helpful nurse-to-client statements using leverage to a therapeutic advantage.

viewing experience. Figure 6-6 illustrates a nurse's use of this leverage to a therapeutic advantage. The nurse can also influence the client to continue in the therapeutic communication process, an involvement that is especially important when harm to self or others is a risk. Since the nurse believes in the client, her leverage, or influence, can help the client begin to hold more favorable views of himself or others. Finally, the nurse's leverage creates potent learning possibilities at the time of termination of the therapeutic relationship. Through communication about the client's concerns and the influence of the nurse, the client is able to understand experientially how one person can allow another to become important and how growth can result from the therapeutic relationship and from coming to terms with the loss of the therapeutic relationship.

Double-Bind Communication

Double-bind communication is the simultaneous communication of conflicting messages. The double-bind theory, developed by the Bateson group[1] (also called the Palo Alto group) was derived from communication theory and the analysis of communication patterns in families in which a member had developed schizophrenia. The original research addressed the analysis of family members' skills with use of various modes of communication, humor, pretending, and learning. One initial belief about the disturbed communication in persons having the symptoms of schizophrenia was that they had difficulty knowing what communication mode they or others were using. For example, they may not recognize the humor in another person's message or they may be comical without knowing it. They also may use metaphors incorrectly or fail to recognize the meaning of a metaphor used by another. A second belief about these persons' communication problems is that they had difficulty recognizing communication modes within themselves. For example, they may have felt pain but were unsure if it hurt or tickled, or may have had an idea and not known whether other people could overhear the thought.

The essential characteristics of double-bind communication are listed in the accompanying box.

The following examples illustrate this pattern of conflicting messages that are characteristic of double-bind communication:

Mother: Come give mother a kiss before going out or she will be angry with you all evening.

Adolescent: Approaches the mother and starts to kiss her good-bye.

Mother: Grimaces and turns head away as if offended, and might say the youngster has bad breath or a dirty shirt collar.

The tertiary, or third, message is implied by the expectation that the child cannot avoid the interaction with the mother, even though no response from the child can prevent the mother's anger or rejection.

A more common type of double-bind communication involves conflicting messages that employ one spoken and one nonverbal message. For example, a friend might complain that no one ever calls her, but she sounds too busy to talk when someone does call, or a supervisor might ask for suggestions about how to solve a problem but then will frown or laugh at each suggestion.

Double-bind communication typically occurs in most types of communication situations at one time or another, so it is not necessarily associated with a disorder such as schizophrenia. Some theorists have argued that it is a necessary ingredient for the disorder but not a sufficient cause. Others suggest that it results from a disturbance in communication originating in the person with the schizophrenic disorder. Others simply respond to the person's disordered communication as best they can, and it turns out to be a conflicting series of messages.

Assessment of this communication pattern involves analysis of the following:

1. The frequency of the double-bind communication pattern
2. The importance of the relationships involved
3. The seriousness of the tertiary messages prohibiting escape
4. The extent to which the victim feels either helpless or capable of coping with or confronting the interactions

Kinesics

The major idea outlined in Scheflen's work on nonverbal communication[30] is that interactions, and inevitably relationships, are controlled by the nonverbal gestures and cues of communications. These gestures are called *kinesic behavior,* or body language. An example of this anthropological approach to analyzing nonverbal behavior is kinesic reciprocals, which deal with *affiliation, dominance,* and *submission.* For example, leaning back, showing the palm

CRITICAL INGREDIENTS OF DOUBLE-BIND COMMUNICATION

1. Two persons must be present; the person with disturbed communication assumes the role of victim or underdog.
2. The two persons engage in a recurring pattern of communication.
3. The victim, or underdog, receives a primary negative message or injunction, such as "Don't do 'X' or I will punish you," or "Do 'X' or I will punish you."
4. The victim receives a secondary injunction that conflicts with the first. This is usually worded in a more abstract way so that the person might realize that there is an implied punishment for not doing "X" despite having been told to do so.
5. The individual also receives a tertiary negative injunction prohibiting escape from the situation.
6. The pattern becomes sufficiently stable and recurring that the person with the disturbed communication comes to expect the conflicting messages and prohibition of escape, even when all three types of injunction are not explicitly communicated.

of the hand, and fussing with another person's collar are all possible courting behaviors conveying an invitation of closeness or affiliation.

Reaching out in the midst of a conversation to poke the other person in the chest is a domineering behavior. Laughing while being poked is a way to submit while at the same time trivializing or eliminating the other's aggressive intent. Reciprocal activities of two people are indicated by the way they place their bodies. For example, two people may lean close together to speak privately, or they may hold their arms in such a way to signal other people not to approach. Other behaviors signify awareness of passing through another's territory, such as a person who has hunched shoulders, hands to the body, and lowered head when passing through a strange neighborhood or when visiting an unfamiliar church. Finally, two people exchanging greetings indicate through their behavior how familiar they are with one another; for example, familiarity is conveyed by a raising of eyebrows, a salutation, and a waving gesture.

Kinesic behaviors also regulate human behavior. Figure 6-7 shows how two different sets of kinesic behaviors instruct about, qualify, or direct human communication behaviors in the same hypothetical situation. This exchange of information about the communication had earlier been described by Ruesch as metacommunication.

Since kinesic behaviors are body movements that convey meaning in communication, it is reasonable to expect that kinesic behaviors vary between cultures and ethnic groups just as spoken language varies.[3,30] One frequently described variation is the use of eye contact in communication. In some cultures, maintaining the gaze for any length of time is inappropriate, whereas others use extended gazing. Typically, the British and Americans who are used to the prolonged gaze mistakenly interpret unwillingness to maintain the gaze as submissiveness or shyness, but because of cultural differences this may not be the case. Chapter 9, covering cultural diversity, discusses these cultural variations in more detail.

Proxemics

The study of *proxemics* focuses on how people use space. Investigators undertook early studies in this subject because they sought to understand how animals achieved and maintained so-called territories. In this context, territories were frequently well defined in terms of physical space. As interest in applying these ideas to human behavior took form, broader conceptions of territory emerged. For example, the definition of a person's territory at one moment may be his room, his home, or the boundaries of his farm. Alternatively, in a busy crowd or an intensely angry confrontation, a person's territory may be an intangible but real boundary surrounding the person beyond which others should not pass. Such boundaries are permeable, and they are usually flexible. More physical closeness is allowed in some instances than in others. Some of the concepts in this area of study include territoriality, social distance, personal space, ego boundaries, and crowding. Humans clearly are territorial (Figure 6-8).

Four different zones of space in human interaction can be defined: intimate, personal, social, and public.[15] Perception of space is a factor in defining the boundaries of these zones. The boundaries expand or contract, depending on the context and the information the person is receiving from the situation.

The *intimate zone* within 18 inches of the body is the space in which physical activity occurs. It permits awareness of the scent and heat of another person's body. It is possible to speak in barely audible terms. Others with

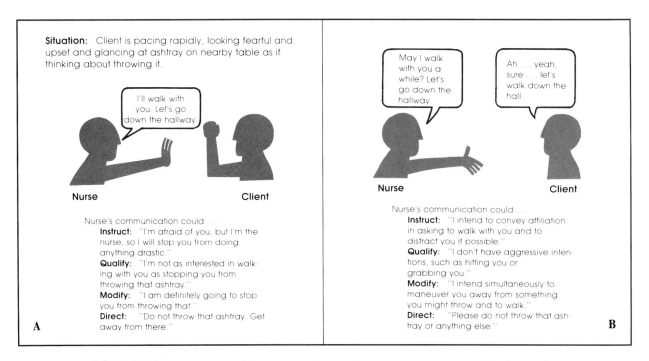

FIGURE 6-7 Metacommunication that instructs, qualifies, modifies, or directs the receiver. **A,** Nontherapeutic communication. **B,** Therapeutic communication.

whom one is close are allowed into this space with ease. The entry of strangers or unwelcome others is an intrusion and creates discomfort. The practice of nursing places people in each other's intimate zone, at times, without the prior establishment of familiarity or trust. Discomfort for client or nurse can result.

From 18 inches to approximately 4 feet is the *personal zone*. It is similar to a protective zone, and it has boundaries that expand and contract according to contextual characteristics. Usually a person wants to limit the entry of others into this space, so that only those with whom there is familiarity can gain entry.

Social space is about 4 to 12 feet from the person. In this zone, no touching is possible. It characterizes such situations as a group therapy session, a small group conference, or a conversation in a living room setting. *Public space* extends outward from approximately 12 feet. This space occurs in large group situations such as between a speaker and a workshop audience. These ideas can be validated by systematically observing human interaction. Behavior evoked by violations of others' boundaries varies with individuals and cultures; aggression might result in one culture and submissive behavior in another.

The use of touch in mental health–psychiatric nursing is related to the concept of space. Mental health–psychiatric nursing differs from most other arenas of nursing practice that require nurses to touch clients to change dressings, give baths, and administer injections. As a result, touch can be defined as optional rather than essential. Thus the appropriateness of touch in mental health–psychiatric nursing has aroused debate over the years.

Before the use of mental health labels, therapy roles, or

psychotropic medications, touch was essential to mental health–psychiatric nursing because nurses fed and bathed their clients when necessary and administered wet-sheet packs to reduce extreme anger or anxiety. In those days, nurses did not wonder whether they should use touch in their practice. The advent of therapeutic roles in nursing meant nurse and client sat and talked in more formal and defined terms, and touching was no longer assumed to be a natural part of practice. The relationship was differentiated as one of oral communication, not physical care and as one of therapeutic, not personal involvement. This distinction changed the way the nurse viewed her relationship with the patient and led some nurses to redefine the patient as a "client."

In therapeutic interactions, the nurse can thoughtfully choose how or when to use touch to increase the effectiveness of her work with the client. Examples of touch that can be used within the context of therapeutic communication are shaking hands, touching the client's hand or arm, a back or neck rub, or a hug. In contemporary practice, even though people commonly greet parents, siblings, spouses, or close friends with a kiss and hug, nurses almost never greet a client with a kiss and hug. Kissing is not a part of therapeutic communication in our culture. Where it is culturally acceptable, it is still made absolutely clear that sexual intimacy is not intended (for example, the light kiss on one or both cheeks often shared by Europeans).

Touch can convey many different kinds of energy or meaning, such as warmth, affection, empathy or understanding, restraint, reassurance, and emphasis. The use of touch is a conscious component of practice. Accordingly, client assessment needs to include evaluation of how the nurse may touch the client, how the client may react, and when touch is appropriate. If touch seems appropriate and consistent with the nurse's conceptual framework for practice, and if contextual factors (agency policy or an instructor's recommendation) are not prohibitive, touching gestures can be incorporated into the client's care plan. Appropriate times are usually defined as special occasions that deserve the added emphasis of touch. The occasions may emerge from the client's need or the nurse's desire to emphasize a point.

Therapeutic touch, or touch with the intent to heal, is a specialized kind of touching that can be learned through training with a clinician already experienced in this approach. The nurse begins with a centering process that is similar to meditation, emphasizing awareness of one's own energies and ability to transmit these energies to other humans. The nurse's motivation is to help heal the client. This motivation creates a conscious intent to heal that combines with the ability to transmit one's energies to another person.[20]

Use of any form of touch in the nursing care of clients in the mental health field must be carefully evaluated in terms of what it will mean to the client. In other words, some clients will be experiencing uncertainty about their body image and sense of boundaries. For these clients, touch may be an intrusion of their personal space or sense of self. Anxiety is heightened in the client who is easily stimulated, overly shy, and/or vulnerable to concerns about sexual contact. As a result of these or other distresses, effective nursing care requires assessment of the client's

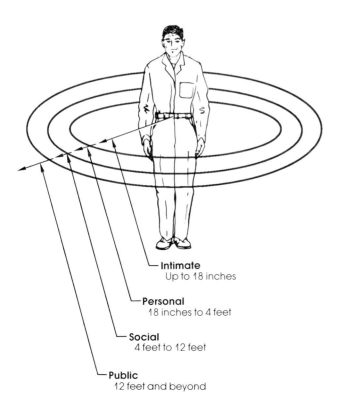

Intimate
Up to 18 inches

Personal
18 inches to 4 feet

Social
4 feet to 12 feet

Public
12 feet and beyond

FIGURE 6-8 Proxemics focuses on four zones of space in human interaction.

▼ **TABLE 6-1**   Description of Communication Channels: Examples of Function, Dysfunction, and Nursing Intervention

Channel	Function and Dysfunction	Nursing Intervention
Physiological	Normal gastrointestinal function versus stomachache and diarrhea in the face of distress	Discussion with client to reveal how gastrointestinal symptoms emerge in response to distress; development of stress management plan to cope with distress
Fine motor (kinesic and proxemic)	Each person in a family discussion speaks for himself or herself versus a family therapy session in which the client never speaks and the mother always speaks for the child	Discussion that brings the communication pattern to the awareness of the family members; if necessary, a request that the child speak for himself or herself
Behavioral	Normal routines versus sharp deviations such as suddenly dropping out of school, marrying, or robbing a bank	If possible—if proximity with the person can be achieved—discussion about how the behavior does not fit with the "expected" routines; inquiry about possible causes
Verbal expression of behavior	Openness about behavior versus unwillingness to see or talk about behavior	Discussion of the client's behavior to achieve shared awareness between client and nurse of the behavior and related problems and need for solutions
Verbal expression of thoughts, opinions, and ideas	Open discussion of ideas versus extreme shyness and reluctance to express thoughts or ideas	Discussion with client in which exploration of thoughts and ideas is pursued to determine (or correct if needed or possible), for example, distortions and error in client's perceptions
Verbal expression of feelings and emotions	Open expression of feelings, including distress, versus withdrawn and flat expression and denial of emotional pain or distress	Discussion with client to achieve openness as well as evaluation of extent of distress; effort to achieve congruence between behavior, thought, and feeling

Modified from Longo DC. In Longo DC, Williams RA, editors: *Clinical practice in psychosocial nursing: assessment and intervention,* ed 2, New York, 1986, Appleton-Century-Crofts.

▼ **TABLE 6-2**   Summary of Theories of Communication

Theory	Dynamics	Major Concepts
Ruesch	Therapeutic communication involves (1) gaining an understanding of the nature of the client's distress; (2) engaging the client in an analysis of his behavior; and (3) reaching agreement about what needs to change and what may bring about this change.	Metacommunication Anticipatory adaptation Momentary adaptation Leverage
Double-bind	The simultaneous communication of conflicting messages results in the recipient's now knowing which message to respond to.	Primary, secondary, and tertiary messages
Kinesics	Behavior is regulated by nonverbal gestures and cues, also called body language.	Affiliation Dominance Submission
Proxemics	Persons have intangible but real boundaries surrounding them that they communicate to others.	Territoriality Social distance Personal space Ego boundaries Crowding Touch
Communication channels	Persons communicate through six "channels"; if one or more channels become dysfunctional, they will communicate through at least one of the other channels.	Congruence across channels

readiness for contact and planning a type of contact that would have therapeutic value.

Communication Channels

Another way to organize observations about human communication is to use the six levels of communication outlined in Longo's "channel construct" of communication (Table 6-1). The need to maintain a sense of relatedness is so great that people have evolved a kind of fail-safe system that ensures the function of communication even if one or more of the others become dysfunctional.[21]

Longo's channel construct provides a focus on the process of communication, which involves the manner in which something is said or done, as in asking a direct question. Longo distinguishes the process from the content. The process is the flow of words and symbols, which is distinguished from the context, which is the setting or circumstances in which communication takes place. The construct offers a framework for assessment and intervention. The six channels provide the nurse with an outline of what to observe and how to classify the data. Evaluation of the congruence of communication across channels is an important part of clinical assessment. For example, the client who says he feels comfortable while squirming about and exhibiting a sad facial expression is demonstrating incongruence across channels.

Intervention is planned and implemented after an analysis of the following four major aspects of the communication:

1. The functional competence
2. The congruence
3. The appropriateness of the findings relative to the client's problem
4. The appropriateness of the findings relative to the context and content

Table 6-1 shows examples of functions and dysfunctions and interventions for the six channels. Table 6-2 summarizes the dynamics and major concepts of the theories of communication.

TECHNIQUES OF THERAPEUTIC COMMUNICATION

This section presents specific techniques for the nurse's use that increase the therapeutic value of nurse-client interactions and facilitate developing learning experiences to help the client achieve greater self-awareness and a higher regard for self. Although each technique is presented separately, the techniques are typically used in combination to facilitate effective nurse-client communication. Table 6-3 provides several examples of some of the most commonly used therapeutic communication techniques. Table 6-4 gives examples of nontherapeutic techniques. A discussion of additional techniques follow.

Conveying Respect

Respect is a point of view that says to another, "You count. You have worth. You matter. You have dignity, and I will treat you in a respectful, polite manner." The nurse may convey respect to the client in several ways. By being on time for appointments and by spending the full time that has been agreed upon with the client, the nurse conveys her respect for the client's time and space. The nurse also conveys respect for the client by treating his room and belongings as private property; permission is requested to gain access to these private spaces. Some people believe that adult clients should never be addressed by first names because it conveys disrespect for their adult status. Although addressing every client with "Mr." or "Ms." may seem extreme, use of first names only when addressing all clients is also extreme and suggests that individual decisions about what to call each client are not being made.

Respect in any society is usually shown through subtle nuances in verbal and nonverbal behavior, for example, calling a person by his or her name. When the client is from a different social class or culture than the nurse, conscious effort permits the nurse to learn how respect is conveyed in the client's culture and how to avoid inadvertently conveying disrespect.

Listening Actively

Listening actively implies that the nurse is an active rather than a passive participant in the interaction. *Active listening* means that the nurse conveys a real desire to hear what the client has to say. Listening actively contributes to the therapeutic value of the communication process in two ways: (1) the client experiences the nurse's active interest and feels reassured of her intention to help, and (2) the nurse is likely to hear more of what the client has to say and to better understand the nature of the client's concerns.

Active listening is apparent to the client in verbal and nonverbal ways. Verbally, the nurse comments or asks questions that relate directly to what the client has been saying. The content of the nurse's questions or comments make it clear that the nurse is listening. Nonverbally, the nurse maintains eye contact (without staring), leans forward in the chair to convey interest and attention, nods to show acceptance, and frowns or smiles to convey an appropriate confusion or understanding about the client's comments.

Defining Boundaries

The boundaries of nurse-client communication are the social, physical, and emotional limits of the interaction. The nurse's efforts to help the client work within these boundaries create opportunities for the client to gain self-awareness. For example, the interaction is defined as therapeutic rather than social, which means it is occurring because of the client's need and is intended to benefit the client. The interaction can be friendly in spirit, but the conversation is not meant to establish friendship. The nurse assists the client to understand and accept that the nurse's purpose is to help the client learn. The client is not expected to help the nurse learn (although the nurse often learns much in working with clients). The nurse cares about the client's well-being, and the client is helped to know that he is not expected to care about the nurse in a personal way. Gentle confrontation of the client's attempts to make the relationship different from therapeutic communication allows the client to understand more about his own motives and to accept the nurse's intentions to be helpful.

▼ **TABLE 6-3**   **Therapeutic Communication Techniques**

Therapeutic Techniques	Examples
Using silence: using absence of verbal communication	
Accepting: indicating reception	Yes.
	Uh-hmm.
	I follow what you said.
	Nodding.
Giving recognition: acknowledging, indicating awareness	You're coughing and breathing deeply.
	You cleaned your house.
Offering self: making one's *self* available	I'll sit with you a while.
	I'll stay here with you.
Giving broad openings: allowing the client to take the initiative in introducing the topic	What would you like to talk about?
	What are you thinking about?
	Where would you like to begin?
Offering general leads: giving encouragement to continue	Go on.
	And then?
	Tell me about it.
Placing the event in time or in sequence: clarifying the relationship of events in time	What seemed to lead up to...?
	This was before or after...?
	When did this happen?
Making observations: verbalizing what is perceived	You appear tense.
	You seem uncomfortable when you....
	I notice you biting your lips.
	I become uncomfortable when you....
Encouraging description of perception: asking the client to verbalize what he perceives	When do you feel anxious?
	What is happening?
	What does the voice seem to be saying?
Encouraging comparison: asking that similarities and differences be noted	This was something like....
	When have you had similar experiences?
Reflecting: directing back to the client's questions, feelings, and ideas; encouraging the client to bring forth his own ideas, which the nurse thereby acknowledges	**Client:** Do you think I should tell the doctor...?
	Nurse: You are wondering if it is important.
Restating: repeating to client what has been said	**Client:** I feel so down and useless since I retired.
	Nurse: You feel down and useless since you retired?
Focusing: concentrating on a single point	This seems like an area we can concentrate on.
Exploring: delving further into a subject or idea	Tell me more about that. Would you describe it more fully? What kind of work?
Seeking clarification: seeking to make clear anything not meaningful or vague	I'm not sure that I follow. What would you say is the main point of what you said? Tell me whether my understanding of it agrees with yours. Are you using this word to convey the idea of...?
Presenting reality: offering for consideration what is real	I see no one else in the room. That sound was a car backfiring. Your mother is not here; I'm a nurse.
Verbalizing the implied: voicing what the client has hinted at or suggested	**Client:** My wife pushes me around just like my mother and sister do.
	Nurse: Is it your impression that women are domineering?
Encouraging evaluation: asking for appraisal of the quality of his experiences	What are your feelings in regard to...? Does this contribute to your discomfort?
Attempting to translate into feelings: seeking to verbalize the feelings being expressed only indirectly	**Client:** I've been in this hospital for 6 weeks. I might as well be dead.
	Nurse: You feel as if you're not getting any better?
Suggesting collaboration: offering to share, to strive to work together with the client for his benefit	Maybe this is something you and I can figure out together.
Encouraging formulation of a plan of action: asking the client to consider behavioral alternatives that may be appropriate in future situations	What could you do to let your anger out harmlessly? Next time this comes up, what can you do to handle it?

Based on data from Hays JS, Larson KH: *Interacting with patients,* New York, 1965, Macmillan.

▼ **TABLE 6-4   Nontherapeutic Communication Techniques**

Nontherapeutic Techniques	Examples
Reassuring: indicating that there is no cause for anxiety	I wouldn't worry about.... Everything will be all right. You're coming along fine.
Giving approval: sanctioning the client's ideas or behavior	That's good.... I'm glad that you....
Rejecting: refusing to consider the client's ideas	Let's not discuss.... I don't want to hear about....
Disapproving: denouncing the client's ideas and behavior	That's bad. I'd rather you wouldn't....
Agreeing: indicating accord with the client	That's right. I agree.
Disagreeing: opposing the client's ideas	That's wrong. I definitely disagree with....
Advising: telling the client what to do	I think you should.... Why don't you...?
Probing: persistent questioning of the client	Now tell me about.... Tell me your life history.
Challenging: demanding proof from the client	**Client:** I feel dead all over. **Nurse:** If you don't need the surgery, then why are you here?
Defending: attempting to protect someone or something from verbal attack	This hospital has a fine reputation. No one here would lie to you. But Dr. B. is a very able psychiatrist. I'm sure that he has your welfare in mind when he....
Requesting an explanation: asking someone to provide reasons for feelings, behavior, and events	Why do you think that? Why do you feel this way? Why did you do that?
Requesting an explanation: asking someone to explain the way he behaves or feels	"How are you different now?" "How did that affect you?" "How do you feel after you drink?"
Indicating the existence of an external source: attributing the source of thoughts, feelings, and behavior to others or to outside influences	What makes you say that? What made you do that?
Belittling feelings expressed: misjudging the degree of the client's discomfort	**Client:** I have nothing to live for. I wish I were dead. **Nurse:** Everybody gets down in the dumps. I've felt that way sometimes.
Making stereotypical comments: offering meaningless clichés and trite expressions	Nice weather we're having. I'm fine, and how are you? It's for your own good. Keep your chin up. Just listen to your doctor and take part in activities. You'll be home in no time.
Giving literal responses: responding to a figurative comment as though it were a statement of fact	**Client:** I feel like my insides are coming out. **Nurse:** Show me where they're coming out.
Using denial: refusing to admit that a problem exists	**Client:** I'm nothing. **Nurse:** Of course you're something. Everybody is somebody. **Client:** I'm dead. **Nurse:** No, you're not.
Introducing an unrelated topic: changing the subject	**Client:** I'd like to die. **Nurse:** Did you have visitors this weekend?

Based on data from Hays JH, Larson KH: *Interacting with patients,* New York, 1965, Macmillan.

The physical boundaries of the nurse-client communication define where the communication will and will not occur. For example, the nurse and client typically meet in a clinic or an office, and meeting in the home of the nurse or client is usually not acceptable unless the contact is structured as a home visit. Alternatively, the nurse and client may appropriately communicate in the home of the nurse if the nurse's home is a private practice setting. At issue here is that the physical space is consistent with the definition of the communication as having therapeutic, not social, purposes.

A further example of defining boundaries is establishing ground rules in the communication process. For example, the nurse can establish such rules as the following: (1) the client may not make phone calls to the nurse's home, and (2) the client may not attempt to meet the nurse in a social situation.

Defining boundaries contributes to the therapeutic potential of the nurse's communication with the client because it maintains a focus on the healing process. The structure is also useful because the nurse can at any point remind the client about the boundaries in a gentle but firm way, stressing the value of keeping the interaction on therapeutic terms. This attention to boundaries also conveys that the nurse continues to care about the client and that the nurse remains committed to the therapeutic purposes of the relationship.

Structuring Time

The therapeutic potential of nurse-client communication can be enhanced when the client knows exactly how much time the nurse has available for the conversation. For example, a 30-minute conversation on an inpatient unit is likely to be disappointing if the client expects the nurse to stay for an hour. Alternatively, the client is likely to feel respected and cared about if the nurse agrees to meet for 30 minutes and keeps that time agreement. For the client who wants extra time, very positive effects can sometimes be achieved by the nurse's occasional decision to make available unexpected extra time with the client.

Pacing

Pacing emphasizes the nurse's ability to recognize the verbal and nonverbal patterns of the client's immediate behavior and levels of tension. Pacing involves following these patterns until the nurse can take the lead in the conversation, directing discussion to needed areas of focus, but doing so in a way consistent with the client's pattern of communication. Pacing also implies that the nurse has a goal. Imagine an example of a client who has been raped who needs to recount what has happened. The client may focus on extraneous information as a means of reducing tension. The nurse, by following and then pacing the client's comments and observing the client's behavioral indicators of tension, can gently lead the client into discussion about the event. The nurse's sensitivity to the client's capacity to tolerate tension is important in maintaining rapport and a sense of alliance with the client. Therapeutic communication is disrupted if the client is overwhelmed. As a client gains confidence and moves through the phases of the relationship, the capacity to experience and profit from intense emotional response increases, and the pace with which the nurse approaches these issues can be much faster.

Using Questions Effectively

Since the assessment process requires nurses to obtain information from clients, the habit of asking clients questions is easy to acquire. In some instances a question is an appropriate way to seek an answer. For example, the easiest way to find out a client's age might be to ask, "How old are you?" or "What is your birth date?" However, an abundance of questions about the client's background tends to make the client feel barraged. Intensive questioning can also convey the message, "You are a statistic." Learning about the effective use of questions is best achieved by examining written verbatim accounts of nurse-client interactions (also called process recordings) to see how often questions are used and what responses clients give. In many instances, information can also be obtained by the use of more indirect invitations to talk, such as "Tell me about your family, brothers, sisters, parents . . . ."

Asking clients "Why did you do that?" or "Why?" can be especially problematic for them. Naturally the nurse wants to know why a particular behavior or event occurred, and the information would also be useful to the client. However, clients frequently do not know why they have done something or felt a certain way. They are "clients" who need to talk about some behavior or event because they are troubled about it in some way and do not understand why it happened. Clients often say, "I don't know why I did that." When asked why, they probably have good reason to say, "If I knew why, I wouldn't be here!" If the nurse seeks a description of how the event took place, that is the question to ask. For example, "Tell me how the argument got started in the first place," or "What were you doing at the time?" are effective questions. "Why did you argue?" is usually nontherapeutic for two reasons: the client is not likely to know, and the question sounds like a demand for explanation or self-defense.

Another very overused question is "How did you feel about that?" This trite question is often heard when a client's nursing care plan recommends "encourage verbalization of feelings." The incorrect belief is that expressing feelings is an end point in therapeutic intervention. However, it is really only a beginning point, and the question often leaves the client consciously experiencing a painful feeling or memory. The expression of feelings is only the first step in the "working through" process of healing or achieving resolution of painful feelings and memories. The steps include:

1. *Verbalization* of the painful feelings or memories
2. *Validation* with another person (such as the nurse) that the feelings or memories are understandable human experiences and that they are acknowledged as sources of pain for the client
3. *Mourning,* or "working through" the pain, by talking about the feelings several times, leading to reexperiencing feelings in a less intense way, feeling more hopeful, and perceiving new alternatives
4. *Restitution,* in which the client has gained a new

perspective on the painful feelings or feels relieved to a sufficient degree that they are no longer a problem

In summary, instead of directly asking the client how he feels, the nurse needs to help the client proceed through the sequence and progress beyond simply expressing and experiencing the pain to resolving the painful feelings and memories as well. As a general rule, questions can be replaced by reflection, by open-ended statements that invite the client to complete the statement, and by declarative statements of what the client may be feeling that contain a slight inflection or implication of a question. Clients can respond to these invitations if they feel comfortable, but are spared the feeling of being interrogated that can be created by a series of questions. These invitations are especially effective if they are offered with a moderate degree of warmth and a spirit of understanding that carefully avoids the excessively sympathetic tones of voice often heard in interactions with clients.

Restating

The client can be aided in his efforts to achieve self-understanding by the judicious use of *restating,* in which the nurse repeats to the client what has been said. For example, the nurse is using restating in the following interaction:

Client: *We are really having a rough time at home.*
Nurse: *You're having a rough time at home . . . . (voice trails off)*
Client: *Well, yes. What I mean is that my teenager is really arguing with me a lot, and I feel like I don't know what to say.*
Nurse: *You aren't sure what to say . . . .*
Client: *Right. I want to really come down hard and say a curfew is a curfew. Instead, I hold back. I don't know why.*

The nurse restates to the client what has been said, using the client's choice of words. The use of restating can be in the form of a question or a statement:

Nurse: *You're having a rough time at home? (Emphasis on the word "home" and voice inflection conveys a question.)*

or

Nurse: *You're having a rough time at home . . . . (Emphasis on the words "rough time" and voice inflection conveys a statement that trails off, as if waiting for the client's response.)*

Restating increases the client's awareness of what he is saying and how it is being said. The approach needs to be used in a calm manner without aggressively confronting the client or trying to pressure the client into greater self-awareness. The nurse needs to incorporate this approach into a larger repertoire of skills so that it is not overused. Excessive reliance on restating is irritating to clients because the nurse sounds unwilling to respond or appears overly reliant on a technique.

Validating

Validating is a technique that can be valuable to therapeutic communication in two important ways: assisting the client to achieve a more realistic view of the world, and creating in the client the experience of feeling understood. *Validation* is the agreement of the nurse with certain elements of the client's communication, as in the following example:

Client: *Boy, you can't believe how bad my boss is. I get hassled all the time for things that aren't even my fault. I really think he has it in for me. Maybe he's even really completely against me because he wants somebody else in the position.*
Nurse: *Yes, it would make sense for you to feel distressed if the boss is against you. I can tell that you feel distressed— that this work situation is uncomfortable. (Pause.) I wonder if we could talk more about what he does and what he says and the circumstances so that I could get a better picture of it.*

Here the nurse has validated the appropriateness of feeling upset about the client's supervisor, although the actual story about the supervisor has not been validated. Instead, the nurse requests further exploration of the topic. The client can feel understood with regard to the distress that he has experienced on the job. The client can also sense the nurse's interest and potential acceptance because of her request to pursue the topic further. At the same time, the nurse's statement also contains a subtle suggestion that the story about the supervisor might not be completely accurate. Use of a subtle hint can be an important first step in casting doubt on a client's perception of experience, which may be all the doubt that is appropriate to show until more information about the situation is obtained. The client is neither totally believed nor totally disbelieved at the outset.

Asking for Demonstrations and Illustrations

Asking for demonstrations and illustrations may involve the client in giving the nurse an example, or the nurse can have the client literally show her what has gone on. For example, a client complained that her mother made her feel guilty every time she talked to her on the phone. The nurse helped the client go through a detailed demonstration of preparing to call her mother, dialing the number, repeating her lines to her mother, and then filling in her mother's responses including mimicking her tone of voice. The client laughed because she identified two aspects of her "guilt": her desire to avoid seeing her mother that day and her anger at her mother for saying it was all right yet sounding very whiny. The client was able to use this information in talking with her mother. Over a period of time, her mother agreed that although she knew it was wrong, she was in fact attempting to make her daughter feel guilty.

Providing Information

Providing information to a client increases the client's resources for solving problems and making decisions. It also conveys the message that the nurse cares and is a giving person. Apprising the client of specific resources that match his needs provides information. Enlisting the assistance of others such as a social worker or rehabilitation counselor can also provide information needed to confront a particular problem. Another significant way of providing information is teaching the client mental health concepts, such as communication skills, to enhance the person's ability to solve problems and relate effectively to others. For example, the nurse may teach problem-solving methods as a way of tackling difficult decisions. The nurse may also teach the concepts of transactional analysis to the client and his significant others as a way to work on communication problems at home and during interactions with her.

Emphasizing Relationships Between Parts and Wholes

Therapeutic nurse-client interaction can assist clients in understanding how their way of thinking about an experience leads to problems or inaccuracies in perception. Some clients generalize too much on the basis of limited experience. Others seem to see only discrete events and fail to learn by generalizing, despite multiple similar experiences. These problems can be addressed in the nurse-client interaction, using the interaction as an illustration when possible. Clients who tend to generalize on the basis of too little experience can be assisted in seeing the gaps in their information.

Client: I know that you don't really like me. People never do like me.
Nurse: That's a pretty big conclusion. How did you arrive at that idea?
Client: You were late today. I know what that means.
Nurse: How is it that my being late makes you think I don't like you?
Client: I just know. It's always been that way.
Nurse: Somebody you wanted to like you was late, and you felt bad because you feared they didn't?

A lengthier example relating specifics to the client's overgeneralization may be needed, but the example illustrates the point that the nurse can lead the client from the general idea (probably a distortion) to certain specifics, some of which confirm the idea and others that do not. The goal of this communication process is to teach the client that general ideas can be formed on the basis of too little or incorrect information. Strengthening skills in inductive thinking enables the client to analyze specific observations to confirm or deny general propositions in his thinking.

Clients who focus too much on specific events need assistance in developing deductive thinking skills so that general propositions (learning) can occur on the basis of discrete experiences or events. The skills of generalizing from experience require an ability to think in more abstract terms. The nurse-client communication can focus on this issue:

Client: Well, I've done it again. I had a huge fight with my wife, and I hate myself for doing it. I'm so depressed.
Nurse: This sounds familiar. I am curious about what led to the disagreement.
Client: It's the same old thing. Every time I forget to do the dishes, it's the same thing—a big fight.
Nurse: You forgot?
Client: Well, see, I was really mad about the house being a mess and having to think about all there was to do, most of which isn't my job, and I just forgot all about the dishes.
Nurse: That sounds like the other day when you were angry with me and forgot to keep our appointment. Is this a
way of doing things that keeps you in trouble—you get angry and fail to do your end of things, say you forgot, and then fight and feel terrible about yourself?

The continuation of this interaction is aimed at helping the client see the relationship between the outcome of feeling bad about himself and the many separate events in which failure to fulfill an obligation is excused as forgetting and a disagreement ensues. Learning that the discrete events are related to the larger undesired outcome is the first step in creating an opportunity for the client to change. All the while, the nurse avoids the message, "You bring this on yourself," which can sound punitive and reinforces the client's self-deprecation. Instead, the nurse emphasizes the relationships between the parts and the whole in an objective manner.

Using Nurse-Client Communication for Experiential Illustrations

As a part of the therapeutic communication process, the nurse provides feedback to the client, which involves the nurse sharing her perceptions of what the client seems to be saying. The following example describes a nurse's response to a client who has described a conflict with a friend. The client described himself as having been unreasonable, ineffective, and overly angry:

Nurse: I have listened to you describe the situation and in my view there was good reason to feel angry. Perhaps it was not such a good idea to threaten to walk out, but the way you describe having stated your concerns sounds like a very reasonable statement.

However, when the nurse-client communication is used as illustration, the nurse provides feedback that directly relates to the communication that has occurred between nurse and client. For example, the nurse could have responded to the same client in the following way:

Nurse: You describe yourself as having been unreasonable, ineffective, and overly angry after expressing your feelings to your friend, feelings you were probably justified in having. I am thinking that may also happen when we talk. Remember the time you were irritated because I answered the phone during our talk and then later berated yourself for having an understandable reaction? (Voice trails off, leaving client the option of responding.)

The major value of using the nurse-client communication to illustrate ideas or conclusions is that both parties have shared the interaction; this means that the client will not think that the nurse failed to understand a situation that had been reported by the client. Another advantage is that this technique says to the client, "What we talk about is very important. You can learn from the way we talk about things and by going back to earlier conversations, which may help you understand yourself better."

Sharing that the Client is Thought About

With most clients, the nurse will think about the client at times other than when the two are engaged in a therapeutic interaction. Sometimes this involves feelings about the client. At other times the nurse is attempting to understand the person or evaluate whether their interactions are helping the client. In any case, a positive statement the nurse can make to the client is "I was thinking about you." This is a common expression of warmth in our society. When a friend or relative calls or is encountered unexpectedly, one often says, "I was just thinking about you the other day." Often an explanation is added in which the person is complimented, such as, "I was remembering how much fun we had that time we went to the theater." With clients, a parallel message that conveys warmth and the feelings of being cared about is, "You know I was thinking yesterday about our last conversation and wondering how that family reunion went." In so doing, the nurse gives the client an unexpected gift of time (the time spent thinking about the client) and also eases the introduction of a potentially painful topic by creating a warm and caring context in which it can be discussed.

Offering Hope

Offering hope is a communication technique frequently used in day-to-day interactions with clients. The issue of hope or the lack of it can also be a major clinical problem to which the nurse addresses therapeutic efforts. (See Chapter 14 on hope and hopelessness.)

Offering hope is a subtle and delicate matter. The nurse needs to simultaneously convey understanding and acceptance of the client's despair or pain. In some instances, hope is an optimistic attitude about the client's potential to return to health. In other instances, it is the belief that the client can become engaged in a therapeutic process that will permit problem solving to begin. Hope is also related to spiritual beliefs, which for some people are directly connected to religious beliefs. Hope in these instances implies some form of faith in a higher power that will support or otherwise lend energy to the healing process. This means that the nurse will either need to support the client's spiritual beliefs or enlist the help of someone who can.

Guidelines that enhance the therapeutic potential of the nurse's offering of hope include the following:
1. Avoid a Pollyanna or overly cheerful attitude.
2. Accept the client's pain or distress as a valid part of the current experience.
3. Avoid urging the client to be more positive.
4. Offer statements calmly and with adequate opportunity for the client to respond.
5. Avoid urging the client to accept the beliefs of any specific religious faith.

Summarizing

Therapeutic nurse-client communication is aimed at creating learning opportunities for the client, and summarizing is an important way in which the nurse can reinforce important ideas or points. Summarizing also provides a check on the nurse's perceptions. By saying, "Now let me try to summarize what we've talked about, and you tell me if it sounds right," the nurse can validate perceptions about the communication. In addition, this is a way of saying, "I have formed certain ideas about you and what you have said here, but I do not just assume I am correct. I value your opinions."

The nurse can also invite the client to summarize, as in saying, "Suppose you were to put what we've talked about in a nutshell. What would you say?" This is another way to check perceptions and determine discrepancies between the views of the nurse and those of the client. It also says, "I am interested in hearing how you sum things up. Your way of looking at things is important, and you are the best person to tell me about it."

ISSUES IN THERAPEUTIC COMMUNICATION

This section reviews the following issues in therapeutic nurse-client interaction:
1. How much self-disclosure by the nurse is appropriate?
2. How much energy and reactivity is appropriate for the nurse to display?
3. How much personal feedback does the client receive?
4. When or how is confrontation of the client therapeutic?
5. To what extent or in what ways is humor appropriate?
6. When is accepting gifts appropriate?

In this discussion, opposing views on the issues as well as the rationale for these views will be presented. Decisions about these issues need to incorporate the client's needs, contextual factors in the clinical setting that impinge on practice, and the nurse's informed judgment.

How Much Self-Disclosure?

Self disclosure is the process of voluntarily revealing information about one's self.[18] Those who believe that self-disclosure by the nurse has therapeutic value argue that if the client views the relationship in personal terms, his problems can be addressed in the therapeutic interaction. When used therapeutically, self-disclosure enables the client to feel secure in revealing information about himself. Self-disclosure provides the client with an opportunity to perceive the nurse as a genuine human being rather than as a mechanical clinician. This approach is believed to be especially helpful when used to reassure the client that other people have the same or similar concerns.

Those who maintain that self-disclosure is inappropriate in nurse-client communication argue that personal disclosures on the part of the nurse encourage the client to view the relationship as one of personal friendship rather than therapeutic involvement. The nurse who uses a great deal of self-disclosure fills the conversation with talk about herself rather than the client. This limits the client's opportunity to gain self-awareness and increases the likelihood that the relationship will focus on the unresolved personal problems of the nurse rather than on those of the client.

Examples of nurse responses to a client's inquiry about where the nurse lives may include the following:

Client: I was wondering, where do you live, anyway?
Nurse: I live out in Ridgewood. (Self-disclosure)
or

Nurse: I'm curious about your reason for asking....
or

Nurse: I live out in Ridgewood (pause). I'm curious about your reason for asking. (Modified self-disclosure)

The client's question does not contain sufficient data for the nurse to make assumptions about why the question is being asked. The nurse may believe that self-disclosure is not acceptable because she perceives that the client's question expresses a wish to become more personally involved with her. If the nurse believes self-disclosure is effective, the client's question can simply be taken at face value. If the nurse wants additional data and sees no problem in answering the question, the third response achieves both purposes.

Clients also frequently remark that the nurse reminds the client of someone, often a person in the client's past or present who is important. For example:

Client: *You're just like my friend J.D.*
Nurse: *Well, I'm certainly not J.D.! (No self-disclosure)*
or
Nurse: *I wonder what about me reminds you of J.D.? (No self-disclosure but invitation to say more)*

The first response indicates surprise or anger at the client's comment. The nurse's response does not imply that any self-disclosure is likely to occur. The second response requests more information and leaves the issue of self-disclosure open.

How Much Emotion and Energy?

Strong emotion and energy conveyed in the nurse's reactions, feelings, or sentiments may have a significant impact on the client. This can be planned or accidental. Examples of strong emotion or energy that the nurse can convey to the client are:

1. Warmth, affection, caring, approval, and love
2. Encouragement, optimism, and hope
3. Irritation, anger, and disapproval
4. Downhearted feelings, despair, and depression
5. Touch, with or without the conscious intent to heal

Traditional approaches in therapeutic communication and psychotherapy have emphasized the importance of the clinician maintaining a neutral and objective stance in responding to the client. This approach precludes the nurse from expressing more than a very mild degree of affection and caring, encouragement, irritation or anger, moodiness, or touch. The rationale for this approach is that the nurse who expresses strong emotion or energy encourages the client to experience the relationship as a personal one, which is thought to be incompatible with the professional goals of the relationship. The client who considers the relationship with the nurse a personal one is more likely to misinterpret the nature of the relationship.

Advocates of the neutral or objective approach view client distortions and errors in interpretation as transference reactions. According to this view, it is nontherapeutic to communicate strong emotion and energy, thus encouraging the client to experience transference reactions. For example, the nurse's enthusiasm toward a client's report of a success may later induce the client to be frightened that a failure would disappoint the nurse. The nurse's expression of feeling downhearted can cause the client to feel responsible, inadequate, or obligated to try to cheer up the nurse. Touching the client may cause fears that the nurse is making sexual overtures. In each of these examples, the client's untoward reaction may be related to a pattern of responding in an earlier relationship with a parent, sibling, or other significant person.

Clinicians who believe the expression of energy and emotion with the client has therapeutic value form the other extreme. They argue that great therapeutic opportunities are created by provoking client reactions, such as when the nurse touches the client or expresses approval, encouragement, anger, or moodiness. The client's reactions are the focus of the therapeutic communication, which can lead to greater self-awareness for the client.

Another somewhat different argument in favor of showing emotion and energy suggests that the client will see the nurse as a more genuine person if feelings are candidly expressed when they occur. If the nurse feels happy, optimistic, angry, or downhearted or wants to touch the client, these reactions are appropriate for the nurse to share. The client has the opportunity to share in how another person experiences and talks about feeling these energies. This sharing is thought to assist the client in becoming more self-aware and better able to communicate effectively with others. When the nurse conveys strong emotion and energy, the client can experience the nurse's approval for a success or the nurse's disapproval for a failure to manage a problem effectively. Some believe that the reality-testing value of such experience far outweighs the dangers of causing excessive transference reactions.

How Much Feedback?

In therapeutic communication, *feedback* refers to the nurse's sharing with the client (1) perceptions of the client's behavior, or (2) interpretations of the client's behavior. The client who storms into the meeting with a tense facial expression, tightened lips, and lack of verbal expressions receives one of the following responses:

Nurse: *Well (softly), I see a person who is tense and not saying very much.... (Pauses after open-ended statement)*
or
Nurse: *You seem upset. (Pauses)*

In the first response, the nurse describes the observed behavior in terms that are as objective as possible. In the second response, the nurse makes no attempt to describe what is observed, instead sharing an interpretation of what has been observed.

Decisions about appropriate use of feedback include whether to use feedback at all, as well as to what degree either type of feedback described should be used. Many nurses use feedback techniques extensively in therapeutic communication, believing that self-awareness is achieved as a result of helping the client learn how he is perceived by others. Assuming that the client is unaware of critical elements of behavior, especially in areas in which problems are reported, the nurse undertakes to bring these elements into the client's conscious awareness.

An alternative view is held by those who do not use feedback techniques very much or at all in therapeutic communication. The rationale is that extensive use of feedback techniques puts the nurse in an excessively directive role with the client. Instead, the nurse's role in therapeutic communication is defined as nondirective in which reflection of the client's thoughts is used to facilitate his responsibility for directing the conversation.

Feedback in which the nurse describes as objectively as possible observed behavior is generally accepted by those who advocate using feedback. However, use of interpretations of these observations is a controversial matter. Some nurses believe that the client can benefit from knowing the nurse's interpretations and conclusions. The client may then respond and offer alternative interpretations for discussion. Other nurses believe that interpretations are too directive, and that they create a risk of bringing to awareness thoughts or feelings for which the client is unprepared. They believe the nurse's role is to facilitate the client's expression of thoughts and feelings, not to impose or force these expressions before the client is ready.

How Much Confrontation?

In mental health work, *confrontation* usually refers to an encounter between two persons in which one person seeks to encourage another to face or acknowledge something presumed to be painful or objectionable. The nurse may confront a client about his resistance evidenced by missing his appointments. The plan to confront the client assumes that the client does not want to face this fact and that the nurse's role is to encourage the client to talk about it. The client may need to be made aware that he is manipulating the staff to get his way or being inconsistent in what he tells the staff are his concerns. The steps used in confrontation are outlined in the accompanying box. Confrontation is often associated with the nurse's being angry, resulting in confrontation of the client in a way that seems to require the client to defend himself against the nurse's anger.

At each point in this sequence, the nurse can decide whether to implement the intervention or whether too much opposition exists for the confrontation to achieve a therapeutic purpose. Since the word "confrontation" often connotes antagonism, following the careful analysis outlined above is necessary. Deliberately antagonistic or retaliatory nursing actions are inappropriate. The potential to provoke anger in the client can create situations of real or potential danger to oneself or others. This risk is only undertaken with careful planning and anticipation of possible outcomes.

There are no rules to guide decisions about when and how much to confront clients in mental health–psychiatric nursing practice. Since there is little research or documentation in this area to guide practice, the decision is often

▼ **STEPS IN USING CONFRONTATION IN CLINICAL PRACTICE**

1. Analyze who needs to be confronted about what.
2. Analyze the appropriate person to be the confronter.
3. Analyze the degree of resistance felt toward the person who is to be confronted.
4. Analyze the degree of defensiveness expected from the person to be confronted.
5. Develop a detailed plan for the confrontation based on specific therapeutic goals.
6. Implement the plan and evaluate the effectiveness of the nursing action.

based on the judgment of the nurse. Some nurses believe a confrontation mode should never be used because it is caused by the nurse's anger, and because it is so likely to sound punitive, provoking self-defensive or aggressive responses. Other nurses use confrontation extensively, believing that it stimulates a real encounter with the added dimension of the willingness of the nurse to talk about the situation with the client (which may not always be possible in real life). Those who use confrontation in their practice believe clients can be held accountable for their behavior and that confrontation is the way to achieve this goal. Opponents of this approach usually agree that clients can be responsible for their behaviors, but they rely on gentler forms of feedback that minimize client's needs to defend themselves or respond forcefully.

How Much Humor?

Humor contributes an essential ingredient to human interaction. It breaks the ice, smooths over stressful moments, and lightens the atmosphere in a great many situations.

The benefits of humor are many. An important consequence in the mental health arena is tension reduction and transcendence of uncomfortable moments or situations. Humor also creates a bond of shared pleasure between people, allowing for enjoyable times that contrast therapeutically with painful problems and distressing feelings that have been shared. Humor is believed to have important physiological effects as well. For example, it has been suggested that humor affects the immune system by promoting the body's ability to combat such health challenges as cancer and diseases of the connective tissue (arthritis, lupus erythematosis, and others).[29]

There is some debate about how much humor should be used in mental health–psychiatric nursing practice. Those who believe the therapist should remain neutral contend that humor is appropriate only in very limited and well-thought-out situations. Others believe that whatever amount of spontaneous humor occurs is probably beneficial. This position is further reinforced by the idea that structuring or limiting humor makes the nurse-client interaction too contrived.

Consideration of why a statement or story is funny can shed light on the problem. For example, one cause of humor is incongruity in human interaction. When an event is so different from what might normally occur, it strikes people as being funny. This is why we laugh when someone loses their dentures or has unzipped pants. Children have a great sense of humor and appreciation of the incongruous, often enjoying wearing costumes with funny faces or telling jokes. These behaviors persist into adulthood in many people.

Anxiety also produces humor. An anxiety provoking situation or conversation is often turned into a joke or something less serious. For example, late in the night at "slumber parties" or on camping trips, people often tell ghost stories and laugh at the story endings, even though they may be frightening. As another example, we often joke about death, sex, and elimination.

Hostility is a third cause of humor. We joke about things or people that evoke angry feelings, particularly when it is not socially acceptable to directly express the anger. The "left-handed compliment" is one example of this type of humor, in which a compliment is extended that clearly contains an insult. This occurs when we say, "You did pretty good for a beginner," or "That's a great looking suit. Isn't that the same one you've worn to the last few presentations?" Another form of this kind of humor occurs when someone says, "Remember when . . . ?" to recall something uncomfortable that has happened to another person. This request typically causes the person being addressed to describe the embarrassing event, resulting in everyone having a good laugh at the person's expense. Our society seems to value the ability of people to "take a joke" or laugh at themselves, suggesting that we are more comfortable with indirect expression of anger. It then follows that if someone chooses to express anger indirectly through a joke, the other person needs to accept it with good spirit as if no hostility were involved.

The clinical use of humor in mental health–psychiatric nursing practice usually includes thoughtful analysis and interpretation of what underlies the expression of humor. This analysis includes examining the nurse's motives in using humor. It also includes evaluation of how humor and the underlying messages may affect the nurse-client interaction.

Laughing at the sheer incongruity of a situation may seem to be a perfectly innocent attempt to help a client develop a sense of humor. However, if calling attention to the incongruity suggests the client looks silly or is acting in a foolish manner, the nurse can reinforce an already negative self-image. In this example, the nurse can also be expressing hostility toward the client, which suggests the nurse needs to resolve some feelings about the client in a more constructive way. Encouraging laughter at incongruity or the unexpected in others may seem perfectly innocent, but it can reinforce the client's denial of anger, or it may encourage the derogation of others to bolster self-esteem.

Use of humor during anxious moments caused by self-disclosure or provocative topics can sometimes be an effective way of lessening the tension for nurse or client. This use of humor is to be carefully evaluated, however, to ensure that it does not trivialize matters that are important to the client. One problem with using humor in such situations is that communication usually has multiple levels. The nurse may be lessening tension on one level but insulting the client on another. With sensitivity and practice, the nurse can learn to use humor effectively in such moments. One important requirement is learning to avoid using humor at times when anger or disapproval toward the client is being experienced.

The nurse may share humor found in movies, books, records, and the like. These offer rich opportunities to promote laughter and a sense of humor in the client. The nurse can achieve therapeutic goals by sharing reactions to a movie, loaning a book, or sharing cartoons with the client. These behaviors provide a "personal touch" to the nurse's work with the client. They require thoughtful use to be sure that the implied friendliness is therapeutic rather than social in nature. In this way, the client knows he is special without the attendant problems of being too special or too close for the client's well-being.

What About Accepting Gifts?

Nurses in every area of clinical practice confront situations in which clients or their family members want to give them gifts. In many settings, gift giving is the simple expression of gratitude for kind and loving care to a client surviving a threatening experience. In the mental health arena, however, other dimensions of gift giving must be considered.

Clients in mental health settings are involved in treatment of their personalities and their relationships with others. As a result, so-called "normal" behavior is typically analyzed to determine the special meaning of behavior for each particular client. Since mental health clients are confronting such difficulties as low self-esteem, inability to feel love, feeling rejected by others, or problems with authority, the impulse to give a gift to a nurse that is appropriate in many social settings is usually not appropriate in mental health settings.

Many experienced clinicians recommend never accepting gifts from clients. They cite as reasons the necessity to avoid implying that the client will not be accepted unless gifts are given, that gifts will secure more attention or better treatment for a client, or that there is a personal relationship between the nurse and client. If the best interests of the client are to be served, then no gift from a client in a mental health setting should be assumed to be "innocent" of added psychological meanings. Instead, the gift is gracefully declined and the client's reasons for wanting to give the gift are explored. In this way, the client can gain in self-awareness and can be reassured that he is accepted, loved, lovable, and safe, without any gifts given to or other special favors done for the staff.

Sometimes a client or family insists on giving a gift after discharge to show appreciation for the care given. In these situations, the best course of action is to suggest a gift that can be shared by all staff members such as food or a monetary gift to a staff fund for refreshments, education, or research. In this way, the nursing staff can avoid reinforcing negative aspects of gift giving, and they can prevent the gift from defining the nurse-client relationship as a personal one.

FRAMEWORKS FOR MODIFYING DYSFUNCTIONAL COMMUNICATION

Two approaches are suggested as frameworks that can be used to guide nursing interventions to modify dysfunctional communication. These two approaches are most effective when the nurse seeks out supervision or consultation from a clinician who has expertise and experience with these approaches. The first approach is called *paradoxical interventions*, and it is an approach that is derived from communication theory. This approach suggests ways of helping people change behaviors that are troublesome or negative for them. The second approach is called *Transactional Analyses*, which is a framework popularized some years ago by Eric Berne,[2] whose theory was published by Thomas Harris in *I'm OK, You're OK.*[16] This approach also emphasizes the role of communication in achieving behavior change.

Use of Paradoxical Interventions

This novel framework for treating dysfunctional communication and interaction specifically addresses problem formation and problem resolution. The framework deals with the concept of change by showing how changes in behavior can let people discover new ways to define problems and new methods for creating solutions.

The paradoxical intervention framework recommends that the practitioner distinguish between *first-order change*, which is change within a system while the system itself remains unchanged, and *second-order change*, in which the system itself is changed. For example, imagine a family that is seeking help with making mealtimes more pleasant by avoiding the fighting and bickering that characterize most mealtime interactions. Further imagine that they do what many people do who are trying to solve a problem; they believe they are trying to solve the problem by eliminating or reducing the fighting. The problem junctions can also be used as intentional nursing interventions. For instance, the nurse may reassure a client by saying, "It is OK for you to talk with your spouse instead of fighting," or "Don't pick a fight when you can start out with talking." In this example, talking instead of fighting is a new behavior. The nurse gives the client permission to try something new in the first example and instructs the person not to use the old behavior in the second. These nursing actions can be helpful if the client has been taught to expect that fighting is the only way to solve problems.

TRANSACTIONAL ANALYSIS

Many clinicians using the TA approach strongly advocate the use of positive rather than negative messages to the client. This means they would never tell the client, "Don't do that." Instead they would offer permission. In one rather unusual example, a nurse tells about encountering a man seeking counseling who was carrying a gun because he was thinking of killing his boss. The nurse had the presence of mind to say calmly to him, "You have my permission to put that gun down on my desk right now, so I can put it in a safe place for you." The man complied.

The TA framework is equally useful to the nurse in professional and personal roles. The approach can guide the nurse to more effective and satisfying communication in interactions with clients, clients' family members, peers, friends, and the general public. The approach is best learned by having supervision or consultation from someone trained in the method. However, many useful applications can be made through independent learning.

BRIEF REVIEW

Communication is the process by which the nurse accomplishes the tasks of the nursing process. Therapeutic communication is the content of the nurse's intervention. Effective implementation of the nursing process requires the nurse to develop knowledge in the following areas: theories for analyzing communication, techniques of therapeutic communication, issues in therapeutic communication with clients, and approaches to modifying dysfunctional communication.

Definitions of communication distinguish verbal and nonverbal forms. The structure of communication can also be analyzed by looking at sentence structure, choice of words, and content. Communication has functions such as disclosure of information, self-disclosure, and achievement of self-awareness.

Communication has been of major interest in many pursuits since the beginning of recorded history. Nursing has formally recognized the importance of communication with the client since the days of Florence Nightingale. In more recent years, nurses in mental health–psychiatric nursing have developed important guidelines for therapeutic communication with clients in one-to-one relationships and with group and family methods of treatment.

Theoretical approaches that facilitate the nurse's understanding of communication processes include the works of Ruesch, Bateson, Scheflen, and theorists studying proxemics and communication channels. Other clinically useful approaches that demonstrate how behavioral change can be effected through communication include paradoxical interventions and transactional analysis.

Therapeutic communication involves mastering techniques such as conveying respect, listening actively, defining boundaries, structuring time, using questions, restating, and validating. Other necessary skills include asking for demonstrations and illustrations, providing information, emphasizing relationships between parts and wholes, using nurse-client communication to illustrate, sharing that the client is thought about, offering hope, and summarizing.

Issues in therapeutic communication include how much self-disclosure is appropriate for the nurse, how much emotion and energy is therapeutic for the nurse to express, how much confrontation is appropriate, and how much feedback and humor to incorporate into the communication process.

REFERENCES AND SUGGESTED READINGS

1. Bateson G and others: Toward a theory of schizophrenia, *Behavioral Science* 1(4):251, 1956.
2. Berne E: *Transactional analysis in psychotherapy*, New York, 1961, Grove Press.
3. Birdwhistle R: *Introduction to kinesics*, Louisville, 1952, University of Louisville Press.
4. Braverman BG: Eliciting assessment data from the patient who is difficult to interview, *Nursing Clinics of North America* 25(4):743, 1990.
5. Clark J: The patient's gift. In Burd SF, Marshall MA, editors: *Some approaches to psychiatric nursing*, London, 1971, Collier-Macmillan.
6. Crowther DJ: Metacommunications: a missed opportunity, *Journal of Psychosocial Nursing and Mental Health Services* 29(4):13, 1991.
7. Douglass T: A real case for non-verbal communication in nursing practice, *Washington Nurse* 19(10):12, 1989.
8. Gagnon L: Customer service: Is the answer better communication? *Journal of Emergency Nursing* 17(2):63, 1991.
9. Garvin BJ, Kennedy CW: Interpersonal communications between nurses and patients, *Annual Review of Nursing Research* 8:213, 1990.
10. Gaze H: Making time to talk, *Nursing Times*, 86(13):38, 1990.
11. Gibb H, O'Brien B: Jokes and reassurances are not enough: ways in which nurses relate through conversation with elderly clients, *Journal of Advanced Nursing* 15(12):1389, 1990.
12. Gibbs A: Aspects of communication with people who have

attempted suicide, *Journal of Advanced Nursing* 15(11):1245, 1990.

13. Greef M: Building blocks . . . effective use of interpersonal and communication skills, *Nursing RSA Verpleging* 5(7):10, 1990.

14. Grensing L: A formula to avoid miscommunicating *Nursing* 20(9):122, 1990.

15. Hall ET: *The hidden dimension,* New York, 1966 Doubleday.

16. Harris T: *I'm OK, you're OK: a practical guide to transactional analysis,* New York, 1969, Harper & Row.

17. Hays JS, Larson KH: *Interacting with patients,* New York, 1965, Macmillan.

18. Johnson MN: Self-disclosure: a variable in the nurse-client relationship, *Journal of Psychiatric Nursing and Mental Health Services* 18(1):17, 1980.

19. Konieczka R: The beginner's attitude . . . good communication, *Journal of Post Anesthesia in Nursing* 5(5):345, 1990.

20. Krieger D: *Therapeutic touch: how to use your hands to help and heal,* Englewood Cliffs, NJ, 1979, Prentice Hall.

21. Longo DC: Communications and human behavior. In Longo DC, Williams RA, editors: *Clinical practice in psychosocial nursing: assessment and intervention,* ed 2, New York, 1986, Appleton-Century-Crofts.

22. Luft J, Ingham H: The Johari window: a graphic model of awareness in interpersonal relations. In Luft J, editor: *Group processes: an introduction to group dynamics,* Palo Alto, Calif, 1963, National Press Books.

23. Mejo SL: Communication as it affects the therapeutic alliance, *Journal of American Academy of Nurse Practitioners* 15(3):329, 1990.

24. Morse J: The structure and function of gift giving in the patient-nurse relationship, *Western Journal of Nursing Research* 13(5):597, 1991.

25. Rothenburger RL: Transcultural nursing: overcoming obstacles to effective communication, *AORN Journal* 51(5):1349, 1990.

26. Ruesch J: *Disturbed communications,* New York, 1957, WW Norton.

27. Ruesch J: *Therapeutic communication,* New York, 1961, WW Norton.

28. Ruesch J, Bateson G: *Communication: the social matrix of psychiatry,* New York, 1951, WW Norton.

29. Ruesch J, Kees W: *Nonverbal communication,* Berkeley, Calif, 1956, University of California Press.

30. Scheflen A: *Body language and social order: communication as behavioral control,* Englewood Cliffs, NJ, 1972, Prentice Hall.

31. Severtsen BM: Therapeutic communication demystified, *Journal of Nursing Education* 29(4):190, 1990.

32. Simonton OC, Matthews-Simonton S: *Getting well again,* Los Angeles, 1978, JP Tarcher.

33. Watzlawick P, Weakland J, Fisch R: *Change: principles of problem formation and problem resolution,* New York, 1974, WW Norton.

34. Woller H: How to face (and difuse) an angry family: a communication skit, *Advances in Clinical Care* 5(2):43, 1990.

35. Williams H: Humor and healing: therapeutic effects in geriatrics, *Gerontion: A Canadian Review of Geriatric Care* 1(3):14, 1986.

36. Wilson DA: My trips over the language barrier, *American Journal of Nursing* 89(12):1718, 1989.

ANNOTATED BIBLIOGRAPHY

Bradley JC, Edinberg MA: *Communication in the nursing context,* ed 3, Norwalk, Conn, 1990, Appleton & Lange.

This text relates theoretical communication concepts to clinical nursing problems. The content is organized around the theories of King, Satir, and neurolinguistics. The text addresses communication between nurses and others in a variety of role relationships as well as in different settings: hospital, ambulatory, and home care. There is a section on communicating with clients with special needs, such as home based communication, AIDS, substance abuse, child abuse, elderly, and cultural and ethnic groups. Attention is given to health promotion. The text includes exercises related to nursing process issues that are a useful focus for group discussion.

Developing a Therapeutic Relationship

Rauda Salkauskas Gelazis
Jackie Coombe-Moore

After studying this chapter, the student will be able to:

- Identify care as the essence of nursing
- Describe the development of the therapeutic relationship in the practice of mental health–psychiatric nursing
- Discuss self-awareness and its role in the nurse-client relationship
- Identify components of the nurse-client relationship

- Describe the use of warmth, empathy, and genuineness in the nurse-client relationship
- Discuss student reaction to psychiatric nursing
- Discuss the therapeutic use of self
- Describe the phases of the therapeutic relationship

The *therapeutic relationship* is the cornerstone of psychiatric mental–health nursing. The therapeutic nurse-client relationship is an interpersonal process between a professional nurse and a client that helps the client. The purpose of the relationship is to foster and promote growth of the personality to help the client improve in constructive and productive ways of living.[28]

Therapeutic relationships require a certain amount of trust between the nurse and the client. The focus of the therapeutic relationship is the achievement of mutually established goals. The therapeutic relationship is limited and progresses through defined stages. The nurse and the client enter the relationship as strangers and progress so that personal details of the client's life, as well as thoughts and feelings can be discussed openly. The nurse is primarily responsible for maintaining the focus, direction, and continuance of the relationship. Termination of a therapeutic relationship needs to be planned and is an integral part of the therapeutic process.

An essential component of nursing is the concept of *caring*. Caring is recognized by many important nurse theorists and researchers as "the essence of nursing."[27] It has been postulated that nursing cannot occur without caring.[21,27] Given the fact that the therapeutic relationship is the basis for psychiatric–mental health nursing, which in turn consists of essential components such as respect, empathy, and genuineness, all of which directly relate to caring. Caring is also viewed as an essential element of the therapeutic nurse-client relationship. (See the research highlight on p. 111.)

RELEVANT NURSE THEORISTS

The therapeutic nurse-client relationship is the core of psychiatric–mental health nursing. This basic tool of the psychiatric nurse was first developed in nursing by Hildegard Peplau.[32] Peplau based her approach on the importance of interpersonal relations and the evolution of various stages of the therapeutic nurse-client relationship.

Other nurse authors and thinkers who added to our current understanding of the therapeutic nurse-client relationship include: Schwartz and Shockley, Orlando, Ujhely, and Travelbee. Schwartz and Shockley were important to nursing because they suggested that nursing practice can be based on nursing observations of client behaviors. They made specific clinical observations of clients who demonstrated withdrawn, demanding behavior and provided nursing care guidelines for such clients.

Orlando[31] proposed the dynamic nurse-client relationship. Orlando introduced two significant concepts for the field of mental health–psychiatric nursing: the importance of the nurses' having self-awareness and the importance of the clients' input in evaluating the relationship.

Ujhely[45] emphasized the nurse as a healing force within the nurse-client context. She established the reciprocal nature of the nurse-client communication in the healing process. Ujhely noted that the nurses' values, problems, and conflicts must not interfere with the clients' work and commitment to the healing process. The area of self-awareness, which is discussed later in the chapter, was thereby established as an important dimension for the psychiatric nurse to explore.

DATES	EVENTS
1900s	Until the early twentieth century the role of the psychiatric nurse largely emphasized care for the physical needs of clients.
1920s	The first major emphasis on the use of interpersonal relationships and milieu as therapeutic tools came from Harry Stack Sullivan.
1950s	Discussion of the relationship between nurse and client developed by Peplau.
1952	Tudor discussed the influence, behavior, and role that the nurse had in relation to the client. Peplau provided the basis for current nursing practice as she emphasized the process of nursing, the nurse's role as a participant-observer, and the importance of understanding the client's subjective experiences.
1954	Schwing placed the nurse in the role of primary therapist and explored the power of the caring practices of the nurse in making therapeutic contact with the psychotic client.
1960s	The concept of a more active role for both nurse and client emerged. Orlando emphasized attention to the client's daily living skills and gentle, consistent feedback. The concept of the mentally ill as clients rather than patients emerged. The emphasis shifted to the client as an active participant in therapy, with responsibility for personal behavior.
1970s	Care as an essential concept in nursing is identified by Leininger and Watson. The first international caring conference is held in the United States. Leininger investigates the meaning of caring in various cultures.
1980s	The current trend is to view the client holistically, emphasizing the relationship of mind and body, along with other dimensions, and the need for the nurse to respect and accept the client, while using the nurse-client relationship to facilitate change. Watson's theory developed; caring is an essential element.
1990s	More emphasis is placed on the biological aspects of psychiatric disorders in psychiatry. Nursing continues to develop and research the importance of caring in the discipline of nursing. Psychiatric mental health nursing will be challenged to demonstrate its effectiveness in the health care system.
Future	Nursing will apply the knowledge of caring within transcultural contexts to strengthen the therapeutic nurse: client relationship.

Travelbee[43] used a comprehensive approach to communication in mental health–psychiatric nursing. She translated ideas about therapeutic communication into the context of everyday psychiatric nursing practice. Travelbee dispelled the myth of "getting too involved" with clients. This was a traditional warning given to students in the past. Travelbee described mental health–psychiatric nursing as incorporating (1) responsibility to the family, the community, and the client; (2) prevention; and (3) support of clients and families during mental suffering. She believed that nurses are skilled in the conduct of therapeutic relationships with clients. She argued that the client's mental suffering provides a rationale for the nurse utilizing an empathic approach to the client. Travelbee also raised the issue of the meaning of the experience on mental illness for the client.

These are a few of the nurse theorists whose work has established the basis of psychiatric–mental health nursing. Research continues to further build the theory base in the field. (See the research highlight on the next page.)

THEORIES OF CARE

Care has been referred to as "human acts and processes that provide assistance to another individual in order to meet an expressed, obvious, or anticipated need."[27] Several models and theories of caring in nursing have emerged during the past several decades. Two important models and theories of care related to the therapeutic relationship are a cultural model and theory of caring, as developed by Leininger, and a humanistic model and theory of caring, as developed by Watson.[46,47]

The cultural model and theory of care has developed from studies of care in various cultures throughout the world. Leininger's research demonstrates that caring is important for the survival of the human race.[27] The care phenomenon is both universal, in that caring occurs in every culture, and specific to each culture and context, in that caring is expressed in unique ways in each different culture. Leininger takes the position that the science of nursing is the science of caring and urges that nursing interventions be based on the application of knowledge of caring within

RESEARCH HIGHLIGHT

Study of Nurse Caring Behaviors in the Neuropsychiatric Setting
• S Bassett

PURPOSE

The purpose of this study was to evaluate and prioritize the neuropsychiatric clients' and the neuropsychiatric nurses' perceptions of caring behaviors.

SAMPLE

The sample consisted of 62 clients and 53 nursing staff from two geropsychiatric and two acute psychiatric units. Clients' diagnoses were mainly schizophrenia, depression, alcoholism, and dementia.

METHODOLOGY

A scaled questionnaire was given to the client and nursing staff participants. The questionnaire consisted of Larson's CARE-Q-II, which was changed substantially to fit the needs of the setting and population.

Based on a study done by Nursing Service Research Committee, Sheridan VAMC, Sheridan, Wyoming, 1989 and presented at Cleveland, Ohio.

FINDINGS

Both clients' and nurses' perceptions of specific behaviors indicating "caring" were very similar with the mean score for clients almost consistently slightly less than the nurses. Specific caring behaviors seemed to convey caring to both groups of participants. Behaviors such as accessibility, monitoring, and comforting were highly valued by both groups.

IMPLICATIONS

If nursing practice is to be based on "caring" behaviors, it is very important that clients and nurses have mutual perceptions of nursing behaviors that convey caring. Only then will effective nursing interventions, which are based on caring—the essence of nursing—occur.

---

various cultural contexts. Hence Leininger proposes that transcultural knowledge, in combination with nursing knowledge, be the basis of transcultural nursing. Nursing in the future will require this broader basis of care.

The humanistic model and theory of care was developed by Jean Watson, a nurse theorist. Watson bases her nursing theory on assumptions about the importance of human caring in the practice of psychiatric nursing and in the development of nursing as a science. Direct application of her model is readily possible to the current field of psychiatric–mental health nursing.

The ten carative factors listed in the accompanying box are the basis for nursing interventions as well as for other elements of the theory.[47] These are useful for the therapeutic process. For example, the third carative factor (sensitivity to self and others) needs to permeate the entire nurse-client relationship.

▼
WATSON'S CARATIVE FACTORS

1. Humanistic-altruistic system of values
2. Faith-hope
3. Sensitivity to self and others
4. Helping-trusting, human care relationship
5. Expressing positive and negative feelings
6. Creative problem-solving caring process
7. Transpersonal teaching-learning
8. Supportive, protective, and/or corrective mental, physical, societal, and spiritual environment
9. Human needs assistance
10. Existential-phenomenological-spiritual focus

From Watson J: *Nursing: human science and human care—a theory of nursing*, New York, 1988, National League of Nursing.

Care is viewed by nurse theorists, Leininger and Watson, as the essence of nursing. The domain of nursing is care and the domain of medical practice is cure. Care is an essential part of all nursing, including psychiatric–mental health nursing.

THE NURSE'S SELF-AWARENESS

The client and nurse bring to the relationship their unique beliefs, behaviors, attitudes, intelligence, and values. How do two very different people interact to help the client gain or regain a sense of worth, energy, and direction? First of all, the nurse increases her own self-awareness. This involves communication with others and self-evaluation. These processes reveal previously unknown aspects of one's personality. Aspects of self-awareness to be explored are self-concept, beliefs, values, and life experiences.

Self-Concept

Self-concept influences the nurse's therapeutic effectiveness. The nurse's feelings about herself influence the way she interprets the communication and behavior of the client. It also affects her ability to interact with the client. Nurses with a positive self-concept have faith in their competence. They believe that they have something useful to offer others. The feeling of self-worth allows the nurse to accept and respect the worth of others. Positive self-worth helps a person accept criticism and ask for help appropriately. Obstacles are seen as temporary and surmountable challenges.

A negative self-concept makes it difficult for the nurse "to see, hear, or think clearly, and therefore she is more prone to step on and depreciate others."[35] The nurse who is uncertain of her self-worth is afraid to be open with clients. She is too timid to risk finding new solutions to problems. She may find it difficult to seek help from peers or supervisors, since they may expose her inadequacy. Finally, a nurse with a negative self-concept is not a good role model for feelings of worth.

Beliefs and Values

Nurse-client relationships are strongly affected by the beliefs and values of the persons involved. Based on beliefs and values, people approve or disapprove of the behavior of others. Some values lead to complete rejection of involvement with persons who have different beliefs. For example, because the nurse values nonviolence, she may not know what to say to a client who is accused of spouse beating. She may request that the case be reassigned. Other values do not prevent interaction. Still others seem insignificant in relationships. A nurse may accept a client with a history of food stamp fraud. Although the nurse's values may define this behavior as objectionable, this does not prevent therapeutic interaction.

Nurses recognize that cultural value differences exist that may cause misunderstandings about how people should think or act. Likewise, misunderstandings may arise when nurses and clients come from different socioeconomic groups. The nurse's awareness of these value differences may help prevent misunderstandings that prevent therapeutic relationships (see Chapter 9).

Peoples' beliefs and values stem from the cultural beliefs and values of the culture and society to which they belong. In the United States many different cultural groups are represented by nurses as well as clients. It is therefore important for the nurse to understand her own cultural background with its particular beliefs and values so that she does not impose these onto clients from different cultures with different belief and value systems. Our beliefs about the nature of humanity, the nature of mental illness, and the nature of change stem from our culture. For example, a nurse who believes that an individual has control over his own behavior and destiny may have difficulty accepting a client who does nothing to change his behavior because he believes that he has no control over the future and has been predestined to behave in a certain manner. This kind of difference can lead to blocked communication and lack of progress in the nurse-client relationship.

To avoid or work out such blocks, the nurse needs to become aware of the differences in belief and value systems and actively seek ways to demonstrate to the client that she is making an effort to understand him. The more open the nurse is to persons with differing values and beliefs, the more likely she is to succeed in establishing a therapeutic relationship with him.

Life Experiences

Nurses can experience the same problems as their clients. Sometimes the nurse has successfully resolved past problems. In other instances, the nurse may be coping with life stresses and problems as serious as those of her clients. The therapeutic effectiveness of the nurse is enhanced by (1) recognition of her problems, (2) an underlying optimism that change is possible, and (3) a nonjudgmental attitude toward herself or the client for having problems. For example, the nurse who takes diazepam (Valium) 6 to 8 times a day may not consciously admit to the seriousness of the problem. She may fear there is no way to stop taking the pills. She may also disrespect herself for taking the pills. This nurse may communicate with chemically dependent clients differently from the nurse who has overcome a similar dependence. As a result, the second nurse has a higher regard for herself.

Young or inexperienced nurses are often unsuccessful in coping with adversity. A nurse who has had a sheltered life may be overwhelmed by the difficulties a client is experiencing. Consultation with a more seasoned nurse may help to ease feelings of inadequacy.

ROUTES TO SELF-AWARENESS

Many opportunities are available to the mental health–psychiatric nurse to foster self-awareness. These opportunities fall into three primary categories—interpersonal relationships, reading, and writing.

Interpersonal Relationships

Involvement in relationships contribute to self-awareness. The family offers the first and probably most lasting lesson in self-awareness. These lessons are modified by later life experiences that usually include other deep, personal relationships. Teachers also play a significant role in developing self-awareness. A teacher's influence is limited by the degree to which the student allows the relationship to develop.

Sometimes an instructor or supervisor becomes a mentor. A mentor is a person who supports, promotes, and guides the intellectual and career development of another person. One does not make a formal contract with a mentor. Rather, this relationship is a process of mutual respect. Its focus is primarily professional and intellectual, and it evolves over time. The mentor's expertise and caring are a powerful combination in guiding the nurse's growth in self-awareness and knowledge.

The nurse can work with a therapist, counselor, or other helping person to learn how to be more effective in therapeutic relationships with clients. Through this exchange, the nurse may achieve greater self-awareness and a more positive regard for herself, which increases her effectiveness in working with clients. By observing how the counselor communicates, the nurse learns to use opportunities to be helpful that arise during interactions. The research highlight on the next page compares the helping styles of nursing students with the styles of other therapists.

Reading

Through formal study of mental health–psychiatric nursing, the nurse is exposed to written ideas about clinical practice. The habit of reading, however, begins long before and, ideally, continues long after one's formal education. Reading fiction and nonfiction helps one learn more about human nature and thus about oneself. Portrayals of people's lives show the range of human emotion, the struggles, and the ways in which people relate to themselves and others.

RESEARCH HIGHLIGHT

A Behavioral Comparison of Helping Styles of Nursing Students, Psychotherapists, Crisis Interveners, and Untrained Individuals

• M Ryden, P McCarthy, M Lewis, and C Sherman

PURPOSE

The purpose of this study was to assess whether nursing students use helping behaviors similar to those of psychotherapists. Specifically, like the psychotherapists, nursing students would talk less and make more responses that reflect the content and feelings of client statements.

SAMPLE

The sample consisted of 30 undergraduate nursing students enrolled in an interpersonal relations course at a large midwestern university. The mean age was 25.3 years.

METHODOLOGY

The Helping Skills Verbal Response System (HSVRS) was used to rate the students verbal behavior. Ten types of responses (thought units) were identified, such as reflects client's feelings and factual self-information. Enrollment in the interpersonal relations course provided autotutorial learning experiences, seminars, and supervised skills practice.

FINDINGS

The nursing students were similar to crisis interveners in their use of thought units and similar to the psychotherapists in their use of affect and content responses. They used significantly less influence than untrained individuals and were similar to the psychotherapists in their use of advice. Nursing students used more self-disclosure than psychotherapists.

IMPLICATIONS

The findings partially support the hypothesis that nursing students display helping behavior similar to psychotherapists. They were similar to psychotherapists in their use of thought content and affective reflections with minimal emphasis on advice and information giving. They resembled crisis interveners in directing the client toward action-oriented plans through influencing responses and by talking more than psychotherapists. Their behavior bore no resemblance to untrained individuals who were verbose, directive, and unhelpful.

The nursing students' behavior was consistent with the values of the nursing profession; for example, their therapeutic reflections demonstrate empathic understanding and acceptance of the client.

From Archives of Psychiatric Nursing 5(3):185, 1991.

Diaries and journals are rich sources of detail about the personal experiences of others. Many books, journals, and diaries have been written by former mentally ill clients, who detail the experience of mental illness and describe health caregivers. In addition, professional publications provide current information and research studies.

Writing

Writing a diary, journal, or log is another significant route to learning about oneself. The nurse can write notes in an unstructured style and may see patterns of behavior, feelings, and evidence of personal growth by reviewing these notes.

Process recording is a formal method of writing that helps the nurse to deal more effectively with clients and to learn about herself. Process recordings are descriptions and analyses of interactions with clients. The record includes a verbatim account of the nurse's and the client's communications. The word-for-word record ensures that complete data about the interaction are available to the nurse for later analysis.

Table 7-1 provides an example of a process recording. Process recordings help the student identify communication techniques, maladaptive behaviors, and beliefs and values. They also show the nurse's strengths and weaknesses. Process recordings improve clinical supervision by instructors, supervisors, or consultants. Over time, at regular intervals, the process recordings can be reviewed and summarized to document major patterns or progress of the relationship. Finally, the nurse with her instructor can use these recordings to analyze her own progress. Process recordings help to develop insight into both client and nurse behaviors.

COMPONENTS OF THE THERAPEUTIC RELATIONSHIP

Rapport

Certain people have qualities that enable them to help others. These people have the ability to understand what the problem is and to help people feel good about themselves. When this happens, *rapport* has been established. Rapport is the key ingredient in the negotiation and maintenance of the therapeutic relationship.

Rapport requires a level of similarity and agreement in the language, body movement, and gestures of two people. Two people in deep conversation may nod their heads in agreement and exhibit similar rates of speech and tonal qualities. Facial expressions often mirror one another. Shifts in one person's body position are reflected by changes in the other person's position. The matching or mirroring of gestures and expressions are usually unconscious (Figure 7-1).

The qualities that help to encourage rapport are warmth,

▼ **TABLE 7-1   Example of a Section of a Process Recording**

Purpose of the interaction: This interview was conducted primarily to explore and overcome resistance exhibited by the client 2 days earlier when he "forgot" our meeting. Based on the outcome of this interview, the contract with the client will either be reestablished or terminated.

Context of the interaction: On the previous clinical day, the client had "forgotten" our meeting and refused to talk when he was found playing pool. Another meeting was set up for the next clinical day. The client did not show up at the time and place agreed on. He was found asleep in his bed. He agreed to accompany me to the courtyard near the unit. This was our fourth interaction. It was a warm, sunny day with few distractions.

Client Behavior	Nurse Behavior	Analysis
Client sat down on a bench, leaned forward with elbows on thighs, and stared straight ahead. He yawned several times and rubbed his eyes.		This client isn't interested in the upcoming interaction. (Metacommunication tells how verbal communication can be interpreted.)
	I sat down on the bench beside the client about 2 feet away. I turned to face the client. I established eye contact. I felt my jaws tighten somewhat before I spoke. I was leaning slightly toward the client with legs uncrossed and hands on my knees. I was breathing faster and deeper than usual.	Observing personal space. Open posture for active listening. Physiological changes secondary to anxiety.
	Thought: What's the best way to approach this resistance thing? Do I ease into it or confront him with my feelings? I'm sure seeing his manipulation, now.	I wanted to reaffirm our contract by breaking down his resistance but not to run him away. (Forcing the client to talk about a painful area may increase his anxiety.)
	Feeling: I felt a little frustrated and angry at the client's resistance.	My feelings of anger and frustration can become a communications barrier if left unresolved. (In an accepting relationship, an individual can deal with resisted material.) I need to be more accepting—student weakness.
	"Joe, I want to talk to you about our agreement." Three second pause.	*Therapeutic:* Defining boundaries by reaffirming contract.
	"We agreed to meet every Tuesday and Thursday at 1 PM for an hour to talk. Today is the second time this week that you weren't where you said you'd be."	*Confrontation:* Pressure another person into facing something objectionable. Perhaps I got into the subject abruptly because of feelings of frustration and anxiety.
	I was still in the same position except that I was gripping my knees with my hands. I quietly sighed after I spoke and relaxed my grip. I looked straight at the client with a serious expression.	I relaxed some after my statement. I had vented my feelings through confrontation. (In many instances this act is associated with the nurse's being angry. The nurse is objective and neutral when confronting.)
	Thought: Well, I wonder how he's going to react to that.	
	Feeling: I felt less frustrated and angry and a little relieved.	
Started moving his feet up and down a little. Ducked his head down slightly. Half-chuckled as he spoke. "Well, I didn't really mean it sincerely."		Foot movement may mean he is anxious about being confronted. Lowered head seems submissive.
In louder tone: "Sometimes I like to talk and sometimes I don't. Maybe I'd rather play pool or sleep."		Voice change may indicate anger.

▼ **TABLE 7-1   Example of a Section of a Process Recording—cont'd**

Client Behavior	Nurse Behavior	Analysis
	I straightened up a little, maintaining eye contact with client. Sighed. Rubbed my chin with right hand and squinted my eyes slightly. *Thought:* I think he's about to get angry. I wonder what he really thinks about me. I hope I can work this out with him. *Feeling:* A little anxious. "Joe, how would you feel if I broke my word to you?" I put my hand back on my knee and half-smiled. I spoke in a slow, low tone.	My behavior, thoughts, and feelings are centered around the client's anger, what to do about the anger, and my own anxiety. *Therapeutic:* Encouraging comparison, asking that similarities and differences be noted. The smile may seem incongruent with the message, but I am trying to be nonthreatening.
Still facing me with eye contact. Serious expression. "I wouldn't like it."		Expression indicates that client's anger hasn't escalated. Absence of previously noted expressions of anger. Client's verbal response is appropriate, an indication of the effectiveness of the question.
	"Well, I don't like it either. My job is to learn about people by meeting with a client who is willing to discuss his problems, and possibly to explore solutions to those problems."	I'm trying to establish rapport by displaying genuineness. "Being myself" is expressing to client my thoughts and feelings. My thoughts probably indicate a low level of warmth. I stated in an informative and matter-of-fact way my intentions and purpose for interaction.
	Thirty-second pause. "I'd like to work with you if you would agree to meet and talk." I spoke slowly and clearly in a low tone. *Thought:* I hope he agrees.	Restating my purpose and recontracting.
Client turns away from me and laughs quickly, looks across courtyard. He puts his elbows on his thighs and looks down.		Behavior indicates a return to submissive state, "lowering head."
	Feeling: I sensed the client's ambivalence and felt uneasy.	*A strength:* Awareness of client's feelings. *A weakness:* Should have communicated my understanding to client.
Client turned his head and was making eye contact. Spoke in a shaky voice. "I want to work with you."	*Thought:* I hope he is not too uncomfortable. I don't want him to just "give in" because he thinks I'm in charge. "Then we will meet every Tuesday and Thursday at the nurse's station at 1 PM as we had originally planned, if that is still a good time for you."	Recontracting complete. Client's resistance may indicate that he had been "testing" me. His behavior may indicate a trend of not fulfilling commitments and being egocentric, which are characteristic of schizophrenia.

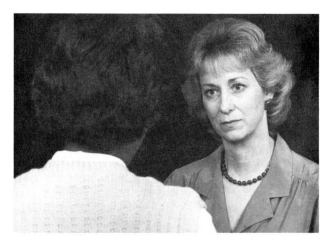

FIGURE 7-1 A therapist demonstrates active listening as she works with a nursing student.

empathy, and genuineness. All of these qualities are based on a caring that the nurse first experiences toward the client.

Warmth

Warmth means the ability to help the client feel cared for and comfortable. It shows acceptance of the client as a unique individual. It involves a nonpossessive caring for the client as a person and a willingness to share the client's joys and sorrows. Warmth can be conveyed by eye contact, an interested, caring tone of voice, a touch on the arm, or a smile. Nonpossessive warmth allows the client to have his own feelings and experiences. It involves appreciating the client for himself, regardless of his behaviors. Below is a scale for measuring nonpossessive warmth in which stage 1 is the lowest level and stage 5 is the highest level. This scale is based on the work of Carl Rogers and others[33] and can be used by beginning students and nurses to grow in the expression and use of warmth with clients.

Empathy

The ability to sense the client's private world as if it were one's own is known as *empathy*. The poem in the box below expresses such an ability. Beyond that, it is the ability to convey this understanding to the client. It is not necessary for the nurse to feel the same emotions the client

▼ **WARMTH**

Stage 1
The nurse:

Offers advice or gives clear negative regard
Tells the client what is "best" for him or approves or disapproves of his behavior
Makes herself the focus of evaluation
Sees herself as responsible for the client

Stage 2
The nurse:

Responds mechanically indicating little warmth
Ignores the client or his feelings
Communicates no unconditional regard

Stage 3
The nurse:

Indicates a positive but semipossessive type of caring
Communicates that what the client does or does not do matters to her

Stage 4
The nurse:

Communicates a deep interest and concern for the client
Communicates nonjudgmental and nonpossessive warmth
Maintains some conditionality in the more personal areas of the client's functioning

Stage 5
The nurse:

Communicates nonpossessive warmth without restriction
Respects the client's worth as a person and his rights as an individual
Gives the client freedom to be himself, to regress, to be defensive, and to dislike or reject the nurse
Cares about and values the client for his potential without allowing her feelings to interfere in evaluations of his behavior
Shares the client's joys, aspirations, sadness, and failures

Modified from Rogers C and others: *The therapeutic relationship and its impact,* Madison, 1967, University of Wisconsin Press.

▼ **EMPATHY**

I feel your pain within my pulse
and beat by beat, and tear by tear, I follow
in my mind and heart your deepest sorrow.
Your anguish rends and wears me down
so in the end, I look at all
and only see the deep, dark, hollow of the world
and think—that's right, that must be all there is!
Then both of us must sink into a hopeless, wallow pit
With no way out—
  No doors
    No windows
      No speck of light
        is left to us in such a state . . .
But no! Do not descend the labyrinths of deep despair!
For if we but *begin*
  we *can* go on!
With comfort from the world
  and one another
That, yes, despite our pain,
There is the hope of triumph
in tomorrow!
  Could we but now begin
    with guarded step!
  Who will be first?
    Come, take hold!
  One hand outstretched
    can only link
    you to the warm
      melodious music of the universe
    and look—the stars unfold!

by Rauda Salkauskas Gelazis, RN, PhC

feels. Rather, empathy is an appreciation and awareness of another person's feelings and the ability to communicate this awareness.

The nurse may demonstrate different levels of empathy as shown in the following case example. The scale in the accompanying box represents nine degrees of empathy. At the lowest level the nurse may be inattentive or misinterpret the client's feelings. At the highest level, the nurse's awareness allows her to sense and respond to feelings the client has only partially revealed (see the research highlight on p. 118). The empathic nurse communicates verbally an understanding of feelings that may be deeply hidden even to the client.

▼ Case Example

Mrs. Jackson has met with the nurse to complete her psychosocial history and explore recent events in her life in greater detail. She has discussed her youth and upbringing fairly calmly. She has described her relationship with her three children as being somewhat strained but satisfying, until her husband's death months earlier. She had sat quietly until she mentioned her husband, maintaining eye contact, speaking in a calm, low voice. As she discussed the current difficulty with her children since his death, she suddenly stopped speaking, lowered her head, and slumped in a limp position, tears running down her cheeks.

The nurse may respond with different levels of empathy. A nurse with low empathy may ignore the change in behavior and go on with history taking by asking: "Mrs. Jackson, you were talking about your children. What ages are they?" (stage 1). A nurse with a higher level of empathy, who is aware of most obvious feelings but is not totally accurate in identifying the hidden feelings of the client, may respond by saying, "Mrs. Jackson, this is upsetting for you. Would you like to end our discussion and resume it later?" (stage 4). A nurse who understands the client's full range of spoken and unspoken feelings may respond by leaning toward Mrs. Jackson, speaking softly, and using touch, saying, "Sometimes you feel so sad and alone. It's like you can't go on anymore." In this manner the nurse is able to respond to Mrs. Jackson's inability to function in her life (stage 9). A mentor or instructor may be helpful to the student or nurse in developing empathic responses to clients. Process recordings can be used to determine at which level of empathy the nurse tends to respond. Self-knowledge and growth can be promoted by frequent reference to the empathy scale.

Sympathy is often confused with *empathy*. Meaningful relationships between close friends include long talks in which each shares feelings with the other. The closeness derived from sharing feelings is enhanced by empathy. Sym-

EMPATHY

Stage 1
The nurse:

Is unaware of the client's feelings
Responses are inappropriate for mood or content of client's statements
May be bored, disinterested, or offer advice

Stage 2
The nurse:

Shows a negligible degree of accuracy in responses to the most obvious feelings
Ignores emotions that are not clearly expressed
Is sensitive to obvious feelings but misunderstands what the client is saying
Responds in a way that inhibits or misdirects the client

Stage 3
The nurse:

Responds accurately to the client's expressed feelings
Shows concern for deeper feelings that she assumes are present, although she does not sense their meaning to the client

Stage 4
The nurse:

Recognizes less obvious feelings
May anticipate feelings that are not current or may misinterpret feelings
Is sensitive and aware but not entirely attuned to the client in the current situation
Desires and makes an effort to understand, but accuracy is low

Stage 5
The nurse:

Responds accurately to the client's readily discernible feelings
Shows awareness of feelings and experiences that are not so evident but tends to be somewhat inaccurate in her understanding of them
Has misunderstandings that may not be disruptive because of their tentative nature

Stage 6
The nurse:

Recognizes most of the client's present feelings, including those not readily apparent
May misjudge the intensity of the feelings with the result that responses may not be suited to the client's mood
Deals directly with what the client is currently experiencing
Is attuned to the client but does not encourage exploration
Is limited in her understanding

Stage 7
The nurse:

Responds accurately to most of the client's present feelings
Shows awareness of the intensity of the client's feelings
Moves slightly beyond the realm of the client's awareness to encourage him to explore currently unrecognized feelings
Moves to more emotionally laden areas

Stage 8
The nurse:

Identifies the client's feelings accurately
Uncovers meanings in the client's experiences of which the client is unaware
Moves into feelings and experiences with sensitivity and accuracy
Is sensitive to her mistakes and alters her responses appropriately
Reflects a rapport with the client
Reflects by her tone of voice a seriousness in her approach to client

Stage 9
The nurse:

Responds unerringly to the client's full range and intensity of feelings
Recognizes each emotional nuance and communicates an understanding of the feelings
Is attuned to the client's feelings and reflects this in her words and voice

RESEARCH HIGHLIGHT

Biopsychosocial Elements of Empathy: A Multidimensional Model

• CA Williams

PURPOSE

The purpose of this study was the analysis of empathy and research approaches to the concept as well as the development of a multidimensional model of empathy.

METHODOLOGY

The author did a metaanalysis of research approaches and literature on empathy.

FINDINGS

Empathy is conceptualized as a multidimensional phenomenon with emotional, cognitive, communicative, and relational components. Researchers have used self-report scales such as the Hogan Empathy Scale to measure empathy. Physiological indicators, such as sensorimotor and limbic brain changes, have also been used to measure empathy.

IMPLICATIONS

Because empirical approaches to empathy can only examine the most easily measured aspects of empathy, the author proposes the need for phenomenological approaches to capture the total construct of empathy. Such a holistic approach to empathy would be useful for nursing research.

Based on data from *Issues in Mental Health Nursing* 11:155, 1990.

---

pathy may also be experienced in a relationship between close friends. Sympathy implies a kind of fusion with the emotional experience of the other. Empathy implies that a degree of emotional separateness exists between the participants. With sympathy, the needs of the other are seen as one's own. With empathy a degree of objectivity is maintained in the relationship. The following example demonstrates the distinction between sympathy and empathy.

Mr. Cosner, a newly admitted client has not seen his doctor since his admission several hours before. He frequently asks the nurse, with increasing irritation, when his doctor is coming. Ms. Rainy, an RN, states that she does not know when he will come and that she wishes he would come and write orders so that she can get her work done. She, too, is annoyed and adds sharply that this is typical of the doctor (sympathy). When Mr. Cosner asks Mr. Petrecelli, another RN, the same question 10 minutes later, Mr. Petrecelli listens to Mr. Cosner express his irritation. He did not dwell on his own feelings about the doctor but verbalized his understanding of Mr. Cosner's feelings of irritation (empathy).

Sympathy is important in human relationships. It feels good to share feelings with another person and to be allied against a common enemy. In helping relationships, however, objectivity is lost when feelings are shared sympathetically. If one person is in need, the sympathizer shares that need and may be unable to provide help in meeting it. Helping people means having a responsibility to the client to assist in solving the problem. To identify and clarify alternatives, the helper needs to be objective.

Genuineness

Genuineness involves being oneself. This implies that the nurse is aware of her thoughts, feelings, values, and their relevance in the immediate interaction with a client. A high level of genuineness does not mean that the nurse expresses her feelings and thoughts at all times—only that she does not deny them. The nurse's response to the client is sincere and reflects her internal response. It is also important that the nurse's verbal and nonverbal communication correspond with each other. The box on p. 119 lists the levels of genuineness. The case example below shows the use of a high level of genuineness.

▼ Case Example

The client, Terry, and nurse have been talking quietly for a few minutes. Terry suddenly becomes angry and shouts, "I don't want to talk to you! In fact I don't ever want to talk to you again! Just get away from me and leave me alone!" The nurse is surprised, hurt, and unsure how to respond. She and the client have had a positive relationship in the past. A possible response that is genuine yet therapeutic would be: "I'm sorry you feel that way. I'm also confused. I value your relationship highly and I'm puzzled that you no longer want to talk to me" (stage 5).

In this example above, although the nurse felt hurt, she chose to respond by expressing her honest confusion. An honest, but more defensive and less therapeutic response is "I don't understand why you're angry at me. I haven't done anything to you, but if you don't want to talk it's OK with me; I have other things to do" (stage 3). It can be seen that various levels of genuineness can be expressed. In moving toward therapeutic responses, the stages of genuineness can be useful to novice and experienced practitioners.

THERAPEUTIC USE OF SELF

The therapeutic use of self means more than just learning general therapeutic techniques and determining which behaviors convey warmth, empathy, or genuineness or those that are perceived as cold or unhelpful. Therapeutic use of self means individualizing the use of therapeutic techniques and using special personality characteristics to an advantage in working with clients. For example, a nurse with a fine sense of humor may be able to tease a client, encouraging him to see some aspect of his behavior. On the other hand,

GENUINENESS

Stage 1
The nurse:

Interacts defensively

Evidences considerable discrepancy between her experiencing and her current verbalization

Contradicts herself

Stage 2
The nurse:

Responds appropriately but responses do not express what she really feels or means

Responses are contrived or rehearsed

Stage 3
The nurse:

Defensiveness is implicit

Stage 4
The nurse:

Is neither implicitly nor explicitly defensive

Does not present a facade

Is genuine

Stage 5
The nurse:

Gives open, honest responses

Is open to feelings and experiences of all types, both pleasant and hurtful

Has no defensiveness

Makes statements that match her feelings and thoughts

---

a nurse who rarely teases will seem insincere if she attempts to use joking as a therapeutic technique.

The therapeutic use of self involves doing what one can do best. Experience reveals the strengths and limitations the nurse brings to the situation, as well as how and when clients are affected by different behaviors. The process requires extensive clinical experience, self-evaluation, and openness to the feedback of others. Trying new techniques and receiving feedback may be uncomfortable at first. In time, the ability to use oneself therapeutically becomes more natural. Therapeutic use of self involves trusting one's instincts. It involves sensitivity to subtle cues about when to act in a certain way with a client.

PHASES OF THE THERAPEUTIC RELATIONSHIP

The phases of the therapeutic relationship are the *preinteraction phase, orientation* (introductory) *phase, working phase,* and *termination phase.*

Preinteraction Phase

The preinteraction phase begins as soon as the student nurse is aware of her intent to interact with a client. For the nursing student this is often a period of anxiety and self-doubt. It is important during this phase to become aware of one's own beliefs, thoughts, and feelings. Recognizing personal values, biases, or fears lets the student develop a greater self-awareness. The student nurse may seek assistance from a more experienced nurse, to avoid feelings

TASKS OF THE PREINTERACTION PHASE

Explore personal beliefs and feelings

Pursue routes to self-awareness

Review appropriate theory

Analyze strengths and limitations in relating to others

Plan for first interactions with client

---

that may interfere with the therapeutic relationship.

The tasks of the preinteraction phase are listed in the accompanying box.

Reactions to the preinteraction phase

Reactions that are likely to surface during the preinteraction phase include anxiety, the need to know client's history, role threat, feelings of incompetency, fear of being hurt or of causing distress, fear of losing control, and fear of rejection.

Everyone brings elements of his or her past experience into any new situation. For the student nurse, this may include rumors about the horror of mental hospitals and psychiatric clients. Mental illness and mental hospitals are often portrayed as frightening in movies and literature. Fears of the unknown cause increased anxiety and make it difficult for the student nurse to hear instruction or accurately assess a situation.

Student nurses often feel incompetent before their first client interaction. They doubt their ability and verbalize fears such as, "How can I help a person just by talking?" The student nurse may be afraid of being asked for advice or feel ill-equipped to give answers.

Feelings of incompetence are worsened because there are fewer traditional nursing tasks associated with the care of psychiatric clients. The staff often do not wear uniforms or stethoscopes or other symbols associated with the nursing role. Clients may be dressed in street clothes, out of their rooms, or off the unit or floor involved in activities. The feeling of role threat may cause a nurse to seek concrete tasks to perform. The nurse may read the client's chart to decrease anxiety. She may also read the chart to avoid the initial contact with a client.

Nursing students often express the fear that they will hurt or be hurt by the client. Students fear that clients are fragile and imagine that an inappropriate comment will "send the client off the deep end" or "set him off." Students fear that the client may do himself harm either physically or psychologically. Moreover, students sometimes believe that psychiatric clients are volatile and may physically or psychologically hurt the nurse at the slightest provocation.

Related to the fear of hurting or being hurt is the fear of loss of self-control. The student fears that the client may say or do something to cause an undesirable reaction in the student. The student may have a history of crying easily, blushing, or even having a quick temper and may be frightened that these behaviors will surface in the clinical setting.

Another fear often expressed by students is that of being rejected by the client. "What if no one wants to talk to me?" This fear is related to shyness or need for approval or gratitude from the client. It is difficult to think of offering oneself as a helper, and then being rejected as unneeded or unwanted.

Strategies for accomplishing the tasks of the preinteraction phase

The student may find it helpful to ask these questions before interaction with the client. "What is my greatest fear about getting to know this client?" "What do I expect this client to be like?" "Is there any type of person or problem that I worry about working with?"

It is helpful to review behaviors associated with the various psychiatric disorders. The nurse may know the client's diagnosis at this point and can read specifically about that disorder. Even if the diagnosis is not known, the basic concepts of anxiety, loss, self-esteem, trust, or dependency apply to most clients.

Self-awareness includes the analysis of personal strengths and limitations in relating to others. At this phase in the relationship the nursing student's list of weaknesses may seem to far outnumber the list of strengths. Interacting with others is not a skill unique to psychiatric nursing. Rather it is a skill that one has practiced daily over a lifetime. The nursing student is preparing to refine, improve, and expand on existing skills.

The fears and expectations of the student nurse need to be examined before the first meeting with the client. It is sometimes helpful just to know that others have experienced similar feelings. Open discussion of fears often makes them less intense. Factual information about the nature of psychiatric illness can reduce the student's fears. Another strategy for decreasing anxiety is to review past situations where the student has successfully dealt with problems such as rejection. It may be helpful for students to imagine a situation and then role play a successful resolution.

Knowledge of the client's history helps the nurse to ask pertinent questions. However, beginning students tend to structure the first interview so that they obtain the same information that is in the chart, rather than the information that the client wishes to discuss. It is helpful to conduct the first interview without having read the chart. This reduces the possibility of preconceived expectations on the part of the nurse and helps the nurse to follow the client's lead during the interview.

After the nursing student has explored personal beliefs, analyzed strengths and limitations, and reviewed psychiatric disorders, it is then helpful to make tentative plans for the first meeting with the client. These plans include when and where to interview the client as well as what initial approach is to be used. The student needs to be aware of the physical structure of the setting in which the interaction will take place and minimize any barriers to communication. It is also helpful to prepare several possible initial questions. These questions may be as simple as, "Tell me what brings you to the hospital?" or "I'd like to get to know you. Tell me something about yourself." Even if the tentative plans cannot be used, having them in mind reduces the student's anxiety before the interaction.

Orientation Phase

The orientation or introductory phase begins when the nurse and client meet. It is essential for the nurse to understand and acknowledge the client's view of the problem and reason for seeking help. Understanding the client's view of the situation is basic to establishing rapport, gathering data, and preparing a contract.

The nurse obtains a psychosocial history, using an organized framework for gathering data and getting to know and understand the client. Telling his history allows the client to describe the current situation and the preceding events as he perceives them. Discussing the past is often less threatening than discussing the present. Discussing behaviors is also less threatening than discussing thoughts and feelings. Initially the client may not be able or willing to discuss feelings. However, the nurse may suppose feelings that can be validated and discussed later in the relationship. Clients often want, even need, to discuss feelings but hold back, waiting for assurance that the nurse is willing to listen. The nurse must be open to cues about the client's willingness to discuss feelings.

During the orientation phase, the nurse and client identify the problems and factors that lead to the difficulty. There may be some differences in perception at this point. While identifying the client's problems, it is also helpful to identify the client's strengths. Each client brings strengths and assets to the situation. It is easy for both nurse and client to overlook these when focusing on the problem.

Collecting data and identifying problems form the basis of a mutual agreement for care, which is called a contract and is an important part of the relationship. It tells the nurse and the client what to expect from each other. Without the contract, the relationship lacks direction. Without direction, misunderstandings are possible. Basic elements of the contract include lengths, location, and time of future meetings. The roles of the nurse and client are defined, including the concept of confidentiality. Later, goals for the relationship are established and criteria for terminating the relationship are discussed.

Establishing mutual goals for the relationship is an important task of the orientation phase. For the severely distressed client, the nurse takes responsibility for goal setting until the client is able to participate. The nurse nurtures the collaborative relationship until joint responsibility is assumed for setting and working toward treatment goals.

The tasks of the orientation (introductory) phase are listed in the accompanying box.

Reactions to the orientation phase

The student nurse sometimes finds it difficult to approach the client and ask to spend time just talking without involving concrete tasks. The student nurse may express guilt about "goofing off" and yet is surprised at how exhausting a clinical day can be.

The client may have no obvious illness, making it difficult

TASKS OF THE ORIENTATION PHASE

Establish rapport, trust, and communication
Determine what help the client desires or needs
Gather data, including client feelings, strengths, and weaknesses
Define client's problems
Formulate a *contract*
Mutually set goals

▼ **TABLE 7-2   Characteristics of a Therapeutic Versus a Social Relationship**

Focus	Therapeutic	Social
Purpose	Help for the client	Mutual enjoyment or need fulfillment
Values	Nurse accepts the client without judging	Often based on shared value systems
Goals	Mutually set to meet client's needs; specific and known	May not have specific goals or may be for mutual satisfaction
Meetings	Planned for regular, specific dates and times	May be erratic, chance, or planned
Responsibility	Nurse keeps relationship focused on goals	Shared
Length	Time limited based on goal attainment or number of meetings	Flexible, may last years
Self-disclosure	Nurse discloses only what will help client; intimate details, thoughts, and feelings of client discussed	Mutual and equal; sometimes remains on a superficial level
Termination	Planned and discussed; an important part of the relationship	Usually gradual and unplanned or caused by outside factors such as relocation; often not discussed

to recognize the symptoms of psychiatric problems. Psychiatric problems are not unique to hospitalized clients. Student nurses may identify with the client. This causes them to deny that the client has problems or even to question their own sanity. There may be an uncomfortable sense that mental illness is contagious. For instance, both the client and student nurse may be experiencing anxiety. At this stage it is very difficult for the student nurse to determine the degree to which the anxiety affects the client.

As the client relates his problems the student nurse may feel overwhelmed. This feeling, combined with her desire to help, causes the student nurse to try to solve all of the client's problems immediately. The student nurse also tends to "do for" the client at this time, doing small tasks that the client can appropriately do for himself.

In contrast to feeling overwhelmed, the nurse may resist entering the therapeutic relationship. The student nurse subconsciously fails to pick up on cues the client sends and continues with a social relationship. The communication remains superficial and often the student nurse reports that the client "doesn't feel comfortable" enough to discuss

▼ **STAGES AND BEHAVIORS OF NURSING STUDENTS IN RELATIONSHIPS WITH CLIENTS**

Stage	Behaviors
1	Selective inattention
	Obsession with detail
	Dissociation of theory from practice
	Avoidance behavior
2	Overidentify with clients
	Unable to identify client's problem because of denial
	Thinking becomes concrete
	Social rather than therapeutic interactions
3	Hostility against staff
	Feelings of anger, frustration, omnipotence
4	Anxiety decreases
	Students accept clients, listen actively, analyze data, plan realistic nursing actions

problems yet. This sometimes leads to the client's rejection of the nurse, since clients often do not wish to enter new social relationships. Table 7-2 discusses the characteristics of a therapeutic versus a social relationship.

Stacklum[41] identified several stages that nursing students go through (see the accompanying box).

Strategies for accomplishing the tasks of the orientation phase

The tasks of the orientation phase are accomplished more easily if the nurse remembers that it is a time of exploration. It is a time to get to know another unique individual. To decrease anxiety about asking personal questions, the nurse remembers that the role of the client is to receive help. Helping relationships by nature include the client's disclosure of personal beliefs and feelings.

The initial interview sets the tone for the orientation phase. This interview deserves particular attention and planning. Communication techniques that allow the client to control the interview are important. These include general leads, clarifying, accepting, and silence. The nurse must be certain that the client's communication is understood. Techniques such as encouraging comparison, paraphrasing, seeking clarification, and exploring ensure that the nurse is accurately interpreting the client's message. The amount and type of self-disclosure the nurse uses is limited, as is the amount and type of confrontation.

During the initial interview the nurse may encounter some resistance from the client. For example, the client may doubt that he can be helped by therapy; ask more of the nurse than is appropriate in a therapy setting; show hostility, dependence, or sexual interest in the nurse; give standard, rote answers to questions; or reveal little if any new information. The nurse may also resist entering the therapeutic relationship. It may be difficult to empathize with the client. The nurse may become irritated at the client's resistive behavior or find it difficult to respect the client as a unique individual. The issue of both client and nurse resistance will be discussed further as transference and countertransference.

Once the initial assessment is concluded, the nurse determines tentative nursing diagnoses. Tentative goals are mutually established. A plan is designed for achieving them. The diagnosis, goals, and plans change as the relationship between nurse and client changes and as the client reveals more of the problem. It may take more than one interview to adequately assess the client's needs. As the nurse and client interact, the dynamics of the problem become clearer. The needs and desires of the client also surface. The therapeutic relationship is not static. When the orientation phase ends and the working phase begins is not always clear. Goals and plans are continually reassessed throughout the relationship. However, once a contract is established, a tentative plan formulated, and the client begins working on identified problems, the relationship enters the working phase.

Working Phase

During the working phase of the relationship, it is necessary to maintain and strengthen the rapport that was established during the orientation phase. There are two overriding goals of the working phase, helping the client develop insight and translating insight into behavioral change. Change is usually painful, and clients often resist at this stage. Data gathering is continuous throughout the therapeutic relationship. Intervention involves having the client rethink his problems and respond differently toward others and himself. The focus of the relationship is the present situation, rather than the past. Transference and countertransference are key issues in resistance. Problems and goals are evaluated and redefined, if necessary, as new data are revealed.

Transference and *countertransference* reactions usually occur during the working phase of the relationship. Transference is the unconscious transfer of qualities or attributes originally associated with another to the nurse. Very often, these are qualities associated with a parent or sibling. Transference occurs because the client brings frustrations, conflicts, and feelings of dependence from a past relationship into the therapeutic relationship. The client expects positive or negative responses of the earlier relationship. These responses are often not even appropriate for the nurse-client relationship. The client may express feelings of affection, rejection, or hostility that are too intense for the current situation. The client may fear rejection by the nurse or feel guilty about perceived inadequacies.

Countertransference is the reverse of transference. The nurse may have unresolved problems from an earlier relationship. This nurse may subconsciously transfer inappropriate attributes to a client that were experienced in that earlier relationship. That is, the client's transference provokes the nurse's countertransference reaction. For example, a client may sulk, thinking the nurse is neglecting him and say, "You are punishing me. You hate me, and that's why you didn't stop to talk to me." This is transference on the client's part. The nurse may then become angry and say, "Your behavior is unacceptable. You are not making a satisfactory effort to get better," thinking that the client is acting just like a younger sibling acted years ago. This is countertransference on the part of the nurse.

Transference carries therapeutic potential as well as a potential barrier to the relationship. Following is a list of transference and countertransference experiences[38]:

1. The client expresses an unreasonable dislike for the nurse.
2. The client describes the nurse as unreal, mechanical, or depersonalized. When the nurse tries to gather more information, the client ignores the point and gives a loosely related response.
3. The client becomes over involved with a personal trait of the nurse that has little or no bearing on the nurse's skill or the client's ability to work with the nurse.
4. The client expresses an excessive liking for the nurse, claiming that no one else could replace her.
5. The client dreads the time spent with the nurse and is persistently uncomfortable during the meeting.
6. The client finds it difficult to focus on his reasons for being with the nurse. He discusses them as if he were consulting the nurse about his "case" as one professional colleague to another.
7. The client is unusually preoccupied with the nurse between sessions. He may find himself imagining remarks, questions, or situations involving the nurse. The nurse may appear in the client's dreams.
8. The client is habitually late for appointments or shows other disturbances regarding time arrangements, such as running past an agreed upon time. Any disturbance about any aspect of the arrangements, once mutually agreed upon and initiated, falls into this category.
9. The client continually argues, seeks love, or remains uninvolved or indifferent about important issues in his life.
10. The client becomes defensive with the nurse. He becomes extremely vulnerable to the nurse's observations, inferences, or interpretations.
11. The client consistently misunderstands or requires further clarification of the nurse's comments. If he never agrees with the nurse's comments, the possibility of transference can be tested by repeating a point made by the client, with which the client will disagree.
12. The client uses provocative remarks, double-edged questions, or dramatic statements to evoke certain responses from the nurse.
13. The client becomes overly concerned with the confidentiality of his work with the nurse.
14. The client begs for sympathy regarding real or imagined maltreatment by an authority figure.
15. The client praises the nurse for improvements in his life that are not direct results of their work together.
16. The client wants to be the nurse's only client.
17. The client reports temporary physical symptoms during contact with the nurse. These symptoms may occur only during the time the client is with the nurse or with certain other people.

The nurse can recognize countertransference by substituting "nurse" for "client" in the preceding list. Also, if client transference is observed, the nurse must examine the relationship and her own feelings for countertransference.

The nurse may find the experience of transference and

countertransference particularly difficult. Since both occur on an unconscious level, the student nurse may not recognize their presence. Besides blocking the therapeutic process, the client may also be blocking the nurse's immediate goals. A goal-oriented nurse may feel successful only to the extent that client goals are met. If the client does not seem to be progressing, the nurse may feel at fault or inadequate. During the working phase the nurse must maintain open communication with a supervisor who can guide the nurse's progress through the resistance.

▼ Case Example

The nurse had been with a group of clients for the whole day. They had all been on a picnic and had returned to the ward. One of the clients, Jane, had attached herself to the nurse when going outside for this first ward outing. Frightened and unsure of herself, she would wrap her arms around the nurse when outside. As she gained confidence, she would gradually separate from the nurse and move on by herself or with other clients. After everyone had returned to the ward, Jane went into the kitchen with the nurse to prepare a cup of coffee. Other clients joined them in the kitchen and began to talk to the nurse. When they left, the nurse asked Jane to hand her the sugar for her coffee. Jane started to scream at the nurse, accusing her of cheating her, taking things from her, and hating her. Jane was most distraught, and when the nurse tried to speak or move toward her, Jane yelled louder. The nurse, keeping some distance, followed Jane to her bedroom, while Jane continued to yell. Another nurse came into the room, moving closer to Jane. Jane did not yell at her and began to calm down. The nurse who was the focus of the outburst removed herself after the other nurse had stepped in. Later that day, Jane came to the first nurse and apologized for her behavior. Together they sat down and talked about what happened. Jane claimed that for a time the nurse had become her mother. In this situation the transference was most dramatic. Jane and the nurse could now talk about Jane's need to be so physically close to the nurse when they first went outside, how it made her feel like a little girl, and how she resented the other clients talking to the nurse in the kitchen.

Reactions to the working phase

During the working phase of the therapeutic relationship the student nurse may experience frustration at not being able to solve the client's problem. She may be overinvolved with the client. Many student nurses become impatient with the client for failing to see solutions that she sees. Some clients even lack willingness to change. Other student nurses become frustrated with the health care system or society for not providing the client with the necessary material or emotional support. For instance, a student nurse may become distraught when placement cannot be found for a pregnant, runaway teenager whose only support is an abusive or rejecting family. The student nurse may focus on what cannot be done and lose sight of what can be accomplished.

Strategies for accomplishing the tasks of the working phase

The first portion of the working phase centers on developing the client's insight and determining the problem. Data gathering focuses on symptoms, feelings, interpersonal relationships, past history, and environmental dissatisfactions. Data gathering is an attempt to identify patterns of behavior.

> ▼
> ## TASKS OF THE WORKING PHASE
>
> Maintain the relationship
> Gather further data
> Promote the client's development of insight
> Facilitate behavioral change
> Overcome resistance behaviors
> Evaluate problems and goals and redefine as necessary

The tasks of the working phase are listed in the accompanying box.

People typically use certain coping mechanisms, defense mechanisms, communication, or behavior patterns in response to perceived threats. The client may not be aware that the current behavior is a pattern that has been used in the past. Once the pattern is identified, the nurse assists the client in discovering the theme underlying the perceived threat. For instance, the nurse may identify a pattern of withdrawal in a client. The withdrawal may be a response to an underlying theme of fear of rejection.

▼ Case Example

Jean, a 39-year-old mother of three, was hospitalized for depression while going through a divorce. She was unable to work, lost interest in friends, and was having difficulty sleeping and eating. On questioning she stated that her husband no longer loved her, her friends thought she was a failure, and she believed that the people at work were laughing at her. Her response to these perceived rejections was to withdraw. When her husband was interviewed, he stated that he still loved his wife and was willing to work on the marriage. Jean's fear of rejection led to her withdrawal and perpetuated the problems she dreaded most. Understanding Jean's withdrawal as a pattern enables the nurse to confront the discrepancy between Jean's perception of the situation and that of her husband, while pointing out the pattern of withdrawal.

Focusing on Symptoms   A thorough analysis of symptoms is useful in linking unconscious psychological patterns to patterns of behavior. In eliciting information from a client regarding a symptom, a nurse may recognize a connection between an event and the response behavior. This does not mean that the client does. Many possibilities exist for the client's lack of awareness, and the nurse decides how and when to make the connection and how and when to use the information. The client must have control over the therapeutic process and function independently of the nurse. Initial efforts to focus on symptoms include introducing the client to the internal psychological processes associated with the behavior. The nurse may explain to the client the possible external triggering events, as in the following example:

Client: I have this pain in my neck. It goes down my arm. (Demonstrates with left hand the pain track in the right arm.) I've had an examination by a doctor, and there is nothing physically wrong with me. He sent me here. (Looks down, silent.)
Nurse: Are you experiencing the pain now?
Client: (Looks at the nurse, raises right hand behind neck.) Well, it hurt more in the waiting room.
Nurse: It hurt more in the waiting room than it does now— hmm. . . . Before I ask you more about this pain, what are

some of your thoughts concerning the doctor's recommendations to come here?

The nurse consciously asks for the client's thoughts. At this point the nurse is operating on a hunch that the client is not used to expressing herself in emotional feeling terms.

Client: Well, I love my kids and husband, and I want to do things—if only the pain would stop. . . . (Looks at nurse, and tears come to her eyes.)

Nurse: It is the pain that stops you? It's difficult to understand how this is related to how you think and feel about things.

Client: Yes, it doesn't make sense, it's not my imagination, but I don't know what else to do. (Looks downward, defeated.)

Nurse: Well, when you have been stuck before, what have you done?

Client: Tried something new. (Looks at nurse and face becomes a bit more animated.)

The nurse has noticed the nonverbal shifts in the client. The client has become more alert, interested, and curious. The nurse decides the client is ready to explore some options.

Nurse: Can I ask you some questions now, and perhaps have you try something?

Client: OK.

Nurse: Take a deep breath and let it out. (Demonstrates more relaxed body posture and shakes her shoulders, loosening tensions in her neck.)

Client: (Mimics nurse's actions.)

Nurse: Now, how is the pain in the neck?

Client: Well, it's not there. Sometimes I'm able to do this at home, but it doesn't last.

Nurse: Sure, now think back to the waiting room. (Observes client as she thinks and remembers.)

Client: (Becomes tense and puts right hand up to back of neck.)

Nurse: What thoughts do you recall?

Client: I was nervous. I felt I shouldn't be here. I thought people would make fun of me. (Looks at the nurse and realizes her hand is behind her neck.)

Nurse: How does the neck feel now?

Client: It's getting a bit tense.

Nurse: Relax yourself. (Makes relaxing body movements.)

Client: (Follows nurse's motions.) This seems too simple. It's more than willpower.

Nurse: I agree with you. What is important is to appreciate that the neck pain, which is very real, is a signal to pay attention to what is going on inside. In the meantime, it's useful to know that you can do some immediate things to reduce the pain, and as you become aware of some of the thoughts and feelings, you will have more options—you won't be stuck.

Focusing on Feeling States Focusing on feeling states helps the client unravel the trends and patterns of interrelationships. Clients often believe that their feeling states come out of the blue or are caused by a specific event. In the following example, the client is not aware of the connection between his emotional arousal and his conscious and unconscious cognitive processes.

Client: I felt fine coming over here today, until I got caught up with all the turtles on the road.

Nurse: Turtles?

Client: Yeah, slow drivers.

Nurse: And now?

Client: I'm just getting over being mad. It was a good day, I thought I was getting a handle on this anger. (Starts to cry.) I'm fine until I get here, then it all comes out. It was a hard weekend. You know Mag and I went to the mountains for the weekend. Plans were for her mother to visit.

Mag has a degenerative brain disease. Mag and the client are in a committed love relationship not approved of by family members. The client has been assuming major responsibilities for Mag.

Client: (Face reddens, clenches fists, tries unsuccessfully to hold back tears.) I don't know how she can do this to her daughter. God, how Mag must feel! Her mother phones at the last minute (we were there Friday). Her mother says she wants to visit with a friend; she'll come Sunday some time. Goddamn her! (Full rage.) She does it all the time.

Nurse: Terribly enraging. (Leans forward.)

Client: Yes, why do I expect things from her when I know they aren't forthcoming? Poor Mag, how upset she must feel.

Nurse: Was Mag enraged, upset?

Client: (Regains some emotional control.) She gets upset when I get angry . . . Then she gets going a bit.

Nurse: Sometimes your anger gets to her.

Client: I almost didn't come today. I was mad at you and all the talk about my mother. I'm mad at her. There's nothing there, like when it's my birthday, there's nothing, not even a card.

Nurse: You are mad at a lot of people. And you were angry with me and almost didn't come.

Client: At times I don't think you are available to me.

Nurse: Like in 2 weeks when I'll be on vacation.

Client: I know, I know, you don't have to tell me (laughing and crying).

Nurse: It seems that to get a handle on the rage it is important to appreciate how it builds up when you feel cut off from what you want and what you need.

Client: Yes, it was a hard weekend with Mag. When I get angry, she says I'm angry with her. I was looking forward to sharing the weekend with other people. I guess I was disappointed.

Focusing on Interpersonal Relationships How people approach relationships with others reflects beliefs, values, and self-esteem. Sometimes clients bring their perceptions of personalities of others into the therapy situation. In this way the nurse sees the client's patterns of projection, expectations, and values.

▼ Case Example

Jill, the client, and Bill married after many years of courtship. After a year and a half they separated. Bill has three teenage daughters, and Jill has a teenage son from previous marriages. Jill left because she believed Bill would not let her be a mother to his daughters and that he wanted her for a housekeeper not a wife. Bill disagrees with this. They are trying to reconcile their relationship. The present situation involves Jill's response to Bill asking her about a blanket he was thinking of sending to his daughter, who has just started college.

Client: Bill wanted the blanket for himself. He didn't want me to have it.

Nurse: How did you arrive at that conclusion?

Client: Well, when Bill phoned me the night before I was going away for the weekend, he asked for it.

Nurse: He wanted the blanket.

Client: Well, he said he phoned to wish me a good time, and then he asked me if I knew where the gold blanket was. I said I had it. I asked why he was asking about it. He said that he was looking for it to give to Juliet to take with her. I asked how he had decided it should be the gold blanket. Here it goes again. He doesn't want me to have the blanket.

Nurse: Did he say that?

Client: No, but why did he phone? We said good night the night before, and he said he would see me next week.

Nurse: What do you think?

Client: Because he wanted the blanket—I know.

Nurse: I'm sure you have reasons for knowing that. But it would be useful to try to make them a little bit more clear.

Jill often assumes what others are thinking. She does this unconsciously. This is a possible pattern of projection. The nurse confronted this possibility. Jill's sense of reality may be challenged, creating anxiety and confusion. The nurse wants to prevent these feelings in Jill.

Client: Well, I guess it's in his tone of voice. I don't want the blanket; I don't want anything that's not mine. I just took the blanket when I left the house because my blankets were on the children's beds, and I didn't want to disturb the household any more than I was.

Nurse: You are sensitive to the needs of Bill and the children.

Client: (Nods yes.)

Nurse: Bill knows this. He doesn't understand it all, but he knows it.

Client: (Continues to nod yes.)

Nurse: Bill said he didn't want the blanket.

Client: Yes, but I don't believe him. There must be something special about the blanket.

Nurse: Did you ask Bill?

Client: Yes. He said there wasn't.

Nurse: Now I'm confused.

Client: Bill said he asked me because he went looking for the blanket and couldn't find it. He wanted to know where it was, so he asked me.

Nurse: What makes it difficult to believe that?

Client: There has to be more to it than that.

Nurse: Like what?

Client: That he doesn't want me to have it.

Nurse: (Gently.) Did he say that?

Client: No. It's hard to believe that I'm assuming all this.

Nurse: It may be more difficult not to realize this. What would Bill have had to do to convince you to keep the blanket?

Client: Not to bring it up. In other relationships in my life I don't do the assuming I do with Bill. In part it is hard to face because it makes me feel that I'm the problem in the marriage.

At this point Jill was beginning to recognize a pattern in her relationship with Bill. She also noticed this pattern at work and in social relationships. However, the breakup with Bill helped her to understand her behavior.

Focusing on the Past Recalling life events helps the client to see patterns of behavior. It also shows how the individual has internalized patterns of coping. The client may be conscious of attitudes toward people important in the past. He may not, however, be conscious of how this affects the present. People and events in the present may resemble those of the past. The individual's responses may be inappropriately based on these past experiences. The client may be aware of unreasonable reactions. However, he may often

justify them, thus preserving past experiences. By contrast, patterns that were important to the person in the past may no longer be necessary. The following is an example.

Client: Well, when I get into those social situations, I feel I've got to make up for something. I figure it isn't right to put such emphasis on dress and things like that. I keep saying I'm better than they are. (Laughs.)

Nurse: Kid from the other side of the tracks, huh? With a chip on her shoulder. Got to make up for something.

Client: (Becomes sober.) Yes. (Silent.)

Nurse: How is it possible that someone so competent is a failure and has to keep making up for something?

Client: (Thoughtful, silent, tears come to eyes.) You know, it's silly . . . (drifting) nothing ever mattered . . . (lost in thought, tearing).

Nurse: To whom?

Client: Nothing I ever wanted for myself meant anything to my mom. Early, I just ignored her. Now I realize I pushed her away, but there are always strings attached. . . . (Silence.)

Nurse: Go on. . . .

Client: Dad and I were close. He always stood up for me. Sure he drank, and he was terrible towards Mom. Limited her on money. Didn't get along with my sister. She just broke away.

Nurse: You were saying that your mother never thought much of what you wanted. (Pulls client back to theme of not being accepted.)

Client: When I got accepted to an outstanding public school, it didn't mean anything to her. Oh, I would hear her brag to her friends, or she would get mad if I got a low grade. (Silent.) One time I got an "F." I was so mad, I was going to quit that damn school. Who were they to give me an "F"? My father agreed. He was going to let me go to private school, even though we didn't have the money. My mother said no. He and I went to make arrangements, and the school said no because I couldn't transfer at that time of year. There we were, caught by my mother. (Laughs.)

The nurse had a choice. She could focus on the client-father alliance. The nurse could also focus on the theme of never being good enough. The nurse chose the latter.

Nurse: Sounds like your mother may have had your best interests at heart by not letting you run from an "F."

Client: (Rather startled.) Well, yes, I suppose so. I know she didn't want me.

Nurse: Didn't want you?

Client: Oh, it's understandable. She had a hard time. Dad was drinking a lot. You know, she left him and then went back to him. She had Dorey, and a year later she was pregnant with me. She had to stay in bed most of her pregnancy because of her heart condition. She was in a long labor with me. I put these things together later. This is why I know she didn't want me.

Nurse: Sounds like she went through a lot to have you.

Client: She went through a lot with my father. He wasn't physically abusive. I was his "chicky." I could have anything. (Laughs.) He never treated me like he treated my mother and sister.

Nurse: Sounds like you were very special to him.

Client: I never thought of that.

Focusing on one's history reveals patterns of behavior and their psychodynamic makeup. The roots of these patterns are locked into internalized beliefs. The organization of these past experiences can be further explored to retrieve unconscious information. One hypothesis is that these unconscious beliefs are factors in repetitive, dysfunctional patterns in the present. Exploring and interpreting these beliefs is therapeutic. Awareness and abreaction (living through these memories) are the working therapeutic tasks of the client and nurse. It is important to determine the relevance of these experiences to current behavior. The preceding example shows how an internal, current state of "having to make up for something in social situations" has roots in past experiences. The first step in helping the client explore patterns of behavior is to bring these patterns to the client's awareness. The nurse and client must link them with past events or internal processes such as emotional states and thought patterns.

Focusing on Environment Dissatisfactions Current dissatisfaction with life in general provides another source of information about existing patterns. Complaints about work, school, which course to choose, which job to take, pressure in a job, the landlord's responsibilities, or living conditions all become relevant focuses of an interview. Patterns interfering with the client's development and sense of satisfaction, control, and growth are revealed.

The first step is to find out from the client whether the attitudes and feelings expressed arise in other situations. The client becomes aware that the attitudes and feelings are present in different situations. Having this awareness, the client explores what he wants, the resources needed to get it, how to pursue it, and other necessary ingredients in decision making. The dilemma regarding the life situation is maintained in part by the client not knowing what he wants. The recurrent attitudes and emotional states block awareness. The following is an example.

Client: I don't know if I want to teach. For 5 years I've been administering special projects. Now I'm going back to the classroom. My wife is mad at me because I'm busy every night planning classes. I don't know if I really like teaching.

Nurse: Has there been a time when you liked teaching? (How does the client identify pleasurable experiences?)

Client: I don't know. I had taught classes for 1 to 2 years and then changed to something else. So, I never get to relax—you know what I mean—I do the hard part of organizing a class, and then I leave the next year.

Nurse: Have you ever worked in a situation in which you felt relaxed?

Client: Well, the time I left teaching for a year and worked in a collective restaurant.

Nurse: How was that for you?

Client: I liked working with the people. We worked together. You knew what to expect.

Nurse: Knew what to expect?

Client: Yeah, you know, I keep thinking I returned to teaching because my parents kept emphasizing security. Dad worked for the city. Mom worked as a nurse. They kept emphasizing, "Get a job for security, benefits, and retirement."

Nurse: What does this have to do with your current concerns?

Client: I don't know. I don't know if I dislike teaching because I'm doing it as a result of my parents' beliefs or because I haven't given myself a chance to enjoy it.

Nurse: How successful are you in giving yourself a chance to enjoy what you do?

Client: Not very. That's what my wife is complaining about; it's hard to do things together that we enjoy. Oh, at times, but it's like we can't decide what to do or I'm worrying about my class preparations. I don't know—life is serious,

hard. You must work; it's like there isn't much I do that I can say I really enjoy.

Nurse: It may be useful to find out what and how you do things when teaching to either experience pleasure or quench it.

Client: Yes, I'm desperate. I find myself worrying about it so much that it's driving my wife away from me.

In the preceding example the nurse agrees with the client that a lack of pleasure is being experienced in many areas of his life. He associates part of this pattern with parental upbringing. He is distressed about his reaction to teaching. The nurse encourages further exploration in this area to determine patterns of thinking responsible for the client's dissatisfaction. The nurse does not focus on changing jobs but rather on identifying the theme of displeasure.

Translating Insights Into Actions Thus far the working phase has been discussed. It emphasized identifying and exploring patterns of dysfunctional behavior. How is this process used for behavioral changes toward positive goals? The process of exploration and identification results in behavioral change by challenging nonproductive beliefs. This process gives the client choices. Clients can expand their basis for making decisions and thus respond differently. They may feel less guilty and more in control of their behavior in responding to others. They are also more open to feedback, and they may be more tolerant of others. A second dimension of the working phase is using insight and knowledge to change behavior and incorporate healthy patterns into the client's responses.

Use of information about patterns requires a model of how in reality behavior can be changed. Regardless of the therapeutic technique. One or more of the following behavioral processes are invoked: combining, separating, sorting, and altering behavioral criteria relevant to values and beliefs or rehearsing new behaviors. For example, when the nurse asks a client to notice how a past event, emotion, or relationship is related to a current behavioral response, the client is forced primarily to *combine* information from seemingly unrelated topics.

Separating occurs when the client *unlinks,* for example, a cause-effect conclusion:

Client: My mother is the cause of my problems with women.

Nurse: How's that?

Client: My mother's nagging when I was little still makes me angry with women.

Nurse: How does that affect you today?

Client: When a woman asks me to do something, I just get mad and say she's not going to tell me what to do.

Nurse: So what you think about being asked to do something makes you mad.

Client: Well, yeah, I learned it from my mother.

Nurse: You learned that when your mother nagged you, you felt angry. Today you've discovered that when a woman asks you to do something and you associate it with the past, you get mad.

Client: Yeah, my mother is dead; so it is the way I think.

Sorting occurs when interventions force a client to select information in a way that differs from an existing pattern. In the preceding example the nurse may ask, "Tell me about a time that a woman asked you to do something and you didn't get mad or angry with her?" This question encourages the client to explore different experiences. If he cannot find any positive examples, the nurse can ask, "How would a woman have to ask you to do something so that you wouldn't get angry?" The client may then outline the behavior necessary for him not to feel nagged.

Altering beliefs about behavior is another powerful way to change behavior. For example, the behavior of a client who is extremely intimidated by authority figures changes when he no longer believes the boss's anger is directed at him. He learns that anger comes from within and represents that person's way of expressing feelings such as frustration. The client learns to replace his original response with a range of possibilities. For example a technique called "chair work" in gestalt therapy has the client perform inner dialogue. The part of himself that is frightened of the boss talks with the part of himself that wants to speak up. The client is encouraged to challenge and change his reasons for being frightened of the boss. The therapist focuses on altering the client's interpretation of his behavior; this is called *reframing*.

Rehearsing new behaviors addresses the use of information about patterns and change. Role playing experiences in self-assertion is one way behavioral changes are accomplished and reinforced. Role playing uses communication techniques to focus interviews on relevant experiential areas. The nurse and client actively participate in strategies that encourage behavioral change. It is important to disrupt the client's dysfunctional behavior patterns during therapy. Distrupting the pattern jolts the client out of habitual behaviors and increases the client's insight and awareness. Experiencing new behaviors during therapy reinforces the concept that the client has control of and makes choices in his life. During the later part of the working phase, the nurse interprets, confronts, and encourages the rehearsal of new behaviors.

Interpretations are aimed at clients who are reframing their view of what is causing dysfunctional behavioral responses. For example, the client who felt something missing in social situations and who believed that her mother could not possibly want her because of the difficult delivery (p. 125) associated much of this feeling with her unilateral relationship with her father. This relationship resulted in part from a fear that he would treat her as he did her mother. Her resentment of her father surfaced, as did her jealousy and love. She understood her father's fear of his children and competition with them for the mother's attention. This understanding was reinforced by the fact that the mother and father "made up" when the kids were out of the house. The client linked the "making-up feeling" to her own need to resolve within herself, and with her mother, their rejection of each other's love. Interpretation was insufficient. The daughter began to communicate with her mother and actively change her behavior toward her mother.

Confrontation is similar to interpretation, except that is is based on the present. A confrontation is usually a direct encounter between nurse and client. For this reason, the nurse is sure of the behavioral patterns she is attempting to change.

▼ **Case Example**

Tabitha, a young social worker, was aware of and had explored at length a strong need to please people and to gain their approval. She had developed a strong self-defeating, self-limiting view and

presentation of herself at work, in her marriage, and with her siblings. She damned herself. She recognized the secondary gain in this behavior, which was obtaining sympathy and attention. The pattern was often directed toward the nurse. The transference aspects were investigated. The behavior decreased but was still obvious. During one particular session, the client was describing her behavior in her new work setting:

Client: *I don't think I'm doing very well. Oh, they like me, but the supervision isn't too good, and I don't think I put enough into my work. I'm not reading; I'm not keeping good notes. My sister, a budding, highly successful psychologist, seems more into her work than I do. I don't know. I think, well, I'm doing all right, but I don't think it's as . . . good as it should be (looks at the nurse). What do you think?*
Nurse: *I agree with you.*
Client: *(Genuine surprise.) What?*
Nurse: *You have been telling me all the things you are not doing and how you appraise yourself. And I believe what you say.*
Client: *Don't you care?*
Nurse: *No. (Silence.)*
Client: *(Looks stunned.)*
Nurse: *I only care that you care.*
Client: *(Silent and thoughtful.) I see what you mean. I wanted you to tell me I was OK.*
Nurse: *And would you believe me?*
Client: *I wouldn't really. It's hard to change and take responsibility for caring, for moving out on my own, and for what I can do.*

In this example, a client's insight into parental issues, sibling rivalry, or transference is of little value unless the client's behavior changes. The nurse assumed a confrontational stance by saying "no." The client had to search for her own sense of worth, regardless of what the nurse thought of her. The next step is to have the client rehearse open, cooperative strategies. The client can now participate in exercises to help her compete more directly.

In addition to behaviors that the client reports to the nurse, problematic behavior patterns also arise within the context of the nurse-client relationship. The nurse seeks to create a balance in maintaining rapport and creating anxiety in the therapeutic process. Anxiety provokes the client to use behaviors that reduce anxiety. Patterns may also surface in relationship to others in the environment, such as staff or other clients. The nurse makes careful observations of the client's relationships with others. She shares these with the client. In this way, the client sees his responsibility within the relationship. In the case example of Jean, who withdrew from her husband (p. 123), it is likely that Jean will withdraw from the nurse (for example, being late, missing appointments, or refusing to share new information), demonstrating in the *here and now* her pattern of withdrawal. She is "transferring" her feelings and behaviors from past relationships onto her current relationship with the nurse.

Bringing old patterns of feeling and behaving into the current situation lets the client alter these behaviors. Also, people who have been important and trustworthy, providing positive past experiences, influence the nurse-client relationship.

Ignoring transference can perpetuate the pattern. For example, being overly critical of the client, withholding information, or being overinvolved in making decisions for the client can encourage the dysfunctional behavior pattern. The nurse and client focus on the client's behavior and its immediate effect. There must be no blame or presumptions on the part of either person.

▼ Case Example

When the nurse asks Jean about her missed appointment Jean becomes angry and states that she knows the nurse is "tired of her" and "really wants to terminate the relationship." After further discussion the nurse asks Jean if the current situation is in any way similar to the situation with Jean's husband or co-workers. Soon Jean develops the insight that the feeling of being unloved and the response of withdrawing is a recurrent pattern and is not necessarily based on a realistic appraisal of the situation. Jean is then in a position to change her behavior with the nurse.

Although painful, the client's acknowledgment of personal responsibility for interpersonal relationships is the first step toward change. The client has the power to change her attitudes, feelings, and behaviors and therefore to change other people's responses to her. It is the client's responsibility to risk trying new behaviors. Behaviors that created problems for the client in the past may surface in the present situation with the nurse. These behaviors can be confronted and new behaviors tried within the therapeutic relationship. Jean's fear of rejection by the nurse is not nearly as important as her fear of rejection by her husband. Thus she can try being on time without missing appointments no matter what her feelings may be. Jean may learn to tell the nurse when she is feeling rejected. She may ask the nurse to confirm her feelings by asking about the nurse's feelings toward her. If Jean can show new successful behaviors without withdrawing from the nurse, this change is possible in more important relationships.

The working phase ends when the initial and any intermediate goals have been addressed, and the client can assess and make changes for himself. If the client desires only a reduction in the symptoms, the nurse accepts this and moves to the termination phase.

Termination Phase

The termination phase begins during the orientation phase and continues during the working phase as progress and outcomes are evaluated. Responsibilities and therapeutic outcomes are defined during the termination phase. The goal of the termination phase is to bring a therapeutic end to the nurse-client relationship. The nurse directs her attention toward making a potentially negative separation a positive one. When the process of termination is complete, it is known as *closure.*

The tasks of the termination phase are listed in the accompanying box.

TASKS OF THE TERMINATION PHASE

Bring a therapeutic end to the relationship
Review feelings about the relationship
Evaluate progress toward goals
Establish mechanisms for meeting future therapy needs

Reactions to the termination phase

Endings are a normal part of life. However, in our society, endings are sometimes equated with failure. Since people usually attempt to avoid failure, the subject of parting is often not discussed. Accordingly, many relationships end badly, leaving scars and unresolved conflicts. Many people never learn the skills needed to terminate a relationship positively. This is true for the nurse as well as the client. The termination phase of the nurse-client relationship reunites past experiences with separation. A sense of disappointment or abandonment may be experienced. Rather than feeling sad about parting, many people get angry and belittle the experience.

Another area of difficulty, particularly for the student or beginning nurse, is letting go of a close and often satisfying relationship. The intimacy and mutual acceptance found in the therapeutic relationship exemplify desirable qualities in personal relationships. During termination, both the client and nurse may be tempted to continue the relationship on a social level. This may simply be a reluctance to say "good-bye," or perhaps a lack of understanding about the nature of the relationship. Failure to terminate the relationship violates the therapy contract established by the two individuals. The nurse who experiences a great difficulty in terminating a relationship can seek the advice of a peer or a more experienced nurse. She may want to sort out the ethical issues involved in converting a therapeutic relationship to a more personal one.

Student nurses who have difficulty teminating a therapeutic relationship may try to delay termination or may fail to adequately say good-bye. Students are often surprised at how difficult it is to say good-bye to clients. Student nurses sometimes fail to recognize how attached they have become to clients until the actual parting. Student nurses may extend the last meeting well beyond the time limits originally agreed on. They may agree to have future contact with clients by phone, letter, or visit. Conversely, the student nurse may avoid saying good-bye by being overly casual with the client during the parting. They may avoid discussing the termination or avoid the last meeting all together.

Strategies for accomplishing the tasks of the termination phase

Termination may occur before or after agreed upon goals have been met. Strategies may differ, depending on the nature of the termination. Termination is an important growth-producing experience for both client and nurse.

Strategies for termination before agreed upon goals have been met

Termination before goals have been met is not unusual. It may result from the nurse's decision, discharge of the client, or the client's request. When a client wishes to terminate prematurely, previous agreements expressed in the contract may ensure a positive ending. The client and nurse should agree in the beginning not to part in anger or to part without discussing the feelings parting evokes. Ideally three sessions are devoted to evaluating and ending the relationship. One session is the minimum time to devote to termination. This allows time for the client and the nurse to negotiate an ending to the relationship or to resolve any conflicts.

The fear of closeness can precipitate an early termination to the relationship. The implied intimacy of the therapeutic relationship can trigger the same fears for the nurse as for the client. The discussion on transference and counter-transference (p. 122) highlights signs that can alert the nurse to these reactions. The nurse may find herself too tense and unable to work through personal reactions to a client. In this case, it is best to terminate the relationship and refer the client to another therapist. This is most effectively done when the nurse assumes responsibility for her behavior and allows the client to express thoughts and feelings of rejection. The emphasis is on the best interests of the client. Often unrealistic attitudes and a sense of pride prevent the nurse from making this reasonable decision. For example, the idea that the nurse can work with everyone is unrealistic. This means that nothing about a client detracts from productive, intimate work. This defies human existence. The mental health–psychiatric nurse constantly examines her personal beliefs and values to gain flexibility, but this does not mean that there are no limits.

Resistance from the client can be expected to surface during the termination phase. This resistance is normal and worthy of attention. Fault finding by either party is a pattern that needs to be disrupted during the last meeting. The client may state that the therapy is not beneficial, or not working. The client may refuse to follow through on something that has been agreed on. The client's resistance does not mean that what is being done is not ultimately useful. It simply means that at this particular point, there has been a loss of appropriateness of therapeutic efforts for the client. The client may ask to terminate the relationship or just refuse to continue.

Resistance often comes in the form of a *flight to health.* This flight to health is exhibited by a client who suddenly declares no further need for therapy. The client claims to be "all right" and wants to discontinue the therapeutic relationship. This may be a form of denial or fear of the anticipated grief over separation.

It is important for the therapist to contact the client and encourage renegotiation of the relationship. As long as the issues surrounding what needs to happen for the therapy to continue are examined, the client can decide to continue or terminate with a sense of direction for the future.

External factors can also cause premature termination, particularly for a nurse in a hospital setting. Discharge decisions may be made without considering the goals the client and nurse have set. It is helpful if discharge decisions are made in advance so that the nurse and client have time to initiate the termination process. Discharge planning is an area for negotiation between the nurse and other health team members. The student nurse, who has a limited number of clinic hours, is particularly susceptible to a sense of loss when a client is discharged on the day that the student is not in the clinic. The lack of closure is compounded if the nurse does not believe the goals that she and the client set were achieved.

Strategies for termination when agreed upon goals have been met

A painful experience with separation can be replaced by a positive experience, but even the termination of a good relationship in which therapy goals have been met can be a difficult process.

If the client or nurse has experienced the loss of an important person, termination may bring back memories and feelings associated with the previous loss. Sorting the past from present becomes a focus of therapy. Both nurse and client discuss their feelings about the separation. The nurse must discuss feelings of sadness or loss about the ending of the relationship as well as her satisfactions. Thus encouraging the client to explore ambivalent feelings honestly. It may be helpful to discuss the grief process as it applies to the nurse-client relationship.

During the exploration of feelings about termination, it is helpful to relate these feelings to past experiences of loss. No new topics are discussed in this phase. Spiritual concerns, if not developed in the early phases of therapy, are most appropriately integrated during termination. Exploration of beliefs about the value of life and the meaning of death flow naturally from discussions of endings and beginnings. This is an extremely valuable experience for both client and nurse.

Flight to illness occurs when a client exhibits a sudden return of symptoms. This is an unconscious effort to show that termination is inappropriate and that the nurse is still needed. The client may disclose new information about himself or more problems in an attempt to delay parting. The threat of suicide is the most extreme symptom of flight to illness. The nurse has a difficult task to remain clam, sensitive, and firm in moving toward termination.

Often the client says that he is unable to function without the nurse's assistance. The client may become increasingly dependent and appear to lose all ability to adapt. The nurse may also believe the client cannot function on his own. The nurse may have particular difficulty if the therapy has gone well. She may overestimate her contribution and underestimate the client's contribution to the success of therapy, unconsciously disrupting termination. Both client and nurse need to examine their beliefs about the ability of individuals to control their own lives, as opposed to being controlled by outside forces. Both the client and nurse need to respect the client's role in achieving the goals of therapy.

The goal of the therapeutic process is for the client to continue to evolve and grow independently of the nurse. However, provisions are made for the client to return to therapy if the need arises. It is helpful for the client and nurse to discuss the future and anticipate possible situations the client may face. The client can project possible solutions to problems and rehearse skills learned in therapy. Client and nurse can assess the client's resources and support systems. Specific signs and symptoms that may denote a recurrence of problems are identified. A plan for meeting future therapy needs is made. Referrals are made where appropriate. The value of an accurate assessment of the phase of the relationship is described in the research highlight on p. 130.

BARRIERS TO THE THERAPEUTIC RELATIONSHIP

In the therapeutic relationship certain barriers have been identified. These barriers may come from the environment, the nurse, or the client. They appear in the form of frustration, discomfort, anger, discouragement, or confusion. Also, the client may change suddenly by expressing hostility or withdrawal.

RESEARCH HIGHLIGHT

Establishing a Nurse-Client Relationship

• C Forchuk and B Brown

PURPOSE

The purposes of the study were to develop an instrument to measure the phases of the nurse-client relationship and also to begin the process of establishing validity and reliability for the tool. The tool was based on Peplau's conceptualization of the nurse-client relationship.

SAMPLE

The convenience sample consisted of 132 situations on which the form was used; 58 were with case management clients, and 74 were with counseling-treatment clients in Ontario, Canada.

METHODOLOGY

The one-page instrument was developed and used by community mental health promotion program nurses for a year, during which nurses identified and plotted the phases of the nurse-client relationships for their clients.

Based on data from *Journal of Psychosocial Nursing and Mental Health Services,* 27(2):30, 1989.

FINDINGS

Contrast and content validity were established for the instrument. Interrater reliability was also established. Limitations of the study were that a small convenience sample was used, and the clients were all in community-based settings and had predominantly chronic health problems.

IMPLICATIONS

The instrument appears to provide an accurate assessment of the phases of the nurse-client relationship. Nurses who used the form found it easy to use as well as clear and practical. Nurses who used the form noted that when the nurse can accurately assess the phase of the relationship, appropriate interventions are more likely to be selected. This development of appropriate instruments for the empirical study of Peplau's theory is a significant step in further developing Peplau's nursing theory.

Environmental Barriers

Barriers to the nurse-client relationship may be external. Many of these, such as lack of privacy, inappropriate meeting place or furniture, and noise, are discussed as barriers to communication. Some of the external barriers to the relationship may be within the nurse's control. The nurse may be able to find a relatively quiet, private place for a one-to-one interaction. However, she may not be able to postpone the serving of lunch if one of her clients feels the need to interact at noon. The nurse can minimize the external barriers with wise scheduling of her time, honest discussion of her duties with each client, and consulting other team members.

Nurse Barriers

Nurses bring their previous experiences and distinct personalities to the nurse-client relationship. Some of these may create barriers to the therapeutic relationship.

Nurses, on the whole, are compassionate and dedicated to helping clients. This trait, however, may lead to becoming too involved with clients, or "rescuing." Nurses sometimes attempt to solve all of the client's problems without allowing the client to make choices or mistakes. This discourages the client from taking personal responsibility. It creates a situation where the nurse is working harder than the client to solve the client's problems. Sometime the client resents the implication that he is not able to mutually or independently solve problems. Usually the nurse who works harder than the client finds herself becoming discouraged and worn out. Changes that the client makes are sometimes temporary since the change was the nurse's idea,

not the client's. The nurse may become more frustrated as her efforts go unrewarded.

A related barrier comes from nurses who have become skeptical about the ability of clients to change. These nurses may have started as rescuers and become discouraged. They may have begun with a pessimistic view of human nature. Such nurses tend to approach the nurse-client relationship by maintaining a certain distance from the client, using a matter-of-fact approach to the exclusion of other techniques. Inherent in this pessimistic view is a tendency to label clients either by diagnoses or as "trouble makers."

Just as nurses bring past experiences to the nurse-client relationship, they also bring current life situations to work. Like many other people, nurses experience divorce, death, sense of loss, job dissatisfaction, problems with children or peers, and other personal situations. These may be difficult to ignore when establishing the nurse-client relationship. Nurses may be preoccupied, interested in socializing with each other, or just plain tired. It takes energy and dedication to switch from the social self to the therapeutic self to focus on the client.

Some nurses are not comfortable with feelings. They prefer that the client think and solve problems without becoming upset or angry. These nurses are disturbed by tears or loud voices. They often fear that the client is "losing control" if he openly expresses any strong emotion. Nurses who are uncomfortable with feelings tend to discourage the client from sharing intimate details. They claim that the client was "getting upset." The nurse who is uncomfortable with feelings is in need of considerable behavioral change to participate therapeutically in the nurse-client relationship.

Client Barriers

Most psychiatric problems can be categorized as difficulties in interpersonal relationships. It is therefore not surprising that these difficulties would surface in the nurse-client relationship. There are certain behaviors that present particular barriers to the relationship. Among these are excessive dependence, hostile aggressiveness, sexual acting out, manipulation, and self-destructive behaviors.

Excessive *dependence* is sometimes difficult to recognize in the early stages of the relationship because the client initially appears to be genuinely seeking help. Dependence is shown in the client's excessive flattery of the nurse and self-deprecation. The client may compare the nurse favorably to others and feel hurt or jealous of the nurse's attention to other clients. The client may constantly ask for the nurse's opinion and advice before making decisions. The client may seek approval and attempt to please the nurse by excessive compliance to the nurse's suggestions or by performing small favors for the nurse.

The pattern of excessive dependence is called *learned helplessness.* It has the effect of creating secondary gains, since the client gets many of his needs for attention, contact, and protection met through this behavior. The client who is initially pleasant and nonthreatening may later become irritating with his excessive demands. The client may feel guilt, anger, and even self-hatred at his dependence.

Hostile aggressiveness is particularly difficult for the nurse to tolerate. Signs may range from challenging, demeaning, and critical remarks to threats of physical violence. Swearing and lewd statements are another form of aggression. The main distinction between anger and aggression is that anger is a feeling and aggression conveys an intent to harm or destroy.

Like excessive dependence, the pattern of hostile aggressiveness is learned and creates a secondary gain for the client. The client may feel more powerful by hurting or intimidating others. The client may use intimidation to drive people away. This decreases the fear associated with closeness. At times, the client is asking for external control such as medication, hospitalization, or seclusion. It is extremely important to assess the underlying reason for a client's aggressive behavior.

Sexual acting out may take the form of excessive flattery, asking the nurse for a date, suggestive remarks, or physical contact. The physical contact may range from excessive casual touching to inappropriate and aggressive acts. Some of the milder expressions of sexual acting out may be a form of dependence, such as a need for approval, attention, or validation of the client's worth. Sexual acting out creates a powerful emotional response on the part of the nurse based on her own past experiences and value system. As with hostile aggressiveness there may a variety of underlying reasons for the sexual acting out.

Overt sexual behavior has more in common with hostile aggressiveness. It may be an attempt to gain power and control over the nurse, or to intimidate and drive the nurse away. In other instances, sexual acting out is a pattern of self-defeating behavior. It is designed to confirm the client's feelings of worthlessness by causing the nurse to reject the client.

Manipulation is an immature pattern of behavior in which the client seeks to obtain personal goals, often without regard for the goals of others (see Chapter 23). The client believes that he is entitled to have his desires met without delay, personal effort, or sacrifice. The manipulative client may cause nurses to become overprotective of him and angry toward other team members who are not being manipulated.

Secondary gains of manipulation include having many needs met without expending much effort, distracting attention from his problems, diverting the attention of the staff, and therefore gaining the freedom to continue old, familiar patterns of behavior. Manipulation decreases anxiety while creating discomfort for those who are being manipulated.

Perhaps the most difficult client barrier is the threat of *self-destruction.* Suicide is the ultimate self-destructive act. Underlying motivations of self-destruction are similar to those of other dysfunctional behaviors such as excessive dependence, hostile aggressiveness, and manipulation (see Chapter 14).

Strategies for overcoming client barriers

Barriers represent patterns of behaviors that the client uses to cope with interpersonal relationships. The real clues to the client's problem are often found in his behaviors rather than his verbalization of the problem. The barriers provide objective data to be considered along with the client's subjective perceptions. For example, a client who verbalizes the need to be close to others, yet refuses to confide in or trust the nurse, is giving the nurse two important pieces of information.

The nurse looks beyond the obvious behavior and tries to see the underlying meaning that it has for the client and the secondary gains that reinforce the behavior. For example, a client asks a nurse for a sexual favor. It is important to assess the context in which the behavior occurred. What was the previous relationship between client and nurse? Had there been any revealing topics discussed recently? Had the relationship changed? Were there any anxiety provoking incidents in the client's life? Are the client's needs for affection and attention being met? Is the client hostile? Does the client have a history of sexual acting out? What was the nonverbal behavior and tone of voice during the conversation? These questions help the nurse to determine the meaning of the behavior.

The nurse also needs to assess the consequences of secondary gain that the client receives from the behavior. What does the client expect to happen as a result of his behavior? Is this a pattern that the client uses in similar circumstances? Why does the client continue to behave in this way? What does he get out of it? In assessing the consequences that the client expects from his behavior, it is sometimes helpful to ask directly, "How do you suppose I'll respond to what you just said?" It is also important for the nurse to be aware of her own feelings in response to the behavior. The nurse's initial response is an indication of how others have responded to the client's behavior and verbalizations in the past.

The nurse should avoid responding emotionally to the barriers the client presents. The most helpful response is one that will break the pattern of reinforcement of the client's behavior. When the nurse remains calm and seeks to clarify the motivation for the behavior, this, in itself, becomes an intervention. The nurse is saying, "You matter. Your feelings matter, and I want to understand you." The client may not be aware of the behavior and its role in his problem. Gently, calmly pointing out the pattern and helping the client explore how it has been used in relationships is therapeutic. Above all the nurse's willingness to continue to work on the relationship, in spite of obstacles, tells the client that he is accepted, valued, and respected. Interventions for specific problem behaviors are covered in other chapters.

BRIEF REVIEW

The historical origins of mental health–psychiatric nursing emphasize the therapeutic potential of the nurse-client relationship. The nurse's therapeutic ability is enhanced by self-awareness as well as knowledge. The nurse establishes rapport through trust, warmth, empathy, and genuineness. The element of caring is central to these aspects of the therapeutic relationship. The nurse creates a climate in which the client can explore personal issues to gain insight and change problematic behavior. The course of the nurse-client relationship progresses through various states, each with tasks, difficulties, and potential rewards. The ultimate goal of the nurse-client relationship is independent functioning of the client.

REFERENCES AND SUGGESTED READINGS

1. Abraham I: Support groups for nursing students in psychiatric rotation, *Issues in Mental Health Nursing* 4:159, 1982.
2. American Psychiatric Association: *Diagnostic and statistical manual of mental disorders (DSM-III-R)*, Washington, DC, 1987, APA.
3. Bandler R, Grinder J: *Frogs into princes: neurolinguistic programming*, Moab, Utah, 1979, Real People Press.
4. Bandler R, Grinder J: *The structure of magic: a book about language and therapy,* vol 1, Palo Alto, Calif, 1975, Science & Behavior Books.
5. Burnard P: *Self awareness for nurses*, Gaithersburg, Md, 1986, Aspen.
6. Campbell J: The relationship of nursing and self-awareness, *Advances in Nursing Science* 2:(4)15, 1980.
7. Cameron-Bandler L: *They lived happily ever after: a book about achieving happy endings in coupling*, Cupertino, Calif, 1978, Meta Publications.
8. Coleman E, Edwards B: *Brief encounters*, New York, 1980, Anchor Press.
9. Colliton M: The history of nursing therapy, *Perspectives in Psychiatric Care* 3(2):10, 1965.
10. Dodds S: A study of influence of role modeling on students' attitude formation during their psychiatric rotation, *Issues in Mental Health Nursing* 2:51, 1980.
11. Donna ME: *Travelbees' intervention in psychiatric nursing,* ed 2, Philadelphia, 1979, FA Davis.
12. Farrelly F, Brandsman J: *Provocative therapy*, Cupertino, Calif, 1981, Meta Publications.
13. Forchuk C, Brown B: Establishing a nurse-client relationship, *Journal of Psychosocial Nursing and Mental Health Services* 22(2):30, 1989.
14. Fry S: The philosophical foundations of caring. In Leininger MM, editor: *Ethical and moral dimensions of care*, Detroit, 1990, Wayne State University Press.
15. Gagan J: Methodological notes on empathy, *Advances in Nursing Science* 5(1):65, 1983.
16. Grinder J, Bandler R: *The structure of magic,* vol 2, Palo Alto, Calif, 1976, Science & Behavior Books.
17. Haley J: *Problem-solving therapy,* San Francisco, 1977, Jossey-Bass.
18. Hughes C: Supervising clinical practice in psychosocial nursing, *Journal of Psychosocial Nursing and Mental Health Services* 23(2):27, 1985.
19. Hutchison C, Bahr SR: Types and meanings of caring behaviors among elderly nursing home residents, *Image: Journal of Nursing Scholarship* 23(2):85, 1991.
20. Kasch C: Toward a theory of nursing action: skills and competency in nurse-patient interaction, *Nursing Research* 35(4):226, 1986.
21. Kelly B: Respect and caring: ethics and essence of nursing. In Leininger MM, editor: *Ethical and moral dimensions of care*, Detroit, 1990, Wayne State University Press.
22. Krieger D: *Foundations for holistic health nursing: the Renaissance nurse,* Philadelphia, 1981, JB Lippincott.
23. Lancaster J: *Adult psychiatric nursing,* New York, 1988, Medical Examination Publishing.
24. Lankton S: *Practical magic: a translation of neuro-linguistic programming into clinical psychotherapy,* Cupertino, Calif, 1980, Meta Publications.
25. LaFrance M, Mayo C: *Moving bodies: nonverbal communication in social relationships,* Monterey, Calif, 1978, Brooks/Cole.
26. Leininger MM: Leininger's theory of nursing: cultural care diversity and universality, *Nursing Science Quarterly* 1(4):156, 1988.
27. Leininger MM: Transcultural care diversity and universality: a theory of nursing, *Nursing and Health Care* 4:209, 1985.
28. Loomis M: Levels of contracting, *Journal of Psychosocial Nursing* 23(3):9, 1985.
29. Mellow J: Nursing therapy as a treatment and clinical investigation approach to emotional illness, *Nursing Forum* 5(3):64, 1966.
30. Mellow J: The experimental order of nursing therapy in the treatment of acute schizophrenia. In *Psychiatric research in our changing world: proceedings of an international symposium,* Montreal, October 3-5, 1968, International Congress Series No 187, New York, 1968, Excerpta Medical Foundation.
30a. Norse V and others: Comparative analysis of conceptualization and theories of caring, *Image: Journal of Nursing Scholarship* 23(2):119, 1991.
31. Orlando IJ: *The dynamic nurse-patient relationship,* New York, 1961, GP Putnam's Sons.
32. Peplau HE: *Interpersonal relations in nursing,* New York, 1952, GP Putnam's Sons.
33. Rogers C and others: *The therapeutic relationship and its impact,* Madison, 1967, University of Wisconsin Press.
34. Satir V: *Conjoint family therapy,* Palo Alto, Calif, 1967, Science & Behavior Books.
35. Satir V: *Peoplemaking,* Palo Alto, Calif, 1972, Science & Behavior Books.
36. Schoffstall C: Concerns of student nurses prior to psychiatric nursing experience: an assessment and intervention technique, *Journal of Psychosocial Nursing and Mental Health Services* 19(11):11, 1981.
37. Schroder P: Recognizing transference and counter-transference, *Journal of Psychosocial Nursing* 23(2):21, 1985.
38. Schwartz M, Schocrisy E: *The nurse and the mental patient,* New York, 1950, Russell Sage Foundation.
39. Schwing G: *A way to the soul of the mentally ill,* New York, 1954, International Press (Translated by R Ekstein and BH Hall).
40. Sechehaye M: The curative function of symbols in a case of traumatic neurosis with psychotic reactions. In Burton A, ed-

itor: *Psychotherapy of the psychoses,* New York, 1961, Basic Books.

41. Stacklum M: New student in psychiatry, *American Journal of Nursing* 81:762, 1981.
42. Sullivan HS: *The interpersonal theory of psychiatry,* New York, 1953, WW Norton.
43. Travelbee J: *Interpersonal aspects of nursing,* ed 2, Philadelphia, 1972, FA Davis.
44. Tudor GE: A sociopsychiatric nursing approach to intervention in a problem of mutual withdrawal on a mental hospital ward, *Journal of Psychiatry* 15:193, 1952.
45. Ujhely G: *Determinants of the nurse-patient relationship,* New York, 1968, Springer.
46. Watson J: Caring knowledge and informed moral passion, *Advances in Nursing Science* 13(1):15, 1990.
47. Watson J: *Nursing human science and human care a theory of nursing,* New York, 1988, National League for Nursing.
48. Williams CA: Biopsychosocial elements of empathy: a multidimensional model, *Issues in Mental Health Nursing* 11:155, 1990.
49. Witherspoon V: Using Lakovic's system of counter-transference classifications, *Journal of Psychosocial Nursing and Mental Health Services* 23(4):30, 1985.
50. Wolstein B: *Transference: its meaning and function in psychoanalytic therapy,* New York, 1954, Grune & Stratton.
51. Yalom I: *The theory and practice of group psychotherapy,* New York, 1975, Basic Books.

ANNOTATED BIBLIOGRAPHY

Coleman E, Edwards B: *Brief encounters,* New York, 1980, Anchor Press.

The authors focus on the potential of short-term relationships— how to achieve meaningful brief relationships and how to terminate successfully.

Forchuk C and others: Incorporating Peplau's theory and case management, *Journal of Psychosocial Nursing and Mental Health Services* 27(2):35, 1989.

The authors built a case management model based on Peplau's interpersonal theory of nursing. A case study demonstrates how a Peplau/Case Management model facilitates movement toward a higher level of functioning and improved quality of life for the client through the interactive interpersonal relationship between the client and the practitioner.

Jourard S: *The transparent self,* New York, 1971, Van Nostrand Reinhold.

This book explores the hypothesis that individuals can attain health and their fullest personal development when they have the courage to be themselves and to find goals that have meaning for them. The author focuses on self-disclosure and on the individual's purpose and meaning for existing, which arises from relationships with others.

Leininger MM, editor: *Ethical and moral dimensions of care,* Detroit, 1990, Wayne State University Press.

This book is the fourth in a series of considerations of care and its importance to nursing by a number of authors who are scholars in the field.

Peplau HE: Future directions in psychiatric nursing from the perspective of history, *Journal of Psychosocial Nursing and Mental Health Services* 27(2):18, 1989.

The author and theorist looks over the progress that has been made in psychiatric mental health and gives her views on what needs to be done to ensure a progressive future.

Ujhely G: *Determinants of the nurse-patient relationship,* New York, 1968, Springer.

This book deals with the many variables that affect the nurse-client relationship, including the data both nurse and client bring to the relationship and the context within which the relationship takes place.

Watson J: Caring knowledge and informed moral passion, *Advances In Nursing Science* 13(1):15, 1990.

In this article the author focuses on the importance of inclusion of caring knowledge into nursing's metaparadigm.

CHAPTER 8

The Nursing Process in Psychiatric Nursing

Ann P Hutton
Alice R Parkinson

After studying this chapter, the student will be able to:

- Correlate Standards of Practice with appropriate phases of the mental health–psychiatric nursing process
- Identify historical phases in development of the nursing process in mental health–psychiatric nursing
- Describe the significance of developing a collaborative interpersonal relationship as a component of the nursing process
- Identify elements that are common helping factors in the nursing process

- Define components of a nursing assessment from a holistic perspective
- Describe the process of analysis and formulation of nursing diagnoses
- Define the elements and purposes of the therapeutic plan
- Discuss holistic interventions for short-term and long-term actual and potential mental health–psychiatric problems
- Identify strategies for evaluating the effectiveness of nursing interventions

Nursing process is the framework for all nursing practice. In psychiatric–mental health nursing, therapeutic use of self is the means for operationalizing helping and healing aspects of the nursing process. Development of a therapeutic alliance with clients is essential to apply effectively the nursing process in caring for clients with mental health problems. Developing and maintaining a therapeutic alliance is central whether the client is an individual, a group, a family, or a community.

The client is an active participant in the nursing process, with varying degrees of control over problem resolution. Determining the extent to which a client is able to achieve autonomy and self-regulation is part of the nursing process assessment.

The nursing process is particularly important in psychiatric–mental health nursing, since it not only forms the basis for interventions but also is itself part of the therapeutic process. It develops on several levels at the same time. First, since information about perceptions, emotional, and behavioral responses are often painful and thus avoided by clients, the nurse must understand the meaning of such defensive processes. Second, the nurse gains information

about possible maladaptive relationship patterns through interactions with the client. The resulting hypotheses about the nature of the client's problems form the basis for nursing diagnoses and decision making. The data base for the nursing process is dynamic, subject to review and change as new understandings regarding the client's problems are gained.

To effectively use the nursing process, knowledge of a number of different theoretical and conceptual frameworks is useful in providing as holistic a view of the client's difficulties as possible. Use of the nursing process is therefore more meaningful, the more one knows about human motivation and development (see Chapter 4 on theoretical approaches).

It is important for the nurse to conceptualize all phases of the nursing process—assessment, analysis, planning, implementation, and evaluation—as therapeutic. Many clients experience considerable relief just through talking, and expressing emotions with someone experienced as caring, empathic, and trying to understand and clarify issues. Concern for the client's emotional state, level of anxiety, and ability to respond to the interviewer guides the length and

	DATES	EVENTS
HISTORICAL OVERVIEW	Before World War II	Mental health–psychiatric nurses depended mainly on experience, rote procedure, and intuitive judgment as a basis for nursing care.
	1940s	Mental health–psychiatric nurses had some awareness of theory but still provided primarily custodial care with no attention to a systematic approach to nursing care.
	1950s	Psychiatric nurses were using nursing care plans as a tool for communicating their practice. Peplau[61] developed a model of nursing care that emphasized a systematic approach to the nurse-client relationship.
	1960s	Orlando[57] was among the first to describe nursing as a deliberative process with a focus on the interpersonal relationship.
	1970s	Psychiatric nursing texts included the nursing process as a method for organizing nursing care within a conceptual framework.
	1980s	Mental health–psychiatric nurses continue to refine their use of the nursing process.
	1990s	With increased understanding, the mental health–psychiatric nurse more deliberately applies the nursing process.
	Future	Psychiatric nurses will engage in more research to systematically examine the effect of the nursing process on the nurse-client relationship.

depth of the initial assessment. As much emphasis should be placed on understanding *how* the client gives information (process) as is placed on the content.

This chapter is organized around the Standards of Practice that provide the basis for discussing each of the phases of the nursing process as applied in psychiatric–mental health nursing. Since the nursing process is facilitated by understanding theoretical concepts and developing skills in therapeutic communication, a group of concepts known as *common helping factors* will also be discussed.[26,81]

COMMON HELPING FACTORS

Helping factors are considered common since they transcend any particular theoretical orientation. These interrelated factors facilitate general goals for nursing interventions, such as increasing client self-understanding and developing client self-care skills, and are therefore useful throughout the nursing process. Their effectiveness depends on the ability of both the nurse and the client to build a collaborative trusting relationship.

Sharing a Common Goal

A general goal for helping clients with psychiatric or emotional problems is to assist the client to achieve self-responsibility, or autonomy, either through gaining self-awareness or learning new skills for living.

Self-responsibility means that an individual recognizes a need to be accountable for his or her thoughts, feelings, and actions. Many psychiatric clients suffer from serious forms of mental illness in which their ability to be self-aware and responsible is greatly compromised. For these

clients, learning daily living skills through psychoeducational interventions keeps the focus on the common goal of increasing self-responsibility to the greatest extent possible.

Activation of Hope and Expectancy of Help

Most clients who seek mental health services are acutely distressed. The nurse and others in the therapeutic milieu offer hope of help by listening and reflecting a realistic perspective to the client. Listening and clarifying the nature of the client's difficulties help reduce anxiety and support expectations of help.[26] A growing body of empirical evidence in the health care field in general supports the positive role played by hope and faith in the healing process.

Anticipatory Guidance and Accurate Expectations

Part of the nursing process involves orienting the client as to what to expect during the treatment process. Just what information is provided depends on the context for treatment (for example, hospitalization or outpatient). Regardless of place of treatment, studies demonstrate that advising the client of what to expect reduces ambiguity and unnecessary anxiety.

Use of Verbal Communication

Apart from the use of psychotropic drugs, electroconvulsive therapy (ECT), and other physical forms of therapy, therapeutic communication is the major vehicle through which the nursing process is operationalized and change mediated. Communication barriers caused by language differences or psychotic processes require special approaches. Nevertheless, communication is an important aspect of all psychiatric nursing interventions.

Provision of New Information

Through interactions with the nurse, clients learn new ways of viewing or managing their problems. These new possibilities for solutions can then be tried out in the relative safety of the treatment environment. As clients experience success in trying out new solutions, they begin to experience themselves as less helpless and more in control of their thoughts, feelings, and behaviors.

Sharing a Set of Guiding Principles

Appropriate use of theory is the basis for clinical decision making. It is therefore important that nurse and client work to develop a shared understanding of the rationale for treatment and that both believe in its effectiveness. Guiding principles include one's theoretical orientation(s), or ways of understanding psychosocial development, maladaptive coping patterns, and strategies that influence the change process.

A variety of theoretical perspectives are generally helpful to our understanding of disturbances in functional health patterns among psychiatric clients. For example, symptoms of mood disorders such as depression and anxiety may be partially explained by each of the following theoretical positions. The individual has:

1. A biological or brain disturbance and is in need of pharmocotherapy
2. A psychodynamic problem stemming from unresolved grief and loss and needs psychotherapy
3. A family systems problem in which symptoms of depression moderate closeness and distance; hence family therapy is needed
4. A social learning problem in which behaviors associated with depression or anxiety are reinforced, and so behavioral, or psychoeducational, therapy is needed
5. Negative automatic thought patterns, and so cognitive therapy is indicated
6. Lost a job as a result of an economic recession and needs vocational retraining

Throughout the nursing process, clients learn to understand their difficulties from these and other theoretical perspectives. By understanding problems from a theoretical perspective, one may correct distortions resulting from self-generated explanations. Many times clients learn to be less judgmental of themselves and others, as they learn to understand and accept human behavior. Using one framework for understanding does not necessarily preclude the validity of another. To develop holistic views of mental health problems, it is best to develop a number of alternative ways of understanding and intervening with psychiatric clients.

Enhancement of Mastery and Maintenance of Improvement

As clients experience success in achievement of goals, increased self-esteem, competence, and a sense of mastery

over conflicts and difficulties need to be reinforced. It is important for the nurse to point out and give credit to the client for positive changes. The dependency that often develops in nurse-client relationships can be gradually confronted by encouraging more independent choices and the development of skills for independent living. The tendency for nurses to feel gratified by clients who appear to need them may lead to overprotectiveness and hence interference with client growth and mastery.

Imitative Behavior

Learning by imitation and identification is an important way by which children develop new skills and a sense of self-identity. These methods of learning are important to keep in mind as the nursing process proceeds. Through imitation and identification with the nurse, the client tries on new attitudes and values that may eventually lead to new ways of coping with problems. Imitation is also a way the client acknowledges the importance of the relationship and the desire to maintain the relationship even when the nurse may not be physically present.

Nurse-Client Therapeutic Alliance

As the nurse and client work to implement the goals identified in the planning phase of the nursing process, the relationship becomes increasingly important. The ability of the nurse to empathize and clarify perceptions and feelings contributes to the development of trust and encourages the client to confide in the nurse. As the nurse accepts the client, the client is more likely to risk trying new behaviors. In general, the more positive the alliance, the more likely change is to occur. Positive alliances are built by collaborating with clients, not by giving advice or imposing beliefs or values.

The alliance with the nurse facilitates release of strong emotions, a process known as *catharsis*. Emotional release promotes healing by reducing anxiety and strengthening the alliance so that the client is more likely to stay motivated for treatment.

Universality

One helpful idea clients learn in psychiatric treatment is that their problems are not unique. Others have similar pain, need help, and experience difficulties in coping too. Since many individuals who seek help are not able to share their pain with others, they develop perceptions about themselves as being alone in a world that does not understand or rejects them. Discovery of universality decreases the distorted view that no one else can possibly understand them or their problems.

NURSING STANDARDS AS PROFESSIONAL PRACTICE GUIDELINES

The American Nurses' Association views the nursing process as a systematic method for organizing the delivery of nursing care. Each phase of the process correlates with a Standard of Psychiatric Mental Health Nursing Practice formulated in 1982 by the American Nurses' Association, Division of Psychiatric and Mental Health Nursing Practice.[4] The phases of the nursing process include assessment of the client's biopsychosocial status, analysis of the data base leading to nursing diagnoses, development of a plan for action, implementation of the plan, and evaluation of the client's responses to nursing actions and interventions.

Throughout all of the steps of the nursing process, the nurse is guided by Standard I, which calls for the application of scientifically sound theories to guide assessment and analysis of data and to support clinical decisions. "Psychiatric Mental Health Nursing is characterized by the applications of relevant theories to explain phenomena of concern to nurses and to provide a basis for intervention and subsequent evaluation of that intervention" (American Nurses' Association 1982, p. 3).

PHASES OF THE NURSING PROCESS

Assessment

Assessment involves the collection of data that reflect the mental health status of the client in relation to all dimensions of the person—physical, emotional, intellectual, social, and spiritual. Clients are the primary sources of data. Other sources include significant others, written records, various legal and social systems, and other health care per-

sonnel. The use of a variety of sources strengthens the assessment by expanding and validating the nurse's perception of the clients and their situations. Data are gathered from these sources through (1) interviews with the client and significant others, (2) observations of the client's behavior, (3) physical and mental status examinations, and (4) diagnostic tools, including psychological tests. (See the accompanying box for Standard 2.)

Interaction, observation, and measurement are the three primary methods used to gather data. Data gathered by interaction and observation are collected during interviews and examinations of mental and physical status. Measurement involves the use of instruments to quantify data.

The assessment data collected during the first nurse-client interaction are particularly important because they provide a baseline for information against which subsequent data may be compared. By making these crucial comparisons, the nurse can determine whether changes occur in the client's condition and may begin to infer factors correlated with these changes. A comprehensive initial assessment also provides a basis for making sound clinical judgments and developing a goal-oriented approach to nursing care rather than random interpretations and reactions to isolated client behaviors. Comparison of subsequent data to the baseline provides a feedback mechanism that links the steps of the nursing process.

For the assessment data to make sense to the nurse, they need to be organized in some way, usually grouped into categories. An assessment format is commonly used to display the data in this way. The design of the format depends on factors such as the client being assessed (individual, family, or community), the nature of the presenting problems (acute crisis or chronic mental illness), the scope of the assessment (limited or comprehensive), and the theoretical orientation of the agency (psychodynamic, behavioral, or family systems). The organization of the format reflects a concept of "the client." Historically, nursing has followed the lead of the medical (illness oriented) model to select data to include in a psychiatric assessment. As nursing becomes more clearly defined and autonomous, the data essential to the development of nursing care become increasingly distinguishable from that of other disciplines. In an agency setting where a predetermined assessment format may be required, the nurse decides whether additional information is needed to satisfy the current concept of nursing practice and profession accountability.

This chapter includes a holistic nursing assessment format (see the box on p. 138) for comprehensively assessing the individual client. It begins by determining the primary problem for which the client seeks services and proceeds through a systematic appraisal of the five dimensions of the person. (For further explanation of these dimensions, see Chapter 2.) Each dimension may be weighed differently in terms of relative importance with each individual client. The nurse must be sensitive to the client's uniqueness and able to adjust the interview focus according to the client's individual needs, strengths, and problems.

Making a holistic assessment involves all the communication, facilitation, and collaboration skills of the nurse to encourage the client to openly share personal information. Throughout the interview the nurse demonstrates re-

ASSESSMENT

Standard 2 of the ANA Standards of Psychiatric and Mental Health Nursing Practice States:

The nurse continuously collects data that are comprehensive, accurate, and systematic.

Structure Criterion

A means by which data are gathered, recorded, and retrieved is available in the practice setting.

Process Criteria

The nurse:

1. Informs the client of their mutual roles and responsibilities in the data-gathering process
2. Uses clinical judgments to determine what information is needed. Health data undergirding the nursing process for psychiatric and mental health clients are obtained through assessing the following:
   a. Biophysical, developmental, mental, and emotional status
   b. Spiritual or philosophical beliefs
   c. Family, social, cultural, and community systems
   d. Daily activities, interactions, and coping patterns
   e. Economic, environmental, and political factors affecting the client's health
   f. Personally significant support systems, as well as unutilized but available support systems
   g. Knowledge, satisfaction, and change motivation regarding current health status
   h. Strengths that can be used in reaching health goals
   i. Knowledge of pertinent legal rights
   j. Contributory data from the family, significant others, the health care team, and pertinent individuals in the community

From *Standards of psychiatric mental health nursing practice,* Kansas City, Mo, 1982, American Nurses' Association. Reprinted with permission.

HOLISTIC NURSING ASSESSMENT FORMAT

Identifying Information

Name? Age? Gender? Marital status? Occupation? Ethnicity? Living arrangements? Source of referral?

How was the client brought to the treatment agency?

Presenting Problem

What symptoms or problems bring the client to the agency at this time?

What is currently causing the client the most discomfort or concern?

For how long has the client had the problem?

How is the problem affecting work and relationships?

Has the problem ever occurred before? When? What was helpful at that time?

What help is the client hoping to receive from the treatment agency?

Physical Dimension
Family health history

Has any family member had any of the following problems:

Physical illness that seemed to be influenced by the person's emotional states, such as stomach ulcers or asthma

Excessive use of drugs or alcohol

Mental retardation

Mental illness

For each "yes" response, inquire about such details such as the relation of the family member to the client and the onset and progression of the illness. A multigenerational family tree or genogram may be constructed as a tool for detecting patterns of mental illness in a family. (See Chapter 29 for example.)

Individual health history

Describe illnesses, injuries, surgeries, and hospitalizations. Include the dates of onset, duration, treatment, resolution, and any sequelae. Note the following:

Are physical health problems currently being experienced?

Do patterns emerge such as recurrent illnesses or accidents?

Were the illnesses mild or serious? Acute or chronic?

Were there any sequelae?

What is the pattern of the client's use of health care services: routine, episodic, frequent?

Growth and developmental history

Explore chronologically the sequence and content of this history, noting points that clients perceive as significant. One approach is to ask clients to describe themselves at typical developmental stages: What were they like? What was the family like? What was it like at school during kindergarten, elementary, junior high, high school, and college? What were their friends like? Construct an image of this person's life.

Activities of daily living

Construct an image of how the client spends a typical 24-hour period. Elaborate as necessary to refine the image of the client's life-style. Focus on the following areas:

DIET AND ELIMINATION

Describe appetite. Any recent change in either weight or appetite?

Food allergies or dietary restrictions?

Describe any use of over-the-counter drugs to affect diet or elimination. How much fluid does the client drink each day? What kind of fluids?

Describe the pattern of diet and elimination for a 24-hour period.

EXERCISE AND ACTIVITY

How often does the client exercise?

What kind of exercise?

How long are the exercise periods?

What effect does it have?

SLEEP AND REST

Describe typical sleep pattern, including hours of sleep, time of resting, time of awaking, quality of sleep, any difficulties falling asleep, staying asleep, or daytime napping.

CAFFEINE, TOBACCO, DRUGS, AND ALCOHOL

Describe use, including kind, amount each day or week, time of day, length, effect, last use, any efforts to stop, and problems associated with use.

LEISURE ACTIVITIES

Describe what the client does for relaxation, pleasure, or peace of mind; include how often, how long, and what effect it has.

Review of body systems

Head, eyes, ears, nose, throat (HEENT); integument; breasts; cardiovascular; respiratory; gastrointestinal; renogenitourinary; reproductive; nervous; musculoskeletal; hematopoietic; and endocrine systems.

Conduct the usual analysis of a symptom for positive responses. It may be helpful to inquire about how the client perceives the symptom and its possible relationship to other factors.

Physical examination findings

Report significant findings from the physical exam including those that are within normal limits and specifically describing those that are outside the normal limits.

Diagnostic test results

Laboratory, x-rays, psychological.

General appearance

What are the client's general physical characteristics, especially unique or unusual features?

Is the client's style of dress neat, untidy, gaudy, or eccentric?

Is the client's posture relaxed, rigid, anxious, or worried?

Does the client engage in appropriate eye contact?

Does the client's motor activity seem to involve excessive or very few body movements?

Does the client have any mannerisms such as a gesture, grimace, or other nonverbal forms of expression?

Does the client have any unusual motor behaviors that suggest a neurological disorder such as static or intention tremors, athetosis, chorea, or dystonia?

Does client have any noticeable deformities?

Does the client appear to be the stated age?

Are there any detectable odors?

Body image

Ask the client:

"What recent changes have you experienced in the appearance of your body?"

"Describe your appearance to me."

"What are your feelings about your body?"

What do you like and dislike about your body?

If you could change your body in any way, what, if anything, would you change?

SEXUALITY

"Are you sexually active?"

"What are some of your sexual complaints?"

If further information is needed the following questions may be considered:

"In what way has the problem that brought you here interfered with the sexual aspect of your life?"

"How satisfied are you with your sex life?"

"How compatible are your needs and those of your partner?"

If not, how do you deal with the problem?

▼

Emotional Dimension

Affect

Observe the following:

Facial expression: Smiling? Frowning? Scowling? Masklike? Fearsome? Anxious?

Motor behavior: Restless? Lethargic? Bizarre posturing? Mannerisms? Gait?

Physical signs: Tears? Flushing? Sweating? Tremors? Respiratory irregularities? Tics?

APPROPRIATENESS OF AFFECT TO THE SITUATION

What is the relationship between the client's affect and thought content?

Does the client convey *ambivalence* expressed in simultaneous, contradictory feelings directed toward the same object?

Is the client's affective response consistent with cultural norms?

Mood

QUALITY OF MOOD

Is the client apprehensive? Anxious? Fearful?

Is there a blunted, apathetic quality to the client's affect—an impoverished, constricted, or flat feeling?

Does the client describe an elevated or depressed mood?

STABILITY OF MOOD

Is the client's affect labile during the interview? That is, do his emotions shift from moment to moment?

How easily do the client's emotional changes occur in response to pleasant or unpleasant stimuli?

Does the client have periodic mood swings from elation to depression or vice versa?

Is the client aware of variations in mood based on time of day?

Emotional patterns

Which emotions predominate in the client's life? How does the client express these emotions? Ask for examples that show how the client deals with anxiety, anger, guilt, or despair. Note the client's level of emotional awareness. Specific areas for assessment are discussed in the related chapters.

Intellectual Dimension

Sensation and perception

Do you ever see or hear things that other people say are not really there?

Do you ever smell or taste things that other people say are not real?

Do you ever have thoughts about something that you believe but that no one else does?

Do you ever believe that your thoughts or actions are under outside control or influence?

Memory

IMMEDIATE MEMORY

Give clients three items of information such as a name, an object, and a color. Instruct them to remember these things since you will be asking them to recall the information later in the interview. Continue the interview for 3 to 5 minutes before asking for recall.

RECENT MEMORY

Ask for the sequence of events leading up to the client's seeking services. If this information was supplied by the client in relating the history of present illness then it can be used for this assessment and not repeated.

REMOTE MEMORY

Note the client's ability to accurately relate past events in sequence with appropriate descriptive detail. As with recent memory, check with other sources of information to validate the accuracy.

Cognition

ORIENTATION

Can the client correctly identify the following: Current time? Place? Other persons? Self?

FUND OF INFORMATION

Ask client to name the five largest cities in the United States or the names of the last three presidents.

JUDGMENT

Social judgment: To what extent is the client aware of social norms and the need for compliance with them or the law?

Family judgment: To what extent does the client appreciate how his behavior affects his family or vice versa?

Financial judgment: Does the client manage money effectively?

Employment judgment: Does the client have unrealistic job expectations or aspirations or fail to recognize his responsibilities to his employer? To what extent does the client plan for the future? Are the plans inappropriate or realistic?

INSIGHT

Does the client recognize that he is ill or that he has emotional problems or symptoms?

To what extent does the client recognize his own contribution to the problem?

Does the client blame other people or circumstances for his difficulties?

Does the client recognize his need for help?

Has the client any desire for help or treatment?

Is the client willing to assume responsibility for changing his behavior?

ABSTRACT THINKING

Ask for interpretation of proverbs, such as "Rome wasn't built in a day," or for identification of similarities between items such as oranges and apples.

ATTENTION

Observe for degree of distractibility and ability to concentrate and cooperate with instructions during the interview. Testing for digit span recall can also be used. Ask the client to repeat some series of digits after you say them. Begin with a series of 3 numbers such as 8, 4, 1, reading them at the rate of about 1 per second, then allowing the client to repeat them. If the client succeeds, increase the number in the series by 1 until the client fails. When this occurs give the client another series of the same length to try again. Stop when the client is unable to succeed in two tries. Do not choose consecutive numbers or numbers that form easily recognized dates such as 1, 9, 8, 8.

Communication

Does the client talk? At what rate? At what volume? With what degree of clarity? In what general tone?

Do ideas flow logically?

Does the client have noticeable speech impediments?

Are there any peculiarities in thought content?

How well are the client's thoughts organized and structured?

Is the client coherent?

Are their particular repetitive words, ideas, or themes?

Flexibility-rigidity

Does the client seem open to ideas different from his own?

Does the client become overly upset when his normal routine is disrupted, or does he adjust with relative ease to change?

Is the client able to make decisions based on logical reasoning, or is he unable to make up his mind on any issue?

Does the client seem too easily influenced by the ideas of others?

Continued.

HOLISTIC NURSING ASSESSMENT FORMAT—cont'd

Social Dimension
Self-concept

Describe yourself as a person, including your strengths and limitations.
Describe the kind of person you would like to be.
How do you compare in relation to other people?
If you could change something about yourself, what would it be?

Interpersonal relations
(family, work, school, community)

How and where does the client fit into these groups?
What roles does the client assume within these groups?
What are the role expectations placed on the client by the others in the groups?
How does the client feel about the expectations?
What are the client's expectations of himself in the various roles?
Is the client overextended or underachieving in these roles?
Who makes up the basic family unit?
Does the family contain the client's "significant other" relationships, or does the client consider people outside the family to be more important.
Within the family, who is supportive of the client? Competitive? Demeaning?
Who interacts with whom in the family? What is the nature of these interactions?
What is the pattern of communication within the family?
What role does the client play within the family?
What roles do the other family members play?
How is conflict handled within the family?
What is the level of trust between family members?
How is the balance of dependence-independence distributed within the family?

Cultural factors

Is the client a member of an identifiable ethnic group?
Is the client from an urban or rural background?
Does the client observe traditions or customs?
Does the client maintain a life-style congruent with the dominant societal culture? With the culture in which the client grew up?
What impact do ethnic and cultural norms have on current illness?

Productivity/Occupation
(employee, student, homemaker)

What is the client's primary work? Is there a secondary job as well?
Does the current health problem affect work status?
To what extent does current work meet financial needs?
Is current work satisfying to the client?
If unemployed does the client possess the education/skills necessary for employment?
Is the client overconforming to the point of sacrificing individuality?
Is the client nonconforming to the point of provoking society's intolerance?
Is the client experiencing difficulties such as legal problems or domestic violence?

Trust-mistrust

Does the client appear to be generally or unusually naive about life, considering his age and developmental level?
Does the client seem to be vulnerable or easily taken advantage of?
Does the client describe a need for self-protection that seems out of proportion to the degree of threat that exists in the client's environment?
Does the client make statements about not trusting anyone? Does the client seem to be suspicious of the interview?

Dependence-independence

Does the client make statements like "I don't need anyone but myself"?
Does the client behave as though he has everything under control?
Does the client profess to be unable to make it through even minor stresses without the presence of certain people or things?
Does the client behave in a clinging manner toward other people?
Does the client frequently resort to whining?
Does the client give the impression of being either more or less dependent than would be expected for his age or developmental level?

Spiritual Domain
Meaningful philosophy of life

Do you spend much time thinking about what's important in your life? Do you worry about the meaning of your distress?
If so
What gives meaning to your life, or makes you want to live?
What are the most important goals in your life?
Who are the most important people in your life?
Do you find yourself preoccupied with past situations you cannot change?
How do you explain (account for) your current problems? What do you think needs to happen so that your situation can improve? What role will you or others play in your recovery?
Do you have any beliefs of a religious or spiritual nature about the cause or treatment of your problems?
Have you ever felt like giving up on life?

Need for transcendence

Where or to whom do you turn in times of need? Has help been available?
Would you consider yourself an optimist or a pessimist?
Is life getting better or worse for you?
Where do you see yourself a month from now? In a year?
What activities (or life experiences) help you to be less self-concerned? Are these activities or experiences currently part of your life?

Need for relatedness with God or higher being

Does belief in God or a Supreme Being play an important role in your life?
If so, in what way(s) has your belief influenced your current situation?
Are you a member of an institutionalized religion (denomination)?
Are any particular religious practices of significance to you? Are there any particular religious practices that provide comfort for you?
Are there conflicts in your family related to differences in religious beliefs or practices that cause you problems now?
Have any "folk remedies" or "alternative healing" methods been of help to you? If so, what are they?
How would you describe your current level of satisfaction with your religious practices and spiritual beliefs?
Have you suffered the loss, through death, of significant relationships? If so, have your spiritual beliefs been of help to you or not?

Need for creativity, inward freedom

Do you tend to welcome new experiences, or prefer your life style to be generally predictable?
Do you believe you make your own choices, or do you sense your choices are strongly influenced by approval or disapproval of others?
What types of activities and relationships help you to feel creative or give you a sense of satisfaction?

spect and concern by teaming with the client to develop a full and accurate picture of his life. To do this requires objectivity and freedom from bias and prejudice. Although guided by a conceptual model, the nurse recognizes and validates the client's uniqueness throughout the collection of data, knowing that in this way the assessment process is in itself therapeutic.

A typical mental health–psychiatric nursing assessment begins by gathering identifying information. This includes name, age, marital status, gender, occupation, ethnicity, living arrangements, and other pertinent data, such as source of referral and how the client was brought to a psychiatric treatment facility. The nurse then begins a thorough exploration with the client into the presenting problem and related physical, emotional, intellectual, social, and spiritual aspects of the client's experiences.

Presenting problem

The client is asked to describe why help is being sought at the present time. The response is recorded in the client's own words. Nonpsychotic clients will usually describe a painful state of mind or circumstances that have lead to emotional suffering. The *chief complaint* is the symptom the client mentions first. A complaint may be embedded in a story the client tells about a troublesome relationship or stressful life experience. Psychotic clients may describe fears of being influenced by bizarre phenomena or of being told by voices to act in inappropriate ways. In an acute psychotic state the client has little insight regarding need for treatment. Although some clients state their complaints specifically, others may report complaints in vague or ambiguous terms such as feeling a little anxious, needing a rest, coming for help because someone else suggested it, or feeling stressed. Symptoms are often reflective of problems in living that are difficult for the client to talk about directly.

It is important to find out when the client first began to experience the presenting problems, their severity, and how long symptoms or problems have persisted. *Dates of onset* give clues to what was going on in the client's life as they began to experience a particular symptom or problem in living. Have the symptoms caused or resulted from disruptions in work, social, or family life? The most recent onset is of particular interest since recall of details and persons involved are likely to be fresher in mind than more remote events. It is also important, however, to assess for previous experiences with the same or similar problems and to determine how the client managed past episodes. The circumstances and events that contributed to the development of symptoms are termed *precipitating events*. The reason precipitating events are significant aspects of assessment is that they relate to the client's underlying problem or difficulties in living and what the client hopes to gain from treatment. In many instances something has occurred in the client's recent past, days or weeks, that can be considered the "straw that broke the camel's back" and motivated the client to seek treatment. Events that are likely to precipitate emotional problems include deaths, separations, serious illnesses, changes in economic status, relationship conflicts, anticipated events, and real or imagined failures. Many times clients do not readily see the connection between an event and onset of symptoms. The nature of the event precipitates psychological pain for the client, and symptoms may develop as a form of protection against that pain.

It is important to determine the *client's perception of the problem*. By asking questions, such as, "What do you think is the cause of your problem?" or "How have you explained the fact that you have these problems to yourself?" the nurse sees how the client interprets his difficulties. Clients may blame others, talk about stressful past events, or deny having a casual opinion. It is important to notice how client's describe relationships with others, as a clue to their attitudes toward and expectations from significant others. Understanding these role expectations about how others should treat them (for example, that others should never criticize them, that they deserve to be hurt or punished, or that they need others to see them as always competent and in control) helps to clarify the client's perception of his problem. This information is useful in determining motivation for change, expectations for improvement, and factors that interfere with self-awareness. Depressed and anxious clients frequently focus on their symptoms and have difficulty explaining the source of their problems. Secondary gains from symptoms, such as freedom from responsibility, seeking unmet needs for attention, or punishing others for perceived injustices, interfere with development of insight and change.

Finally, in assessing the client's presenting problem, the nurse determines what the client hopes to gain from treatment providers at the present time. Why has the client arrived for treatment at this time and in what way is he hoping that the staff will be helpful? Responses to these questions will help the staff determine if the client's needs and desires match the available resources.

Physical dimension Clients who have been diagnosed as mentally ill need to have thorough physical assessments, since they may have both related and unrelated medical problems that need care. Often changes in behavior are the first signs that something is physically wrong. These changes may be associated with physical conditions, such as brain tumors, or metabolic disturbances, such as hyperthyroidism and hypothyroidism. Such conditions are often overlooked when the predominant symptoms are related to a mental illness. Nurses on inpatient units have the opportunity to observe symptoms and subtle changes in behavior that can contribute to the diagnosis, which could have tremendous consequences for the client. Assessment of the physical dimension focuses on family health history, the client's current and past history of physical problems and the client's body image.

A family history is the first method of assessment and reveals a profile of the familial strengths and risk factors for the client. The client is questioned about illness in family members, both living and deceased. Information is elicited to determine the presence of stress disorders, substance abuse, mental retardation, and mental illness.

Assessing for physical problems is the second major concern in the physical dimension. At the time of data collection, the determination of whether a physcial examination is done and who does it depends on the clinical setting and the role of the nurse. In some instances, the physical examination data are gathered from written records or through consultation with a physician or other health care professional. This does not prohibit the nurse from ongoing assessment of physical health processes.

The objective findings of a physical assessment need to be compared with the client's perception of the problem. Discrepancies between findings and the client's reported symptoms may indicate a need for further evaluation and validation either with other health professionals or through more comprehensive medical testing. Inconclusive findings also require further evaluation and monitoring. The client's health and medical histories are explored to include an overview of the client's growth and developmental history and a chronological record of illnesses, injuries, and medical care received.

The client's normal daily routines and health practices are assessed. These practices include nutrition and elimination patterns, exercise routines, leisure activities, sleep patterns, and use of tobacco, caffeine, alcohol, and drugs. When all systems function smoothly, the client may take them for granted. However, one may abuse body systems for some time without developing apparent symptoms. Thus in reviewing daily health practices the nurse notes potential for future difficulties as well as presenting problems. This aspect of the assessment also affords the nurse an opportunity to identify and reinforce positive health promotion practices.

Many clients who are anxious or depressed search for the source of their discomfort in somatic problems. Clients needing psychiatric treatment may be first seen by their family physician or in a medical clinic. Specific physical complaints that are often associated with emotional distress include chronic fatigue, diarrhea, allergic symptoms, constipation, emesis, enuresis, loss of appetite, weight loss or gain, impotence, frigidity, decreased amount of sleep, early morning awakening, restless sleep, and repetitive or disturbing dreams. If the client's current problem focuses on somatic symptoms, questions are asked to determine whether the client perceives the somatic difficulties as the primary source of the problem or as an associated factor of the problem.

Observation skills are essential in assessment. A general survey of the client's overall appearance provides information regarding grooming, self-care, general demeanor, and the presence of unique or unusual features. These initial impressions provide a baseline for comparison in future observations of the client.

The final component of the physical dimension to be assessed is body image. *Body image* is the composite of conscious and unconscious attitudes one has toward one's physical body. It includes present and past perceptions as well as feelings about appearance, size, function, and potential. It forms part of the larger self-concept and is closely related to self-esteem. Although body image is largely formed by the end of adolescence, it remains to some degree dynamic throughout life and, therefore, subject to modification by new experiences. The occurrence of physical or mental illness can impact body image.

Feelings and perceptions about one's body are also related to sociocultural influences from which one derives standards of perfection, referred to as one's *body ideal.* In determining the healthiness of a client's body image the nurse is alert not only to the client's perceptions, but also to their congruence with reality and discrepancies between body image (how I look) and body ideal (how I want to look or think I should look).

Sexuality is encompassed in multiple dimensions of the person, thus requiring a comprehensive assessment of related physical, psychosocial, and cultural factors. The World Health Organization (WHO) has defined sexual health as the "integration of the somatic, emotional, intellectual, and social aspects of sexual being in ways that are positively enriching and that enhance personality, communication and love."[80] There is no universally "normal" sexual behavior. It is an individually expressed and highly personal phenomenon. Sexual normalcy may be best described as whatever behaviors give sexual pleasure and satisfaction to those involved without threat of coercion or infringement upon the rights of others.

Because of the entwinement of body image and sexual identity, sexuality is assessed in this section. In conducting this aspect of the assessment the nurse is sensitive to discomfort the client may experience when asked questions of a highly personal nature. She moves from general to specific questions as the client develops trust and rapport. Beginning the interview with a brief, clear explanation of the nurse's purpose in asking about sexuality may facilitate open responses (for example, "People often have difficulties with sexual activities related to problems with their health. Therefore I would like to ask you a few questions about your sexuality"). Self-awareness and respect for individual differences are essential for the nurse to be able to objectively assess a client's sexual health. Specific questions regarding medication use are warranted if the client reports problems with sexual desire or functioning.

Emotional dimension The emotional status of the client is assessed in terms of affect, appropriateness of affect to the situation, quality and stability of mood, physical signs of emotion, and emotional response patterns. *Affect* is the feeling tone or emotion accompanying a thought. It is determined by those observable characteristics of a client that usually indicate an emotional state. It includes facial expression, posture, body movements, and physical signs of emotion such as crying. It is the emotional picture that a client presents to observers. The appropriateness of affect to the situation is based on the congruency between the affect the client is displaying and the client's culturally expected affective response in a particular situation. Both affect and appropriateness of affect are culturally determined in part, and this is considered in any interpretation by the nurse.

Mood is a prolonged emotional state that colors one's whole psychic life. Mood includes both the particular emotional state being experienced, such as anxiety, anger, or euphoria, as well as the range and intensity of the emotional experience. Stability of mood simply refers to the degree of constancy or fluctuation in mood. When the mood changes very abruptly and suddenly it is considered labile. When the mood continues with little change over time it is considered stable.

Physical signs of emotion include expressive signs, such as tears, and observable signs indicative of autonomic nervous system (ANS) activity, such as flushing, sweating, and tachycardia. Observation of these signs by the nurse should not be misinterpreted as conclusive of a particular emo-

▼ **TABLE 8-1** Disorders of Perception

Disorder	Definition	Example
Illusions	Common experiences everyone has at one time or another when they misinterpret a sensory experience. A stimulus in the environment sparks the experience, but the person does not interpret it correctly.	An elderly client mistakes a chair for a person. An inebriated client mistakes cracks in the floor for snakes.
Hallucinations	False sensory perceptions that have no identifiable source outside the individual.	A client sees doors, hears voices, feels bugs crawling on him, or sees snakes where none exists.
Delusions	Fixed false beliefs out of keeping with reality or the client's level of knowledge, and not shared by their subculture. The beliefs are "fixed" in that they are not amenable to reason and do not change.	A client insists that a general in the Pentagon has been telephoning him and accuses the nurse of not calling him to the phone when in fact, the client has received no telephone calls.
Deja vu	The sensation that what one is experiencing has been experienced before. The experience is paradoxical, since the client cannot recall any previous experience that corroborates the feeling of recognition.	A client enters a room for the first time and remarks that it seems as though an identical experience has happened before.

tional state, but should instead be viewed as clues which need to be explored further and consensually validated with the client.

Patterns of emotional response include the client's most common or prominent emotional experiences and how the client deals with and expresses emotions. If a particular emotional response pattern such as anxiety, anger, guilt, or dispair is established, further exploration of the depth, intensity, and persistence of this emotional reaction is pursued. Clients may also be asked to describe their feeling tone as it exists for that moment and to compare it with how they have felt in the past. In this way the nurse gets a glimpse of the client's baseline before seeking services.

Emotional status is commonly altered in acute and chronic illness. The entire range of affect may be encountered, both qualitatively and quantitatively. Exhilaration, giddiness, and an exaggerated sense of well-being are displayed in mania; melancholy and despondency are seen in depressive states; the organic brain syndromes are generally characterized by lability; "flat," "uncanny," and "bizarre" are terms used to describe schizophrenic affect.

The emotional dimension of the person is open to inaccurate interpretations by others. Because of this possibility, it is imperative that the nurse exercise great care to avoid interpretations based on incomplete data and personal biases. Interpretations of data that occur during assessment are considered tentative and reviewed during analysis when a more complete understanding is possible.

◤ **Intellectual dimension** Assessment of the intellectual dimension includes collecting data regarding the client's perceptions, memory, cognitions, communication, and flexibility-rigidity.

Because perception is the process by which the client makes meaningful and adaptive interpretations of sensory, emotional, and intellectual stimuli, perceptual disorders markedly affect the individual's ability to function. Disorders of perception commonly include illusions, hallucinations, delusions, and *deja vu.* Table 8-1 presents the definitions and examples of these disorders.

Memory is divided into three areas: immediate, recent, and remote. Immediate memory affects the client's ability to attend and retain information presented in the current situation, such as the interview. Mental retardation, high levels of anxiety, or organic brain syndromes may contribute to difficulties with immediate memory function.

Recent memory reflects the client's ability to recall events of the past few days, such as those leading up to the need for service. The inability to give a coherent picture of these events suggests a recent memory problem. Remote memory involves the client's ability to recall events of the distant past and can be assessed by asking about life milestones, such as birth date. The inability to give an answer is highly suggestive of memory dysfunction. When it is difficult to determine the actual dates of occurrence, outside information such as a relative or an old medical chart may be consulted for validation. When there are discrepancies between reports by the client and other sources, additional observation and information are needed to determine the status of memory.

Cognition includes the functions of orientation, fund of knowledge, judgment, and insight, abstract or concrete thinking, and attention. Orientation encompasses the clarity of the client's conscious processes and his ability to ascertain the significance of his present situation. Orientation is tested for person, place, and time. Orientation to person is judged on the basis of whether or not the person knows who he is and can accurately identify others. Orientation to place is judged by whether or not the client knows where he is. Orientation to time includes knowing the year, month, season, day, date, and time of day. Does he know how old he is or his birth date?

The client's general fund of information will optimally include commonly known facts. This is somewhat determined by the person's educational experience and interests and may be influenced by gender and culture. Modification of the traditional testing procedure is advisable to ascertain this. For instance, a person with little formal education from a rural subculture may not respond to questions of a political or geographical nature by may have a considerable knowledge of herbs and gardening.

Judgment is the end result of the client's ability to assess a situation, analyze it, come to an appropriate conclusion, and make sound decisions. Judgment can involve decisions in the areas of social, familial, financial, and occupational situations. The nurse can assess judgment by listening as the client relates actual life events that required gathering and interpreting data, formulating decisions, and carrying out a plan. Judgment can also be assessed by asking the client to make decisions about hypothetical problems such as, "If you were stopped for speeding, what would you do?"

Insight enables clients to understand and relate the significance of their symptoms and illness. It is common for clients to initially have limited, if any, insight into their problems. For some clients, the development of insight becomes a focus for treatment; for others, it is of secondary importance. However, it is useful for the nurse to establish a baseline from which to measure change in insight.

Abstract reasoning involves the ability to think beyond a concrete level. Communication is severely affected when the client thinks mostly on concrete terms. Questions and comments need to be phrased so that abstraction is not relied upon. Client education is planned, keeping in mind that the client may take what is said literally. For example, a client who was preoccupied with the effect of his medication inquired about the term "half-life" of the drug by asking if it meant that half his life was gone.

Abstract reasoning is tested by the interpretation of proverbs or the identification of similarities between items. The person is asked to restate a common saying in general, nonpersonalized items. Any number of proverbs can be used. The following is an example of a proverb and possible interpretations, both abstract and concrete.

Proverb:
"Don't cry over spilled milk."
Interpretation:
Concrete—Persons shouldn't cry if they spill some milk.
Abstract—Persons should not waste time regretting what has already happened.
Other commonly used proverbs are:
"People who live in glass houses shouldn't throw stones."
"A rolling stone gathers no moss."
"Rome wasn't built in a day."
The nurse may test the client's ability to abstract by asking him to identify similarities between items such as oranges and apples, a coat and a dress, and a table and a chair. If he cannot respond, the client is given the answer as an example and then asked about another set of items. This is a test of the client's ability to consider general relationships as opposed to dealing at a sensory level.

Attention refers to the degree of distractibility that the client shows during the interview. If his attention is drawn easily from the conversation by unimportant or irrelevant stimuli, it may indicate a high level of anxiety, a response to illusion or hallucinations, or an inability to focus or process material because of organic defects.

As the client communicates thoughts the nurse attends to content, thought processes, structure and rate of associations, quantity and flow of ideas, and any peculiarities. People under stress typically are preoccupied by intrusive thoughts. The client is asked to describe any major preoc-

cupations. In listening to the client communicate, the nurse can assess for the following abnormalities in thought content or processes:

Blocking is a sudden cessation of a train of thought that occurs in the middle of a sentence. Blocking happens to everyone occasionally. Its clinical significance, however, is seen when the person repeatedly blocks on the same theme.

Tangentiality is the loss of goal direction in communication; it is a failure to address the original point by digressing to another end point.

Circumstantiality occurs when the person includes nonessential details in a message, eventually coming to the point, but doing so through a long, circuitous route.

Fragmentation is the communication of incomplete ideas. Thinking is disrupted, haphazard, and scattered. Ideas appear to shift from one subject to another in an unrelated manner, lacking logical ordering of content. This is also called *loose association*. For example, the client may say, "I can't go to the store, no money . . . fat, fat is not good on beef . . . but grass needs to be cut in September . . . it's hot today, isn't it?" This is seen most often in schizophrenic psychosis.

Flight of ideas is verbal skipping from one idea to another. The ideas appear to be continuous but are fragmentary and determined by chance association. This disturbance is characteristic of acute manic states.

Word salad is the most extreme form of fragmentation of thought processes, appearing as a totally incoherent mixture of words and neologisms. For example, the client may say, "Store . . . time . . . queen bee . . . codwakalls . . . pancakes . . . football."

Neologisms are new words or condensations of words created by the client. Although the word may have meaning to the client, its meaning is not known to others. In the client statement above "codwakalls" is a neologism. Such coined words are often part of the client's delusional system.

Clang associations are characterized by rhyming of words. For example, the client may say "Goose, loose, moose."

Autistic thinking is highly self-centered; the client attaches personalized meanings to words he uses.

Confabulation involves fabrication of experiences, often recounted in a detailed and plausible way to fill in and cover up gaps in memory. The client realizes to some extent that he cannot remember but tries to cover up memory loss to avoid embarrassment. This is most often seen in organic conditions such as Korsakoff's psychosis.

Perserveration involves involuntary persistent, rigid repetition of a word, phrase, or theme even if the subject is changed by the interviewer. For example, a client may repeatedly say, "Ring a bell, doggie" regardless of what is said to him.

Ideas of reference involve incorrectly interpreting incidents as having direct reference to oneself. The client who watches television and thinks the news announcer is reporting a story about him is demonstrating ideas of reference.

Paranoid ideation involves feelings of suspiciousness stemming from the belief that one has been singled out for unfair treatment. These are also referred to as *ideas of persecution*.

Depersonalization is the loss of one's identity as a person or the feeling that one does not occupy one's body. For example, the client may say, "I look at my body and it is not mine. I don't live in it. I live outside of it."

Grandiosity is an overappraisal of one's worth and ability beyond what is supported by reality. For example, the client may present himself as the president of a very large company, whereas in reality he is junior clerk.

Religiosity refers to excessive concern with spiritual and religious matters. This may reach delusional intensity, as in the client who reports, "I am on a mission from God to see into the brains of all those who are thinking evil thoughts."

Mutism refers to the total absence of verbal response from the client despite indications that the interviewer's questions have been heard.

Echolalia is repeating exactly the words just said by the interviewer, much like an echo.

The client's ability to communicate in writing can be assessed from samples already available, or the client can be asked to write a brief autobiographical sketch, a creative story, or a daily journal. The writing can be examined for flow, order, and thought content.

Finally, the client may be asked to draw himself, his family, his home, or something abstract such as a feeling or his illness. This is a particularly useful communication modality with children. The drawing can be examined for content, form, color, and dimension. Great expressive value also stems from the client's subsequent verbal explanation of the drawing. The nurse can prompt this by asking, "Tell me about your picture."

The final area of assessment in the intellectual dimension is the client's degree of flexibility-rigidity. Here the nurse is exploring the client's openness to new ideas, ability to respond to change, and ability to accommodate behavior as new conditions arise.

Social dimension Assessment of the social dimension involves the client's self-concept, interpersonal relationships, socialization, cultural factors, productivity, and location of the client on the trust-mistrust and dependence-independence continuums. It is helpful to gather information from the client and the significant others and social systems with which the client interacts. These sets of data can be compared to detect areas of conflict or agreement.

Self-concept is the individual's mental composite of all the aspects of self of which one is aware. It includes all of one's self-perceptions, including physical, emotional, intellectual, social, and spiritual dimensions. It is assessed on a continuum from positive to negative. *Self-esteem* is one's judgment of personal worth. It is derived from two primary sources—the self and others. It is assessed on a continuum from high to low. After adolescence, self-concept is less amenable to changes and is more constant than self-esteem. It is more internally regulated. However, in general self-concept and self-esteem are correlated. That is, a person with a positive self-concept usually has a high level of self-esteem, while the person with a negative self-concept has a low self-esteem. Based on the client's description of himself, and the nurse's observations of the client's grooming, body language, and other pertinent data, the nurse formulates an idea of how the client views himself and to what degree he values himself. The extent to which the client's views are realistic and congruent with other's perceptions influences the assessment.

It is important to explore the client's social relatedness in a broad context, developing a picture of the client's interaction patterns in the various environment in which he works, studies, and plays. Sources of stress and support can be identified in these areas. It may also be helpful to know about the social and cultural influences that contributed to the client's early development.

Regarding the client's level of socialization, the nurse notes the degree to which the client conforms to the norms and values of both the family of origin and the larger society. Because of changing sex roles and alterations in norms for social behavior, socialization is a significant area for assessment. The nurse understands that clients may experience conflict in their social environments because of these changes. For example, the woman who is socialized to the traditional female role as homemaker, but who needs to enter the job market, may experience considerable conflict in adjusting to the new role.

The ability to be productive and derive satisfaction from work is often identified as an indicator of mental health. Individuals may be productive within or outside the home by engaging in traditional and nontraditional work, attending school, homemaking, and/or childrearing. The nature of the activity, the skills involved, the degree of personal satisfaction derived from the activity, and the degree of interference imposed by the current illness is assessed. If the client is employed, the nurse explores the extent to which the job meets financial needs and, if unemployed, how are these needs met.

As the nurse listens to the client describe his interpersonal world she also looks for clues about the client's level of trust-mistrust and dependence-independence. The level of trust-mistrust can be assessed by determining whether the client is excessively naive or suspicious. The level of dependence-independence can be assessed by determining how the client is able to function emotionally and behaviorally with regard to support systems. Does the client have the ability to function autonomously as well as the ability to receive support and assistance from others when needed?

Acutely ill clients may experience severe disturbances in their ability to communicate with and relate to others. The desire to express needs and feelings and to participate in social interactions may remain intact, although ability to do so may be impaired. Some clients may exhibit pervasive mistrust and dependency conflicts that contribute to impaired interpersonal relating.

Throughout the interview, clients display certain attitudes toward the interviewer. The nurse notes these attitudes, since they offer clues as to how the client relates to other people as well. Some individuals appear to be indifferent toward the nurse. They may simply lack any interest in those around them. Some are passive: they take no part in the process, offer no opposition, and act submissive. Other clients may be aggressive, using direct physical assault or verbal aggression. Some clients are hostile, unfriendly, and antagonistic; some are suspicious and will not trust the interviewer. They check around the room and challenge the motives of the interviewer or give false information. The antiauthoritarian person expresses contempt for parents, legal authorities, or social organizations and is likely to include the interviewer in his devaluing. Other clients are dramatic, telling vivid tales in the history they give and finding satisfaction in the effect they achieve. The nurse needs to note these unique attitudes and any changes that occur related to specific topics or variations in approach by the nurse.

Spiritual dimension Assessment of an individual's spiritual life is often overlooked or neglected entirely in psychiatric nursing.[31,38] Psychotherapists tend to give limited attention to the client's perception of his spiritual world.[60]

Our neglect of spiritual processes relates in part to three factors.[62] First, nursing shares a common theoretical heritage with psychiatry wherein religious beliefs are often seen as causing or contributing to symptomatic behavior such as excessive guilt, religious delusions, or the performance of bizarre acts directed by God. Second, in much of the psychiatric literature, particularly psychoanalytically oriented literature, religion is perceived as serving a defensive function by maintaining repression of unconscious conflicts that inhibit rather than foster self-understanding. Third, there is strong educational emphasis in nursing to be nonjudgmental, not to impose personal beliefs on clients. Hence nurses may have tendencies toward avoiding discussions of religion and spiritual values altogether or to experience conflicts between their personal beliefs and psychiatric practices.[43] Clarifying ones own spiritual beliefs is a step toward helping clients who may express confusion and religious symptomatology.

More recent trends incorporating the healing dimensions of spirituality, are creating openness among nurses to not only respect differences in belief systems but also to develop appropriate interventions. Therefore, it is important to differentiate between spiritual needs and symptoms of psychopathology.

Spirituality refers to the search for meaning in life and one's values and belief system, which may include a belief in a power or powers greater than oneself. Part of the nature of being human is to experience longing for relationships or a need to feel connected with others. Many are convinced that humans also experience an innate *spiritual* need to search for and find meaning in life through developing ethical and moral values or maintaining a belief in a higher being greater than the self.

In assessing the spiritual dimension, the nurse uses all of her interpersonal skills—listening, attending, clarifying, and empathizing. Spiritual needs and beliefs are often expressed indirectly and in the context of explaining life experiences or problems; hence careful observation and sensitivity to underlying beliefs is important. Cues that indicate a readiness to talk about spiritual issues may include (1) direct references to religion; (2) inquiries about the nurse's own practices and beliefs; (3) quotations from religious works; (4) expressions of guilt or fears of punishment or retribution; (5) ambivalent attitudes toward religious practices; and (6) despair, frustration, or anxiety regarding life's meaning or obsessive preoccupation with failures and lack of accomplishments. The spiritual assessment may thus be partly extrapolated from other assessment dimensions through understanding and observing phenomena such as, thought and speech patterns, cultural background and social relationships, and patterns of relating that only become apparent as a nurse-client relationship develops. Assessment of the spiritual dimension is guided by an understanding that many clients will deny religious or spiritual needs. It is, therefore, important to differentiate whether or not the client ever perceived himself to have had strong spiritual commitments or has experienced a change or disillusionment in spiritual beliefs or religious practices. In addition, espousal of a religious affiliation does not necessarily mean the individual entirely agrees with the practices of that particular church or denomination.

Assessment of the spiritual dimension can be approached in a variety of ways. Subheadings under spiritual assessment that are recommended[62,74] include a (1) meaningful philosophy of life, (2) need for transcendence, (3) need for relatedness with God or higher being, and (4) need for creativity and inward freedom.

Meaningful Philosophy of Life One of the greatest needs we have is to make sense of our lives. Failure to see purpose in life or to finding meaning in our experiences contributes to psychological and physical distress.

Many individuals are not able to directly articulate a philosophy of life. Assessment is therefore dependent on inferential data, often in the form of negative statements and behaviors. For example, lack of goal-oriented behaviors, feelings of purposelessness, rage over injustices in life, failure to mourn past losses, engaging in addictive behaviors, failure to develop commitment in relationships or career goals, and blaming others can all be manifestations of failure to develop a coherent sense of self-direction and meaning in life. Individuals who accept their own vulnerabilities, painful experiences that cannot be changed, and responsibility for change and who experience a sense of relatedness with others are less likely to express concerns about life's meaning and purpose.

Assessment of beliefs about faith, health and healing, and the causality of emotional problems may reveal distortions in belief systems that have spiritual implications (for example, sins of omission or commission, violence, hatred, sexual or physical abuse, primitive beliefs about supernatural forces, miracles, and faith healing). Attributions regarding illness causality that involve guilt and diminish self-esteem are likely to result in feelings of helplessness and depression.

Assumptions regarding illness causality have been categorized under five different belief systems[72] or models (Table 8-2). The importance of identifying a belief system is that it implies the method by which an individual anticipates being helped or healed. Respecting the healing powers of an individual's belief systems should not be overlooked as a potential source of support.[18]

Need for Transcendence By and large, psychology has focused on theories that explain the development of a sense of identity, self, or individual ego. Assisting individuals in obtaining a coherent sense of self, a sense of self in space and time, and a sense of self-harmony or congruence are fundamental goals of traditional psychotherapy approaches. Moving from self-absorption to concerns for the welfare of others, relinquishing unhealthy self-attachments, and experiencing the self as only a small part of the connectedness of all matter involves a shift from the exclusive focus on the self to goals that transcend concerns about the self.

▼ **TABLE 8-2** Belief Systems Regarding Illness Causality

Model	Cause	Recovery
PERSONAL/HISTORICAL		
Judeo-Christian	Sin, suffering, impulses, faults,	Salvation, analysis, insight
Psychoanalysis	limitations	
Buddhist		
SELF-REGULATION		
Chinese medicine	Imbalance in bodily processes	Medical treatment acupuncture
Western medicine		
EXISTENTIAL		
Eastern religions	Anxiety, failure to make choices	Enlightenment, insight, transcendence
ECO-SPIRITUAL		
Native American	Upset in ecological balance	Healer, appease spirit world
Shamanic healers		
REVITALIZATION		
Native American	Social order out of balance	Social connectedness, spiritual renewal
Subcultures		
Cults		

Modified from Simpkinson CH: Healing in altered states, *Common Boundary* 9(2):47, 1991.

Many individuals who are emotionally disabled feel alone and isolated. Concern for the natural world and building human connections cannot occur when individuals experience themselves as fragmented, disconnected, chaotic, or alienated from self and others. The need for self-transcendence is masked by emotional pain and interpersonal conflict. Assessment of feelings of estrangement, fears that no one one can truly understand their inner experience, rejection of caring and help, and holding negative expectations about the future indicate clients are stuck in seeing others as responsible for their unhappiness, failures, or problems.

Need for Relatedness With God or Higher Being In assessing the need for a trusting relationship with a deity or external power, the nurse determines in whom or what a client believes and the nature of his experience with a divine being. Belief in a loving and forgiving God, or higher being, sets expectations of strength and support that are quite different from expectations of punishment stemming from belief in a harsh and vengeful deity. Many clients with emotional problems perceive themselves to be alienated from others and from God and to be unloveable, defective, or bad. Individuals may experience guilt or anxiety and fear punishment for perceived sins. Seriously mentally ill individuals may have experienced painful rejections that leave them mistrustful of all relationships, even doubting that God, or a supreme being, could care about them.

Spiritual practices such as prayer, reading the Bible, meditation, confession, and attending church services are known to be stabilizing forces for many individuals.[74] For some nurses, understanding spiritual practices may help them assess the nature of their own relationship with God or a higher being.

Many family rituals develop around religious holidays and rites of passage. Disruption in these practices often occurs as a result of stress, conflict, and family dysfunction. It is important to determine what practices, if any, were ever helpful to the individual and what meaning they have in the light of present circumstances. Stress and crises may generate renewed interest in spiritual practices or for some bring negative attitudes and feelings of being betrayed or disillusioned by God or religion. Since religious practices vary widely from traditional to nontraditional, it is useful to assess beliefs and practices that may promote or impede spiritual healing and affect the individual's response to emotional problems.

Need for Creativity and Inward Freedom Creativity can be thought of as a spectrum "from mundane acts of habit and memory to miraculous instances of revelation and prophecy."[33] However defined, the capacity for creativity and inspiration can be a meaningul part of everyone's life. Emotional distress may divert energy away from creative pursuits and into maintaining emotional security. Creativity is nurtured in an environment in which the person feels accepted and valued and is permitted freedom to experiment with ideas and symbolic forms of self-expression.

Assessment of creative needs is achieved by both observation and history. According to Harman and Rheingold,[33] in addition to psychological security and freedom, three additional inner conditions contribute to constructive creativity. First, is the individual *open to new experiences,* ideas, and concepts, or is he rigid and defensive, believing that there is a right and wrong way to do everything? Second, does the individual have an *internal locus of evaluation,* or do the praises or criticisms of others strongly restrict freedom of choice? Third, does the individual have the ability to *play with ideas, colors, shapes, and relationships?* Being able to tolerate uncertainty, trying out alternative solutions to problems, and learning from what does not work can promote creativity and a sense of inner freedom.

Helpful Versus Unhelpful Belief Systems Spiritual beliefs may be sorted into three categories of influence,[13] inspiring, ineffectual, and deleterious. Inspiring beliefs lead to growth, peace of mind, and strong inner directedness. Ineffectual beliefs are colorless. They do not harm, but neither are they of much use as a source of support. Deleterious beliefs cause distress because they are associated with emotions such as fear, anger, guilt, and anxiety or physical and interpersonal disturbances. Habitual styles of responding such as judging, fearing, doubting, controlling, worrying, or detachment are likely to be based on unhelpful or deleterious belief systems.

Through the spiritual assessment, the nurse differentiates beliefs that sustain the client from those that are a source of conflict. Problems with spirituality many be a sign of other problems with authority figures. People may form an alliance with religious beliefs that is used defensively to set themselves above other mortals and to distance themselves from people whom they fear. At the same time the alliance with a particular religion or Godlike figure gives the individual an illusion of great power and control that masks feelings of weakness and powerlessness. Psychotic delusions of being the Messiah, or Jesus Christ, are believed to be based on the need to compensate for feelings of inferiority and powerlessness.

Similarly, psychiatric clients may also attempt to resolve interpersonal conflicts through excessive preoccupation with religiosity and reliance on religious practices. Close inspection reveals that such individuals use religion to buffer themselves from dealing with painful family and life conflicts.

Responses to some general questions help to differentiate ineffectual from effectual spiritual coping.[62] For example, (1) Do spiritual beliefs facilitate or inhibit relationships? (2) How do spiritual beliefs foster autonomy versus dependency and conflicts with authority? (3) What is the relationship between spiritual beliefs and a mature or immature sense of moral values? (4) Do the individual's spiritual beliefs strengthen or weaken self-esteem? (5) Do spiritual practices encourage self-centeredness? (6) Studying why some spiritual or cult groups end up hurting rather than helping individuals is useful in making a spiritual assessment.[67]

The box on pp. 138-140 gives ideas for completing a comprehensive holistic assessment. Not all areas of assessment may be included in an initial assessment. The assessment is guided by client needs, presenting symptoms, and condition.

Analysis

Analysis is the step of the nursing process in which the nurse uses diagnostic reasoning, theoretical knowledge, and clinical judgment to examine, organize, and synthesize the data collected during assessment (see the accompanying box for Standard 3). Information derived from the client and collateral sources is compared to documented norms of health and wellness, social and cultural standards, and theories of adaptation and dysfunction. As the data are

---

▼ **ANALYSIS**

Standard 3 of the ANA Standards of Psychiatric and Mental Health Nursing Practice States:

The nurse utilizes nursing diagnoses and/or standard classification of mental disorders to express conclusions supported by recorded assessment data and current scientific premises.

Structure Criterion

In the practice setting, opportunities are provided for validation of diagnosis by peers and for exchange of information and research findings regarding the scientific premises underlying nursing diagnosis among peers.

Process Criteria

The nurse:
1. Identifies actual or potential health problems in regard to—
   a. Self-care limitations or impaired functioning whose general etiology is mental and emotional distress, deficits in the ways significant systems are functioning, and internal psychic and/or developmental issues
   b. Emotional stress or crisis components of illness, pain, self-concept changes, and life process changes
   c. Emotional problems related to daily experiences, such as anxiety, aggression, loss, loneliness, and grief
   d. Physical symptoms that occur simultaneously with altered psychic functioning, such as altered intestinal functioning and anorexia
   e. Alterations in thinking, perceiving, symbolizing, communicating, and decision-making abilities
   f. Impaired abilities to relate to others
   g. Behaviors and mental states that indicate the client is a danger to self or others or is gravely disabled
2. Analyzes available information according to accepted theoretical frameworks
3. Collects sufficient data to verify a diagnosis
4. Makes inferences regarding data from phenomena
5. Formulates a nursing diagnosis subject to revision with subsequent data

From *Standards of psychiatric mental health nursing practice*, Kansas City, Mo, 1982, American Nurses' Association. Reprinted with permission.

---

viewed collectively, significant patterns are identified. The end result of nursing analysis is the nurse's statement of the client's health status. Any given client may require numerous problem statements to fully describe his condition. These statements are known as the nursing diagnoses.

Utilizing nursing diagnoses

A nursing diagnosis is a statement of a client's actual or potential health problems that nurses by virtue of their education and experience are capable and licensed to treat.[38] It is a clinical judgment derived through the application of a systematic process of assessment and analysis. It is through the formulation of nursing diagnoses that nurses can develop goals and interventions specific to the nursing discipline and can thus identify the specific contributions of nurses to the treatment team. In developing nursing diagnoses, the nurse validates clinical impressions with the client or the client's significant others whenever possible. Consideration is given to the client's wishes, values, and culture as well as to standards established by society and theoretical models.

▼ **NANDA DIAGNOSTIC LABELS COMMONLY USED IN PSYCHIATRIC–MENTAL HEALTH NURSING**

Adjustment, impaired	Noncompliance (specify)
Anxiety	Nutrition, altered (less than or more than body requirements)
Bowel elimination, altered (constipation or diarrhea)	Parenting, altered: actual/potential
Caregiver role strain	Post-trauma response
Communication, impaired verbal	Powerlessness
Coping, family: potential for growth	Rape-trauma syndrome
Coping, ineffective family: compromised	Relocation stress syndrome
Coping, ineffective family: disabling	Role performance, altered
Coping, ineffective individual	Self-care deficit (bathing/hygiene, dressing/grooming, feeding, toileting)
Diversional activity, deficit	Self-concept, disturbance in body image
Family processes, altered	Self-concept, disturbance in personal identity
Fear	Self-concept, disturbance in self-esteem
Grieving, anticipatory	Sensory/perceptual alterations (visual, auditory, kinesthetic, gustatory, tactile, olfactory)
Grieving, dysfunctional	
Growth and development, altered	Sexual dysfunction
Health maintenance, altered	Sexuality patterns, altered
High risk for caregiver role strain	Sleep pattern disturbance
High risk for self-mutilation	Social interaction, impaired
Home maintenance management, impaired	Social isolation
Hopelessness	Spiritual distress
Injury, high risk for	Thought processes, altered
Knowledge deficit (specify)	Violence, high risk: self-directed or directed at others

Modified from McFarland GK, Wasli EL, Gerety EK: *Nursing diagnoses and process in psychiatric mental health nursing*, ed 2, New York, 1992, JB Lippincott.

Two groups have provided leadership at the national level for the development of classification systems for nursing diagnoses. The first is the North American Nursing Diagnosis Association (NANDA), originally called the National Group for the Classification of Nursing Diagnosis. The group has held a series of national conferences on nursing diagnoses since its inception in 1973. The work of this group has focused on the development of a basic taxonomy of nursing diagnoses without regard to specialty areas. The accompanying box lists NANDA diagnostic labels commonly used in mental health nursing to identify problems. Other nursing diagnoses more commonly associated with physical health conditions may also be applicable to the psychiatric client and would be included in diagnosing and planning care.

The second major group working to develop a nursing diagnosis system is a task force of the Council of Specialists in Psychiatric/Mental Health Nursing of the American Nurses' Association. The task force first convened in 1984 to study and make recommendations on the phenomena of concern for psychiatric–mental health (PMH) nurses. The outcome of the work of this task force is the development of a Classification System for the Human Responses of Concern for PMH Nursing Practice (PND-I). The classification system is organized according to three generic response classes: individual, interpersonal/family, and community/environment. Each response class has human response patterns. (See the box on the next page for classifications.)[46]

Comprehensive information gathering is a prerequisite of the development of accurate diagnoses. Once the necessary data are gathered and organized, the nurse identifies specific problems and patterns and establishes a causal, or etiological, relationship by exploring the factors that are influencing or contributing to the client's health problems.

Gordon has suggested three necessary components of an actual nursing diagnosis.[29] These components include the following:

- Problem or health state
- Etiology or related risk and contributing factors
- Signs and symptoms or defining characteristics that show evidence of the problem

The second part of the diagnosis suggests etiology or factors contributing to the actual or potential problem. This causative factor is often the focus of nursing care. Successful treatment of the cause often results in elimination of the problem and associated signs and symptoms. Early in the nurse-client relationship it may be difficult to determine etiological factors, in which case "unknown etiology" may be used until this aspect can be further explored. As the therapeutic alliance develops and more data are available, an etiological statement is added to the diagnosis. For example:

- Altered thought processes
- Related to discontinuation of phenothiazines
- As evidenced by hallucinations

In addition to developing actual nursing diagnoses in which the problem, etiology, and symptoms can be identified, nurses also develop diagnoses to describe potential health problems when known risk factors are present. Since the problem is only potential and has not actually occurred, only the first two steps of this diagnostic system are used (problem and etiology); there are no identifiable symptoms. For example:

- At risk for self-directed violence
- Related to feelings of hopelessness

Carpenito suggests that the qualifier "possible" preceeding the nursing diagnosis "describes problems (and areas of growth) that may be present but require additional data to be confirmed or ruled out."[17] When this qualifier is used,

▼

CLASSIFICATION SYSTEM FOR THE HUMAN RESPONSES OF CONCERN FOR PMH NURSING PRACTICE (PND-I)

01. Human Response Patterns in Activity Processes

*01.01 Altered motor behavior
*01.02 Altered recreation pattern
*01.03 Altered self-care
*01.04 Altered sleep/arousal patterns
01.97 Undeveloped activity processes
01.98 Altered activity processes not otherwise specified (NOS)
01.99 Potential for altered activity processes

02. Human Response Patterns in Cognition Processes

02.01 Altered decision making
02.02 Altered judgement
*02.03 Altered knowledge processes
02.04 Altered learning processes
*02.05 Altered memory
*02.06 Altered orientation
*02.07 Altered thought content
*02.08 Altered thought processes
02.97 Undeveloped cognition processes
02.98 Altered cognition processes NOS
02.99 Potential for altered cognition processes

03. Human Response Patterns in Ecological Processes

*03.01 Altered community maintenance
03.02 Altered environmental integrity
*03.03 Altered home maintenance

04. Human Response Patterns in Emotional Processes

*04.01 Abuse response patterns
*04.02 Altered feeling patterns
04.03 Undifferentiated feeling pattern
04.97 Undeveloped emotional responses
04.98 Altered emotional processes NOS
04.99 Potential for altered emotional processes

05. Human Response Patterns in Interpersonal Processes

*05.01 Altered communication processes
*05.02 Altered conduct/impulse processes
*05.03 Altered role performance
05.04 Altered sexuality processes
*05.05 Altered social interaction
05.97 Undeveloped interpersonal processes
05.98 Altered interpersonal processes NOS
05.99 Potential for altered interpersonal processes

06. Human Response Patterns in Perception Processes

*06.01 Altered attention
*06.02 Altered comfort patterns
*06.03 Altered self-concept
*06.04 Altered sensory perception
06.97 Undeveloped perception processes
06.98 Altered perception processes NOS
06.99 Potential for altered perception processes

07. Human Response Patterns in Physiological Processes

*07.01 Altered circulation processes
*07.02 Altered elimination processes
*07.03 Altered endocrine/metabolic processes
*07.04 Altered gastrointestinal processes
*07.05 Altered neurosensory processes
*07.06 Altered nutriton processes
*07.07 Altered oxygenation processes
*07.08 Altered physical integrity processes
*07.09 Altered physical regulation processes
*07.10 Altered body temperature
07.97 Undeveloped physiological processes
07.98 Altered physiological processes NOS
07.99 Potential for altered physiological processes

08. Human Response Patterns in Valuation Processes

*08.01 Altered meaningful
*08.02 Altered spirituality
*08.03 Altered values
08.97 Undeveloped valuation processes
08.98 Altered valuation processes NOS
08.99 Potential for altered valuation processes

*For additional subheadings see ANA Classification of Individual Human Responses by M Loomis and others, 1986, published by the American Nurses' Association.

one or more etiological factors or symptoms may be vaguely present, but sufficient information is not available to warrant a conclusion. In these instances the nurse's actions are focused on further evaluation.

Proper utilization of the nursing diagnostic system enables nurses to make clear, concise statements regarding client conditions that nurses can identify and treat. It provides the basis for planning nursing care.

Utilizing psychiatric diagnosis

The Standards of Psychiatric and Mental Health Nursing Practice recognizes the usefulness of both the nursing diagnostic system and the current psychiatric diagnostic system, DSM-III-R in expressing conclusions drawn from assessment.

The *Diagnostic and Statistical Manual of Mental Disorders* (DSM-I) was originally introduced by the American Psychiatric Association in 1952 to organize symptoms of mental disorder into recognizable syndromes and to label the syndromes in a way that facilitated communication among professionals. In the years since its inception, the system has undergone numerous revisions. The most recent revision, in 1987, resulted in the DSM-III-R, which remains the most commonly used interdisciplinary classification system for mental disorders in clinical use. Nurses encounter the use of the DSM-III-R system in clinical practice and thus need to understand how it is used.

DSM-III-R lists 313 mental disorders in the following 17 major categories:

1. Disorders usually first evidenced in infancy, childhood, or adolescence
2. Organic mental syndromes and disorders
3. Psychoactive substance use disorders
4. Schizophrenia
5. Delusional disorders
6. Psychotic disorders not elsewhere classified

7. Mood disorders
8. Anxiety disorders
9. Somatoform disorders
10. Dissociative disorders
11. Sexual disorders
12. Sleep disorders
13. Factitious disorders
14. Impulse control disorders not elsewhere classified
15. Adjustment disorder
16. Psychological factors affecting physical condition
17. Personality disorders

Each category is further subdivided into more specific disorders with associated behavioral indicators (see Appendix A).

As the current form of this psychiatric diagnostic system has been developed, perhaps the most outstanding new feature is the multiaxial approach in which each client is assessed on each of five different axes. This approach encourages the clinician to keep related factors in mind when making a psychiatric diagnosis. In this way it has become more compatible with the holistic nursing perspective. Briefly described the five axes are:

Axis I: Clinical syndromes
    Conditions not attributable to mental illness (for example, interpersonal problems) that will be the focus of treatment
Axis II: Personality disorders
    Developmental disorders
Axis III: Physical disorders and conditions
Axis IV: Psychosocial stressors (type and severity) experienced within the past year or that pertain to the disorder
Axis V: Global assessment of functioning in psychological, social, and occupational aspects of life during the past year

Advantages of having a system such as the DSM-III-R include the utility of organizing symptoms into identifiable patterns and labeling those patterns as disorders with specific defining features. With standardization of nomenclature, communication between clinicians is facilitated. The DSM-III-R is strictly a phenomenological approach to mental illness; it does not attempt to propose etiology or suggest treatment. It is an atheoretical system of classification. As a member of the treatment team, the nurse can contribute observations and relevant information provided by the client and significant others. In developing a plan for care, the nurse can benefit from knowing the client's psychiatric diagnosis. The diagnostic label guides the nurse's review of pertinent literature regarding the identified disorder and thus contributes to the theoretical base essential to effective nursing practice. However, this information, though essential, is not sufficient for carrying out the nursing process. It is an incomplete data base because it does not address the unique responses of the individual client to the medically diagnosed disorder.

The practices of psychiatry and psychiatric nursing are different but complimentary. While the psychiatric diagnosis labels the identified disorder, the nursing diagnosis acknowledges that clients differ in their response to and manifestations of the disorder. Based on diagnosis of these individualized response patterns, nurses plan their interventions.

Planning
Purposes of the therapeutic plan

The plan of care guides nursing actions. It consists of two aspects. First, it sets forth the client outcomes to be achieved and defines the outcomes in terms of the behaviors that will help achieve them. Second, the outcome statements are recorded into a total plan, called the *nursing care plan* (see the accompanying box for Standard 4).

Formats for developing a plan of care vary, but generally consist of a brief summary of pertinent assessment data, and the following: (1) nursing diagnoses, including problem statements, etiology, and signs and symptoms from assessment domains; (2) DSM-III-R diagnosis; (3) long-term criteria reflecting desired outcomes based on needs that are expected to persist beyond the immediate period of treatment; (4) short-term outcome criteria are statements that are measurable or observable and often include expected dates of accomplishment; (5) nursing interventions selected to meet short- and long-term outcome criteria with the rationale for the interventions; and (6) documentation of evaluation according to outcome criteria. Some client care plans are developed by a treatment team; therefore the plan reflects interventions that are primarily the responsibility of nursing and those that are shared with or referred to others (see the box on p. 152).

Just as the assessment experience can be therapeutic for some clients, the process of planning, clarifying, and working through the decision-making process can also be helpful. Planning offers an opportunity for clients to learn about

PLANNING

Standard 4 of the ANA Standards of Psychiatric and Mental Health Nursing Practice States:
The nurse develops a nursing care plan with specific goals and interventions delineating nursing actions unique to each client's needs.

Structure Criteria
1. The practice setting is one in which the nurse has opportunities to collaborate with others in the development of nursing care plans compatible with overall treatment plans.
2. Within the practice setting, mechanisms exist for nursing care plans to be recorded, communicated to others, and revised as necessary.

Process Criteria
1. The nurse collaborates with clients, their significant others, and team members in establishing nursing care plans.
2. In the care plan, the nurse:
  a. Identifies priorities of care.
  b. States realistic goals in measurable terms with an expected date of accomplishment.
  c. Uses identifiable psychotherapeutic principles.
  d. Indicates which client needs will be a primary responsibility of the psychiatric and mental health nurse and which will be referred to others with the appropriate expertise.
  e. Stresses mutual goal setting and shared responsibility for goal attainment at the level of the client's abilities.
  f. Provides guidance for the client care activities performed by others under the nurse's supervision.
3. The nurse revises the care plan as goals are achieved, changed, or updated.

▼ **COMPONENTS OF A NURSING CARE PLAN**

Pertinent Data from Assessment Domains
1. Nursing diagnoses:
   1.1. Problem statements with identification of high-risk problems (for example, violence, suicide, wandering)
   1.2. Etiology (related to)
   1.3. Signs and symptoms from assessment data that support defining characteristics
2. DSM-III-R diagnoses
3. Long-term client outcome criteria
4. Short-term client outcome criteria
5. Nursing interventions with rationale
6. Evaluation of expected outcomes; dated review
7. Delegation of responsibility when appropriate

their personal health, emotions, thoughts, and behaviors. The nurse discusses the purpose of identifying and clarifying goals with the client by exploring the meaning of change. Most clients can identify and share perceptions regarding their current level of functioning and expectations about how they wish they were functioning. Clients may wish to change the way they think, feel, or behave, or the way others react to them.

The extent to which the nurse can expect the client to participate in planning and goal setting is contingent on the client's coping resources, maturational level, intellectual ability, and degree of insight. Psychotic clients are often perceived as being out of touch with reality and therefore not capable of participating actively in setting goals and planning treatment. However, even acutely psychotic clients may express desires for life changes that can be translated, with some help, into goal statements. Some clients may remain uninvolved because they lack insight, blame others for their problems, or have been ordered into treatment by some aspect of the legal system. Whenever possible, planning should also involve significant others in the client's network, such as family members, social workers, vocational counselors, and other mental health professionals currently involved in the client's care.

The ultimate goal of the plan is to guide the proposed interventions. In situations involving a number of staff members, the plan coordinates efforts and protects the client from random or conflicting interventions. The plan also provides the baseline for evaluation. The long-term and short-term outcome criteria may be built around general psychiatric nursing care plans, but each plan is individualized based on assessment data, acuity of problems, and intervention resources.

Outcome statements

To be realistic, outcome statements: (1) are formulated from well-grounded nursing assessments and diagnoses, (2) are stated clearly in terms of client behaviors, (3) arise from an awareness of current client coping deficients, and (4) arise from an awareness of the client's potential for growth, capacity for insight, and need for behavioral changes. An example of a general nursing care plan is given in Table 8-3.

Completeness of outcome statements

An outcome is a statement of a desired, achievable behavior or expression of feeling, to be attained within a predicted period of time, that is based on the client's current status and available resources.[29] Nursing interventions are designed to impact client outcomes. Unless outcomes are realistic and obtainable, direction is lost, the purpose for intervening is obscured, and evaluation of effectiveness is meaningless.

Initially, a client may state that he has a goal of thinking more positively about himself or of being less dependent or passive. These goals need to be translated into actual behaviors that can be observed, counted, or monitored by both the client and the nursing staff.

For ensuring completeness in composition of outcome statements, reliance on the investigative process is useful. This process involves stipulating the "who, what, when, where, and how" of the outcome statement.

Who is *always* the client. Outcome statements refer to the client; nursing interventions are the measures undertaken by the nursing staff to facilitate client outcome attainment. Stating outcomes using the client's name reminds the nurse to ask:
1. Is it in fact an outcome for the client?
2. Is it in fact individualized for this specific client?
Asking these questions safeguards the client-centered integrity of the outcome statement. Other persons may be involved in an outcome statement, depending on the circumstances and setting for treatment.

What is the behavior to be undertaken by the client. Terms for the behavior need to be chosen carefully to minimize subjectivity and increase the chances for consensual validation of what is to happen; for example, *understand*, *appreciate*, *feel*, or *realize*, are easily misinterpreted. Whereas *identify*, *state*, *describe*, or *demonstrate* are less likely to be misunderstood, are observable, and therefore permit evaluation.

How and *how much* reflect the manner in which the client will carry out the behavior and allow for greater accuracy and precision by identifying, if necessary, any conditional requirement or restriction of the behavioral outcome. Defining the level of change means setting criteria for determining progress in therapy and specifying the amount and direction of desired or expected change. Type, degree, or amount are the usual considerations to further describe the action to be taken.

It is important to remember to include *how* or *how much* only if it adds clarity and enhances the meaning and focus of the action. It is confusing to say, "Client will eat heartily," since the nurse may wonder if interventions should be directed at the amount of food eaten or the client's mood when eating. To clarify this outcome, the statement might read, "Client will eat three fourths of food served at mealtimes."

Where also serves the purpose of clarifying specific restrictions or requirements of the desired outcome behaviors. Again, specifying where may not be relevant to all outcomes. For example, a client may be working on assertive verbalizations, which are expected to be initiated in a particular group setting before the behavior is expected to generalize to relationships outside the group.

When represents specification of the time interval or

▼ TABLE 8-3   NURSING CARE PLAN Example of a Nursing Care Plan

OUTCOME CRITERIA

NURSING DIAGNOSIS: Severe anxiety with panic attacks

Related to: Fear of separation
DSM-III-R Diagnosis: Axis I: Panic disorder, with agoraphobia, 300.21

LONG TERM:

Verbalizes significant decrease in physiological, cognitive, behavioral, and emotional symptoms of anxiety (for example, decrease in palpitations, shortness of breath, diarrhea, fear of loss of control or dying, inability to problem solve, and avoidant behaviors)

Discusses relationship between anxiety symptoms and fears of abandonment

Utilizes anxiety reducing strategies (for example, meditation, relaxation, Yoga, exercise, support network)

SHORT TERM:

Identifies early warning signs of increasing anxiety levels and reports to appropriate nursing staff

Practices relaxation and visual imagery strategies for 20 minutes twice a day

Verbalizes irrational fears in group therapy

Decreases intake of caffeine to no more than equivalent of 2 cups of coffee per day

Attends mildly threatening outing with support by _____ (date) _____

Attends mildly threatening outing without support by _____ (date) _____

NURSING INTERVENTIONS WITH RATIONALES

LISTEN ACTIVELY TO CLIENT'S FEARS AND CONCERNS

Listening conveys respect and validates the need to be accepted and understood; helps client clarify nature and development of panic attacks

ASSIST THE CLIENT IN IDENTIFYING AND DESCRIBING SYMPTOMS OF ANXIETY

Helps identify anticipatory anxiety in early stages when client can learn to implement alternative anxiety reduction strategies rather than use denial and avoidance

TEACH THE CLIENT EFFECTS OF STIMULANTS SUCH AS CAFFEINE AND EFFECT ON INCREASING SYMPTOMS OF ANXIETY

CNS stimulants increase heart rate and interfere with sleep and relaxation responses

HELP THE CLIENT ASSOCIATE ANXIETY ATTACKS WITH UNMET EXPECTATIONS, FEARS OF LOSING CONTROL, OR PAST UNMASTERED SEPARATIONS

Developing insight regarding source of anxiety, may lead eventually to more realistic expectations, and identifying alternative sources of support and satisfaction

---

target date for completion of the outcome behavior. When may refer to a particular date, a time of day, or to the occurrence of particular circumstances, such as "when the client experiences symptoms of anxiety (anger, sadness, boredom), he will initiate relaxation techniques."

Not all outcome criteria, however, are easily translated into specific amounts, times, and exact conditions for measurement. Whenever possible it is useful to plan in terms of gradually increasing desirable behaviors or decreasing undesirable ones. For example, an outcome statement for a client with dependency problems may be that the client will initiate contact with nursing staff only for appropriate reasons such as for medications or to engage in planning care and activities. Or the client will decrease the number of inappropriate contacts (where a baseline average is known), for example, from six times a shift to three times per shift.

Outcome statements in relation to verbalizations, such

as expressing self-confidence, can be made specific to the individual client by modifiers such as, the client will verbalize self-confidence in relation to self-care activities, being a student, completing a project, applying for a job, going shopping alone, or handling a conflictual relationship. Having the client participate in setting realistic outcome expectations helps ensure that the outcomes are meaningful to the client and that ultimate responsibility for their success also rests with the client.

Short-term and long-term outcome criteria

Outcome statements are generally divided into two categories—short-term and long-term. Short-term outcomes are typically considered to be more immediate, of smaller proportion, and involve the sequential steps necessary for achievement of the broader long-term outcomes. Long-term outcomes are achieved by intermediate, short-term outcomes that can be equated to a learning sequence, such as making progressive changes in life-style habits, activities of daily living, compliance behaviors, changes in thought and feeling patterns, or behavioral modification programs.

Months and years are usual measurement intervals for long-term goals, the directional indicators for the more tangible short-term goal statements. Outcomes to be achieved during a shift, day, or week are thought of as being short-term.

Reliance on sound problem-solving approaches adds credence to outcome formulation. However, one of the most frequently committed errors of omission is setting outcome criteria. For example, if the nurse assesses the client to be disoriented regarding time and place, the outcome statement may read:

Outcome A: The client will respond correctly when questioned regarding time and place by 3/19.

or

Outcome B: The client will locate the orientation board when questioned regarding time and place by 3/19.

The difference between these outcome statements is contingent on the accuracy of the nursing diagnosis. If the client's disorientation is a transient, acute condition, then outcome A is appropriate. However, if the client's disorientation is the result of organic mental disorder of a chronic nature, then outcome B is more applicable.

Outcome statements that are not realistic or that are not based on current assessment data will inhibit client progress. The following example illustrates the relevance of discerning the client's level of functioning before designating outcome criteria.

NURSING DIAGNOSIS	SHORT-TERM OUTCOME
Alteration in thought processes related to depressive ideation	A. *Unrealistic:* Client will verbalize enjoyment in completing a project within 3 days. B. *More realistic:* Client will work on a project for at least 10 minutes a day for 3 days.

Outcome A is unrealistic primarily because it calls on the client to be able to verbalize a feeling state incompatible with a chronic state of depression. It is also unrealistic to assume the client with a thought disorder would be capable of finishing a project within such a short period during an acute stage of illness. Unrealistic expectations of a depressed client result in frustration and heightened feelings of inadequacy.

Outcome criteria are relevant when they are based on the client's ability to achieve the desired behavior. In the following example, the nurse underestimates the client's ability for self-care and minimizes his reliance on routine by setting a 6-day deadline for achievement of outcome. Based on data available from the client's history and an awareness of the client's functional capacity, it is likely the client will achieve the self-care outcome in 2 days.

NURSING DIAGNOSIS	SHORT-TERM OUTCOME
Self-care deficit related to depressed motivational level	A. *Unrealistic:* Within 6 days the client will shave, shower, and brush teeth daily before 9 AM without prompting. B. *Realistic:* Within 48 hours, the client will shave, shower, and brush teeth daily before 9 AM without prompting.

Outcome statements provide target dates for the client and nurse. Timing is indicated by the statement that reflects an individualized, directional course of action. The desired behavior is identified, and all measures are geared toward attainment of the specific outcome. The nurse's ability to conduct a triage of client problems greatly aids in the maintenance of current outcomes and the pace at which the therapeutic efforts proceed, for example:

NURSING DIAGNOSIS	SHORT-TERM OUTCOME
Ineffective individual coping related to knowledge deficit about stress reduction techniques	A. *Unrealistic:* 1. The client will use autogenic relaxation exercises immediately after recognizing anxiety symptoms by 6/20. B. *Realistic:* 1. The client will learn steps in autogenic relaxation training in a workshop (6/20, 6/21, 6/22). 2. The client will identify two prodromal symptoms, experienced repeatedly before onset of severe anxiety states, in discussions on 6/21. 3. The client will use autogenic relaxation exercises immediately after recognizing anxiety, symptoms of restlessness, and tremulousness by 6/22.

The preceding exemplifies the obvious way in which outcomes have an impact on the pace and currency of therapeutic endeavors. Outcome A represents an overwhelming abstract conglomeration of several concrete, sequential goals, whereas outcome B specifically defines a pace and course of action and increases the chance of accomplishment for the client.

The type of clinical setting influences the formulation of goal statements. The acute care facility uses time intervals from a much different perspective than does the extended care facility or the outpatient clinic. The average length of hospitalization on an acute care unit may be 3 to 10 days, whereas the length of stay in an extended care facility may average months to years.

The focus of the setting affects the content and direction of the outcome statement. Stabilization of a client experiencing a psychotic state or crisis is often the primary aim in an acute care unit, whereas the maintenance of optimal functioning, although at a reduced level, may be the focus in the long-term facility.

The cultural and social framework of the client influences the formulation and design of outcomes. Congruence with cultural expectations and norms is essential for effective action. For example, many Native Americans avoid eye contact when conversing. Without knowledge of their traditions and culture, the novice may assess this downward casting of eyes as indicative of low self-esteem. An expected outcome may then be devised related to increased eye contact and social interaction as two behavioral indicators of an improved self-concept. However, in reality this custom conveys respect to the person with whom the conversation is being held. The appropriateness of outcome statements clearly depends on the cultural values of the society in which the client was reared or currently resides.

In addition to determining outcomes that are realistic, individualizing outcomes will also involve assessment of *feasibility*. What will make it difficult for the client to change? What are the risks that may be precipitated by change. For example, overcoming panic attacks or agoraphobia may mean loss of a special relationship with the person(s) who always had to accompany the client on outings. Suicidal impulses or acting out behaviors may be precipitated by abrupt demands for change? Planning includes thinking through how circumstances will be different for the client if the desired change is accomplished? What are the rewards or gains that maintain the change? For a client involved in an abusive relationship to become self-assertive will be self-defeating if she has not developed skills for coping in other areas of managing her life.

Discharge planning

Discharge planning is a special area of planning that begins during the assessment phase of the nursing process with the first nurse-client contact. Discharge planning is generally understood to mean discharge from the hospital. Recent trends toward brief hospitalization stress the importance of discharge planning. Clients discharged too rapidly, without time for appropriate discharge planning, may increase readmission rates and thus overall costs of care.[20]

Along with allowing time for discharge planning is the importance of involving the client's social network in the planning process. Research on relapse prevention among schizophrenic clients demonstrates that family psychoeducational support groups that start during hospitalization and continue after discharge significantly reduce readmission rates.[6,21,35,44] Client's who have a supportive friendship network also tend to be rehospitalized less frequently than those who do not.[36] Other important factors that appear to help clients adapt to community living include developing a positive self-image and healthy life-style and acceptance of their illness.[36] Knowledge of these factors that favor successful adjustment are useful in guiding discharge planning.

It is, for example, important that nurses involve family members, friends, and other team members in the client's treatment in preparing for discharge (see the research highlight below). A few principles are suggested as guidelines for family involvement in care[11]:

1. View relatives who desire to participate as empowered members of the caregiving network.
2. Provide adequate orientation.
3. Provide multiple channels for communication.
4. Aim interventions toward reducing family burden.
5. Include the family in the individualized care plan.
6. Respond to changing needs.
7. Involve staff in training experiences on collaboration, consultation, and support of families.

The overall goal for discharge planning is that the client reach his optimal level of functioning as stipulated by the outcome criteria. Analysis of the following information

---

RESEARCH HIGHLIGHT

Discharge Planning for Psychiatric Clients: The Effects of a Family-Client Teaching Program
• FA Youssef

PURPOSE

The purpose of the study was to determine the effect of a family-client education program on the functional level of psychiatric clients and their readmission rate.

SAMPLE

The sample consisted of 30 clients hospitalized on a psychiatric unit with a diagnosis of schizoaffective disorder and who ranged in age from 28 to 52 years. To be included in the study the clients' families had to agree to participate in the study, join three education sessions, and be available for follow-up interviews after discharge.

METHODOLOGY

The subjects were randomly assigned to two groups, an experimental group and a control group. Fifteen were assigned to each group. Each client was rated on the Global Assessment Scale (GAS) to describe his or her level of functioning. The scale was given to all clients included in the study on the second day of admission and the day of discharge. Clients assigned to the experimental group participated in the teaching program with their families. Clients in the control group did not receive education. The sessions were held twice a week during visiting hours in the psychiatric unit. Participants were required to attend three consecutive sessions, each lasting 1 hour. The sessions were co-led by the investigator and unit nurse. At the time of discharge all clients were given a card indicating the time and place of the follow-up visits. Clients were followed by the investigator for a period of 12 months after discharge. Lectures and question-and-answer format were used for the program sessions. Topics for the sessions were: the meaning of illness, causes, and treatments of the disease, and a variety of treatment modalities, with emphasis on pharmacotherapy and its side effects.

FINDINGS

Results revealed a marked increase on the GAS scores between the time of admission and the time of discharge, with subjects in the experimental group having the greatest increase. The majority of those subjects who kept clinic appointments (subjects in the experimental group) had a lower rate of readmission.

IMPLICATIONS

Client-family education is an effective means of reducing the readmission rate among psychiatric clients. Nurses must continue to develop knowledge and skills needed to conduct family-client education. Nurses also need to plan for client's discharge from the day of admission.

Based on data from *Journal of Advanced Nursing* 12:611, 1987.

▼ **IMPLEMENTATION**

Standard 5 of the ANA Standards of Psychiatric and Mental Health Nursing Practice States:

The nurse intervenes as guided by the nursing care plan to imple- ment nursing actions that promote, maintain, or restore physical and mental health, prevent illness, and effect rehabilitation.

Structure Criteria

1. Independent nursing interventions are promoted within the practice setting.
2. Professional staffing patterns in psychiatric and mental health care settings are determined by the documented health care needs of the population served.
3. A mechanism exists to review and revise nurse-client ratios on at least a biennial basis to ensure implementation of the standards of psychiatric and mental health nursing practice.

Process Criteria

The nurse:
1. Acts to ensure that health care needs are met either by using nursing skills or by obtaining assistance from other health care providers when indicated.
2. Acts as the client's advocate when necessary to facilitate the achieve- ment of health.
3. Reviews and modifies interventions based on client progress.

▼ **TABLE 8-4** Classification of Interventions

Category	Dimensions
1. Nursing diagnoses	Actual, at risk for
2. Functional	Domains of health
3. Theoretical	Psychodynamic, behavioral, cognitive, existential, social, systemic
4. Focus	Individual, family, group, com- munity
5. Setting	In hospital, community, home, jail, homeless shelter
6. Responsibility	Independent, nursing collabo- rative, team referred, other
7. Developmental level	Trust versus mistrust; auton- omy versus shame; initiative versus guilt; identity versus identity diffusion; industry versus inferiority; intimacy versus stagnation; ego integ- rity versus despair
8. Priority	Risk of harm to self or others; Maslow's hierarchy of needs
9. Capacity for insight	Continuum, denial of prob- lems to self-awareness

guides the planning process. Understanding the client's:

1. Ability to function independently before hospitaliza- tion; highest level of functioning during the past year (DSM-III-R, Axis V diagnosis)
2. Home or living environment, including the nature of his relationship with significant others
3. Resources and support system (personal, social, eco- nomic, community)
4. Need for involvement in follow-up care (for example, psychotherapy, psychosocial rehabilitation, day treat- ment, residential living, family support or therapy, vocational rehabilitation, transfer to another institu- tion)
5. Current level of functioning and mental status
6. Expectations for help from others
7. Expectations for the outcome of treatment
8. Motivation to remain hospitalized or to be discharged
9. Expectations of family for involvement in client's care

Using the assessment data outlined above, the nurse col- laborates with the client, family, and other team members to establish realistic discharge goals. Early interventions that increase the client's independent living skills will also increase options for discharge planning. Like all planning, discharge planning is based on ongoing evaluation and changes are needed as the client responds to care.

As part of a multidisciplinary team, the nurse may assume responsibility for coordinating the discharge plan. Team conferences are a means for sharing information, establish- ing goals, involving the client, and assigning responsibilities.

Implementation

Nursing interventions are directives, orders, or prescrip- tions for specific nursing behaviors aimed at influencing

and changing client response patterns. Implementation therefore involves both a nursing action and the client's response to that action. Psychiatric nursing interventions are highly individualized and grounded in biopsychosocial theories. Most nursing interventions address the sequela of primary psychiatric disorders, that is, what happens to an individual's functional capacity as a result of the psychiatric disorder. (See the accompanying box for Standard 5.)

All nursing interventions are tied to objectives and goals. For example, implementation of measures to reduce fear and anxiety among psychiatric clients is expected. Some of these measures are generic, such as orienting clients to the unit and discussing expectations, and some measures are specific to the client's particular situation, such as im- plementing a behavioral desensitization or relaxation pro- gram for a client with anxiety or panic attacks. So, under- standing to what the anxiety is related determines the in- tervention to be implemented.

Skills and strategies for implementing change in func- tional health patterns are derived from nursing as well as other schools of psychological and social therapy. Since intervention begins with initial client contact, implemen- tation may not appear to be a discrete phase. However, implementation is best thought of as planned nursing ac- tivities that serve to mobilize the client's own resources and facilitate adaptive coping.

Some basic considerations for design of nursing actions include restrictions in the setting, supplies, resources, and the qualifications and skills of the nurse. The best laid plans are of little relevance if the equipment or personnel nec- essary are not available or if costs prohibit implementation.

Nursing interventions can be categorized in a variety of ways (Table 8-4). Each category can be considered a variable that influences selection of nursing interventions.

▼
MASLOW'S HIERARCHY OF NEEDS

VII. *Aesthetic Needs*
- Appreciation of beauty and art

VI. *Desire to Know and to Understand*
- Curiosity and search for meaning and order

V. *Self-actualization Needs*
- The need for self-actualization
- The ability to utilize one's potential to accomplish and achieve

IV. *Esteem Needs*
Need for self-respect and self-esteem and respect and esteem from others
- Ability to satisfy wants
- Self-control
- Meaningful communication
- Be productive
- Meet self-expectations
- Gain approval of others

III. *Belongingness and Love Needs*
- Need to give and receive love, warmth, and affection

II. *Safety Needs*
- Safety needs for physical security and avoidance of danger

I. *Physiological Needs*
- Physiological needs to satisfy hunger, thirst, sex, and maintain homeostasis

Psychiatric nursing actions may be selected from various types of intervention modalities. The rationale for selecting a particular nursing action is based on theoretical understanding of the client's psychiatric and nursing diagnoses and on the effectiveness of particular interventions in modifying the problem. In psychiatric nursing, as in all aspects of nursing, general principles are used to guide development of creative solutions to problems. Since most mental health problems are multicausal, there is generally no single nursing action that determines resolution.

Maslow's hierarchy of needs is a helpful framework for determining the focus and priority of interventions. For example, meeting basic physiological and safety needs take priority over esteem needs.[49,50] Although Maslow considered most human needs and drives to be interrelated, in many acute psychiatric conditions priority is given to interventions that are lifesaving, such as suicide precautions, rest, fluids and nutrition, and providing a safe environment. (See the accompanying box for Maslow's Hierarchy of Needs.)

By increasing understanding and knowledge of psychiatric disorders and their treatment, nurses can expand their repertoire of potentially helpful interventions.

Some of these interventions will be discussed in more detail as they pertain to specific nursing and psychiatric diagnoses. For illustrative purposes, these interventions are summarized in the accompanying boxes, Standards 5A through 5F.

Intervention

Most psychotherapeutic intervention strategies are designed to help clients alter dysfunctional relationship patterns and to develop more effective problem-solving skills. Development of insight, or awareness of factors that motivate feelings, thoughts, and behavior, is generally seen as

▼
INTERVENTION: PSYCHOTHERAPEUTIC INTERVENTIONS

Standard 5A of the ANA Standards of Psychiatric and Mental Health Nursing Practice States:

The nurse uses psychotherapeutic interventions to assist clients in regaining or improving their previous coping abilities and to prevent further disability.

Structure Criterion

The nurse who engages in psychotherapeutic interventions is minimally prepared as a generalist in psychiatric and mental health nursing.

Process Criteria

The nurse:
1. Identifies the client's responses to health problems.
2. Reinforces those responses to health problems that are functional and helps the client modify or eliminate those that are dysfunctional.
3. Employs principles of communication, interviewing techniques, problem solving, and crisis intervention when performing psychotherapeutic interventions.
4. Uses knowledge of behavioral concepts such as anxiety, loss, conflict, grief, and anger to assist the client in coping, adapting, and dealing constructively with feelings.
5. Demonstrates knowledge about and skill in the use of psychotherapeutic interventions specifically useful in the modification of thought, perception, affect, behavior, and motivation.
6. Utilizes health team members to help evaluate the outcome of interventions and to formulate modification of psychotherapeutic techniques.
7. Reinforces useful patterns and themes in the client's interactions with others.
8. Uses crisis intervention to promote growth and to aid the personal and social integration of clients in developmental, situational, or suicidal crisis.

From *Standards of psychiatric mental health nursing practice,* Kansas City, Mo, 1982, American Nurses' Association. Reprinted with permission.

a necessary precondition for change. However, clients vary in their capacity for insight, so some interventions serve to stimulate client change even when the need for change is not recognized or resisted. (See the accompanying box for Standard 5A.)

Some of the psychotherapeutic interventions nurses use belong to *cognitive-behavioral* methods such as those used in operant and classical conditioning strategies (for example, systematic desensitization, relaxation training, meditation, and biofeedback) and cognitive therapies (for example, thought stopping, recognition of automatic negative thoughts, Rational Emotive Therapy, positive reframing, problem solving, and assertiveness training). Other intervention strategies are derived from *experiential* techniques used to provoke heightened emotional awareness through guided imagery, art and music therapy, risk-taking experiences (for example, rope and rock climbing exercises and outdoor survival schools), and various forms of role-playing and psychodrama.

Underlying all psychotherapeutic strategies is the therapeutic *nurse-client relationship*.[24] Use of therapeutic communication in the context of developing a relationship with the client is the primary means for influencing client change in most psychiatric nursing settings. *Social networking*, *crisis intervention*, and use of *supportive ther-*

apies all involve therapeutic communication and problem-solving strategies.

There are many opportunities for both formal and informal health education in psychiatric settings. Some of these teaching strategies are termed *psychoeducation* because they involve elements of both education and psychological support and counseling. Psychoeducational models for working with families of seriously mentally ill clients begin with the first hospitalization and continue through discharge and community adjustment, placement, and follow-up care. Psychoeducational strategies are also effective in group work where such factors as drug management, developing support networks, identifying and managing symptoms of mental illness, stress management and coping, learning to communicate effectively, management of anger, aggression, and physical and sexual abuse can be discussed from the perspective of each group member and strategies for coping developed (see the accompanying box for Standard 5B).

Health education strategies that address behavioral risk factors for coronary heart disease, stroke, cancer, chronic lung conditions, and HIV infection are often overlooked in psychiatric clients. Seriously mentally ill clients frequently do not understand the relationship between behavioral risk factors and physical illness. Educational strategies can help clients link the two by providing experiential opportunities, such as grocery shopping, cooking, exercise classes, and stress management techniques.

Helping clients who experience problems with the activities of daily living is a primary nursing responsibility in residential and acute care settings. This role is now being operationalized under the title of psychosocial rehabilitation and extended to community living clients who are seriously mentally ill. Like principles underlying physical rehabilitation, psychosocial rehabilitation focuses on helping clients learn new skills or regaining those that have been lost secondary to a psychiatric disorder. Learning to take care of one's daily living tasks, coping with stress, personal hygiene, nutrition, money management, and acquiring appropriate social and vocational skills are all aspects of the rehabilitation model. The overall goals are to maximize self-care skills, and to improve self-esteem and quality of life. Learning or reinforcing self-care activities may begin when clients are hospitalized and ideally continues after discharge. (See the accompanying box for Standard 5C.)

The most common type of somatic therapy used in psychiatric settings is psychotropic medication treatment. In most settings nurses are responsible for administering medications and/or monitoring clients for medication responses and side effects. Nurses also have considerable responsibility for client and family education concerning the expected effects of medications and management of unpleasant side effects. Maintaining long-term adherence to a prescribed medication regimen is a common problem among seriously mentally ill clients. Education and helping clients identify early warning signs of impending problems are useful nursing interventions.

Other somatic therapies include electroconvulsive treatments (usually for severe depressive disorders), forms of physical therapy, biofeedback techniques, and some forms of mind-body healing, such as acupressure and therapeutic touch (see the box on p. 159 for Standard 5D).

Structuring for a therapeutic environment, or milieu, is an important part of the psychiatric nursing role regardless of whether the treatment setting is residential, community based, or hospitalization. Providing for a safe, clean, and supportive environment is a more obvious aspect of nursing interventions under this standard of care. Less apparent in milieu therapy is the importance of collaboration with the whole treatment team in developing a client-centered philosophy of treatment and establishing policies and practices

---

▼
INTERVENTION: HEALTH TEACHING

Standard 5B of the ANA Standards of Psychiatric and Mental Health Nursing Practice States:

The nurse assists clients, families, and groups to achieve satisfying and productive patterns of living through health teaching.

Structure Criteria

1. Opportunities to use varied and appropriate teaching methodologies are available.
2. Appropriate teaching facilities and resources are provided within the practice setting.
3. Health teaching by nurses is specified in job descriptions.

Process Criteria

The nurse:
1. Identifies health education needs of clients.
2. Employs principles of learning and appropriate teaching methods.
3. Teaches the basic principles of physical and mental health.
4. Teaches communication, interpersonal, and social skills.
5. Provides opportunities for clients to learn experientially.

From *Standards of psychiatric mental health nursing practice,* Kansas City, Mo, 1982, American Nurses' Association. Reprinted with permission.

▼
INTERVENTION: ACTIVITIES OF DAILY LIVING

Standard 5C of the ANA Standards of Psychiatric and Mental Health Nursing Practice States:

The nurse uses the activities of daily living in a goal-directed way to foster adequate self-care and physical and mental well-being of clients.

Structure Criteria

1. A policy specifies a time frame in which an initial appraisal of self-care needs is made.
2. A method of communicating information about the client's self-care needs that ensures consistency in approach is established and utilized within the practice setting.
3. Nurses are authorized to prescribe self-care activities in the practice setting.

Process Criteria

The nurse:
1. Respects and protects the client's rights.
2. Encourages the client to collaborate in the development of a self-care plan.
3. Sets limits in a manner that is humane and the least restrictive necessary for ensuring safety of the client and others.

From *Standards of psychiatric mental health nursing practice,* Kansas City, Mo, 1982, American Nurses' Association. Reprinted with permission.

▼
INTERVENTION: SOMATIC THERAPIES

Standard 5D of the ANA Standards of Psychiatric and Mental Health Nursing Practice States:

The nurse uses knowledge of somatic therapies and applies related clinical skills in working with clients.

Structure Criteria

1. There are policies and guidelines for provision of nursing care in somatic therapies.
2. Organizational policies regarding the client's rights for treatment or refusal of treatment are congruent with applicable laws.

Process Criteria

The nurse:

1. Utilizes knowledge of current psychopharmacology to guide nursing actions.
2. Observes and interprets pertinent responses to somatic therapies in terms of the underlying principles of each therapy.
3. Evaluates effectiveness of somatic therapies and recommends changes in the treatment plan as appropriate.
4. Collaborates with other team members to provide for safe administration of therapies.
5. Supervises the client's chemotherapeutic regimen in collaboration with the physician.
6. Provides opportunities for clients and families to discuss, question, and explore their feelings and concerns about past, current, or projected use of somatic therapies.
7. Reviews expected actions and side effects of somatic therapies with clients and their families.
8. Uses prescribing authority for medications as congruent with the state nursing practice act.

From *Standards of psychiatric mental health nursing practice,* Kansas City, Mo, 1982, American Nurses' Association. Reprinted with permission.

▼
INTERVENTION: THERAPEUTIC ENVIRONMENT

Standard 5E of the ANA Standards of Psychiatric and Mental Health Nursing Practice States:

The nurse provides, structures, and maintains a therapeutic environment in collaboration with the client and other health care providers.

Structure Criteria

1. Within the practice setting are mechanisms that govern the establishment and maintenance of settings that are clean, safe, humane, and attractive.
2. Written policies and procedures that govern the safe use of seclusion, restraint, or aversion measures are utilized when staff institute such activity.
3. The environment is characterized by features that facilitate therapeutic gains on the part of clients.

Process Criteria

The nurse:

1. Makes certain that clients are adequately oriented to the milieu and are familiar with scheduled activities and rules that govern behavior and daily living.
2. Observes, analyzes, interprets, and records the effects of environmental forces on the client.
3. Assesses and develops the therapeutic potential of the practice setting on behalf of clients through consideration of the physical environment, the social structure, and the culture of the setting.
4. Fosters communications in the environment that are congruent with therapeutic goals.
5. Collaborates with others in the development and institution of milieu activities specific to the client's physical and mental health needs.
6. Articulates to the client and staff the justification for use of limit setting, restraint, or seclusion and the conditions necessary for release from restriction.
7. Participates in ongoing evaluation of the effectiveness of the therapeutic milieu.
8. Assists clients living at home to achieve and maintain an environment that supports and maintains health.

From *Standards of psychiatric mental health nursing practice,* Kansas City, Mo, 1982, American Nurses' Association. Reprinted with permission.

that are clear to both clients and staff (see the accompanying box for Standard 5E).

Nurses who engage in the practice of psychotherapy are qualified through graduate education, and advanced ANA certification, or state licensure as a psychiatric–mental health nurse specialist or practitioner. Aspects of the nurse-psychotherapist role are incorporated in other psychotherapeutic interventions, such as using the nursing process for completing a psychiatric nursing assessment, diagnoses, setting goals, and, also, in the use of therapeutic communication (see the box on p. 160 for Standard 5F).

Nurse psychotherapists may specialize in working with particular populations such as adult, children, adolescents, or the elderly; with clients who have particular types of disorders, such as addictions, serious mental illness, or who are victims of sexual or physical abuse; and may use a variety of theoretical treatment modalities in therapy with individuals, groups, or families.

One intervention not included in the general standards of psychiatric–mental health nursing practice is that involving *consultation-liaison*. Psychiatric nurses use their skills in helping individuals and families cope with emotional responses to stressful events and physical illness. Separate standards of practice have been developed for consultation-liaison nursing (see Chapter 45).

Documentation is an important part of implementation, and includes writing nursing interventions in the care plan

to encourage consistency of approach. These intervention statements are in effect, *nursing orders*. Each nursing order is dated and initialed by the nurse when added to the therapeutic plan. The nursing order statements include enough specificity and description so that all involved understand the plan. The following questions are helpful to keep in mind when composing implementation statements:

- Does the intervention address *who, what, how, where,* and *when*?
- Is the intervention written *specifically* so that another team member is able to carry out the action effectively?
- Is a target *date* for completion indicated?
- Does the intervention allow for *outcome evaluation*?
- Is the intervention tied to client *goal attainment*?
- Are interventions periodically *reviewed, revised,* and *updated*?

Consideration of the five dimensions of the person and age-appropriate tasks for each client underlies all nursing actions. To maximize success, interventions are built on the client's strengths and effective coping skills.

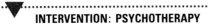

INTERVENTION: PSYCHOTHERAPY

Standard 5F of the ANA Standards of Psychiatric and Mental Health Nursing Practice States:

The nurse utilizes advanced clinical expertise in individual, group, and family psychotherapy, child psychotherapy, and other treatment modalities to function as a psychotherapist, and recognizes professional accountability for nursing practice.

Structure Criteria

1. The nurse who engages in psychotherapy shall be qualified as a psychiatric and mental health nurse specialist.
2. An agency policy specifies the educational and experiential qualifications required of the nurse who functions as a psychotherapist.
3. Job descriptions of nurses expected to function as psychotherapists and to use specific treatment modalities shall include educational and experiential qualifications.
4. Work assignment and staffing patterns provide adequate time for conducting psychotherapy when that responsibility is included in the job description.
5. A mechanism for peer review exists within the agency or is established by the nurse in solo or group practice.
6. The psychiatric and mental health nurse specialist who conducts psychotherapy in private practice maintains an ongoing, regular, formal consultative relationship with a professional colleague.
7. The psychiatric and mental health nurse specialist in private practice utilizes physician services when needed.

Process Criteria

The nurse:

1. Structures the therapeutic contract with the client in the beginning phase of the relationship, including such elements as purpose, time, place, fees, participants, confidentiality, available means of contact, and responsibilities of both client and therapist.

2. Engages in interdisciplinary and intradisciplinary collaboration to achieve treatment goals.
3. Engages the client in the process of determining the appropriate form of psychotherapy.
4. Identifies the goals of psychotherapy.
5. Uses knowledge of growth and development, psychopathology, psychosocial systems, small group and family dynamics, and knowledge of selected treatment modalities as indicated.
6. Articulates a rationale for the goals chosen and interventions utilized.
7. Fosters increasing personal and therapeutic responsibility on the part of the client.
8. Provides for continuity of care for client in the therapist's absence.
9. Determines, with the client when possible, that goals have been achieved and facilitates the termination process.
10. Refers clients to other professionals when indicated.
11. Respects and protects the client's legal rights.
12. Avails self of appropriate opportunities to increase knowledge and skill in the therapies utilized in nursing practice.
13. Obtains recognized educational preparation and ongoing supervision for types of psychotherapy utilized, for example, individual psychotherapy, group and family psychotherapy, child psychotherapy, and psychoanalysis.
14. Uses clinical judgment in determining whether providing physical care (especially procedures prone to misinterpretation, for example, injections, enemas) will enhance or impair the therapist-client relationship and delegates such care as needed.

From *Standards of psychiatric mental health nursing practice,* Kansas City, Mo, 1982, American Nurses' Association. Reprinted with permission.

Evaluation

Evaluation begins in the assessment phase of the nursing process as the nurse compares the client's functional health status and coping patterns with developmental norms and healthy patterns of adjustment. It continues throughout the nursing process as the nurse monitors the client's responses to interventions and determines the impact of any changes on overall functioning. So, although evaluation is considered the final phase in the nursing process, it is more helpful to think of evaluation as providing essential, corrective feedback in all phases of the nursing process. Through interaction with the client, new information is gained. At the same time behavioral changes may be occurring. Both these factors may indicate need for reassessment and review of the original nursing diagnostic statements, client goals, and nursing interventions (see the box on the next page for Standard 6).

The nurse evaluates how the client responds to professional attention, to the opportunity to be heard and to share feelings. The client's perceptions of changes in thoughts, feelings, and behavior serve to corroborate observations the nurse or others make. Symptomatic relief (for example, reduction in anxiety, restoration of balance in sleep-wake patterns, increase in ability to enjoy life, decrease in hallucinations) is measured by the client's reports as well as nursing observations. Thus evaluation includes observing the frequency and severity of symptomatic behaviors.

Behavioral change is a slow process. Although, in a real sense, only clients can change their behavior, the process of change is dynamic and reciprocal, since the nurse alters her interventions to reflect new aspects of the client's response to treatment. In situations that provoke emotional crises, opportunity for change, for learning new ways of viewing past and present events, and for trying alternative coping strategies are created. Nurses depend on client feedback to evaluate the effectiveness of the nursing care plan.

Other sources of evaluative data include other professionals, family members, teachers, and friends. The family has the advantage of knowing the client over time. They frequently can detect small changes that reflect progress or regression. For some psychiatric populations (children, the seriously mentally ill, and elderly), family members are part of the focus of intervention and are included in treatment planning and goal setting.

Rapid assessment and evaluation are familiar aspects of all nursing roles regardless of setting. However, in this time of high client acuity and emphasis on cost containment, issues of efficiency and efficacy in all phases of the nursing process are becoming enormously important in managing nursing care.

Two types of evaluation are particularly pertinent in determining the efficacy of clinical practice: formative evaluation and summative evaluation. *Formative evaluation* describes judgments made about the effectiveness of nurs-

▼ EVALUATION

> **Standard 6 of the ANA Standards of Psychiatric and Mental Health Nursing Practice States:**
>
> *The nurse evaluates client responses to nursing actions in order to revise the data base, nursing diagnoses, and nursing care plan.*
>
> **Structure Criteria**
>
> 1. Supervision and/or consultation with psychiatric and mental health nurse specialists is available within the practice setting to enable the nurse to analyze the effectiveness of nursing actions.
> 2. The client or those of necessity acting in behalf of the client are asked to participate in evaluating the nursing process.
>
> **Process Criteria**
>
> The nurse:
> 1. Pursues validation, suggestions, and new information.
> 2. Evaluates observations, insights, and data with colleagues.
> 3. Documents the results of evaluation of nursing care.

From *Standards of psychiatric mental health nursing practice*, Kansas City, Mo, 1982, American Nurses' Association. Reprinted with permission.

ing interventions as they are implemented. These judgments are used to make immediate modifications in nursing care of the client, when necessary. *Summative evaluation* involves judgments about the effectiveness of nursing care when it is terminated. This evaluation involves a retrospective review of the entire course of care and measures the extent to which the goals for the client's care are or are not achieved. Summative evaluation is based on the outcome criteria established in the planning phases of the nursing process. Outcome criteria statements describe aspects of client or family behaviors that can be observed, and that reflect movement toward goal achievement. Outcome criteria become the standard against which effectiveness of nursing interventions are measured. If favorable changes do not occur, then a reevaluation of the nursing care plan is indicated.

During the past several decades the role of evaluation in nursing has expanded as higher treatment costs are pressuring providers to be accountable for both effective and efficient quality care. *Quality assurance* indicators reflect efficacy of care. The focus of quality assurance is on the *structure of care*, the *process of care*, and the *outcome of care*. These three factors comprise the published nursing standards of care as outlined in this chapter. Quality assurance involves a process of systematically evaluating the extent to which client care meets the designated standards of care. See Chapter 44 for a discussion of quality assurance.

Utilization management is another type of evaluation that involves assessing efficiency of care. Efficacy and efficiency are interrelated; for example, underutilization of discharge planning will result in quality of care problems.[28] Nursing care costs in psychiatric settings are often less visible than in other forms of nursing. It is crucial that psychiatric nurses expand their evaluation skills to include documentation of both the effectiveness and efficiency of nursing interventions. New indicators of quality psychiatric nursing care need to be developed and studied for cost-effectiveness if psychiatric nursing is to demonstrate accountability for practice to the public and other mental health professionals.

Evaluation of effectiveness and efficiency are based on process and outcome criteria embedded in answers to the following questions:

1. Is the assessment data base comprehensive?
   a. Are there unanswered questions?
   b. What does the client want or wish, and is there a fit between wishes and capacity to achieve them?
   c. What hinders goal achievement?
   d. What emotional purposes are served by behavior that hinders goal achievement?
   e. What factors make it difficult for the client to work positively in a nurse-client relationship?
   f. What facilitates the development of a relationship with the client?
   g. If the client cannot participate in data gathering, are other sources of information included?
   h. Is the assessment data available in a standardized format?
2. Are there problems with analysis and decision making?
   a. Is there a need to alter diagnostic statements based on additional contributing factors?
   b. Are nursing diagnoses recorded so that planning and research are facilitated?
3. Is the nursing care plan functional in guiding nursing actions?
   a. Are the client's responses reflected in short- and long-term goal setting?
   b. Are outcome criteria clear and realistic?
   c. Is the nursing care plan recorded and available for review?
   d. Is there evidence that the plan has been revised as goals are achieved?
4. Are modifications in nursing actions and interventions indicated?
   The following four criteria are used for evaluating nursing interventions:
   a. *Adequacy.* Are the interventions sufficient to meet the specific needs for which the plans were developed?
   b. *Appropriateness.* Are the interventions relevant for the problems arising in the five dimensions? Were the interventions started in a timely manner? Does the client agree on the goals? Are the goals related to the problem?
   c. *Effectiveness.* Do the interventions allow the goals to be achieved? To what extent have the goals been achieved?
   d. *Efficiency.* Are evaluative data obtained from relevant souces, such as clients, health team members, or family members? Are interventions evaluated in a timely manner?
5. Additional questions:
   a. Is there a theoretical connection between interventions and outcome criteria?
   b. Are interventions being implemented consistently?
   c. Is there opportunity to validate interventions and client responses with others?
   d. Is there a record of interventions derived from the nursing care plan?
   e. Are health teaching activities documented?

f. Do the clients and family members demonstrate acquisition of knowledge?

g. Is the client's level of self-care ability recorded?

h. Are specific self-care skills and abilities delineated?

i. Are the client's responses to drugs and other therapies recorded?

j. Is there evidence that the client understands the rationale for compliance with taking drugs and reporting side-effects?

k. Is there documentation of client orientation to new settings or treatment modalities?

l. If restraint and seclusion are used, does the client understand the rationale and the conditions for release, unless unusual circumstances exist?

RECORDING

Documentation is a written record of the nursing process and an important tool for the nurse. The recording provides a visible baseline and feedback mechanism for the nurse engaged in using the nursing process. It also offers a means of communicating about nursing practice with other professionals involved in the client's care.

Many methods and formulas have been designed for recording, including the nursing care plan, the narrative record, and the problem-oriented record (POR). Factors such as setting, role function, and client population determine which method the nurse uses. Whichever one is used, each component of the process—assessment, analysis, planning, implementation, and evaluation—is addressed.

Narrative Record

The narrative record is constructed according to chronological order beginning with an admission entry and continuing with entries that are written at least once each shift or after any significant occurrence. The notes include observations or other important client data collected, nursing interventions that are implemented, and client responses to the interventions. The narrative record is contained within the client's larger chart in a section commonly entitled "nurse's notes." A major disadvantage of this approach is the lack of structure and organization of information to facilitate the recording of the nursing process. In recent years, the narrative record has been replaced by the more structured problem-oriented record.

Problem-Oriented Record (POR)

The problem-oriented method of recording is being used more frequently as a method for documenting nursing care. Following are the primary advantages of the POR:

1. It complements use of the nursing process.
2. It provides organization and coordination of information.
3. It facilitates evaluation of the quality of care.

Regardless of variance in terms and organizational detail, the POR has the following four basic components that parallel the five steps of the nursing process:

1. The *data base* comprises the information collected during the assessment step of the nursing process. The assessment data may be compiled in the format of the holistic nursing assessment tool composed of the five dimensions of the client (see the box on pp. 138-140).

2. The *comprehensive problem list* is formulated during the analysis step of the nursing process. Each entry on the list is dated, numbered, and titled. The problem titles form the nursing diagnoses, which represent a more thorough process of analysis.

DATE	NUMBER	TITLE
2-25-92	1	Depressed mood
2-25-92	2	Anxiety
2-25-92	3	Ineffective individual coping

3. *Initial plans* reflect the planning step of the nursing process. The plans are written for each problem on the problem list. Each entry is dated, numbered, and titled to match the corresponding problem in the problem list. The initial plan for each problem is subdivided into the following five parts:

a. *Subjective data* include verbal information from the client and significant others. The data are recorded as direct quotes or as paraphrases with the source of the information indicated. The letter *S* is used to index the entry of subjective data:

S *Client states, "I feel so nervous and shaky inside."*

b. *Objective data* include information about the client collected through observation, measurement, and sources such as written records of other health care workers. The source of the data is indicated. The letter *O* is used to index the entry of objective data:

O *Client is observed to be fidgety and restless with shortened attention span and narrowed perceptual field during the initial interview.*

c. *Assessment statement* is a succinct analysis of the subjective and objective data. The most concise form of assessment statement is the nursing diagnosis. It may also include more detail, such as the reason for the problems and interpretation of the data. The letter *A* is used to index the entry of the assessment statement:

A *Client's anxiety is related to his inability to express feelings and is exhibited as constricted, controlled affect.*

d. *Plans* include the long-term outcomes and the short-term outcome statements with accompanying outcome criteria and planned nursing interventions. The letter *P* is used to index the entry of the plans.

P *Assist client to identify negative thoughts that precede anxiety symptoms.*

4. *Progress notes* reflect the implementation and evaluation steps of the nursing process as well as a recycling to earlier steps of the process such as further assessment, analysis, or revision of plans as they pertain to a particular problem. The entry of each prog-

ress note is dated, numbered, and titled to correspond with the matching problem from the problem list and initial plans. Progress notes consist of four parts, which are titled and indexed in a form identical to that of the initial plans—*SOAP*.

S *Update on subjective data included in the initial plans or new subjective data pertaining to the problem*

O *Update on objective data included in the initial plans or new objective data pertaining to the problem*

A *Substantiation of the analysis included in the initial plans, revision of the analysis, and factors such as interpretations of the effects of medication, nursing interventions, and progress or prognosis of the client*

P *Intent to follow the plans as outlined in the initial plans or a revision or proposal of plans*

The format of a progress note is as follows:

DATE	NUMBER	TITLE
2-25-92	2	Anxiety

S *Client states, "I don't feel quite so nervous and shaky today."*

O *Client was observed to engage in a 30-minute period of task-oriented activity without notable restlessness. Attention span and ability to perceive the requirements of the task were adequate.*

A *Client's anxiety level is beginning to decrease. As yet, there is no indication of any change in client's inability to express other emotional states.*

P *Continue with nursing care as outlined in initial plans.*

BRIEF REVIEW

The nursing process is a holistic, systematic, dynamic, problem-solving method for gathering and analyzing data and planning, implementing, and evaluating care. Although the nursing process is discussed as though one stage neatly follows another, in reality the process is nonlinear. Each stage is impacted by shifts and changes in the client's functional health status and response to interventions. The five phases of the nursing process—assessment, analysis, planning, implementation, and evaluation—follow the ANA Psychiatric/Mental Health Standards of Practice.

The development of psychiatric problems are viewed as multicausal, and therefore a number of psychosocial and psychiatric theoretical models are needed to understand the psychiatric client's current level of coping.

The nursing process begins with assessment that involves the collection of data from the five health dimensions: physical, emotional, intellectual, social, and spiritual. Data from these dimensions are categorized and collated to provide the bases for analysis, the second phase of the process.

During the analysis phase, data are interpreted to determine developmental gaps, incongruities, patterns of coping and relating, motivational problems, unresolved conflicts, and stressful life experiences. Data from each dimen-

sion contribute to the overall understanding of the client's total health status. Problems are then identified, nursing diagnoses are formulated. Diagnostic statements reflect actual or potential health concerns, response to the concern or problem, and probable related or etiological factors associated with each nursing diagnosis.

The planning phase is based on results of analyses and nursing diagnosis. Planning includes establishing expected long- and short-term expected outcome criteria, prescribing nursing interventions designed to facilitate or promote desired outcomes, identifying the theoretical rationale for the interventions, determining the overall plan of treatment in collaboration with other team members, assigning responsibility for implementation and coordination of the plan of treatment, and discharge planning.

Long-term and short-term outcome statements are based on the nursing assessments and diagnoses. Effective outcome statements are specific, realistic, and complete. They reflect an understanding of the client's capabilities and level of functioning. The client is involved in planning and determining the outcomes.

Discharge planning begins during the assessment phase of the nursing process. The overall goal of discharge planning is to assist the client to achieve an optimal level of functioning as defined by the outcome criteria. To be effective, the client, family members, friends, and health team need to participate in the discharge planning.

Implementation involves carrying out nursing interventions. It is through implementing various interventions that nurses help to influence or modify client behaviors. Interventions include those classified as psychotherapeutic, health teaching (psychoeducation), promotion of activities of daily living, psychosocial rehabilitation, somatic therapies, management of the therapeutic environment, or milieu therapy, and all modalities of psychotherapy.

Although the final phase of the nursing process is evaluation, it is really an ongoing process involving feedback and updating or making changes in other phases of the nursing process as indicated. Evaluation at its simplest level means comparing the client's actual behaviors with expected outcome criteria. Determining the extent to which outcomes are achieved within a projected time frame is a measure of the effectiveness of nursing and team planning and interventions.

Evaluation is a collaborative process involving nurse, client, other team members, and in many instances the client's family or support network. Evaluation questions address the adequacy, appropriateness, effectiveness, and efficiency of nursing interventions. Evaluation may be relatively informal, such as when psychiatric clients are treated daily in the hospital, or evaluation may involve a more formal collection of data using questionnaires or standardized measures.

Quality assurance is a systematic way to collect data on the structure, outcome, and process of nursing care. Accurate recording such as the use of problem-oriented records (POR), and other forms of systematic documentation are important aspects of evaluation. Cost-containment measures and managed care restrictions are pressing psychiatric nurses to become more accountable and responsible for documenting the efficacy of their practice.

REFERENCES AND SUGGESTED READINGS

1. Aidroos NI: Use and effectiveness of psychiatric nursing care plans, *Journal of Advanced Nursing* 16(2):177, 1991.
2. Alfaro R: *Application of nursing: a step-by-step guide*, Philadelphia, 1986, JB Lippincott.
3. American Nurses Association: *Nursing: a social policy statement*, Kansas City, 1980, American Nurses' Association.
4. American Nurses Association, Division of Psychiatric and Mental Health Nursing Practice: *Standards of psychiatric and mental health nursing practice*, Kansas City, 1982, American Nurses Association.
5. American Psychiatric Association: *Diagnostic and statistical manual of mental disorders* (DSM-III-R), Washington, DC, 1987, American Psychiatric Association.
6. Anderson CM and others: Family treatment of adult schizophrenic patients: a psycho-educational approach, *Schizophrenia Bulletin* 8(3):490, 1980.
7. Arnold K and others: Writing and using standards of nursing care, *Nurse Practitioner* 4(1):25, 1990.
8. Atkinson LD, Murray ME: *Understanding the nursing process*, ed 4, New York, 1990, Pergamon Press.
9. Austad CS and others: Treatment implication of the post discharge contact, *Hospital and Community Psychiatry* 37(8):839, 1986.
10. Bauer BB, Hill SS: *Essentials of mental health care: planning and intervention*, Philadelphia, 1986, WB Saunders.
11. Bernheim KF: Principles of professional and family collaboration, *Hospital and Community Psychiatry* 41:1353, 1990.
12. Berry KN: Let's create nursing diagnoses pysch nurses can use, *American Journal of Nursing* 87:707, 1987.
13. Brallier L: *Transition and transformation: successfully managing stress*, San Francisco, 1982, National Nursing Review.
14. Carlson JH and others: *Nursing diagnosis: a case study approach*, Philadelphia, 1991, WB Saunders.
15. Capra F: *Uncommon wisdom*, New York, 1989, Bantam Books.
16. Carpenito LJ: *Nursing diagnosis: application to clinical practice*, ed 3, Philadelphia, 1989, JB Lippincott.
17. Carpenito LJ: Actual, potential, or possible? *American Journal of Nursing* 85:458, 1985.
18. Carton G and others: Teaching the nursing process, *Nursing Standard* 5(8):23, 1990.
19. Childs-Clarke A, Sharpe L: Keeping the faith: religion in the healing of phobic anxiety, *Journal of Psychosocial Nursing* 29(2):22, 1991.
20. DeFrancisco D and others: The relationship between length of stay and rapid readmission rates, *Hospital and Community Psychiatry* 3(3):196, 1980.
21. Falloon IRH: Expressed emotion: current status, *Psychological Medicine* 18:269, 1988.
22. Farkas M: Utilizing the nursing process in the development of a medication group on an inpatient psychiatric unit, *Perspectives in Psychiatric Care* 26(3):12, 1990.
23. Fauman MA: Monitoring the quality of psychiatric care, *Psychiatric Clinics of North America* 13(1):73, 1990.
24. Forchuk C, Brown B: Establishing a nurse-client relationship, *Journal of Psychosocial Nursing* 27(2):30, 1989.
25. Fortinash KM, Holoday-Worrett PA: *Psychiatric nursing care plans*, St Louis, 1991, Mosby—Year Book.
26. Frank JD: Therapeutic components of psychotherapy, *Journal of Nervous and Mental Disease* 159(5):325, 1974.
27. Fraser R: The nursing process: a core concept for mental handicap nursing, *Nursing* 2(37):1096, 1985.
28. Goldstein LS: Linking utilization management with quality improvement, *Psychiatric Clinics of North America* 13(1):157, 1990.
29. Gordon M: *Nursing diagnosis: process and application*, ed 2, New York, 1986, McGraw-Hill.
30. Gordon M: The nursing process and clinical judgment. In McFarland GK, Thomas MD, editors: *Psychiatric mental health nursing: application of the nursing process*, Philadelphia, 1991, JB Lippincott.
31. Green R: Healing and spirituality, *The Practitioner* 230:1087, 1986.
32. Griffith JW, Christensen PJ, editors: *Nursing process: application of theories, frameworks, and models*, ed 2, St Louis, 1986, Mosby—Year Book.
33. Harman W, Rheingold H: *Higher creativity*, New York, 1984, St. Martin's Press.
34. Hogstel MO: Assessing mental status, *Journal of Gerontological Nursing* 17(5):4, 1991.
35. Hughes L and others: Does the family make a difference? *Journal of Psychosocial Nursing* 25(8):8, 1987.
36. Joyce B and others: Staying well: factors contributing to successful community adaptation, *Journal of Psychosocial Nursing* 28(6):18, 1990.
37. Karshmer J: Expert nursing diagnoses: the link between nursing care and patient classification systems, *Journal of Nursing Administration* 2(1):31, 1991.
38. Kennison MM: Faith: an untapped health resource, *Journal of Psychosocial Nursing* 25:10:28, 1987.
39. Kim M, McFarland G, McLane A: *Pocket guide to nursing diagnoses*, ed 4, St Louis, 1991, Mosby—Year Book.
40. Kim M, McFarland G, McLane A: *Classification of nursing diagnoses: proceedings of the fifth conference*, St Louis, 1984, Mosby—Year Book.
41. Kitson A: Standard of care in psychiatric nursing, *Nursing Times* 82(52):51. 1987.
42. Larkins PD, Backer BA: *Problem-oriented nursing assessment*, New York, 1977, McGraw-Hill.
43. Lederach NK, Lederach JP: Religion and society: cognitive dissonance in nursing students, *Journal of Psychosocial Nursing* 25(3):32, 1987.
44. Liberman RP: Behavioral family management. In Liberman RP, editor: *Psychiatric rehabilitation of chronic mental patients*, Washington, DC, American Psychiatric Press.
45. Long LG, Higgins PG, Brady D: Psychosocial assessment, Norwalk, Conn, 1988, Appleton & Lange.
46. Loomis ME and others: Development of a classification system for psychiatric/mental health nursing: individual response class, *Archives of Psychiatric Nursing* 1(1):16, 1987.
47. Malone JA: Health assessment of individuals with mental illness. In Maurin JT, editor: *Chronic mental illness: coping strategies*, Thorofare, NJ, 1989, Slack.
48. Malone JA: The DSM-III-R versus nursing diagnosis: a dilemma in interdisciplinary practice, *Issues in Mental Health Nursing* 12(3):219, 1991.
49. Maslow AH: *Motivation and personality*, New York, 1954, Harpers & Brothers.
50. Maslow AH: *Toward a psychology of being*, New York, 1962, Van Nostrand.
51. Marriner A: *The nursing process*, St Louis, 1986, Mosby—Year Book.
52. McFarland G, Wasli E: *Nursing diagnoses and process in psychiatric mental health nursing*, Philadelphia, 1986, JB Lippincott.
53. McLane A: *Classification of nursing diagnoses: proceedings of the seventh conference*, St Louis, 1988, Mosby—Year Book.
54. Morrison EG: Nursing assessment: What do nurses want to know? *Western Journal of Nursing Research* 11(4):469, 1989.
55. Mirowsky J, Ross CE: Psychiatric diagnosis as reified measurements, *Journal of Health and Social Behavior* 30:11, 1989.
56. Newman M: Nursing diagnosis: looking at the whole, *American Journal of Nursing* 84:1496, 1984.
57. Orlando IJ: *The dynamic nurse-patient relationship: function, process, and principles*, New York, 1961, Putnam.

58. O'Sullivan A and others: Discharge planning for the mentally disabled, *Quarterly Review Bulletin* 12(3):90, 1986.

59. Parsons PJ: Building better treatment plans, *Journal Psychosocial Nursing and Mental Health Service* 24(4):8, 1986.

60. Peck MS: *The road less traveled*, New York, 1978, Simon & Schuster.

61. Peplau HE: *Interpersonal relations in nursing: a conceptual frame of reference for psychodynamic nursing*, New York, 1952, Putnam.

62. Peterson EA, Nelson K: How to meet your clients' spiritual needs, *Journal of Psychosocial Nursing* 255:34, 1987.

63. Pinnell NN, DeMeneses M: *The nursing process: theory, application and related processes*, Hartford, Conn, 1986, Appleton-Century-Crofts.

64. Reighley JW: *Nursing care planning guides for mental health*, Baltimore, 1988, Williams & Wilkins.

65. Richards DA and others: The nursing process: the effect on patient's satisfaction with nursing care, *Journal of Advanced Nursing* 12(5):559, 1987.

66. Rittman MR and others: Nursing diagnosis in psychiatric nursing, *Florida Nurse* 34(9):16, 1986.

67. Sanders J: Why spiritual groups go awry, *Uncommon Boundary* 83:24, 1991.

68. Savage P: Patient assessment in psychiatric nursing, *Journal of Advances in Nursing* 16(3):311, 1991.

69. Schultz JM, Dark SL: *Manual of psychiatric nursing care plans*, ed 3, Glenview, Ill, 1990, Scott, Foresman/Little, Brown Higher Education.

70. Sebastian L: Psychiatric hospital: admissions, assessing patients' perceptions, *Journal of Psychosocial Nursing* 25(6):25, 1987.

71. Shoemaker JK: Essential features of a nursing diagnosis. In Kin MJ, McFarland GK, McLane AM, editors: *Classification of nursing diagnosis: proceedings of the fifth national conference*, St Louis, 1984, Mosby–Year Book.

72. Simpkinson CH: Healing in altered states, *Common Boundary* 9(2):47, 1991.

73. Stark JL: Streamline your discharge planning, *Nursing* 21(5):32, 1991.

74. Stoll R: Guidelines for spiritual assessment, *American Journal of Nursing* 79:1574, 1979.

75. Townsend MC: *Nursing diagnoses in psychiatric nursing*, ed 2, Philadelphia, 1991, FA Davis.

76. Valentine NM and others: A collaborative approach to clinical development. Psychiatric and psychiatric nursing in a changing world, *Psychiatric Clinics of North America* 13(1):171, 1990.

77. Watson AC: Use of nursing diagnosis in group work with Vietnam veterans, *VA Nursing* 54(1):34, 1986.

78. West PP, Pothier PC: Clinical applications of human responses classification system: child example, *Archives of Psychiatric Nursing* 3(5):300, 1989.

79. Williams J, Wilkson H: A psychiatric nursing perspective on DSM-III, *Journal of Psychosocial Nursing and Mental Health Services* 20(4):15, 1982.

80. World Health Organization: *Education and treatment in human sexuality*, The training of health professional World, Health Organization Technical Report Series, No 572, 1975, WHO.

81. Yalom I: *The theory and practice of group psychotherapy*, ed 3, New York, 1985, Basic Books.

82. Yura H, Walsh M: *The nursing process*, ed 4, New York, 1983, Appleton-Century-Crofts.

ANNOTATED BIBLIOGRAPHY

Carpenito LJ: *Nursing diagnosis: application to clinical practice*, Philadelphia, 1990, JB Lippincott.

The book is a detailed guide to the use of nursing diagnosis in clinical nursing practice. It describes the most highly developed approach to implementing a conceptual framework for nursing process. Beginning with a historical perspective on nursing process, the author proposes a method for distinguishing between nursing diagnoses and other problems in which nurses intervene. The steps of the nursing process are described. The major portion of the book is devoted to a manual of nursing diagnoses consisting of 43 diagnostic categories. Each category is described according to definition, etiological and contributing factors, defining characteristics, focus assessment criteria, nursing goals, and principles and rationale for nursing care.

Rawlins RP, Heacock P, editors: *Psychiatric nursing: a manual for clinical practice*, St Louis, 1992, Mosby–Year Book.

The third edition of this clinical manual is a useful guide for writing psychiatric nursing care plans. It includes plans for a variety of behaviors that are seen in a psychiatric setting and guidelines for taking a history. Case examples depict the various behaviors.

Cultural Considerations in Mental Health– Psychiatric Nursing

Toni Tripp-Reimer
Sonja H Lively

After studying this chapter, the student will be able to:

- Trace the historical relationship of culture and mental health–psychiatric nursing practice
- Describe the nature of culture
- Discuss dysfunctional aspects of both positive and negative stereotyping
- Distinguish between the concepts of ethnocentrism and cultural relativity

- Identify important cultural variables in mental health nursing
- Describe cultural influences on values and patterns of communication in the nurse-client relationship
- Identify culturally sensitive intervention strategies

A case of suspected child abuse was reported recently at a county mental health facility. The case involved a Vietnamese refugee family newly arrived in the United States. The referral was made by a school nurse who, while conducting routine physical assessments, identified long bruised areas on the chest and back of a girl in the second grade. The marks were determined to be the results of a standard home remedy for the symptoms of fever, chills, and headaches. This practice consists of applying oil to the back and chest of the child with cotton swabs. The skin is massaged until warm and then rubbed with the edge of a copper coin until marks (bruises) appear. Thus the parents had not been abusing the child but rather were following a culturally prescribed and sanctioned mode of folk therapy.

In a neighborhood mental health clinic, a nurse therapist misread a Navajo client's body language. The nurse knew that good counseling skills include direct eye contact. She had been taught that when clients do not engage in direct eye contact they are disinterested or have something to hide. In fact, this Navajo client was being polite by averting his eyes, as might a person from Asia or Appalachia.

These two vignettes illustrate the importance of knowing about the client's culture in mental health–psychiatric nursing. The potential for misunderstanding is accentuated when the nurse and recipient are from different cultural or ethnic groups. Misunderstandings may arise from variations in values, beliefs, and customs or patterns of behavior. Sensitivity to these cultural variables is a requisite for quality health care in multiethnic situations.

THE NATURE OF CULTURE

Culture is defined as learned patterns of values, beliefs, customs, and behaviors that are shared by a group of interacting individuals. It is a set of rules or standards for behavior. The sharing of a common culture allows members of the group to predict each other's actions and react accordingly.

Culture is learned. Although all humans have basic biological needs (such as elimination and safety), they respond to these biological needs in cultural ways. For example, every individual has a need for food, but culture determines the patterns of behavioral responses to this need, including what, where, when, and with whom one eats. Culture is transmitted from one generation to the next by the process called *enculturation*. It may be learned formally, as in highly structured religious instructions, such as Roman Catholic catechism, or informally by observing the behaviors of various individuals within the culture. By watching different persons, modeling their behavior, and observing the reactions of others to this behavior, appropriate and acceptable behavior is learned.

The term *cultural group* is sometimes used imprecisely. People who share some common characteristics do not necessarily share a culture. Groups of individuals who share values, beliefs, and behaviors that differ from those of the dominant society are referred to as a *subculture*, for example, Appalachians, Haitian Americans, or Vietnamese Americans. Elderly Americans are often referred to as a subculture. However, this is an inappropriate designation

HISTORICAL OVERVIEW

DATES	EVENTS
1910s	Emil Kraepelin traveled to Indonesia, found that the frequency of mental disorders in Java differed from that of his native Germany, and attributed this difference to heredity rather than culture. He is considered one of the earliest pioneers in the study of the relationship between culture and mental disorder.
1914	In his book, *Totem and Taboo,* Freud attempted to use anthropological sources to substantiate his psychoanalytical theories. Using cultural data, Freud erroneously argued that the Oedipal complex is universal.
1927	Malinowski[46] studied natives of the Trobriand Islands in the Pacific Ocean and convincingly demonstrated the errors in Freud's theory of a universal Oedipal complex.
1928	In her hallmark book *Coming of Age in Samoa,* Mead documented that the adolescence experience is largely influenced by one's culture.
Late 1920s–Early 1930s	The culture and personality school in anthropology was founded by Margaret Mead, Ruth Benedict, Ralph Linton, Clyde Kluckholn, Gregory Bateson, and Irving Hollowell, who initiated extensive investigations of psychiatric problems in a cross-cultural perspective.
1930s–1940s	Transcultural data highlighted the effects of culture on psychopathology, and there was an overemphasis on the exotic manifestations of psychopathological conditions among Third World peoples.
1950s	Peplau introduced the idea that culture is an important client variable in mental health. Leininger spearheaded the transcultural nursing movement.
1960s	Transcultural nursing was established as a legitimate field of study.[42] The civil rights movement led many nurses to emphasize the necessity for specialized knowledge and skill in providing care for minority clients.
1962	King[32] concluded that psychopathology is universal, its prevalence across culture groups is similar, but manifestations of psychopathological behaviors differ among cultures.
1969	The Council on Nursing and Anthropology was established to investigate the integration of cultural content into nursing practice.
1970s	A new perspective emerged that identified the ways in which culture influences mental disorders and characteristics of health systems.
1974	The Transcultural Nursing Society was established.
1970s–1980s	Investigators in the field of mental health began to identify methods for working with culturally distinct clients in pluralistic societies.
1981	The American Nurses' Association Council on Cultural Diversity in Nursing Practice was initiated to promote minority rights and improve care for minority clients.
1990	The *Journal of Transcultural Nursing* was initiated.
Future	Because the United States is a pluralistic society and continues to have high rates of immigration, cultural variables will increasingly be viewed as crucial factors in holistic assessment of and intervention with clients in mental health settings.

of the term subculture, since it erroneously categorizes the elderly after life patterns that only superficially indicate homogeneity.[52,67] In fact, their "shared" characteristics do not represent an aged subculture but only features that are dictated by specific life circumstances, such as mandatory retirement laws and declining physical integrity. Similarly, socioeconomic level or social class does not determine a cultural group. Consequently, the "culture of poverty or the aged" is a misnomer.

Integration is the tendency for all aspects of a culture to function as an interrelated whole. Universal aspects of culture include kinship, education, diet, religion, art, politics, economics, health, and patterns of communication. It is difficult to study a single aspect of a culture because these categories are so closely interrelated.

Culture contains both ideal and real components. The way people think they should behave often differs from their actual behavior. Every society has ideal cultural patterns, *norms* that represent what most members of the society say they ought to do in a particular situation. These norms may be enforced through legal or social means. However, actual behavior may differ from the ideal and still be acceptable.

Cultural identity differs from race. Cultural identity concerns shared values, beliefs, and patterns of behavior, whereas racial identity refers to biological inherited characteristics that may be observed in physical traits. Ethnicity is a more ambiguous term and may refer to geographical origin, race, language, culture, or religion.

Because each individual tends to view his culture as correct, many people have the misconception that only other people have a culture. It is important to remember that all people are under the influence of their own cultural system. The material below summarizes what culture is and what it is not.

WHAT CULTURE IS AND WHAT IT IS NOT

CULTURE IS:	CULTURE IS NOT:
• The total way of life of a people	• Genetically inherited or determined
• The values, beliefs, and norms of a population	• Individualistic, idiosyncratic behavior
	• Racial or biological characteristics
	• Deterministic

WHAT CULTURE IS AND WHAT IT IS NOT

CULTURE IS:	CULTURE IS NOT:
• Transmitted from generation to generation	• Easily changed
• Stored in memories, books, and objects of the people	• Static
• Exhibited in actions	
• Dynamic, constantly changing, and adaptive	
• Ideational and real	
• Integrative	

STEREOTYPING

Because each client is an individual, it is imperative not to overgeneralize or *stereotype* on the basis of cultural or ethnic affiliation. Sensitivity to cultural differences in clients is essential, but ethnic and cultural affiliation serve only as a clue to assist in assessment and intervention in mental health–psychiatric nursing.

Most stereotyping is the result of misconceptions about another culture. For example, among members of the dominant American culture, Anglos,* the Hispanic concept *machismo* is surrounded by misconceptions. In Hispanic cultures machismo is a combination of the culturally de-

*The term "Anglo" is used throughout this chapter to refer to Americans of northern European descent. This use of the term is a purposeful strategy to highlight the point that all people, not only members of minority groups, are influenced by their culture.

RESEARCH HIGHLIGHT

Barriers to Health Care: Perceptual Variations of Appalachian and Non-Appalachian Health Care Professionals

• T Tripp-Reimer

PURPOSE

The purpose of this study was to identify the way in which health professionals characterized Appalachian clients.

SAMPLE

The study sample included health professionals who worked in a variety of clinical settings witth a high proportion of Appalachian migrant clients.

METHODOLOGY

The health professionals were asked to identify and interpret characteristic Appalachian behaviors. Subsequent analysis was conducted that divided the professionals into two groups: those who grew up in Appalachia and those who grew up elsewhere.

FINDINGS

Both groups generally identified the same five areas of Appalachian behavior: (1) Appalachians tend to have large families, (2) Appalachian migrants tend to move back and forth between the urban areas and the "hills," (3) Appalachian migrants tend to quit school at an early age, (4) many Appalachians use welfare services, and (5) Appalachian migrants tend to be oriented to the present.

Although the same objective facts were noted by both groups, there was a dichotomous interpretation of the behavior based on the background of the health professional. Non-Appalachians tended to view the behaviors negatively, from an ethnocentric perspective, whereas Appalachian professionals generally interpreted the same behavior as adaptive, from a relativistic perspective.

IMPLICATIONS

This study illustrates the difference between a culturally relativistic and an ethnocentric perspective. Mental health nurses need to understand client behavior in the context of the client's culture and not to interpret client behavior from personal standards.

Based on data from *Western Journal of Nursing Research* 4:179, 1982.

sirable traits of courage and fearlessness is a man. The man is the head of his family and the protector of his honor. As an authority figure, he must be just and fair. The misuse of authority results in loss of respect. The machismo ethic also allows a father to be more openly expressive of his love for his children than is generally seen in Anglo culture. However, the dominant American culture has generally emphasized the dysfunctional aspects of machismo (heavy drinking, seduction of women, and domineering and spouse abuse behaviors, for example). These aspects of machismo have also been overemphasized by health care workers.

Even stereotypes that characterize people in a positive way may be misleading. For example, there is evidence that Anglos stereotype blacks as providing more care for the elderly than is true.[26] Similarly, investigations of the elderly in San Francisco's Chinatown have revealed a serious erosion of Chinese patterns of kinship and community.[7,30] These findings contradict stereotypes of Asians as always revering their elders. As a result of this "positive" stereotyping, actual problems of elderly blacks and Chinese Americans may be overlooked.

Sometimes stereotyping is done unconsciously, simply because client behaviors are interpreted within the health professional's own value system. This practice, documented in a study concerning health professionals working with Appalachian migrants, is reported in the research highlight on p. 168.

Indiscriminately characterizing all members of minority populations as traditionalists leads to another stereotype. Each ethnic groups has members who are more or less acculturated to the dominant society.

An exception is a tendency for more adherence to tradition by recent immigrants, because economic, religious, political, and social acculturation may be restricted in American society. Furthermore, every ethnic or minority group has a historical memory of prejudice that is evident in all immigrant experiences. This memory affects even second- and third-generation members so that they never feel quite comfortable with the dominant cultural group in America.[20,63,64,79]

The degree to which any individual in a subculture adheres to the traditional culture depends on a number of different factors, including age, sex, education, and generation of immigration. The research highlight below demonstrates the importance of realizing that traditional health beliefs and behaviors may not be retained, even in individuals with high ethnic affiliation.[75]

ETHNOCENTRISM AND CULTURAL RELATIVITY

Ethnocentrism and *cultural relativity* are complementary concepts. Each denotes the perspective from which cultural characteristics are interpreted. From an ethnocentric perspective a nurse judges the behaviors of clients of a different culture by the standards of her own culture. From a culturally relativistic perspective the nurse attempts to understand the behavior of clients within the context

---

RESEARCH HIGHLIGHT

Retention of a Folk Healing Practice (Matiasma) Among Four Generations of Urban Greek Immigrants

• T Tripp-Reimer

PURPOSE

The purpose of this study was to delineate specific facets of *matiasma*, the configuration surrounding the evil eye, and to trace the retention of knowledge and use of this configuration over a four-generation population.

SAMPLE

The study sample included 328 individuals of Greek descent from 102 extended family units living in Columbus, Ohio.

METHODOLOGY

Data were collected during a field investigation over an 11-month period through the use of semistructured interviews and participant observation.

FINDINGS

The data yielded results indicating the Greek community's beliefs and practices concerning the cause, prevention, diagnosis, and treatment of the evil eye. Although the Greek community was politically, economically, and geographically integrated into the larger metropolitan community, it remained culturally distinct. However, the retention of beliefs and practices concerning the evil eye varied dramatically by generation of immigration. In the first generation, virtually all the members knew about the evil eye and nearly 90% had used practices concerned with the evil eye. However, by the fourth generation, although 46% were still knowledgeable about the evil eye, none had actually used practices concerning it.

IMPLICATIONS

This study demonstrates the importance of the generation depth as a variable in the health beliefs and behaviors of clients. It points out the importance of not stereotyping individuals on the basis of their cultural background.

Based on data from *Nursing Research* 32:91, 1983.

of their culture. Cultural relativity stresses cultural acceptance over cultural imposition.

CULTURAL VARIABLES IN MENTAL HEALTH–PSYCHIATRIC NURSING

Knowledge of cultural variables is important for the practice of mental health nursing for three major reasons. First, culture patterns how mental illness is defined, influences the perception of the mentally ill by their reference groups, and identifies appropriate health-seeking behaviors. Second, culture itself may act as a stressor for the client. Third, cultural differences between the nurse and client may lead to misunderstandings and a nontherapeutic relationship.

Influence of Culture on Mental Illness

The client and the nurse may come to the health care setting with different belief systems of how mental disorder is defined, how it is caused, and how it can best be treated. The question that emerges is "What do we mean when we say the behavior is abnormal or pathological?"

Each individual's definition of mental illness is part of a belief system and is largely determined by cultural factors. There is wide variation in the way mental disorders are defined and identified. These differences can be better understood by using the framework that distinguishes *emic* and *etic* perspectives devised by Pike.[48] This framework differentiates how members within a culture group define normal and abnormal behavior (emic) as opposed to the way individuals outside that culture group define the same behavior (etic).

An emic definition seeks to discover the perspective of individuals within a particular culture. The main aim of emic study is to discover native principles of classification and conceptualization. The result is sometimes called "subjective culture."[2,16,59,65]

Etic categories are culturally universal. An etic analysis generally includes observing behavior without regard for the viewpoint of those being studied. Using externally derived criteria, the etic investigator examines and compares several cultures.[2,16,48,59] Because these etic categories can be applied across cultures, Pike calls them culture-free features of the real world. The categories of mental disorder in the scientific diagnostic system (DSM-III-R) can be viewed as an etic classification system. This etic approach imposes a classification system that may be external to that of the client.

A nurse whose client indicates that he has been in contact with a dead relative or that he has been possessed by a spirit may consider this to be a sign of mental disorder, without recognizing that it may be an accepted occurrence in his culture. Many culture groups encourage altered states of consciousness that may indicate mental disturbance to an Anglo nurse. Altered states of consciousness are universal phenomena that are experienced in a number of forms by all humans.[3,4] In addition to normal waking consciousness, there are other states of consciousness, such as dream states and states of alcohol or drug intoxication. Mental health–psychiatric nurses normally recognize these states.

However, other altered states of consciousness are less familiar to nurses but are found in the majority of the world's societies.

Two other states of consciousness are *trance* and *possession trance*. Trance is generally interpreted as the detachment of the soul from the body and is frequently linked to hallucinations or visions. Possession trance, on the other hand, involves the belief that the body has been taken over by a spiritual entity. These two altered forms of consciousness are generally considered sacred, ritual states. They involve cultural patterning and therefore are influenced by learning and tradition.

Possession is described in Biblical scripture. In Matthew 12:22, Jesus "drove out devils and healed possessed persons." Among American Pentecostal groups, and more recently among the charismatic religious movements, the Holy Ghost is believed to possess individuals. This possession is sometimes called "baptism of the Holy Spirit."

From an etic perspective a client claiming to be possessed by a spirit may be seen as expressing symptoms of mental disorder. From an emic perspective the client may be seen as engaged in normal, culturally sanctioned behavior.

Emic and etic definitions of mental disorder involve factors other than altered states of consciousness. A study of Indo-Chinese refugees in Los Angeles found that only individuals exhibiting psychotic, endangering behaviors were regarded as requiring professional help. Other problems, such as depression, were not considered serious enough to merit professional help. Another study[14] found significant differences between Appalachian clients and Anglo mental health professionals in their identification of problematic behaviors. Behaviors that were identified as indicative of mental illness by the mental health professionals were labeled as lazy, mean, immoral, criminal, or psychic by Appalachians. The study concluded that nursing can provide a better framework for understanding client behavior by incorporating the study of culture as a concept central to determining which behaviors indicate mental disorders and which do not.[14]

In Western scientific practice there is generally a split between mental and physical symptoms. However, many other cultures view the mind and body more holistically. For example, Hispanics tend to conceptualize mental illness as a physical disease of the nervous system. Affective responses such as anxiety or depression are reported in psychophysiological concomitants; dizziness, fatigue, headaches, and various gastrointestinal disturbances.[1] Similarly, Chinese people also tend to express their emotional distress in somatic rather than emotional terms. Instead of identifying stress or tension, Chinese may speak of headaches, dizzy spells, stomach troubles, or insomnia.[41] In discussing emotional problems, Greeks refer to "nerves." This perspective is mirrored in Greek clinical practice in which most psychiatrists are also neurologists. Consequently, Greek psychiatric clients usually experience neurophysiological symptoms.[56]

There are many instances in which emic and etic classification systems may be incongruent, such as when the emic classification systems attribute mental disorders to nonscientific causes. Illnesses that are attributed to nonscientific causes are generally termed *folk illnesses*. Folk illnesses have been divided into two major categories of illness: naturalistic and personalistic.[15]

Naturalistic illnesses

Naturalistic illnesses are caused by impersonal factors without regard for the individual. Generally, naturalistic illnesses are based on an equilibrium model; when the balance is disturbed, illness results. The equilibrium theory is common throughout the world. Three of the most prevalent examples are the yin and yang model of Chinese culture, the Navajo model of balance and harmony with nature; and the hot and cold model of Hispanic cultures.

Among the Indo-Chinese, health is based on the balance of yin and yang forces. Yin forces are characterized as cold, weak, female, and small. Yang forces are characterized as hot, strong, male, and large. An excess of biological or emotional states is a yang illness. A deficiency results in a yin illness. Treatment for yin and yang conditions is based on the principle of opposition. Yin illnesses are treated by yang foods, medications, or techniques; yang illnesses are treated by yin foods, medications, and techniques. Examples of cold, or yin, treatments are acupuncture and consumption of herbal teas and vegetables. Examples of hot, or yang, treatments are moxibustion (burning a cone of mugwort, a lichen, on the skin) and consumption of foods that are spicy or high in protein or fat content. Lin and Lin[41] have identified one Chinese theory in which mental illness results from the imbalance of yin and yang. Excesses or deficiencies in physiological functions are thought to affect the balance of yin and yang, leading to mental illness. For example, sexuality, climatic changes, diet, and exercise are thought to cause some mental illness.

Personalistic illnesses

Personalistic illnesses result from punishment or aggression and are specifically directed toward an individual. Two examples of personalistic illnesses are evil eye and witchcraft.

The evil eye, discussed in the research highlight on p. 169, is a pervasive folk illness throughout Mediterranean and Spanish-speaking cultures. The evil eye is usually unintentionally caused and may result simply from envy or admiration. For example, a woman may unintentionally cast the "eye" simply by admiring another woman's child. The child may later feel lethargic, have a headache, or be irritable. Cultural groups differ in the way they determine if the eye has been cast. Among Mexican Americans, casting of the eye *(mal ojo)* is detected by rubbing an uncooked, unshelled egg over the abdomen of the affected individual. The egg is then broken into a glass of water; if it assumes a sunny-side up position, it indicates that the eye has been cast. Greeks determine whether the eye *(matiasma)* has been cast by dropping oil into a glass of water; dispersion of the oil over the water indicates presence of the evil eye. Generally, diagnosis of the eye is sufficient to remove the affliction.

Groups believing in the evil eye also have methods of protecting against it. For example, Hispanic girls may wear gold crosses or have tiny spiders embroidered on their dresses. Greek children may wear a blue stone to "reflect" the eye. In addition, after complimenting a child, the Hispanic admirer may touch a child gently on the forehead to thwart any unintentional effects of envy. Greeks may invoke the name of the Virgin Mary after admiring a child.

Belief in witchcraft as a cause of illness also falls into the personalistic category. This belief is widespread among Puerto Ricans, Haitians, and black Americans. In a specific southern psychiatric center a third of black clients treated believed that they were victims of witchcraft.[62] Terms commonly used to describe such occurrences are roots, root work, witchcraft, voodoo, a fix, a hex, and *mojo*. Regardless of the term used, the common theme is that someone has done something to cause another person illness, injury, or death.

In summary, there is wide variation in the way different cultural groups define mental disorder. It is important to understand both the etic Western diagnostic systems, and the client's emic perspective in defining normal and abnormal behavior.

Influence of Culture on Illness Behaviors

Cultures differ in the expression of symptoms and in perception and treatment of the ill person by others.

Psychotic disorders are found in every culture, and primary manifestations of these disorders are common to people in any culture. On the other hand, secondary features of these disorders are highly conditioned by culture. For example, in many groups guilt and suicidal ideation do not accompany depression. In addition, somatic rather than emotional symptoms may be most dominant, as with the Chinese expression of depression. Finally, the content of delusions and hallucinations is largely culturally patterned.[31]

There is also wide variation in the way that clients with the same disorder may be perceived and treated by their cultural group. This variation is most evident in tracing the treatment of individuals with one disorder from culture to culture. For example, persons with epilepsy are shunned in Uganda, while they are treated charitably by Hutterites.

Influence of Culture on Health-Seeking Behaviors

For some minority clients seeking mental health care, consulting mental health professionals may not be the first or only course of action. Mental health services may be seen as inappropriate or inaccessible for reasons of distance, finances, or language.

A study of the traditional Chinese on the west coast of the United States revealed that the majority of families made early, intensive, and prolonged efforts to cope independently with members having psychiatric difficulties. These efforts included advice, diet and herbal therapies, and faith healing. Secondarily, community leaders and family physicians were called in for consultations. Only as a last resort did these traditionally oriented families turn to social service agencies. This delay in seeking psychiatric help was in large part the result of the family's genuine concern for the well-being of its sick members.[33]

Among groups with beliefs in folk illness, mental health professionals may not be immediately sought for treatment of a disorder. In these instances clients may first seek assistance from a person trained in the use of folk treatments. For example, depending on the specific cultural background, Hispanic clients may use the services of a *curandero*, *santero*, or spiritist. Blacks who believe they have a folk illness may use the services of a root worker or spiritualist. Similarly, Navajo clients may first use the services of a hand trembler, who diagnoses the client's problem, and then a medicine man, who uses chants, songs, and sand paintings to affect a cure.

It is also important to know that the client may have used the services of a folk practitioner before or in conjunction with mental health therapy. Sue[66] promotes the idea that individuals who believe in folk remedies may regard biomedical treatment as only palliative because the condition can be cured only by a specially skilled folk healer.

Influence of Culture on Client Stress

All societies classify persons according to age and sex. Each society ascribes differential status and norms of behavior in terms of this classification. That is, people are expected to behave and to be treated differently on the basis of their age and their sex. These expectations result in stress at one or more stages in the life cycle. Knowledge of these high-stress periods may assist mental health nurses in anticipating client problems.

For example, although all societies define a certain group as elderly, there is wide variation in the way members of

each society perceive the aged person. The elderly as a group may be highly regarded or largely disvalued. In some societies old age is a time of high prestige and power, whereas in others it is a period of insecurity, alienation, and high stress. Old age may be the period when people enjoy the greatest respect or when they endure emotional and physical abandonment.

In the United States, the aged are typically stereotyped as nonproductive, physically and mentally deteriorating, poverty stricken, disengaged, and burdensome. Among other culture groups the aged may be the most powerful, the most engaged, and the most respected members of the society. In a study of 102 noninstitutionalized retired urban blacks, findings suggested that emotional adjustment to aging may be easier for black than for white middle-class Americans.[27] The role of the elderly black woman in black families as a source of love, strength, and stability is described frequently.[27,43,45] Often black grandmothers share in the responsibility for child care or informally adopt children whose parents are experiencing economic hardship or are temporarily seeking employment opportunities away from home. This ability of elderly black women to maintain the family unit provides them with a functional role and assists in promoting a positive aging experience. Religious orientation also effects the elderly black womens' adjustment to aging as the accompanying research highlight describes.

Similarly, adolescence seems to be an especially troubled time for most Americans. This has been viewed as stemming from a number of factors[51]:

RESEARCH HIGHLIGHT

Ethnic Differences in Intrinsic/Extrinsic Religious Orientation and Depression in the Elderly
• P Nelson

PURPOSE

The purpose of the study was to determine if black and white individuals differ in religious behaviors and if there is a relationship between their religious behaviors and depression.

SAMPLE

The purposive sample consisted of 68 elderly persons living in the community and attending day-care programs in five senior citizen centers with 46.9% white, 50% black, and 3.1%, Mexican American.

METHODOLOGY

The Age Universal Religious Orientation Scale was used to measure religious behaviors. The Geriatric Depression Scale (GDS) was used to measure depression. In addition, selected demographic information was collected. The scales were compiled into a questionnaire and administered to prearranged groups. Questionnaires were administered individually to subjects with special needs.

FINDINGS

Results suggested that black elderly persons had a higher intrinsic orientation score than did white elderly persons ($\chi = 30.32$, $df = 18$, $P = 0.03$). There was no significant difference between black and white persons in extrinsic religious orientation ($\chi = 23.45$, $df = 25$, $P = 0.55$). Results also indicated that black persons were more depressed than white persons. A negative correlation was found between depression and intrinsic orientation in the total sample ($r = 0.23$, $P = 0.026$).

IMPLICATIONS

The findings from the study suggest that black and white elderly persons do differ in religious orientation and that their religious orientation does not necessarily determine their success in coping with depression. However, the results do suggest that the religious orientation of the elderly may play an important role in adjustment to aging. Nurses should be aware of these differences, respect the elderly person's use of religion in meeting the day-to-day demands of adjustment to aging, and assess the environment for opportunities for the elderly to practice their religion according to their religious orientation.

From *Archives of Psychiatric Nursing* 3(4):199, 1989.

1. The lack of a clear termination point of adolescence
2. The prolongation of the education process and subsequent social role fulfillment
3. The variety of cultural choices open to the adolescent in the areas of life-style, occupation, and religion

On the other hand, compared to these dominant American cultural norms, old-order Amish adolescents have fewer stressors. Their education is completed after the eighth grade and the choices available at that point are limited. It is likely that the adolescent boy will become a farmer like his father and that the adolescent girl will become a mother and homemaker like her mother.

Sex role differences may also lead to differential stress periods. Schlegel[57] investigated situational stress among the Hopi. Historically, Hopi women were farmers who owned their own land and passed it from mother to daughter.[13] These activities required a great deal of skill and role development that may have been stress producing. She concluded that the role of the adult Hopi woman and the socialization she undergoes for this role places the adolescent Hopi girl in a position of high stress.

As previously noted, cultures are not static; they evolve through time. However, when culture change is rapid and extensive, the change may produce stress. Culture change may occur when an individual from one culture moves into another. The immigrant undergoes acculturation, the process in which the customs, knowledge, attitudes, values, and material choices of one culture or way of life become adopted in whole or in part by the people of another.[10] A number of stressors have been identified for new immigrants:

1. The strain involved in expending effort on adaptation, speaking a new language, abiding by unfamiliar customs, and following a variety of new rules of behavior
2. A sense of loss at being uprooted, which is particularly prevalent among involuntary or forced migrants such as refugees
3. The rejection of the newcomer by the host population
4. The confusion of one's roles, values, and feelings
5. Rejection of the host's culture by the newcomer with accompanying feelings of discomfort, anxiety, or disgust
6. The feeling of helplessness in dealing with the new culture

A national study of the mental health needs of Southeast Asian refugees found a high incidence of mental health problems.[47] Data from more than 1000 agencies working with refugee populations indicate that the age group 19 to 35 years is most at risk. This group contains the majority of single adults who are most excluded from the traditional family support system. Those aged 36 to 55 years comprise the second most frequently reported group at risk. Stress for this group tends to result from the loss of traditional roles and status and a marked degree of intergenerational conflict. Common mental health problems of Southeast Asian refugees are, in descending order of importance: depression, anxiety, marital conflict, intergenerational conflict, and school adjustment. The study also indicated that all smaller ethnic groups that lacked an ethnic community support system were more at risk of mental health problems that those with community support.

Role Expectations of the Nurse

To be effective, the nurse needs a clear, solid understanding of the client's culture. Because role expectations of the nurse vary from one culture to another, the nurse needs to be alert to different world views and preferred behavior styles.

The middle-class, white, American client characteristically views a helpful nurse as democratic, passive, and concerned with emotions. Clients with other backgrounds, such as Asian or Hispanic, may expect the nurse to be an authority figure who provides interpretations and suggestions for problem solutions.[10] The latter two groups may perceive nurses as persons who warrant respect and deference—an expert who will provide answers. Out of respect for authority, some clients, such as Native Americans, do not speak until spoken to. They expect the therapist to be directive and provide solutions to their problems.

Values and Health Behaviors

A variety of approaches have been used to examine the values of different cultural groups. One of the most basic is simply to describe the dominant values of a specific group. For example, Hicks[24] identified a dominant value of Appalachians as the ethic of neutrality. He found that these mountaineers typically demonstrate this ethic, which is composed of four behavioral imperatives.

1. One must not be assertive or aggressive.
2. One must avoid argument and seek agreement.
3. Unless otherwise requested, one should mind one's own business. Asking direct, personal questions is taken as an attempt to interfere in a person's private matters.
4. One must not assume authority over others. To do so would violate the presumption of equality.

This ethic of neutrality has important implications for mental health nurses working with Appalachian clients. In a study investigating traits that made practitioners unsuccessful with Appalachian clients, it was noted that those who were authoritarian had little success with Appalachian clients.[73] Counseling and health teaching given in an authoritarian manner are not readily accepted. The following topics are generally avoided by successful Appalachian practitioners:

1. Income and how it was spent. (This can be used against the client by welfare agencies.)
2. Questions about how often their children go to school. (This can be used against them by truant officers.)
3. Questions about who is living with the Appalachians. (This can be used against them by welfare workers and landlords.)

If the information listed above is absolutely necessary, successful practitioners suggest approaching sensitive topics with indirect questions and refraining from using coercion. Finally, they emphasize that the Appalachian client may be sensitive to perceived criticism.

A second approach to value orientations is to compare several cultures. Kluckhohn and Strodtbeck[35] identified various problems with which all societies must cope: time, personal activities, interpersonal relations, and relationship to nature. These value orientations are described here and related to health behaviors in the next section.

Temporal orientation

The temporal orientation is divided into three time frames: past, present, and future. Although all societies consider all three domains, their emphasis differs. While lower economic, agricultural cultures tend to emphasize a present orientation, highly industrialized cultures tend to be future oriented.

Activity orientation

The activity orientation identifies whether a given culture is primarily oriented toward "doing" or "being." Middle-class America has been characterized as doing oriented; each person is valued for his or her accomplishments. On the other hand, in societies with a being orientation, each person is valued for his or her very existence. The being pattern is typical of lineage societies (such as the Chinese) in which the person is valued as a link in the chain of continuity between generations.

Relational orientation

The relational orientation distinguishes among interpersonal patterns and deals with the ways in which the society sets goals for its individual members. It is characterized by collateral, lineal, and individualistic modes.

When the collateral principle is dominant, the goals and welfare of the siblings or members of the same age groups are of prime importance. Collectivistic societies such as Russia and Israel typically demonstrate a collateral orientation in the ideal. In these societies, the goals of the individual are subordinated to those of the group, and the group maintains responsibility for all its members.

The lineal mode parallels the collateral mode in that group goals and welfare have primary importance. However, with the lineal orientation, continuity of the group and ordered succession within the group are important. In virtually all societies with emphasis on lineality, as in Samoa, kinship is the basis for maintaining the lineage with the oldest male of the family the head of the lineage.

When the individualistic principle is dominant, individual goals supersede the goals of specific collateral or lineage groups. Each person's responsibility to the total society and his or her place in it are defined by autonomous goals. Most industrialized Western societies, including the United States, emphasize the individualistic orientation. The individual alone is held responsible for personal behavior and is judged on the basis of personal accomplishments.

People-to-nature orientation

The orientation of people to nature identifies whether humans dominate nature, live in harmony with nature, or are subjugated to nature.

The dominating nature orientation holds that humans can master or control natural events. Most middle-class Americans believe that, given sufficient time, science and technology will prevail over nature. The concept of harmony with nature denotes a sense of holism among humans and nature. Many Native American and Asian philosophies promote this integrated approach. Subjugation to nature is

often presented as fatalism. Among many Moslems, for example, it is believed that a person's ultimate fate is considered inevitable.

Because of its diverse ethnic populations, the United States exhibits greater heterogeneity than most other Western cultures; no dominant value system can be identified. Although a dominant orientation can be identified for middle-class Americans of northern European descent, the orientation of other American culture groups may vary considerably from this. Table 9-1 illustrates the diversity in value orientations of selected American ethnic groups.

Values and Mental Health Nursing Practice

Clients' behaviors are generally consistent with their cultural values. A discussion of the potential influence of value orientations on client behaviors follows.

As illustrated in Table 9-1, the dominant American culture perceives the relationship of people to nature as one of control. These clients believe that humans, through science and technology, can control nature. They tend to actively seek the assistance of mental health practitioners, believing that these practitioners can, through the application of scientific knowledge, alleviate their problems. On the other hand, Appalachian clients tend to feel subjugated to nature. This may result in a fatalistic approach to mental disorder and skepticism regarding the benefits of counseling.[78] In contrast, Navajos have been identified as feeling in harmony with nature, society, and the world of the supernatural. Correspondingly the Navajo religion is a design in harmony, a striving for rapport between humans and every phase of nature.[50] Thus health care may be seen as a religious activity and mental health practitioners as adjuncts to a more holistic therapy.

In the relational value orientation, middle-class Americans tend to be individualistic, seeking self-actualization through vocational and personal improvement. This contrasts with the traditional Asian relational orientation, in which the lineal mode is dominant. The welfare and integrity of the family is of prime importance to traditional Asian-Americans. Family members may be expected to put aside their own behaviors and feelings to further the welfare of the family. Furthermore, the behavior of each individual member of the family is expected to be a credit to the entire family. Similar qualities of the Hispanic culture are (1) family being one of the most proud and valued aspects of life, and (2) the need for preserving the family's unit, respect, and loyalty.

A number of studies have indicated that traditional Asian-Americans prefer to use family or friends as a primary source of help for mental health problems. Families may deny that members have emotional problems until they become unmanageable. This results in part because mental disorders are viewed as shameful.[81] In these cultures, for example, extreme psychotic symptoms are tolerated it they are not accompanied by destructive behavior.[41] Mental health nurses working with traditional Asians may find that their clients experience strong feelings of guilt and shame when admitting that problems exist. Issues of confidentiality are therefore crucial in dealing with traditional Asian clients. Furthermore, it may be the relatives, more than the clients, who need to be convinced of the importance of

▼ **TABLE 9-1**   Dominant Value Orientations of Selected American Ethnic Groups

Ethnic Group	Temporal Orientation	Activity Orientation	Relational Orientation	People-to-Nature Orientation
Dominant American	Future over present	Doing	Individualistic	Over-with-subjugated
Southern black	Present over future	Being	Collateral-lineal	Subjugated-over-with
Puerto Rican	Present over future	Doing	Individualistic	With-subjugated-over
Southern Appalachian	Present	Being	Lineal-collateral	Subjugated
Native American	Present	Being	Collateral-lineal	With
Mexican American	Present	Being	Lineal-collateral	Subjugated
Traditional Chinese American	Present	Being	Lineal	With

From Tripp-Reimer T: In *Nursing assessment: a multidimensional approach* by J Bellack and P Bamford, Monterey, California, 1984, Wadsworth Health Sciences Division.

treatment before the client can start or continue a therapeutic program.[71] In some instances, greater benefit may be derived from family therapy than from individual therapy. Consequently, it is particularly important to consider an Asian or Hispanic client as an integral member of the family constellation. The family should be included in the therapy plan and treatment goals.

In temporal orientation, middle-class Americans tend to be future oriented. This future orientation may be seen in examples of deferred gratification, such as an emphasis on the importance of extended education. In addition, members of the dominant American culture tend to structure time rigidly. Adhering to time schedules is a way of life. In a clinical setting this may mean that they will be punctual and may carefully watch the clock during therapy. In contrast, individuals with a present time orientation may be less concerned with adherence to schedules. An Anglo nurse should avoid labeling missed appointments or tardiness as signs of disrespect, laziness, or lack of interest. Present time orientation may be one reason Hispanic clients may be late for appointments.[25] Carter[8] stressed the need for awareness of differences in values regarding time for blacks from low socioeconomic groups. Instead of labeling tardiness as a blatant disregard of time, problems of health, economics, and transportation need to be considered. The Native American's flexible sense of time contrasts sharply with the dominant middle-class American value of time schedules. The Native American is able to focus on the present and enjoy it and is not bound by time constraints. In mental health practice, a focus on the present may result in a crisis orientation rather than a preventive approach. It also promotes a more flexible adherence to schedules. Consequently, mental health nurses need to be aware that clients with a present orientation who are deeply engaged in a counseling situation may be reluctant to leave the appointment simply because "the time is up."

Patterns of Communication

Communication of emotional states is strongly influenced by culture. Many Indo-Chinese emphasize self-control because they believe it is one's duty to maintain an even temper. Hostility is not expressed toward persons who are considered "superior," such as parents, elders, or health professionals. A client's smile of "yes" may not necessarily indicate compliance or agreement as much as it indicates an unwillingness to be disrespectful or impolite.

Volume, speed, and directness in conversation is influenced by cultural values. Health practitioners may be viewed as loud and boisterous by minority clients. Likewise, the softer volume of Asian or Native American speech may be interpreted by the mental health nurse as shyness.

Many cultures value indirectness and subtlety in communicating. The frankness of the American mental health professional may alienate some minority clients. For example, Asian clients may interpret this communication style as rude, immature, and lacking finesse. On the other hand, Asian clients may be perceived as evasive and afraid to confront their problems by Anglo health professionals.[66]

Nurses need to be aware of the role of language in intercultural therapy. In working with Hispanic groups, group process is greatly facilitated when members and leader can speak both English and Spanish. Likewise, both Asians and Hispanics believe language is a vital issue. Treatment in the native language is essential when working among unacculturated groups. Being fluent in the client's native language greatly facilitates discussion and understanding of emotionally charged topics. Clients can spontaneously express feelings in words that are most comfortable to them. However, when a bilingual nurse is not available, interpreters can be used effectively.

The meaning of silence may also vary considerably among various cultures. For some groups silence is extremely uncomfortable, and they attempt to fill every gap in the conversation. In contrast, many Native Americans often consider silence essential to understanding because a persons needs to fully consider what another has said before responding. Silence by traditional Chinese and Japanese clients does not necessarily indicate that they have nothing more to say. They may wish the nurse to consider the content of what they said before continuing. Other cultures may use silence much differently. The Russians, French, and Spanish, for example, may read it as a sign of agreement among parties, while Asian cultures may view silence as a sign of respect for an elder.

Many ethnic groups, such as Native Americans, Southeast Asians, and Appalachians, may view direct eye contact differently than do Anglos. For example, Navajos consider direct eye contact hostile. They therefore tend to use more peripheral vision. Lack of eye contact among Japanese and Mexican Americans is a sign of politeness and respect. This nonverbal behavior may be misunderstood by professionals.

Cultural norms dictate differences in personal space. Hall,[21] in his research on territoriality, identifies the following four interpersonal distance zones used by middle-class adults from the northeastern United States:

INTERPERSONAL DISTANCE ZONES

Intimate	Contact-1½ feet
Personal	1½-4 feet
Social	4 feet-12 feet
Public	Greater than 12 feet

Nurses and clients from the population group that includes Native Americans, Appalachians, Japanese, and Mexican Americans would comfortably position themselves between the personal and social distance. Positioning is done unconsciously until, "It just feels right." The Anglo counselor may feel uncomfortable with Latin Americans, Africans, black Americans, or Indonesians whose cultures generally dictate closer personal space.[78] Blacks engage in eye contact more often than whites when they are speaking, and they have a closer personal space and greater body activity. Thus Anglo nurses working with black clients may misinterpret their nonverbal behaviors as indicating anger or aggression.

The psychotherapy situation is often ambiguous and unstructured. Consequently, a number of cross-cultural therapists* have suggested that many minority clients prefer a logical, rational, structured approach over an effective, reflective, or ambiguous one. They further point out that nondirective, client-centered approaches may not work well with many minority clients. They recommend that the nurse use a directive approach that is highly goal oriented. For example, short-term therapy that deals with immediate concrete concerns is preferable to the long-term insightful approach. Behavioral therapy, such as contracting for targeted problems and goals or teaching assertiveness or relaxation, can be most helpful.[82]

However, it is crucial to remember that the client's cultural background serves only as a cue for assessment and intervention. For example, "talk therapy," acceptable to a client from the dominant American middle-class, is an enigma for the client who is less verbally oriented and who believes life events are determined by luck or fate. As a general approach to therapy with minority clients, Draguns advises the following[12]:

Be prepared to adapt your techniques (general activity level, mode of verbal intervention, content of remarks, tone of voice) to the cultural background of the client; communicate acceptance of and respect for the client in terms that are intelligible and meaningful within his cultural frame of reference; and be open to the possibility of more direct intervention in the life of the client than the traditional ethos of the counseling profession would dictate or permit.

Culturally Sensitive Intervention Strategies

For a nurse involved in transcultural counseling, a variety of treatment approaches needs to be explored, depending on the characteristics of the client. There is an increasing acceptance of the efficacy of specific therapeutic modalities for clients with certain behavioral characteristics.

Ethnotherapy (family therapy and ethnicity)

As previously stated, the family unit of varying ethnic groups may determine individual behavior. Restoring a greater sense of identity may require resolution of cultural conflicts within the family, between the family and the outside community, or in the larger society in which the family exists. Nurses may need to help families sort out strong convictions from values asserted for emotional reasons. Often families need to decide which traditional ethnic values they wish to retain. Those ethnic values that are retained play a significant role in family life and personal development throughout the life cycle by influencing family patterns and belief systems.[44]

Families who are experiencing cultural transition when migrating to the United States may experience numerous stresses, such as loss of support systems, decrease in health status, or economic difficulties. These factors lead to isolation (fear of new environment), enmeshment (imposing strict traditional values, avoiding any support in adapting to new demands), and disengagement (no longer accepting family values and life-style, vulnerability to new environmental stressors).[38] However, some families may negotiate the acculturation process without difficulty if adaptation factors are positive.

For those families seeking assistance, there are several approaches to cultural transition in a new environment.

Transitional mapping

When the migratory process is considered in terms of patterns instead of specific content, a model emerges that describes specific stages through which each migrating family passes: preparatory stage, act of migration, period of overcompensation, period of decompensation, and transgenerational phenomena.

During the first interview, the nurse needs to establish which phase of the migration process the family is experiencing and their previous experiences in migration phases. A comprehensive map is created that includes the position of each family member, the entire family's life-cycle stages, cultural origin, family form, and current status with other family members and the community. Factors that support adaptation and rates of adaptation by family members as a whole are considered.

The majority of families needing counseling are in the period of decompensation, which occurs some 6 months after the move. At this unsettling time, the family is reshaping its reality as it attempts to both retain its identity and become compatible with the new culture. For example, children may adapt to the new culture and language faster than the parents. This change in the children's roles and values can cause family upheaval. When this differential adaptation rate exists, the impact of transcultural conflict can be assumed and therapy begun.[61]

Link therapy

This therapeutic process involves having a single family member represent the "link" between the mental health nurse and the extended family. Although not characteristic

---

*References 5, 33, 55, 66, 68, 69, 72.

of family therapy approaches, this therapy may be appropriate for East Indians, Africans, or Iranians, in whose cultures parents cannot discuss issues in the presence of children. The family member acting as the link therapist is trained to initiate interventions with the guidance and supervision of the family counselor. The most successful link therapist is a person experiencing unresolved transitional conflict, because a fully acculturated or entrenched traditionalist would dictate the transitional direction to be taken by the family.[47]

The key to treating families who are in cultural transition is to recognize that their problems arise because different family subsystems adapt at different rates. Transitional therapy clarifies the differential rates of adaptation and facilitates the family's resolution of transitional conflict. The nurse must not presume that the values of the new or dominant American middle-class culture are right for everybody and that a nuclear family structure is the correct family system. Ethnic families need to be encouraged to make their own choices.

BRIEF REVIEW

Culture includes the learned patterns of values, beliefs, customs, and behaviors that are shared by a group of individuals. Knowledge of the client's culture assist the nurse in predicting the client's actions and acting accordingly; it allows her to assume a culturally relativistic perspective. At the same time, it is important not to overgeneralize or stereotype clients on the basis of cultural or ethnic affiliation.

The definitions of mental illnesses, the perceived role of the mental health nurse, as well as the secondary characteristics of these illnesses are largely determined by cultural factors. The client's culture itself can serve as a stressor to the individual.

When the client and nurse are from different cultural groups, misunderstandings can rise from differences in values and patterns of communication. Thus a key component is to assess and treat the client from his ethnic perspective. This involves assessment of cultural variables related to illness behaviors and health seeking behaviors. It is important for the nurse to develop culturally sensitive interaction strategies that focus on immediate, concrete solutions to mental health problems. Emphasis is on family involvement as a major asset to supporting the client's acceptance of clinical interventions. It is also crucial for nurses to assess their own cultural background and how it influences therapeutic interventions with ethnic minority clients. The preferred outcome is to have both the nurse and client be enriched from the cultural interaction.

REFERENCES AND SUGGESTED READINGS

1. Arce A, Torres-Matrullo C: Application of cognitive behavorial techniques in the treatment of Hispanic patients, *Psychiatric Quarterly* 54:230, 1982.
2. Berry JW, Dasen PR, editors: *Culture and cognition: readings in cross-cultural psychology*, London, 1974, Methuen & Co.
3. Bourguignon EE: *Culture and varieties of consciousness*, Reading, Mass, 1974, Addison-Wesley.
4. Bourguignon EE: *Possession*, San Francisco, 1976, Chandler & Sharp.
5. Bush M, Ullom J, Osborne O: The meaning of mental health: a report of two ethnoscientific studies, *Nursing Research* 24:130, 1975.
6. Campbell B: Family paradigm theory and family rituals: implications for child and family health, *Nurse Practitioner* 16(2):22, 1991.
7. Carp F, Kataoka E: Health care problems of the elderly of San Francisco's Chinatown, *Gerontologist* 16:30, 1976.
8. Carter J: Frequent mistakes made with black clients in psychotherapy, *Journal of the National Medical Association* 71:10, 1979.
9. Dancy J: *The black elderly: a guide for practitioners*, Ann Arbor, Mich, 1977, Institute of Gerontology, University of Michigan.
10. Delgado M: Hispanics and psychotherapeutic groups, *International Journal of Group Psychotherapy* 33:4, 1983.
11. Doku J: Approaches to cultural awareness, *Nursing Times* 86(39):69, 1990.
12. Draguns J: Common themes and distinct approaches. In Pedersen PB and others, editors: *Counseling across cultures*, Honolulu, 1981, University of Hawaii Press.
13. Farris L: The American Indian. In Clark AL, editor: *Culture, childbearing, and health professionals*, Philadelphia, 1978, FA Davis.
14. Flaskerud J: Perception of problematic behavior by Appalachians, mental health professionals and lay non-Appalachians, *Nursing Research* 19:140, 1980.
15. Foster G, Anderson B: *Medical anthropology*, New York, 1978, John Wiley & Sons.
16. French D: The relationship of anthropology to studies in perception and cognition. In Kotch S, editor: *Psychology: a study of science*, New York, 1963, McGraw-Hill.
17. Frye B: Cultural themes in health care decision making among Cambodian refugee women, *Journal of Community Health Nursing* 8(1):33, 1991.
18. Geiger J: Culture and space, *Advanced Clinical Care* 5(6):8, 1990.
19. Giordano J, Giordano GP: *The ethnocultural factor in mental health: a literature review and bibliography*, New York, 1977, Institute on Pluralism and Group Identity.
20. Greely AM: *Why can't they be like us?* New York, 1969, Institute of Human Relations.
21. Hall E: *The hidden dimension*, New York, 1969, Doubleday.
22. Hansen M: Health beliefs, health care, and rural Appalachian subcultures from an ethnographic perspective, *Family and Community Health* 13(1):1, 1990.
23. Henkle J: Cultural diversity: a resource in planning and implementing nursing care, *Public Health Nursing* 7(3):145, 1990.
24. Hicks G: *Appalachian valley*, New York, 1976, Holt, Rinehart and Winston.
25. Hoppe S, Heller P: Alienation, familism, and the utilization of health services by Mexican-Americans, *Journal of Health and Social Behavior* 15:304, 1974.
26. Jackson JS: Aged Negroes, their culture departures from statistical stereotypes and rural-urban differences, *Gerontologist* 10:140, 1970.
27. Jackson JS, Bacon J, Peterson J: Life satisfaction among black urban elderly, *Journal of Aging and Human Development* 8:169, 1971.
28. Johnson R: The culturally diverse student, *Nursing Health Care* 10(7):402, 1989.
29. Jones FC: The lofty role of the black grandmother, *The Crisis* 80:19, 1973.
30. Kalish R, Yuen S: Americans of East Asian ancestry: aging and the aged, *Gerontologist* 11(suppl):36, 1971.
31. Kiev A: *Transcultural psychiatry*, New York, 1972, Free Press.

32. King S: *Perceptions of illness in medical practice*, New York, 1962, Russell Sage Foundation.

33. Kitano H, Matsushima N: Counseling Asian-Americans. In Pedersen PG and others, editors: *Counseling across cultures*, Honolulu, 1981, University of Hawaii Press.

34. Kleinman A: Major conceptual and research issues for cultural (anthropological) psychiatry, *Culture, Medicine and Psychiatry* 4:3, 1980.

35. Kluckhohn F, Strodtbeck F: Variations in value orientations, Evanston, Ill, 1961, Row, Peterson & Co.

36. Knab S: Polish Americans: historical and cultural perspectives of influence in the use of mental health services, *Journal of Psychosocial Nursing and Mental Health Services* 1(24):31, 1986.

37. Landau J: Link therapy as a family therapy technique for transitional extended families, *Psychotherapeia* 7:382, 1981.

38. Landau J: Therapy with families in cultural transition. In McGoldrick M, Pearce JK, and Giordano J, editors: *Ethnicity and family therapy*, New York, 1982, Guilford Press.

39. Lazarus A: *The practice of multidimensional therapy*, New York, 1981, McGraw-Hill.

40. Leininger M: *Nursing and anthropology: two worlds to blend*, New York, 1970, John Wiley.

41. Lin T, Lin M: Service delivery issues in Asian-North American communities, *American Journal of Psychiatry* 135:454, 1978.

42. Martin EP, Martin JM: The black extended family, Chicago, 1978, University of Chicago Press.

43. McAdoo HP, editor: *Black families*, Beverly Hills, Calif, 1981, Sage Publications.

44. McGoldrick M, Pearce JK, Giordano J: *Ethnicity and family therapy*, New York, 1982, Guilford Press.

45. Nobles W: African philosophy: foundations for black psychology. In Hones R, editor: *Black psychology*, ed 2, New York, 1980, Harper & Row.

46. Pedersen PB and others, editors: *Counseling across cultures*, Honolulu, 1981, University of Hawaii Press.

47. Pennsylvania Department of Public Welfare, Bureau of Research and Training, Office of Mental Health: *National mental health needs assessment of Indochinese refugee populations*, Harrisburg, 1979, The Bureau.

48. Pike KL: *Language in relation to a unified theory of the structure of human behavior*, ed 2, 1967, New York, Humanities Press International.

49. Reeves K: Hispanic utilization of an ethic mental health clinic, *Journal of Psychosocial Nursing and Mental Health Services* 24(2):23, 1986.

50. Richardson E: Cultural and historical perspectives in counseling American Indians. In Sue D, editor: *Counseling the culturally different: theory and practice*, 1981, New York, John Wiley & Sons.

51. Ridley C: Clinical treatment of the nondisclosing black client, *American Psychologist* 39:11, 1984.

52. Rose A: The sub-culture of the aging. In Rose A, Peterson W, editors: *Older people and their social world*, Philadelphia, 1965, FA Davis.

53. Ruiz M: Open-closed mindedness: intolerance of ambiguity and nursing faculty attitudes toward culturally different patients, *Nursing Research* 30:177, 1981.

54. Ruiz R: Cultural and historical perspectives in counseling Hispanics. In Sue D, editor: *Counseling the culturally different: theory and practice*, New York, 1981, John Wiley & Sons.

55. Ruiz R, Cassas J: Culturally relevant and behavioristic counseling for Chicano counseling students. In Pedersen PB and others, editors: *Counseling across cultures*, Honolulu, 1981, University of Hawaii Press.

56. Samouilidis L: Psychoanalytic vicissitudes in working with Greek patients, *The American Journal of Psychoanalysis* 38:223, 1978.

57. Sehlegel A: Situational stress: a Hopi example. In Datan N, editor: *Life span developmental psychology*, New York, 1975, Academic Press.

58. Scaffa M, Davis DA: Cultural considerations in the treatment of persons with AIDS, *Occupational Therapy Health Care* 7(2/3/4):69, 1990.

59. Segall M: *Human behavior in cross-cultural psychology: global perspectives*. Monterey, Calif, 1979, Brooks/Cole.

60. Silver M: Focus on health care: Vietnamese in Denver. In Van P, Arsdale P, Pisarowicz J, editors: *Processes of transition: Vietnamese in Colorado*, Austin, Tex, 1980, High Street Press.

61. Sluzki CE: Migration and family conflict, *Family Process* 18:379, 1979.

62. Snow L: Sorcerers, saints and charlatans: black folk healers in urban America, *Culture, Medicine and Psychiatry* 2:69, 1978.

63. Sowell T: *Ethnic America*, New York, 1981, Basic Books.

64. Stein HF: The Slovak-American "swaddling-ethos": homeostat for family dynamics and cultural persistence, *Family Process* 17:31, 1978.

65. Sturtevant W: Studies in ethnoscience, *American Anthropologist* 66:99, 1964.

66. Sue D: *Counseling the culturally different: theory and practice*, New York, 1981, John Wiley & Sons.

67. Sullivan T: Values beliefs, and practice of the elderly in the United States: implications for health and nursing care, *Transcultural Nursing Care* 2:13, 1977.

68. Sundberg N: Research and research hypothesis about effectiveness in intercultural counseling. In Pedersen PB and others, editors: *Counseling across cultures*, Honolulu, 1981, University of Hawaii Press.

69. Toupin E: Counseling Asians: psychotherapy in the context of racism and Asian-American history, *American Journal of Orthopsychiatry* 50:76, 1980.

70. Tousignant M, Mishara B: Suicide and culture: a review of the literature from 1969 to 1980, *Transculture Psychiatric Research Review* 18:5, 1981.

71. Triandis H, Draguns J: *Handbook of cross-cultural psychology*, vol 6, Psychopathology, Boston, 1980, Allyn & Bacon.

72. Trimble J: Value differentials and their importance in counseling American Indians. In Pedersen PB and others, editors: *Counseling across cultures*, Honolulu, 1981, University of Hawaii Press.

73. Tripp-Reimer T: *Appalachian health care: from research to practice*, Proceedings of the Fifth National Transcultural Nursing Conference, 44, 1980, Salt Lake City, University of Utah.

74. Tripp-Reimer T: Ethnomedical beliefs among Greek immigrants: implications for nursing intervention. In Morley P, editor: *Developing, teaching and practicing transcultural nursing*, Proceedings of the Sixth National Transcultural Nursing Conference, 126, 1981.

75. Tripp-Reimer T: Barriers to health care: perceptual variations of Appalachians and non-Appalachian health care professionals, *Western Journal of Nursing Research* 4:179, 1982.

76. Tripp-Reimer T: Retention of a folk healing practice (matiasma) among four generations of urban Greek immigrants, *Nursing Research* 32:97, 1983.

77. Tripp-Reimer T: Cultural assessment. In Ballack J, Bamford P, editors: *Nursing assessment: a multidimensional approach*, Monterey, Calif, 1984, Wadsworth.

78. Tripp-Reimer T, Friedl M: Appalachians: a neglected minority, *Nursing Clinics of North America* 12:41, 1977.

79. Tseng WS, McDermott JF: *Culture, mind, and therapy: an introduction to cultural psychiatry*, New York, 1981, Brunner/Mazel.

80. Tung M: Life values, psychotherapy and East-West integration, *Psychiatry* 47:8, 1984.

81. Van Deusen J: Health/mental studies of Indochinese refugees: a critical overview, *Medical Anthropology* 4:231, 1982.

82. Yamamoto J, Acosta F: Treatment of Asian Americans and Hispanic Americans: similarities and differences, *Journal of the American Academy of Psychoanalysis* 10:4, 1982.

83. Yuki T: Cultural responsiveness and social work practice: an Indian clinic's success, *Health and Social Work* 11(3):223, 1986.

ANNOTATED BIBLIOGRAPHY

Giger J, Davidhizar R: *Transcultural nursing: assessment and intervention*, St Louis, 1991, Mosby—Year Book.

This is an excellent resource for nurses and nursing students interested in developing knowledge of transcultural concepts to apply to client care. Theory and six cultural phenomena that have been identified in all cultural groups are addressed in part one of the book. The second part applies the six cultural phenomena to care of individuals in a variety of specific cultures.

Pedersen PB and others, editors: *Counseling across cultures*, Honolulu, 1981, University of Hawaii Press.

This book is an edited volume of articles that deal with a variety of aspects of cross-cultural mental health. Specific chapters address issues concerning racial and ethnic barriers in counseling, themes and approaches in cross-cultural counseling, and special considerations for working with the following minority clients: foreign students, Native Americans, Asian-Americans, and Chicano college students.

Sue D: *Counseling the culturally different: theory and practice*, New York, 1981, John Wiley & Sons.

This book presents a more unified approach to cross-cultural counseling. The book is divided into three parts. Part One deals with broad concepts and theoretical foundations that serve as a base for counseling minority clients. It covers politics of counseling, barriers to effective cross-cultural counseling, value differences between health professionals and clients, and issues such as whether a counselor who is culturally different can work effectively with a minority client. Part Two focuses on issues and techniques when working with specific ethnic populations including Asian-Americans, blacks, Hispanics, and Native Americans. Part Three presents a series of case studies depicting a variety of cross-cultural counseling situations. These vignettes reveal how traditional mental health approaches may be at odds with cultural values and suggest alternative ways of dealing with the critical incident.

PART II

Behavioral Concepts

Part II focuses on concepts that represent commonly seen behavioral patterns in mental health and illness. Each chapter includes a discussion of the medical and nursing diagnoses related to the behaviors. Manifestations of the behaviors within each of the five dimensions of the person are presented, with the focus on both the healthy and the unhealthy aspects of the behavior. Using the five dimensions of the person—physical, emotional, intellectual, social, and spiritual—as an organizing framework, the five-step nursing process is applied. Tools for measuring behaviors are presented. Each chapter includes key interventions for each behavior, current research as it relates to the specific behavior, and guidelines for primary/tertiary prevention.

Chapter 10, Anxiety, provides the groundwork for understanding the behavior of clients, as it is the primary emotion from which most other emotions are generated. Anger, guilt, and loss are discussed in Chapters 11, 12, and 13. The next four chapters, Hope-Hopelessness, Flexibility-Rigidity, Dependence-Independence, and Trust-Mistrust (Chapters 14 to 17) describe behaviors on a continuum. Chapters 18 and 19 examine addictive and somatizing behaviors.

Part II concludes with a discussion of pain, loneliness, boredom, and manipulation (Chapters 20 to 23), behaviors often seen in inpatient and clinical settings today.

The behavioral and holistic approach to the organization of basic content is intended to provide the student with a foundation for understanding mental health–psychiatric nursing and for intervening therapeutically with clients using theory as a base for practice.

CHAPTER 10 Anxiety

Margery Menges Chisholm

After studying this chapter, the student will be able to:

- Define anxiety
- Trace the historical perspectives of anxiety
- Describe theories of anxiety
- Use the nursing process in caring for anxious clients
- Identify current research findings related to anxiety
- Discuss the psychopathology of selected anxiety disorders as described in the DSM-III-R

The term *anxiety* conjures up images of someone pacing the floor and wringing his hands, with pounding heart and rapid breathing. Personal descriptions include a feeling of uneasiness, "weak knees," a queasy feeling in the stomach, and lightheadedness. Popular use of the term also refers to anticipation of dreaded possibilities. Words such as *worry, care, concern,* and *solicitude* are often associated with the term anxiety.

Anxiety can also have a positive meaning implying eagerness. Being anxious can enhance experiences such as performing a piano recital or completing a final term paper. Anxiety is a healthy response to novel, unique, and unfamiliar experiences. Being slightly anxious initiates a heightened state of perceptual, emotional, and physiological arousal. These responses increase the person's perception and performance and enhance learning, problem solving, satisfaction, and pleasure. Healthy anxiety is a cue to the person to attend to himself and his environment. If anxiety is accepted as a signaling response, it c n motivate the individual to engage in coping strategies. Just as pain is a cue and response to physical danger, anxiety can serve as a cue and response to emotional, social, and spiritual danger. Mental health is enhanced by appreciating the importance of anxiety as a normal, facilitating response to initiate coping strategies. If anxiety is viewed and accepted as a personal resource, it can provoke movement toward self-actualization.

Anxiety often occurs as a response to life stressors of a personal and financial nature, such as divorce or loss of a job, and to changes in home and living environments, such as hospitalization, geographical relocation, and natural disasters.

An individual may be uncomfortable with the sensations accompanying anxiety in these situations. If he wishes to avoid the feeling altogether, he may engage in unhealthy practices. Unfortunately, our society has encouraged the use of certain substances, such as drugs, alcohol, and even medications, as aids to remove, extinguish, or cover up unpleasant feelings. When healthy coping strategies are ineffective or even culturally discouraged as means for adjusting to anxious feelings, the person's development of unhealthy responses can lead to illness. Agoraphobia, simple and social phobias, post-traumatic stress disorder, sleep disorders, and depersonalization responses are medical diagnoses pertaining to unhealthy coping responses to anxieties.

Anxiety has objective and subjective qualities. One's previous subjective experience with anxiety provides a basis

▶ DIAGNOSES Related to Anxiety

MEDICAL DIAGNOSES	NURSING DIAGNOSES
Agoraphobia	**NANDA**
Simple phobia	
Social phobia	Anxiety
Post-traumatic stress dis-	Sleep pattern disturbance
order	Post-trauma response
Sleep disorders	
Depersonalization	**PMH**
Psychophysiological disorders	Anxiety
	Altered sleep/arousal patterns
	Altered abuse response

	DATES	EVENTS
HISTORICAL OVERVIEW	Pre-1900s	In early Greek literature responses to anxiety were described as accepting fate, appealing to a higher being, or stoicism.
		During the Middle Ages emphasis was placed on the identification and categorization of emotions. Anxiety was identified as a disagreeable feeling.
		The use of reason to control anxiety, which led to denial and repression, was emphasized during the Renaissance.
	1900	Kierkegaard described the direct confrontation of anxiety as a way to open possibilities of freedom and self-development.
		Freud identified anxiety as central to the development of the personality.
	1950s	Peplau linked nursing actions directly to the security of clients. She developed a theory of anxiety characterized by levels of anxiety that ranged from mild to panic levels.
	1960s	The twentieth century is described as the "age of anxiety" because of the advent of the atom bomb and other profound, anxiety producing situations, such as economic insecurity, nuclear warfare, political upheaval, and changing values and standards of behaviors related to family, church, and school.
	1980s	Nursing today emphasizes the relationship between anxiety and physical conditions such as heart attacks, ulcers, hypertension, pregnancy, and response to accidents and surgical procedures. Additional emphasis is placed on the effect of anxiety on clients' ability to receive information and to learn.
	Future	Sharper diagnostic categorization of anxiety disorders through continued investigation and the rapid discovery of new medications to treat anxiety will require the nurse to keep current with these advances and incorporate them into her practice.

for understanding the anxious client. Objective signs and symptoms displayed by the client also become important areas of nursing observation.

Anxiety differs from *fear*. Fear is viewed as more specific, having a definite referent, and capable of being contained through reasoned action. Anxiety originates from an uncertain source or cause and can border on the nonrational. In contemporary thinking, anxiety is viewed as the condition of a person's existence and as a continual experience that cannot be easily denied or defended against.

DSM-III-R DIAGNOSES

The DSM-III-R indicates that Anxiety Disorders are those most frequently found in the general population, with *Simple Phobia* the most commonly occurring and Panic Disorder the most common Anxiety Disorder in those people seeking treatment. Avoidance behaviors usually develop as a form of coping or mastery of the fears.

Agoraphobia, one type of anxiety disorder, is an intense fear of being in public places such as busy streets, stores, elevators, or crowds, from which escape may be difficult or help may not be available. Agoraphobia may be mild, moderate, or severe. When mild, some avoidance occurs, but the person maintains a relatively normal life-style (e.g., travels alone when necessary [to work, shop] but otherwise avoids travel). Those with moderate agoraphobia constrict their life-style. They may leave the house only when accompanied by another person. Those with severe agora-

phobia remain completely housebound. The disorder most commonly begins during the person's twenties or thirties. It is more common in women and persists for years.

Simple phobia is characterized by a fear of a particular object or situation. The most common of the simple phobias involves animals, particularly dogs, snakes, and mice; closed spaces; heights; and air travel. The fear significantly interferes with the person's usual routine, with social activities, and with relationships with others. There is marked distress about having the fear. At the same time, the person recognizes that the fear is excessive and unreasonable. Table 10-1 lists some of the most common phobias.

Psychophysiological disorders can be viewed as a group of illnesses in which the dominant feature is emotional maladaptation that leads to irreversible organ or tissue damage. The emotional disorder leaves the person vulnerable to severe physiological dysfunction. These disorders differ from the commonly occurring response of increased susceptibility to illness as a result of an emotional upset and from the emotional turmoil resulting as a reaction to disease.

An example of a psychophysiological disorder is the proneness of some clients to migraine headaches. Usually the client is aware of high stress in his life but is unable to divert the onset of the aura and painful throbbing, which are symptoms of the migraine response. The headache and its aftermath produce intense physical responses and a groggy, hangover feeling. Other clients when stressed emotionally may develop a psychophysiological skin response,

▼ **TABLE 10-1**   **Clinical Names of Some Phobias and Their Meanings**

Name	Meaning (Fear of . . .)
Acrophobia	Height
Agoraphobia	Open spaces
Ailurophobia	Cats
Anthophobia	Flowers
Anthropophobia	People
Aquaphobia	Water
Arachnophobia	Spiders
Astraphobia	Lightning
Brontophobia	Thunder
Claustrophobia	Closed spaces
Cynophobia	Dogs
Dementophobia	Insanity
Equinophobia	Horses
Herpetophobia	Lizards, reptiles
Mikophobia	Germs
Murophobia	Mice
Mysophobia	Dirt, germs, contamination
Numerophobia	Number
Nyctophobia	Darkness
Ophidiophobia	Snakes
Pyrophobia	Fire
Thanatophobia	Death
Trichophobia	Hair
Xenophobia	Stranger
Zoophobia	Animal

such as "hives" in which welts and intense itching occupy the person's attention while the life stressors continue.

A hypochondriacal response differs from psychophysiological reactions and may occur as a response to anxiety. The client's excessive anxiety is displaced from its unconscious origins to one or more body organs that become the center of preoccupation. Frequent complaints include insomnia, irritability, and alternating aches and pains. The client with a hypochondriacal response focuses on these body sensations, which are often unique to the anxious state. The worry and preoccupation distract the client's attention from unpleasant anxiety-producing feelings (see Chapter 19).

Social phobia is a fear of humiliation or embarrassment in certain social situations. Exposure to the feared conditions causes an anxiety attack. Many phobias begin in childhood or early adulthood. Some phobias, such as fear of heights, driving, closed spaces, and air travel, begin most frequently in the fourth decade of life. The phobias occur most frequently in women.

The essential feature of post-traumatic stress disorder is the reexperiencing of symptoms of distress after a psychologically traumatic event. The event is usually outside the range of common human experience and may be experienced alone (rape or assault) or with groups of people (military combat or natural disasters). The characteristic symptoms involve a numbing of general responsiveness, increased arousal, and avoidance of stimuli associated with the event. The disorder can occur at any age and impairment can affect all areas of life.

Sleep disorders are divided into two major subgroups: those involving a disturbance in amount quality or timing of sleep (dyssomnia) and those involving excessive daytime sleepiness or sleep attacks (hypersomnia). Sleep disorders are more common in persons with increased levels of stress and those who seem to lack awareness of their own emotions. Insomnia often occurs in other mental and physical disorders and occurs in about 15% of the population. It can begin at any age, but appears more frequently with advancing age.

Hypersomnia occurs in 1% to 2% of the population and is more common among biological relatives of persons with these disorders. Sleep attacks can occur at any time and the person can suffer from sleep drunkenness during which he requires a prolonged transition from sleep to be fully alert and oriented.

Depersonalization disorder is characterized by an experience of feeling detached from one's body or mental processes. The person feels like an automaton, as if in a dream, and as if outside himself as an observer. The experience is very distressing to the person; however, reality testing remains intact. The disorder usually begins in adolescence and early adult life. Severe stress may predispose a person to this mental disorder, and the symptoms recur when there is mild anxiety or depression. Brief episodes are fairly common, with as many as 70% of young adults experiencing them at some time.

THEORETICAL APPROACHES

The theoretical definitions of anxiety are wide ranging, but generally theorists recognize the uneasiness that is experienced and make distinctions in terms of the source of the anxiety (internal or external), the process or dynamics of the feeling, the signs and symptoms of the feeling, and the appropriate intervention to relieve the anxious condition. In various theoretical perspectives, anxiety is viewed as a normal aspect of the developing personality when one is exposed to new situations. Anxiety is the key concept in various theories of personality and behavior and in the determination of illness arising from stressors in all dimensions of the individual.

Biological

Anxiety is the uneasy, uncomfortable feeling aroused by a threat or danger and is accompanied by physiological symptoms. This response prepares the person for anticipatory fight or flight. The fight response to anxiety (sympathetic stimulation) causes a variety of physiological reactions primarily due to changes in the cardiovascular and neuroendocrine systems (see Chapter 4). During the flight response (parasympathetic stimulation), as occurs in acute fear states, an effort is made to conserve body resources.

Several other explanations suggest a biological basis for anxiety; however, more specific information about the highly complex aspect of brain functioning is needed before conclusive evidence can be determined. Evidence increasingly points to the metabolism of the monamines and the function of the limbic system as being central to the expression of emotions such as anxiety. The discovery of the benefits of the benzodiazepines for chronic anxiety and of the tricyclics and the monamine oxidase inhibitors (MAOIs) for panic attacks contributed to the division of anxiety into two different components mediated by different underlying neuronal mechanisms. Further clinical observations suggest that panic anxiety is closely related to a disruption of a relationship that provides nurturance and support. The anxiety resulting from such a disruption is based on innate biological mechanisms that preserve the life-sustaining relationship. This innate biological alarm mechanism may indicate that some individuals, whether as a result of a genetic factor or adverse early life experiences, react unduly to environmental stimulation.

Other clinical evidence suggests that lactate metabolism has implications for anxiety. Experimental studies demonstrated that the infusion of sodium lactate in persons suffering from panic anxiety induces anxiety attacks; clients whose panic disorder is controlled by MAOIs are protected from experiencing panic attacks following lactate infusion.[39]

Research has indicated a genetic predisposition for anxiety neurosis. Some identical twins with anxiety neurosis have been found to have the same diagnosis and marked anxiety traits.[17] Some persons with anxiety neurosis have a previous family history of anxiety.[24]

Psychoanalytical

This theoretical orientation to anxiety is based on a psychodynamic explanation of its etiology. Within this framework anxiety represents a person's struggle with the demands and prohibitions in his environment. It also arises from an internal struggle among the person's instinctual drives (id), the realistic assessment of the possibility for need fulfillment (ego), and the person's conscience (superego).

Anxiety is a signal of the ego that an unacceptable drive is pressing for conscious discharge. It alerts the ego to take defensive action against the pressures of the drive because the person fears that its expression will lead to forbidden and unacceptable actions. A conflict results between the drive, usually of a sexual or aggressive nature, and fear of punishment or disapproval arising as a consequence of its expression. The feared punishment may be an actual threat in the environment (parents will spank the child) or a fear of retribution from one's conscience (felt as guilt, self-doubt, and self-reproach).

The environment provides the means for the person to fulfill biologically driven needs for food, water, shelter, and sexual expression. These resources become the means for reducing tension and providing pleasure. The environment also confronts the individual with danger and insecurity and can threaten and disturb as well as provide satisfaction of needs. Repression of the unacceptable drive generally results in restoring emotional equilibrium. When repression is not effective, *defense mechanisms* are called into play to reduce the anxiety. If the defense mechanisms are successful the anxiety is dispelled or safely contained.

The significance and meaning of anxiety depend on the nature of the underlying conflict. The conflict may be a legacy of the individual's experiences during early stages of growth and development. Stimulation from the adult environment activates the conflict.

Phobias are fears that are disproportionate to the demands of the situation and cannot be explained or reasoned away. A phobia leads to avoidance of the feared situation. The phobic stimulus produces profound feelings that reach panic proportions, with physiological symptoms such as palpitations, sweating, rapid breathing, diarrhea, and urinary frequency.

According to psychoanalytical theory, phobias originate in the oral stage of development. Intense conflicts give rise to basic impulses that need to be repressed and denied conscious expression. As repression fails, the original source of the anxiety is displaced to some other object, person, or situation. This source of anxiety may be only loosely or indirectly related to the original conflict. *Displacement* is an essential dynamic in phobias. Displacement allows conscious impulses such as forbidden, aggressive, or sexual needs to be denied in the self and placed on other objects or persons. Displacement thus eliminates awareness of the relationship between the self and the forbidden impulse. If displacement does not succeed in binding all of the anxiety, the range of fears may increase so that more phobias appear or more complicated defenses are enlisted.

Freud's classic case of Little Hans typifies the dynamics of displacement. Freud treated a 5-year-old boy for a phobia of horses. The boy's fear of his father was displaced to horses, a symbolic object that he could avoid. Freud determined that Hans' aggressive feelings toward his parents, especially his father, were repressed, resulting in a mental conflict that emerged as a fear of horses.

Several different forms of anxiety described by Freud are listed in the box on p. 186.

Interpersonal

Interpersonal theorists believe that anxiety arises from experiences in relationships with significant others throughout a person's development. The child develops a sense of his worth and security through positive exchanges with others.

If the child is treated malevolently or is mystified by or not encouraged in his own uniqueness, the foundation is laid for the child to become basically insecure and anxious in future interpersonal situations.

Karen Horney and Harry Stack Sullivan share the beliefs that (1) social interaction is imperative in human development, (2) the origin of anxiety lies in interaction with others, and (3) the development of a self-system serves to provide security and to protect the person from anxiety.

Horney[18] believed that multiple adverse factors in the environment can produce insecurity in the developing child, resulting in basic anxiety. Basic anxiety is a profound insecurity and vague apprehensiveness. Because the world is viewed as hostile, the pressure from basic anxiety prevents children from relating spontaneously. The child is forced to find ways to relate to others that can allay basic anxiety. In doing so, the child develops coping strategies: moving toward other people for fulfillment of dependency needs, moving away from other people because of the need for independence, and moving against people in response to the need for power.[18]

As the child matures these strategies become an aspect of the personality style of the adult. The learned behaviors

▼ FORMS OF ANXIETY DESCRIBED BY FREUD

Primary anxiety	The sudden stimulation and trauma of birth is the first experience of anxiety. The environment is perceived as threatening, and this threat predisposes the person to anxiety later in life.
Subsequent anxiety	Emotional conflicts depend on the maturation of the ego and superego. As the ego develops it protects the individual from instinctual demands of the id, from attack and frustration by the external world, and from rebuke by the superego.
Reality anxiety	Often equated with fear and is based on the perception of danger in the environment. Either some important object is absent or the person's existence is threatened.
Neurotic anxiety	Arises when the perception of danger is from the instincts of the id. The anxiety is based on the fear that the ego is unable to prevent an instinctual urge from getting out of control and that the person will engage in acts for which he will be punished. The ego then resorts to maladaptive defense maneuvers.
Free-floating anxiety	A type of neurotic anxiety characterized by general apprehensiveness and pessimism.
Phobic anxiety	A type of neurotic anxiety that is an intense reaction to fear of some object that can be avoided.
Panic state	A type of neurotic anxiety accompanied by acute anxiety, intense physiological arousal, and disorganization of personality and functional abilities.
Moral anxiety	Fear of the superego; danger to the ego coming from the superego is experienced as guilt or shame. The ego is punished for doing or thinking something that is contrary to the parental standard or moral code.
Castration anxiety	Refers to a variety of anxieties having in common a fear of bodily damage or of some kind of diminution of one's capacities. Confusion about sexual identity is often associated with castration anxiety.
Separation anxiety	Represents the fearful anticipation of the loss of a significant person.

to allay anxiety when relating to others become the basis for inner conflict when needs for security continue to be unmet. Normally, a person can resolve these conflicts between unmet needs and the learned strategies complicating their attainment; however, the neurotic person develops irrational solutions because of intense basic anxiety. The neurotic person creates an idealized, unrealistic self-image and attempts to live up to it. His pride reinforces the basic anxiety and leads him to overvalue other people (to help to maintain the idealized image) and to feel hatred or contempt for himself. Basic anxiety and the resulting conflicts can be avoided if the child is raised in security, respect, warmth, and love.

Sullivan[50] makes distinctions among several states of anxiety (Table 10-2). He believes that severe anxiety produces confusion and forgetfulness and inhibits learning. Less severe anxiety or mild anxiety promotes learning. Although fear and anxiety may be experienced in much the same way, Sullivan makes a distinction between these two states. Fear results from tension arising from the danger of actual physical harm. It is an adaptive response that heightens the individual's sensitivity, resulting in increased alertness and

▼ TABLE 10-2   Sullivan's States of Anxiety

State	Description
Primitive	A fearlike state induced by the anxiousness of the mothering person
Mild	An uneasy, uncomfortable state commonly occurring in interpersonal relationships
Severe	State in which the individual negates aspects of himself and attunes to disapproving comments from important people

increased energy available for bodily responses for self-preservation. Anxiety, on the other hand, arises from threats to personal security.

Sullivan believes that all human behavior is oriented toward the pursuit of satisfaction and security. The attainment of satisfaction is closely related to the physical needs of the human body and includes meeting the needs for sleep, food, and sexual fulfillment. The feeling of security arises from fulfillment of these biological needs according to culturally approved patterns. An individual experiences intense and painful uneasiness, insecurity, and anxiousness when he meets his needs through culturally disapproved means.

Rank[45] believes that the central problem in human development is individuation and the repeated separations that occur throughout a person's life. Each separation creates not only greater independence for the person, but also increases anxiety when conditions of relative security and unity are disrupted. In Rank's view, anxiety is also experienced when the individual refuses to be separated, thus threatening the development of autonomy. There is the continually revolving dilemma of fear of becoming an individual and fear of losing individuality. This view is poignantly represented in adolescent struggles with authority.

Adler[2] suggests that anxiety arises from feelings of inferiority. In his view, anxiety provides the means for adopting a helpless stance and the basis for avoiding decisions and responsibility. In addition, anxiety can be an aggressive weapon or a means of dominating others. This use of anxiety provides a means of controlling others in an attempt to rid oneself of basic feelings of inferiority. For example, a child has anxiety attacks as a means of controlling his parent and decreasing his feelings of inferiority.

Learning-Behavioral

In the learning theorist's view, anxiety can motivate behavior. For example, if a student is anxious about the consequences of failing a test, the anxiety may motivate studying behavior. Anxiety may also be a response to an unpleasant experience; for example, a child who has touched a stove and been burned becomes anxious about exposure to hot objects. Anxiety also may be the predominant feeling accompanying a behavioral sequence. For example, a person who wants to stop smoking may become very anxious when reaching for a cigarette.

In this theory, the development of fear and anxiety as learned drives are based on the primary drive of pain. Dollard and Miller[7] believe that fear and anxiety are learned because (1) neutral cues can evoke feelings associated with pain, (2) fear and anxiety can motivate the person to avoidance behavior, and (3) fear and anxiety can reinforce behavior because their reduction prompts similar behavioral responses to eliminate pain in the future. An example is a child's fearful response to receiving injections. Originally the needle is a neutral cue, but after the first injection the child's behavior alters. The sight of the needle (stimulus cue), previously associated with pain (innate drive) and now fear (learned drive), evokes crying, running, or combative behavior (responses) that serve to reduce fear (reinforcement). If the behavior is successful, the learned response becomes a learned drive as well, and the child will habitually experience fear and engage in avoidance thoughts or actions at the sight of a needle.

Conflicts occur when a stimulus evokes competing behavioral reactions (Table 10-3). The stimulus cue may evoke tendencies for the individual to engage in behaviors that involve incompatible and mutually exclusive goals. The ensuing conflicts may involve two positive goals, two undesirable goals, a desire to obtain and avoid a single goal, or a tendency to see desirable and undesirable aspects of two alternative goals.

Dollard and Miller[7] identify four basic assumptions in analyzing conflict behavior: (1) the nearer a person is to a goal, the stronger the tendency to approach it, (2) the nearer a person is to a feared goal, the stronger the tendency to avoid it, (3) avoidance desires increase more rapidly nearer the goal than do approach desires, and (4) whether the tendency to avoid or approach is stronger depends on the strength of the drive. For example, a very hungry man may approach dangerous situations more readily to fulfill this drive.

Dollard and Miller[7] believe that the resolution of conflicts may produce several outcomes. The individual usually makes choices easily between desirable alternatives and can resolve avoidance conflicts by escape or by lessening the negative aspects of one of the choices. Approach to avoidance conflicts appear to cause the greatest indecision and ensuing anxiety. When a person is far from the goal, the tendency to approach is stronger. As the goal is approached, the avoidance desires increase and the person is immobilized by the indecision evoked by the competing tendencies. For example, a child feels hungry and sees a cookie jar. As he approaches the container he remembers that he is not allowed to eat cookies before meals. The child may stop movement toward the cookies because his desire to eat cookies and to please his mother are equally strong; he is indecisive. Should he satisfy himself and risk punishment? He can talk himself into taking the cookies anyway, feeling he deserves them and thus increasing the approach tendencies, or he may try to reduce his fear of punishment by asking permission and negating avoidance tendencies. He may also develop symptoms, such as a stomachache, that would protect him from the original conflict. Usually resolving the conflict through increasing one's motivation to approach the goal ("I'll take the cookies anyway") results in increased anxiety. Attempts to reduce the avoidance tendencies, the fearful aspects of the situation, usually result in less painful alternatives.

Existential

According to existentialist writers, anxiety is a fact of life. It arises from being situated or thrust into the world as a finite being who is faced with eventual death or nothingness. Anxiety is a continuous, underlying current throughout life. Anxiety becomes more evident in situations such as confrontation with one's values, freedom and authority, other persons, one's need to be authentic, and impending death.

May[35] defined anxiety as apprehension caused by a threat to some value that an individual holds essential to his existence. Situations that precipitate anxiety usually involve choice. Individuals choose what they value. This freedom to choose can precipitate anxiety because of the possibility of choosing unwisely or erring in one's choices.

Consideration of others is important in making choices. Tension between personal freedom and commitment to the group or social context of one's life can cause anxiety. To become oriented primarily to the group may mean the individual becomes inauthentic or loses the self. The anxiety arising from an inauthentic existence comes from the inability to face and accept oneself. Ultimately, the greatest anxiety comes from the threat of nothingness, death, and the realization of life's limitations.

Table 10-4 reviews the main theories of anxiety, illustrating the meanings attached to its causes as well as the different dynamics involved. These theories orient the nurse to differing observational data and suggest a variety of models for nursing intervention for anxiety states.

▼ **TABLE 10-3**   **Behavioral Reactions to Conflict**

Conflict	Reactions
Approach to approach	The individual is motivated to pursue two equally desirable but incompatible goals
Approach to avoidance	The person wishes, at once, to obtain and avoid a goal
Avoidance to avoidance	The person must choose between two undesirable goals
Double approach to avoidance	The person sees the desirable and undesirable aspects of either alternative (ambivalence)

▼ **TABLE 10-4**   **Theories of Anxiety**

Theorist	Types of Anxiety	Source of Anxiety	Dynamics	Observational Cues	Nurse's Role in Anxiety
INTRAPSYCHIC					
Freud	Developmental anxiety Primary Subsequent Ego anxiety Realistic Neurotic Moral	Ego overwhelmed by excessive stimulation; biological and instinctual needs paramount	Development of defensive mechanisms— unconscious maneuvers related to repression of instinctual demands	Development of symptoms	Sounding board or screen for projection of transference feelings
INTERPERSONAL					
Horney	Basic anxiety	Hostile environment	Development of coping strategies and idealized self-image	Patterns of behavior in relation to others	Passive participant in experience; a source of support and approval
Sullivan	Primitive anxiety Mild anxiety Severe anxiety Fear	Interpersonal relations and fear of disapproval by significant others	Development of security operations	Areas of vulnerability in interpersonal relations	Reflective participant-observer in experience of anxiety to provide security base
LEARNING-BEHAVIORAL					
Dollard and Miller	Fear Anxiety	Learned drive acquired by association with a primary drive	Development of strategies in response to conflict	Antecedent environmental stimulus; consequent behavioral response	Active reinforcer; model of response options, cognitive reframer
EXISTENTIAL					
Kierkegaard and May	Lived anxiety (normal and basic)	Conditions of life; threat of nothingness; threats to something valued	Development of accepting attitude, leading to authenticity, freedom, and taking responsibility for one's choices; or nonaccepting attitude, leading to inauthenticity and despair	Inability to live with uncertainty or ambiguity, to flee situation; refusal to actively participate	Active participant in dialogue regarding fears, uncertainties, and values; makes assessment of life review and encourager of client decision making

NURSING PROCESS

Assessment

An assessment of the level of a person's anxiety is a priority in working with anxious clients (Table 10-5). The nurse collects data about the duration, intensity, and appropriateness of the anxiety and also attends to its progression from one level to another. Because anxiety interacts with other dimensions of the person, the physical, intellectual, and social responses are also included in the assessment.

Physical dimension   Clients experiencing anxiety can be assessed in three primary systems: musculoskeletal, cardiovascular, and gastrointestinal. Table 10-6 lists characteristics of responses in each system.

There may also be a direct relationship between the increase in physiological responses to anxiety and the intensity of a person's emotional state. For example, in a client experiencing a significant loss, physiological responses— such as flushing; irritability; headache; and fastidiousness about his surroundings, clothing, and other personal items—are used to distract attention from any concerns or anxious feeling. If the source of stress continues or increases, additional symptoms may emerge as the client's threshold for anxiety continues to be tested. More prolonged and intense physiological arousal due to anxiety can lead to difficulty sleeping, dilated pupils, and urinary urgency and frequency.

Clients may exhibit a particular sequence of symptoms in stressful situations.[28] Knowledge of the client's symptom pattern is helpful in planning interventions. If the symptom

▼ TABLE 10-5   Levels of Anxiety

Severity of Anxiety	Physical	Intellectual	Social and Emotional
Minimal (near 0)	Basal levels of: Blood pressure Pulse Respiration rate O_2 consumption Pupillary constriction Muscles relaxed; little or no resistance to passive range of motion	Cognitive activity minimal Disregard for external environmental stimuli; no attempt to actively process information Focus typically on single, nonthreatening mental image States of altered consciousness	No social interaction No attempt to deal with environmental stimuli Minimal emotional activity Feelings of indifference, invulnerability, and contentment prevail
Mild (+1)	Low-level sympathetic arousal Moderate to low skeletal muscle tension Body relaxed; movements smooth, directed, and purposeful Makes and holds eye contact easily Voice calm, well-modulated	Perceptual field open; able to shift focus of attention readily Passively aware of external environment Self-referent thoughts positive; low concern for unexpected or negative outcomes	Behavior primarily automatic; habitual patterns and well-learned skills Positive feeling of security, confidence, and satisfaction dominate Solitary activities
Moderate (+2)	Sympathetic nervous system activation ↑ Blood pressure ↑ Pulse rate ↑ Respiratory rate Pupillary dilation Sweat glands stimulated Peripheral vascular constriction Increased muscular tension, mixed sense of tension and excitement; may experience "jitters" Heightened performance of well-learned skills Voice suggests interest and concern with problem analysis; rate of speech increased, pitch heightened Increased alertness	Narrowing of perception; attentional focus on specific internal or external stimuli Conscious effort in processing of information; optimal level for learning Self-referent thoughts ± mixed; some concern about personal ability or available resources necessary to solve problems; probability of positive outcomes increasingly uncertain	Increased skill in learning and refining of skills; analyzing problematic situations; integrating cognitive and motor domains Feelings of challenge; drive to resolve problems or dilemmas Mixed sense of confidence/ optimism with fear, lowered self-esteem, and potential inadequacy
Severe (+3)	Fight-flight response Generalized sympathetic nervous system discharge Stimulation of adrenal medulla ↑ Catecholamines, accelerated heart rate, palpitations ↑ Blood glucose ↓ Blood flow to digestive system ↑ Blood flow to skeletal muscles Muscles extremely tense, rigid, fixed Hyperventilation Physical actions increasingly agitated, random, and disorganized; pacing, wringing of hands quivering, fidgeting, trembling, immobilization	Perceptual capacity restricted; exclusive attention to singular stimuli (internal or external) or multifocal, fragmented processing of stimuli Problem solving inefficient, difficult Some threatening stimuli disregarded, minimized, denied Disorientation in terms of time and place Expected likelihood of negative consequences or outcomes high; estimates of personal self-efficacy low	Flight behavior may be manifested by withdrawal, denial, depression, somatization Feelings of increasing threat, need to respond to situation are heightened Dissociating tendency; feelings are denied

Modified from Longo D, Williams R: *Clinical practice in psychosocial nursing: assessment and intervention*, New York, 1986, Appleton-Century-Crofts.

Continued.

▼ **TABLE 10-5   Levels of Anxiety—cont'd**

Severity of Anxiety	Physical	Intellectual	Social and Emotional
	May experience loss of appetite, nausea, "cold sweats" Verbal effects: stammering, blocking, rapid, high-pitched speech, fragmented sentences, hesitations Facial expression: poor eye contact, fleeting eye movements; may fix gaze if preoccupied with internal thoughts; gnashing of teeth, jaw clenching		
Panic (+4)	Continued physiological arousal Actions disorganized, directionless; unable to execute simple motor tasks; fumbling, gross motor agitation, flailing May strike out verbally or physically; may attempt to withdraw from situation Eventual depletion of sympathetic neurotransmitters Blood redistributed throughout body Hypotension May feel dizzy, faint, or exhausted Appears pale, drawn, weary Facial expression: aghast, grimacing, eyebrows raised, mouth agape, eyes fixed; may hide face Voice louder, higher pitched; may ramble incessantly; may falter or be speechless; gasping	Perception severely restricted, may be impervious to external stimuli Thoughts are random, distorted, disconnected, logical processing impaired Unable to solve problems; limited tolerance for processing novel stimuli (verbal, auditory, or visual) Preoccupied with thoughts of highly probable negative outcomes; conclusion may be drawn, negative consequences seen as inevitable	Emotionally drained, overwhelmed Reliance on earlier, more "primitive" coping behaviors: crying, shouting, curling up, rocking, freezing Feelings of impotence, helplessness, agony and desperation dominate; may be experienced as horror, dread, defenselessness; may be converted to anger, rage

pattern of a particular client involves physical changes or develops into compulsive behavior the nurse may expect this same sequence of symptoms when the client experiences anxiety in the future.

Environmental stressors can precipitate or exacerbate the physiological symptoms of anxiety. These stressors include caffeine consumption, use of opium and hallucinogenic drugs, reaction to an epinephrine medication, loss of sleep, fatigue, premenstrual edema, poor nutrition and hypoglycemia, threats to body integrity as a result of surgery or injury, blood loss, hyperthyroidism, and hyperventilation.

Anxiety can appear after ingestion of 500 to 600 mg of caffeine, the equivalent of 5 or 6 cups of coffee. Caffeine can produce symptoms indistinguishable from anxiety, such as nervousness, irritability, agitation, tremors, rapid breathing, palpitations, and dysrhythmias. In addition, even a brief abstinence from caffeine by persons who are moderate users may produce anxiety. It is important to review the use of caffeine by anxious patients.[45] Foods high in caffeine include coffee, tea, cola drinks, cocoa, over-the-counter analgesics, stimulants, and appetite suppressants.

In summary, assessment of the physical dimension of the client includes identifying physiological symptoms in the musculoskeletal, cardiovascular, gastrointestinal, and other systems; compulsive behaviors; and environmental stressors.

Emotional dimension Although anxiety appears to be distinguished from other unpleasant affective states, such as anger, grief or despair, and guilt, it is closely related to these emotional experiences. Anxiety is a mixed feeling state and includes negative components (fear, distress, shame, shyness, guilt, and anger) and positive elements (interest and excitement). As illustrated in Figure 10-1, anxiety during test taking could be associated with guilt regarding poor preparation, despair related to memory recall, and/or interest and excitement related to doing well. The emotions associated with anxiety, such as anger, guilt,

▼ **TABLE 10-6**   **Physical Characteristics of Anxiety**

System	Characteristics
Musculoskeletal	Increased tendon reflexes
	Rigid, tense muscles
	Knee and ankle clonus
	Muscular tremors
	Increased generalized fatigue
	Increased weakness
	Clumsiness
	Jerking of limbs
	Tics
	Unsteady voice
	Tightening of throat
	Unsteadiness
	Inability to move
Cardiovascular	Palpitations
	Precordial pressure
	Throbbing sensations
	Increased pulse, respiration, blood pressure
	Flushing and heat sensations
	Cold hands and feet
	Sweating
Gastrointestinal	Nausea
	Belching
	Heartburn
	Cramps
	An "empty stomach" feeling
	Bad taste in mouth
Others	Difficulty sleeping
	Dilated pupils
	Urinary urgency
	Urinary frequency

and despair, are mentioned briefly here to illustrate the ways in which they differ from anxiety.

Guilt is closely tied to feelings of anxiety, whether one views it from the initial personality development of the child or in the treatment of emotional disturbances. According to psychoanalytical theory, during early development, prohibitions from the parents lead to hostility in the child who then feels guilty. It is difficult for the child to accept his anger; in attempts to repress it the child may develop self-derogatory feelings. Guilt is experienced as a feeling of unworthiness by someone who has violated the dictates of his conscience. As a person develops and the discrepancies between the actual and ideal self are increased, there is usually an increasing capacity for self-derogation, which can lead to increasing anxiety when the person sees himself as inadequate. A person who feels guilty usually has a desire for punishment as well as a fear of punishment. Guilt may be viewed as a form of anxiety and depression and involves a personal, self-oriented internal struggle. Anxiety in guilty states appears to be related most to the fear of punishment. Anxiety may also be an effect rather than a cause of guilt feelings. This effect is illustrated when a person attempts to repress guilt-provoking incidents or attitudes and begins to feel anxious. To the person with a guilty conscience, the physiological responses to guilt may feel the same as those to anxiety. These responses include heavier breathing, heaviness in the chest, muscular laxness, stooped posture, and slowed gait. A troubled conscience therefore has implications for the physical health of the individual. The relation of guilt to the genesis of anxiety and to the person's interpersonal world is important.

Shame as a component of guilt refers to the person's fear of being discovered unworthy; like guilt, shame can lead to avoidance of important interpersonal support. In Freud's view, guilt can be identified as moral anxiety.[12] Sullivan[50] identifies shame as social anxiety.

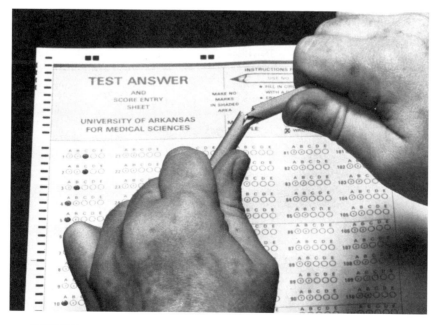

FIGURE 10-1 Anxiety during test taking is often expressed as seen in this illustration.

Grief is a response to the loss of some important resource for the satisfaction of one's needs. Psychoanalytical theorists describe the reactions of infants who were separated from their parents. Initially the child was seen as protesting and crying a great deal, followed within a week by withdrawal characterized by a sad facial expression and loss of interest in the environment. Separation is characteristically viewed as the precipitant to anxiety in the developing child; it quickly leads to anger and later to depression. A study of reactions of individuals to the loss of relatives in the 1942 Coconut Grove fire in Boston[33] noted the same response of initial disbelief and shock followed by insomnia, irritability, and loss of appetite. These studies help illustrate the intimate relationship between anger (as protest) and grief, which are often the sequelae of an intense anxiety producing life event. The dynamics of the loss of important loved objects can also be applied to the individual's loss of aspects of the self. For example, an important source of anxiety for combat soldiers is the threat of losing the self as a loved object through physical damage and injury.

Anxiety can be linked to the experience of sadness and fear. Throughout development the individual may tend to become afraid and want to escape instead of dealing with the source of sadness. This linking of sadness and anxiety can lead to panic reactions in response to pain, hypochondriasis, or lack of physical courage. The fear/sadness bind can prevent the person from empathizing and from sharing problems with others and can lead to denial of sickness, defeat, and loneliness.

According to interpersonal theorists, anger, as an emotion related to anxiety, appears to arise in interpersonal situations that are viewed as hostile and demanding and occurs as a protest in response to loss. Anger is a learned behavior in response to the authority of parents in punishing, prohibiting, and redirecting the child's behavioral strivings. As an adult the person may respond with anger if he feels that his personal authority has been violated. This anger response can be called forth by mild degrees of anxiety. Anger toward others becomes a way of coping with the feeling of uneasiness. Resentment develops in situations in which the person is punished when anger is displayed. The individual then learns to conceal his actual feelings, and the potential for the development of psychosomatic illnesses is seen. When anger is evoked in response to anx-

iety, the person may feel a surge of energy, heightened alertness and readiness for action, pounding heart, and generalized muscular tension. These reactions are similar to reactions in an anxiety episode and thus are not distinguishing features in themselves. There may be little actual change in the heart rate during anger, but both the diastolic and systolic blood pressure increase; the diastolic blood pressure does not appear to increase during a fear reaction. Additional changes during anger appear to be a decrease in blood flow to the skin and viscera and an increase in blood vessel constriction in the skin and skeletal muscles.

The preceding discussion of similarities in physiological expression of emotions and their independence from any particular source or stimulus indicates the need to individualize assessment of anxiety based on the client and the situation. A client's physiological reaction can change over time, representing either a greater emotional response or the signal that a client is in emotional transition and shifting from anxiety to anger, guilt, or depression, thus the nurse assesses these emotions, as they may indicate the presence of anxiety. Astute assessment is based on alertness to the process occurring over time. Table 10-7 provides a summary of the source, manifestations, physiological responses, and relation of anxiety to other emotions.

◥ **Intellectual dimension** Anxious persons are usually preoccupied by the anticipation of unpleasantness, although it is not occurring presently. There appear to be exceptions to this future time orientation in clients experiencing anxiety after involvement in traumatic situations such as combat, rape, or near avoidance of actual physical danger. However, using learning–behavioral theory, when the anxiety response recurs, the person, on recalling the event, appears to experience the trauma in the present through a flashback process.

Interference with realistic thinking can be readily observed in the anxious person, as reflected in (1) repetitive thinking or rumination about the danger; (2) reduction in the ability to reason and to evaluate and reappraise objectively one's thoughts (see the research highlight on abused women); (3) overreaction, psychologically and emotionally, to stimuli that are perceived as dangerous; (4) difficulty with short-term recall and blocking on words; (5) difficulty in concentrating on immediate tasks; and (6) hypervigilance to dangerous stimuli through constant scanning of

▼ **TABLE 10-7   Relationship of Anxiety to Other Emotions**

Source	Manifestation	Physiological Response	Relation to Anxiety
Guilt—violation of conscience	Feeling of unworthiness in relation to self	Parasympathetic response	Fear of punishment
Shame—disapproved action or wish exposed to others	Feeling of unworthiness in relation to others	Parasympathetic response	Fear of being discovered and disapproved
Grief—loss of loved object	Feeling of sadness, aloneness	Mixed sympathetic (in protest) and parasympathetic (weeping, depression) response	Fear of separation
Anger—hostile and demanding interpersonal situation	Feeling of frustration, resentment	Sympathetic response	Fear of control by authority

RESEARCH HIGHLIGHT

Self-Esteem and Anxiety: Key Issues in an Abused Women's Support Group
• ML Trimpey

PURPOSE

This descriptive study was conducted to determine the extent of high anxiety and low self-esteem in abused women participating in a support group. The levels of reported self-esteem and anxiety facilitate the designing of group activities to meet the needs of the members. Interventions to increase self-esteem and lower anxiety are proposed.

SAMPLE

1. Subjects consisted of 36 new members.
2. Recruitment of subjects occurred during a 5-month period during which each new member was asked to voluntarily participate. Subjects ranged in age from 20 to 69 years (mean age = 33.7). Fifteen women were married, 16 women were separated or divorced, and four were single. Eight women indicated they were still living with the abuser. Twelve women were employed full or part-time, whereas 18 reported incomes of $10,000 or less. Twelve subjects lived in the community and 25 subjects were residents in the shelter. The sample comprised women who actively sought out or were referred for services in a private agency for abused women.

METHODOLOGY

Data were collected at the end of the first group session. Each study participant was requested to complete an information sheet and two self-report questionnaires: the State Trait Anxiety Inventory (STAI) and the Culture Free Self-Esteem Inventories for Adults (CFSEI). The mean scores for the subject group on the Self-Esteem Inventory and State Trait Anxiety Inventory were calculated. The mean scores of the subjects were compared to the normed groups of working women, college women, and male patients with anxiety and depressive reactions. T-tests were used to explore group differences in state trait anxiety between abused women and the normed groups.

FINDINGS

The sample group self-esteem scores ranged from 6 to 30 out of a possible score of 32. The mean score of 16.12 (SD = 6.09) was in the eleventh percentile for women. The

Based on data from *Issues in Mental Health Nursing* 10:297, 1989.

scores of the subjects in this study indicated 35.2% of the women classified in the low self-esteem category and 41.1% in the very low category. This represents 26 women with low to very low self-esteem scores. Only three women had scores in the high self-esteem range.

The mean state trait anxiety scores for the sample of abused women were higher than the normed groups of working and college women and for male patients with depressed and anxious reactions. T-test analysis revealed significant difference ($P = 0.001$) between the anxiety mean scores of the abused women and working women, college women, and men with anxiety reactions. Nonsignificant difference was found between the scores of the abused group and depressed men.

IMPLICATIONS

Three fourths of the women in the study suffered from low self-esteem that may have preceded or resulted from the abuse or was a combination of preexisting and current life events. They also exhibited high trait anxiety, which may represent chronic and pervasive anxiety that results from living in an abusive situation. In planning support groups of abused women, an important goal becomes one of reducing state anxiety to a level where problem solving can occur. In addition self-esteem can be enhanced by introducing new ways of thinking about oneself, supplying new information, and increasing coping skills. These measures include the use of relaxation techniques and consciousness raising in regards to personal rights and choices. Information on the cycle of violence helps members understand the process of abuse and their own anxious responses. Support for independent choice in the decision to separate from the abusive spouse and reinforcement of positive contributions to others in the group through sharing knowledge, encouragement, and leadership contribute to self-esteem. Finally, encouragement to recognize negative personal statements and mental images and change them to positive assertive self-statements is important in helping an abused woman internalize a different, more positive sense of herself.

---

his surroundings. In addition, anxious persons who dwell on negative outcomes may see every situation as catastrophic; they assume that potential threats are actual threats. They are not able to discriminate, and the tendency to avoid the threat does not lead to increased confidence or ability to cope.

A person can attach dangerous meanings to the experience of anxiety itself. In this situation, a vicious cycle of escalation can occur. A threatening thought produces anxiety that causes the person to evaluate the situation as even more threatening, thus producing even more anxiety. Anxiety becomes a type of preoccupation characterized by increased self-awareness, self-doubt, and self-depreciation.

This preoccupation with self interferes with attention to environmental cues and information processing; the person may respond with irrelevant responses pertaining mainly to himself. The worry that arises from this self-focus interferes with problem solving because attention is diverted to emotionally demanding self-issues. Highly anxious clients appear to be nondiscriminatory in terms of the situations to which they respond with anxiety. For example, a client, overhearing nurses talking about a blood transfusion, assumes it is for him, even though he is scheduled to be discharged.

Highly anxious clients also experience difficulty in learning complex and difficult tasks. For example, a client who

▼ **TABLE 10-8   Defense Mechanisms**

Defense Mechanism	Purpose	Definition	Example
FIRST LEVEL: CONSCIOUS ATTEMPTS AT COPING			
Suppression	Helps keep forbidden drives and wishes out of one's conscience	Voluntary and intentional exclusion from conscious level of ideas, feelings, and situations that produce anxiety	A student receives a poor report card and "forgets" to give it to his parents
Substitution	Helps reduce frustration by disguising motivations	Replacement of an unacceptable need, attitude, or emotion with one that is more acceptable	A woman feels unattractive physically, so she puts her energy into sports and competitive trials
Rationalization	Helps raise self-esteem and social approval by disguising motivations	An attempt by the ego to make unacceptable feelings and behavior tolerable and acceptable	A nurse fails to do a procedure correctly and justifies her feeling of incompetence by stating that there is too much work on the ward
Fantasy	Provides a way to resolve conflict and meet needs in a symbolic way	A conscious creation or distortion of unacceptable fears, wishes, and behaviors	A nurse fails an important test and daydreams about her heroic attempts to save a client
SECOND LEVEL: CHARACTER DEVELOPMENT AS A WAY OF COPING			
Identification	Helps preserve the ego of the person while allowing concealment of inadequacies	An attempt to emulate oneself to resemble an admired, idealized person	A little girl dresses like her mother and mimics her behavior
Internalization or introjection	Attempts to deny or disguise by changing the ego to avoid threat	Assimilation (often symbolic) of loved or hated wishes, values, and attitudes	A child scolds his toys while playing, similar to the prohibitions of his parents
Restitution	Attempts to assuage guilt feelings by making reparation	Going back or attempting to resolve unconscious guilt feelings	A boss is short tempered with an employee and then gives her the rest of the afternoon off
THIRD LEVEL: REPRESSIVE ATTEMPTS AT COPING			
Compensation	Helps relieve fears of failure in one activity by emphasizing another can result in one-sidedness caused by over-compensation	An attempt to make up for real or imagined deficiences	A girl feels socially unattractive or inept, is responded to this way by peers, and becomes an honor student
Reaction formation	Serves as a protective device to prevent painful or unacceptable attitudes from being expressed	The assumption of attitudes, motives, and needs that are opposite those repudiated consciously	An adolescent struggles with hostile feelings, but presents herself in an ingratiating way
Sublimation	Helps channel forbidden instinctual impulses into constructive activities	Diversion of unacceptable instinctual drives into personally and socially accepted areas	A young man who struggles with rebellion against authority becomes a policeman who enforces law and order
Displacement	Helps the person disguise feelings by using a less threatening object to release feelings	Redirection of an emotional feeling from one idea, person, or object to another	A physician berates a nurse, and, when a visitor enters the client's room, the nurse harshly tells the person to wait for visiting hours
Projection	Helps the person avoid awareness of his undesirable impulses	Rejecting and imputing to others unpleasant aspects of oneself; attributing intolerable wishes, feelings, and motivations to others	A student suspects other classmates of being jealous of her good grades and thereby avoiding her
Symbolization	Serves to help compensate for and disguise true feelings	Disguisement of an object as a representation of a hidden idea	In a busy family, a child creates a picture of all family members on a Ferris wheel
Conversion	Channels and contains unbearable feelings through body expression	Symbolic expression of intrapsychic conflict through physical symptoms	A student develops headaches before taking an important test for which she feels unprepared

▼ **TABLE 10-8**   Defense Mechanisms—cont'd

Defense Mechanism	Purpose	Definition	Example
Repression	Helps provide a forgetting and protective function for the ego	Involuntary and automatic regulation of unbearable ideas and impulses; submersion of these to subconscious realm	After the recent death of a spouse the surviving spouse cannot remember the marriage date
Undoing	Disguises and attempts to repair feelings or actions that have led to anxiety or guilt	An attempt to actually or symbolically take away a previously intolerable action or experience	A mother who has just lost her temper and beaten her children develops compulsive hand-washing and child-checking behaviors
FOURTH LEVEL: REGRESSIVE ATTEMPTS AT COPING			
Denial	Helps the person escape unpleasant reality	Disownment of intolerable ideas and impulses; refusal to perceive conflict	A terminal cancer client appears not to be aware of impending death
Dissociation	Helps the person put painful feelings aside and isolate, compartmentalize them	Separation and detachment of emotional significance and affect from an idea or situation	A client relates a tale of victimization on the street in a matter-of-fact manner, even jokingly at times
Regression	Helps the person retreat from the present situation and become dependent and less anxious	Retreat to an earlier and more comfortable level of adjustment	A wife refuses to drive a car even though it causes the family much disorganization; her refusal necessitates that her husband take her everywhere

is learning diabetic care may appear unable to understand the steps in sterile technique or be unable to calculate dosages and insulin preparation.

Three conditions are necessary for anxiety to occur: (1) overstimulation by thoughts or by environmental cues, (2) expectations that are incompatible with abilities, and (3) inability to act. Anxiety continues because of this inability to engage in purposeful action. Indecision, conflict, and external restraint limit the person's behavioral options; make them unclear; and contribute to an anxious reaction.

Anxiety is precipitated by threatening external events occurring outside the person's control and by drives and impulses from within the person that threaten for expression. Anxiety that is aroused internally may evoke responses that are different from those caused by an external danger. When anxiety arises from a thought or internal cue, its reduction depends on avoidance of this thought or memory. According to psychoanalytical theorists, this avoidance need initiates a defense mechanism.

There are four levels of defense against anxiety. The first is considered normal and involves conscious efforts at controlling anxiety by changing the environment or one's perspective. The efforts directed toward *external* dangers may include removing oneself from stressful situations, indulging in substitute physical satisfactions, such as eating or sex, and engaging in social or recreational activities to divert one's attention from the external threat. These are examples of conscious coping strategies. The concept of defense mechanism refers to coping strategies used to confront the threat arising from dire thoughts and emotions *internal* to the person (Table 10-8). These include primarily substitutive strategies for needs such as daydreaming and fanta-

sizing, suppression of real needs through other activities, and disguising actions or motivations through rationalization. These are examples of normal first level defense mechanisms.

The second line of defense against internal anxiety involves character changes and development. Character development occurs through repetitive behaviors that provide a socially approved means of meeting ones needs. These coping strategies can become consistent behavioral styles (through which the person attempts to meet his needs). For example, through internalization of certain values and beliefs and imitation of idealized significant others, a person could become a follower of a religious group or a hard rocker. Either choice requires adherence to certain forms of personal expression and behavior as means for coping with anxiety arising in relationships. This level reflects the understanding of Horney's theory in which the individual adapts through a consistent behavior of moving against, toward, or away from others in relationships. These second line defenses often involve manipulation of relationships with others and may lead to personality disorders if prolonged or exaggerated and to difficulties in the interpersonal areas of work, marriage, and parenting.

The third line of defense comprises the repressive defenses, which involve further changes in the intrapsychic process. These repressive defenses fall into four main categories: (1) those aimed at keeping conflicting ideas out of one's awareness; (2) those aimed at inhibiting attention, concentration, conscious awareness, memory, emotions, sensory stimulation, and motor and visceral functioning; (3) defenses of displacement and phobic avoidance; and (4) undoing through compulsive rituals.

The fourth line of defense uses regressive defenses and involves a return to a state of helplessness, withdrawal from reality through psychotic maneuvers, internalization of hostility with suicidal thoughts, and acting out of repressed sexual or hostile impulses.

In summary, assessment of anxiety in the intellectual dimension includes the following:

1. Distorted or impaired thinking, e.g., ruminations, overreaction, preoccupation, difficulty problem solving
2. Difficulty learning, remembering
3. Evidence of flashbacks following a traumatic event
4. Evidence of conflict, indecision
5. Use of defense mechanisms

Social dimension Anxiety arising from social situations appears to be related to loss of self-esteem and affection and fears of rejection. Throughout the life cycle, physiological growth and decline precipitate changes in the person's social and emotional environments as well as presenting challenges for personal integration and adaptation.

From a developmental and psychoanalytical perspective, anxiety is essentially related to changes in individual and environmental expectations as the person develops. These changes can lead to anxiety because of uncertainty about the future. Generally, developmental anxiety refers to particularly stressful stages, such as the separation and stranger anxiety of the young infant and adolescent and death anxiety in the elderly. These stages, although normal, can precipitate anxiety and necessitate adaptive coping strategies. When coping leads to an alleviation of anxiety and fosters problem solving, successful development occurs. However, the transition stage can lead to unsuccessful coping, and clients may present with symptoms and delays in development and adaptation and require assistance in the form of individual or family counseling. When assessing an anxious person, it is important to consider normal life crises and transitions as possible sources of anxiety (see the research highlight on the next page).

Children often become anxious in response to a parent's anxiety. According to learning theorists, this learned response can be repeated later in life when the person identifies with and reacts to the emotional responses of another person.

Social anxiety refers to the discomfort experienced in the presence of others. This discomfort creates uncertainty regarding the scrutiny or remarks of others. Social anxiety is caused by specific characteristics of social situations as well as the behavior of others.

It is important for the nurse to assess social contexts that can cause anxiety for the client, such as (1) the number of persons present, (2) the amount of attention the client receives or expects to receive when in a large group, (3) familiarity with the persons present, (4) the degree of formality in the social exchange, and (5) the client's expectation of evaluation by others. Large groups of people and being the focus of attention make most individuals nervous. New people or situations as well as highly formal situations also tend to raise anxiety.

The nurse assesses the degree of attentiveness the client receives. Overattentiveness or underattentiveness by others can affect a person's social anxiety. Socially anxious persons may withdraw when they are ignored or receive less attention than anticipated. Statements that direct attention to the socially anxious person may induce shyness. Intrusions into the domain of another person, such as too much self-disclosure, overhearing private conversations, or witnessing private acts can also lead to social anxiety. Conspicuousness, novelty, disclosure, and fear of evaluation all contribute to the experience of social anxiety.

Sociocultural variables related to anxiety are important to consider during assessment. Women have scored higher than men in general anxiety, and the sex differences appear to be even more pronounced when considering women in lower socioeconomic and minority groups.[13] Similarly, lower-class children appear to be more anxious than middle-class children. In his study of Scandinavian countries, Kata[22] reported lower levels of anxiety in persons working in high prestige occupations; anxiety also decreased with an increase in family and individual income.

Other social stressors that can lead to anxiety include decreased self-esteem through job loss, change in social status through retirement, and loss of love relationships through death, separation, or divorce. In addition, unexpected events such as illness, changes in living conditions or financial status, loss of ability to care for oneself, and threats to independence increase anxiety. Highly anxious family members or significant others, a lack of supportive relationships, an inability to meet the expectations of important others, and nonacceptance by significant others of the person's emotional needs can also cause anxiety.

When a person has an organized, well-thought-out plan for dealing with an important aspect of his life and this plan is interrupted with no available alternative, helplessness and anxiety may result.[33] For example, an ailing elderly person desires to stay in his own home among familiar and important belongings and has made arrangements for a relative to visit and check on him daily. When the family moves out of town, the elderly client becomes extremely anxious and feels helpless, unable to focus on ways to maintain his independence.

Spiritual dimension The values one holds become important sources of support and self-definition. Throughout life, normal growth as well as crises provide the opportunity to assess values, to give up old ones, and to aspire to new ones. Relinquishing old values and the creativity needed to view things differently can generate anxiety.

Love requires giving as well as receiving and the autonomous, mature adult chooses, affirms, and participates in the experience of love. Anxiety can arise when the person is denied the opportunity to give love to a valued partner through separation of death.

Fear and guilt about the ethical nature of one's actions may also lead to anxiety. For example, a client, resenting his wife's anger and rejection of their son, may choose to have nothing to do with the son. The father experiences anxiety about this choice because he has strong beliefs about the value of parental support.

Using existential theory, the nurse is concerned with assessing the client's search for meaning in life and overcoming his alienation through communication with others. The client's capacity to respect his own individuality and uniqueness and that of others will help him face the normal anxieties of life and live with commitment, love, and hope.

Religious Behavior and Death Anxiety in Later Life

• HG Koenig

PURPOSE

This study was designed to examine the association between death anxiety and the use of (1) religious beliefs and prayer during stress, and (2) socially oriented behavior of religious community activity. The influence of both the intrapsychic cognitive behaviors (religious belief and prayer) and the more socially oriented behaviors (church attendance and involvement in a religious community) on death anxiety were studied separately and together in two age groups of elderly subjects. Involvement in nonreligious community activity as a coping response for death anxiety was also investigated. The study sought to discover association between these variables within sex and age groupings and to provide an exploratory approach to the coping behaviors of the elderly.

SAMPLE

The sample was chosen from 708 persons (aged 60 and over) attending senior lunch programs sponsored by the Missouri State Division of Aging. Seven communities in mid-Missouri were selected as sites for questionnaire distribution.

The study sample comprised two subsamples of seniors who participated in the lunch program. The subsamples consisted of 630 ambulatory lunch program participants and 78 homebound elderly to whom lunch was delivered. Study results were based on 263 (42%) of the ambulatory participants and 41 (53%) of the home bound participants. The over all response rate was 43%.

METHODOLOGY

No religious organizations were associated with any of the lunch programs included in the study. Lunch program staff members handled the distribution of the questionnaires at each site. A 26-item questionnaire assessed religious beliefs and activities, feelings about death, stress and coping levels, and health.

The variable "use of prayer and religious beliefs" (UPRB) was developed from scores addressing the use of these intrapsychic behaviors when facing a difficult situation and in coping with their most recent stressful experience.

Involvement in community activities was measured by questions addressing subject participation in general community activities and religious activities. A combined religious variable (CRB) was developed from these responses to questions addressing use of prayer and religious beliefs during difficult times and involvement in religious community activity.

The death anxiety variable was developed from responses to feelings about death, with a range of scores from "no fear or anxiety" to "fearful and anxious."

Subjects were also asked to provide a subjective health assessment ranging from "sick and disabled" to "very healthy, not disabled." They were also asked to assess the amount of stress in their lives and their ability to cope with it.

For purposes of anaylsis, the sample was dichotomized into two age groups: 60 to 74 years and 75 to 94 years. Possible associations between religious behaviors and feelings about death were explored for the entire sample and then among stratified subgroups based on age and sex.

Chi-square analysis was used to examine statistical significance, and Pearson's correlation was included to show the strength of association between variables.

Based on data from *The Hospice Journal* 4(1):3, 1988.

FINDINGS

1. When compared to the 1980 US Census of the elderly population of Missouri with respect to age, sex, race, and living situation and religious characteristics, the study population was moderately skewed toward older, white Protestant women of lower middle socioeconomic class who lived alone.

2. Little or no fear of death was reported by 84% of the sample.

3. Respondents who were very likely to use religious beliefs and prayers during stressful situations were significantly more likely to report low or no fear and death anxiety. Likewise, 59.3% of respondents reporting use of prayer and religious beliefs (high UPRB) reported no fear or death anxiety compared with 37.8% with low UPRB scores. Older respondents (aged 75 to 94) and women with high UPRB were only about one third as likely to report fears about death. There was a tendency for those with higher levels of involvement in the religious community to also experience lower death anxiety.

4. Respondents reporting both the use of prayer and religious beliefs during stress and active involvement in the religious community were approximately 2.5 less likely to report fear about death than those less likely to use religious behaviors for coping.

5. Greater anxiety and fear about death was noted in those respondents reporting a low ability to handle stress and in those who reported being sicker.

6. A distinctive pattern emerged by examination of the sample in the two age subgroupings. Older respondents (aged 75 to 94) showed: a strong association between high use of prayer and religious beliefs and low levels of death anxiety; less death anxiety in those older respondents more actively involved in the religious community; and older respondents were less likely to report no fear or anxiety about death than the younger respondents.

IMPLICATIONS

As people reach their 80s and 90s, religious behaviors may function as a coping response to fears about death as death becomes more real. Women in this study were more likely to use religious behaviors and more likely to benefit in terms of lower anxiety and fear concerning death. Because two thirds of the U.S. population over 75 years is composed of women, this observation is particularly germane to the coping responses of women. The presence of high death anxiety appears to be a good indicator of poor coping ability in general, since respondents reporting high amounts of stress and possessing little ability to handle stress were noted to have greater fears about death.

Religious beliefs and anxieties may serve as a buffer against anxiety by conveying hope and reassurance that death does not end everything, that there is a continuity between life and death. Death may be seen as a reward for earthly struggles.

Religious beliefs may also help in developing a positive coping style of denial and aid in adaptive personality adjustment when dealing with the anxiety associated with old age. Finally, involvement in religious community activity may create an age-matched peer support group and distraction from anxieties through social activity. Religious activities may also contribute to a greater sense of peace through involvement in activities of choice in the face of the inevitability of death.

▼ TABLE 10-9 Measurement Tools for Anxiety

Instrument	Measures
Manifest Anxiety Scale[50]	Global measure of anxiety
S-R Inventory of Anxiousness[9]	Proneness to anxiety in interpersonal, dangerous, and ambiguous situations
S-R Inventory of General Trait Anxiousness[10]	Anxiety in innocuous, daily routines with potentially dangerous objects or things
State Trait Anxiety Inventory[49]	Measures how persons generally feel (trait) and how they feel at a particular moment in time (state)
Affect Adjective Checklist[58]	Measures of feeling states including anxiety
Fear Survey Schedule[3]	Fears associated with small animals, death, physical pain, surgery, aggression, and interpersonal events
Sexual Anxiety Scale[40]	Cognitively experienced sexual and social anxieties
Total Anxiety Scale[56]	Feelings about death, mutilation, separation, guilt, shame, and diffuse sources of fears in the chronically ill
Lewis et al Anxiety Scale[30]	Developed for use with cancer patients
Fear Thermometer[57]	Rating of level of anxiety
IPAT Anxiety Scale Questionnaire[6]	Measures apprehension tension, low self-control, emotional instability, and suspicion
Death Anxiety Scale[52]	Death anxiety

A significant source of anxiety in the spiritual dimension is the person's fear and distrust of himself and his abilities. No matter how extreme situations may be, if the client is maintaining the faith in himself and courage in terms of his convictions, anxiety will be more bearable. This belief in oneself and one's capacities can be fostered in a caring environment and is particularly important to preserve in nursing situations.

Measurement Tools

Several scales are available to assess anxiety. Table 10-9 summarizes the most common ones.

Analysis
Nursing diagnosis

Anxiety, sleep pattern disturbances, and post-traumatic response are three of the nursing diagnoses approved by the North American Nursing Diagnosis Association (NANDA) that apply to the anxious person. The defining characteristics of these nursing diagnoses are listed in the accompanying boxes. The following list provides examples of NANDA-accepted nursing diagnoses with causative statements:

1. Severe anxiety related to irrational thoughts of guilt

▼ ANXIETY

DEFINITION
A subjective feeling of apprehension and tension manifested by physiological arousal and varying patterns of behavior. The source of anxiety is often nonspecific or unknown to the individual.

DEFINING CHARACTERISTICS

- **Physical dimension**
  - Increased heart rate
  - Elevated blood pressure
  - Insomnia
  - Increased respirations
  - Diaphoresis
  - Dilated pupils
  - Voice quivers
  - Hand tremors/trembling
  - Palpitations
  - Dry mouth
  - Restlessness
  - Poor eye contact
  - Glancing about
  - Extraneous movements
  - Increased tension

- **Emotional dimension**
  - Apprehension
  - Fearful/scared
  - Uncertainty
  - Rattled
  - Overexcited
  - Distressed
  - Jittery
  - Shakiness

- **Intellectual dimension**
  - Regretful
  - Self-focus
  - Increased wariness
  - Worried

- **Social dimension**
  - Helplessness

Modified from McFarland G, McFarlane E: *Nursing diagnosis and intervention: planning for patient care,* ed 2, St Louis, 1993, Mosby–Year Book.

2. Ineffective individual coping related to altered ability to constructively manage stressors secondary to marital discord
3. Ineffective individual coping related to irrational avoidance of objects
4. Ineffective individual coping: irritability related to anxiety about surgery
5. Social isolation related to irrational fear of social situations

The following case example illustrates the nursing diagnosis anxiety.

▼ Case Example

Gary has been preparing for an upcoming examination for several months and is confident that he will do well. As the date of the examination approaches, the possibility that he will not do well enters his mind. The examination begins to pose a serious threat to him as he considers the consequences of failure: a blow to his self-esteem, an obstacle to future plans, personal defeat, disgrace in the eyes of his friends, and a disappointment to his family. He then turns his attention to possible weaknesses, omissions in studying material, deficits in comprehension, and difficulty in expressing what he has learned. These flaws tend to overshadow his previous accomplishments and abilities. On the day of the examination he is concerned about his weaknesses and the possibility of encountering questions that he may be unable to answer. As he looks at the questions his mind goes blank and his reasoning ability seems paralyzed. He is unable to recall information. The test becomes overwhelming and he further berates himself.

▼ SLEEP PATTERN DISTURBANCE

DEFINITION

State in which disruption of sleep time causes discomfort or interferes with desired life-style.

DEFINING CHARACTERISTICS

- **Physical dimension**

  Difficulty awakening
  Awakening earlier or later than desired
  Interrupted sleep
  Hand tremors
  Ptosis of eyelid
  Dark circles under eyes
  Frequent yawning
  Thick speech
  Lethargy
  Restlessness
  Listlessness

- **Emotional dimension**

  Agitation
  Irritability

- **Intellectual dimension**

  Verbal complaints of difficulty falling alseep
  Verbal complaints of not feeling well rested

Modified from McFarland G, McFarlane E: *Nursing diagnosis and intervention: planning for patient care,* ed 2, St Louis, 1993, Mosby—Year Book.

The following case example illustrates the nursing diagnosis of sleep pattern disturbance.

▼ Case Example

Leslie, 31 years old, has recently been promoted to an executive position in a small, but growing investment agency. Having functioned at a high level in her previous position, she is now increasingly anxious about dressing appropriately for her new position, making a mistake, and being fired. These fears interrupt her sleep at night, lead to increased fatigue during the day, and increase her anxiety about making mistakes. She drinks several cups of coffee each day to help combat the fatigue, which, in turn, intensifies her inability to sleep at night.

The following case example illustrates the nursing diagnosis of post-traumatic response.

▼ Case Example

Marty, 17 years old, witnessed the death of her father during a robbery of their family-owned store. Since then she has been unable to sleep and has recurring nightmares about the robbery. Much of her day is spent replaying what she might have done to prevent her father's death. In addition to blaming herself, she feels that she is being punished for not having done things during the robbery that could have saved her father's life.

Planning

Table 10-10 lists examples of long- and short-term goals, outcome criteria, interventions, and rationales related to

▼ POST-TRAUMATIC RESPONSE

DEFINITION

An intense, sustained emotional response to a traumatic experience or natural or man-made disaster.

DEFINING CHARACTERISTICS

- **Physical dimension**

  Alcohol and drug abuse
  Suicidal actions

- **Emotional dimension**

  Emotional numbing
  Generalized fear and anxiety
  Guilt
  Helplessness
  Hopelessness

- **Intellectual dimension**

  Nightmares
  Flashbacks of traumatic event
  Intrusive thoughts
  Impaired cognition, memory, concentration
  Denial of impact of trauma
  Suicidal thoughts

- **Social dimension**

  Impaired interpersonal relationships
  Social withdrawal
  Impaired occupational or academic functioning

Modified from McFarland G, McFarlane E: *Nursing diagnosis and intervention: planning for patient care,* ed 2, St Louis, 1993, Mosby—Year Book.

anxiety. These serve as examples of the planning stage in the nursing process.

Implementation

 Physical dimension Simply encouraging the client to focus on physical symptoms and to describe them can be supportive in anxiety-related disorders. The client can learn that the symptoms are related to anxiety and are not the result of a physical disease after physical factors are ruled out. The box below gives helpful steps in working with an anxious client.

▼ HELPFUL STEPS IN WORKING WITH THE ANXIOUS CLIENT

Steps	Rationale
Observe for behaviors characteristic of anxiety	To identify anxiety
Ask: "What are you feeling?"	To help client name the feeling
Connect the feeling with behavior	To help client understand that when he gets anxious, he behaves in a characteristic way
Explore with client what happened before he felt anxious	To discover the cause
Discuss alternatives for dealing with the situation (cause)	To improve patterns of handling anxiety

▼ **TABLE 10-10   NURSING CARE PLAN**

GOALS	OUTCOME CRITERIA	INTERVENTIONS	RATIONALES
NURSING DIAGNOSIS: Severe anxiety related to loss of husband			
LONG TERM			
To cope with loss of husband with less anxiety	Manages anxiety effectively Gains insight into effects of anxiety on behavior		
SHORT TERM			
To express anxious feelings about loss of husband	Expresses feelings about loss	Assist with identification and expression of anxious feelings: conveying empathy, validating and reflecting impressions, acknowledging feelings as normal	Labeling feelings as normal reduces the intensity of the feeling
To identify effects of anxious feelings on behavior and functioning	Identifies effects of anxiety on behavior and functioning	Discuss effects of anxiety: tension, insomnia, decreased cognitive abilities	Providing information reduces the level of anxiety; information on the physiological basis of anxiety makes symptoms more acceptable
To identify effective coping skills for dealing with losses	Identifies and demonstrates effective coping skills	Discuss effective coping skills: exercise, deep breathing, talking, problem solving	Increase ways to manage anxiety in future

Helping clients find palliative relief through natural sources of anxiety reduction is another important nursing intervention. Activities that focus the client's attention on self-help include a warm bath, back rub, a walk, or a regularly scheduled workout.

Physical means of anxiety reduction also include emphasis on slower breathing, meditation, and relaxation techniques (Figure 10-2). Relaxation procedures can be either passive or active. In the passive approach the client is encouraged to relax completely to encourage him to let his defenses down, open his mind, and become receptive to suggestions about how to deal with stressors. Active relaxation involves a conscious and deliberate relaxation of one muscle group after another, while the mind remains alert. This procedure works by focusing the client's mind on physical relaxation rather than anxious thoughts (see box).

Desensitization therapy is the use of the relaxation response as a counter response to stimuli that previously elicited anxiety. This is accomplished through (1) relaxation training, (2) construction of a hierarchy of situations that elicit anxiety, and (3) working through each situation in the hierarchy by maintaining relaxation until the most anxiety producing situation can be approached and relaxation maintained. The anxiety hierarchy may be approached through imagery or through real-life situations.

Another form of desensitization involves the use of a model whom the client observes approaching the feared object. The model assists the client's approach and then gradually leaves as the client approaches the feared object on his own.

Implosive therapy or flooding avoids the use of relaxation; rather the client is presented with the stimulus at the top of the hierarchy. The client is shown that the resulting anxiety is not unbearable by repeated exposure to the feared object.

If symptoms do not abate through any of these means, antianxiety medication may be used (see Chapter 24). The

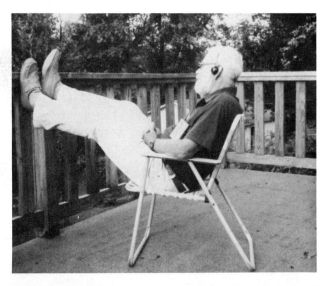

FIGURE 10-2 Listening to music in the quiet of one's home at the end of a busy day is relaxing.

ALPRAZOLAM

(al-pray'zoe-lam)
Xanax
Func. class.: Antianxiety
Chem. class.: Benzodiazepine

Controlled Substance Schedule IV
Action: Depresses subcortical levels of CNS, including limbic system, reticular formation
Uses: Anxiety, panic disorders, anxiety with depressive symptoms
Dosage and routes:
▶ *Adult:* PO 0.25-0.5 mg tid, not to exceed 4 mg in divided doses/day
▶ *Geriatric:* PO 0.25 mg bid-tid
Available forms include: Tab 0.25, 0.5, 1 mg
Side effects/adverse reactions:
CNS: Dizziness, drowsiness, confusion, headache, anxiety, tremors, stimulation, fatigue, depression, insomnia, hallucinations
GI: Constipation, dry mouth, nausea, vomiting, anorexia, diarrhea
INTEG: Rash, dermatitis, itching
CV: Orthostatic hypotension, ***ECG changes, tachycardia,*** hypotension

---

Italic indicates common side effects.
Bold italic indicates life-threatening reactions.

EENT: Blurred vision, tinnitus, mydriasis
Contraindications: Hypersensitivity to benzodiazepines, narrow-angle glaucoma, psychosis, pregnancy (D), child <18 yr
Precautions: Elderly, debilitated, hepatic disease, renal disease
Pharmacokinetics:
PO: Onset 30 min, peak 1-2 hr, duration 4-6 hr, therapeutic response 2-3 days, metabolized by liver, excreted by kidneys, crosses placenta, breast milk, half-life 12-15 hr
Interactions/incompatibilities:
—Increased CNS depression: anticonvulsants, alcohol, antihistamines, sedative/hypnotics
—Decreased action of alprazolam: disulfiram, cimetidine
—Decreased action of: levodopa

NURSING CONSIDERATIONS
Assess:
—B/P (lying, standing); pulse; if systolic B/P drops 20 mm Hg, hold drug, notify physician
—Blood studies: CBC during long-term therapy; blood dyscrasias have occurred rarely
—Hepatic studies: AST, ALT, bilirubin, creatinine, LDH, alk phosphatase

—I&O; may indicate renal dysfunction
—For indications of increasing tolerance and abuse
Administer:
—With food or milk for GI symptoms
—Crushed if patient is unable to swallow medication whole
—Sugarless gum, hard candy, frequent sips of water for dry mouth
Perform/provide:
—Assistance with ambulation during beginning therapy; drowsiness/dizziness occurs
—Safety measures, including side rails
—Check to see PO medication has been swallowed
Evaluate:
—Therapeutic response: decreased anxiety, restlessness, sleeplessness
—Mental status: mood, sensorium, affect, sleeping pattern, drowsiness, dizziness
—Physical dependency, withdrawal symptoms: anxiety, panic attacks, agitation, convulsions, headache, nausea, vomiting, muscle pain, weakness
—Suicidal tendencies

Teach client/family:
—That drug may be taken with food
—Not to be used for everyday stress or longer than 3 mo, unless directed by physician; not to take more than prescribed amount, may be habit forming
—Avoid OTC preparations unless approved by physician
—To avoid driving, activities that require alertness, since drowsiness may occur
—To avoid alcohol ingestion or other psychotropic medications, unless prescribed by physician
—Not to discontinue medication abruptly after long-term use
—To rise slowly or fainting may occur
—That drowsiness might worsen at beginning of treatment
Lab test interferences:
Increase: AST/ALT, serum bilirubin
False increase: 17-OHCS
Decrease: RAIU
Treatment of overdose: Lavage, VS, supportive care

Modified from Skidmore-Roth L: *Mosby's nursing drug reference,* St Louis, 1993, Mosby–Year Book.

▼ RELAXATION EXERCISE

Before proceeding with this exercise, provide the following conditions:
A quiet environment
A passive attitude
A comfortable position
A mental device to control distracting thoughts, such as "one" or "breathe in, breathe out"

1. *Hands.* First the fists are tensed and relaxed, then the fingers are extended and relaxed.
2. *Biceps and triceps.* These muscles are tensed and relaxed.
3. *Shoulders.* The shoulders are pulled back and relaxed and then pushed forward and relaxed.
4. *Neck.* The head is turned slowly as far to the right as possible and relaxed, turned to the left and relaxed, and then brought forward until the chin touches the chest and relaxed.
5. *Mouth.* The mouth is opened as wide as possible and relaxed. The lips form a pout and are then relaxed. The tongue is extended as far as possible and relaxed, and is then retracted into the throat and relaxed. It is pressed hard into the roof of the mouth and relaxed and then is pressed hard into the floor of the mouth and relaxed.
6. *Eyes.* The eyes are opened as wide as possible and relaxed and then closed as tightly as possible and relaxed.

7. *Breathing.* The person inhales as deeply as possible and relaxes and then exhales as much as possible and relaxes.
8. *Torso.* The buttock muscles are tensed and relaxed.
9. *Back.* The trunk of the body is pushed forward so that the entire back is arched, and then it is relaxed.
10. *Thighs.* The legs are extended and raised about six inches off the floor and then relaxed, and backs of the feet are pressed into the floor and relaxed.
11. *Stomach.* The stomach is pulled in as much as possible and relaxed and is then extended and relaxed.
12. *Calves and feet.* With legs supported, the feet are bent with the toes pointing toward the head and then relaxed. The feet are then bent in the opposite direction and relaxed.
13. *Toes.* The toes are pressed into the bottom of the shoes and relaxed. They are then bent to touch the top of the shoes and relaxed.

The final part of the exercise involves becoming completely relaxed, beginning with one's toes and following the sensation up through the body to the eyes and forehead. When learning the procedure, the person can eliminate some of the exercises and employ them only on the muscles that usually become tense. The muscle groups involved (shoulders, forehead, back, neck) depend on the individual.

Modified from Rimm D, Masters J: *Behavior therapy,* New York, 1974, Academic Press.

accompanying profiles for alprazolam (Xanax) and lorazepam (Ativan) describe nursing care appropriate to their administration. The treatment team should discuss the client's level of anxiety and determine appropriate medication. The use of a one-to-one relationship with the caregiver, seclusion, or restraints may be indicated to provide a safer, less stimulating environment. Table 10-11 lists additional antianxiety medications with daily dose ranges.

Emotional dimension One of the most important contributions the nurse can make is to encourage the open expression of feelings according to psychoanalytical theorists. Clients can be taught to distinguish anxiety from other emotions, to recognize causes of their anxiety, and to identify the sequence of emotions they experience when exposed to anxiety producing situations.

Unnecessary sources of anxiety can be eliminated by including the client in treatment plans and by informing him about matters that affect care. In addition, the nurse can model appropriate behavior (learning theory), demonstrate decisive behavior without being coercive, and provide encouragement and support by changing the environment for clients with disabling anxieties.

Intellectual dimension Guidance and education are nursing interventions that help promote adaptive and growth experiences for the anxious individual. The educational approach uses supportive coaching to enhance the person's coping abilities.

Anticipatory guidance provides the client with both knowledge of a potentially stressful situation and techniques he can use to cope with it. Helping the client to anticipate an expected challenge and to consider the accompanying unpleasant emotions and fantasies reduces the threat stemming from uncertainty. Supporting and guiding the client with techniques he can use to deal actively and constructively with the stressful situation provides a means of coping. Both aspects of this approach help reduce the anxiety of stressful events.

Other coping strategies include the *work of worrying* and *positive thinking*. Worrying can help to relieve the painful effects of anxiety by warding off an anticipated trauma or reliving a recent trauma. Positive thinking, as a defense against environmental obstacles and as a pursuit of happiness, can lead to excessive generality and ineffectiveness as a coping tool. However, the encouragement of repetitive "good thoughts" can be a way of inhibiting and thwarting negative, anxiety producing thoughts. This tech

nique can be illustrated by statements such as "I can do it," or "I did that well."

A cognitive approach to anxiety reduction essentially involves the following stages: (1) recognizing ideas that are irrational and that lead to anxiety, (2) establishing a relationship between thoughts and the anxiety attack, (3) distancing by viewing one's thoughts objectively and not necessarily as identical to reality, (4) testing the validity of one's thought in actual situations, (5) identifying the assumptions that lie behind the thoughts, and (6) reviewing the belief system underlying the ideas and changing the behaviors that have evolved from the irrational, incorrect beliefs.[5]

Another cognitive approach that is helpful in dealing with anxiety related to situational crises is the use of the problem-solving method. The aim of this approach is to help clients recognize that problematic situations are a normal part of life and that a person can attempt to cope with the situation. In defining the problem, the nurse helps the client identify the various issues involved in the situation. This aids in determining a focus and direction for the problem solving. In generating alternatives, clients need to be encouraged to defer immediate judgment and to identify as many options as possible. The nurse can then help the client identify which course of action will be most likely to resolve the problem. This review can lead to further problem solving or to resolution of the disturbing situation.

Stress inoculation procedures have been developed to help the client control physiological responses and to substitute positive coping statements that reduce anxiety. Education and rehearsal are used as part of the technique. During the education phase the client is alerted to body reactions, thoughts, and images associated with emotional arousal. The client is encouraged to view the reaction in phases that include preparing for a disturbing event, confronting or handling the situation, possibly being overwhelmed, and finally praising oneself after dealing with the situation.

During rehearsal the client is provided with a variety of coping strategies that can be employed in each of the preceding phases. These include relaxation, designing escape routes, and collecting more information about the feared objects and situations. Statements are generated to help the client relabel the experience, motivate himself for successful coping, and reinforce himself after coping successfully with the situation. Imagery procedures can be used to help the client develop a model of behavior, rehearse responses to self-doubt, and serve as a cue to initiate coping statements.

Social dimension The nurse becomes important in the world of the client and is a role model to demonstrate effective coping skills. Using behavioral-learning theory the nurse provides calm reassurance and helps the client reengage in social situations and learn to tolerate his fears in the unfamiliar setting of the clinic or hospital. Through involvement with the nurse, the client redirects his attention from excessive rumination to engagement in grooming, games, reading, or social activities. Clients often need guidance in focusing attention on new ways of responding to events and people and in identifying satisfying activities and avoiding stressful ones.

According to existential theorists, the key aspect of the

▼ TABLE 10-11 **Antianxiety Medications**

Generic Name	Trade Name	Daily Dose Range (mg)
Alprazolam	Xanax	0.5-4
Chlordiazepoxide	Librium	10-100
Diazepam	Valium	2-30
Hydroxyzine	Atarax	75-400
Lorazepam	Ativan	0.5-9
Meprobamate	Equanil	1200-1600
Oxazepam	Serax	30-120

LORAZEPAM

(lor-a'ze-pam)
Ativan, Novolorazem*
Func. class.: Antianxiety
Chem. class.: Benzodiazepine

Controlled Substance Schedule IV
Action: Depresses subcortical levels of CNS, including limbic system and reticular formation
Uses: Anxiety, irritability in psychiatric or organic disorders, preoperatively, insomnia, acute alcohol withdrawal symptoms, anticonvulsant, adjunct in endoscopic procedures
Dosage and routes:
Anxiety
▶ *Adult:* PO 2-6 mg/day in divided doses, not to exceed 10 mg/day
Insomnia
▶ *Adult:* PO 2-4 mg hs; only minimally effective after 2 wk continuous therapy
Preoperatively
▶ *Adult:* IM/IV 2-4 mg
Available forms include: Tab 0.5, 1, 2 mg; IM/IV inj 2, 4 mg/ml
Side effects/adverse reactions:
CNS: Dizziness, drowsiness, confusion, headache, anxiety, tremors, stimulation, fatigue, depression, insomnia, hallucinations, weakness, unsteadiness

*Available in Canada only.
Italic indicates common side effects.
Bold italic indicates life-threatening reactions.

GI: Constipation, dry mouth, nausea, vomiting, anorexia, diarrhea
INTEG: Rash, dermatitis, itching
CV: Orthostatic hypotension,
ECG changes, tachycardia,
hypotension
EENT: Blurred vision, tinnitus, mydriasis
Contraindications: Hypersensitivity to benzodiazepines, narrow-angle glaucoma, psychosis, pregnancy (D), child <12 yr, history of drug abuse, COPD
Precautions: Elderly, debilitated, hepatic disease, renal disease
Pharmacokinetics:
PO Peak 1-3 hr, duration 3-6 hr metabolized by liver, excreted by kidneys, crosses placenta, breast milk, half-life 14 hr
Interactions/incompatibilities:
—Decreased effects of lorazepam: oral contraceptives, valproic acid
—Increased effects of lorazepam: CNS depressants, alcohol, disulfiram, oral contraceptives

NURSING CONSIDERATIONS
Assess:
—B/P (lying, standing), pulse; if systolic B/P drops 20 mm Hg, hold drug, notify physician; respirations q5-15 min if given IV
—Blood studies: CBC during long-term therapy, blood dyscrasias have occurred rarely
—Hepatic studies: AST, ALT, bilirubin, creatinine, LDH, alk phosphatase

Administer:
—With food or milk for GI symptoms
—Crushed if patient is unable to swallow medication whole
—Sugarless gum, hard candy, frequent sips of water for dry mouth
—IV after diluting in an equal volume of compatible sol; give through Y-tube or 3-way stopcock; give at 2 mg or less over 1 min
—Deep into large muscle mass (IM inj)
Perform/provide:
—Assistance with ambulation during beginning therapy since drowsiness/dizziness occurs
—Safety measures, including side rails
—Check to see PO medication has been swallowed
Evaluate:
—Therapeutic response: decreased anxiety, restlessness, insomnia
—Mental status: mood, sensorium, affect, sleeping pattern, drowsiness, dizziness
—Physical dependency, withdrawal symptoms: headache, nausea, vomiting, muscle pain, weakness, tremors, convulsions, after long-term, excessive use
—Suicidal tendencies

Teach client/family:
—That drug may be taken with food
—Not to be used for everyday stress or used longer than 4 mo unless directed by physician, not to take more than prescribed amount, may be habit forming
—Avoid OTC preparations (cough, cold, hay fever) unless approved by physician
—To avoid driving, activities that require alertness, since drowsiness may occur
—To avoid alcohol ingestion or other psychotropic medications, unless prescribed by physician
—Not to discontinue medication abruptly after long-term use
—To rise slowly or fainting may occur
—That drowsiness might worsen at beginning of treatment
—Use birth-control method if childbearing age
Lab test interferences:
Increase: AST/ALT, serum bilirubin
Decrease: RAIU
False increase: 17-OHCS
Treatment of overdose: Lavage, VS, supportive care

Modified from Skidmore-Roth L: *Mosby's nursing drug reference,* St Louis, 1993, Mosby–Year Book.

self-management approach is the client's development of a sense of responsibility for his behavior, for changing the bothersome or worrisome aspects of his environment, and for planning for his future. This participant model relies on the client's motivation to accept a program for change and involves his active cooperation in defining treatment objectives. Emphasizing self-help skills places the burden of engaging in the process of change on the client; the nurse provides only as much assistance as needed to enable the client to gain control over his life. Within this model the nurse is an instigator or motivator to help the client start a program for change. The nurse is also a consultant and expert adviser who negotiates ways of changing and defines the goals of treatment with the client through modeling, work assignments, and helping the client to analyze problems and determine their solutions. This process is future oriented and focused on the development of behavioral repertoires for dealing with anxiety. Attention is also given to the transfer of new behaviors to the environments of home, work, and social situations so that the learning has

immediate applicability and the results of intervention can extend beyond the treatment situation.

Several steps are involved in establishing a self-regulation process: (1) standard setting or identification of performance criteria; (2) a self-monitoring or self-observation phase in which clients are encouraged to carefully scrutinize their behavior; (3) self-evaluation in which the information obtained from self-observation is compared to the identified standards; and (4) self-reinforcement through rewards, self-validation, and praise.

Spiritual dimension An essential nursing intervention with the anxious client is to instill hopefulness and a sense that the anxiety can be mastered. The nurse can help accomplish this goal by permitting expression of negative feelings and by helping the client plan future outcomes and alternatives. One way for a person to find relief from anxiety is to transcend everyday life and find importance in objects or events outside himself. For example, doing something for others such as volunteer work or becoming politically active can help relieve anxiety. This abil-

GUIDELINES FOR PRIMARY/TERTIARY PREVENTION

Anxiety

Primary Prevention

Teach person to be kind to self and to appreciate self
       to be less critical of self
       to maintain high self-esteem
       to restore self-esteem when lowered
       to identify bodily symptoms of anxiety
       to share feelings when upset or anxious with a supportive person
       to manage stress with diet, exercise, rest/sleep, relaxation
       that some anxiety is part of living
       to problem solve
       information about prescribed antianxiety medications; name, dosage, side effects, and addictive effects
Teach family to lessen demands on person when upset or anxious
       listening skills
       ways to be supportive

Tertiary Prevention

Community Resources
   Mental Health Centers
   PTSD Groups for Vietnam veterans, rape victims, battered women
Self-help Groups
   Phobia Groups

KEY INTERVENTIONS FOR THE ANXIOUS CLIENT

Mild Anxiety
- Give information on the physiological responses accompanying anxiety.
- Help client find relief through natural means (i.e., bath, walk, workout).
- Encourage expression of anxious feelings.
- Connect the feeling with behavior.
- Discuss alternatives for dealing with the causes.
- Teach client passive relaxation through slower breathing, loosening of muscle groups.

Moderate Anxiety

Teach client active relaxation techniques throughout systematic muscle groups.
- Teach positive thinking.
- Help client identify thoughts that are irrational.
- Encourage client to test the accuracy of thoughts and assumptions when irrationally based.
- Teach client problem solving.
- Encourage client to defer judgment and choice until thorough review is made.
- Encourage client in rehearsing before an anticipated anxious situation.
- Use value clarification to resolve conflicts and reduce anxiety.
- Prepare client for dreaded events, loss of love relationships, or death.

Severe Anxiety
- Provide information and calm reassurance.
- Encourage deep breathing exercises.
- Encourage client to describe the feeling of relaxation.
- Ask client to describe the extreme feared images in detail.
- Encourage client that the intensity of feelings is time limited, can be tolerable, and will subside.
- Change immediate environment of client.
- Administer antianxiety medication.

ity to transcend the mundane aspects of life provides the client with the opportunity to entertain new life choices and to create new possibilities.

The nurse can help the client find meaning in his life and his problems; the client can thus be helped to acknowledge things of importance and to commit himself to chosen values. Facilitating the resolution of conflict in values may help reduce anxiety as well as help the client meet ethical and moral obligations. Open, frank discussion of religious and spiritual needs and attitudes can facilitate the client's use of spiritual beliefs as a means of coping with anxiety.

Preparation for anticipated, dreaded events, such as loss of love relationships and death, can provide a source of strength and protection against anxiety in the face of the unknown.

The nurse initially intervenes to relieve the client's acute anxiety by helping him to relax with deep breathing exercises. Once the acute phase has subsided she asks the client to describe his feelings. This helps the client to identify his relaxed state, acknowledge that he is alive and well, and indicates his readiness to discuss the incident further. The nurse pushes the client to describe the most extreme aspect of his feared image—that he is dying. She then guides him through a discussion that helps him see that the outcome of each incident is less catastrophic than he imagined.

The nurse understands that the anxious person's image usually stops where the feared image occurs. He tends to exaggerate the event and believes it is real—that he will die. The nurse does not attempt to dissuade the client from his prediction. Instead, she conveys a belief that the discomfort, however intense, does not last long, is tolerable, and involves some choice regarding outcome. The accompanying boxes provide key interventions for anxiety and guidelines for prevention. Table 10-10 is a sample nursing care plan for a client experiencing anxiety.

INTERACTION WITH AN ANXIOUS CLIENT

Client: *I'm choking. I can't breathe. I think I'm having a heart attack.*

Nurse: *Relax. Take some deep breaths. Breathe in. Breathe out. Slowly. Breathe in. Breathe out.*

Nurse: *(After a brief period of time.) What is happening now?*

Client: *I'm okay. I guess I'm not having a heart attack. But I keep getting this picture of myself having a heart attack.*

Nurse: *What happens after you have the heart attack?*

Client: *I see myself helpless and dying. That's all I can see. I feel it is a premonition or ESP. Something like that.*

Nurse: *You have these pictures and nothing happens?*

Client: *Yes, I have them all the time and nothing happens.*

Nurse: *This is not unusual. Yet the imagined event rarely takes place. You might keep a record of your images of having a heart attack and see what happens.*

Client: But what if it does happen?
Nurse: The fantasy is usually worse than the reality. You may want to work at not treating the fantasy as an actual event.

Evaluation

Several criteria can be applied to evaluate the process as well as the specific interventions. Some of these criteria follow:

1. *Adequacy:* Did the interventions mainly provide relief of symptoms of anxiety? Did they also include self-learning and management of anxiety?
2. *Appropriateness:* If the client was in severe anxiety, was intervention started immediately, with formal data gathering suspended until the client could participate? Did the client agree on the goals? Were the interventions relevant for the identified level of anxiety and problems arising in the five dimensions?
3. *Effectiveness:* To what degree were anxiety behaviors relieved and self-learning accomplished? Were the goals and interventions specifically related to anxiety?
4. *Efficiency:* Were interventions sufficient to assuage anxiety? Were sources of help and support coordinated to increase the impact on the client's problem with anxiety?

The client needs to be included in evaluation throughout the assessment and treatment phases. This involvement aids in the teacher-learning process for the anxious client and provides important information for the nurse's growth in her care-giving activities.

BRIEF REVIEW

Anxiety is a common experience among the general population, with physical manifestation being easily identified by the individual and others observing the anxious person. Nurses have studied the concept as an aspect of normal development and life crises and as a reaction to procedure. The DSM-III-R categories provide a means for classifying the anxiety related disorders.

Biological, psychoanalytical, interpersonal, learning theorists, and existential frameworks provide definitions of anxiety and identify the source, dynamics, and observational cues of anxiety and the role of the nurse. These frameworks provide a means for specifying clinical activities.

Self-reports, nursing observation, and standardized tests aid in identifying anxiety, leading to a nursing diagnosis and subsequent care plan. During assessment the nurse must identify the level of anxiety that the individual is experiencing. These levels range from mild anxiety to panic.

Anxiety differs from fear because the source of anxiety is nonspecific, whereas fear has an identifiable source.

Anxiety affects the intellectual capabilities of the individual by distorting perception, concentration, recall, and reasoning. Helplessness may result from these intellectual changes. The individual develops ego defense mechanisms to protect himself from anxiety.

Anxiety arising in social situations appears to be related to a loss of self-esteem and affection and fear of rejection.

Families develop characteristic means of dealing with anxiety individually and in groups. Certain sociocultural variables appear to be related to the development and level of experienced anxiety.

Anxiety appears to be related to maturation and the development of conflict in values, a lack or loss of love relationships, commitments, and self-definition and autonomy.

Measurement tools are primarily based on the use of self-reports and ask the client to rate his present and usual feeling states and to identify the descriptive aspects of being anxious. Measures have been developed to identify fears associated with death, physical pain, surgery, aggression, and interpersonal events.

Analysis involves coordinating observational, self-reported, and standardized measures with the duration of the anxiety response and the effect on the life adjustment of the client. The DSM-III-R categories provide a means of classifying the anxiety-related illnesses. Nursing analysis takes into consideration the level of anxiety and assessment data from the five dimensions of the person. During the planning stage the short- and long-term goals are established according to the specific nursing diagnoses.

Implementation of goals is effected by application of specific interventions, with consideration for the client's readiness to learn. Suggestions for intervention in each of the five dimensions were discussed along with their rationale.

REFERENCES

1. Adams, MF: Post traumatic stress disorder, *American Journal of Nursing* 82:1704, 1982.
2. Adler A: *The practice and theory of individual psychology,* Totowan, NJ, 1959, Littlefield, Adams & Co. (Translated by P Radin.)
3. Akutagawa D: *A study in constant validity of the psychoanalytic concept of latent anxiety and a test of projection distance hypothesis,* doctoral dissertation, Pittsburgh, 1956, University of Pittsburgh.
4. Beck A: *Cognitive therapy and the emotional disorders,* New York, 1976, International Universities Press, Inc.
5. Beck A, Emory G: *Anxiety disorders and phobias,* New York, 1985, Basic Books.
6. Cattell RB, Scheier IH: *IPAT Anxiety Scale Questionnaire: Manual,* Champaign, Ill, 1963, Institute for Personality and Ability Testing.
7. Dollard J, Miller NE: *Personality and psychotherapy: an analysis in terms of learning, thinking, and culture,* New York, 1950, McGraw-Hill.
8. Eaton WN and others: Consumption of coffee or tea and symptoms of anxiety, *American Journal of Public Health* 74:66, 1984.
9. Endler N, Hunt J, Rosentstein A: An S-R inventory of anxiousness, *Psychological Monographs* 76:536, 1962.
10. Endler N, Odada M: A multidimensional measure of trait anxiety: the S-R inventory of general trait anxiousness, *Journal of Consulting and Clinical Psychology* 43:319, 1975.
11. Erickson E: *Identity and the life cycle,* New York, 1959, International Universities Press.
12. Freud S: Inhibitions, symptoms and anxiety. In *Standard edition of the complete psychological works of Sigmund Freud,* vol 20, London, 1959, The Hogarth Press, Ltd. (Translated by J Strachey.)
13. Furey JA: Post traumatic stress disorders in Vietnam veterans, *American Journal of Nursing* 82:1694, 1982.
14. Gomez EA, and others: Anxiety as a human emotion: some basic conceptual models, *Nursing Forum* 21:38, 1984.

15. Goodwyn J: Post-traumatic symptoms in abused children, *Journal of Traumatic Stress* 1:4, 475, 1988.

16. Grainger RD: Anxiety interrupters, *American Journal of Nursing* 90:2, 14, 1990.

17. Haack MR: Collaborative investigation of adult children of alcoholics with anxiety, *Archives of Psychiatric Nursing* 4:1, 62, 1990.

18. Horney K: *Our inner conflicts, a constructive theory of neurosis*, New York, 1945, WW Norton.

19. Huppenbauer SL: PTSD: a portrait of the problem, *American Journal of Nursing* 82:1169, 1982.

20. Kanfer FH: Self-management methods. In Kanfer FH, Goldstein AP, editors: *Helping people change*, New York, 1980, Pergamon Press.

21. Kanfer FH, Goldstein AP: *Helping people change*, ed 2, New York, 1981, Pergamon Press.

22. Kata K: On anxiety in the Scandinavian countries. In Sarason IG, Spielberger CD, editors: *Stress and anxiety*, vol 2, New York, 1975, Halstead Press.

23. Katon W, Sheehan D, Whole T: Panic disorder: a treatable problem, *Patient Care* 2:6, 148, 1988.

24. Kell D: *Anxiety and emotions*, Springfield, Ill, 1980, Charles C Thomas.

25. Kierkegaard S: *The concept of dread*, Princeton, NJ, 1944, Princeton University Press. (Translated by W Lowrie.)

26. Koenig HG: Religious behaviors and death anxiety in later life, *The Hospice Journal* 4:1, 3, 1988.

27. Kreitler S, Kreitler H: Trauma and anxiety: the cognitive approach, *Journal of Traumatic Stress* 1:1, 35, 1988.

28. Lesses S: *Anxiety: its components, development, and treatment*, New York, 1970, Grune & Stratton.

29. Levinson H, Carter S: *Phobia free*, New York, 1986, M Evans and Co.

30. Lewis F, Firsich S, Parsell S: Clinical tool development for adult chemotherapy patients: process and content, *Cancer News* 2(2):99, 1979.

31. Long CG, Bluteau P: Group coping skills training for anxiety and depression: its application with chronic patients, *Journal of Advanced Nursing* 13:3, 358, 1988.

32. Lyons JA, Keane M: Implosive therapy for the treatment of combat-related PTSD, PTSD, *Journal of Traumatic Stress* 2:2, 137, 1989.

33. Mandler G: Helplessness: theory and research in anxiety. In Spielberger, CD, editor: *Anxiety: current trends in theory and research*, vol 1, New York, 1972, Academic Press.

34. Martin P: A feeling that needs expressing: helping patients manage their anxiety, *Professional Nurse* 5:7, 374, 1990.

35. May R: *The meaning of anxiety*, rev ed, New York, 1977, WW Norton and Co.

36. May R: Value conflicts and anxiety. In Kutash IL, editor: *Handbook on stress and anxiety*, San Francisco, 1980, Jossey-Bass, Inc.

37. McNally R: Preparedness and phobias: a review, *Psychological Bulletin* 101(2):283, 1987.

38. Mowrer OH: Pain, punishment, guilt, and anxiety. In Hock P, Zubin J, editors: *Anxiety*, New York, 1950, Grune & Stratton.

39. Nemiah J: Anxiety states. In Kaplan H, Dadock B, editors: *Comprehensive textbook of psychiatry*, ed 4, Baltimore, 1985, Williams and Wilkins.

40. Obler M: Systematic desensitization in sexual disorders: *Journal of Behavioral Therapy and Experimental Psychiatry* 4(2):93, 1975.

41. Pasnau R: *Diagnosis and treatment of anxiety disorders*, Washington, DC, 1984, American Psychiatric Press.

42. Peplau H: *Interpersonal relations in nursing*, New York, 1952, G.P. Putnam's Sons.

43. Phillips BN, Martin RP, Meyers J: Interventions in relation to anxiety in school. In Spielberger CD, editor: *Anxiety: current trends in theory and research*, vol 2, New York, 1972, Academic Press.

44. Pilette WL: Caffeine, *Journal of Psychosocial Nursing* 21:19, 1983.

45. Rank O: *Will therapy*, New York, 1936, Alfred A. Knopf.

46. Runck B: *Biofeedback—issues in treatment assessment*, NIMH Science Monograph, US Department of Health and Human Services, Washington, DC, 1980, US Government Printing Office.

47. Slater E, Sheilds J: Genetical aspects of anxiety. In Lader M, editor: *Studies of anxiety*, Ashford, Kent, England, 1969, Headless Brothers.

48. Sluckin A: Psychotherapy with an acutely anxious six year old, *Health Visitor* 61:6, 184, 1988.

49. Spielburger CD: *STAI-self evaluation questionnaire*, Palo Alto, Calif, 1977, Consulting Psychologists Press.

50. Sullivan HS: *The interpersonal theory of psychiatry*, New York, 1950, WW Norton & Co.

51. Taylor J: A personality scale of manifest anxiety, *Journal of Abnormal and Social Psychology* 48:235, 1953.

52. Templer DI: The construction and validation of a death anxiety scale, *Journal of General Psychology*, 82:165, 1970.

53. Titlebaum HM: Relaxation, *Holistic Nurse Practitioner* 2:3, 17-25, 1988.

54. Trimpey ML: Self-esteem and anxiety: key issues in an abused women's support group, *Issues in Mental Health Nursing* 10:297, 1989.

55. Valente SM: Children, adolescents and nuclear war anxiety, *Journal of Child and Adolescent Psychiatric and Mental Health Nursing* 1:1, 36, 1988.

56. Viney LL, Westbrook MT: Patterns of anxiety in the chronically ill, *British Journal Medical Psychology* 55:87, 1982.

57. Walk R: Self-rating of fear in a fear-invoking situation, *Journal of Abnormal and Social Psychology* 52:171, 1956.

58. Zuckerman M: The development of an affect adjective checklist for the measurement of anxiety, *Journal of Consulting Psychology* 24:456, 1960.

ANNOTATED BIBLIOGRAPHY

Barlow D: *The anxiety disorders: the nature and treatment of anxiety and panic*, New York, 1988, Guilford Press.

This book presents a comprehensive overview of the anxiety disorders and methods of treatment.

Haack M: Collaborative investigation of adult children of alcoholics with anxiety, *Archives of Psychiatric Nursing* 4(1):62, 1990.

Because of the increased incidence of anxiety in alcoholic families, the author explored the interaction between the etiological factors that led to anxiety and substance abuse. The study was a collaborative effort between psychiatric medicine and nursing.

Karl G: Survival skills for psychic trauma, *Journal of Psychosocial Nursing and Mental Health Services* 27(4):15, 1989.

This article discusses behavioral responses to severe stress with emphasis on coping and adaptation processes.

May R: *The meaning of anxiety*, New York, 1950, Ronald Press.

This book is a classic in the field of anxiety. Various theories are described and methods for managing anxiety are discussed.

Whitley G: Anxiety: defining the diagnosis, *Journal of Psychosocial Nursing and Mental Health Services* 27(10):7, 1989.

This article discusses the nursing diagnosis, anxiety, and includes areas for further study.

CHAPTER

11 Anger

James L Harris
Ruth Parmelee Rawlins

After studying this chapter, the student will be able to:

- Define anger
- Discuss the psychopathology of intermittent explosive and passive-aggressive personality disorders as described in DSM-III-R
- Trace the historical perspectives of anger
- Describe theories of anger
- Use the nursing process in caring for angry clients
- Identify current research findings related to anger

Anger, a strong feeling of annoyance or displeasure, is part of each person's everyday life. Words such as *indignation, wrath, ire, frustration, resentment,* and *fury* all describe feelings of anger.

Closely related to anger are *aggression, hostility, violence,* and *rage.* Aggression arises from innate drives or occurs as a defense mechanism and is manifested either by constructive or destructive acts directly toward self or others. Hostility is characterized by destructive behavior secondary to feelings of anger or resentment. Acting out of destructive aggression by assaulting people or objects in the environment is characteristic of hostility. Violent, intense, and short-lived anger describe rage. Viewing anger on a continuum with mild irritation at one end and rage at the other helps the nurse determine the point at which the person feeling anger moves from health to illness or from constructive to destructive behavior. When angry, people momentarily lose their intellectual clarity and feel consumed by the emotion. Subsequently, episodes of assault, destruction of property, or the indirect expression of anger occurs. The consistent exhibition of such individual behaviors can result in a diagnosis of intermittent explosive and passive-aggressive personality disorders.

Anger is a warning that needs attention. For many reasons people have learned to reject, mistrust, and deny this warning device. They look on it at best as a suspect part of themselves and at worst as a sinful, destructive element. People learn to couch their anger in euphemisms: *out of sorts, put out, frustrated, insulted,* and countless other socially acceptable ways that attempt to describe the inner experience of anger as something completely different, such as anxiety or dread, because the label anger is so objectionable.

Viewing anger as a natural and valuable aspect of each person is a relatively new concept. To see anger in this light, anger needs to be separated from its violent counterpart, rage. Rage results when the natural pathway to a spontaneous expression of anger has been cut off. Rage is a physical experience and requires a physical release like pounding, hitting, banging, running, or pushing. It is intent on destruction and interested only in its own reduction. Anger can be expressed verbally, and its *catharsis* propels the individual to a creative solution. Anger provides the foundation for relationships, whereas rage destroys them.

All persons become angry. Understanding the dynamics of anger from a personal and a client perspective is essential if nurses are to help clients gain insight into what is happening.

The psychiatric nurse may find it helpful to discuss with clients how to recognize anger and its triggers and to express it in ways that are not injurious to self or others. Further, teaching families of clients diagnosed with inter-

> **DIAGNOSES Related to Anger**

MEDICAL DIAGNOSES	NURSING DIAGNOSES
Intermittent explosive disorder	**NANDA**
Passive-aggressive personality disorder	High risk for violence
	PMH
	Altered feeling state—anger
	Altered conduct/impulse processes

▶ DATES	EVENTS
Before Christ (BC) and After the Death of Christ (AD)	Frequent documented accounts of violence, anger, and rebellion in the Bible: Exodus, Kings, Job, Matthew, Acts
1564-1616	Anger and rebellion evidenced throughout the works of William Shakespeare
Early 1900s	Institutions (prisons and mental health facilities) created that removed people from the mainstream of life because of *violent* and *aggressive* behavior
1950s	Introduction of psychotropic medications reduced angry behavior in clients in inpatient settings; patients able to learn more easily new coping skills
1960s-1970s	Conflicts such as the Civil Rights movement and antiwar demonstrations resulted in hostility, anger, and aggressive acts
1980s	*Violence* pervasive: increasing numbers of children, spouses, and elderly abused and battered: murders, rapes, suicides increased; terrorist attacks increased; nuclear weapons readily available to several nations
1990s	Nursing offered many opportunities for helping clients channel their anger into constructive acts, both in inpatient and community mental health settings
Future	Because of the increase in violent acts and international conflicts, nursing will need to become more politically involved with prevention of violence in individuals, families, communities, and nations

mittent explosive or passive-aggressive disorder about the behaviors associated with each and how to relate to their significant others is essential to reduce or eliminate ineffective patterns of behavior.

DSM-III-R DIAGNOSES

The DSM-III-R diagnoses related to anger are intermittent explosive and passive-aggressive personality disorders. Essential features, predisposing factors, and behavioral responses associated with each disorder follow.

Intermittent Explosive Disorder

The essential feature of the disorder is the display of discrete episodes of loss of control of aggressive impulses, resulting in serious assaultive acts or destruction of property. The degree of aggressiveness expressed during the episodes is grossly out of proportion to any psychosocial stressors. Further, there are no signs of impulsiveness or aggressiveness between episodes. The episodes of loss of control do not occur during the course of a psychotic disorder such as organic personality syndrome, antisocial or borderline personality disorder, conduct disorder, or intoxication with a psychoactive substance. Behavioral responses include episodes described as spells or attacks. These behaviors appear within minutes and, regardless of duration, remit quickly. There is evidence of genuine regret

and self-reproach about consequences of action and inability to control the aggressive impulse.[1]

Passive-Aggressive Personality Disorder

The essential feature of this disorder is the demonstration of a pervasive pattern of resistance to demands for adequate social and occupational performance, in a variety of social and occupational contexts, beginning by early adulthood. Oppositional defiant disorder in childhood or adolescence is a predisposing factor to the development of the disorder. At least five of the following behaviors must be present for diagnosis: procrastinating; sulky, irritable, or argumentative when asked to do something that is undesirable; deliberately working slowly or doing a bad job on tasks that are undesirable; argumentative; forgetful; resentful toward authority figures; obstructing efforts of others; and unreasonably critical or scornful behavior.[1]

THEORETICAL APPROACHES

Theories of anger include biological, psychoanalytical, interpersonal, behavioral, and existential (Table 11-1).

Biological

Recent studies of the anatomy of the brain identify the limbic system as the regulator of aggression. Any lesion of

▼ **TABLE 11-1**   **Summary of the Theories of Anger**

Theories	Theorist	Dynamics
Biological Biochemical		Lesions or disease in the limbic system (which regulates aggression) may cause aggressive acts. Chemical imbalances and endocrine disorders may lead to aggression.
Genetic	Lorenz	Aggression is an inborn response pattern and is genetically influenced.
Psychoanalytical	Freud	Anger is instinctual and seeks expression through aggressive acts of self-destruction. Anger may be displaced onto an object resembling the original object of anger. Some disease conditions are indications of internalized anger.
Interpersonal	Sullivan	Any anxiety producing situation has the potential for evoking anger and aggression. The emotion of anger gives one a feeling of power that compensates for an underlying anxiety. Anger attempts to destroy the object or situation that produced the anxiety.
Behavioral	Dollard and Miller	Aggression results from frustration in achieving a goal.
	Bandura, Moreno	Anger is learned through the socialization process, by observation and modeling. Anger is energy that propels people to new learning, thus enhancing feelings of adequacy as a person.
Existential	Frankl	Anger in suffering gives people an opportunity to find new meanings in life.

the hypothalamus and amygdala may increase or decrease aggressive behavior. Advances in neurophysiology and neuroanatomy are identifying specific areas of the brain that may be responsible for particular emotional responses. Areas have been identified that, when stimulated, cause aggressive outbursts; other areas have been identified that inhibit these emotional responses.

Biochemical studies suggest that the release of norepinephrine by the adrenal medulla is directly related to aggressive behavior. Modification of the aggressive behavior can be achieved by adjusting the rate of metabolism of the biogenic amines norepinephrine, dopamine, and serotonin. Other chemical and endocrine disorders such as hypoglycemia and allergies may lead to aggression. Studies of increased blood levels of male sex hormones, particularly testosterone, correlate with increased aggressiveness. In women, premenstrual decrease in blood levels of progesterone may result in irritability and increased hostility.[36]

Lorenz,[40] a physician and naturalist, perceived aggression as an inborn response pattern originating from a type of instinctual force similar to that of animals. When an appropriate stimulus occurs, the individual's instinctual response is to fight. According to Lorenz, individuals suffer from an inability to discharge aggression drives. This inability may result in self-destructive events such as accidents and suicide. Conversely, it may produce behavior that appears

superficially as intense kindness but actually is motivated by an underlying current of anger.

Psychoanalytical

Freud[24] described aggression as evolving from thanatos, the death wish. According to Freud, individuals are born with a given amount of death drive (aggression) that seeks expression. Because of the strength of the death drive, individuals are prone to behave destructively. When the death drive predominates destructive behavior such as suicide occurs.

Aggression is hostile, destructive behavior. The energy of aggression is diminished through direct expression (catharsis). When direct expression is blocked, indirect expression may result and the person directs the anger toward self. Depression, for example, is anger directed toward self. Some diseases may be indications of internalized anger, including rheumatoid arthritis, asthma, ulcers, migraine headache, hypertension, colitis, angina, and chronic back pain. Disowning or behaving the opposite of what is expected is another form of inwardly expressed anger. Being overly polite, exceptionally kind or "killing with kindness" are examples of disowning. Withdrawal may be an avenue to escape from one's anger. Abuse of drugs or alcohol provides an escape from reality. Running away, overeating, and inappropriate silence are also forms of escaping reality and withdrawing from anger.

Anger also may be displaced onto an object or person resembling the original object of anger. Safe objects that lack authority or power to retaliate are generally selected. For example, the worker who cannot express feelings to a boss will direct anger toward a spouse. The spouse, being unable to talk to her husband, may yell at a child, and the child, in frustration, may kick the door. Another indirect expression of anger is passive aggression. The individual is inhibited from expressing actual feelings.

▼ Case Example

Pat is angry with her husband for his preoccupation with activities outside the home. Instead of directly confronting him, she responds with sugary sweetness and indicates she "doesn't mind" his involvement elsewhere. However, she expresses her resentment by such actions as taking the car when she knows he needs it and leaving him alone with the children when he is busy at home. These subtle acts are substitutes for the direct expression of anger.

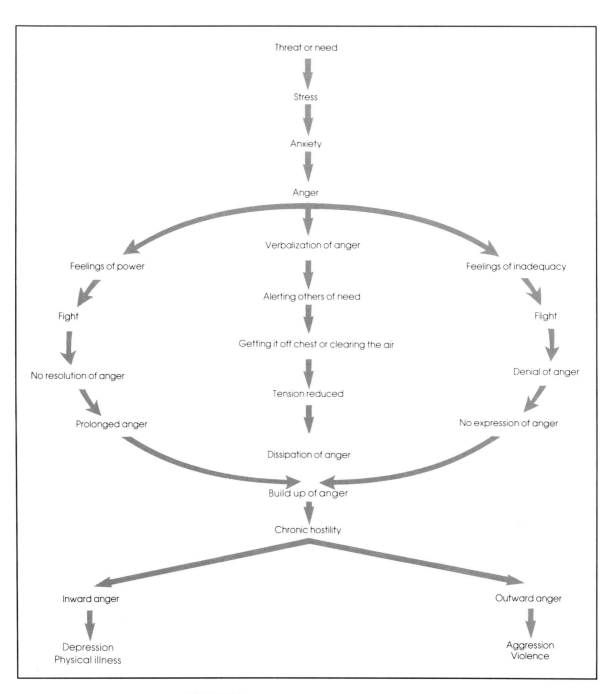

FIGURE 11-1 The development and expression of anger.

Interpersonal

Sullivan[63] believed that people use anger to avoid experiencing anxiety. An angry response pushes the threat away; that is, anger is used to destroy the object or situation that produced the anxiety. Any threat to self-esteem or security results in frustration and produces feelings of inadequacy and anxiety. A person experiences a situation in which expectations of oneself or others are not met. The resulting anger gives the person a feeling of power that compensates for the underlying anxiety (Figure 11-1).

▼ Case Example

Seven-year-old David sits helplessly clutching the tiny bridle of his new toy stallion, Silver. He has managed to get on the saddle but has trouble buckling the strap. He screams, "Silver, stand still, you dumb horse!" and even louder, "Silver!" His mother, trying to rest on the sofa, screams, "David, that's no reason to get mad! Now, if you can't buckle the bridle, bring it here!" David promptly bursts into tears and throws Silver against the wall. Mothers puts a pillow over her head and prays for him to grow up; then she screams, "Your temper really bugs me!" Her response only escalates David's rage, and he starts kicking the floor.

Sullivan[63] states that the suppression of anger produces three probable outcomes: conforming, rebelling, or malevolent behaviors. For example, David may conform to his mother's expectations. (After his mother screams, he may pick up his horse, smile sweetly, hand her the horse, and ask her if she is tired.) The behavior does not represent his real self, but it alleviates the interpersonal threat with his mother. David then learns to deny his anger and develops a behavioral pattern based on pretense. On the other hand, David may choose to become enraged and rebel. He may throw the horse and scream at his mother. The pattern can persist into adulthood. David will then deal with his anxiety by becoming enraged. The third alternative is to neither rebel nor conform but to develop a malevolent or evil disposition. In response to his mother's scream, David may stare coldly at her, pick up his horse, and go outside to play with 4-year-old Michelle in her sandbox. David may then sneak up behind Michelle, hit her on the head with the horse, grab her shovel and bucket, and run away laughing.

Behavioral

Dollard and Miller,[15] in their development of the frustration-aggression theory, suggest that all aggression results from an experience of frustration. Frustration occurs when the individual is blocked from attaining a desired goal. This leads to anger, which produces an aggressive drive. When the goal is highly valued, the sense of frustration and the ensuing aggression increases. The aggressive drive is reduced by an act of belligerence.

The social learning theorists believe that the impulse to behave aggressively is subject to the influence of learning, socialization, and experience. According to Bandura,[3] aggression is learned behavior under voluntary control. The learning of aggressive behavior occurs by observation and modeling. For example, a child watches an angry parent strike out at another person. Learning aggressive behavior also takes place by direct experience. The person feels anger and behaves aggressively. If behaving aggressively brings rewards, the behavior is encouraged.

Modeling also demonstrates aggression and can be purposeful or unintentional. Purposeful modeling of aggression occurs when the nurse is angry and makes statements such as, "I get upset when you let others continue to tell you what to do about your problems." Aggression is unintentionally demonstrated when a physician yells at a nurse in the presence of interns and clients or when a parent spanks a child while angry.

Moreno[44] believed that anger is a natural by-product of the learning process; it is the signal that a person needs to learn something. The more inadequate a person feels, the more anger may be present. Moreno also believed that anger is spontaneous energy that propels an individual into new learning. Those who have learned a wide variety of adequate responses to anger value their anger, express it, and see it as an emotion that promotes greater feelings of adequacy. The expression of anger frees one to reach out, to love, and to remain connected to vital people.

▼ Case Example

Nineteen-year-old Sally rushes home because she expects a call from her boyfriend, John, at 5 PM. He is free from 5 to 5:15 PM and will be calling to let her know if he can go out that night. Once inside the front door, she hears her 16-year-old brother David talking to his girlfriend, Jane. Sally glares at the kitchen clock; it is 4:55 PM. She whispers to her brother that John is calling at 5 o'clock, and he annoyingly nods back. With tears in his eyes, he angrily continues talking. Sally realizes that David is having a fight with Jane. Sally knows that Jane is on the verge of breaking up with David and that he has been extremely upset about it. Sally glances at the clock again; it is 4:58 PM. She is worried that this fight could go on for another half hour.

Sally feels stirring inside her stomach, flushing of her face, and sweating in her underarms and palms. She feels fidgety and says to herself, "Oh damn, I've got to know if we're going out tonight!" But David looks terrible. He simply has got to talk this through; he's been waiting to talk with Jane about this for 3 days. Sally paces around the living room, frequently glancing at the clock; it is 5:06 PM. She remembers other times when David has been furious, and she is a little afraid to invite him to unload all this on her. She gets David's attention and points to the clock; he is unimpressed with her dilemma. The excited feeling she had when she came home has completely vanished, and a burning pressure is building inside her. The thought occurs to her that John will think she is talking to someone else! Finally, her own concerns and needs overshadow her concern for her brother and she screams, "I want to talk to John, David—get off the phone!" David hollers, "I had the phone first, get lost. Who do you think you are, coming in like this?"

David swears, tells Jane he will call her back in 10 minutes, and turns to Sally and says, "Get off my back! I hate it when you pull stuff like this!" He hands her the phone and storms out of the room. Sally feels immediate relief, and, after she talks with John, she finds her brother in his room. There is a heavy silence before she says, "Things are pretty bad between Jane and you—huh?"

David (*Nods.*) *You could have waited. I was on the phone first.*
Sally: *No . . . John could only call between 5 and 5:15 PM.*
David: *You shouldn't count on the phone being free.*

Sally: Yeah—I suppose I got mad when you ignored me. (Pauses, notices the tension is gone, and smiles.) Sorry and good luck!

David: (Smiles and shakes his head.) I'm going to call her now.

Sally tousles his hair, and they both grin. Sally walks away and reflecting, "Sure feels good to clear the air. It was a little presumptious of me to believe that in a family of five the phone would be free for those 15 minutes.

The preceding example illustrates a spontaneous, creative, and integrated expression of anger. Sally felt anger, expressed it, and made sense out of the experience. In fact, it brought her closer to her brother and taught her something about herself.

Existential

According to Frankl,[22] people need to find meaning in and from their suffering. Suffering includes the emotion of anger and gives people the opportunity to develop deeper meaning in their lives.

Frankl draws from his experiences as a prisoner in a German concentration camp during World War II to explain his theory. He noted that the men who lost hope for a future, who occupied themselves with memories of the past and ignored the present, were angry. They could find no meaning in their suffering, and they became aggressive toward fellow inmates. Those who created dreams of the future with family, friends, and job were more sensitive to others and better adjusted.

Frankl believes that humans are truly free to choose their attitudes when confronted with infuriating situations. People can transcend these situations with humor and curiosity. They can develop more encompassing meanings of situations and finally activate thoughts and images that produce love. Frankl sees anger as a vehicle to new understanding, meaning, and love.

NURSING PROCESS

Assessment

Physical dimension The nurse assesses the client's overall posture and appearance. Nonpurposeful motor symptoms such as agitation and pacing may indicate increasing tension. A flushed face, tightened jaws, flared nostrils, and protruding neck veins indicate intense efforts of control. The fists may be clenched, posture tense, and the voice louder. Eye contact that is directed and glaring or staring also indicate anger.

People sometimes use their bodies to make a defiant statement to the world. The "I don't care what you think" attitude can be conveyed through unconventional clothing, jewelry, and hairstyles.

Physiological responses to anger result primarily from the action of the autonomic nervous system in response to the secretion of epinephrine. Blood pressure increases, and tachycardia is present. Blood composition is altered with increased fatty acids and fewer lymphocytes. Gastrointestinal changes include nausea, increased salivation, increased hydrochloric acid secretion, and decreased gastric peri-

▼ ·····
MESSAGES OF ANGER

Sight

Body tense	Lowered eyebrows	Shaking fist
Shoulders tight	Pounding	Kicking
Flushed face	Stomping	Hands on hips
Slashing	Arms crossed	Holding breath
Pacing	Index finger pointed	Eyes staring
Turning away	Direct, glaring eye contact	Accidents
Nostrils flared	Fist hitting hand	Tight lips

Taste

No taste to food

Touch

Pushing	Hitting	Slapping
Tight fist	Elevated body temperature	Shoving

Hearing

Change in voice tone	Chewing food loudly	Pounding
Accusing words	Deep sighs	Hitting
Statements of anger	Breaking of objects	Slamming
Heavy footsteps	Drumming of fingernails	doors
		Cursing

stalsis. Symptoms similar to those of anxiety are noted, such as increased alertness, increased muscle tension, and rapid reflexes. Urination is frequently increased, pupils are dilated, and the person has difficulty relaxing and sleeping.

Disorders known to have an anger-related source include hypertension, rheumatoid arthritis, ulcers, colitis, asthma, migraine headaches, angina, and chronic back pain. Based on biological theories, it is equally important for the nurse to be aware that trauma or brain lesions may be a contributing factor in explosive, violent behavior. Because of the relationship of these conditions to anger, the nurse collects data about the client's past and present illnesses.

A person's sensory receptors receive messages of anger (see box). The messages are subsequently transferred into observable client behaviors and physiological responses. Because these behaviors and responses are important to understand the client's anger, the nurse collects data about their frequency and documents the findings.

Laboratory tests are scheduled to rule out a physical basis for the angry behavior. These include x-ray examinations of the skull; computerized axial *tomography* (CT scan); arteriography; tests for metabolic abnormalities, chemical imbalances, and endocrine disturbances; and electroencephalogram (EEG). According to Lorenz,[40] genetic studies may also be helpful to determine whether others in the family have exhibited similar behavior.

Emotional dimension Expressions like the following describe the discomfort of anger. "I feel . . . "

Out of sorts	Irritated	Angry
Disappointed	Upset	Furious
Annoyed	Hurt	Enraged

Based on the theories of Freud[24] and Sullivan,[63] being alert to the many expressions of anger and anxiety is a necessary nursing action. Other feelings that the nurse may observe in an angry person include powerlessness, annoyance, frustration, resentment, belligerence, rage, fury, hostility, hurt, depression, humiliation, vengeance, defensiveness, domination, blaming, and demanding (Table 11-2). For some, the loss of control and negative effects associated with the expression of anger produce guilt or embarrassment. The energy released in anger may create additional problems such as greater tension rather than relief. The nurse needs to be sensitive to the influences that affect the person's expression of anger and look for signs of guilt or embarrassment. For others, a sense of power comes with anger.

In despair and depression, anger is denied and turned inward on the self. The energy of anger is used to maintain the depression. Further assessment of anger as it relates to depression is found in Chapter 14.

It is important for the nurse to assess the intensity of the client's expression of anger. In addition, the appropriateness of the anger to the anger-provoking situation provides data about the client's anger threshold. A person with a low tolerance for frustration is easily provoked to anger;

▼ **TABLE 11-2** **Types of Anger and Examples**

Hostility Type	Example
Assault	I get into fights about as often as the next person.
	If I have to resort to physical violence to defend my rights, I will.
Indirect hostility	I sometimes slam doors when I am mad.
	I sometimes pout when I don't get my own way.
Irritability	It makes my blood boil when people make fun of me.
	Sometimes people bother me just by being around.
Negativism	Unless somebody asks me in a nice way, I won't do what they want.
	When people are bossy, I take my time just to show them.
Resentment	Other people seem to get the breaks.
	At times I feel I get a raw deal out of life.
Suspicion	I know people tend to talk about me behind my back.
	My motto is, "Never trust strangers."
Verbal hostility	When I disapprove of my friend's behavior, I let him know.
	When I get mad I say nasty things.
Guilt	The few times I have cheated I have suffered unbearable feelings of remorse.
	It depresses me that I do not do more for my parents.

one with a high tolerance may demonstrate self-control and adequacy in handling anger.

Intellectual dimension At first glance, it seems that intellect plays little or no role in anger. The emotion itself seems to push aside rationality and any semblance of an orderly progression of thought. The strength and intensity of the anger may cause a person to misinterpret information that affects perceptions, conclusions, memory, judgment, and actions. By listening the nurse can determine the amount of anger present through repetitive thoughts. Long after anger dissipates, thoughts about the incident often regenerate the anger. Individuals can work themselves into a rage without the presence of the original stimulus. Repetitive thoughts keep the anger flowing. The following case example shows one way of keeping anger alive with repetitive thoughts.

▼ **Case Example**

Daniel sits slumped in his third-grade arithmetic class shortly after recess. His best friend, Steve, did not choose him for the recess soccer team, and he is scheming how to get even. He certainly is not going to walk home from school with Steve; he will walk right past his friend, pretending not to see him. He doesn't need him anyway. His mind flashes on how he stood there as the teams were being chosen. So what if he can't play soccer? Steve could have chosen him anyway. The big-shot soccer captain, he'd show him! He glares at the back of his friend's head. He imagines himself the captain of the soccer team choosing his friend last. By the end of the arithmetic class Daniel's stomach is in a knot, and he is convinced that Steve is a stupid slob. He believes Steve doesn't want to be his friend anymore, so he marches straight up to him after class and says, "I think your mother eats worms!"

The nurse assesses the methods the client uses to express anger. Some persons express anger by scolding, sarcasm, humor, and gossiping. Others deny their feelings of anger and express it by forgetting appointments, being late, misunderstanding, procrastinating, and failing to learn.

The associative processes influence the development and expression of anger. People conceptually link cause to effect. For instance, because most parents are angry when punishing children, people learn to associate anger with bad and wrong. Peoples' beliefs dictate their experience; if they believe anger is wrong, an experience involving anger will be blocked from expression as in the following case example.

▼ **Case Example**

June, a 29-year-old teacher, mother, and wife, came for help when she could not generate the optimistic and loving feeling that she had once possessed for her family. The family had recently moved into a new community because of her husband's promotion. John's job now entailed 2 weeks' travel every month, and the isolation of staying home with their 5-year-old son, Jacob, and the 2-year-old twin daughters in a rural neighborhood was defeating June. She had not wanted the house in the country, but it had been a dream of her husband for years. She also had not wanted John to take the job because of the travel, but she understood the potential promotions that would be available for him in a couple of years. She always had been one to "make-do" and not cause a fuss. She could not remember having a fight with anyone, but now it concerned her when she would yell at the children for the "smallest things," kick the cat when it got underfoot, and be visibly irritated at John if he was 10 minutes late. She did not like herself this way. She asked the therapist to help her be more loving and accepting. When asked how she felt about anger, she replied, "I really don't think it's right. John gets mad at me and the kids, and it just makes us feel bad. Jacob gets mad back, which makes matters worse. I think people should try to be positive if they do get annoyed and keep it to themselves until it passes. There's no sense in making other people feel bad, too; they generally do not mean to insult you. When I find myself blaming John for putting me and the kids in the country, I just tell myself to be positive—John's doing the best he can—but I'm finding it hard to do."

In therapy, June revealed that when she was young her mother had angrily accused her of being bad and evil whenever she did something wrong. June then felt as if she were completely evil and bad. She paired anger with evil and wrongdoing. As an adult she had to learn to separate these two and to slowly learn to voice her frustrations to her husband.

Individuals with good verbal and social skills are less likely to resort to expressing anger by physical means. A person may preserve self-esteem by using verbal skills such as pacification, persuasion, and humor. The mind can be used to consider alternative actions and consequences. If individuals have learned to perceive the situation from a number of vantage points, they are less likely to attack physically. The presence of verbal skills implies a cognitive process. The nurse needs to assess the client's verbal skills to determine his ability to perceive situations and to consider options for dealing with them.

An assessment by the nurse of the client's readiness for change is essential before establishing goals. By observing and listening, the nurse can identify those clients who have developed fixed, rigid views of the world that do not allow for growth. They are often angry, and the fixed beliefs do not allow them to accommodate to change and thus lead to frustration. A rigid belief is, "People will abandon me if I express my anger, and I will end up all alone. I must not express anger." If people can develop beliefs that stimulate and initiate a new learning process, they are less likely to live in a state of anger. A flexible belief is, "If I express my anger directly, some people will interact with me directly, some will retreat for a short time and reengage later, and some will terminate the relationship entirely. Each person has a belief about and a style of expressing anger, and I will just have to get to know the person and find out what it is. One thing is sure—we all have anger."

Social dimension Using behavioral theory the nurse assesses the client's patterned responses to the anger of others; particular attention is paid to passive or aggressive responses. Passive responses include self-denying; being inhibited, hurt, or anxious; allowing others to choose for one; and not achieving desired goals. Aggressive responses include self-enhancing at expense of another; depreciating others; choosing for others; and achieving desired goal by hurting others.

Some people express anger in a way that stimulates rejection. They say to themselves, "It is not fair that I should feel this way." They channel their anger into judgments and look for someone to blame. They angrily critique the behaviors of others as wrong, unfair, or unethical and expect them to do penance. This process alienates the individual from himself and from others. The individual loses the opportunity to learn because the original source of anger is no longer the focus. People react negatively to the critique and distance themselves from the angry person.

The following are ways to express anger that distance others:

- Projecting self-anger onto another ("I know you hate it when I feel inadequate.")
- Blaming another for pain that resulted from a prior non assertive stance of self ("You made me cook this meal for you, and you had better enjoy it.")
- Being consistently late
- Screaming and shouting at others' mistakes
- Belittling and ridiculing
- Using sarcasm
- Rejecting (A person may "say," through nonverbal behavior, "You were supposed to be home half an hour ago, so I won't talk to you for a day.")
- Being angry at one incident and reiterating past grievances
- Talking to another (An angry person talks to John about anger at Bill, so both are angry at Bill.)
- Breaking or throwing objects, or hitting a wall
- Moralizing or preaching
- Covering anger with sweetness
- Hitting a person

According to interpersonal theory, some individuals need a relationship in which the other person serves specific, seemingly vital, functions. Because these relationships seem essential to one's sense of well-being, anger directed at these persons is threatening to experience and express. To maintain these relationships, people are likely to lie about their anger, sacrifice their integrity, and pretend. Pretense kills the essence of the vital relationship. Fear of anger and its consequences can be overwhelming, as the threat of losing important relationships is powerful. Isolation, no matter how brief, can be devastating to some.

Other people take more risks with their anger. Some maintain social relationships through intimidation, and the emotion of anger dominates. Their love, sexuality, joy, and sadness are minimally acknowledged; and they berate these emotional experiences in others. Although their anger makes them appear strong, their fragility is evident when one realizes how limited their emotional repositories actually are. Thus it is essential to assess the client's self-esteem, self-concept, and feelings of adequacy.

Anger plays a vital role when terminating significant relationships. It can be used constructively to let go, or it can be used destructively to cling. Anger allows one to focus on the self in a new light. It encourages separateness. When disentangling from people, places, and roles, a person, through anger, considers new perspectives and alternatives. When new people, places, and roles are required to facilitate a change, the old ends as the new begins. Beginnings are difficult, however, because they highlight people's inadequacies. Often people angrily cling to memories of more fulfilled times and do not risk the process of letting go. Clinging is a form of anger that says, "I don't want change in my life. I'm angry about it, and so it's not going to happen!"

The nurse needs to consider culture when assessing anger. According to behavioral theorists, anger is culturally defined as part of certain roles. People in some roles have the right to be angry, whereas people in others do not. The boss can express anger toward an employee, but the employees cannot express anger toward the supervisor. Parents can express anger at their children, but if children express anger at their parents, it is disrespectful. The client can express anger at a nurse, but the nurse cannot exhibit anger to a client.

The emotion of anger is expressed in different ways in various cultures. In some cultures, to express anger is to risk rejection and isolation; in others it brings favor. When assessing cultural differences of anger, one needs to consider the influence of prejudice and fear. Groups with a minority status may fear the intensity of anger generated from the prejudice they encounter in their daily lives. They develop norms for its expression in public life that differ from those used within their own subculture. In public life they may fear that direct expression of anger may jeopardize their position. Therefore they may express anger indirectly or passively with overly compliant or passive-aggressive behavior, anger directed against themselves, or aggression directed into creative outlets, such as writing, sports, music, and art.

All interactions contribute to a person's style of expressing anger. According to Bandura[3] and Moreno,[16] people learn about their anger from those around them. They are socialized to behave in a way that fits the pattern developed by their family and culture. The messages may be contradictory; for example, the family may yell at each other, whereas the teacher may teach polite behavior. The individual quickly becomes socialized to behave accordingly in the various contexts.

Anger is also expressed differently at different ages. Infants' rage can be heard loudly and clearly when needs are unmet. The toddler's tantrums and the loud "no's" from 3- and 4-year-olds are age appropriate. The expressions of anger progress from physical to verbal and decrease in frequency as the child matures. Adult expressions of anger reflect this trend; that is, typically the adult expresses anger verbally or indirectly.

Finally, it is important for the nurse to see that the client's behavior is, in part, a reflection of a life situation and the present interaction. If someone appears angry "all the time" and is disagreeable to be around, it may be a response to a status of isolation or rejection in a primary group. Anger may be the energy that helps the person survive.

Spiritual dimension Clients' beliefs about anger are integral to their philosophy of life and spirituality. If the client belongs to an organized religion, the nurse needs to investigate how that religion views anger. If it is seen as sinful and the nurse is encouraging its expression, clients may experience considerable turmoil.

According to existential theory, the absence of a meaningful philosophy engenders frustration and anger. People who have no framework within which to act make their way through life impulsively, much like a boat in a storm. They may value neither their acts nor ultimately themselves. They feel disparaging toward life's demands and resent giving to others. People may experience a lack of meaning at transition points in their life, for example, as they change their focus from school to employment to retirement. What once was considered vital now has little or no significance, yet nothing else has filled the void; irritation and frustration are present. For others, finding a meaningful existence has been a continual problem, and they feel en-

raged. They believe they are justified in inflicting their anger on the world, either openly or privately.

Beliefs about oneself evolve from one's concept of how one has met the challenges of life. Some people are angry and disappointed about their performances. They have been unable to meet their own or others' expectations and direct their anger against themselves. A person cannot be angry and simultaneously transcend the limitations of human experience. To transcend is to leave the self behind and identify with the whole, knowing that the self will continue to exist and that it has value. In these moments there is no place for the emotion of anger.

People strive to be spontaneous and creative beings and to develop meaningful existences. Anger indicates that the creativity is inhibited, preventing greater self-actualization.

Spiritual conflicts, absence of a meaningful philosophy, and contradictory beliefs may generate anger. The following questions are a guide to determine the effects of a client's spiritual life on dealing with anger.

- As an adult, what is the role of anger in your spiritual development?
- How do you value anger?
- In your current situation, what strong beliefs seem contradictory of one another?
- At what time in your life have you felt resentment and alienation from God, a supreme power, or other persons?
- When have you expressed the need to suffer?

Measurement Tools

Numerous instruments exist to measure anger. Table 11-3 summarizes the more common instruments.

▼ **TABLE 11-3** **Instruments to Measure Anger and Hostility**

Instrument	Measures
Anger Expression Scale (AX)[61]	Expression of angry feelings
Anger Inventory (AI)[51]	Extent to which a broad range of situations provoke anger reactions
Buss-Durkee Hostility Inventory[8]	Different types of hostility
Cook-Medley Hostility (Ho) Scale[11]	Relationship among hostility and health consequences
Framingham Psychosocial Survey[31] (Anger section)	Response to anger arousal
Reaction Inventory (RI)[18]	Extent to which situations evoke anger reactions
Self-Statement and Affective State Inventory (SSASI)[30]	Self-reporting of anger, anxiety, depression, suspiciousness, and rationales in response to interpersonal scenarios involving conflict
State-Trait Personality Inventory (STPI)[60]	Self-reporting levels of anger, anxiety, and curiosity

Analysis

Nursing diagnosis

Examples of anger-related nursing diagnoses approved by the North American Nursing Diagnosis Association (NANDA) are listed below.

1. Ineffective individual coping: inappropriate anger related to loss of job
2. Ineffective individual coping; anger related to financial problems
3. High risk for violence related to delusions of persecution
4. High risk for violence: self-directed related to suicide attempt
5. Impaired social interactions related to hostile, threatening statements
6. Noncompliance related to anger over physical limitations
7. Sleep pattern disturbance related to anger
8. Altered parenting: child neglect related to frustration and dissatisfaction of parenting role

The accompanying box lists the defining characteristics of the nursing diagnosis *high-risk for violence*, and the case example illustrates this nursing diagnosis.

Planning

The care plan (Table 11-4) shows examples of long- and short-term goals, outcome criteria, interventions, and ra-

---

▼ DEFINING CHARACTERISTICS OF POTENTIAL FOR VIOLENCE

DEFINITION

A state in which an individual experiences behaviors that can be physically harmful to self or others.

DEFINING CHARACTERISTICS

- **Physical dimension**

  History of aggressive acts
  Poor impulse control
  History of self-harm attempt
  Withdrawal from drugs
  Rigid/taut body
  Increased pacing

- **Emotional dimension**

  Increased agitation
  Increased anxiety, panic
  Low tolerance for frustration
  Temper tantrums

- **Intellectual dimension**

  Delusions
  Verbal threats of physical assault
  Confusion
  Boasting about previous violent episodes
  Defiance
  Argumentation

- **Social dimension**

  Bullying others

Modified from McFarland G, McFarlane E: *Nursing diagnosis and intervention: planning for patient care,* ed 2, St Louis, 1993, Mosby–Year Book.

---

tionales related to anger. These serve as examples of the planning stage in the nursing process.

▼ Case Example

Terry, aged 25, attempted to kill herself by taking an overdose of a combination of medications including Valium, Librium, Dalmene, and Xanax. She had a fight with her husband of 9 months as well as with her mother who lived next door. She has no other close relationships. On returning from work, she became angry about her situation and labeled it as hopeless. She searched the house for medications she could find and swallowed them. Thirty minutes later her husband returned from work, and on learning what Terry had done, had her admitted to an adult psychiatric unit.

Implementation

Physical dimension Interventions include providing constructive outlets for the energy of anger. Physical activity is helpful. The nurse can encourage jogging, swimming, weight lifting, dancing, using punching bags, and activities that allow large muscle involvement and socially accepted expressions of aggression (Figure 11-2).

Other activities often offered in occupational therapy include sanding and hammering to offset the energy of anger. Use of a punching bag may dissipate feelings of anger. Providing distraction and channeling angry behavior through games like volleyball, tennis, and badminton are therapeutic. Constructive tasks and challenging activities such as painting and trivia games at which the client is proficient also dilute anger and provide socially acceptable outlets for expressing it. In addition, feelings of self-esteem are fostered, and feelings of accomplishment are promoted.

External controls can be applied as a last resort by physical restraints or by use of a seclusion room until the client is able to gain self-control. Indications for application of physical restraints include the following:

1. Physical assault to self, others, and environment
2. Physical and verbal threats
3. Hypersensitivity and responsiveness to environmental stimuli

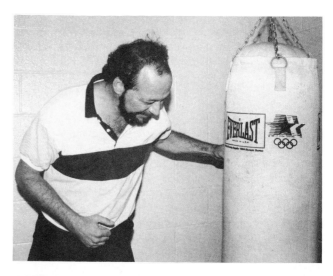

FIGURE 11-2 Punching bags are effective ways to express one's anger.

▼ **TABLE 11-4   NURSING CARE PLAN**

GOALS	OUTCOME CRITERIA	INTERVENTIONS	RATIONALES
NURSING DIAGNOSIS: Ineffective individual coping related to: Inability to express anger appropriately			
LONG TERM			
To express anger in ways that are not injurious to self or others	Expresses anger assertively		
SHORT TERM			
Will not harm self or others	Does not harm self or others	Observe for agitation, restlessness	Indicators that anger may be escalating
		Set limits on behavior	Provides external controls when client loses control, promotes a sense of security that is important for people to feel while they are confronting their own disturbing behaviors
Will express angry feelings	Describes angry feelings verbally	Encourage to verbalize angry feelings in safe situations (group therapy, with nurse)	To gain skill and confidence in managing anger
		Help client identify consequences of anger	To develop awareness of effects of anger on self and others
		Give positive reinforcement for appropriate expression of anger	To reinforce appropriate behavior and increase self-esteem, confidence in self
Will tell others when angry	States angry feelings to others	Teach assertive skills	To communicate when angry without interfering with the rights of others
Will cope with threats and life disappointments	Manages anxiety and anger	Instill confidence that life can improve when responsibility is taken to improve it	To build confidence in self and help client to take responsibility for own behavior

Behaviors that are considered clinical justifications for seclusions are the following:

1. Increasing agitation from ward stimuli
2. Destructiveness to the physical environment
3. Hyperactivity
4. Need for protection of self and others in the environment

If physical restraints are used, nursing documentation that supports a sufficient risk of harm to self or others is essential. Restraints are applied under the supervision of a registered nurse and with a physician's order using an adequate number of staff members for quick, efficient action. When a client is secluded, the procedure also requires nursing documentation that supports the need for the intervention. A concern for the client's dignity and value as a person is essential.

Whether the intervention is restraint or seclusion, a room is prepared in advance and the purpose of the procedure is explained to the client using short, simple, direct statements. Potentially dangerous articles are removed, and the client is monitored at designated times according to established policies. Food and fluids are provided, and bathroom use is permitted with supervision. Medications may be given to calm the client (see Chapter 24). The profile for Haldol (p. 219) describes nursing care appropriate to its administration. The nurse suggests socially acceptable behavior in a supportive, nurturing manner and helps the client regain control of behavior. Throughout the restraint or seclusion period, the nurse documents the client's response and all nursing care given. Upon release from restraint or seclusion, nursing documentation of the client's behavior and any teaching offered on appropriate behavior for return to the unit community is recorded. The research highlight on p. 218 explores precipitants of violence in a psychiatric inpatient setting.

Emotional dimension Reducing sources of undue anxiety or high levels of anxiety is a way of preventing anger from developing or escalating. Frequently, hospitalization removes the client from overwhelming stress and anxiety and the subsequent anger and allows the person time to place life situations in a more tolerable perspective.

The nurse can help angry clients by observing and acknowledging their anger. Empathic statements such as "You're upset" or "You're angry" provide validation for ob-

RESEARCH HIGHLIGHT

Precipitants of Violence in a Psychiatric Inpatient Setting
• M Sheridan, R Henrion, L Robinson, and V Baxter

PURPOSE

The study was designed to examine events preceding restraints of clients due to threatening or aggressive behavior.

SAMPLE

The sample included 73 clients from an acute and chronic psychiatric division in a Veterans Affairs Medical Center during a 12-month period. Only two of the participants were women.

METHODOLOGY

Semistructured interviews were conducted concurrently with nursing staff and clients who had been placed in four-point leather restraints due to threatening or aggressive behavior within 72 hours of release. Staff members were asked to state any knowledge of past aggressive behavior by the client, recount any behavioral clues exhibited preceding application of restraint, elaborate on events from a staff perspective, and describe how the aggressive behavior was managed short of actual restraint. Clients were asked to relate what occurred before application of restraints, thoughts and feelings at that time, their view of the restraint experience, and suggestions for how future episodes requiring restraints could be prevented. Also, the researchers rated behaviors that had occurred before restraint as moderately to severely aggressive using an Overt Aggressive Scale. Demographic characteristics, diagnosis, and history of aggressive behavior were collected from the medical record.

Data from *Hospital and Community Psychiatry* 41(7):776, 1990.

FINDINGS

The majority of participants in the study had a diagnosis of paranoia schizophrenia. Behaviors exhibited most frequently by clients during the events leading to restraint were physical aggression (86%), verbal threats (58%), and threats directed toward an object (8%), with 71% directed toward staff, 53% toward other clients, and 27% toward objects. The most frequent external event leading to restraint was client-staff conflict. Staff's most frequent response to the aggression was to talk down the client. A comparison of clients with a positive response to the restraint experience with those who had a negative response revealed no differences between the two groups. Clients' suggestions for preventing events leading to restraint included better communication with staff, discharge from the hospital, a better attitude toward treatment, taking medications, and avoiding drinking.

IMPLICATIONS

Because the findings revealed that events preceding episodes of restraint were frequently external to the client and often involved client-staff conflict underscore the need for staff to establish a working alliance with clients early in the hospitalization, provide an opportunity for conflict resolution, and educate clients on appropriate responses to anger and frustration. Further, opportunities for staff to discuss emotional reactions toward clients who are aggressive are justified. Such discussions could result in new and innovative approaches to prevent violence.

---

servations and help the client recognize the feeling of anger. If the client denies the anger, the nurse can rephrase the statement by saying, "You sound annoyed" or "You look distressed." These statements clarify and verify observations about the behavior and facilitate recognition of angry feelings. Encouraging description of the feelings prevents the client from avoiding or denying them. "What do you mean when you say you're feeling frustrated?" or "Tell me more about your feeling of disappointment" focuses attention on the feeling. The nurse needs to communicate to the client that it is normal to feel angry and that the expression of the feeling can be constructive or destructive. Constructive expressions of anger include talking about the feeling or withdrawing until some of the anger is dissipated and then talking about it. Time can be crucial when anger is intense; for example, a period of withdrawal can provide a cooling-down time until the person regains control.

Feelings associated with anger, such as guilt and depression, are also explored. Interventions for guilt or depression are addressed in Chapters 12 and 13.

Intellectual dimension According to behavioral theorists, when people are angry, they require limits, a here-and-now orientation to circumstance, and people who

can facilitate a more adequate response. The case example illustrates the process of setting a limit.

▼ Case Example

It is 4 PM, time for change of shift. John has just been told that he must receive one-on-one care because he is suicidal. He is 50 years old, 5 feet 10 inches tall, and weighs 175 pounds.

John paces down the hall hitting his fist into the palm of his hand. Periodically, he strikes the wall, obviously injuring his hand, but he feels no pain. He swings around then heads toward the dayroom. The other people stop talking and remain motionless; John kicks a metal trash can and swears. He looks menacingly at the nurse who has just told him he will have to remain on one-on-one care for 24 hours.

The nurse elicits the support of two male employees and alerts the reporting staff members to stand by. She approaches John but maintains a safe distance from him.

Nurse: (Loudly and firmly.) Get control of yourself, John. We will not let you hurt yourself.
John: (Stops and trembles as face turns ashen.)
Nurse: (Firmly.) What are you angry about? Use your words. I want to hear from you.
John: You bitch, what do you know? (Turns to walk away.)

HALOPERIDOL/ HALOPERIDOL DECANOATE

(ha-loe-per′idole)

Haldol, Peridol/Haloperidol Decanoate

Func. Class.: Antipsychotic/ neuroleptic

Chem. class.: Butyrophenone

Action: Depresses cerebral cortex, hypothalamus, limbic system, which control activity and aggression; blocks neurotransmission produced by dopamine at synapse; exhibits strong α-adrenergic, anticholinergic blocking action; mechanism for antipsychotic effects is unclear.

Uses: Psychotic disorders, control of tics, vocal utterances in Tourette syndrome, short-term treatment of hyperactive children showing excessive motor activity, prolonged parenteral therapy in chronic schizophrenia

Dosage and routes:

Psychosis

▶ *Adult:* PO 0.5-5 mg bid or tid initially depending on severity of condition; dose is increased to desired dose, max 100 mg/day; IM 2-5 mg q1-8h

▶ *Child 3-12 yr:* PO/IM 0.05-0.15 mg/kg/day

▶ *Decanoate:* Initial dose IM is 10-15 × daily oral dose at 4 wk interval; do not administer IV, not to exceed 100 mg

Chronic schizophrenia

▶ *Adult:* IM 10-15 times the PO dose q4 wk (decanoate)

▶ *Child 3-12 yr:* PO/IM 0.05-0.15 mg/kg/day

Tics/vocal utterances

▶ *Adult:* PO 0.5-5 mg bid or tid increased until desired response occurs

▶ *Child 3-12 yr:* PO 0.05-0.075 mg/kg/day

Hyperactive children

▶ *Child 3-12 yr:* PO 0.05-0.075 mg/kg/day

Available forms include: Tabs 0.5, 1, 2, 5, 10, 20 mg; conc 2 mg/ml; inj IM 5 mg/ml

Side effects/adverse reactions:

RESP: **Laryngospasm,** dyspnea, **respiratory depression**

CNS: Extrapyramidal symptoms: pseudoparkinsonism, akathisia, dystonia, tardive dyskinesia, drowsiness, headache, **seizures neuroleptic malignant syndrome**

INTEG: Rash, photosensitivity, dermatitis

EENT: Blurred vision, glaucoma

GI: Dry mouth, nausea, vomiting, anorexia, constipation, diarrhea, jaundice, weight gain

GU: Urinary retention, urinary frequency, enuresis, impotence, amenorrhea, gynecomastia

CV: Orthostatic hypotension, hypertension, **cardiac arrest,** ECG changes, **tachycardia**

Contraindications: Hypersensitivity, blood dyscrasias, coma, child <3 yr, brain damage, bone marrow depression, alcohol and barbiturate withdrawal states, Parkinson's disease, angina, epilepsy, urinary retention

Precautions: Pregnancy (C), lactation, seizure disorders, hypertension, hepatic disease, cardiac disease

Pharmacokinetics:

PO: Onset erratic, peak 2-6 hr, half-life 24 hr

IM: Onset 15-30 min, peak 15-20 min, half-life 21 hr

IM (Decanoate): Peak 4-11 days, half-life 3 wk

Metabolized by liver, excreted in urine, bile, crosses placenta, enters breast milk

Interactions/incompatibilities:

- Oversedation: other CNS depressants, alcohol, barbiturate anesthetics
- Toxicity: epinephrine
- Toxicity: with lithium, neurotoxicity and brain damage possible
- Decreased effects of: lithium, levodopa
- Increased effects of both drugs: β-adrenergic blockers, alcohol
- Increased anticholinergic effects: anticholinergics

NURSING CONSIDERATIONS

Assess:

- Swallowing of PO medication; check for hoarding or giving of medication to other patients
- I&O ratio; palpate bladder if low urinary output occurs
- Bilirubin, CBC, liver function studies monthly
- Urinalysis is recommended before and during prolonged therapy

Administer:

- Antiparkinsonian agent, to be used if extrapyramidal symptoms occur
- IM injection into large muscle mass, use No. 21G needle; give no more than 3 ml/injection site
- Oral liquid use calibrated dropper, do not mix in coffee or tea
- PO with food or milk

Perform/provide:

- Decreased noise input by dimming lights, avoiding loud noises
- Supervised ambulation until stabilized on medication; do not involve in strenuous exercise program because fainting is possible; patient should not stand still for long periods of time
- Increased fluids to prevent constipation
- Sips of water, candy, gum for dry mouth
- Storage in tight, light-resistant container

Evaluate:

- Therapeutic response: decrease in emotional excitement, hallucinations, delusions, paranoia, reorganization of patterns of thought, speech
- For depression in bipolar patients; rapid mood swings may occur with this drug
- Affect, orientation, LOC, reflexes, gait, coordination, sleep pattern disturbances
- B/P standing and lying; take pulse and respirations q4h during initial treatment; establish baseline before starting treatment; report drops of 30 mm Hg

- Dizziness, faintness, palpitations, tachycardia on rising
- Extrapyramidal symptoms including akathisia (inability to sit still, no pattern to movements), tardive dyskinesia (bizarre movements of jaw, mouth, tongue, extremities), pseudoparkinsonism (rigidity, tremors, pill rolling, shuffling gait)
- Skin turgor daily
- For neuroleptic malignant syndrome: hyperthermia, muscle rigidity, altered mental status, increased CPK
- Constipation, urinary retention daily; if these occur, increase bulk, water in diet

Teach client/family:

- That orthostatic hypotension occurs often, and to rise from sitting or lying position gradually
- To remain lying down after IM injection for at least 30 min
- To avoid hot tubs, hot showers, or tub baths since hypotension may occur
- To avoid abrupt withdrawal of this drug or extrapyramidal symptoms may result; drug should be withdrawn slowly
- To avoid OTC preparations (cough, hayfever, cold) unless approved by physician since serious drug interactions may occur; avoid use with alcohol or CNS depressants, increased drowsiness may occur
- To use a sunscreen during sun exposure to prevent burns
- Regarding compliance with drug regimen
- About EPS and necessity for meticulous oral hygiene since oral candidiasis may occur
- To report impaired vision, jaundice, tremors, muscle twitching
- In hot weather, heat stroke may occur; take extra precautions to stay cool

Lab test interferences:

Increase: Liver function tests, cardiac enzymes, cholesterol, blood glucose, prolactin, bilirubin, PBI, cholinesterase, ^{131}I

Decrease: Hormones (blood, urine)

False positive: Pregnancy tests, PKU

False negative: Urinary steroids

Treatment of overdose: Induce emesis, activated charcoal lavage, if orally injested, provide an airway; *do not induce vomiting*

Italic indicates common side effects.

Bold italic indicates life-threatening reactions.

DRUG PROFILE

Modified from Skidmore-Roth L: *Mosby's nursing drug reference,* St Louis, 1993, Mosby–Year Book.

Nurse: Nothing until you tell me. Now talk about how you feel.
John: (Stops and screams.) I feel like going home, and I don't want to be here!
Nurse: (Loudly.) I know. So say it again.
John: (Looks at nurse, not trusting what he has heard.)
Nurse: I'm serious—say it again.
John: (Shouts.) I don't want to be here. I want to go home, and I don't want to live!

John bursts into tears, falls to his knees, and covers his face with his hands. The three staff members slowly move toward him and stand close by. When the nurse sees John's body relax and soften, she gently places a hand on his shoulder and tells him that she can feel how hard the struggle is for him. He nods, and the nurse suggests that he stay in the dayroom with the assigned staff member for one-on-one and other clients. She motions for others to come over and stands by with the one-on-one staff member as they invite him to join them in a conversation.

In this incident, the nurse (1) established the limits while protecting self, (2) encountered the client's intensity, (3) encouraged the client's verbalization of feelings, (4) made physical contact with the client, and (5) integrated the client with the group although one-on-one for suicidal precautions was enforced.

Anger is aroused when conflicts between persons are encountered. The following steps assist in conflict resolution:

1. State, "I have a problem or I am feeling . . . "
2. Describe the situation and areas of conflict.
3. Tell the person what you need.
4. Ask if the person is willing to give you what you need.
5. If the answer is no, ask what the person is willing to do. Acknowledge the person's response and offer thanks.
6. Listen to what the other person is willing or not willing to do. You do not have to agree or accept thoughts and feelings.
7. State what you are willing to do to reach a workable compromise and give feedback about the other person's communication.
8. The process of communication has begun, and you are now in negotiation for the resolution of the conflict. Repeat your needs as often as necessary. Keep your communication honest, direct, and free from attempts to manipulate and control. Keep your voice calm, steady, self-assured, and firm.

Social dimension Because anger is a response to a threat to the self-concept, it is essential to help the client identify the source of the threat, as well as his feelings of inadequacy, and deal with the accompanying anxiety. See Chapter 10 for interventions with anxiety.

Using interpersonal theory, the nurse helps the client to see the consequences of the angry behavior: rejection, abandonment, alienation, and isolation. The client is helped to explore other options for handling anger that do not result in rejection and alienation from others. Withdrawing from others temporarily may help prevent harsh words or action that are regretted later. Physical activity dilutes the intensity of the emotion, and talking with another person may relieve some of the anger. However, it is important to discuss the situation later with the person to whom the anger was initially directed when thinking is more rational.

Because anger may be caused by resentment toward a person on whom the client depends, the client can be assisted to function more independently. Ways to increase independence include learning a skill, becoming financially independent, becoming less dependent emotionally on another, and learning problem-solving skills. When the client has no option other than being dependent, the nurse assists the client to accept the situation without anger and resentment and to develop attitudes that enhance personality and relationship building with others.

Role-playing allows clients to explore their anger by acting out a realistic problem situation. According to behavioral theory, the role-playing process includes providing the leadership that allows those involved to feel spontaneous. The nurse provides leadership by:

1. Providing parameters to ensure safety
2. Keeping the focus in the here-and-now
3. Ensuring that the focus is in keeping with the norms and purposes of the group
4. Establishing a permissive atmosphere that encourages experimentation within the parameters and by supporting novelty; suspending judgments and criticisms
5. Setting the expectation that the goal of the experience is to be creative.

Immediately following the role-playing, the process is analyzed. Because emotions may become highly charged during role-playing, the nurse must be sensitive to both the topic and the topic's effect on the client(s).

The nurse can model how to express and resolve anger. Styles of expressing anger that allow people to stay and hear the anger and engage in dialogue are vital if clients are to benefit from role modeling. Make "I" statements about the feeling, such as the following:

- "I feel angry because I wanted breakfast ready on time."
- "I feel angry because I don't think you love me."
- "I feel angry when you are late."
- "I feel angry and I don't know why; I just do."

Feel the anger, express it, and verbalize the nature of the inadequacy, for example, "I feel so angry when I can't make my feelings clear to you." As evidenced here, "I" statements place the responsibility for the behavior on the client. "You" statements such as "You make me angry" project the blame or responsibility to another.

Role-playing helps the client experience the anger, withdraw, and come back to report what was learned to another. Clients often need to talk with a nurse about anger directed at others. The nurse encourages catharsis and understanding of the anger with the client. The nurse then supports the client in expressing the anger and understanding the other person.

Spiritual dimension Clients need to clarify their values and beliefs about anger in their lives. When anger is directed toward God or a supreme power, as sometimes happens when illness is viewed as punishment, the nurse helps the client identify the resentment, hostility, and alienation. Encouraging the client to talk about the feelings or calling in a religious leader to assist in this process is appropriate and can be spiritually uplifting. Clients can move beyond the anger and resentment and learn from the experience of anger. The nurse must have an accepting atti-

▼
KEY INTERVENTIONS FOR THE ANGRY CLIENT

1. Ensure safety and dignity of client and safety of staff members.
2. Provide constructive outlets for expressing anger.
3. Set limits on behavior.
4. Acknowledge anger with empathic statements.
5. Assist in conflict resolution and problem solving.
6. Assist in seeing consequences of anger.
7. Model expression and resolution of anger.
8. Listen actively.
9. Support effective coping mechanisms.
10. Promote description of angry feelings.
11. Teach assertiveness.
12. Provide information about effects of anger on self and others.
13. Provide positive feedback when anger is expressed appropriately.

▼
GUIDELINES FOR PRIMARY/TERTIARY PREVENTION

Anger

Primary Prevention

Teach person: to like, respect self
to accept limits
to manage threats to self without defensiveness, anger
to identify bodily symptoms of anger (e.g., tenseness)
to learn to control impulses (to think before acting)
to handle frustrations, disappointments, rejections effectively
to avoid substances such as alcohol or drugs that impair judgment
to acknowledge healthy aspects of anger
to reduce anger through exercise or sports
to talk with person who provoked anger after emotion of anger subsides
to withdraw from situation provoking anger
assertive skills
conflict resolution
to have realistic and attainable goals for self; do not have to be perfect, can make mistakes without anger
Teach family signs and symptoms of escalating anger
ways to help client reduce/control anger

Tertiary Prevention

Community resources
Mental health centers
Self-help groups
Parents Anonymous

tude to help the angry person who is questioning the meaning of illness or suffering. Attentive listening and skillful communication facilitate a discussion of spiritual values that includes how well one has fulfilled life goals, the loss of significant people, and beliefs about one's own life and death. The box provides key interventions for the angry client. Table 11-4 lists nursing interventions and rationales for the client experiencing anger.

INTERACTION WITH AN ANGRY CLIENT

The following dialogue provides strategies for interacting with an angry client.

Client: (Loudly.) Someone stole my cigarettes!
Nurse: Your cigarettes are missing?
Client: No. (Louder.) Someone stole them. I had them on my table, and now they are gone.
Nurse: I'll go back with you to be sure you haven't misplaced them. (Walks toward bedroom.)
Client: No, I didn't misplace them. I told you someone stole them. Rodney did; he's always after me for a cigarette. (Sees Rodney.) Give them back to me, you thief! (Starts toward Rodney angrily.)
Nurse: Stop! Jeff. (With authority.)

Two other staff personnel hear the interaction and enter the room. They calmly and quietly walk Jeff to another room where no others are present. Rodney sits down.

Nurse: We cannot let you hurt anyone, Jeff.
Client: I wasn't going to hurt him. I just want my cigarettes back. (Voice is calmer, appears less tense.) (Silence.)
Nurse: What are you feeling now, Jeff?

Jeff is convinced that Rodney stole his cigarettes. Aware of this, the nurse refrains from further discussion and offers to help him look for them. On seeing Rodney, Jeff becomes increasingly angry and heads for him in a threatening manner. The nurse, along with a strong and authoritative voice, tells Jeff to stop. She is aware that a short command works better with an angered client than a lengthy explanation. Two other staff members enter, having heard the conversation, and escort Jeff from the room to eliminate further stimulation, to help decrease his anger, and to prevent him from losing control and perhaps hurting another person. A calm statement from the nurse that he cannot hurt anyone helps Jeff to understand the reason he was removed from the room. Later, when Jeff is calmer, he is asked to describe his feelings. It will then be important to help Jeff talk about the incident and more healthy and constructive ways to channel his anger. Timing is crucial because the angry client cannot talk about anger while it is being experienced. Only after the episode can the feelings be discussed more rationally.

Evaluation

The following criteria can be used to evaluate the process and specific interventions with the angry client:

1. *Adequacy*: Did the interventions reduce or eliminate anger? Did they include self-learning and management of anger?
2. *Appropriateness*: Were interventions started immediately, with formal data gathering suspended until the client's anger lessened? Did the client agree to the goals? Were the interventions relevant for the anger expressed and problems arising in the five dimensions?
3. *Effectiveness*: This criterion addresses questions related to the degree to which anger is reduced, behaviors altered, safety ensured, and self-learning accomplished. Were the goals and interventions specifically related to anger?
4. *Efficiency*: Were interventions enough to reduce the anger? Were sources of help and support coordinated

to increase the impact on the client's problem with anger?

The client needs to be involved in evaluation throughout the assessment and treatment phases. This involvement aids in the teaching-learning process and provides important information about the nurse's interventions with the angry client. The box on p. 221 provides guidelines for primary/tertiary prevention.

BRIEF REVIEW

Anger is a natural response to provocative situations or events. It has both constructive and destructive components. Because anger is a frightening emotion, people tend to deny, devalue, and avoid its expression. The adequate expression of anger promotes and adds depth to relationships; inadequate expression of anger destroys relationships.

Several theorists explain the dynamics of anger. Biologically, anger may result from brain impairment or may be genetically influenced. Psychoanalytical theorists suggest that anger is inborn and seeks expression through aggression and self-destruction. Those with an interpersonal approach describe anger as a response to anxiety. Behaviorists view anger as resulting from frustration when goals are blocked or as being learned from observations or the modeling of others. The existentialists approach anger as a way to find new meanings for life or as a signal that the individual is inadequate and in need of learning.

Working with the angry client offers the nurse many challenges. Using the nursing process, the nurse assesses the client's anger and plans actions that help the client manage anger in socially acceptable ways. Research findings provide a sound basis for the assessment and management of violent clients.

REFERENCES

1. American Psychiatric Association: *Diagnostic and statistical manual of mental disorders (DSM-III-R)*, Washington, DC, 1987, The Association.
2. Babich K, editor: *Assessing patient violence in the health care setting*, Boulder, Colo, 1981, Western Interstate Commission for Higher Education (WICHE).
3. Bandura A: *Aggression: a social learning analysis*, Englewood Cliffs, NJ, 1973, Prentice-Hall.
4. Barile L: A model for teaching management of disturbed behavior, *Journal of Psychosocial Nursing and Mental Health Services* 20(11):9, 1982.
5. Beaty J and others: Anger generated by unmet expectations, *Maternal-Child Nursing Journal* 10(5):324, 1985.
6. Burrows R: Nurses and violence . . . psychiatric ward, *Nursing Times* 80(4):56, 1984.
7. Bushman P: Anger in the clinical setting, *Maternal-Child Nursing Journal* 10(5):313, 1985.
8. Buss A, Durkee A: An inventory for assessing different kinds of hostility, *Journal of Consulting and Clinical Psychology* 21(4):343, 1957.
9. Carlson NRL: *Physiology of behavior*, Boston, 1977, Allyn & Bacon.
10. Clunn P: Nurses' assessment of violence potential. In Babich K, editor: *Assessing patient violence in the health care setting*, Boulder, Colo, 1981, Western Interstate Commission for Higher Education (WICHE).
11. Cook WW, Medley DM: Proposed hostility and pharisaic-virtue scores for the MMPI, *Journal of Applied Psychology* 38:414, 1954.
12. Coutant NL: Rage: implied neurological correlates, *Journal of Neurosurgical Nursing* 14(1):28, 1982.
13. Csernansky J and others: Pharmacologic treatment of aggression, *Hospital Formulary* 20(10):1091, 1985.
14. Davidhizar RE: Managing the passive-aggressive student nurse, *Nurse Educator* 8(2):34, 1983.
15. Dollard J, Miller N: *Frustration and aggression*, New Haven, Conn, 1939, Yale University Press.
16. Duldt BW: Anger: an occupational hazard for nurses, *Nursing Outlook* 29:510, 1981.
17. Dunne K: Anger: normal, appropriate, and justifiable, *Maternal-Child Nursing Journal* 10(5):316, 1985.
18. Evans DR, Stangeland M: Development of the reaction inventory to measure anger, *Psychological Reports* 29:412, 1971.
19. Ferguson M: *The aquarian conspiracy*, Los Angeles, 1980, Jeremy P Tarcher.
20. Fernandez T: Classic: how to deal with overt aggression, *Issues in Mental Health Nursing* 8(1):79, 1986.
21. Frankl VE: *Man's search for meaning*, New York, 1959, Pocket Books.
22. Frankl VE: *The will to meaning: foundations and applications of logotherapy*, New York, 1969, The New American Library.
23. Friedman M, Roseman RH: *Type A behavior and your heart*, New York, 1981, Fawcett.
24. Freud S: Mourning and melancholia. In *The complete works of Sigmund Freud*, vol 14, London, 1957, The Hogarth Press, Ltd. (Translated by J Stachey and A Tyson).
25. Gesell AL, Ilg FL, Ames LB: *Youth: the years from ten to sixteen*, New York, 1956, Harper & Row.
26. Gessell AL and others: *Infant and child in the culture of today: the guidance of development in home and nursery school*, rev ed, New York, 1974, Harper & Row.
27. Gesell AL and others: *The child from five to ten*, New York, 1977, Harper & Row.
28. Goldstein MJ, Baker BI, Jamison KR: *Abnormal psychology experiences, origins, and interventions*, Boston, 1980, Little, Brown.
29. Golub Z and others: The ripple effect of anger, *Maternal-Child Nursing Journal* 10(5):333, 1985.
30. Harrel TN, Chambless DL, Calhoun JF: Correlational relationships between self-statements and affective states, *Cognitive Therapy and Research* 5:159, 1981.
31. Hayes SG and others: The relationship of psychosocial factors to coronary heart diseases in the Framingham Study. I. Methods and risk factors, *Journal of Epidemiology* 107:362, 1978.
32. Heck, P: How to keep your poise under pressure, *RN* 49(6):15, 1986.
33. Herbener G: How to control anger, your own and other's, *Nursing Life* 2(6):42, 1982.
34. Holden R: Aggression against nurses, *Australian Nurses Journal* 15(3):44, 1985.
35. Hollander SL: Spontaneity, sociometry and the warming process in family therapy, *Psychodrama and Sociometry* 34:44, 1981.
36. Johnson R: *Aggression in men and animals*, Philadelphia, 1972, WB Saunders.
37. Johnson-Saylor M: An exploratory study of the experience of resentment, *Western Journal of Nursing Research* 81(1):49, 1986.
38. Lee I: Getting things under control: angry nurses, *Nursing Life* 5(4):26, 1986.
39. Lindgren K and others: Avoidance of anger, *Maternal-Child Nursing Journal* 10(5):320, 1985.
40. Lorenz K: *On aggression*, New York, 1966, Harcourt Brace Jovanovich.

41. Madow L: *Anger,* New York, 1972, Charles Scribner's Sons.
42. Millon T: *Disorders of personality; DSM-III: Axis II,* New York, 1981, Wiley-Interscience.
43. Moran J: Aggression management, responses and responsibilities, (Part 1), *Nursing Times* 80(4):28, 1984.
44. Moreno JL: *Who shall survive?* New York, 1953, Beacon House.
45. Moreno JL: Sociometric school and science of mankind. In Moreno JL, editor: *Sociometry and the science of man,* New York, 1956, Beacon House.
46. Moreno JL: *The sociometry reader,* Chicago, 1960, The Free Press of Glencoe.
47. Moreno JL: *Psychodrama,* vol 1, New York, 1970, Beacon House.
48. Mullahy P: *Psychoanalysis and interpersonal psychiatry: the contributions of Harry Stack Sullivan,* New York, 1970, Science House.
49. Needs A: Making sense of violence, *National Association of Theatre News* 23(1):19, 1986.
50. Neizo B and others: Post violence dialogue: perception change through language restructuring, *Issues in Mental Health Nursing* 62:45, 1984.
51. Novaco RW: Stress inoculation: a cognitive therapy for anger and its application to a case of depression, *Journal of Counseling and Clinical Psychology* 45:600, 1977.
52. Pisarcik G: Danger: you are facing the violent patient, *Nursing '81* 11(9):63, 1981.
53. Rubin TL: *The angry book,* New York, 1969, Macmillan.
54. Sadalla E, Burroughs J: Profiles in eating, sexy vegetarians and other sex-based social stereotypes, *Psychology Today* 15(9):10, 1981.
55. Sanford K: How to cope with verbal abuse, *Nursing Life* 5(5):52, 1985.
56. Scott J: *Aggression,* Chicago, 1975, The University of Chicago Press.
57. Sheridan M and others: Precipitants of violence in a psychiatric inpatient setting, *Hospital & Community Psychiatry* 41(7):776, 1990.
58. Smeaton W: The nature and management of hostility, *Nursing* 2(35):1033, 1985.
59. Smitherman C: *Anger in nursing actions for health promotion,* Philadelphia, 1981, FA Davis.
60. Spielberger CD: *Preliminary manual for the State-Trait Personality Inventory,* Tampa, The University of South Florida Human Resources Institute, 1987.
61. Spielberger CD and others: The experience of anger: construction and validation of an Anger Expression Scale. In Chesney MA, Roseman RH, editors: *Anger and hostility in cardiovascular and behavioral disorders,* New York, 1985, McGraw-Hill.
62. Stuart R: *Violent behavior: social learning approaches to prediction, management, and treatment,* New York, 1981, Brunner/Mazel.
63. Sullivan HS: *The interpersonal theory of psychiatry,* New York, 1953, WW Norton.
64. Tarvis C: Feeling angry? Letting off steam may not be enough, *Nursing Life* 45(5):58, 1984.
65. Throwe A: Families and alcohol, *Critical Care Quarterly* 8(4):79, 1986.
66. Valzelli L: *Psychology of aggression and violence,* New York, 1981, Raven Press.

ANNOTATED BIBLIOGRAPHY

Grainger RD: Anger within ourselves, *American Journal of Nursing* 90(7):12, 1990.

The author highlights the importance of analyzing the threat behind anger. Questions to assist a person interpret the meaning of anger are presented.

Green CP: How to recognize hostility and what to do about it, *American Journal of Nursing* 86(11):1230, 1986.

The author discusses how to recognize hostility, its relationship to anger, and ways to intervene with hostile clients.

Hamburg D, Trudeau M: *Biobehavioral aspects of aggression,* New York, 1981, Alan R. Liss.

This book presents many perspectives on aggression: biochemical, pharmacological, genetic, psychoendocrinological, as well as views concerning adolescent violence and violence in mental illness and alcoholism

Lanza M: Origins in aggression, *Journal of Psychiatric Nursing and Mental Health Services* 21(6):11, 1983.

The author discusses various theories of aggression and develops a model suggesting that both innate and environmental factors interact to contribute to a person's potential for aggression.

Meddaugh DI: Reactance. Understanding aggressive behaviors in long-term care, *Journal of Psychosocial Nursing* 28(4):28, 1990.

This study suggests the need for the nurse to discover ways in which choice and participation can be safely introduced into the care plan. Reactance theory is offered as a direction in understanding aggressive behaviors by recognizing the need for choice in everyday life, the role of institutional constraints, and staff interaction behaviors.

Munns D: A validation of the defining characteristics of the nursing diagnosis "potential for violence," *Nursing Clinics of North America* 20(4):711, 1985.

This descriptive survey attempts to provide validation for the characteristics that define the diagnosis, "potential for violence." The study validates seven of the characteristics.

Turnbull J and others: Turn it around. Short-term management for aggression and anger, *Journal of Psychosocial Nursing* 28(6):7, 1990.

The authors offer practical and specific guidelines for controlling anger and aggression. Results from a training course on managing potentially violent situations are presented.

Louise Bradford Suit

After studying this chapter, the student will be able to:

- Define guilt
- Discuss the historical perspectives of guilt
- Describe theories of guilt

- Apply the nursing process to clients experiencing guilt
- Use current research findings related to guilt

Guilt is the emotion that occurs when a person does something wrong and expects to be punished or expects that someone will be displeased. It is an internal process, a voice within the conscience that tells people that their behavior is inconsistent with their own value system. It is accompanied by sudden pain that can range from mild affect to intense feeling.

Guilt can be healthy and appropriate to the situation, or it can be absent or excessive for a given situation and can thus be unhealthy (Figure 12-1). Healthy guilt helps a person see the effects of wrongdoing and make amends by apologizing or making restitution. A person who feels no remorse for wrongdoing (absence of guilt) or one whose guilt is out of proportion or unrealistic (excessive guilt) for the situation demonstrates unhealthy guilt.

Many situations evoke strong feelings of guilt, including ill health, unsanctioned sexual activity, abortion, giving birth to a child with birth defects, surviving a person who has committed suicide, a tragedy in which others died, and contracting acquired immunodeficiency syndrome (AIDS).

Guilt occurs before, during, and after events inconsistent with one's value system. It may be brought on by one's thinking, acting, or feeling. The following common situations represent the emotion of guilt:

- A couple divorces after their child dies from sudden infant death syndrome (SIDS).
- A family spends their entire savings for the care of a son who became disabled as a result of a car accident that happened while the father was driving.
- A middle-aged recovered alcoholic works for years in Alcoholics Anonymous helping others stay sober.
- A teenage girl who becomes pregnant while unmarried becomes active in her church group.
- A husband commits suicide after discovering that his "one night stand" with a prostitute contributed to giving his wife AIDS.
- A young woman gives up her baby for adoption.

In these situations, people feel guilt about something they should not have done or something that happened. Each person feels remorse about the past while living in the present. Sometimes guilt is such a powerful emotion that it limits the person's functioning in the present because of ruminating about situations and events of the past.

Nurses are challenged to identify the disruptions guilt feelings may cause within clients. The nurse seeks to help clients learn to forgive themselves and others and move forward with renewed enthusiasm for life.

THEORETICAL APPROACHES

Psychoanalytical

Freud[16] believed the unconscious superego uses guilt or anxiety from guilt in the conscious mind to limit the individual's immoral behavior. The superego can be harsh, punitive, and blaming or mild, lenient, and without responsibility. A harsh, punitive superego can lead to the extreme punishment of the self through behaviors such as placation, self-deprecation, self-destruction, or self-mutilation.

> ▶ **DIAGNOSES Related to Guilt**

NURSING DIAGNOSES
NANDA
   Spiritual distress

PMH
   Altered feeling state—guilt/shame
   Altered spirituality
   Altered values

The superego that develops from parental conditioning functions within the person as a special internal monitoring agency. The agency maintains balance or self-regulation. The superego houses the internalized parental and social standards of behavior. It uses guilt to cause the person to act in accordance with this internalized standard of behavior. If this internalized standard of behavior is extremely rigid and punitive, the person's response to violations of the standard may be guilt that is disproportionate to the act. If the person has no internalized standard of behavior, the person feels no guilt.

According to psychoanalytical theory, guilt is seen as a signal that alters instinctual (id) behavior. It is used by the superego to alter the activity of the person's instincts. When guilt is disproportionate to the act, it is called *neurotic* guilt. People who are guilt ridden display behavior to rid themselves of guilt. To deal with a guilty conscience, they may accept or provoke abuse or seek rejection from others. Some people relieve a sense of guilt by giving things or time to others, by trying to please others, or by exhibiting a strong need to be liked. Another response to guilt is emotional blackmail, in which the individual acts as a target for exploitation by others.

Two types of guilt have been identified: *leftover guilt* and *self-imposed guilt*.[8] Leftover guilt results from early parental conditioning. It is shaped by emotional patterns of thinking, feelings, and behaving within the family. For example, a mother took extra allowance from her husband to give to her son, who knew this. As an adult, the son believed he could not indulge himself. He felt inferior and guilt toward his father and toward other honest, hardworking men. He struggled between indulging himself as his mother had done and being the responsible worker and family man his father was.

Self-imposed guilt is guilt felt within the individual when a rule or moral code is broken. A person such as a "working mother" may have a strong internal sense of what being a wife and mother entails. She may become anxious when

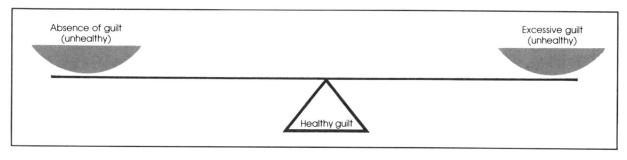

FIGURE 12-1 Guilt continuum.

RESEARCH HIGHLIGHT

Employed Mother's Concerns About Separation from the First- and Second-Born Child
- M Pitzer and E Hock

PURPOSE

The study was conducted to determine the concerns of mothers with first-born and second-born children and to determine if the concerns of the mother were the same for both children.

SAMPLE

Forty employed mothers were assessed when their first-born children were 7 months old and again when their second-born children were 7 months old.

METHODOLOGY

The Maternal Separation Anxiety Scale and Interview-Based Rating Scale were administered to the 40 mothers when their first-born child was 7 months old and again when the second-born child was 7 months old.

Based on data from *Research in Nursing and Health* 12:123, 1989.

FINDINGS

Mothers reported feeling less guilt and anxiety about separation from their second-born child than they had felt about their first-born child at the same age.

IMPLICATIONS

Many mothers need the support of the nurse if they work outside the home while raising their children. Often working mothers experience guilt and anxiety and especially when the child becomes ill.

Nurses comprise a great deal of the working mother work force and need help and support as they resolve child-raising issues for themselves.

---

she is unable to enjoy her child and her husband, feel restricted in her activities, and experience difficulties in the homemaker role. Both her husband and friends sense what is happening as does the young woman herself. They urge her to obtain some help with the house and baby, to go out more, and to achieve more balance in her life. She reacts by denying herself the relief from the responsibilities and she protests. She becomes caught in a vicious cycle of self-imposed frustration, anger, and guilt (see the accompanying research highlight).

During the phallic stage of psychosexual development, children vividly fantasize. They have many wishes and desires that they do not understand. Boys fear castration; girls fear retaliation for fantasies, desires, and wishes. If the child learns self-control, a sense of moral responsibility develops through the superego. The superego uses guilt to keep the child's behavior consistent with the intended value system.

Improper parental guidance can lead to a superego with an overdeveloped or underdeveloped conscience. With either extremely harsh or permissive parental conditioning, the conscience may not develop freely. The child may become either overly permissive or restrictive with himself and experience little guilt, no guilt, or too much guilt. A moral sense is lacking or is painfully present. A lack of moral sense leads the child into antisocial behavior in which disregard for social mores and norms is displayed by acting out behavior. On the other hand, with the moral sense painfully present, the child experiences too much guilt when minor offenses are committed.

A healthy conscience is formed by helpful feedback from parents. Through positive reinforcement, the child is motivated to control primitive emotions and desires within the norms of society. Trust develops within the child from a yielding, accepting, and predictable environment created by parents. Guilt felt by the child develops in healthy degrees. An excessively punishing conscience formed by parental feedback that is harsh, unfeeling, and unbending with inconsistent limits for the child may not help the child change undesirable behavior. Instead, the child may feel extreme guilt and may use ineffective behaviors in dealing with underlying feelings. The child may engage in self-defeating behavior as the need for punishment grows out of the excessive guilt.

Erikson[11] presented a developmental approach to guilt. In the developmental stage of autonomy versus shame and doubt, from 18 months to 3 years of age, the child internalizes a standard of law and order consistent with family and societal values. During the child's quest for autonomy, a beginning conscience emerges. If the child develops a conscience that is oversensitive during this time, it may lead to shame and doubt within the child.

In Erikson's stage of initiative versus guilt, from ages 3 to 6, the child begins to be curious about the surrounding world. The child seeks new experiences and explores new situations. If guilt does not dominate this stage, successful development of initiative occurs. Mastering the initiative stage produces a child who can cooperate, plan, solve problems, and relate to other people. Guilt occurs when the child does something for which he can be punished or incur parental displeasure (Figure 12-2).

Guilt can be differentiated from *shame*. When a person is found out and exposed to other people while doing something inconsistent with his self-concept, the resulting feeling is shame. Shame, then, is external exposure of one or more aspects of oneself to others. Shame supposes that one is exposed and is aware of being looked at (i.e., self-conscious).

Shame is related to feelings of inadequacy and insecurity. Although it is an individual experience within the person, shame has external consequences. Shame is reflected in the character of the person; that is, in what one is; a lack of shame is referred to as insensitivity to oneself and others.

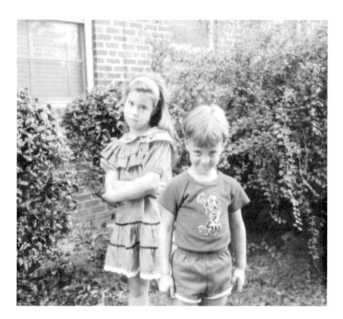

FIGURE 12-2 Children experiencing guilt.

Guilt feelings, on the other hand, tell people that their own internal code of behavior has been transgressed. Both shame and guilt assure society of acceptable behavior from its members.[17]

Bradshaw[5] views shame as the warning light that tells people when they have gone beyond their boundaries. *Healthy shame* gives people information about their limits. *Toxic shame* is a painful experience in which people feel flawed and worthless. Feelings related to toxic shame block people from revealing their inner selves to others. Bradshaw described a shame-based identity that gives rise to distorted thinking within the person.

Embarrassment is an emotion that is usually incorporated within shame. It is the initial feeling of shame before the person deals with the shame. The physiological reactions of blushing, feeling warm, and feeling as if the heart has skipped a beat are reactions to embarrassment. Situa-

tions that produce embarrassment can be explored to help people identify embarrassing situations and gain a better understanding of themselves.

Guilt is different from worry. Guilt occupies present moments with thoughts about the past. *Worry* involves being concerned in the present about something in the future. In each case, the person's ability to focus on the present is diminished because of preoccupation with either the past or future.

Guilt can be distinguished from guilty fear.[17] *Guilty fear* is the intense feeling that occurs when the individual is doing something that is disapproved of, illegal, or immoral. It is associated with the fear of getting what is deserved. Guilty fear seeks to avoid punishment, whereas guilt needs forgiveness and exposure. However, guilt can promote self-hate to such a degree that forgiveness by punishment does not eliminate the feeling.

Table 12-1 summarizes terms related to guilt.

Interpersonal

In his interpersonal theory, Sullivan[41] said that guilt follows a violation of one's moral code or ideal system. Sullivan viewed guilt as a conscious process. Guilt is in the person's awareness. It occurs when the person knows what he is doing or at least knows soon afterward that he has done something wrong. It is a form of anxiety. A person's internal regulating system is the "ideal system"; it houses the standard of behavior and guilt functions as a policeman.

Sullivan described "crazy guilt" as a form of anxiety used to escape one's conscious awareness and thus the pain of guilt. With crazy guilt, through the process of rationalizing one's behavior to oneself, the person avoids the anxiety that accompanies guilt. The antisocial person fits the category of crazy guilt. Antisocial persons have failed to develop a conscience. These people manipulate and use others for personal gain. They lack an appropriate internal value system and sense of responsibility. Guilt does not regulate their behavior in accordance with society's norms.

Unhealthy guilt can range from mild to severe. A person may seek punishment that ranges from inciting verbal abuse

TABLE 12-1 Terms Related to Guilt

Term	Definition
Guilt	Feeling evoked when one does something wrong or is possibly going to be punished or provoke another's displeasure
Leftover guilt	Feeling of guilt shaped from patterns of behavior as a result of early parental conditioning
Self-imposed guilt	Feeling of guilt a person brings on oneself
Shame	Feeling of exposure of one or more aspects of oneself to others
Healthy shame	Feeling within people that gives them input about their own limits and boundaries
Toxic shame	Painful experience in which the person feels flawed and worthless; inner aspects of the person is hidden from others
Embarrassment	Initial feeling of shame that produces a behavior such as blushing or feeling warm all over
Worry	Concern in the present about something in the future
Guilty fear	Intense flood of feeling when one is in the process of doing something immoral, disapproved of, or illegal
Survivor guilt	Guilt experienced by people who survive combat experiences during war, are left behind after suicide, or survive mass tragedies

from significant others to suicide. People who feel guilty may see their wrongdoings and shortcomings as deserving punishment. A strong need for punishment may lead clients to do anything to invite people to punish them. Self-punishment may lead to self-destruction. Guilt may become a self-defeating spiral, and the person may attempt suicide if the nurse cannot successfully intervene in this unhealthy spiral and help the client lessen the guilt.

Cognitive

According to Piaget,[35] moral judgment goes through a series of stages. An internalized standard of behavior develops during these stages. Moral values from the parents are internalized by the child, and conscience develops. As cognitive processes develop, the adolescent and young adult examine their own moral sense of right and wrong. They go through the process of choosing values for themselves. Meanwhile, the trained or overtrained conscience is at work within the person keeping behavior in line with one's moral values.

Guilt is both a motivator and a product. It can motivate one to behave in certain ways, and it can be the resultant emotional state produced by certain events (see the research highlight). For example, a teenage girl's anticipation of guilt for violating her internal moral standard of behavior during dating can cause her to act in harmony with her values. Guilt occurs if she violates her standard of behavior. Conflicts may also occur for her if she does not know what her beliefs are. In the process of discovering her beliefs, she may act in a way that is inconsistent with her beliefs. She may not discover until afterward that she holds a particular belief. Regardless of whether she thinks beforehand that her actions will bother her or whether she becomes aware of the conflict between her values and her behavior,

the resulting painful feeling is guilt.

As a motivator guilt has healthy and unhealthy components. Healthy guilt can keep one's behavior in line with one's value system. Guilt can signal violations of conscience. Like anxiety, healthy guilt can motivate one to positive actions depending on one's life orientation. Healthy guilt may cause one to visit a sick friend, go to school, study for a test, go to church, or speak when spoken to in a social situation. A person wanting to be liked by other people may be motivated by feelings of guilt.

Ellis and Harper[9] theorized that people can organize and discipline their thinking to make inner thoughts more rational. Individuals feel the way they think. The person's internal feeling state can be influenced and changed by changing the way a person thinks about situations and events. For example, a nursing student who makes a medication error may feel certain emotions, possibly shame and guilt. The student nurse may feel shame when her instructor becomes aware of her error and guilty because of her error and the possibility of punishment. Every time she is asked to give medicine after this incident, the student may feel guilt associated with making the first medication error. However, the student may also think through the problem and thus relieve her guilt by the cognitive process. Four things may happen: (1) the medication error occurs, (2) the student internally evaluates the event, (3) her evaluation results in the emotion of guilt, and (4) the guilt is relieved by reexamination of irrational thoughts about the error (Figure 12-3). The resultant emotions are individual reactions. In the same situation, some student nurses may have felt anger at the instructor for allowing the error to be made, disgust with themselves for the error, or worry over their progression in the nursing program. Each student has a characteristic response according to the student's personality and life experience.

RESEARCH HIGHLIGHT

Guilt and Grief: When Daughters Place Their Mothers in Nursing Homes
• V Matthieson

PURPOSE

This study examines the emotional impact on adult daughters who became responsible for continued supervision of their mothers as they were placed in nursing homes.

SAMPLE

The sample consisted of 36 adult daughters whose mothers had been placed in nursing homes. All participants were over age 35, white, and English-speaking.

METHODOLOGY

Interviews lasting approximately 2 hours were conducted with each subject. Interviews were taped, numbered for confidentiality, and coded for conceptual categories. Grounded theory was the selected method for analyzing the data.

From *Journal of Gerontological Nursing* 15(7):11, 1989.

FINDINGS

Two basic social processes related to adult daughters were identified: (1) becoming the chosen daughter who was responsible for the mother before and after placement and (2) redefining roles during the transition process. Two emotional themes that emerged were emotional responses of guilt and grief.

IMPLICATIONS

Nurses can assist daughters during the transitional process from home to nursing home by collaborating with daughters in providing continuity of care for the mother, facilitating reasonable visiting schedules, helping daughters work through their grief and guilt, and offering support services.

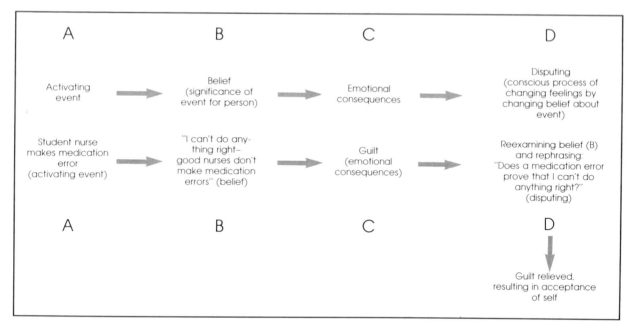

FIGURE 12-3 Application of Ellis' theory of guilt.

Communication

Transactional analysis, developed by Berne,[3] depicts the person as having three ego states: (1) the Parent, (2) the Adult, and (3) the Child. The *Parent ego state* stores all of the messages a child receives from the family, such as "Do this," "Do that," "Hurry up," and "You should." Parents set the parameters of behavior for children by telling them what they "should" and "should not" do. These messages register in the child's mind and are rehearsed. As the child encounters situations, these *should*'s and *should not*'s are recalled. If the person has excessive "should" or "should not" messages stored up, the person may experience guilt feelings. Critical messages come from the part of the Parent called the *Critical Parent*.

The *Child ego state* is the part of the personality responsible for free feelings and primitive emotions. Anger, sadness, gladness, and fear are examples of feelings arising from the child ego state.

The *Adult ego state* is the center for regulation, mediation, and decision making between the Child and Parent ego states. It is like a computer processing center with information from the Parent and Child coming in and going out. The Adult takes the *should not*'s from the Parent and the *go ahead*'s and feelings from the Child and renders a decision about the person's behavior.

Guilt is self-punishment and represents a trial between the parent and the child. The parent functions as the judge and the child functions as the defendant as if a trial were going on in the person's head.[23] Guilt may also be a result of parental programming to live out one's life in a certain way. This life script guides the actions of a person.[3]

Guilt may be based on a script in which a person feels

TABLE 12-2   Theories of Guilt

Theory	Theorist	Dynamics
Psychoanalytical	Freud	Healthy guilt motivates one to control primitive emotions and drives. Guilt is used by the superego to alter instinctual activity and limit the individual's behavior.
	Erikson	Successful completion of the initiative versus guilt stage of development results in a person who is curious, can solve problems, and can relate to others without excessive guilt.
Interpersonal	Sullivan	Guilt occurs when a person does something for which he can be punished or receive parental disapproval. Some persons with guilt have a need to be punished. Those without guilt are seen as persons with antisocial behavior.
Cognitive	Piaget	Guilt follows a violation of one's moral code or ideal system. Guilt motivates one to behave in certain ways.
	Ellis	The person's internal feeling state (guilt) can be influenced by changing the way a person thinks about events or situations.
Communication	Berne	Guilt may be the result of parental programming to live one's life in a certain way. Parental messages of "should" and "ought" act as one's conscience and an internalized standard of behavior.

responsible for other people.[20] This person rescues people rather than allowing others to solve their own problems or care for themselves. For example, a mother may rescue her son in a divorce. She may bail him out of financial trouble or take care of his home, meals, and laundry. Her actions may be motivated by feeling guilty that she did not give her son what he needed while growing up or that in some way she was responsible for the divorce because of her nonparental guidance.

Table 12-2 summarizes various theories of guilt.

NURSING PROCESS

Assessment

Physical dimension The physical manifestations of guilt are much like those of anxiety. Guilt may produce changes in physiological processes such as tachycardia, palpitations, dry mouth, sweaty palms, loss of appetite, nausea, fainting, nervousness, hyperventilation, diarrhea, and urinary frequency and urgency (see Chapter 10).

People who feel guilty may avoid eye contact, fidget, sit motionless, stare, shuffle feet, or blush. Some phrases the client may use to describe the somatic symptoms associated with guilt are "tightness in the chest," "chest pain," "heart flip-flops," "butterflies in the stomach," "heart feels like it's running away with me," "can't sit still," and "skin feels like it's crawling."

Guilt may trigger the stress ("fight or flight") response in the body.[43] In response to a threat to the person, such as guilt, the general adaptation syndrome is activated to help the body deal with stress. To handle stressors, the sympathetic nervous system prepares the person to take action in dealing with the stressor. Thus the sympathetic nervous system is responsible for the physical manifestations of guilt. Guilt may be accompanied by symptoms in the intestinal region and disturbances of circulation and breathing that are similar to those produced by anxiety.

The person who feels guilty may use drugs and alcohol to decrease the intensity of the guilt feelings.

Emotional dimension An assessment of guilt involves both subjective and objective observations about the client's feelings. Clients may describe guilt as a vague, diffuse, uncomfortable feeling (the pangs of conscience) much like anxiety. They may simply look, act, and state that they are not happy. Individuals may describe feelings of heaviness or burden that are commonly seen as a significant aspect of the grieving process.

Clients may feel ashamed or embarrassed; or they may indicate a lack of self-forgiveness and a feeling of unworthiness and self-condemnation. The affect may be subdued, depressed, or inappropriate; or it may be intensified. Flooded with internal feelings, clients may cry a lot. Internally, people may experience pain from an unknown source and describe it as "just not feeling right." Disguised forms of guilt are sadness, despair, hopelessness, helplessness, and limited capacity to enjoy life.

Based on Freud's theory, anger or aggression may be a disguised form of guilt. The open expression of aggression serves as a release of guilt feelings. Setting up situations in which clients can be punished by others is also a disguised form of dealing with the anger associated with guilt feelings.

Feelings of inferiority may indicate guilt feelings within the client. Both are related to anxiety and represent tension between the ego and superego according to Freud. Guilt, as discussed earlier, relates to wrongdoing, whereas feelings of inferiority relate to weakness and inadequacy. Guilt feelings may lead to submission, subordination, and dependence. With shame, people may feel a tendency to hide their faces or flee the situation.

Intellectual dimension According to cognitive theory, persons experiencing guilt are usually preoccupied with the guilt-producing situations and cannot forgive themselves. This preoccupation produces a shortened attention span and decreased capacity to learn new things. The person may block intellectual content from conscious awareness and be forgetful and confused; decision-making and problem-solving skills become less effective. For example, the depressed person is often preoccupied with guilt and has difficulty with attention and decision making.

Preoccupation with guilt alters a person's perception into tunnel vision, in which perception of the world is narrowed. Instead of seeing the world optimistically, the person sees the world pessimistically.

With selective inattention, individuals perceive negative feedback as acceptable, process this sensory information, and ignore additional sensory input. Compliments only add to the feelings of guilt, increasing the need for punishment for wrongdoing. Thus compliments are filtered out or ignored as a protective mechanism. For example, if a man feels guilt about the care he is giving to his elderly parents, he may not accept any compliments that he receives about the care.

Guilt may also cause obsessive thoughts. These thoughts result in compulsive acts to cancel the obsessive thoughts. A high degree of punctuality, rigid adherence to rules, and orderliness are all compulsive behaviors that the person uses to undo guilt.

Compulsive actions are used to cancel out obsessive thoughts. For example, a woman who thinks sexual thoughts and feels guilty about them may keep her house excessively clean. This reaction can be a symbolic way of cleaning up her thoughts. The obsessive thought motivated by guilt is cancelled by the actions of cleanliness. Based on Freud's theory, defense mechanisms such as undoing, displacement, regression, projection, reaction formation, rationalization, and somatization may be used to manage guilt.

Perfectionism is another characteristic that may result in guilt feelings. It is the obsessive desire to maintain high standards that people set for themselves. Guilt results when individuals cannot live up to their own high standards. Clients may limit their striving for perfectionism, or they may impose their own standards of perfectionism onto others. Guilt arises when the standard is violated.

Guilt-ridden people may wish for self-punishment. Using communication theory, clients may make recriminating statements such as "It's my fault" or "I'm to blame" and statements containing words like "should" and "should not," "ought to" or "ought not to," or "I must." Clients also communicate a sense of disgrace. Behavior that seeks negative criticism from others is likely. Other indicators of guilt include a tendency to argue one's point, blaming or unjustly criticizing another, being rude or defiant, and offering excuses for failures or forgetfulness.

A person may also show guilt by defending a friend or a cause. Whatever is defended is what the person experiences guilt over. Kidding is a mild form of criticism. It may represent something about which the kidder is sensitive. Kidding may thus be an expression of guilt.

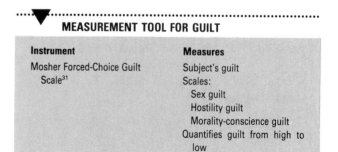 **Social dimension** Interactions and relationships with others are disrupted for the person with guilt feelings, according to interpersonal theory. Some clients act as if they are seeking pity or sympathy from the nurse. This is exemplified in the "poor defenseless me" attitude or "I feel sorry for myself" attitude. Arguing with others may be an attempt to cover up guilt. Withdrawing from others may be a method used to avoid and deny one's guilt.

Clients with excessive guilt feelings may be dependent in relationships. They may intentionally overrely on others to compensate for feelings of inadequacy. Anger, hostility, resentment, and ambivalence about the relationship indicate underlying guilt feelings.

An assessment of family relationships and child-rearing practices may provide data about the client who feels guilty. In general, parents assume moral responsibility for their children, punishing disapproved acts and rewarding approved acts. A child may show guilt by submitting without protest to the wishes of the parents.

Children learn to feel guilt as a result of transgressing the parent's standard of behavior. Through adherence to limits set by the parents, children give up self-will and learn that their behavior has limits. Children adopt an internal standard of behavior. The locus of control moves from outside (parental) to internal (the child's).

People who experience guilt may not fully develop their potential. They may have jobs with less responsibility than their abilities indicate because feelings of guilt hold them back. For example, an 18-year-old boy with asthma goes to a vocational school to study drafting rather than to a college to study architecture, which is his lifetime dream. His family has overprotected him because of the physical illness and has tried to rescue him from failure in life by telling him he could not do things because of his numerous asthmatic attacks. Although the message from the family was "If you fail, it is because of your physical limitations; be careful with your health," the adolescent boy heard the message as "You can't do anything." The guilt felt by the parents in producing an unhealthy child was transferred to the boy and incorporated as his own feeling of guilt. The boy's guilt was manifested as lowering his goal in life. The boy now feels further guilt for not living up to his potential (Figure 12-4).

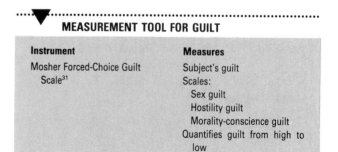 **Spiritual dimension** The nurse also looks at the client's personal philosophy and spiritual and religious beliefs. The nurse looks for any discrepancies and conflicts between the client's beliefs and behavior as a potential source of guilt. Persons who lead highly moral and religious lives or who are overly polite, courteous, and proper may have put aside tendencies to resist, rebel, or defend against attacks of others. The purer the life, the more painful the feelings of guilt that result from not adhering to high moral standards.

People's level of self-forgiveness needs to be assessed. Lack of self-forgiveness may be observed as constant helplessness, doing religious or volunteer work in an attempt to undo some feelings of guilt, or berating oneself as unworthy. Lack of self-forgiveness may also result in leaving the religious group if one's level of guilt feelings becomes too high or in self-destructive behavior such as suicide.

The nurse inquires about the client's religious beliefs and tries to identify tension or conflict between the beliefs and the client's practice of the beliefs. For example, the hospitalized client with a strong religious faith may feel guilty about his lack of participation in religious activity or ritual, such as communion, prayer, or eating kosher food.

Behaviors that demonstrate guilt and shame include wishing to undo or relive the past. The person may express regret, sinfulness, bitterness, or recrimination. One's illness may be seen as a punishment from God. Persons experiencing guilt limit their ability to enjoy and appreciate life. The burden of negative feelings of guilt reduces energy to create satisfactions in day-to-day living. The nurse explores with clients at an appropriate time their views about how life in general has treated them.

Measurement Tools

Guilt can be measured using the Mosher Forced-Choice Guilt Scale (see the box below). See the research high-

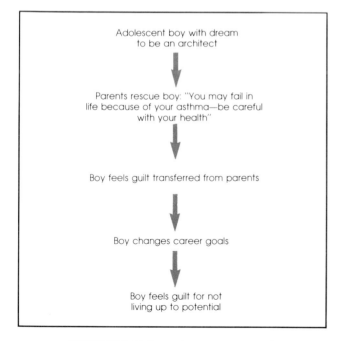

FIGURE 12-4 Adolescent boy experiencing guilt.

▼ **MEASUREMENT TOOL FOR GUILT**

Instrument	Measures
Mosher Forced-Choice Guilt Scale[31]	Subject's guilt Scales: 　Sex guilt 　Hostility guilt 　Morality-conscience guilt Quantifies guilt from high to low

RESEARCH HIGHLIGHT

Guilt in Alcoholics: An Evaluation of the Mosher Forced-Choice Guilt Scale
• L Fehr

PURPOSE

The study was implemented to test the Mosher Forced-Choice Guilt Scale with an alcoholic population. The scale has three subscales that measure sex guilt, hostility guilt, and morality-conscience guilt.

SAMPLE

The sample consisted of 25 men who had voluntarily admitted themselves to an alcoholism treatment center and a control group of 25 men. Subjects ranged from 28-61 years of age. There were no differences in the two groups for age or education.

METHODOLOGY

The forced-choice version of the Mosher Guilt Scale was given to both groups. The instruments were scored according to the standardized procedure.

Based on data from *Psychological Reports* 62:92, 1988.

FINDINGS

Higher sex guilt and higher morality conscience-guilt was found in the alcoholic group than in the control group. There were no significant differences between the groups for hostility guilt.

IMPLICATIONS

The findings of higher sex guilt and higher morality conscience-guilt in the alcoholic group suggests that this group is especially at risk for experiencing guilt. Nurses in alcoholism treatment centers need to recognize guilt within these clients and assist alcoholic clients in finding effective ways of dealing with guilt.

---

light for an application of the measurement tool to an alcoholic population.

Analysis
Nursing diagnosis

The following list provides examples of NANDA-accepted nursing diagnosis with causative statements.
1. Ineffective individual coping: guilt related to inability to live up to own expectations
2. Ineffective individual coping: guilt related to error in judgment
3. Ineffective individual coping: guilt related to inability to deal effectively with being a working mother
4. Ineffective individual coping: guilt related to excessive drinking
5. Altered thought processes related to preoccupation with guilt
6. Powerlessness related to self-defeating pattern of guilt
7. Social isolation related to painful feelings of guilt
8. Self-esteem disturbance related to guilt associated with feelings of inadequacy
9. Spiritual distress related to guilt about past life experiences.

The defining characteristics of spiritual distress are listed in the box.

The following case example demonstrates the characteristics of the nursing diagnosis spiritual distress.

▼ Case Example

Ada Stephensen, a 51-year-old woman, recently placed her mother, age 73 in a nursing home. Her mother lived with her until 3 months ago when her mother underwent exploratory surgery and was diagnosed with cancer. Her mother returned home after

▼ SPIRITUAL DISTRESS

DEFINITION

Disruption of a person's life that pervades one's entire being and integrates and transcends one's biological and psychosocial nature

DEFINING CHARACTERISTICS

• **Physical dimension**

Refusal to participate in usual religious practices
Somatic complaints (loss of appetite, muscular tension, headaches, sleep disturbances)

• **Emotional dimension**

Anger toward God, other supreme power, self, or others
Powerlessness
Crying
Hostility

• **Intellectual dimension**

Expressions of concern over meaning of life, death, or belief system
Regards illness as a punishment
Self-blame
Denial of responsibility for problems

• **Social dimension**

Withdrawal

• **Spiritual dimension**

Questions significance of existence and suffering
Seeks spiritual assistance
Inability to accept self
Questions relationship with God

Modified from McFarland G, McFarlane E: *Nursing diagnosis and intervention,* ed 2, St Louis, 1993, Mosby–Year Book.

the surgery. In the last month, her mother's condition has become worse. She is now bedfast and requires constant and total care. During her daily visit to her mother Ms. Stephensen expresses to the nurse feelings of guilt at placing her mother in a nursing home. The nurse observes Ms. Stephensen wringing her hands as she speaks and notices her loss of weight. She states that her mother took good care of her when she was a child and now she has abandoned her when she needed her most.

Ms. Stephensen's belief that she should care for her mother has been violated. She feels guilty about placing her mother in a nursing home as evidenced by her body language, weight loss, and daily visits to see her mother. While the care of her mother is too complicated for her to manage, she feels like she is letting down her mother in her time of need.

Planning

Table 12-3 lists examples of long- and short-term goals, outcome criteria, interventions, and rationales. These serve as examples of the planning stage in the nursing process.

Implementation

Physical dimension Because the physical characteristics of guilt are similar to those of anxiety, interventions aimed at reducing anxiety are helpful for the client experiencing guilt (see Chapter 10). The nurse identifies and acknowledges the presence of physical symptoms (avoiding eye contact, fidgeting, restlessness, staring, blushing, and nail biting) to help clients identify their feelings of guilt, promote awareness, and understand the cause of the feelings.

Shame associated with perceived unpleasant aspects of one's physical appearance (e.g., birth marks or being overweight) can be relieved by the use of empathic statements. The nurse needs to help clients realistically appraise the aspect of themselves that causes shame or embarrassment and focus on attractive aspects of his body (e.g., one's smile or skin). This approach fosters positive attitudes about body image and over time may lessen the client's shame or embarrassment.

For the client with excessive guilt who may be self-destructive, hospitalization with suicide precautions is indicated. Removing sharp objects and monitoring possessions are essential, especially for the client prone to self-mutilation who feels the need for punishment. For these persons, antidepressant medications may be prescribed, for example, amoxapine (Asendin). The profile for amoxapine (p. 235) describes the nursing care appropriate to its administration.

Emotional dimension The nurse assists the client in identifying feelings of guilt, embarrassment, or shame. Naming the feelings by discussing the situation that initially prompted them enables the nurse to help the client become aware of the feeling and to link the feeling to the behavior. The nurse then encourages the client to express these feelings and acknowledge them as acceptable or consider other ways of responding to the situation. The process of naming feelings is essential for the client to gain self-awareness and for the nurse to intervene therapeutically.

Gradually, as the intensity of the feelings diminishes and the client accepts the feelings as appropriate and realistic, other positive areas of the client's life can be emphasized. Building on the client's strengths and coping techniques emphasizes the client's positive characteristics. The nurse's

---

▼ **TABLE 12-3 NURSING CARE PLAN**

GOALS	OUTCOME CRITERIA	INTERVENTIONS	RATIONALES
NURSING DIAGNOSIS: Ineffective coping: guilt related to past unacceptable behavior			
LONG TERM			
To accept self and past behavior	Verbalizes acceptance of self and past behavior		
SHORT TERM			
Identify source of guilt feelings	Verbalizes source of guilt	Discuss situations/events that precipitated guilt feelings	Examining the source of guilt and its irrational aspects provides opportunity for behavioral change
Express feelings of guilt	Verbalizes feelings of guilt	Help client express guilt feelings	Verbal expression of guilt helps identify feeling and promotes self-awareness
Explore ways to relieve guilt	Verbalizes ways to relieve guilt Apologizes or makes restitution for wrongdoing	Encourage admission of wrongdoing if realistic	Wrongdoing may be denied, or there may be no conscious awareness of guilt
		Help client to assume responsibility for wrongs	Accepting responsibility for wrongs promotes dealing with guilt in an acceptable way; restores self-esteem
		Limit self-punishing statements	To interrupt irrational aspects of self-reproach

acceptance of the client who cries or expresses anger, guilt, and resentment indicates that this response is appropriate.

Self-awareness by nurses can help them deal constructively with their own responses to clients experiencing guilt. Sad stories may promote a feeling of sadness or pity within the nurse. Awareness of these feelings helps nurses to respond effectively to the client.

Nurses need to develop sensitivity in relating to people who feel embarrassed, shamed, or guilty. One of the most difficult aspects of dealing with guilt is the private nature of the things one feels guilty about. They are the very things one wants to hide and not talk about. Respect, acceptance, and empathic understanding by the nurse help the client establish contact with and confidence in the nurse. Clients are then able to discuss guilt feelings openly.

Based on Berne's[3] communication theory, guilt may be a lifelong pattern that is not easy for clients to change. Nurses may become frustrated. They need to recognize that change is slow. Clients who feel excessive guilt can be difficult to deal with, especially if they refuse to give up ingrained guilt responses and when secondary gain is a factor. Often nurses become insensitive and frustrated and feel helpless. Responding to the helplessness, nurses may flee the situation and avoid the client. The role of nurses is to stay with clients and work through these difficult situations. If necessary, nurses can seek the counsel of the head nurse, a colleague, supervisor, or counselor to gain assistance in dealing with these uncomfortable situations and clients.

Intellectual dimension Preoccupation with guilt about past experiences may trap some clients into being unwilling and inflexible about learning new ways of coping. They believe they have no choice about the situation and that guilt about the past cannot change. Using Ellis'[9,10] cognitive theory, nurses can help clients understand that they can choose to change and thus free themselves from guilt feelings about the past, as in the following case example.

▼ Case Example

Jeannie came to counseling because she was nervous and anxious and blamed herself for her parents' divorce 8 years ago. She was now 45 years old, and both parents were dead. By examining the futility of blaming herself during the course of therapy and being helped to see her ineffective coping behaviors, Jeannie began to believe in her own ability to choose other ways of coping with the guilt. Rather than continuing to feel guilty, she chose to believe that she was not the cause of her parent's divorce and left the guilt feelings in the past.

Persons feeling guilt label themselves negatively, for example, "I'm at fault" or "I'm to blame." Nurses can help clients promote realistic expectations for themselves. Using cognitive theory, nurses explore with clients the reasons for the self-blame, what they think causes it, whether others important to them agree with the negative label, and whether it is realistic. Through cognitive restructuring nurses can help clients change negative "self-talk" and form positive perceptions of themselves. Skillful communication techniques such as validation and clarification assist clients in discussing self-criticisms. In addition, behavior modification in the form of *thought stopping* helps clients limit negative thoughts about themselves. The accompanying box lists the techniques of thought stopping.

Thought substitution is another technique that deals directly with clients' negative thinking and dwelling on guilt-producing thoughts. Clients are instructed to replace negative thoughts with positive ones. For example, the alcoholic who feels guilty for all of the problems that he has caused for his family may find himself preoccupied with thoughts of guilt. Interventions include teaching him to think of a pleasant, calming place in nature and mentally remove himself to that spot. A favorite poem or scripture may also be used for thought substitution. The idea is for the guilt-producing thought to be replaced by a predetermined pleasant thought.

By disputing, another technique, nurses confront clients with irrational ideas upon which they have formed their conclusions. For example, the mother of a retarded child may feel guilty because she believes she has caused the retardation. It is therapeutic to confront her belief and assist her in exploring more rational explanations for her child's condition.

Imagery is another therapeutic technique to help clients who experience guilt. The nurse helps the client imagine how it would be and what it would feel like to be free of excessive guilt. She then explores what the client would like to think and feel. Then, she helps the client relax by giving positive suggestions that help them to experience freedom from excessive guilt. The session is taped and clients are asked to listen to the tape at home.

Social dimension Interventions for guilt in the social dimension focus on relationships according to interpersonal theory. The nurse explores methods of interrupting patterns of withdrawal, dependence, and alienation or isolation. For example, when a person avoids a friend because he owes the friend some money, simply paying back the money provides restitution and can relieve guilt. The estrangement of the two friends may also be restored. Nurses assist clients by showing them how to make restitution and provide support for clients as they make amends. Nurses rehearse with clients what to say and prepare clients for possible responses from the other person. Clients may write letters, provide monetary compensation, or make an apology as examples of restitution. In other situations, in which the guilt feelings are more intense and clients isolate themselves from others, nurses become a support system for the client. Eventually, members of the family replace nurses in this role.

While interacting with the client, nurses may feel guilt

▼
THOUGHT-STOPPING TECHNIQUE

1. Sit in a comfortable chair and bring to mind the unwanted thought (concentrate on only one thought per procedure).
2. As soon as the thought forms, give the command, "STOP!" Follow this with calm and deliberate relaxation of muscles and diversion of thoughts to something pleasant.
3. Repeat the procedure. Memorize the sequence: thought—STOP!—calm—muscle relaxation—diverting thought.
4. Use the technique in real-life situations *as soon as* and *every time* unwanted thinking occurs.

Modified from Fensterheim H, Baer Jr: *Stop running scared!* New York, 1977, Dell Publishing Co.

AMOXAPINE

(a-mox′a-peen)
Asendin
Func. class.:
Antidepressant—tricyclic
Chem. class.:
Dibenzoxazepine
derivative—secondary
amine

Action: Blocks reuptake of norepinephrine, serotonin into nerve endings, increasing action of norepinephrine, serotonin in nerve cells

Uses: Depression

Dosage and routes:

▶ *Adult:* PO 50 mg tid, may increase to 100 mg tid on 3rd day of therapy; not to exceed 300 mg/day unless lower doses have been given for at least 2 wk, may be given daily dose hs, not to exceed 600 mg/day in hospitalized patients

Available forms include: Tabs 10, 25, 50, 75, 100, 150 mg

Side effects/adverse reactions:

HEMA: **Agranulocytosis, thrombocytopenia, eosinophilia, leukopenia**

CNS: Dizziness, drowsiness, confusion, headache, anxiety, tremors, stimulation, weakness, insomnia, nightmares, EPS (elderly), increased psychiatric symptoms, paresthesia

GI: Diarrhea, dry mouth, nausea, vomiting, *paralytic ileus,* increased appetite, cramps, epigastric distress, jaundice, hepatitis,

stomatitis

GU: Retention, *acute renal failure*

INTEG: Rash, urticaria, sweating, pruritus, photosensitivity

CV: Orthostatic hypotension, ECG changes, tachycardia, hypertension, palpitations

EENT: Blurred vision, tinnitus, mydriasis, ophthalmoplegia

Contraindications: Hypersensitivity to tricyclic antidepressants, recovery phase of myocardial infarction, convulsive disorders, prostatic hypertrophy

Precautions: Suicidal patients, severe depression, increased intraocular pressure, narrow-angle glaucoma, urinary retention, cardiac disease, hepatic disease, hyperthyroidism, electroshock therapy, elective surgery, elderly, pregnancy (C)

Pharmacokinetics:

PO: Steady state 7 days; metabolized by liver, excreted by kidneys, croses placenta, half-life 8 hr

Interactions/incompatibilities:

–Decreased effects of: guanethidine, clonidine, indirect-acting sympathomimetics (ephedrine)

–Increased effects of: direct-acting sympathomimetics (epinephrine), alcohol, barbiturates, benzodiazepines, CNS depressants

–Hyperpyretic crisis, convulsions, hypertensive episode: MAOI (pargyline [Eutonyl])

NURSING CONSIDERATIONS

Assess:

–B/P (lying, standing), pulse q4h; if systolic B/P drops 20 mm Hg hold drug, notify physician; take vital signs q4h in patients with cardiovascular disease

–Blood studies: CBC, leukocytes, differential, cardiac enzymes if patient is receiving long-term therapy

–Hepatic studies: AST, ALT, bilirubin, creatinine

–Weight qwk, appetite may increase with drug

–ECG for flattening of T wave, bundle branch block, AV block, dysrhythmias in cardiac patients

Administer:

–Increased fluids, bulk in diet if constipation, urinary retention occur

–With food or milk for GI symptoms

–Crushed if patient is unable to swallow medication whole

–Dosage hs if over-sedation occurs during day; may take entire dose hs; elderly may not tolerate once/day dosing

–Gum, hard candy, or frequent sips of water for dry mouth

Perform/provide:

–Storage at room temperature, do not freeze

–Assistance with ambulation during beginning therapy since drowsiness/dizziness occurs

–Safety measures, including side rails, primarily in elderly

–Checking to see PO medication swallowed

Evaluate:

–EPS primarily in elderly: rigidity, dystonia, akathisia

–Mental status: mood, sensorium, affect, suicidal tendencies; increase in psychiatric symptoms: depression, panic

–Urinary retention, constipation; constipation is more likely to occur in children

–Withdrawal symptoms: headache, nausea, vomiting, muscle pain, weakness; do not usually occur unless drug was discontinued abruptly

–Alcohol consumption; if alcohol is consumed, withhold dose until morning

Teach client/family:

–That therapeutic effects may take 2-3 wk

–Use caution in driving or other activities requiring alertness because of drowsiness, dizziness, blurred vision

–To avoid alcohol ingestion, other CNS depressants

–Not to discontinue medication quickly after long-term use, may cause nausea, headache, malaise

–To wear sunscreen or large hat since photosensitivity occurs

Lab test interferences:

Increase: Serum bilirubin, blood glucose, alk phosphatase

False increase: Urinary catecholamines

Decrease: VMA, 5-HIAA

Treatment of overdose: ECG monitoring, induce emesis, lavage, activated charcoal, administer anticonvulsant

---

Italic indicates common side effects.

Bold italic indicates life-threatening reactions.

Modified from Skidmore—Roth L: *Mosby's nursing drug reference,* St Louis, 1993, Mosby—Year Book.

---

within themselves because of *overidentification* with clients. For example, a divorced nurse during an interaction with a client who is in the process of divorce listens. The client expresses guilt about his part in contributing to the divorce. The nurse finds it difficult to concentrate on the client's conversation. Her mind drifts to her own failed marriage and her feelings of guilt about the divorce. The nurse's effectiveness is hampered by her overidentification with the client. Nurses who use active listening skills to understand the situation from the client's viewpoint can set limits on their overidentification. Nurses monitor their own empathic response. They search within themselves to allow full understanding of the client's problem from the perspective of the client. This awareness prevents their own feelings from influencing their response.

Assertiveness helps clients who feel guilty by restoring control and power within their relationships. In addition,

clients who can assert themselves strengthen their self-concept. Ways in which clients can become assertive are discussed in Chapter 16.

Spiritual dimension Interventions for clients experiencing guilt primarily promote a sense of being forgiven for wrongdoings. For many clients, the church performs the role of forgiver; members can confess, chant, pray, or repent and have their transgressions forgiven. The church forgives and is seen as a deterrent for wrongdoings. The fear of punishment of God's wrath for disobeying the scriptural teachings is emphasized in many religions.

Some clients who experience guilt have no ties to organized religion. Nurses ask them to explore what they have stopped doing because of guilt feelings and the reason for their self-imposed punishment. In this way, nurses can help clients to forgive themselves and to be more forgiving of others.

According to Borysenko,[4] forgiveness is the process by which clients convert the suffering brought on by making a mistake into a growth experience. First it is recognizing that clients have done something wrong and are holding on to guilt as a result of the incident. Next, forgiveness is taking the responsibility for the action and letting go of guilt through self-forgiveness. The box lists the steps of forgiving oneself.

Guilt is a separating experience. Interventions are aimed at reconciling the estrangement. The person can eventually be relieved of guilt, can learn to live with his guilt, or can transcend the discomfort and conflict and become a more fully functioning, creative, whole person. The box lists the key interventions for dealing with guilt in patients.

INTERACTION WITH A CLIENT EXPERIENCING GUILT

Nurse: (In nurse's office counseling a college student.) *Connie, what's on your mind today?*
Client: I've lost my boyfriend. I really can't believe that I said what I said. It's just not like me at all.
Nurse: Connie, tell me what happened.
Client: Well, I told him he wasn't good enough for me and I would always have a better job than him and other things. Now, after being away for the summer, I realized that it was wrong, especially after seeing him with someone else. I can't believe that I was so cruel to him.
Nurse: It sounds like you are feeling guilty and ashamed of your treatment of your boyfriend.
Client: Oh yes, I'm feeling guilty. I'm having trouble getting it off my mind.
Nurse: It sounds like you haven't forgiven yourself.
Client: Oh no! How can I forgive myself for being so cruel?
Nurse: Connie, what you did comes from a side of you that you are not proud of; nonetheless, it is a part of you. All of us have those things in our lives that we are not proud of. The past cannot be changed. Perhaps, when you've had a chance to talk with him and make your peace with him, you will be able to forgive yourself.
Client: I'd like to forgive myself if I could.
Nurse: It sounds to me like you are saying, "I'd like to forgive myself if I 'should.'"
Client: Yes, I guess I am.
Nurse: It's OK to forgive yourself. Would you do the same thing today?
Client: No.
Nurse: Then, you've learned from the situation.
Client: Yes, I have. I've learned that I feel awful when I hurt people. I just don't know what to say to him.
Nurse: Let's take some time to practice talking to him.

Evaluation

To evaluate the effectiveness of nursing interventions, nurses assess the clients' level of guilt and analyze the achievement of the outcome criteria. Nurses also assess the methods used by clients to cope with guilt and evaluate their effectiveness in lessening the guilt feelings. Clients may still have feelings of guilt, but these feelings are in proportion to the situation and do not severely limit the client.

Interventions are successful when clients make positive statements about themselves and are free of excessive preoccupation with guilt in their conversations. Use of words like *should* and *ought* is minimal. Self-critical statements and self-destructive behavior are limited. Clients verbalize self-acceptance and self-forgiveness. Clients identify feelings of guilt as their own and deal positively with them.

Other criteria indicating that interventions have been therapeutic include eye contact, less spontaneous crying, an ability to enjoy life, creative endeavors, minimal blushing, and the ability to relax and to view situations realistically. See the accompanying box for guidelines for primary/tertiary prevention.

BRIEF REVIEW

Guilt is an emotion that occurs when a person does something wrong and expects to be punished. Guilt arises in people when their actions conflict with their internalized value system. Guilt can be healthy, which means that it is appropriate for a given situation, or it can be unhealthy, as when it is excessive or absent.

The experience of guilt is central to human experience. It is like anxiety: it can cripple a person for life if it is not dealt with appropriately. Guilt has far-reaching and devastating consequences; therefore nurses need to recognize guilt in clients and help them successfully deal with feelings of guilt.

Nurses function with clients experiencing guilt to help them express their guilt and deal with it realistically and successfully. The experience of guilt can be painful. Nurses assess clients to determine how the experience feels and what caused the feeling. Through establishing and building a therapeutic nurse-client relationship, nurses set goals and plan interventions to help clients deal with feelings of guilt. Nursing interventions are evaluated by measuring their effectiveness in lessening guilt feelings.

REFERENCES

1. American Psychiatric Association: *Diagnostic and statistical manual of mental disorders,* Washington, DC, 1987.
2. Berne E, Steiner C: *Beyond games and scripts,* New York, 1981, Grove Press.
3. Berne E: *Transactional analysis in psychotherapy,* New York, 1986, Grove Press.
4. Borysenko J: *Guilt is the teacher, love is the lesson,* New York, 1990, Warner Books.
5. Bradshaw J: *Healing the shame that binds you,* Deerfield Beach, Fla, 1988, Health Communications, Inc.
6. Chase D: The nurse responds: weak excuses and persistent guilt, *Journal of Christian Nursing* 1:9, 1988.
7. Dobson J: *Emotions: can you trust them?* Ventura, Calif, 1981, Regal Books.
8. Dryer W: *Your erroneous zones,* New York, 1977, Avon Books.
9. Ellis A, Harper R: *A guide to rational living,* Englewood Cliffs, NJ, 1971, Prentice Hall.
10. Ellis A: *Reason and emotion in psychotherapy,* New York, 1984, Citadel Press.
11. Erikson EH: *Childhood and society,* ed 2, New York, 1986, WW Norton.
12. Fehr L: Guilt in alcoholics: an evaluation of the Mosher Guilt Scales, *Psychological Reports* 62:92, 1988.
13. Firestone R: The "voice": the dual nature of guilt reactions, *American Journal of Psychoanalysis* 47:210, 1987.
14. Fersterheim H, Baer J: *Stop running scared,* New York, 1977, Dell Publishing Co.
15. Freeman L, Stean H: *Guilt: letting go,* New York, 1986, John Wiley & Sons.
16. Freud S: Mourning and melancholia, In *The complete works of Sigmund Freud,* vol 14, London, 1976, The Hogarth Press, Ltd. (Translated by J Strachey and A Tyson.)
17. Gaylin W: *Feelings: our vital signs,* New York, 1988, Ballantine Books.
18. Gerrard M, Gibbons F: Sexual experience, sex guilt, and sexual moral reasoning, *Journal of Personality* 50:345, 1982.
19. Glasser W: *Reality therapy: a new approach to psychiatry,* New York, 1990, Harper & Row.
20. Harris T: *I'm OK—you're OK,* New York, 1969, Avon Books.
21. Jampolsky G: *Goodbye to guilt,* New York, 1985, Bantam Books.
22. Krozek C: Free yourself from guilt, *Nursing* 20:88, 1990.
23. James M: *Born to win,* Reading, Mass, 1985, Addison-Wesley.
24. Johnson S: Counseling families experiencing guilt, *Dimensions of Critical Care Nursing* 3:238, 1984.
25. Kubler-Ross E: *On death and dying,* New York, 1970, Macmillan.
26. Labun E: Spiritual care: an element in nursing care planning, *Journal of Advanced Nursing* 13:314, 1988.
27. Lewis H: *Shame and guilt in neurosis,* New York, 1971, International Universities Press, Inc.
28. Limandri B: Disclosure of stigmatizing conditions: the discloser's perspective, *Archives and Psychiatric Nursing* 3(2):69-78, 1989.
29. Menninger K: *Whatever became of sin?,* New York, 1988, Hawthorn Publishing Co.
30. McGraw K: Guilt following transgression: an attribution of responsibility approach, *Journal of Personality and Social Psychology* 53:247, 1987.
31. Mosher D: The development and multitrait-multimethod matrix analysis of three measures of three aspects of guilt, *Journal of Consulting Psychology* 30:25, 1966.
32. O'Toole A: The phenomenon of shame: part 2, *Archives of Psychiatric Nursing* 1:308, 1987.
33. O'Toole A, Rouslin S: *Interpersonal theory in nursing practice: selected works of Hildegard Peplau,* New York, 1989, Springer Publishing Co.
34. Peplau H: *Interpersonal relations in nursing,* New York, 1952, GP Putnam's Sons.
35. Piaget J: *The moral judgment of the child,* New York, 1965, Macmillan Publishing Co.
36. Pitzer M, Hock E: Employed mothers' concerns about separation from the first- and second-born child, *Research in Nursing and Health* 12:123, 1989.
37. Potter-Efron R, Potter-Efron P: *Letting go of shame,* New York, 1989, Harper & Row.
38. Rubin T: *Emotional common sense,* New York, 1986, Harper & Row.
39. Steiner C: *Scripts people live,* New York, 1975, Bantam Books.
40. Subby R: *Co-dependency: an emerging issue,* Pompano Beach, Fla, 1984, Health Communications.
41. Sullivan H: *The interpersonal theory of psychiatry,* New York, 1968, WW Norton.
42. Weiss L, Weiss J: *Recovery from co-dependency,* Deerfield Beach, Fla, 1989, Health Communications.
43. Wilson E: Spiritual care: helping a guilt-ridden patient, *Journal of Christian Nursing* 5:10, 1988.

ANNOTATED BIBLIOGRAPHY

Engel L, Ferguson T: *Hidden guilt: how to stop punishing yourself and enjoy the happiness you deserve,* New York, 1990, Pocket Books.

The authors provide several sources of hidden guilt experienced by people. Control Mastery Theory is used with clients displaying hidden or overt sources of guilt. The ultimate goal of this approach is to absolve clients of their sources of guilt and live happy and productive lives.

Bradshaw J: *Healing the shame that binds you.* Deerfield Beach, Fl, 1988, Health Communications, Inc.

Dr. Bradshaw discusses the healthy and unhealthy aspects of shame. He presents methods to liberate the inner child and experience spiritual awakening.

Borysenko J: *Guilt is the teacher, love is the lesson,* New York, 1990, Warner Books.

Dr. Borysenko discusses healthy and unhealthy guilt. She discusses how to heal painful guilt and to acquire spiritual growth. She discusses forgiveness and the essential steps in forgiving one's self and others.

Ann Mabe Newman

After studying this chapter, the student will be able to:

- Define loss, grief, mourning, and uncomplicated bereavement
- Discuss historical perspectives of loss
- Discuss the diagnosis of uncomplicated bereavement as described in the DSM-III-R
- Describe theories of loss and grief
- Apply the nursing process to clients experiencing loss and who are grieving
- Identify current research findings related to clients responding to loss

Loss is an inevitable dimension of the human experience: loss of hearing, mobility, job, friends, health, one's own life. Loss is the essence of dying. Although death represents the ultimate loss, losses that span the life cycle may produce grief responses as intense and painful as those observed in the death experience. Loss is an actual or potential state in which a valued object, person, or body part that was formerly present is lost or changed and can no longer be seen, felt, heard, known, or experienced. The loss may be temporary or permanent, complete or partial, real or perceived, physical or symbolic. The manner in which each individual views the loss, however, depends on past experiences with loss; the value placed on the object lost; and the cultural, psychosocial, economic, and family supports available for dealing with the loss. Loss of a significant other, loss of some part of one's physiopsychosocial well-being, and loss of one's possessions are three forms of loss.

The most intense loss is the loss of a significant individual. Loss by death is a permanent and complete loss that one experiences at the end of life of friends or loved ones. Divorce implies a permanent loss in that both parties are no longer legally or emotionally committed to each other. However, when there are monetary or legal requirements, as seen in visitation rights with children or property settlements, the loss may be partial. Loss by separation can result from numerous situations, such as work, travel, hospitalization, estrangement, imprisonment, or war. Everyone contends with separation at some time. Separation may be temporary, if contact occurs with the other person through letters or telephone calls.

The loss of one's physiopsychosocial well-being includes three components: the individual's physical state, self-concept, and social roles. Changes in physiological functioning occur at any point during the life cycle and may represent

a loss. Changes may occur in vision or hearing or through limb amputation, chronic illness, or renal failure. Changes in a person's self-concept or any alteration in individuals' ideas and feelings about their worth, attractability, or desirability may represent a loss. A traumatic injury that results in a disability may cause a person to doubt his capabilities and view himself as undesirable. With rehabilitation, however, the individual usually restores his feelings of worthiness and desirability. The loss of one's occupation or profession, status in family, or position in the community comprises the final component of one's physiopsychosocial well-being. Job layoffs, additional family responsibilities, or lost elections are examples of changes in social roles that may precipitate feelings of loss.

Loss of one's possessions is the third form of loss. Personal possessions consist of items such as money, clothing, jewelry, home, and country. Because these possessions may represent an extension of one's being, their loss may demonstrate a true personal threat (Figure 13-1).

▶ **DIAGNOSES Related to Loss**

MEDICAL DIAGNOSES	NURSING DIAGNOSES
Uncomplicated bereavement	**NANDA**
	Anticipatory grieving
	Dysfunctional grieving
	PMH
	Altered feeling state-grief/ sadness
	Potential for altered feeling state

HISTORICAL OVERVIEW

DATES	EVENTS
Ancient Times	In the biblical account of the Garden of Eden, Adam and Eve experienced the loss of innocence as result of eating of the tree of life. Most religions incorporate the concept of eternal life to decrease fears of death and dying.
Middle Ages 1700s	Shakespeare and others wrote tragedies about the loss of a love and the devastating effects on the survivor.
1800s	Freud's concept of anxiety as the primary motivator of behavior as it relates to loss of self-image served as a basis for understanding unresolved grief.
Early 1900s	With the increase in the number of hospitals, the role of nursing and medicine as professionals who worked with the dying became more prominent.
1940s	Lindemann's work focused on symptomatology and grief work.
1950s	Before 1950, most people died at home with a member of the clergy in attendance. After 1950, hospitals and institutions became the place where most people died.
1960s	Erikson theorized that the success or failure of responding to developmental crises will influence the ability to deal with the next stage. For example, the transition to adolescence entails the loss of childhood security behaviors. Kübler-Ross identified the stages of death and dying. Engel identified the importance of life events that elicit feelings of loss to an individual.
1970s	Changes in life-styles led to a focus on dealing with losses other than death and the inherent stress created by these changes: seminars and research on sensitivity to loss associated with divorce, single parenting, adoption, miscarriage, infertility. The Hospice movement was recognized in the United States as a method of caring for the dying. The American Nurses Association addressed nursing care for dying clients in the Code for Nurses.[1]
1980s	Active involvement in the management of the dying process began to be encouraged. Grief therapy was recognized as a way of helping clients manage loss.
1990s	Issues concerning the right to die and living wills are being addressed by the courts, ethicists, consumers, nurses, and other health care providers.
Future	Because of increased public awareness, clients will experience increasing control over situations related to loss. Nurses working in home health care will assist families in securing a peaceful death for their significant others at home.

Loss results in change. The response to loss, the effective or ineffective resolution of feelings surrounding the loss, determines one's ability to deal with the resulting changes.

Regardless of what is lost, grief is the emotional response that accompanies changes. *Grieving, mourning,* and *bereavement* are the processes one uses to work through the response to loss and are healthy responses to loss. The resolution of the process ultimately leads to the investment of energy in new relationships and to positive self-regard. The process of adapting to a loss can take a day or several months, depending on the meaning of the loss to the one experiencing it (see the research highlight on p. 240). Although each person experiences loss in a different manner, there are guidelines to assist the nurse in assessment, diagnosis, and intervention.

The nurse's role in the grieving process is to provide an atmosphere for clients to accomplish the painful work of grieving. The psychiatric–mental health nurse who has knowledge and skills appropriate for application to the response of loss can assist clients in coming to terms with the loss. The issues inherent in loss affect many other responses seen in psychiatric–mental health nursing practice. Therefore the psychiatric–mental health nurse plays a vital role in assisting the individual or family as they work through the loss experience. The client and family need to deal successfully with each loss as it occurs since prior

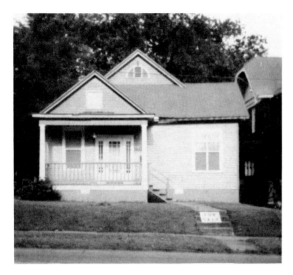

FIGURE 13-1 Selling the family home, as occurs when an elderly person moves to a nursing home or to the home of adult children, is often a traumatic loss for the person.

losses and how they have been resolved affect the client and family's ability to cope with the current loss. This chapter discusses clients who have experienced losses, grief, and the grieving process.

DSM-III-R DIAGNOSIS

Uncomplicated Bereavement

According to the DSM-III-R, the diagnosis of uncomplicated bereavement is made when the client is experiencing a reaction to the death of a loved one. Depression frequently is a reaction to a loss, with symptoms such as poor appetite, weight loss, and insomnia. However, preoccupation with worthlessness, prolonged and marked functional impairment, and psychomotor retardation is not uncommon and suggests that bereavement is complicated by a major depression.

In uncomplicated bereavement, guilt, if present, is mostly about actions taken or not taken by the survivor at the time of death; thoughts of death are usually limited to the person's thinking that he would be better off dead or that he should have died with the deceased person. The person may seek help for relief of symptoms such as insomnia or anorexia. The duration of bereavement varies considerably among different cultural groups. The client experiencing a grief reaction beyond the criteria established for uncomplicated bereavement is further assessed for symptoms of other conditions not attributable to a mental disorder or for mood disorders before a differential diagnosis is established.[2]

THEORETICAL APPROACHES

Psychoanalytical

Freud,[19] in his classic paper "Mourning and melancholia," discussed grief and mourning as reactions to loss. His work provided valuable insights in structuring the subject of grief. Freud described the mourning process as one in which the individual makes a gradual withdrawal of attachment from the lost object or person. With normal grieving this withdrawal of attachment is followed by readiness to make new attachments. In comparing melancholia with the "normal emotions of grief, and its expression in mourning,"

RESEARCH HIGHLIGHT

Vietnam: Resolving the Death of a Loved One
- P Provost

PURPOSE

The purpose of this study was to explore the grief process of individuals who suffer the loss of family member in the Vietnam War.

SAMPLE

A convenience sample of five subjects was used; two sisters, two wives, and one brother of five men killed in action in Vietnam.

METHODOLOGY

Open-ended questions eliciting memories at six consecutive time periods were used. Data were analyzed according to Giorgi's phenomenological research model, modified to extract themes and patterns from interviews.

FINDINGS

Patterns and themes that emerged included the following: (1) denial, (2) anger, (3) isolation, (4) sadness, (5)

frustration, and (6) ambivalence. The study shows the effects of loss and crises within a setting of inadequate supports. The emerging themes indicated a prolonged grief reaction.

IMPLICATIONS

Findings from the study indicated that the grief experienced by individuals who suffer a stigmatized or socially unsanctioned loss is complicated and each grief stage may be prolonged. The nurse must gain a sensitive awareness of the needs of individuals coping with a taboo grief. She needs to be alert to the possibility of unresolved grief even years after the loss has occurred. A need exists for further investigations to add to the foundation for a theoretical framework that will be useful for understanding various types of unsanctioned grief such as death from AIDS, suicide, or drugs. Such knowledge will facilitate the resolution of grief and promote wellness.

From *Archives in Psychiatric Nursing* 3(1):29, 1989.

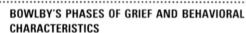

BOWLBY'S PHASES OF GRIEF AND BEHAVIORAL CHARACTERISTICS

Protest

Lack of acceptance of loss, all energy is directed toward protesting the loss; feelings of anger toward self and others, and feelings of ambivalence toward lost object. Crying and angry behaviors characterize this phase.

Despair

Behavior becomes disorganized; despair mounts as efforts to deny the loss compete with acceptance of permanent loss. Crying and sadness, coupled with a desire for the lost object to return, result in disorganized thoughts as the reality of the loss is recognized.

Detachment

As the permanency of the loss is realized and attachment to the lost object is gradually relinquished, a reinvestment of energy occurs. Both the positive and negative aspects of the relationship are remembered. Expressions of hopefulness and readiness to move forward are characteristic of this phase.

Freud observed that the "work of mourning" is a nonpathological condition that reaches a state of completion after a period of "inner labor." He differentiated melancholia as a pathological state from grieving as a nonpathological state.

Bowlby[5,6] continued to develop the psychoanalytical theory of mourning by examining the grief process in infancy and childhood and its relationship to grief of adults. He believed that the successful grieving process initiated by a loss or separation from a loved object or person ends with feelings of emancipation from the lost object. Bowlby divided the grieving process into three phases and identified behaviors characteristic of each phase (see box).

Cognitive

Like Bowlby, Engel[17] also identified stages of mourning, but delineated grief as acute and long term. Engel observed that after a stage of shock a realization of the loss occurs, which grows stronger and is followed by restitution. Influenced by stress theory, Engel perceived the grief process as coping with stress, in which, after perception and evaluation of the event, adaptation results. For Engel, the cognitive factors impact the grieving process.

The acute stage of mourning as identified by Engel lasts 4 to 8 weeks. The first phase of the acute stage, beginning immediately after receiving the news of the loss, is characterized by *shock and disbelief.* The initial response is that of denial, which may occur in order to cope with the overwhelming pain. Bereaved persons may even appear to accept the loss by making statements such as "it was for the best," while emotionally repressing their feelings. The stage of shock usually lasts only for a few hours; normally after 1 or 2 days it is over. A second stage of *developing awareness* begins as the denial fades. As the finality of the loss becomes a reality, pain and anguish begin to surface. Crying is the most frequently observed behavior. It is during this time that the greatest degree of anguish, within the limits imposed by cultural patterns, is experienced. During this stage culturally patterned behavior determines whether one is stoic in public or weeps openly. Anger, guilt, and blame surface. There is a need to make someone responsible for the loss. "If only"... or "why" frequently punctuates the expressed or inner dialogue of the mourner. The stage of *restitution* is described by Engel as one in which the institutionalization of mourning occurs. Friends and family gather to support the bereaved through participation in the rituals dictated by the culture. A painful void is felt by the mourner who is frequently preoccupied with thoughts of the loss. Engel[17] observed that after a period of restitution, the mourner begins to come to terms with the loss. Interest in people and activities are renewed during this *long-term phase.* The lost relationship is put in perspective as the bereaved person begins to form new relationships. According to Engel, this phase of mourning may last 1 to 2 years.

Sociocultural

The study by Lindemann[36] of grieving after the Coconut Grove fire in 1944 has contributed to the current understanding of the grieving process. The response to loss results in a defined sequence of behaviors experienced by bereaved individuals after a catastrophic event. Lindemann described *anticipatory grief* as a response to an anticipated loss. These are the range of feelings experienced by the individual or family in which a heightened preoccupation with the anticipated event occurs. The client or family reviews the details of the expected loss and anticipates all of the adjustments that will be needed to cope with the loss. Lindemann used the term *morbid grief reaction* to describe delayed and dysfunctional reactions to loss. A variety of debilitating health problems were observed by Lindemann in individuals who displayed excessive or delayed responses to loss. Five categories of symptoms were delineated by Lindemann in describing normal grief:

1. Somatic distress
2. Preoccupation with the image of the deceased
3. Feelings of guilt
4. Hostile reactions
5. Loss of patterns of conduct

Bugen[9] developed a model of grief that has contributed significantly to the understanding of the grief process as a response to loss. This model can be used to predict the outcomes of the grieving process based on the significance of the relationships involved. If the relationship is viewed as central, the grieving process will be the most intense and the survivor feels that life cannot be pursued in a meaningful way. When the relationship is peripheral, the grieving may be less intense and progress more rapidly to resolution. If the loss is viewed as preventable, the bereaved may feel directly or indirectly responsible. The intensity and length of the grieving process are increased under these circumstances. If the loss is viewed as unpreventable, the lack of guilt feelings and sense of responsibility for the loss may produce a milder and briefer period of mourning.

Behavioral

Kübler-Ross[30,31] developed a framework of death and dying that provides an understanding of the stages of coping

KÜBLER-ROSS' STAGES OF GRIEVING

Denial

A person's reaction may be shock and disbelief after receiving word of an actual or potential loss. Typically, after receiving a terminal diagnosis, notification of a death, or other serious loss, statements, such as "This can't be happening to me" or "This can't be true," are common. This initial stage of denial serves as a buffer in helping the individual or family mobilize alternative defenses.

Anger

The loss is resisted and the anger, behaviorally described as "acting out," is often directed toward family and health care providers.

Bargaining

This stage is an attempt to formulate an agreement to postpone the reality of the loss. A secret bargain is made with God in which the individual is willing to do anything to postpone the loss or change the prognosis. Model behavior or being a "good patient" is the individual's plea for an extension of life or the chance to "make everything right" with family and friends.

Depression

This stage occurs when the full impact of the actual or perceived loss is realized. The depression stage allows the individual to prepare for the impending loss by working through the struggle of separation. Grieving over "what cannot be" is manifested behaviorally either as talking freely about the loss or withdrawal.

Acceptance

This stage is reached by some individuals who are dying. When the dying person has reached peaceful acceptance, the stage is almost void of emotion. The struggle is past and the emotional pain is gone. If the loss is of a loved one or other valued object, the bereaved individual begins to come to terms with the loss and resumes activities with an air of hopefulness for the future.

with an impending loss. Some or all of these reactions are observed during the grieving process and may reappear as the loss is experienced (see box).

Kübler-Ross stresses that not all individuals go through these stages, and those that do may experience them in varying sequences. Her goal in identifying stages was to describe her observations of how people come to terms with situations of loss.

Glaser and Strauss[22] identified the concept of *awareness* in describing the relationships between the dying person and family. Several types of awareness contexts are observed as the dying person and family relate to each other:

1. *Closed awareness:* Efforts are made to keep the terminally ill person from being aware of the impending death.
2. *Suspicious awareness:* The dying person becomes suspicious that information is being withheld.
3. *Mutual pretense:* The dying person and others know the condition is terminal but pretend otherwise.
4. *Open awareness:* The dying person and others know the condition is terminal and relate to each other openly.

Developmental

Understanding of and reaction to loss are affected by age. Individual differences occur in each age group and are

TABLE 13-1   Development of the Concept of Death

Age (years)	Beliefs and Attitudes
3	Fears separation; does not comprehend permanent separation
3-5	Believes death is reversible; sleeping Curious about what happens to body Does not understand the concept of death
6-10	Understands that death is final Views own death as avoidable Associates death with violence Believes wishes can be responsible for death
11-12	Reflects views of death expressed by parents Expresses interest in afterlife as understanding of mortality develops Recognizes death as irreversible and inevitable
13-21	Usually has a religious and philosophical view of death, but seldom thinks about death Views own death as distant or a challenge, acting out defiance through reckless behavior Previously held developmental awareness of death may still be present
22-45	Does not think about death unless confronted Emotionally distances self from death Attitude toward death influenced by religious and cultural beliefs
46-65	Experiences the death of parents or friends Accepts own mortality Experiences waves of death anxiety Puts life in order to prepare for death and decrease anxiety Fears lingering, incapacitating illness Views death as inevitable but from a philosophical viewpoint: freedom from pain, illness, or as a spiritual reunion with deceased others.

affected by the growth and development stage of the individual. As people experience life transitions, they generally gain greater understanding and acceptance of the accompanying losses associated with the transitions. The development of the concept of death as a loss proceeds rapidly from the age of 3 years. Table 13-1 outlines the development of the concept of death throughout the life span.

Humanistic-Holistic

The work of Carter,[11] a nurse researcher, has contributed to the understanding of grief through the identification of themes of bereavement expressed by grieving persons. She identified themes disclosed by people who had experienced the death of a loved one and compared them with the theoretical perspectives of Freud, Kübler-Ross, and an existential-phenomenological theory based on the work of Frankl, Tillich, and others. Carter identified features of bereavement that are dissimilar or unaddressed by the other theoretical perspectives:

▼ **TABLE 13-2 Summary of Theories of Loss**

Theory	Theorist	Dynamics
Psychoana-lytical	Freud	Grief and mourning are reactions to loss. Grieving is the inner labor of mourning a loss. Inability to grieve a loss results in depression.
	Bowlby	The successful grieving process initiated by a loss or separation during childhood ends with feelings of emancipation from the lost loved object.
Cognitive	Engel	Following perception and evaluation of the loss, adaptation to the event results. Shock and disbelief, developing awareness, and restitution occur during the first year after the loss; in subsequent months, the lost relationship is put in perspective.
Sociocultural	Lindemann	A sequence of responses is experienced after a catastrophic event.
	Bugen	The outcome of the grieving process can be predicted based on the significance of the relationship and whether the death was viewed as preventable.
Behavioral	Kübler-Ross	Five stages define the response to loss: denial, anger, bargaining, depression, and acceptance.
	Glaser and Strauss	Differing levels of awareness related to dying influence communication patterns: closed awareness, suspicious awareness, mutual pretense, and open awareness.
Develop-mental	Erikson	Individual reactions to loss and death differ in each age group.
Humanistic-Holistic	Carter	Themes of grief are expressed as the response to a loss: waves of intense pain years after a death, holding as a process of preserving the meaning of the loss, expectations, and personal history.

1. Grief's changing character, including "waves" and intense pain, which may be triggered years after the death
2. Holding, an individual process of preserving the fact and the meaning of the loved one's existence
3. Expectations, both social and personal, as to how the bereaved should be coping with the experience
4. The critical importance of personal history in affecting the quality and meaning of individual bereavement.

Table 13-2 summarizes the theoretical approaches to loss and grieving.

NURSING PROCESS

Assessment

Physical dimension Assessment of the expected physical reactions to loss provides the nurse with a basis for further assessment. The category of grief symptoms developed by Lindemann[36] and the stages of grief and mourning described by Engel[17] can be used to assess behaviors associated with the physical dimensions of loss. As the client becomes aware of the loss, somatic symptoms are frequently observed.

The nurse asks questions about sleeping patterns, eating patterns, activities of daily living, general health status, and pain to assess the extent of somatic distress. The normal routines of sleeping and eating may be disrupted by the grief process. Somatic symptoms reported by grieving clients include gastrointestinal disturbances such as indigestion, nausea or vomiting, anorexia, weight gain or loss, constipation, or diarrhea. The shock and disbelief that accompany a loss may cause shortness of breath, a choking sensation, hyperventilation, and loss of strength. Insomnia, preoccupation with sleep, and fatigue (decreased or increased activity level) are also subjectively reported by clients.[10]

Crying is often observed during normal grief states. A person who is unable to cry may have difficulty completing the mourning process. In addition reports of overindulgence in alcohol or drugs by the grieving person may signal dysfunctional grief.

When the loss is associated with body image, the nurse assesses behaviors associated with altered body image in the grieving client. Loss of hair, weight gain or loss, the loss of a body part, or other mutilations from surgery or trauma can make it difficult for the client to accept the physical aspects of the loss. Children and adolescents, in particular, are concerned with the loss of hair.

Concerns about pain need to be assessed, especially in clients with cancer and other painful terminal illnesses. Knowledge of pain theories and pain assessment are helpful to the nurse in assessing the need for pain medication. During the last stages of dying, the client usually becomes very weak and sensations and reflexes decrease, requiring careful assessment of the client's physical needs.

Reactions to loss are not always obvious when the nurse is assessing the client's physical dimension. For example, assessment of a client admitted for a medical or surgical illness after a serious loss may reveal somatic complaints related to the grief state as well as the illness. Patterns of increased illness in a person who has been healthy may signal dysfunctional grieving.

Emotional dimension Anxiety and fear of the unknown are commonly observed in the client responding to an actual or perceived loss. The client's well-being can be threatened by extreme levels of anxiety. An assessment in the emotional domain includes helping the client identify the fears associated with the loss such as loneliness, abandonment, or loss of control.

The most common sources of loss that clients fear are the following:
1. Health
2. Social status
3. Possessions
4. Life-style
5. Sexual functioning
6. Body part
7. Death

8. Divorce
9. Reproductive functioning
10. Changing relationships

Assessing which losses are of greatest concern to the client is part of the nurse's initial assessment. The fear and anxiety may not be of the actual loss as much as it is of the feelings experienced while proceeding through the grieving process. The fears associated with the loss and the changes it will produce can be a serious threat to the client working through the grief process.

Focusing on the meaning of the loss originating out of the total experience of the person during the assessment phase of the emotional dimension is more important than attempting to place the client in a sequence or phase of grief. However, the protest phase identified by Bowlby[5,6] can be used to explain the disorganized behavior observed in grieving clients. In addition the altered sensorium observed during the stage of shock and disbelief described by Engel provides parameters for assessment: feelings of numbness, unreality, emotional distance, intense preoccupation with the lost object, helplessness, loneliness, and disorganization. As the client begins to develop an awareness of the loss, an increased preoccupation with the lost object, self-accusation, and ambivalence toward the lost object may be manifested.

The model of grief developed by Bugen[9] can be helpful in assessing the anger, ambivalence, and guilt felt toward the lost object. As trust is built with the nurse, the client may reveal the significance of the relationship and the circumstances surrounding the loss. These factors assist the nurse in posing sensitive questions in assessing the impact of the loss. If the relationship was central, the nurse will observe the most intense grief and the client may state, "I can't go on without him/her." As with any love relationship, the client may simultaneously express feelings of anger toward the love object. The grieving person may feel angry at the lost person for having left, whether through death, divorce, or separation. The losses associated with body image changes and changes in work roles may produce similar feelings.

Younger children have more difficulty expressing grief. The nurse may find the anger and sadness identified by Bowlby[5,6] helpful in assessing children experiencing a significant loss. The despair and detachment behaviors especially deserve careful assessment.

Although anger is a part of the normal grieving process, assessment of the extent, duration in the grieving process, and effect on the client help the nurse determine whether the anger is functional or dysfunctional. Within Engel's framework of developing awareness of the loss, the client's expression of anger can be a positive sign of working through the grief process. Anger helps the grieving client get past the "why me" feeling. It may be helpful in giving the client a sense of control in managing the events surrounding the loss.

Anger may be manifested as guilt in the grieving client. The "if only" element of grief identified by Engel is an expression of guilt by the mourner. Clients may blame themselves for what is happening. Subjective statements such as "If only I had done more, this might not have happened" provide the nurse with assessment data confirming the client's feelings of guilt. A direct assessment question such as "Do you feel your loss is the result of something you did or didn't do?" may be necessary to determine the extent of the guilt. If guilt is not resolved, it may become dysfunctional anger as the client continues to lash out at friends, family, and caregivers. For example, guilt can destroy a marriage if parents blame each other for the death of a child.[21] Guilt and anger, as a part of the normal grieving process, subside as the mourner begins to deal with the permanency of the loss.

Anger is often replaced by preoccupation with thoughts of the loss. Engel[17] identified this stage as a period of restitution in which the work of mourning continues. Careful assessment of the symptoms of depression is needed because the client's unresponsiveness to visitors and decreased physical activity normally seen during this time may be assessed incorrectly as symptoms of clinical depression. Kübler-Ross[30] described this stage of depression in grief and dying and identified it as grieving over "what cannot be." In the normal grieving process this stage is characterized as either withdrawal or the ability to talk openly about the loss.

Acceptance of the loss is assessed by subjective or objective data indicating the client has dealt with the strong emotional components associated with grieving. The dying client may appear to be almost completely devoid of emotions. Carter[11] noted that persons responding to the death of a loved one reported "waves" of intense emotional pain years after the loss. Thus careful ongoing assessment of the emotional dimension of loss is required by the nurse.

Intellectual dimension Although most people can intellectualize the inevitability of eventual loss, all aspects of the intellectual dimension of the client can be altered in the process of responding to an actual loss. On becoming aware of the loss, the client is likely to experience an altered sensorium. Changes in sensory processes may occur in response to the shock, denial, and disbelief created by the loss according to Engel.[17] In the dying client debilitated by the illness, hearing and sight are sometimes diminished as the client nears death. Although decreased hearing is thought to be more common, increased sensory perception is observed in some dying clients. Because responses are highly individual, assessment of responses to sensory stimulation may vary widely.

The awareness contexts described by Glaser and Strauss[22] can be used by the nurse to assess the client's and others' desires to talk about the actual or perceived loss. Although it is widely accepted that clients know they are dying whether they are told or not, the same is true of clients dealing with other losses. The nurse assesses the client's desire for knowledge and the family's beliefs about how much and what knowledge needs to be shared. In initially dealing with the shock and disbelief surrounding the loss, the client needs the emotional protection provided by denial and mutual pretense. Bereaved persons may even appear to accept the loss by making statements such as, "It was for the best," while emotionally repressing their feelings. In spite of apparent intellectual and verbalized acceptance of the loss, a state of developing awareness must follow for successful grieving to be accomplished. The client who overtly continues to behave as if nothing had happened is at risk for developing the delayed or morbid grief reactions identified by Lindemann. The nurse may feel that open awareness promotes acceptance of the loss; the client and family may need to deal with the loss through closed awareness or mutual pretense. Thus an assessment of the desired awareness context is imperative.

The use of defense mechanisms is beneficial in initially helping the grieving client deal with the shock of loss. The most common defense mechanism used by clients is denial. The nurse needs to assess the extent and usefulness of the defense mechanisms as a basis for assessing their prolonged use.

Denial may help the dying client preserve hope, but it becomes dysfunctional when used to avoid making decisions that affect the family's future. Research on the maternal bereavement experience in intrauterine fetal death reveals that denial may be used to support hope until the stillborn is delivered. No matter how overwhelming the information that the fetus has died, as long as the fetus remains in the uterus, the mother will use various sources of data to support her hope that the diagnosis is wrong.[26] Denial initially gives the client and family time to mobilize and respond in healthier ways, but if it is used to refuse health care because "nothing is wrong," it becomes an ineffective way of coping. The criteria that most clearly distinguishes healthy forms of defenses from pathological ones (as in dysfunctional grieving) are the length of time during which they persist and the extent to which they influence mental functioning or come to dominate it completely.[6] Thus information about the length of time since the loss occurred will provide additional data for the nurse's assessment.

The use of imagery and art is helpful in assessing the intellectual dimension in children and some adults. Imagery can be described verbally or through art to help the client explore feelings and fears related to the loss. It helps to express what the client may not be able to convey directly. Through drawings, dying children are often able to express their knowledge of their impending death. In descriptions of images or art, the client may use symbolic language to speak of feelings that are too painful to name.

To determine whether a client has reached the acceptance or resolution stage of grieving, the nurse assesses the degree to which the client is able to put the loss in perspective. The client is able to acknowledge that the loss has created a painful void in life, but is able to verbalize the positive and negative qualities of the loss.

Social dimension Because of its positive influence on the successful resolution of grief, assessment of the client's social support system is important. Social isolation may be experienced more with some losses than with others. For example, a move or a divorce, or even the death of a pet can cause a person to feel extremely isolated, and yet, the person does not ordinarily receive the same social support as a person mourning the death of a person. The woman who undergoes an abortion or places a child for adoption seldom receives the same support as the mother of a child who dies at birth. Thus the nurse should refrain from placing a value on the client's loss in assessing the need for support.

The painful nature of grief can cause the client to withdraw from a normal social support system, increasing the feelings of loneliness caused by the loss itself. The client's needs for social interaction remain similar to those established before the loss. Assessment of the social dimension includes previous styles and frequency of interactions as well as the members of the client's social network. Asking clients to name significant people in their lives gives the nurse the opportunity to encourage contact with them when the client experiences the loneliness and isolation of grief. The wish not to burden people is often expressed by clients who have lost a spouse. For example, a new widow may refuse invitations from her circle of married friends with whom she had socialized when her husband was alive.

After the initial stage of shock and disbelief, a well-functioning family is able to shift roles, levels of responsibility, and ways of communicating to provide support for each other during all phases of the grieving process. Assessment of the family patterns of interaction include the following:

1. Family structure and usual roles
2. Family norms, values, and attitudes
3. Level of trust among family members
4. Perceptions of relationships with extended family
5. Willingness to use outside supports

The family may have a negative as well as a positive effect on the grieving client. Well-meaning family members may try to shield the client from the pain of grieving. The nurse assesses the family's individual reactions to the loss because no two people grieve alike. Anger, denial, and acceptance are experienced by both the client and the family. For example, while one member is in denial, another may be expressing angry accusations because "not enough is being done."

When the nurse assesses a pattern of changes in relationships with friends and family and behavior detrimental to physical and social existence, dysfunctional grieving may be suspected. If the grief of the family becomes dysfunctional, family members may begin missing work or school, getting in trouble with the law, or abusing alcohol or drugs.

The dying client may be unresponsive to most family members. He may seem withdrawn and unapproachable. Nurses often mislabel this behavior as depression. To help the nurse identify depression, assessment of responses to direct questions may help:

1. What are you feeling right now?
2. What are you thinking about?
3. Whom do you need at this time?

Responses such as "It's hopeless," or "What's the use" may indicate clinical depression (see Chapter 14).

Every culture has ceremonies that help people acknowledge loss. The ceremonies may not be as obvious or sad as a funeral, but they are designed to allow family and friends to give social support during the process of grieving. The retirement or graduation party, for example, although varying in intensity of feeling, represents a sense of closure to one phase of life and the beginning of another, essentially what the funeral means after a death. Culture primarily dictates the rituals of mourning a loss. The nurse's observations of the planning and participation in ceremonies add to the assessment of the impact of the loss on the client.

Spiritual dimension According to Engel's theory, the institutionalization of mourning occurs in the stage of restitution and is an important part of the actual work of mourning. Religious ceremonies such as baptism, confirmation, and bar and bat mitzvah are joyous occasions for celebrating progression to a new stage of life and loss of another. The funeral ceremony serves many of the same purposes. People gather to share loss. Through the ceremony people symbolically express triumph over death and deny the fear of death.[12] Publically adapting to the loss does not decrease the suffering the bereaved will continue to feel, but moves them toward reinvesting emotionally in new relationships.

Because spiritual beliefs and practices greatly influence people's reaction to loss, it is important to explore them with the client.[34] The spiritually healthy client has inner resources that help in working through the grief process. Faith, prayer, trust in God or a superior being, perception of a purpose in life, or belief in immortality are examples of the inner resources that may sustain the client during an actual or perceived loss. In assessing the spiritual dimension of the client's life, church, synagogue, or other spiritual affiliation and its significance to the client and family are explored to help identify spiritual support systems. Although addressing the spiritual dimension is an area with which some nurses are uncomfortable, it can effectively be assessed by exploring questions such as the following:

1. What are the spiritual aspects of the client's philosophy about life? death?
2. Are the values and beliefs about life and death congruent with those of individuals important to the client?
3. Which spiritual resources and rituals have significance for the client?

Incompatible beliefs about death among family members can be an additional source of stress for clients dealing with a loss, for example, hospital or home care, burial or cremation. Assessment of the potential impact of differing beliefs may prevent the anger and resentment often observed among families when decisions need to be made about dying members.

Clients dealing with a loss may feel that it is a punishment from God because of past misdeeds or not being faithful to religious practices. According to Lindemann,[36] it would be important to assess the level of guilt the client or family expresses. In Kübler-Ross' stage of bargaining, the grieving person attempts to make a pact with God in order to postpone the loss.[30] Assessing the client's comments about responsibility for the loss will help the nurse focus on themes of guilt or punishment as an expected phase of grieving or an indicator of dysfunctional grieving.

Clients who would not have considered themselves religious before the actual or perceived loss event may turn to religion as a way to seek comfort and to deal with the fear of going crazy because of felt despair, helplessness, hopelessness, and guilt. They may cry out in anguish, "Why, God," or "Please help me, God." Recognizing feelings related to finding spiritual comfort during the assessment phase allows the nurse time to help the client explore them.

Analysis
Nursing diagnosis

Two nursing diagnoses approved by the North American Nursing Diagnosis Association (NANDA) pertaining to loss are anticipatory grieving and dysfunctional grieving. The definition and defining characteristics are presented in the accompanying boxes.

▼ ANTICIPATORY GRIEVING

DEFINITION
The state in which an individual grieves before an actual loss

DEFINING CHARACTERISTICS

- **Physical dimension**

  Physiological symptoms:
  Changes in eating habits
  Emptiness in stomach
  Choking sensation
  Decreased muscular power
  Alterations in sleeping patterns
  Alterations in activity level
  Altered libido
  Difficulty/disinterest in carrying out ADL

- **Emotional dimension**

  Distress at potential loss
  Guilt
  Hostility/irritability toward others
  Anger
  Feelings of loss, loneliness
  Hope for prevention of loss

- **Intellectual dimension**

  Perceived potential loss of significant object of value:
  Significant other
  Impending death of self
  Physiopsychosocial well-being
  Social role
  Body part
  Body function(s)
  Personal possessions
  Pet animal
  Altered communication patterns
  Preoccupation with self
  Self-accusation of negligence
  Ambivalence
  Realization or resolution of impending death or loss
  Denial of potential loss; shock, disbelief, avoidance of focus on loss
  Sense of unreality

- **Social dimension**

  Social withdrawal

Modified from McFarland G, McFarlane E: *Nursing diagnosis and intervention: planning patient care,* ed 2, St Louis, 1993, Mosby–Year Book.

The following case example illustrates the characteristics of a client with a diagnosis of anticipatory grieving.

▼ Case Example

Lara, a 35-year-old mother of three young children, was diagnosed with breast cancer. She was informed by the physician that with a modified radical mastectomy and chemotherapy her chances for survival were excellent. She verbalized that she knew she should be grateful that her life would be spared but she could not imagine what life would be like without her breast. Lara ad-

▼ DYSFUNCTIONAL GRIEVING

DEFINITION

A maladaptive process that occurs when grief is intensified so that a person is overwhelmed, becomes stuck in one phase of grieving, and demonstrates excessive or prolonged emotional responses to a significant loss

DEFINING CHARACTERISTICS

- **Physical dimension**

  Loss of significant person, animal, or prized possession
  Interference with life functioning
  Developmental regression
  Alterations in eating habits, sleep and dream patterns, activity level, or libido
  Choking sensations
  Difficulty breathing
  Physical distress
  Somatic symptoms representing identification of person who died

- **Emotional dimension**

  Inhibiton, suppression, or absence of emotional reactions
  Delayed emotional reactions
  Feeling that loss occurred only yesterday
  Extreme anger or hostility
  Excessive guilt
  Severe hopelessness
  Prolonged depression
  Prolonged panic attacks

- **Intellectual dimension**

  Difficulty expressing loss
  Excessive relieving of past experiences
  Prolonged alterations in concentration
  Prolonged denial
  Excessive idealization of dead person
  Excessive self-blame
  Suicidal thoughts
  Refusal to follow treatment regimen

- **Social dimension**

  Low self-esteem
  Identity loss
  Social isolation
  Inadequate social supports

- **Spiritual dimension**

  Diminished participation in religious and ritual acitivties

Modified from McFarland G, McFarlane E: *Nursing diagnosis and intervention: planning patient care,* ed 2, St Louis, 1993, Mosby–Year Book.

mitted that she had not had sex with her husband since she discovered the lump several weeks ago. "I'm preparing for the worst," she stated. "I know my husband will find me unattractive and I just couldn't bear that."

The following case example illustrates the defining characteristics of a client with a diagnosis of dysfunctional grieving.

▼ Case Example

Stephanie is a 52-year-old unmarried school teacher who lived much of her adult life estranged from her mother. When her mother died 2 years ago, Stephanie arrived just in time to attend the funeral and left immediately afterward. Over the past year and a half, Stephanie has suffered increasingly from GI disturbances, has become unable to sleep, and has begun missing school 2 or 3 days a week. Her principal's mother died about the same time as Stephanie's. She called Stephanie into the office to discuss the absences. In trying to be supportive of Stephanie, the principal mentioned that she had a difficult time getting over her mother's death and had experienced some guilt because she hadn't been able to spend as much time with her mother as she wanted to before her death. Stephanie became hostile and defensive and told the principal that this certainly wasn't her problem.

Following are other examples of NANDA diagnoses with causative statements related to grieving and loss:
1. Powerlessness related to loss of independence
2. Pain related to grief over loss of spouse
3. Social isolation related to perceived abandonment by friends
4. Ineffective individual coping related to awareness of impending death
5. Self-esteem disturbance related to altered body image
6. Ineffective family coping related to role change
7. Spiritual distress related to separation from religious ties
8. Social isolation related to separation from family
9. Altered nutrition: less than body requirement related to grieving
10. Sleep pattern disturbance related to fear of death
11. Altered family processes related to the loss of spouse, child, or parent
12. Altered sexuality patterns related to impaired relationship with or lack of a significant other
13. Fear of loneliness related to lack of social support
14. Anxiety related to perceived threat to self-concept associated with changing health status

Planning

The nursing care plan (Table 13-3) lists examples of long- and short-term goals, outcome criteria, interventions, and rationales related to loss and grieving.

Implementation

Physical dimension Knowing that the client's grief is affected by many factors such as personality, previous losses, intimacy of the relationship, and personal resources provides a constant reminder of the necessity for interventions based on the specific needs of the individual client experiencing loss.[10] The client or family may collapse in tears and anguish or lose control when the news of a loss is received. During this stage of shock and disbelief, crying helps provide relief from feelings of acute pain and tension. Whether verbally or nonverbally, the nurse needs to convey acceptance of the client's grief reaction. No attempt should be made to suppress the crying during this time. When the client cries, the nurse quietly remains to offer comfort, rather than leaving the client at the time of greatest need.[48]

▼ **TABLE 13-3   NURSING CARE PLAN**

GOALS	OUTCOME CRITERIA	INTERVENTIONS	RATIONALES
NURSING DIAGNOSIS: Dysfunctional grieving related to loss evidenced by inability to grieve			
LONG TERM			
To express grief appropriately	Describes meaning of loss Shares grief with significant other Participates with decision-making for future Verbalizes stages of grief process Expresses feelings associated with each stage Carries out ADL independently		
SHORT TERM			
To express feelings about loss	Expresses feelings of sadness, anger over loss	Facilitate expression of feelings by empathy and caring	Expressing feelings helps bring them to awareness and prevent delayed grief In a nonthreatening environment client can verbalize feelings
		Demonstrate respect for client's culture	Cultural groups differ in ways of showing grief
		Discourage blunting feelings with medications	To promote grief work
To describe relationship with loss	Identifies reality of loss	Encourage talk about the loss and its meaning	The significance of the relationship influences the grief response
		Offer support and reassurance	To reduce feelings of aloneness and instill hope
		Foster environment in which loss can be placed in a spiritual context by discussing philosophy, beliefs, values	Participation in spiritual practices and rituals helps client to reaffirm life
To identify appropriate ways of coping with current loss	Uses healthy coping skills	Explore previous losses and ways client coped	Grief is affected by previous losses and personality style
		Explain grief reactions	Knowing the feelings associated with grieving helps to acknowledge them as normal and acceptable and helps to understand anger and guilt, if present
		Refer to community agency or self-help group	Contact with others who have experienced a similar loss decreases feelings of isolation and loneliness

The silent presence of the nurse is often the most effective intervention in communicating caring to the client.

While the agony and crying provide relief, they can be physically exhausting. The client's energy level can fluctuate daily or even hourly. The nurse should help the client maintain as regular a sleeping pattern as possible. Restful sleep is promoted when clients maintain their usual bedtimes. Although clients may complain of lethargy, encouraging them to stay awake during the day and engaging in as much physical activity as possible helps to ensure they will be tired enough to sleep at night. Many of the GI symptoms reported by the grieving client can be ameliorated by encouraging the client's normal sleep, eating, and activity patterns.

When the loss is associated with body image, through the loss of a body part, weight gain or loss, loss of hair, or other effects of illness or treatment, interventions are focused on these physical manifestations of loss. The nurse encourages clients to wear their own clothing, put on makeup, or wear a wig or turban to minimize body changes. Children's and adolescents' self-images can often be enhanced by encouraging the wearing of headgear associated with their favorite media or sports hero. Wearing a temporary prosthesis can help a woman who has had a mastectomy feel less self-conscious. If the woman has begun to accept the loss of her breast, the nurse introduces her to a program such as Reach for Recovery, which gives information about breast prostheses, clothing, exercise, and other ways to help her resume normal activities.

When a diagnosis of dysfunctional grieving is made, the nurse intervenes to help the client establish a more functional pattern of grieving. Persistent absence of any emotion, inability to cry, or ruminations beyond a period of time culturally established for dealing with the loss may signal a delay in the work of mourning or a delayed grief reaction. The nurse intervenes by providing positive reinforcement of behaviors observed in normal grief reactions. For example, in a trusting relationship, the nurse can intervene simply by stating, "sometimes crying helps." The nurse offers support and reassurance that grieving is normal and painful and that the nurse will be available if the client fears losing control. When the interventions directed toward the physical aspects of normal grief and anticipatory grieving are ineffective in promoting relief of dysfunctional grieving, interventions directed toward depression may be necessary (see Chapter 14).

Interventions for the dying client require special attention to physical needs. The dying client needs to be kept as comfortable as possible. Nursing measures instituted to maintain attention to the physical care of the client are essential:

1. Wrinkle-free sheets
2. Bowel and bladder care
3. Prevention of skin breakdown
4. Positioning
5. Turning
6. Mouth care
7. Nutrition and hydration
8. Pain management

All dying clients do not experience pain, but most fear it. Open communication during the assessment phase of the nursing process allows the client to express this fear; the nurse then can explain ways to control pain. Parents' grief about their dying child goes beyond comprehension but often surfaces as concerns about the suffering and pain experienced by the child. The nurse assures the client or family that all possible ways of managing pain will be used. She addresses the client's or family's unrealistic fear of addiction by explaining the appropriate use of the medication in relieving the client's pain.

The nurse instructs the family member who wants to assist in the dying client's care in the use of therapeutic massage. If they are not comfortable massaging the upper body or trunk, or if the massage is painful for the client, the feet can be massaged. The foot is usually relatively free of pain; achieves similar results as body massage; and the massage promotes increased comfort, touching, and feelings of togetherness.

Emotional dimension Therapeutic communication with the client experiencing an actual or perceived loss begins with acceptance of the client's feelings, attitudes, and values related to the loss. When the client does not want to talk, sitting quietly conveys an understanding and acceptance without expecting the client to interact. If touch is acceptable to the client, it can be used as a nonverbal expression of caring and acceptance; stiffening or pulling away may indicate that touching is unacceptable. This client may be more comfortable with the nurse sitting close to the bedside. Spending time listening to clients, as opposed to interacting with them only to provide physical care, is an effective intervention in conveying acceptance of the client's emotional response to loss.

The nurse's role in the grieving process is to provide an atmosphere for clients to accomplish the painful work of grief. Being an active, nonjudgmental listener is essential to assure clients that their feelings are being accepted and no value judgments are being made. The nurse can acknowledge the client's grief by an empathic statement such as, "It must be very difficult for you." If the client is ready to talk about the loss, listening is the most appropriate intervention. Verbalizing fears and anxieties is helpful for the client. Forcing the client to talk, however, may increase discomfort rather than be therapeutic. Allowing clients experiencing a loss to verbalize when they choose provides sensitive comfort.

When a client is dealing with a loss, anger and guilt are normal feelings that need to be expressed to facilitate the work of mourning. Anger toward the loss object that is expressed near the time of the loss will not likely be turned inward later. The nurse understands that anger usually replaces denial and as such represents a progression in the grieving process. If nurses react defensively to the anger, they are telling clients that they are only acceptable when they are "good." When the family is upset by the client's anger, it may be helpful to explain to them that anger is a mechanism to try to control the environment more closely when one cannot control the loss.[10] It is difficult not to take the client's anger personally. Knowing that these expressions of anger are normal, however, the nurse may respond by saying, "I see you are really upset. I just want to let you know I'm available to talk if you'd like."[48]

Criticizing the client's anger or expressions of guilt will become barriers to communication, and the client may become less willing to share feelings related to the loss. For example, well-intentioned remarks such as, "At least you're alive" or "You're young, you can have other children," may make the client feel more guilty or increase the anger.

When clients indicate they are moving toward the awareness stage of grief, the nurse can intervene by helping them examine the guilt feelings and determining if they are realistic. The following is an example:

Client: *If I had gone to the doctor earlier this would not have happened.*
Nurse: *Did you have any reason to suspect something was wrong?*
Client: *Not really, but....*
Nurse: *Then how would you have known to go to the doctor earlier?*

Even if symptoms were ignored or the client engaged in health habits that led to the condition, pointing them out now is not helpful and serves as a barrier to communication.

When the client is dying, the nurse can respond to the need to work through any unfinished business, whether it be financial or social (e.g., saying good-bye to family and friends). By saying to the client, "You seemed sad after your husband left," the nurse is not invading the client's privacy, but expressing concern. Communicating openly will give the client the opportunity to deny or confirm the nurse's observations. The nurse provides acceptance and support by attentive listening to the client.

Kübler-Ross[30] noted that the nurse's fear of death frequently interferes with being able to provide support for the dying client and family. The statement, "Please God, don't let him die on my shift," expresses the nurse's emotional turmoil in dealing with the task. If nurses have worked through their own feelings about death and dying, they will be more at ease in assisting the dying client toward a peaceful death. Nurses who recognize their limitations in providing appropriate interventions to the dying client can seek support from nurses who are more experienced or have had special training. Nurses who genuinely care about the client as an individual should remember that their presence is likely to be more comforting than words to the dying client and his family.

Intellectual dimension The clouded sensorium and numbness clients experience may cause them to think they are going crazy, so the nurse should assure them that these are normal expressions of grief. After observing the response to the loss, the nurse intervenes by helping the client identify strengths in dealing with past losses as a way to deal with the current loss. The nurse should encourage the client to talk about the loss and the changes it will bring. This dialogue will provide the opportunity for the client to become aware of the impact of the loss, and encourages the client to plan for the necessary changes. Open-ended and reflective statements by the nurse are more helpful than direct questions in helping the client move through the grieving response. When the client has demonstrated a readiness to move to the awareness or restitution stage, explaining recognized grief reactions is an appropriate intervention.[18]

Involving the client in decision making and working on specific tasks will give the client a sense of control and help to diminish the feelings of hopelessness related to the loss. The nurse can help the client make informed decisions by answering the client's questions honestly and directly. Keeping in mind the contexts of awareness described by Glaser and Strauss,[22] information about the actual or perceived loss is given to clients as they request it. For example, if the client asks, "Am I going to die?" answering "Yes, the doctor says you have about a month to live," is inappropriate. An appropriate reflective response is "Do you think you are dying?" This allows the client to express thoughts and allows the nurse to respond based on an assessment of the client's desired awareness context. The nurse is responding with honest concern without taking away the client's hope. When and what information to disclose presents a dilemma for many nurses because of their difficulty weighing the client's "right to know" against withholding information under the guise of "protecting the client." Regardless of the nurse's stance, the client must be allowed to set the pace. Due to the client's altered sensorium from pain, medications, or the emotional response to the loss, information may have to be repeated frequently. Using language the client understands and having the client repeat it allow for clarification and ensure that the message is understood. When clients have the information, they can exercise control as to how, when, and by whom a task is to be accomplished. Encouraging clients to do what they can for themselves says to them, "I think you are a capable person." Gaining an intellectual understanding of the loss and what they can do to help themselves is often empowering for the client.

If dying clients imagine death negatively, the nurse can help them engage in activities to gain a sense of control. Visualization and imagery can be used to help the client explore fears and concerns by altering the image and ultimate reality. For example, the client whose image of death is darkness can be helped to imagine lights and soft music. The nurse can ask the client to imagine that he is with family and friends, free of pain, and surrounded by favorite music playing. If the client expresses a desire to die at home, the nurse works with the family to achieve that goal. If this goal is not possible, the nurse helps the client to amend the goal by visualizing the hospital room as a safe, comfortable place to die by surrounding the client with familiar articles from home. In addition dying children and adolescents, as well as adults, may benefit from drawing pictures, which the nurse can use to facilitate discussions of images of death.

Successful grief work in children through exploring actual or anticipated loss must be accomplished at the appropriate maturational level. The nurse encourages the parents and staff to be truthful and offers explanations that can be understood. Correcting misperceptions about death, illness, and rituals (funerals) is approached with the same sensitivity and caring as with an adult. Reducing fears of separation may be accomplished by allowing the grieving child to remain at home with significant others who are grieving rather than sending the child to a friend or neighbors to "protect" the child. Providing the child with close contact and holding may also reduce fears of separation.[10] Providing accurate explanations for sibling illness or death in terms the child can understand will help to dispel the child's fantasy that the death resulted from being bad or because the well child wished it.

The nurse needs to allow and accept the client's intermittent use of denial. If the client's denial is destructive, however, the nurse needs to help the client examine the purpose of the behavior. When the client's denial is manifested by going from one physician to another or postponing or prematurely terminating treatment, the nurse explores with the client the reasons for the behavior. Rather than criticizing or trying to talk the client out of some behavior, the nurse may ask what the client expects to be told about his illness, or what will happen when the client hears the same thing again.

If the client decides to return home to die, the nurse may need to teach the family the physical skills to enable them to care for the client. Positive and negative aspects of returning home to die are explored with the client and

RESEARCH HIGHLIGHT

Home Care for Children Dying of Cancer

• IM Martison, DG Moldow, G Armstrong, WF Henry, ME Nesbit, and JH Kersey

PURPOSE

This study was designed to explore the provision and process of home care for the dying child. It examined (1) the family's ability to provide good care at home until the child's death; (2) the family's willingness to provide such care; (3) the degree of nurse and physician involvement in care; and (4) the nurse's and family's abilities to secure adequate medication, equipment, and supplies.

SAMPLE

The subjects were 58 children diagnosed as dying from cancer who were being cared for at home. The children were 17 years of age or younger.

METHODOLOGY

Data were collected from questionnaires and semistructured interviews. The questionnaires and interview schedules were developed during a pilot study using health records, records completed by home care nurses, questions from standard demographical and personal characteristics questionnaires, grief support lists, care ratings, and progress records. After the initial data collection, interviews were conducted with the family 1 month and 1 year after the

Based on data from *Research in Nursing and Health* 9:11, 1986.

death of the child. A home care nurse directed the care with a consultant physician. Parents were given the option of readmitting the child to the hospital at any time.

FINDINGS

Of the 58 children in the study, 46 (79%) died at home, 11 died in the hospital, and 1 child died on the way to the hospital. Only 2 of the parents whose children died at home expressed uncertainty about choosing home care again, when interviewed at 1 month. Of the parents whose children did not die at home, 6 (37.5%) said they would choose home care again, 6 parents (31.5%) expressed uncertainty, and 4 said they would definitely choose hospital care. A year after their child's death, 56 families (96.5%) said they would definitely choose home care again.

IMPLICATIONS

Home care is a viable alternative for children dying from cancer. Families from diverse backgrounds were satisfied with their choice. Additional studies are needed to examine the economics of home care and criteria for children and parents who can and cannot benefit from the home care alternative.

---

family. If the dying client is a child, the parents often make the decision and need support and counseling in weighing all of the factors (see the research highlight).

In addition to information about physical skills, teaching may include signs of deterioration and how to identify additional sources of support. Hospice, home health care agencies, and public health departments provide nursing care services. Families also are encouraged to identify friends and other family members who can help out either routinely or occasionally.

Because a client near death may have an altered sensorium, the nurse stands near the bedside, speaks clearly and distinctly, and tells the client what is happening. Various levels of consciousness may be observed just before death. Clients may be alert, drowsy, stuporous, or comatose. Since hearing is thought to be the last sense a dying client loses, the nurse should never whisper or engage in conversation with the family as if the client were not there.

Educating the client and family about grief and grieving as a normal response to loss can promote understanding of what to expect when a loss occurs and may help to prevent the development of serious health problems associated with unresolved grief. General teaching guidelines for health care providers are provided in the box on p. 252.

Social dimension Among other factors, an individual's reaction to loss is affected by personal resources, primarily the perception of social support. Because of the positive influence of the social support system, nursing interventions based on the assessment of the client's percep-

tion of support are implemented to facilitate the successful resolution of grief. The nurse works with the client's significant others to help the client achieve social interaction patterns similar to those before the loss.

Grieving is painful and lonely. Lack of a support system has been identified as one of the causative and contributing factors that may delay grief work.[10] Even if the client is reacting to loss in an expected manner, feelings of isolation and withdrawal behaviors are often observed. Interventions, then, focus on helping clients reestablish contact with significant others in their lives to allow them to share their grief. Or, if the client is not making progress in grief work, the nurse may need to intervene by explaining the influence of the significant other's responses on the client. Using open-ended questions, reflection, and silence, the nurse facilitates expression of feelings.[8] For example, in the case of a 28-year-old woman with no children who is experiencing loss following a hysterectomy, the nurse gives the significant other information about the grief process, what to expect, and how long each stage might last.[8] In the case of body image disturbance after ostomy surgery, the nurse tells the significant other what to expect about the care and appearance of the ostomy. The nurse then listens to the significant other's responses, answers questions, and prepares the person to be supportive of the client with the ostomy.[8]

Because no two people grieve alike, the nurse promotes family cohesiveness by recognizing and supporting the stage of grieving and strengths of each family member. The

GUIDELINES FOR PRIMARY/TERTIARY INTERVENTIONS

Loss

Primary Prevention

Provide anticipatory guidance in dealing with an anticipated loss
Teach problem-solving skills
Identify persons at risk for dysfunctional grieving; those who:
    present a brave, stoic front
    have a history of multiple loss
    are socially isolated
    perceive their social network as unsupportive
    have a history of ineffectively dealing with loss
Teach ways to support a person dealing with an impending loss
Explain what to expect with a loss: sadness, fear, rejection, anger, guilt, loneliness
Teach signs of grief resolution:
    griever no longer lives in past but is future oriented
    griever breaks ties with lost person/object; time varies but acute stage
      shows signs of resolving in 6 to 12 months
    griever may have painful waves of grief years after the loss
Teach signs of exaggerated responses requiring treatment, especially persons at risk: hallucinations, delusions, isolation, egocentricity, overt hostility

Tertiary Prevention
Community resources:

AIDS Project Los Angeles, Inc
American Association of Retired Persons
    Widowed Persons Service
Committee on Pain Therapy

The Hemlock Society
National Council on Aging, Inc
National Hospice Organization
Parents Without Partners, Inc
Resolve, Inc
Dying With Dignity
The Compassionate Friends
The Candelighters Foundation
Survivors of Suicide (SOS)
Bereavement Outreach Network
Growing Through Grief
Widow to Widow Program
The National SIDS Foundation
Pregnancy and Infant Loss Center
Share

Self-help groups:

Parents Without Partners
Survivors of Suicide
Pregnancy and Infant Loss Groups
Widow Groups

---

nurse explains the need to discuss behaviors that interfere with relationships in the family and encourages self-exploration of feelings related to the loss with each family member. She encourages family members to talk directly to each other and to listen to each other. The trusting relationship the nurse has built with the client and family will help to facilitate the process.

Assisting clients and families to seek support from concerned others in their environment decreases feelings of loneliness and helplessness in managing the loss. The nurse should identify appropriate community resources to which the client or family can be referred to provide group support from others who have experienced a similar loss (see list of community resources in the accompanying box).

In addition to the promotion of comfort discussed in the physical dimension, nursing care of clients who are dying involves maintaining independence. The nurse promotes independence and maintains self-esteem by allowing the client to remain as self-sufficient as possible. For example, if the client cannot perform complete care, the nurse allows the client to do the things that will maintain self-esteem and dignity, such as face washing and holding a cup.

Even though the family wants to participate in the client's physical care, the client should maintain as much independence as possible. The role of the nurse may be to be gently, but firmly, the client's advocate in encouraging the family to allow the client to be as self-sufficient as pos-

sible. The nurse explains that clients need to feel some sense of control over the loss and that making the client dependent robs them of their dignity. Conversely, the nurse must remember that the family's role is not to provide nursing care for the client. The family may develop hostility and mistrust of the nursing staff if they perceive that they are performing all of the care for the client.

Some groups are particularly vulnerable to the development of dysfunctional grieving. One such group is that of persons with acquired immune deficiency syndrome (AIDS). When fears about caring for dying clients are compounded by fear of AIDS, the nurse may avoid the dying client with AIDS and the client experiences an overwhelming loneliness. Developing self-awareness becomes an imperative for the nurse in providing sensitive care to the client and family. Although AIDS affects all segments of the population, the realities of grief for the single, gay, bereaved partner are just beginning to be recognized as legitimate and as overwhelming as those of other individuals experiencing a loss. During the course of grief work, the gay client dying from AIDS and his lover are supported by the nurse in the same way as other clients in dealing with loss.[45] Interventions to decrease loneliness and isolation that involve the family include the following:

1. Providing meaningful environmental stimulation
2. Helping the family learn how to interact with the dying client
3. Providing information on the client's condition

4. Before death, encouraging the family to stay in communication through caring, silence, touch, and telling the client of their love for him[48]
5. Refering to appropriate support groups

Another group at high risk for developing dysfunctional grieving is that of clients dealing with loss related to miscarriage, stillbirth, and neonatal death. Interventions for assisting these clients include recognizing the grief and loss that the parents are experiencing, no matter how short the infant's life. For example, maternal-child nurses at one hospital initiated a formal procedure for helping grieving parents. It includes a card placed on the mother's door explaining the situation and a packet of information given to the parents by the nurse. Included in the packet are a booklet for parents whose child has died; a letter expressing sympathy and offering assistance; a memento card on which the baby's name, length, footprints, and date of birth are recorded; and suggestions for dealing with grief and a list of support groups.[44]

The nurse supports clients' adaptation to loss and assists them in restructuring their life-style to promote a meaningful existence. This goal is encouraged by helping the client remain involved in established relationships, particularly the most significant ones. Encouraging the client to renew meaningful interests, such as a hobby, can be therapeutic and contributes to a sense of accomplishment. The nurse may need to encourage the client and family to maintain current roles, personal interests, and life-styles as long as possible. As the client accepts the reality of the loss, there is a tendency to abandon prematurely jobs, hobbies, vacations, and social interests. Discussing subjects that span the past, present, and future allows clients to affirm their being. By encouraging the celebration of birthdays, anniversaries, and other special events, the nurse offers assistance to the client and family in the resolution phase of the grieving process.

The resolution of grieving begins with the acceptance of the loss. After the death, the family is encouraged to acknowledge the pain of loss. The nurse's presence and support as the bereaved express their sorrow, anger, or guilt can facilitate the resolution of grief. It is important to avoid suppressing the pain of grieving with drugs. In allowing for variations in expressing grief, the nurse is acknowledging acceptance and support of the family's grief reaction as a necessary part of preventing dysfunctional grieving.

As the client's condition deteriorates, the nurse's knowledge of the client's and family's awareness context guides the interventions. For example, if there is an open awareness, the nurse assists the client in exploring the impact of the client's death on the survivors. It may also be necessary to provide opportunities for clients to talk about where they want to die and what preferences they have for funeral and burial arrangements. If the family expresses that these topics are morbid, the nurse explains that the discussion helps clients to maintain a sense of control when they feel so overwhelmed by their impending death.

Likewise, talking about the past may be helpful for the dying client. Life review is an intervention the nurse uses to encourage the client and family to talk about past accomplishments, pleasures, and hardships. Past recollections of successes or overcoming setbacks offer affirmations of

the self. The past represents control that dying clients may feel they are losing. The past is something that cannot be taken away. Framing memories is another effective technique the nurse can use to encourage the client and family members to review the past and envision the future. Using this technique, the client and family reminisce about a happy experience. The nurse then asks the client to give the family members meaningful information to pass on to future generations. The family members, in return, share what the client means to them and their future aspirations.

Nurses and family members often avoid discussing present events because they fear upsetting dying clients with talking about plans in which the client may not be able to participate. The opportunity for communication and sharing may be lost if the nurse or family assumes that talking about the past or future in present terms will make the dying client uncomfortable. Feelings of loneliness, isolation, and abandonment are increased when clients feel that significant others are excluding them from conversations about topics that are a meaningful part of their lives.

The client needs the opportunity to say good-bye to others. The nurse encourages and supports the client and family as they terminate relationships as a necessary part of the grief process. The nurse acknowledges that termination is painful and, if the client or family desires, stays with them during this time. Being present at the moment of death is a common fear expressed by nurses and family members alike, and dying alone is the greatest fear expressed by clients.[30,31] In recognizing this common fear, the nurse can reduce the possibility of client abandonment as death approaches by participating in and encouraging client's and family's participation in support groups that offer help in dealing with this fear.

Grief work cannot begin until the loss is acknowledged. The nurse can encourage this process by open honest dialogue and by providing the family with the opportunity to view the dead person.[10] After making the body appear as natural and comfortable as possible, the nurse prepares the family for what to expect. As the finality of the death is realized, families are often comforted by the presence of the nurse who cared for the client during the dying.

Termination may be difficult for the client and the nurse. The client may view it as yet another loss. If the nurse has developed a close relationship with the family of the client who has died, the termination phase of the relationship may activate feelings of unresolved grief on the part of the nurse. Supporting the effects of the grieving family after the death of a loved one helps the nurse to resolve her own feelings related to loss. In addition to self-reflection, nurses who work with clients experiencing reactions to loss also need support from peers and other professionals to work through the often overwhelming feelings that result from dealing with death, grief, and loss.

Spiritual dimension Spirituality is at the core of human existence, integrating and transcending the physical, emotional, intellectual, and social dimensions.[34] The principles, values, personal philosophy, and meaning of life by which the client has pursued goals and self-actualization, however, may be called in to question when the client is responding to an actual or perceived loss. Because of a fear of intruding on the personal spiritual beliefs and practices of the client, the nurse often feels at a loss in implementing interventions that would be helpful to the client responding to a loss. The responses to the questions that guided the assessment help the nurse meet the spiritual needs of the client. The trusting relationship the nurse has developed with the client and family help to get past the initial discomfort in dealing with the spiritual aspects of care, even though the client and nurse have different views.

During the initial stages of grief, the nurse is accepting and nonjudgmental when the client expresses a belief that the loss is related to some past misdeed or failure "to do right" for which punishment is being dealt out. Even spiritually healthy clients need time to challenge their beliefs and values before moving on to the next stage of grieving. Although the nurse is aware that the progression is rarely sequential, as the client becomes aware of the loss, spiritual beliefs and rituals help to find meaning in the loss. The nurse provides spiritual support by listening as a client analyzes beliefs and values related to a philosophy of life. The client gradually begins to put the loss in perspective and expresses renewed interest in getting on with life. When the nurse perceives blocks in the client's grief work due to spiritual distress, interventions to help the client remove the barriers to finding spiritual comfort may be needed. For example, providing a client with spiritual comfort may involve role-playing with the client who feels the need to seek forgiveness from someone it is not possible to confront directly.

Regardless of the stage of grieving, the nurse demonstrates continued acceptance of the client and the client's beliefs. Meeting the client's spiritual needs may take many forms, including involvement by the clergy. If the client requests the nurse's participation in religious practices such as communion or prayer, the nurse should do so if she is comfortable with the request. The clergy can be a valuable resource to the nurse who needs guidance in meeting the client's specific requests. Even though clients who do not consider themselves to be religious often turn to religion as a way to seek spiritual comfort, especially when they are dying, nurses have a responsibility not to impose their own religious beliefs on clients when they are most vulnerable.

▼
KEY INTERVENTIONS FOR LOSS

Allow crying
Promote adequate sleep, activity, nutrition, hydration
Enhance body image and improve self-esteem
Alleviate pain
Touch, if appropriate
Facilitate expression of feelings about the loss: anger, guilt, fears
Listen nonjudgmentally
Identify strengths (e.g., past coping skills)
Increase feelings of control by encouraging participation in making decisions about care
Allow denial, when not destructive
Promote a support system to decrease isolation, loneliness
Support family members in their grief
Encourage life review
Refer to clergy and/or community resources

If the client expresses comfort in prayer or the reading of religious material, the nurse provides opportunities and privacy for the activities with members of the client's religious group or members of the health care team who feel comfortable with these activities. Whether through direct intervention or arranging access to spiritual care, the nurse ensures that the client's spiritual needs are met with the same care and concern given to their physical, emotional, and intellectual dimensions.

Key interventions for loss are summarized in the accompanying box. See the accompanying box for primary and tertiary interventions for a client experiencing a loss. Table 13-3 is a sample nursing care plan.

INTERACTION WITH A CLIENT EXPERIENCING A LOSS

Nurse: Did they tell you what the biopsy report said?
Client: No.
Nurse: Do you want to know?
Client: No.
Nurse: Okay. I'll be back tomorrow and we can talk about it, if you are ready.

The nurse allows and accepts the client's temporary use of denial. She is truthful and does not force him to hear information or discuss subjects that he resists.

Evaluation

Resolution of grief related to an actual or perceived loss may require months or years. Evaluation of nursing care for a client diagnosed with grieving, anticipatory grieving, or dysfunctional grieving is measured within the context of the expectations stated in the goals and the outcome criteria. Because the nurse will usually encounter the grieving client for a relatively short time, establishing small, measurable goals will give the nurse the opportunity to evaluate progress toward meeting the goals and to reassess and establish new goals with the client when the feedback indicates the client is not progressing toward grief resolution.

Bugen's model can be used to evaluate the predicted outcomes of grief based on the significance of the relationship and whether the loss was viewed as preventable. Observations of behaviors in Engel's stages of grief can be evaluated and used to establish additional goals when anticipatory or dysfunctional grieving patterns are assessed. Additional criteria to evaluate the process as well as the specific interventions include the following:

1. *Adequacy:* Did the interventions address only the symptoms of grief, or did they also include teaching the client what to expect throughout the grieving process?
2. *Appropriateness:* Were short-term goals established with the client to identify outcome criteria that allowed the client to feel some control over the grief process? Were long-term goals established to prevent the client from feeling overwhelmed when experiencing waves of despair associated with the length of the grief process?
3. *Effectiveness:* Were the interventions successful in providing relief from the somatic symptoms of grief

while helping the client accept the necessity of the pain of grief work?

4. *Efficiency:* Were the interventions enough to help the client deal with the immediacy of the loss? Were sources of support by others experiencing similar losses identified and made available to the client for later use?

BRIEF REVIEW

Loss is experienced throughout the life cycle. Each person responds to loss in a different way by asking, "What is happening to me? How can I live through this? How can I get over my loss?" While death is viewed as the ultimate loss, other losses produce grief reactions as intense and painful as those of the death experience.

The concept of loss is receiving increased attention as the critical role of resolution of the response to loss is recognized as a major factor in mental health and illness. Theories of loss and grief developed by practitioners in a variety of disciplines provide a basis for understanding the process an individual goes through in the work of grieving and mourning a loss.

Working with clients responding to loss can be both difficult and rewarding for the nurse. Loss is painful and can be viewed as a crisis in people's lives. Changes required in adjusting to the loss can influence the successful resolution of the loss. Knowledge and understanding of the grieving process offer the nurse the potential for self-growth as well as the opportunity to provide effective nursing care for clients responding to loss.

REFERENCES

1. American Nurses' Association: *Code for nurses,* Kansas City, 1976, American Nurses' Association.
2. American Psychiatric Association: *Diagnostic and statistical manual of mental disorders (DSM-III-R),* Washington, DC, 1987, American Psychiatric Association.
3. Baumer J, Wadsworth J, Taylor B: Family recovery after death of a child, *Archives of Disease in Childhood* 63:942, 1988.
4. Bloom-Feshbach J and others: *The psychology of separation and loss,* San Francisco, 1987, Josey-Bass Publishers.
5. Bowlby J: *Attachment and loss, separation, anxiety, and anger,* vol 2, New York, 1973, Basic Books.
6. Bowlby J: *Attachment and loss, loss, sadness and depression,* vol 3, New York, 1980, Basic Books.
7. Browning M, Lewis E: *The dying patient: a nursing perspective,* New York, 1972, American Journal of Nursing Co.
8. Buck M: The physical self. In Roy C, Andrews H, editors: *The Roy adaptation model—the definitive statement,* Norwalk, Conn, 1991, Appleton & Lange.
9. Bugen L: Human grief: a model for prediction and intervention, *American Journal of Orthopsychiatry* 46(2):196, 1977.
10. Carpenito L: *Nursing diagnosis application to clinical practice,* Philadelphia, 1989, JB Lippincott.
11. Carter S: Themes of grief, *Nursing Research* 38(6):354, 1989.
12. Castles M, Murray R: *Dying in an institution: nurse/patient perspectives,* New York, 1979, Appleton-Century-Crofts.
13. Cody W: Grieving a personal loss, *Nursing Science Quarterly* 4(2):61, 1991.
14. Collison C, Miller S: Using images of the future in grief work, *Image* 19(1):9, 1987.
15. Demi A, Miles M: Bereavement, *Annual Review of Nursing Research* 4:105, 1986.
16. Dracup K and others: Using nursing research findings to meet the needs of grieving spouses, *Nursing Research* 27:212, 1978.
17. Engel G: Grief and grieving, *American Journal of Nursing* 64:93, 1964.
18. Epstein C: *Nursing the dying patient,* Reston, Va, 1975, Reston.
19. Freud S: Mourning and melancholia. In *The complete psychological works of Sigmund Freud,* vol 14, London, 1957, The Hogarth Press, Ltd. (Translated from the German under the general editorship of J Strachey and A Tyson.)
20. Furman E: Children's patterns in mourning the death of a loved one, *Issues in Comprehensive Pediatric Nursing* 8(6):185, 1985.
21. Gifford B, Cleary B: Supporting the bereaved, *American Journal of Nursing* 90(2):49, 1990.
22. Glaser B, Strauss A: *Awareness of dying,* Chicago, 1965, Aldine Publishing.
23. Gordon M: *Manual of nursing diagnosis 1991-1992,* St Louis, 1991, Mosby—Year Book.
24. Granstrom S: Spiritual nursing care for oncology patients, *Topics in Clinical Nursing* 7(1):39, 1985.
25. Gullo S, Church S: *Loveshock,* New York, 1988, Simon and Schuster.
26. Grubb-Phillips C: Intrauterine fetal death: the maternal bereavement experience, *Journal of Perinatal Neonatal Nursing* 2(2):34, 1988.
27. Horsley G: Baggage from the past, *American Journal of Nursing* 88:60, 1988.
28. Kavanaugh R: *Facing death,* Kingsport, Tenn, 1972, Kingsport Press.
29. Kim M, McFarland G, McLane A: *Pocket guide to nursing diagnoses,* ed 3, St Louis, 1991, Mosby—Year Book.
30. Kübler-Ross E: *On death and dying,* New York, 1969, Macmillian.
31. Kübler-Ross E: *To live until we say good-bye,* Englewood Cliffs, NJ, 1978, Prentice Hall.
32. Lake M and others: Evaluation of a perinatal grief support team, *American Journal of Obstetrics and Gynecology* 157(5):1203, 1987.
33. Lambert V, Lambert C: *Psychosocial care of the physically ill,* ed 2, Englewood Cliffs, NJ, 1985, Prentice-Hall.
34. Landrum P, Rawlins R, Beck C, Williams S: The person as a client. In Beck C, Rawlins R, Williams S, editors: *Mental health—psychiatric nursing,* ed 2, St Louis, 1988, Mosby—Year Book.
35. Lewis C: *A grief observed,* New York, 1961, The Seabury Press.
36. Lindemann E: Symptomatology and management of acute grief, *American Journal of Psychiatry* 32:141, 1944.
37. Lunden T: Long-term outcome of bereavement, *British Journal of Psychiatry* 145:424, 1984.
38. McFarland G, Gerety E: Grieving, anticipatory. In Kim M, McFarland G, McLane A: *Pocket guide to nursing diagnosis,* ed 3, St Louis, 1989, Mosby—Year Book.
39. McFarland G, and Wasli E: *Nursing diagnosis and process in psychiatric mental health nursing,* Philadelphia, 1986, JB Lippincott.
40. Melges F: *Time and the inner future,* New York, 1982, John Wiley.
41. Morris D: Management of perinatal bereavement, *Archives of Disease in Childhood* 63:870, 1988.
42. Murray R, Zentner J: *Crisis intervention: a therapy technique, nursing concepts for health promotion,* ed 3, Englewood Cliffs, NJ, 1985, Prentice-Hall.
43. Neeld E: *Seven choices: taking the steps to new life after losing someone you love,* New York, 1990, Clarkson N Potter.
44. Null S: Nursing care to ease parents' grief, *Maternal Child Nursing* 14:84, 1989.
45. Oerlemans-Bunn M: On being gay, single, and bereaved, *American Journal of Nursing* 80(4):472, 1988.

46. Paquette M, Neal M, Rodemich C: *Psychiatric nursing diagnosis care plans for DSM-III-R,* Boston, 1991, Jones and Bartlett.

47. Parks R: *Bereavement: studies of grief in adult life,* London, 1972, Tavistock.

48. Potter P, Perry A: *Fundamentals of nursing concepts, process, and practice,* ed 2, St Louis, 1992, Mosby–Year Book.

49. Ptalum M and others: Understanding the final message of dying, *Nursing* 16(6):26, 1986.

50. Polanyi M: *The tacit dimension,* Garden City, NY, 1967, Anchor Books, Doubleday.

51. Sahler O, editor: *The child and death,* St Louis, 1978, Mosby–Year Book.

52. Schneider J: *Stress, loss, and grief,* Baltimore, Md, 1984, University Park Press.

53. Shipes E: Sexual functioning following ostomy surgery, *Nursing Clinics of North America* 22(2):303, 1987.

54. Shneidman E, editor: *Death: current perspectives,* Palo Alto, Calif, 1976, Mayfield.

55. Stewart R, Eoyang T: Grieving. In Kozier B, Erb G, editors: *Concepts and issues in nursing practice,* Menlo Park, Calif, 1988, Addison-Wesley.

56. Strother A: Drawing the line between life and death, *American Journal of Nursing* 91(4):24, 1991.

57. Townsend M: *Nursing diagnoses in psychiatric nursing: a pocket guide for care plan construction,* ed 2, 1991, Philadelphia, FA Davis.

58. Weisman A: *The realization of death: a guide for the psychological autopsy,* New York, 1974, Jason Aronson, Inc.

59. Wilcox S, Sutton M: *Understanding death and dying: a multidisciplinary approach,* Port Washington, NY, 1977, Alfred Publishing Co.

60. Wilkes E: Quality of life: effects of the knowledge of diagnosis in terminal illness, *Nursing Times* 73:1506, 1977.

61. Worden W: *Grief counseling and grief therapy,* New York, 1982, Springer.

62. Zlsook S, editor: *Biophysical aspects of bereavement,* Washington, DC, 1987, American Psychiatric Press.

ANNOTATED BIBLIOGRAPHY

Cody E: Grieving a personal loss, *Nursing Science Quarterly* 4(2):61, 1991.

The author reports research on grief from a nursing perspective. Through engaging in dialogue with the researcher, four subjects described their experience of grieving a personal loss. The research findings are compared with those of theorists commonly found in the literature.

Neeld E: *Seven choices,* New York, 1990, Clarkson N Poter.

The author uses the subtitle of her book, taking the steps to new life after losing someone you love, to describe the choices people can make in resolving grief. The author uses true stories of individuals and her own to describe the significance and progression of the mourning process.

Peck R, Stefanics C: *Learning to say good-bye,* Muncie, Ind, 1987, Accelerated Development, Inc.

The authors provide helpful information for those delivering health care services as well as individuals who question the meaning of death and who struggle to handle their own emotional problems when a loved one dies and when confronted with their own deaths.

After studying this chapter, the student will be able to:

- Define hope, hopelessness, depression, manic behavior, and suicide
- Discuss the psychopathology of major depression and bipolar disorder as described in the DSM-III-R
- Discuss historical perspectives of hope and hopelessness

- Describe theories of hope and hopelessness
- Apply the nursing process to clients who have feelings of hope and hopelessness
- Identify current research findings related to hope and hopelessness

With *hope* a person acts, moves, and achieves. Without hope the person becomes dull, listless, despairing, and hopeless. Hope defends against *hopelessness*; it enables an individual to tolerate difficult situations and maintain motivation. However, hope can also decrease a person's contact with reality. With hopelessness there is a loss of confidence. A sense of entrapment and futility prevails, convincing the person that what is wanted is beyond reach. Energy to think and act is lacking, and passiveness immobilizes the individual. Hopeless individuals feel like giving up and sometimes do. They decide that there is no use, no good, no sense, or meaning to life.

The idea of hope and hopelessness as a continuum is useful in discussing these entities. On one end of the continuum is hope, including confidence, faith, inspiration, and determination. At the other end of the continuum is hopelessness, including despair, helplessness, doubt, grief, apathy, sadness, *depression*, and *suicide*.

Hopelessness is a feeling experienced by persons who are depressed. Depressed persons are described as having a mood or affective disturbance that affects their behavior. Behaviors commonly seen in persons with mood disturbances include depression, mania, and suicide. This chapter focuses on the concept of hope-hopelessness and its application to clients who have feelings of hope or hopelessness evidenced in depression, mania, and suicide. The chapter begins with a discussion of the psychopathology of major depression and bipolar disorder so that students can have the knowledge base essential for giving care to clients with these disorders.

DSM-III-R diagnoses. Major depression and *bipolar disorder* are classified in the DSM-III-R as mood disorders. A distinguishing characteristic of major depression and bi-

polar disorder is a disturbance in mood that is not due to any other physical or mental disorder. Major depression may occur as a single episode or as recurring episodes. The essential feature of a major depression is either a depressed mood or a loss of interest in activities for a period of at least 2 weeks. The symptoms represent a change from the person's usual functioning. The degree of impairment to the individual varies, but there is usually severe interference with social and occupational functioning. Associated

▶ DIAGNOSES Related to Hope-Hopelessness

MEDICAL DIAGNOSES	NURSING DIAGNOSES
Major depression	**NANDA**
Bipolar disorder	Body image disturbance
Seasonal affective disorder	Personal identity disturbance
	Self-esteem disturbance
	Chronic low self-esteem disturbance
	Situational low self-esteem
	High risk for violence
	Self-care deficit
	Hopelessness
	PMH
	Altered self-concept
	Altered body image
	Altered personal identity
	Altered self-esteem
	Suicide ideation
	Altered self-care

DATES	EVENTS
600 BC	Early chronicles describe Nebuchadnezzar as suffering from wild, erratic moods (probably manic activity), followed by profound depression.
460 BC	Hippocrates related depression to the humidity of the brain. His theory of body substances, called humors, determined physical and mental health. Depression was blamed on a surplus of melancholy (black bile).
300 BC	Early Greek philosophers viewed fate as unchangeable and hope as an illusion or curse distorting reality, prolonging agony, and promoting a reliance on faith rather than action.
5 AD	Attitudes about hope changed with the spread of Christianity when St Paul declared that hope stands with love.
1500s	During the Elizabethan period, people prided themselves on being melancholic and came to view it as a superior malady and mark of refinement among those deeply touched by the pathos in life. The writings of Shakespeare and Robert Burton included depressive themes.
1800s	Dostoyevsky, Poe, and Hawthorne expressed inner anguish and despair in their writings. Later poets, such as Shelley, accepted the fatalistic cynical view of the Greeks. Nietzsche wrote, "Hope is the worst of evils, for it prolongs the torment of man."
1900s	Winston Churchill, by frequent referral to his "black dog" of depression, suggested how familiar a companion his despair was.
1930s	Electroconvulsive therapy (ECT) was introduced in Rome by two physicians who observed that epileptic clients showed no evidence of schizophrenia. Thinking that seizures prevented schizophrenia, they promoted the use of artificially induced seizures to treat schizophrenia and depression.
1950s	Introduction of the first clinically effective antidepressants, Imipramine and monoamine oxidase inhibitors (MAOIs).
1980s	An age of depression exists, generated by the rising expectations for standards of living after World War II, coming up against the harsh realities of the population explosion, limited resources, inflation, unemployment, and the possibility of nuclear warfare. The anxieties of the mid-1960s have given way to despair as a dominant mood. Suicide is a major health problem in the United States.
1990s	The antidepressant Prozac shows promise in treating depression without having the side effects associated with other antidepressants.
Future	The "Decade of the Brain" emerges with an emphasis on biological causes of depression such as disruptions in circadian rhythms, brain dysfunction, and the role of genetics. The stigma of depression and mental illness may diminish as biological causes are emphasized and replace the psychological causes for depression. Nurses are challenged to contribute to the expanding knowledge of the biological aspects of mental illness by collaborative research with other disciplines. Legal and ethical issues will emerge as individuals commit suicide with help from family.

HISTORICAL OVERVIEW

symptoms include appetite disturbance, change in weight, sleep disturbance, psychomotor agitation or retardation, decreased energy, feelings of worthlessness, excessive or inappropriate guilt, difficulty thinking or concentrating, recurring thoughts of death, or suicide attempts. Criteria for the severity of a depressive episode include the following:

1. *Mild*: Symptoms result in minor impairment in occupational functioning, in usual social activities, or in relationships with others.
2. *Moderate*: Symptoms of functional impairment are between mild and severe.
3. *Severe*: Symptoms markedly interfere with occupational functioning, with usual social activities, or relationships with others.
4. *Severe with psychotic features*: Client experiences delusions or hallucinations.

A person with a chronically depressed mood for a period of at least 2 years is described as having *dysthymia* (depressive neurosis). Symptoms are similar to those of major depression but persist over a longer period and are less severe. Symptoms do not represent a change from the person's usual functioning. The impairment in social and occupational functioning is mild to moderate because of the chronicity rather that the severity of the depressive symptoms.

The distinguishing characteristic of bipolar disorder is the occurrence of one or more manic episodes with or without depressive episodes. The essential feature of a manic episode is a predominant mood that is elevated, expansive, or irritable. Associated symptoms include inflated self-esteem, or grandiosity; decreased need for sleep; *pressure of speech; flight of ideas*; distractibility, increased involvement in activities, psychomotor agitation, and excessive involvement in pleasurable activities that have a potential for painful consequences. The disturbance is sufficiently severe to cause impairment in social and occupational functioning or in relationships with others, or to require hospitalization to prevent harm to oneself or others.

Cyclothymia is a chronic mood disturbance of at least 2 years' duration that involves numerous manic episodes alternating with depressive episodes. The symptoms are not severe enough to meet the criteria for major depression or bipolar disorder. There is no marked impairment in social or occupational functioning. Some persons are socially effective and particularly productive in occupational situations during hypomanic episodes.

A diagnosis of *seasonal affective disorder* (SAD) is made when a regular temporal relationship between the onset of the depression and a particular 60-day period of the year occurs, for example, between the beginning of January and the end of February. The diagnosis of SAD does not apply to persons with obvious seasonally related stressors such as being unemployed every winter. In addition, there will have been at least three episodes of mood disturbance in three separate years and at least two of the years were consecutive.

DEPRESSION

Theoretical Approaches

Feelings of hopelessness generate depressed behavior. This section addresses theoretical approaches to the behavior, depression, which encompasses feelings of hopelessness.

Biological

Recent studies indicate that the biological view of depression is replacing the psychological view. Advances in technology have made it possible to explain the functioning, purposes, and interconnections of the brain with other body systems such as the nervous, endocrine, and immune systems with the environment. This technology has advanced our knowledge of depression.

Genetic Studies have shown that depression is more likely to occur in a person with a family history of depression. From twin, family, and adoption studies, it is certain that mood disorders are heritable. However, the number of twins with affective disorders is limited and studies cannot exclude environmental influences. Adoption studies lend support to the concept of heritable transmission since researchers separate genetic and environmental contributions to depression.[86]

Biochemical With the expansion of knowledge in neurophysiology, a biochemical model of depression has emerged. This model concerns physiological chemical changes that take place during depressed states. Whether these chemical changes cause depression or are a result of depression is not clearly understood. However, significant functional abnormalities have been found in several body systems during a depressive illness. Studies of biogenic amine metabolism have indicated that a deficiency of particular biogenic amines at receptor sites in the brain may be related to depression. For example, lower levels of norepinephrine have been found in depressed persons. Serotonin, another biogenic amine, is also deficient in depressed persons. Measuring the concentration of the amine metabolites in the urine of depressed clients helps determine the relationship between biogenic amines and depression. However, variables such as diet, activity, endocrine factors, and anxiety levels may alter the excretion rates of amines and their metabolites. Investigations indicate an increased steroid output in depression. Electrolyte metabolism studies showed increased sodium levels in depression and a lowering of sodium levels after recovery.

The following list includes other approaches to understanding depression from a biological framework:

1. Depression is associated with disruptions in circadian rhythms such as the sleep-wake cycle. Depressed clients frequently complain of insomnia, having either difficulty falling asleep or difficulty waking up. Another circadian disruption involves the light-dark cycle. Low levels of melatonin, a hormone secreted during sleep, are associated with depression. Light enhances melatonin output, changes neuroendocrine imbalances, and relieves symptoms.[71]

2. Depression is linked to brain function. Dietary components of common foods, for example, caffeine, salicylates, food preservatives, and sugar, can influence brain function.[25]

3. Depression is also associated with limbic seizure activity as seen in EEG changes, with neuroendocrine dysfunctions such as hypothyroidism, and with defects in the immune system, for example, decreased numbers of disease-fighting immune cells. Although research in the biochemical model is inconclusive, there is evidence that a variety of factors can produce changes in body chemistry that may contribute to depression.[25]

Psychoanalytical

A sense of hope develops from early childhood experiences, especially those related to formation of trust. According to Erikson,[31] hope emanates from a successful resolution of the conflict between trust and mistrust. The child learns to hope if the environment is suitable to the development of trust. Children first learn trust from the mothering person. The probable basis of trust is the knowledge that help is forthcoming when needed. Hope in this framework then is not a solitary activity but is related to the expectation of assistance from other people.

Freud[38] viewed depression as the aggressive instinct turned inward. The anger is not directed at the appropriate

▼ **TABLE 14-1** Bibring's Model of Depression

Developmental Stage	Ego Ideals	Characteristics of Depression
Oral	To be loved and taken care of, to get affection, to be worthy	Excessive hunger for love, affection, warmth, appreciation
Anal	To be obedient, good, kind, humane, clean, loving	Guilt, weakness, lack of control
Phallic	To be strong, secure, superior	Inadequacy, inferiority, helplessness
Latency	To be valued and important, to achieve	Powerlessness, low self-esteem

object, but displaced onto the self and accompanied by feelings of guilt. Initially, there may be a loss of a loved person or object. The person feels both angry and loving toward the lost object (ambivalence) but is unable to express his angry feelings because of repression. Thinking that these feelings are inappropriate or irrational, or having developed a pattern throughout life of containing feelings, particularly negative ones, the individual then directs his angry feelings inward.

Bibring[10] believed that the ego may fail to achieve its narcissistic goals at any stage of development, and this failure impairs the development of self-esteem. Low self-esteem, helplessness, and powerlessness are characteristic features of depression. Because infants are helpless and dependent on others to meet their needs, it was suggested that many depressions have their predisposing roots in trauma during the oral phase of development. As a result of early trauma, the individual has an excessive hunger for affection, warmth, and appreciation. A loss of affection and love reactivates earlier feelings of helplessness. This theory explains depression as also having predisposing roots in other stages of development (Table 14-1).

Behavioral

Lewinsohn's behavioral model[56] proposed that a low rate of reinforcement predisposes one to depression. Two variables are important to this model: (1) the individual may fail to initiate the appropriate responses to receive positive reinforcement, and (2) the environment may fail to provide the reinforcement. These variables may occur when people find the behavior of the depressed person distressing, negative, or offensive.

The model of *learned helplessness*,[84] as described by Seligman, proposed that it is not the situation itself that produces depression but the belief that one has no control over the situation. He defined *helplessness* as a belief that no one will do anything to aid you and *hopelessness* as a belief that neither you nor anyone else can do anything. Learned helplessness is both a behavioral state and a personality trait of persons who believe that they have lost control over their environment. These negative expectations lead to hopelessness, passivity, and an inability to assert oneself.

The object loss model of depression proposed by Bowlby[13] referred to the person's traumatic separation from significant objects. Two factors are important in this theory: (1) a loss during childhood predisposes one to adult depression, and (2) a loss or separation in adult life acts as a

stressor in depression. A child ordinarily has formed a bond to a mothering person by 6 months of age. If this bond is broken, the child experiences separation anxiety and grief. According to Bowlby, unfavorable personality development is often attributed to unsatisfactory responses to loss during infancy and childhood, resulting in a predisposition to respond to all losses in a similar way.

Cognitive

Beck[3] described depression as an altered style of thinking characterized by negative expectations. This approach emphasizes the role that disturbances in thinking play in determining emotional states. Hopelessness and helplessness represent the central features of depression and reflect a negative conception of self, negative interpretation of one's experiences, and a negative view of the future. The depressed person finds that the world presents insurmountable obstacles to carrying out goals, views the self as helpless to surmount these obstacles, and has given up any hope of exercising future control over his life.

Sociological

Becker[6] defined depression as a social phenomenon. He proposed that the ego is rooted in social reality, and the ego ideal is composed of socially learned symbols and motives. Becker stated that a breakdown of self-esteem may involve, in addition to object losses, the individual's symbolic possessions such as power, status, roles, identity, values, and purpose for existence. Particularly susceptible to depression are individuals with upward social mobility and women who strongly identify with the role prescribed to them by their culture. The rigid sex role stereotyping that characterizes a woman as a faithful and loyal wife, a dedicated and loving mother, a competent and diligent housewife, and a supporter of moral and religious values effected through the socialization process may be detrimental to women's emotional health and personal growth. One study of female depression indicates that conflicts inherent in the changing roles of women increase their chances of experiencing depression during role transition periods.[93]

Holistic

A holistic approach to depression reflects aspects of each of the previously described models. Depression is explained by the integration of genetic, biological, psychoanalytical, behavioral, cognitive, and sociological models.

Table 14-2 summarizes the different theoretical approaches to depression.

▼ **TABLE 14-2   Summary of Theories of Depression**

Theory	Theorist	Dynamics
Biological	—	Depression is associated with disruptions in circadian rhythms, brain dysfunction, limbic seizure activity, neuroendocrine dysfunction, biogenic amine deficiencies, defects in the immune system, and genetics.
Psychoanalytical	Freud	Depression originates as a response to a loss, disappointment, or failure. Anger is displaced and turned inward on the self. Inability to mourn or grieve for a loss results in depression.
	Bibring	When the ego fails to achieve goals during developmental stages, loss of self-esteem, helplessness, and powerlessness may result.
Behavioral	Lewinsohn	Failure to receive positive reinforcement from others and from the environment predisposes one to depression.
Cognitive	Beck	A negative conception of self, experiences, others, and the world contributes to depression.
	Seligman	The belief that one has no control over a situation contributes to depression.
	Bowlby	Loss during childhood predisposes one to adult depression.
Sociological	Becker	Loss of power, status, identity, values, and purpose for existence creates susceptibility for depression.
Holism	—	Depression is the result of genetic, biological, psychoanalytical, behavioral, cognitive, and sociological experiences.

NURSING PROCESS

Assessment

Physical dimension In general, an individual with a sense of hope has energy and drive and generates *joie de vivre*, or an excitement about life. Overall well-being and optimism are projected. An assessment of the client's nutrition, exercise, habits such as smoking and alcohol intake, and self-care can determine the quality of overall health. Personality traits such as assertiveness and love of adventure frequently are seen in these individuals.

Identifying hope in an individual includes observing facial expression (affect) and behavior in general. Persons with a sense of hope feel and look vital, vibrant, alert, and have a sense of humor.

Clues to the client's depression can be observed. Sitting slumped with eyes lowered, quietly and alone, and looking sad and dejected are characteristic of the depressed person. The face may appear tired and drawn, with deep circles under the eyes, and with little change in expressions. The client may appear disheveled and unkempt. Hair is uncombed, and clothes may be worn several days without a change. Motor activity is decreased. The person moves as if each action requires a special effort. Walking, talking, and activities of daily living are generally slowed down. Because of the reduced activity level *(psychomotor retardation)* and the slowing down of body processes, a cluster of *vegetative symptoms* can be identified, which include weakness and fatigue, insomnia, anorexia and weight loss, gastrointestinal disturbances (commonly constipation), and a lack of interest in food, sleep, activities, and sex. These symptoms are the classic manifestations of depression.

Some depressed clients demonstrate *psychomotor agitation*, which includes restlessness, sobbing, and excessive verbalizations. Recognizing the agitation, which resembles anxiety, is crucial because the client may be a high risk for attempting suicide. In agitated depression, motor activity may include pacing a given route and repetitive movements such as hand wringing. In anxiety, motor activity proceeds in random, unpredictable movements.

In depression, as the physiological processes are slowed down, body responses are altered, and metabolism decreases. The depressed client complains of a loss of appetite and weight. A loss of 15 to 30 pounds is not uncommon in a 2- to 3-month period. Epigastric distress, nausea, vomiting, indigestion, and constipation occur frequently.

Neurological symptoms include headaches, dizziness, and blurred vision. Occasionally, clients complain of cardiovascular symptoms such as mild chest pain, dyspnea, and palpitations. Alterations in the reproductive system include amenorrhea, impotence, and a decreased sex drive. Alterations in the immune system lead to increased susceptibility to illness, such as colds, urinary tract infections, viral infections, and pneumonia. Thus frequent infections may be a clue to a depressed state.

Symptoms of depression may accompany physical illness. The box on p. 262 shows a list of illnesses that often coexist with depression.

Hypochondriacal complaints that have no organic basis but that mimic a physical illness may be present. This morbid preoccupation with one's state of health can range from a series of minor complaints to the conviction that one has some serious disease. Minor complaints include frequent headaches, gastrointestinal disturbances, constipation, and vague aches and pains. Other complaints may involve the client's belief that he has a serious physical illness. This needs to be taken seriously and evaluated medically, because the complaint may be masking depression.

Based on biological theory, it is important to assess disturbances in sleep patterns, the effects of medications, and the family for a history of depression. Depressed persons have sleep disturbances, so determining sleep habits is essential. Some wake early, between 4 and 5 AM, and cannot go back to sleep. Others sleep only for short periods. For some who sleep for long periods, sleep is neither restful nor refreshing. Severely depressed clients who have a pat-

ILLNESSES OFTEN COEXISTING WITH DEPRESSION

AIDS
Addison's disease
Amyotrophic lateral sclerosis
Brain tumors
Cancer
Cardiac illnesses
Brucellosis
Diabetes
Hepatitis
Lingering influenza
Subacute bacterial endocarditis
Tuberculosis
Cushing's disease
Diseases of the pancreas
Diseases of the parathyroid glands
Failure to thrive
Hypothyroidism
Leukemia
Lupus erythematosus
Migraine headaches
Multiple sclerosis
Parkinson's disease
Pernicious anemia
Renal diseases
Sleep disturbances

tern of early morning wakefulness combined with despondency may be at risk for attempting suicide.

Certain medications are often responsible for the development of depression, the aggravation of a preexisting depression, or the production of depressive symptoms such as sedation, apathy, and lethargy. Medications that may produce depressive symptoms include digitalis, antihypertensives, antiparkinson medications, estrogens, neuroleptics, hypnotics, sedatives, and cortisones.

Because of the genetic predisposition to affective disorders, it is essential to determine the presence or absence of depression in other family members.

Some persons have a pattern of becoming depressed during specific seasons, particularly winter when daylight is shortened. A relationship between a specific period of time and depression that occurs over several years may indicate a seasonal type of depression.

Emotional dimension The nurse assesses the client's state of contentedness and optimism. With hope, there is inner buoyancy, internal peace, harmony, serenity, and a general freedom from overpowering anxiety, anger, guilt, and despair. The individual feels relaxed, secure, and safe. Tensions and conflicts are lessened and life is worth living. The individual is confident and feels an inner strength.

In depression, sadness is the major affect. Other characteristics to look for include irritability, agitation, hostility, anger, guilt, and lack of pleasure *(anhedonia)*. Feelings of emptiness, worthlessness, and a lack of self-respect and confidence can be identified. The client may be emotionally labile, crying easily one moment and laughing the next. Determining how the client feels early in the morning provides clues about the type of depression. Generally, the client with a major depression feels worse early in the

morning and improves as the day goes on. The client with dysthymia (neurotic depression) may begin the day optimistically but feel progressively worse as the day wears on.

Based on psychoanalytical theory, the depressed person is angry. The anger may not be clearly observable because it commonly is turned inward on the self. When anger is repressed, physical symptoms such as headaches, backaches, and diarrhea may be present. (See Chapter 11 for further assessment of anger.)

In depression, persons frequently express feelings of guilt. The guilt may be related to a real situation, such as being fired from a job for drinking, or to an imagined situation, for example, a mother may feel guilty for some supposed wrongdoing to her adult children. In either situation the expressions of guilt are reiterated over and over to anyone who will listen. The client is inappropriately feeling guilt. (See Chapter 12 for further assessment of guilt.)

An assessment of depression needs to include whether or not the client feels a sense of powerlessness, helplessness, or hopelessness. Powerlessness is seen when the client feels no control over life events and remains unmotivated and passive. A fatalistic viewpoint is taken—what happens, happens. The harsh, rigid thinking of the despairing person allows no way to change or take control of events. Helplessness is identified in the client by lack of energy and staunch pessimism. Clients are convinced that everything that can be done has been done and will attempt to convince others of this. Hopelessness may accompany helplessness in a client. The client accepts the fact that it is of no use to continue treatment. There is no hope of ever feeling better. Feelings of futility, entrapment, and the impossible are expressed when the client is without hope.

Intellectual dimension Positive experiences remembered from earlier times and reinforced through learning generate optimism and hope. The person with hope is oriented, exercises reasonable judgment, explores alternatives, and generally understands the situation realistically.

Assessing hope means looking at the individual's motivation and determination. The client who does not deny the problem or run away from the difficulty experiences hope. He comes to believe that in the future another obstacle can be conquered. Armed with this knowledge, clients will not lack courage when they again need this sustaining quality.

Closely related to motivation is the ability to set or change goals when the original goal is no longer feasible. A person who is able to be flexible and adapt to changes is more likely to maintain hope against overwhelming stress. Having other options in a difficult situation gives a person a sense of autonomy. Although the choices may not be directed toward the desired goal, the person retains the freedom to decide for himself. This can provide a feeling of control.

Another aspect of hope includes differentiating hope from wishing. The difference between hope and wishing is the probability of attaining the object of one's desire. A wish is closely related to "magic hope." A person using magic hope realizes that the possibility of obtaining the wish is highly improbable, such as wishing for a million dollars. The person knows he is not likely to ever have the million dollars, but the fantasy is a pleasant one. The person who hopes has a sense that he will obtain what he hopes for. The hoping person makes a concrete plans to gain what is desired, while the person who wishes (for example, for the million dollars) does not because it is so unlikely that the wish can be achieved.

In summary, an optimistic outlook, motivation to change, ability to think of options, recognition of freedom to choose alternatives, and a sense of the possible are indicators of hope within the individual.

Depressed persons have little interest in activities around them. Because they are preoccupied with their own unhappy condition, their minds are filled with unrelenting thoughts about their misery. Negativism permeates their thinking about themselves, others, and the world. Ruminating over past events and self-blame leaves no time for communication with others.

Cognitive abilities are impaired, and the client has difficulty concentrating and making decisions. Judgment, insight, and memory are also impaired. Thoughts may become rigidly fixed and expressed over and over, particularly critical, self-blaming, or self-accusing thoughts about personal failure and guilt.

Based on cognitive theory, an assessment of the client's type of thinking is essential. The depressed client's thought processes may be distorted, and misinterpretation of reality is evident at times. The presence of delusions or hallucinations in a depressed client is important to assess (see Chapter 17).

Social dimension Assessment of hope includes observing the individual's interactions with others and his involvement in life experiences. Persons with hope are gregarious and actively involved with others. For some, approaching others who have had a similar loss may indicate hope within the individual. For example, a woman who has had a mastectomy may want to talk to others who have had mastectomies, or parents who have lost children to sudden infant death syndrome may spend time with other parents who have lost children under similar circumstances. The nurse observes whether the client reaches out to initiate interactions and notes the amount of touching, holding, and wanting to be close to another person. What is the depth of the interaction? Is it shallow and superficial, or does the interaction proceed at a deeper level with ideas and feelings being discussed? When interactions are maintained over time, relationships become meaningful, and the individual receives a positiveness from the relationship and a sense of hope that this is a person who can be counted on in times of distress. Hope then is related to the expectation of assistance from others at a time when the person's resources are inadequate or diminished. When ill, a person depends on others and hopes for help from them. Trust generated from meaningful relationships between persons enhances hope. Thus it is vital to identify significant persons in the client's life.

Through the process of socialization, attitudes develop. Nurturing families tend to foster positive, optimistic attitudes toward life. Assessing family attitudes toward life events such as marriage, child rearing, male and female roles, education, work, and the larger society is useful in determining hope in an individual.

The depressed person withdraws from interactions with others and from life experiences, resulting in a self-imposed isolation. The nurse determines the nature and severity of the withdrawal and isolation by observing the client's participation in social interactions and activities. Which persons and activities are resources for interactions and relationships that can be strengthened? Because of increased preoccupation with oneself *(narcissism)*, the client's withdrawal may be self-perpetuating and may increase distancing within the family. Data regarding the client's relations to family members are helpful, since clients feel alienated even though family members take an active interest and are caring.

The nurse determines the degree of dependence and helplessness the client demonstrates. Are basic activities of daily living met? Does the client need assistance with appropriate dress and grooming, hygiene, meal preparation, and personal safety?

The nurse identifies the client's needs for reassurance, support, and acceptance from others. Persons who have not had basic needs met in childhood tend to lack inner strengths and resources for trusting their own abilities and decisions. A thorough history of the client's infancy, childhood, and early school years yields information on how well his needs were or are being met.

Being emotionally needy, the depressed client may be demanding. When needs cannot be met or satisfied, more demands are made, resulting in further rejection by others. The client sees others as unable or unwilling to meet demands and becomes distrustful and passive in relationships. Assessing the kinds of demands will provide information about the client's unmet needs.

Some depressed clients obtain *secondary gains*, such as additional attention, from their symptoms of depression. If they get narcissistic gratification from their illness, clients may exploit the kindness and attentiveness of others, shirk responsibilities, and avoid the demands of interpersonal interactions. The nurse carefully assesses whether the client is receiving secondary gains from the depression.

Assessing cultural background adds important information about the client's roles and functions, according to sociological theory. For example, in some cultures women are expected to be subordinate and passive. Depressive symptoms may occur when individuals are in conflict with the roles and functions assigned them by the culture, for example, when a woman chooses a career that is heavily male-dominated, such as medicine. Identifying conflicts in roles and functions of the client provides valuable information in the assessment of depression.

Spiritual dimension A client with hope has a meaningful philosophy of life and feels a purposeful sense of direction. The individual demonstrates courage to face up to the unexpected, no matter how grievous or disastrous, and feels a sense of challenge that provides the stamina to survive disaster and resist despair. Hope is a sense of the possible. The client believes that if the object of his desire is obtained, life will be changed in some way or be more comfortable, meaningful, or enjoyable. Hope is future oriented. Feelings of satisfaction, security, and serenity emanate from the individual who hopes. Questions such as "How satisfied are you with your life right now?" and "What are your feelings about your life situation?" may determine how meaningful the person's life is at present.

RESEARCH HIGHLIGHT

Assessment of Hope in Psychiatric and Chemically Dependent Patients
• C Holdcraft and C Williamson

PURPOSE
The purpose of this study was to measure hope in psychiatric and chemically dependent inpatients during the initial phase of treatment and at discharge. A second purpose was to add to the validation of the Miller Hope Scale with clinical populations.

SAMPLE
A convenience sample of 192 patients on the mental health and chemical dependency units of a large Midwestern hospital were studied. There were 48 chemical dependency clients and 144 mental health patients.

METHODOLOGY
After consent was obtained, the Miller Hope Scale, a 40-item, 5-point Likert-type response tool based on critical elements of hope, was administered. Patients on the mental health unit were surveyed within the first 3 days after admission. Patients on the chemical dependency unit were surveyed during the transition from the detoxification phase of their treatment. Subjects completed the questionnaire a second time, either on the day before or on the day of their discharge.

From *Applied Nursing Research* 4(3):129, 1991.

FINDINGS
First administration scores were indicative of lower levels of hope, as was expected. Just after detoxification, the chemical dependency group had a mean hope score of 145.31. The mental health group had a mean hope score of 132.49. The difference between the two groups was significant ($P = 0.002$). At the time of discharge, the chemical dependency group had a mean hope score of 165.50. The mental health group had also increased in level of hope to 156.79.

IMPLICATIONS
The study supported the expectation that psychiatric and chemically dependent patients would express lower levels of hope during the initial phase of treatment. The study also provided a known groups comparison that adds to the construct validity of the Miller Hope Scale. Hope is an essential element in providing care for mental health and chemically dependent patients. More research is needed on testing hope inspiring interventions in clinical populations.

▼ TABLE 14-3   Measurement Tools for Hope-Hopelessness

Instrument	Measures
HOPE SCALES	
Gottschalk[40]	Optimism that a favorable outcome is likely to occur
Erikson, Post, Paige[32]	Perceived importance and perceived probability of attaining desired goals
Obayuwana and others[69]	Hope resulting from the outcome of ego strength, perceived family support, religion, education, and economic assets
Miller Hope Scale[65]	Eleven critical elements of hope
Staats[88]	Level of hope
HOPELESSNESS SCALES	
Beck's Depression Inventory[3]	Feelings and behavior demonstrated by the depressed person
Beck's Hopelessness Scale[5]	Hopelessness
Seasonal Pattern Assessment Questionnaire[91]	Seasonal changes in mood and behavior
Zung's Self-Rated Depression Scale[95]	The level and pervasiveness of depression

A person who hopes, perseveres. Perseverance is the ability to keep on working toward solutions that will ease distress or change one's condition. Perseverance enables one to confront a difficult situation over a long period without losing courage or giving up. To persevere requires strength of will. Related to perseverance is courage, the ability to persist toward a goal even though there is no certainty the goal will be reached.

Assessing the client's religious beliefs and values is essential. Participation in usual religious activities may strengthen hope in some clients. Questions such as "Who comforts you?" or "What is it that sustains you, when all else fails?" will elicit information about the individual's spiritual beliefs.

A person with hope receives strength from a relationship with God, a supreme being, other people, or nature. Assessing these relationships provides data for determining the client's strengths and resources. A person with hope is in the process of becoming a fully functioning human being. One sees in this person a blending of inner peace as a result of his sense of purpose and a conscious recognition of his ability to live life fully. Observation and sensitive listening reveal the client's sense of hope in difficult life situations.

Measurement tools

Numerous tools exist to measure hope and hopelessness. The accompanying research highlight shows the use of the Miller Hope scale in psychiatric and chemically dependent clients. Table 14-3 summarizes the more common ones.

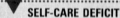
SELF-ESTEEM DISTURBANCE

DEFINITION

Negative self-evaluation or feelings about self or self-capabilities, which may be directly or indirectly expressed.

DEFINING CHARACTERISTICS

- **Physical dimension**

  Hesitant to try new things or situations

- **Emotional dimension**

  Feelings of inferiority

- **Intellectual dimension**

  Self-negating verbalization
  Expressions of shame or guilt
  Evaluates self as unable to deal with events
  Rationalizes away or rejects positive feedback and exaggerates negative feedback about self
  Denial of problems obvious to others
  Projection of blame and responsibility for problem
  Rationalizes personal failures
  Hypersensitive to criticism
  Grandiosity

Modified from Kim M, McFarland G, McLane A: *Pocket guide to nursing diagnoses*, ed 5, St Louis, 1993, Mosby—Year Book.

Analysis
Nursing diagnosis

The following list provides examples of NANDA-accepted nursing diagnoses with causative statements.

1. Self-esteem disturbance: feelings of worthlessness related to hopelessness
2. High risk for violence directed toward self related to hopelessness
3. Self-care deficit: neglect of personal grooming related to being depressed
4. Hopelessness related to multiple losses
5. Decisional conflict: unable to make decisions related to impaired judgment associated with being depressed

The defining characteristics of the nursing diagnoses: self-esteem disturbance, self-care deficit, and hopelessness are listed in the accompanying boxes. Case examples for self-care deficit and hopelessness may be found on the following page.

▼ Case Example: Self-Esteem Disturbance

Nancy, who is 46 years old, has been depressed since her youngest child left for college 2 months ago. She has little to do at home now that all her children are away. Her husband works long hours at his business and is inattentive to her when he is home. Her children have been an important part of her life for the past 20 years. She feels unimportant and unneeded now as she perceives that her homemaking skills are no longer useful and that her childrearing responsibilities are over. She lacks confidence in herself and her ability to participate in community activities. She sees herself as having no job skills, and her husband is not supportive of her working outside the home.

SELF-CARE DEFICIT

DEFINITION

The state in which an individual experiences an impaired ability to perform or complete dressing and grooming activities for oneself.

DEFINING CHARACTERISTICS

- **Physical dimension**

  Impaired ability to put on or take off necessary items of clothing
  Impaired ability to obtain or replace articles of clothing
  Impaired ability to fasten clothing
  Inability to maintain appearance at satisfactory level

Modified from Kim M, McFarland G, McLane A: *Pocket guide to nursing diagnoses*, ed 5, St Louis, 1993, Mosby—Year Book.

HOPELESSNESS

DEFINITION

A sustained emotional state in which an individual sees limited or no alternatives or personal choices available to solve problems or achieve what is desirable and is unable to mobilize energy on his own behalf to establish goals.

DEFINING CHARACTERISTICS

- **Physical dimension**

  Profound apathy
  Closing eyes
  Turning away from speaker
  Decreased appetite
  Decreased/increased sleep
  Shrugging in response to speaker
  Decreased response to stimuli

- **Emotional dimension**

  Helpless
  Decreased affect

- **Intellectual dimension**

  Decreased verbalizations
  Despondent verbalizations (sighing)
  Decreased problem-solving and decision-making capabilities

- **Social dimension**

  Passivity
  Lack of initiative
  Lack of involvement in care
  Social withdrawal

Modified from Kim M, McFarland G, McLane A: *Pocket guide to nursing diagnoses*, ed 5, St Louis, 1993, Mosby—Year Book.

▼ Case Example: Self-Care Deficit

Ted, 64 years old, recently lost his wife after a brief illness. They had been married 42 years and had no children. He was quite dependent on her for care and for his day-to-day activities since his retirement 2 years ago, even though he was in good physical health. After her death he became despondent, had no appetite, was extremely fatigued, and had difficulty sleeping. He stopped shaving, forgot to change his clothes, and made no attempts to clean his home or care for his yard and garden, which had been a source of great pleasure to him before her death.

▼ Case Example: Hopelessness

Chris, who is 26 years old, lost his wife of 7 months in an automobile accident. He has been despondent since her death and unable to be consoled by friends or parents. He neglects his personal care and becomes less and less involved in his usual activities. He thinks life no longer has any meaning for him, and he feels hopeless about it ever improving.

Planning

Assessment of the depressed client frequently results in goals that are related to the following client needs:
1. Physical health and safety
2. Expression of anger and other painful feelings
3. Positive thinking
4. Meaningful, satisfying social relationships
5. Pleasurable experience

The nursing care plan (Table 14-5) lists examples of long-term and short-term goals, outcome criteria, interventions, and rationales related to depression. These serve as examples of the planning stage in the nursing process.

Implementation

Physical dimension A healthy life-style that provides for sound nutrition, adequate sleep, exercise and activity, satisfactory sexual relations, and appropriate management of stress contributes to a sense of well-being and a *joie de vivre*, all essential components in hope. Diet and health counseling by the nurse may contribute to the client's sense of well-being, but generally the client assumes responsibility for maintaining a healthy life-style when hope and optimism are present. Genetic counseling for couples considering whether to have children may be indicated when there is a family history of depression.

Helping the depressed client with activities of daily living is essential because the client has little energy or interest in caring for himself. Although interest in appearance and hygiene is negligible during depression, feelings of esteem and worth are related to appearance and cleanliness. Encouraging a neat, clean appearance seems to enhance recovery.

The nurse sees that attractive meals with small portions are served to help stimulate the client's appetite. For the hospitalized client, between-meal feedings provide additional nourishment and indicate a caring attitude when served unhurriedly with time taken to sit with the client. Having relatives bring favorite foods from home may increase the pleasure of eating.

Research is being conducted to relate diet to depression. Studies show that some vitamin deficiencies are produced by certain long-term medication therapy. For example, isoniazid and cycloserine, used to treat tuberculosis, can bring on a pyridoxine deficiency and produce symptoms of euphoria or depression. Women taking oral contraceptives that contain estrogen sometimes exhibit low levels of vitamin B_6, and supplements of B_6 relieve the symptoms of depression. A balanced diet is the best treatment to prevent vitamin deficiencies.

Physical symptoms need to be relieved promptly. Providing laxatives for constipation and medications to relieve headache assures the client that the nurse cares and promotes physical comfort. Because of the client's body preoccupation, the nurse does not become overly concerned with the complaints. The nurse evaluates the validity of the complaint, relieves it when possible, and does not focus on it.

Disturbances in sleep patterns are treated with comfort measures such as warm baths, quiet music, back rubs, or a glass of warm milk. A few minutes with a concerned and attentive person at bedtime to talk over the events of the day, with a focus on pleasant happenings, may promote sleep.

When the client is agitated, the nurse needs to initiate regularly scheduled contacts to demonstrate acceptance of the client as a person. Providing distraction and channeling the agitated behavior through activities or constructive tasks such as housekeeping or physical exercise is helpful.

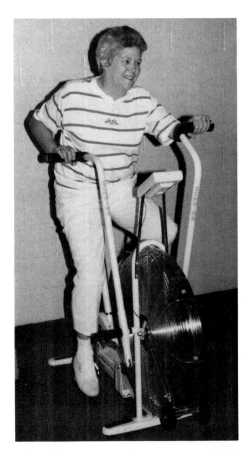

FIGURE 14-1 This woman is enjoying her exercise. An exercycle is an excellent way to increase muscle tone and cardiovascular activity and to relieve depression.

FLUOXETINE

(floo-ox'e-teen)
Prozac
Func. class.: Bicyclic antidepressant

Action: Inhibits CNS neuron uptake of serotonin, but not of norepinephrine

Uses: Major depressive disorder

Dosage and routes:

▶ *Adult:* PO 20 mg qd in AM; after 4 wk if no clinical improvement is noted, dose may be increased to 20 mg bid in AM, afternoon, not to exceed 80 mg/day

Available forms include: Pulvules 20 mg

Side effects/adverse reactions:

CNS: Headache, nervousness, insomnia, drowsiness, anxiety, tremor, dizziness, fatigue, sedation, poor concentration, abnormal dreams, agitation, **convulsions,** *apathy, euphoria, hallucinations, delusions, psychosis*

GI: Nausea, diarrhea, dry mouth, anorexia, dyspepsia, constipation, cramps, vomiting, taste changes, flatulence, decreased appetite

INTEG: Sweating, rash, pruritus, acne, alopecia, urticaria

RESP: Infection, pharyngitis, nasal congestion, sinus headache, sinusitis, cough, dyspnea, bronchitis, asthma, hyperventilation, pneumonia

CV: Hot flashes, palpitations, angina pectoris, **hemorrhage,** hypertension, tachycardia, first-degree AV block, bradycardia, *MI,* thrombophlebitis

MS: Pain, arthritis, twitching

GU: Dysmenorrhea, decreased libido, urinary frequency, urinary tract infection, amenorrhea, cystitis, impotence

EENT: Visual changes, ear/eye pain, photophobia, tinnitus

SYST: Asthenia, viral infection, fever, allergy, chills

Contraindications: Hypersensitivity

Precautions: Pregnancy (B), lactation, children, elderly

Pharmacokinetics:

PO: Peak 6-8 hr; metabolized in liver, excreted in urine; half-life 2-7 days

Interactions/incompatibilities:

—Do not use with MAOIs
—Increased agitation: L-Tryptophan
—Increased side effects: highly protein bound drugs (i.e., fluoxetine)
—Increased half-life of: diazepam

NURSING CONSIDERATIONS

Assess:

—Mental status: mood, sensorium, affect, suicidal tendencies, increase in psychiatric symptoms, depression, panic

—B/P (lying/standing), pulse q4h; if systolic B/P drops 20 mm Hg, hold drug, notify physician; take vital signs q4h in clients with cardiovascular disease

—Blood studies: CBC, leukocytes, differential, cardiac enzymes if client is receiving long-term therapy

—Hepatic studies: AST, ALT, bilirubin, creatinine

—Weight qwk, appetite may decrease with drug

—ECG for flattening of T wave, bundle branch, AV block, dysrhythmias in cardiac clients

Administer:

—Increased fluids, bulk in diet if constipation, urinary retention occur

—With food or milk for GI symptoms

—Crushed if client is unable to swallow medication whole

—Dosage hs if over-sedation occurs during the day; may take entire dose hs; elderly may not tolerate once/day dosing

—Gum, hard candy, frequent sips of water for dry mouth

Perform/provide:

—Storage at room temperature, do not freeze

—Assistance with ambulation during therapy since drowsiness, dizziness occur

—Safety measures including side rails, primarily in elderly

—Checking to see PO medication swallowed

Evaluate:

—EPS primarily in elderly, rigidity, dystonia, akathisia

—Urinary retention, constipation

—Withdrawal symptoms: headache, nausea, vomiting, muscle pain, weakness; do not usually occur unless drug was discontinued abruptly

—Alcohol consumption; if alcohol is consumed, hold dose until morning

Teach client/family:

—That therapeutic effect may take 2-3 wk

—Use caution in driving or other activities requiring alertness because of drowsiness, dizziness, or blurred vision

—Not to discontinue medication quickly after long-term use, may cause nausea, headache, malaise

—To avoid alcohol ingestion or other CNS depressants

—To notify physician if pregnant or plan to become pregnant or breast feed

Lab test interferences:

Increase: Serum bilirubin, blood glucose, alk phosphatase

Decrease: VMA, 5-HIAA

False increase: Urinary catecholamines

Italic indicates common side effects.

Bold italic indicates life-threatening reactions.

Modified from Skidmore-Roth L: *Mosby's nursing drug reference,* St Louis, 1993, Mosby–Year Book.

Challenging activities at which the client is proficient promote the constructive expression of aggressive behavior. As a last resort, applying external controls such as medications, seclusion, or restraints may be necessary.

Exercise is vital in the treatment of depression. Research shows that depressed persons become more responsive if they exercise every day[70] (Figure 14-1). Although the client may have no desire, it is important to strongly encourage him to participate in some form of exercise daily. Exercise heightens a sense of well-being by increasing the production of body endorphins. Developing an exercise program is effective in treating depression because it represents an achievement and success for many people. Running or swimming improves one's physical health and appearance, consequently increasing self-acceptance. In addition, depressive thoughts are difficult to maintain during exercise. If the individual is not inclined to physical sports, some other strenuous activity, such as washing the car or kitchen floor or raking leaves, has similar benefits.

A change in the environment may reduce stress and tension, particularly when the individual is unable to perform activities of daily living. A leave of absence from work or school and the milieu therapy offered in hospitalization are often indicated during the acute phase of depression. The structured daily activity program provided in the hospital leaves the depressed client with little time to brood over problems. It also prevents the client from sleeping during the day, thus promoting sleeping at night.

Touch has therapeutic value. A handshake or touch on the shoulder establishes contact and promotes a sense of worth and acceptance.

Medications also are frequently used for depressed clients (Table 14-4; see also Chapter 24). The accompanying profiles for fluoxetine (Prozac) (above) and isocarboxazid (Marplan) (p. 269) describe nursing care appropriate to their administration.

Electroconvulsive therapy (ECT)

Electroconvulsive therapy (ECT) is found to help some depressed clients. Symptom reduction from antidepressant

▼ **TABLE 14-4**   **Antidepressant Medications**

Generic Name	Trade Name	Daily Dose Range (mg)
TRICYCLICS		
Amitriptyline	Elavil	75-300
Amoxapine	Asendin	75-300
Desipramine	Norpramin	75-200
Doxepin	Sinequan	75-300
Imipramine	Tofranil	75-300
Nortriptyline	Aventyl, Pamelor	20-100
Protriptyline	Vivactil	15-60
Fluoxetine	Prozac	20-80
Maprotiline	Ludiomil	75-300
Trazodone	Desyrel	75-600
MAO INHIBITORS		
Isocarboxazid	Marplan	20-30
Phenelzine	Nardil	45-90
Tranylcypromine	Parnate	20-30

medications generally requires 2 to 4 weeks. Responses to ECT are often effective in a short period of time. For these reasons, ECT may be the treatment of choice, particularly when the risk of suicide is high.

ECT involves the passage of an electrical stimulus of 70 to 150 volts to the brain for 0.1 to 1 second to produce a seizure. The voltage and the length of application vary with each client. The least amount of electrical current necessary to produce a seizure is used. Individual seizure thresholds vary and are generally higher in women and older people.

The client must experience a seizure for symptoms to improve. The seizure is thought to result from change in the postsynaptic response to the neurotransmitters in the central nervous system (CNS). Because ECT stimulates synaptic remodeling, the number of vesicles that contain synaptic protein increases. This results in increased neurotransmitters, which are associated with relief of depressive symptoms.

The client receives atropine sulfate before the procedure to decrease oropharyngeal secretions. At the beginning of the treatment, sodium pentothal or methohexital sodium (Brevital) is given intravenously as a sedative. Electrode jelly is applied to both temples or to just the nondominant hemisphere, and padded electrodes are applied. An airway or soft mouth gag is put in the client's mouth. Succinylcholine chloride (Anectine) is given as a muscle relaxant.

The use of a muscle relaxant permits CNS features of a seizure while keeping muscle spasms minimal. The resulting grand mal seizure closely resembles one having a spontaneous origin, with a *tonic* phase (tightening of muscles) for approximately 10 seconds and a *clonic* phase (rhythmic movement of muscles) for 30 seconds. The movements are slight and often limited to plantar flexion of the feet, followed by rhythmic twitching of the toes and clenching of the jaw. The client's EEG is monitored during the procedure.

The seizure is accompanied by a short period of *apnea* and then snoringlike respiration. Because the muscle re-

laxant paralyzes the respiratory muscles, an anesthetist is present to administer oxygen to the client and assist respiration by mechanical means if necessary. Usually the client sleeps for 5 to 10 minutes after the seizure, slowly awakens, and does not remember the treatment.

The number of treatments varies according to the severity of the disorder and therapeutic response. Response varies widely, and sometimes only three to five treatments are needed. A risk of manic reaction or short-term confusion exists if a client is treated excessively.[36] Clients benefiting most from ECT generally show mild improvement after the first several treatments.

Treatments are usually given two or three times a week, with 48-hour intervals most desirable. Clients over 65 years of age given ECT more than twice a week are confused significantly longer after the treatment.[37]

Indications   Clinical indications for ECT are major mood disorders with pronounced physical deterioration and risk of suicide, severe mania uncontrolled by neuroleptics or lithium, and some forms of schizophrenia (such as acute, catatonic, and paranoid) that have not responded to medication. Clients most likely to receive therapeutic benefits from ECT are those who have a history of depressive episodes.

ECT is preferred to antidepressant therapy in some cases, such as for pregnant clients, in whom antidepressants place the fetus at risk for congenital defects. ECT does not help neurotic clients and those with a personality disorder or grief reactions.

Contraindications   ECT is not recommended for clients with histories of cardiovascular disease, because elevated hormone levels contribute to transient hypertension and tachycardia that may increase the risk of stroke or coronary thrombosis. It is contraindicated for clients with a brain tumor. Clients must have a complete system review and physical examination before treatment.

Complications   The most common side effects include headache, nausea, and muscle aches. Life-threatening complications of ECT are rare.[48] Back pain occasionally results and may persist for a few days or weeks. Fractures sometimes occur in elderly clients with osteoporosis. The aged with a history of coronary disease also may develop cardiac dysrhythmia, which is reversible. The potential for self-neglect and suicide of the depressed elderly client is far more hazardous than the possible side effects.

Memory loss during ECT treatment, both short and long term, is commonplace. Memory loss reaches its peak approximately halfway through a full course of treatments (12 to 15) and then gradually subsides over the next several months. Some studies have demonstrated no long-term ill effects of ECT on cognitive functioning, while others have demonstrated more potentially lasting effects on memory. The consensus of neuropsychological literature suggests that the majority of studies examining long-term residual effects of ECT on memory have demonstrated no lasting effects.

Nursing Roles   ECT treatments can be administered in a hospital, clinic, or physician's office. Nursing responsibilities, which are similar to those preceding a surgical procedure, are found in the box on p. 270.

The following case example describes a client and her response to ECT.

ISOCARBOXAZID

(eye-soe-kar-box'a-zid)
Marplan
Func. class.:
Antidepressant—MAOI
Chem. class.: Hydrazine

Action: Increases concentrations of endogenous epinephrine, norepinephrine, serotonin, dopamine in storage sites in CNS by inhibition of MAO; increased concentration reduces depression
Uses: Depression, when uncontrolled by other means
Dosage and routes:
▶ *Adult:* PO 30 mg/day in divided doses, reduce dose to lowest effective dose when condition improves
Available forms include: Tabs 10 mg
Side effects/adverse reactions:
HEMA: Anemia
CNS: Dizziness, drowsiness, confusion, headache, anxiety, tremors, stimulation, weakness, hyperreflexia, mania, insomnia, fatigue, weight gain
GI: Constipation, dry mouth, nausea, vomiting, *anorexia,* diarrhea, weight gain
GU: Change in libido, frequency
INTEG: Rash, flushing, increased perspiration, jaundice

CV: Orthostatic hypotension, hypertension, dysrhythmias, hypertensive crisis
EENT: Blurred vision
ENDO: SIADH-like syndrome
Contraindications: Hypersensitivity to MAOIs, elderly, hypertension, CHF, severe hepatic disease, pheochromocytoma, severe renal disease, severe cardiac disease
Precautions: Suicidal clients convulsive disorders, severe depression, schizophrenia, hyperactivity, diabetes mellitus, pregnancy (C)
Pharmacokinetics:
PO: Duration up to 2 wk; metabolized by liver, excreted by kidneys
Interactions/incompatibilities:
—Increased pressor effects: guanethidine, clonidine, indirect acting sympathomimetics (ephedrine)
—Increased effects of: direct acting sympathomimetics (epinephrine), alcohol, barbiturates, benzodiazepines, CNS depressants, levodopa
—Hyperpyretic crisis, convulsions, hypertensive episode: tricyclic antidepressants, meperidine
—Hypoglycemic effect: increased insulin

NURSING CONSIDERATIONS
Assess:
—B/P (lying, standing); pulse; if systolic B/P drops 20 mm Hg hold drug, notify physician
—Blood studies: CBC, leukocytes, cardiac enzymes if client is receiving long-term therapy
—Hepatic studies: ALT, AST, bilirubin, creatinine, hepatotoxicity may occur
Administer:
—Increased fluids, bulk in diet if constipation, urinary retention occur
—With food or milk for GI symptoms
—Crushed if client is unable to swallow medication whole
—Dosage hs if over-sedation occurs during day
—Gum, hard candy, or frequent sips of water for dry mouth
—Phentolamine for severe hypertension
Perform/provide
—Storage in tight container in cool environment
—Assistance with ambulation during beginning therapy since drowsiness/dizziness occurs
—Safety measures including side-rails
—Checking to see PO medication swallowed

Evaluate:
—Toxicity: increased headache, palpitation; discontinue drug immediately; prodromal signs of hypertensive crisis
—Mental status: mood, sensorium, affect, memory (long, short), increase in psychiatric symptoms
—Urinary retention, constipation, edema, take weight weekly
—Withdrawal symptoms: headache, nausea, vomiting, muscle pain, weakness
Teach client/family
—That therapeutic effects may take 1-4 wk
—To avoid driving or other activities requiring alertness
—To avoid alcohol ingestion, CNS depressants or OTC medications: cold, weight, hay fever, cough syrup
—Not to discontinue medication quickly after long-term use
—To avoid high tyramine foods: cheese (aged), sour cream, beer, wine, pickled products, liver, raisins, bananas, figs, avocados, meat tenderizers, chocolate, yogurt; increase caffeine
—Report headache, palpitation, neck stiffness
Treatment of overdose: Lavage, activated charcoal, monitor electrolytes, vital signs, diazepam IV, NaHCO₃

Italic indicates common side effects.
Bold italic indicates life-threatening reactions.

Modified from Skidmore-Roth L: *Mosby's nursing drug reference,* St Louis, 1993, Mosby–Year Book.

▼ Case Example

A 73-year-old widow with severe recurrent affective illness since age 38 was admitted. The reason was a progressive 3-month deterioration demonstrated by social withdrawal, poor hygiene, agitation, feelings of hopelessness, extreme fatigue, sleeplessness, poor concentration and memory, and anorexia. The diagnosis was a major mood disorder with delusional features. She was unresponsive to tricyclic antidepressants, lithium, and monoamine oxidase inhibitors; ECT was indicated. She was informed and signed the consent form. The procedure and its common side effects were explained, and she was encouraged to ask questions and express her fears and feelings. The client's daughter was included in the discussion for her information and emotional support. After five treatments in 12 days the client's depressive symptoms improved markedly. After ten treatments her depressive symptoms disappeared, and she returned to her usual level of functioning.

Ethical and Legal Considerations The use of ECT has provoked criticisms about informed consent and the determination of competence (see Chapter 42). The American Psychiatric Association (APA) task force addressed these issues and recommended that the consent form include the following:

1. Information on the nature and seriousness of the disorder
2. Probable course without ECT
3. Description of the procedure
4. Risks and side effects
5. Possibility of alternative treatments
6. Reason why ECT is recommended
7. Statement of the individual's or guardian's right to refuse or revoke consent
8. Statement that a new consent form will be obtained for additional treatment series

The task force also suggested documentation in the clinical record specifying that the information was given to the client and that the consent giver is competent, able to understand the information, and able to act responsibly. It also stated that a competent client who refuses ECT cannot be forced to receive it. It suggested that when competence is in question, the client be evaluated by a group including the client's attorney and psychiatrist. A treatment committee of one or preferably two psychiatrists, a neurologist, an internist, and an attorney can also review the case if any

▼ **NURSING RESPONSIBILITIES WITH ELECTROCONVULSIVE THERAPY**

Before Treatment

1. Check the record for recent physical examination and routine laboratory work (blood count, blood chemistries, and urinalysis). Results of pre-ECT evaluations of memory capability are helpful.
2. Check for a signed consent form. It is best to have a relative read the informed consent also. If the client's ability to understand the information is questionable, additional medical and legal opinions may be needed.
3. Involve the family as much as possible to inform them and relieve their fears.
4. Communicate positive feelings about the procedure to the family and client.
5. Discourage cigarette smoking just before the procedure, since smoking makes pulmonary secretions more difficult to manage during treatment.
6. Omit liquids 6 hours and solids 8 hours before treatment.
7. Remove dentures, glasses, and jewelry (rings may be taped) and dress the client in loose clothing.
8. Have the client evacuate bladder and bowels.
9. Monitor vital signs before, during, and after treatment.
10. Give atropine as ordered before treatment. It may also be given intravenously just before the treatment.
11. Make sure that oxygen, suction, and endotracheal intubation are accessible and functional in case of a cardiorespiratory emergency.
12. Display a warm, supportive attitude to reduce apprehension. Clients receiving ECT are somewhat anxious (especially about the first treatment). Although the procedure is painless, some feel a sense of dread. The idea of shock and subsequent seizure can be frightening.

During Treatment

1. Maintain the airway and remove pharyngeal secretions with suction as necessary.
2. Observe the client continuously until he is fully recovered. He is allowed up when awake, alert, and able to ambulate.
3. Give the client a mild sedative for restlessness, if prescribed.

After Treatment

1. Touch the client as he awakens to demonstrate care, establish your presence, and allay fear.
2. Orient the client to time, place, and events as he awakens.
3. Give medications for minor discomforts, such as headache or nausea.
4. Provide opportunities for the client to express his feelings about the treatment.
5. Promote normal activity after the treatment to discourage incapacity.
6. Document client responses during and after treatment.

---

of the initial evaluators find the client to be incompetent. The treatment committee interviews each client and determines competence.

Emotional dimension Promoting healthy feelings contributes to a person's sense of hope. The nurse encourages the client to share both positive and negative feelings in a healthy manner. The following statement is a healthy expression of a positive feeling: "I feel good knowing my daughter wants me to stay with her after I leave the hospital." The healthy expression of a negative feeling is demonstrated in the following example: "I resent it that my kids don't want me involved in their lives." Expressing feelings about disappointments, losses, and death can help the client accept a situation that cannot be changed.

Interventions for depressed clients include helping them unburden themselves of feelings associated with a loss (see Research Highlight). Some of the feelings are anger, anxiety, guilt, loneliness, worthlessness, uselessness, powerlessness, and despair (see Chapters 10 to 12 and 21). According to psychoanalytical theory, expressing these feelings helps a client to develop an awareness and understanding of his predominant feeling. The nurse facilitates the expression of feelings with statements that communicate empathy and understanding, such as "You're feeling angry," "You're anxious," "You think maybe you are a burden to your family," or "You wish you could be more useful at your son's house." Willingness to listen, nonjudgmental acceptance, and support are essential. Once the feeling has been identified and acknowledged, other ways of coping with the situation can be explored. While the client cannot change the situation, he can be helped to change his feelings about it.

Severely depressed clients often feel powerless. Having clients make decisions about their treatment procedures, food choices, self-care, schedules, and activities helps restore feelings of power and significance.

Intellectual dimension Interventions that promote hope include providing the individual with information about depression, its incidence, causes, signs and symptoms, and prevention. Knowledge about depression gives the individual power to make choices, to think positively about himself, to be able to assume responsibility for himself among available options, and to maintain a sense of hope and optimism.

For the depressed client, interventions include allowing time for the client to respond. The psychomotor retardation and verbal inactivity require the rate of conversation to slow down to give the client time to think and respond.

The nurse can help depressed clients distinguish between thoughts and feelings, thus permitting them to analyze their perceptions of an experience and make the perceptions more tolerable. A feeling can be explained to the client as an emotion, such as sadness or anger; thoughts are explained by the use of such phrases as "I see no way out" or "There is no hope." Once the distinctions are established, the client can proceed to the next step, which is identifying the facts leading to a conclusion. Usually the only facts are the client's severely painful emotions. Emotions as such, however, are not facts. Painful feelings are real and the pain is acknowledged, but the pain is not a sufficient cause for concluding that all is hopeless. Although the feelings are indeed painful, the conclusion is not logical. By leading the client through these steps, a way of recognizing the nature of the pain, tolerating the pain, and avoiding illogical or irrational conclusions is possible.

Cognitive theory directs interventions for negative thinking. The negative thinking of depressed clients, which includes self-doubt, self-pity, resentment, worrying, self-criticism, and self-accusations, can be made more positive by having the client focus on personal strengths and assets. The nurse can ask clients to list positive attributes about

RESEARCH HIGHLIGHT

Preventative Intervention Following Accidental Death of a Child
- SA Murphy

PURPOSE

The purpose of this study was to describe the rationale, development, and pilot testing of a preventative intervention program for bereaved parents whose adolescent and young adult children died as a result of an accident.

SAMPLE

The sample consisted of bereaved parents; 5 were 2 to 6 months past the death of their child; 10 were 7 to 13 months past the death of their child; and 19 were for the nonintervention comparison group.

METHODOLOGY

Six sessions providing informational and emotional support were conducted by a professional nurse clinician. In addition, eight written tests were administered, including The Grief Experience Inventory (GEI), The Rosenberg Self-Esteem Scale (RSE), The Parent Bereavement Scale (PBS), The Marital and Parent Role Strain Scale, The Life Event Questionnaire, The Symptom Check List, and The Perceived Support Network Inventory.

Based on data from *Image: Journal of Nursing Scholarship* 22(5):174, 1990.

FINDINGS

Parents in the 2- to 6-month group rated both informational and emotional support as useful. Parents in the 7- to 13-month group rated emotional support consistently more useful. Timing and type of support were both considered important intervention factors.

IMPLICATIONS

This study attempts to respond to the supportive needs of persons who are victimized by loss. The intervention principles incorporated in this research could be part of any community intervention program. Identifying a specific need, designing treatment protocols for high-risk groups, training group leaders, conducting the intervention according to protocols, and evaluating results systematically are essential components of any support program.

---

themselves to enhance positive thinking. Negative thinking can be controlled by the client's consciously stating, "I am going to stop thinking about that now." Another technique involves wearing a rubber band around one's wrist. As soon as the client is aware of a negative thought, he snaps the rubber band. Doing this consistently promotes awareness of the negative thought. Studies show that an act that is brought into awareness consistently will show a reduction in frequency.

For clients who worry excessively, setting aside a precise time for mulling over negative thoughts helps. The client decides the best time to devote to this negative thinking. The client may say, for example, "My worrying time will start at 11:00 and last 20 minutes." Clients are not avoiding worrying—they are deciding how long to worry. It is agreed that the client will not worry at other times.

Visualization and *guided imagery* are other interventions that help when the client is preoccupied with negative thoughts. Clients are helped to focus on happier times or peak experiences or to imagine they are in a place they love, such as the beach, the mountains, or wherever they feel fully alive, comfortable, and healthy. They are asked to imagine the area is filled with bright, clear light and to let the light flow into their bodies, making them brighter and filling them with the energy of health. Or they can visualize using a heavy black marker to draw a circle around their negative thoughts so that these thoughts are contained. Visualization and imagery are both healing and liberating, and they help the person let go of negative thinking.

The ability to make decisions is difficult for depressed clients. The nurse can limit the clients' choices to simple ones, such as what suit or dress to wear. The nurse makes decisions for the client in more complex situations. If the problem of choosing between the plaid dress and the green dress is too difficult, the nurse simply hands the client a dress to prevent her from being overwhelmed by the decision.

The depressed client's judgment may be impaired. Being subject to extreme pessimism, a client may be convinced of the need to liquidate a business or quit a job. The nurse may encourage the family to assume responsibility for business affairs while the client is recovering from depression. Clients also need protection, since many are accident prone because of their decreased concentration and poor judgment.

When delusions or hallucinations are present, the nurse helps orient the client to reality (see Chapter 17). Because depressed clients often tend to be perfectionistic, rigid, and compulsive, the nurse helps them accept flaws in themselves and others without persecuting and blaming.

Social dimension Nursing behaviors that foster meaningful relationships and promote independence are essential. Involving family members or friends and neighbors in the client's care enlarges the client's social network. Support persons are important in maintaining an attitude of hopefulness.

Hope is fostered when the nurse helps the client successfully adapt or adjust to changes. The client comes to trust the nurse, and the feelings of trust and safety enhance hope and optimism.

A healthy environment free from pollution, excessive noise, overcrowding, and undue violence also assists in maintaining a sense of hope. Encouraging personality traits such as assertiveness, love of adventure, and risk-taking promotes hope and optimism.

Promoting active involvement in life activates a sense of hope for the future. For example, a person who campaigns for conservation of natural resources demonstrates hope that his or her efforts are not futile. Generally, people who demonstrate hope and optimism assume responsibility for creating situations that foster such attitudes.

Interventions for depressed persons include preventing them from being alone. The nurse needs to seek out the client, since depressed people tend to withdraw from others. An initial approach that does not pressure the client to talk is an important step in building trust. Short, frequent interactions exemplify a caring attitude and produce less anxiety than do longer interactions. A one-to-one relationship provides security, trust, and support until the client's own support system is reestablished. Activities that allow the client to interact with others, such as cards, puzzles, crafts, or small group projects, prevent further preoccupation with self and provide positive reinforcement for appropriate behavior, according to behavioral theory. Group therapy provides interactions with others and promotes a sense of belonging as well as allowing time to solve problems. Encouraging family members to stay in contact with the client is essential. Frequently, depressed persons view the family as hostile and uncaring. when actually the family is caring and concerned about the client but is at a loss as to what to do.

Working with the family to rebuild broken relationships can be rewarding for the nurse. When the nurse can help families enjoy life more fully and without guilt about the depressed member, satisfaction is achieved by the nurse, the client, and the family.

Encouraging interdependence, whereby the client reaches out to others to give or receive help, is therapeutic for the depressed person. For example, pushing another client confined to a wheelchair to meals each day may increase the depressed client's sense of independence and feelings of being needed and important. Assertiveness training provides the dependent client with the skills to become independent. Learning how to ask for what one wants, to take risks, and to gain confidence in oneself are skills that the depressed person can learn in an assertiveness course (see Chapter 16).

Because despair over loss and death is expressed differently in various cultures, the nurse needs to be knowledgeable about the client's cultural background. She can refer the client to a more knowledgeable person when she lacks the resources to deal with cultural responses to losses, separations, and death.

Occupational therapy, activity therapy, and music therapy are effective treatments for the depressed client. Activities that clients find pleasurable, as well as those that foster interactions with others, are beneficial. The nurse strongly encourages depressed clients to participate in these activities. In addition, involving the client in activities is an important way of increasing self-esteem and fostering responsibility for personal health care. Other interventions that enhance the client's self-esteem and help alleviate depression include exploring the client's feelings about himself, identifying where the feelings may have come from

and whether or not they are realistic, and helping the client choose between continuing to have these miserable feelings or focusing on finding more positive feelings.

Using sociological theory, which suggests that losses in status, roles, and power contribute to a breakdown in self-esteem, the nurse assists clients in identifying sources of pleasure and in planning activities that provide pleasure and success, a vital component for increasing self-esteem. For some depressed persons, working in the kitchen provides pleasure and a sense of worth and competence. For retired office workers, an assignment in the greenhouse may enable them to learn a new skill, thereby increasing their self-esteem. Such diversional activities also prevent brooding and self-centeredness and promote self-confidence.

Spiritual dimension The person with hope and optimism needs minimal support and encouragement from the nurse. Reinforcing inner strengths such as courage and self-worth is a primary intervention within the spiritual dimension. With inner strengths identified and reinforced, individuals are free to strive for maximal potential and creativity. If individuals can be freed from inner conflicts, opportunities for them to grow in hope, to create, and to become more self-actualized persons can result. Clarifying values contributes to a person's feelings of hope by reducing conflicts within that value system. For some individuals, belief in life after death is a vital component in sustaining a sense of hope. Encouraging and providing ways for clients to worship may fulfill the need to demonstrate and practice their beliefs.

Listening attentively to cues may tell the nurse when the depressed client is willing to discuss his hopelessness and his belief that there is no way that his life will get better. He may see death as a relief from despair and unbearable guilt and may consider suicide. The nurse, alert to the possibility of suicide, initiates a one-to-one relationship so that close observation can be maintained. A chaplain, minister, or other religious leader can be helpful for the client who needs assistance in forgiving himself or others.

Through creative opportunities in art, poetry, sculpture, or music, clients can move away from their self-centeredness toward the freedom often experienced in these pursuits. They can learn to value themselves as unique individuals.

▼..
KEY INTERVENTIONS FOR DEPRESSED PERSONS

1. Help with ADL when client is unable to perform them.
2. Ensure adequate nutrition and sleep.
3. Relieve physical complaints.
4. Encourage exercise.
5. Promote expression of sad, angry feelings.
6. Allow time to respond.
7. Emphasize positive thinking.
8. Limit decision making.
9. Promote assertiveness.
10. Prevent client from being alone.
11. Encourage participation in group activities.
12. Increase self-esteem to enhance personal competence and power.
13. Provide information about diagnosis, medications, and treatment of depression.

▼ **TABLE 14-5   NURSING CARE PLAN**

GOALS	OUTCOME CRITERIA	INTERVENTIONS	RATIONALES
NURSING DIAGNOSIS: Hopelessness related to multiple losses			
LONG TERM			
To share suffering with others	Shares suffering with others		
To express positive expectations about the future	Verbalizes positive expectations about the future		
SHORT TERM			
To reminisce and review life positively	Verbalizes positive aspects of life	Allow time to reminisce	To gain insight about losses and place in perspective
To express feelings of optimism about the present	Verbalizes optimistic feelings about present	Assist to identify and express feelings by: Conveying empathy Validating and reflecting impressions Accepting negative feelings, for example, hurt or anger Encouraging verbalization of ways hope is significant in life	To assist client to identify feelings and form a baseline for planning interventions
To express confidence in self and desired outcome	Verbalizes confidence in self and desired outcome	To assess and mobilize external resources (significant others, support groups, God, and higher power): Involve family and significant others in care Convey a caring attitude Provide staff support Support client's belief system	To promote confidence To emphasize importance of supportive relationships
		To assess and mobilize internal resources (autonomy, spirituality, cognitive abilities: Emphasize client's strengths and interests Compliment on appropriate appearance Promote motivation Identify areas of hope Assist to develop short-term goals	To focus on positive aspects of life that promote hope and optimism To restore esteem and confidence in self
		Assist with problem solving and decision making	To help client move away from the impossible and hopeless to deal with what is realistic and hopeful
		Assist to learn new coping skills	To increase ways to deal with problems
		Identify if client is at risk for self-harm	To prevent possible suicide

When depressed clients question the meaning of their suffering and the purposelessness of their lives, the nurse needs to encourage and facilitate further expression of feelings. Once the client's feelings have been identified, the nurse can assist the client in considering other options available, and the client can move beyond the pain of depression with integrity, a greater awareness of self, personal value, and a relatedness to another. The helpless, despairing client may find meaning in or accept suffering when the nurse is available, accepting, and empathetic. This satisfies the need for relatedness so that the client finds the strength to come to terms with life, gain confidence, and live a more enriched life. See the box on p. 272 for key interventions for depressed persons.

See Table 14-5 for a sample nursing care plan.

INTERACTION WITH A DEPRESSED CLIENT

Nurse: Betty, it's time to go to O.T.
Client: I'm not going today.
Nurse: You're not going?
Client: No.
Nurse: You seemed to enjoy working on your cup yesterday.
Client: No, I didn't.
Nurse: It was beginning to look real pretty.
Client: I didn't like it.
Nurse: (Pause.) You may not feel like going to O.T., but I would like for you to go for a short time. It is part of your treatment plan to participate in activities while you are here.
Client: (Silence.)
Nurse: I'll be back in 10 minutes, and we will walk down together. (Ten minutes later the nurse returns.)
Nurse: I'll walk down to O.T. with you now, Betty.
Client: (Silence, gets up and starts walking.) Why do you make me do things I don't want to do? I wish you would leave me alone, all of you.
Nurse: You are irritated because you are going to O.T.?
Client: No, I just don't want to go. It's not helping me. (She keeps on walking.)

Betty is severely depressed. She prefers to stay alone, responding minimally to others and with negativism. Because Betty is depressed, the nurse speaks slowly and allows ample time for Betty to respond to her requests.

The nurse uses restatement to encourage Betty to expand on her reason for not wanting to go to O.T. When this approach fails, she states an observation that she made of Betty in O.T. the previous day. A positive statement such as this helps to elevate Betty's self-esteem.

The nurse follows this statement with another positive one to help Betty alter her negative thinking. Because Betty's thinking is so deeply negative, she screens out any positive statements about herself. The nurse is aware that Betty will probably continue to do this and is supportive and empathic at the same time, letting her know what is expected of her (to go to O.T.). She gives Betty some time to get ready and returns 10 minutes later, as she stated, with the expectation that Betty will go. She accepts Betty's expression of her annoyance with her and the staff for asking her to do what she does not want to do and continues walking with her to O.T.

It will be important for the nurse to provide some positive feedback to Betty on her return from O.T. about her behavior, such as "I know you didn't want to go, but I'm pleased that you did. I think you are trying to help yourself feel better."

MANIC BEHAVIOR
Theoretical Approaches

Table 14-6 summarizes theories of manic behavior.

NURSING PROCESS
Assessment

Physical dimension Manic behavior is the opposite of depressed behavior. Motor activity is increased; the client is hyperactive, restless, and involved in many activities, such as buying sprees, reckless driving, foolish business investments, and sexual behavior unusual for the individual. Dress is flamboyant and colorful. Women may wear excessive and inappropriate jewelry for the situation. Makeup may be excessive and poorly applied. Men may dress in an exaggerated fashion with little or no attention to personal hygiene. Because of disruptions in circadian

▼ **TABLE 14-6** **Summary of Theories of Manic Behavior**

Theory	Dynamics
Genetic	Behavior is transmitted in families in which one or more members have had a manic episode as well as a depressive episode.
Biological	Excesses in biogenic amines, norepinephrine, and serotonin predispose one to periods of elation.
	Chromosomal abnormalities contribute to manic behavior.
	Defects in cell membranes are found in clients with bipolar disorder.
	Disruptions in circadian rhythms, the sleep-wake cycle, and the light-dark cycle are associated with mood changes.
	Psychopharmacological substances such as the anticonvulsants effect neurotransmitter synthesis, resulting in mood changes.
	Mood changes are related to EEG changes, neuroendocrine dysfunctions, and may follow closed head traumas.
Psychoanalytical	Loss, real or imagined, may precipitate a manic episode and defend against depression. Anxiety and tension are denied, resulting in elated and uninhibited behavior.

rhythms, there is a decreased need for sleep. The individual awakens several hours before the usual time, full of energy, and may go for days without sleep and without feeling tired. Appetite is decreased, and the client does not take time from his unceasing activities to eat. Lack of sleep and failure to eat may become life threatening. The client also fails to notice minor ailments or physical complaints and may become susceptible to infection and illness.

An assessment of the family's history of mental illness is essential to determine if a genetic basis for the behavior is present. A thorough physical examination is important for ruling out dysfunctions in the neurological, endocrine, or immune systems.

Emotional dimension During manic episodes, the client's mood is euphoric. He is overly cheerful, excessively enthusiastic, and appears "high." According to psychoanalytical theory, he may exhibit a wide range of mood swings, becoming irritable and angry easily when his desires are thwarted. There is an infectious quality about his mood and an unwarranted optimism, but feeling of inadequacy and inferiority lurk beneath his euphoria.

Intellectual dimension Thought processes in the manic client are accelerated, and he is easily distracted. As a result of responding to various environmental stimuli (noises, movements, pictures, colors, temperature, other people, activities), his speech becomes pressured. He has flight of ideas resulting from his thoughts racing ahead of his speech. Communication may be humorous—full of jokes, puns, plays on words, and amusing irrelevancies. The client may become theatrical, with singing and dramatic mannerisms. Sounds rather than meanings govern word choice (clanging). Thoughts may become grandiose and delusional, with the client thinking he is a well-known entertainer, writer, or political or religious figure. Judgment and insight are impaired, and the client may give away valued possessions or very expensive belongings.

Social dimension Self-esteem is unrealistically inflated during manic episodes. Overconfidence in one's self and one's abilities is exhibited. Increased sociability may result in calling old friends and acquaintances at all hours of the day and night. The intrusive, domineering, demanding, and meddling nature of his interactions is unrecognized by the manic client. He is often involved in excessive planning and participation in multiple activities—sexual, political, religious, and occupational.

Spiritual dimension Clients with recurring episodes of manic behavior may come to value the "highs" in their lives. As a way to avoid the painful realities in their own lives, they may choose not to adhere to their medication regimen to maintain their high. Life may become far more bearable and pleasurable when the individual is elated and euphoric than when he is depressed. It then becomes important to assess the meaning and value of the illness to the client.

Analysis
Nursing diagnosis

The following list provides examples of NANDA-accepted diagnoses that may relate to manic behavior.

1. Self-esteem disturbance related to exaggerated sense of self-importance.
2. Impaired social interactions related to demanding, meddling behavior.
3. Sleep pattern disturbance related to hyperactivity.
4. Altered thought processes related to delusions of grandeur.
5. Noncompliance related to thinking that medications are no longer needed.

The following case example describes characteristics of a client with manic behavior.

▼ Case Example

Sondra, a 39-year old opera singer, is admitted to a psychiatric hospital after keeping her family awake for several nights with prayers and a song marathon. She is flamboyantly dressed in a floor-length red skirt and peasant blouse and is adorned with heavy earrings, numerous necklaces and bracelets, and medals pinned to her bosom. She speaks rapidly and is difficult to interrupt as she talks about her intimate relationship with God. She often breaks into song, explaining that her beautiful singing voice is a special gift that God has given her to compensate for her insanity. She uses it to share the joy she feels with others who are less fortunate.

Planning

Assessment of clients with manic behavior frequently results in goals that are related to the following client needs:

1. Physical health and safety
2. Outlets for tension and energy
3. Expression of painful feelings
4. Expression of realistic presentations
5. Compliance with medication regimen

The nursing care plan (Table 14-8) lists examples of long-term and short-term goals, outcome criteria, interventions, and rationales related to disturbance in self-esteem. These serve as examples of the planning stage of the nursing process.

Implementation

Physical dimension The client who exhibits manic behavior needs external controls until he is able to set limits on his own physical activity. A structured, subdued environment helps to limit the restlessness and hyperactivity. A private room with minimal furnishings and neutral colors is helpful. The nurse selects noncompetitive, solitary activities, such as walking, swimming, gymnastics, raking leaves, writing, finger painting, and jogging, that help the client direct energy appropriately. By providing activities or projects that can be completed in a short time, the nurse gives the client opportunities to experience success, reduce feelings of inadequacy, and develop self-control. It is important to assist the client with his grooming so that clothing is in good repair and appropriate for the season, activity, and time of day. An appropriate appearance helps the client maintain his identity and prevents ridicule from others. The nurse reduces environmental stimuli as much as possible, particularly at bedtime, to promote sleep.

Comfort measures such as warm bath, darkness, and administering prescribed medications prevent fatigue and exhaustion. The nurse must closely supervise the administra-

▼ **TABLE 14-7**   Antimanic Medications

Generic Name	Trade Name	Daily Dose Range (mg)
Carbamazepine	Tegretol	600-1600
Lithium	Eskalith	600-2100

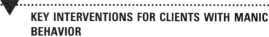

KEY INTERVENTIONS FOR CLIENTS WITH MANIC BEHAVIOR

1. Set limits on inappropriate behavior.
2. Reduce environmental stimuli.
3. Supervise administration of medications.
4. Ensure adequate nutrition and sleep.
5. Help client focus on one topic during conversation.
6. Ignore or distract client from grandiose thinking.
7. Present reality.
8. Have consistent nurse assigned to care for client.
9. Provide information about diagnosis, medications, and treatment.
10. Promote a realistic self-esteem.

tion of medications, because the client may "cheek" it and dispose of it later. Changing to the liquid form of medication may alleviate this problem.

A high-calorie, high-vitamin diet with supplemental feedings and adequate fluids prevents excessive weight loss. Finger foods such as sandwiches, fruits, and milkshakes, which can be eaten when the client is too restless to sit down and eat, ensures healthy nutrition.

Because the client tends to ignore physical ailments, the nurse needs to carefully monitor vital signs, weight, and any signs of injury.

Medications help stabilize the client's emotional state (Table 14-7; see also Chapter 24). The nurse observes the administration of medications carefully to ensure that the client takes them as prescribed. The profile for lithium (p. 277) describes nursing care appropriate to its administration.

Emotional dimension When the client's mood is euphoric and elated, he is pleasant to be with; however, staff and others do not encourage behavior that promotes or accelerates his elation and euphoria. According to psychoanalytical theory, helping the client to express his feelings of inadequacy and inferiority may minimize his constant state of threat and reduce psychomotor activity. The irritability and anger that erupts easily when his desires are not met can best be handled with a kind, firm, and persuasive approach that promotes external controls before the anger escalates and becomes destructive.

Intellectual dimension Listening quietly and attentively provides a sounding board for the verbally active client. It is helpful to attempt to interrupt the constant stream of conversation and encourage him to focus on one topic at a time, to direct his attention to real concerns and limit his flight of ideas. It is also helpful to focus on the idea being expressed rather than attempting to process each word. Laughing at or encouraging jokes, puns, and humorous anecdotes tends to escalate the behavior and has little therapeutic benefit. The nurse may ignore grandiose thinking or distract him by focusing his attention on real activities and events. Short, simple, direct requests and explanations for activities and procedures are more easily heard and may elimiate some of the arguing, belligerence, and impetuousness of the manic client. The nurse promotes opportunities for the client to see himself realistically. Simply stating "You are Gary Johnson," when the client claims to be the well-known singer Michael Jackson, helps reorient the client to reality.

Social dimension Realistic self-esteem is promoted by simple, matter-of-fact reality statements. It is essential to avoid arguing or being irritated by the client's persistence and repetitiveness in proclaiming his competence and achievements. Ignoring his remarks or directing to an-

other topic can be helpful. Scheduling short, frequent interactions helps maximize the client's short attention span. Reducing the number of contacts with others and assigning the same person to work with the client each day promotes a meaningful relationship with a consistent person and may prevent attempts to dominate, meddle, manipulate, and demand from others. Setting limits on involvements in business investments and political and religious activities is crucial during a manic episode to prevent future negative consequences and embarrassent. Involving the family in setting limits in these areas is an important part of the treatment. Manic-depressive self-help groups are available in some communities for clients to receive additional support and information about the illness.

Spiritual dimension A client with manic behavior needs to learn to value himself realistically. Promoting self-worth reduces the underlying feelings of inadequacy and inferiority and lessens his need to inflate ideas about himself. Helping the client see himself as a unique individual with realistic, positive attributes and as a member of a family or larger community increases the client's valuing himself in spite of the limitations caused by his illness. It is also imporant to help the client discuss the meaning of his illness. Avoiding painful realities by becoming "sick" (manic) may be seen as a pleasant way to handle life stress, and he may come to enjoy the feeling rather than face life's problems. The client needs to accept his illness as one that is treatable so that he can function effectively througout his lifetime.

See the accompanying box for key interventions for the client with manic behavior.

See Table 14-8 for a sample care plan.

SUICIDE

Suicide is the intentional action taken by a person to end his or her own life. The ultimate level of self-destruction, suicide, is a perplexing problem in a culture that teaches the value of life and abhors death. The term *suicide* is used to describe a thought, a threat, a gesture, an attempt, or a completed act. *Suicidal ideations* are thoughts a person may have about killing himself. Many people harbor ideas about suicide without ever verbally expressing the idea. A *suicidal threat* is a verbal indication that the person is considering a self-destructive act. A *suicidal gesture* is an act of self-harm that generally is not a threat to the

LITHIUM CARBONATE

(li'thee-um)

Carbolith,* Lithane, Eskalith, Lithonate, Lithotabs, Lithobid, Lithium Citrate, Lithonate-S

Func. class.: Antimanic
Chem. class.: Alkali metal ion salt

Action: May alter sodium, potassium ion transport across cell membrane in nerve, muscle cells; may balance biogenic amines of norepinephrine, serotonin in CNS areas involved in emotional responses

Uses: Manic-depressive illness (manic phase), prevention of bipolar manic depressive psychosis

Dosage and routes:
▶ *Adult:* PO 600 mg tid, maintenance 300 mg tid or qid; SLOW REL TABS 300 mg bid, dose should be individualized to maintain blood levels at 0.5-1.5 mEq/L

Available forms include: Caps 150, 300 mg; tabs 300 mg; tabs ext rel 300, 450 mg; oral sol 8 mEq/5 ml

Side effects/adverse reactions:
CNS: Headache, drowsiness, dizziness, tremors, twitching, ataxia, seizure, slurred speech, restlessness, confusion, stupor, memory loss, clonic movements

GI: Dry mouth, anorexia, nausea, vomiting, diarrhea, incontinence, abdominal pain
GU: **Polyuria, glycosuria, proteinuria, albuminuria,** urinary incontinence, polydipsia, edema
CV: Hypotension, ECG changes, dysrhythmias, **circulatory collapse**
INTEG: Drying of hair, alopecia, rash, pruritus, hyperkeratosis
HEMA: **Leukocytosis**
EENT: Tinnitus, blurred vision
ENDO: Hyponatremia
MS: Muscle weakness

Contraindications: Hepatic disease, renal disease, brain trauma, OBS, pregnancy (D), lactation, children <12 yr, schizophrenia, severe cardiac disease, severe renal disease, severe dehydration

Precautions: Elderly, thyroid disease, seizure disorders, diabetes mellitus, systemic infection, urinary retention

Pharmacokinetics:
PO: Onset rapid, peak ½-4 hr, half-life 18-36 hr depending on age; crosses blood-brain barrier, 80% of filtered lithium is reabsorbed by the renal tubules, excreted in urine, crosses placenta, enters breast milk, well absorbed by oral method

Interactions/incompatibilities:
–Increased hypothyroid effects: antithyroid effects, calcium iodide, potassium iodide, iodinated glycerol
–Brain damage: haloperidol
–Increased effects of: neuromuscular blocking agents, phenothiazines
–Increased renal clearance: sodium bicarbonate, acetazolamide, mannitol, aminophylline
–Increased toxicity: indomethacin, diuretics, nonsteroidal antiinflammatories
–Decreased effects of lithium: theophyllines, urea, urinary alkalinizers

NURSING CONSIDERATIONS

Assess:
–Weight daily, check for edema in legs, ankles, wrists; report if present
–Sodium intake; decreased sodium intake with decreased fluid intake may lead to lithium retention; increased sodium and fluids may decrease lithium retention
–Skin turgor at least daily
–Urine for albuminuria, glycosuria, uric acid during beginning treatment, q2 mo thereafter

–Neuro status: LOC, gait, motor reflexes, hand tremors
–Serum lithium levels weekly initially, then q2 mo (therapeutic level: 0.5-1.5 mEq/L)

Administer:
–With meals to avoid GI upset
–Adequate fluids (2-3 L/day) to prevent dehydration during initial treatment, 1-2 L/day during maintenance

Teach client/family:
–Symptoms of minor toxicity: vomiting, diarrhea, poor coordination, fine motor tremors, weakness, lassitude; major toxicity: coarse tremors, severe thirst, tinnitus, dilute urine
–To monitor urine specific gravity
–That contraception is necessary since lithium may harm fetus
–Not to operate machinery until lithium levels are stable

Lab test interferences:
Increase: Potassium excretion, urine glucose, blood glucose, protein, BUN
Decrease: VMA, T₃, T₄, PBI, ¹³¹I
Treatment: Induce emesis or lavage, maintain airway, respiratory function; dialysis for severe intoxication

*Available in Canada only.
Italic indicates common side effects.
Bold italic indicates life-threatening reactions.

Modified from Skidmore-Roth L: *Mosby's nursing drug reference,* St Louis, 1993, Mosby–Year Book.

person's life. The suidical gesture is seen as a cry for help in many situations. A *suicidal atttempt* may follow a gesture and occurs when the person believes his behavior will result in death. Many times the attempt is unsuccessful because the person is unexpectedly rescued; for example, someone returns home and interrupts the suicide attempt or takes the person to the hospital. Suicide attempts and gestures may be used to communicate anger, frustration, and despair to significant persons in his life. Completed suicide results when a person takes his own life with conscious intent.

A controversial type of suicide known as *rational suicide* proposes that individuals carry out their death wish in a planned manner, using a method of choice and with the cooperation and participation of family members and friends at a time selected by the individual. Although not widely accepted, it is subject to much discussion today (see the following case example).

▼ Case Example

John and Delores, both 81, were found dead of gunshot wounds in the front seat of their auto in a pasture 5 miles from their home. On investigation, the double suicide was found to be a deliberately planned act by both people. Delores' failing vision, heart congestion, and stroke had forced her husband to place her in a nursing home earlier. He brought her home when she complained bitterly and wanted to be at home with him. A note found on the floorboard of their car had type-written funeral instructions and the telephone number of their son. The note said, "Dear Eric, we know this will be a terrible shock and embarrassment. But as we see it, it is one solution to the problem of growing old. We greatly appreciate your willingness to try to take care of us. After being married for 60 years, it only makes sense for us to leave this world together because we loved each other so much. Don't grieve for us, as we had a good life and saw you turn out to be a fine person. Love, Mother and Dad." Eric, their son, shocked and horrified, looked at the options they could have chosen and sadly stated that he could find none that would have been satisfactory to his parents.

▼ **TABLE 14-8** **NURSING CARE PLAN**

GOALS	OUTCOME CRITERIA	INTERVENTIONS	RATIONALES
NURSING DIAGNOSIS: Self-esteem disturbance related to feelings of self-importance associated with manic behavior			
LONG TERM			
To have a realistic perception of self and abilities	Perceives self and abilities realistically		
SHORT TERM			
To express realistic ideas about self and abilities	Verbalizes no grandiose ideas	Present reality without arguing or disapproving	To help client maintain contact with reality without criticism or belittling
	Makes realistic statements about self and abilities	Set limits on attention-seeking behaviors	To prevent reinforcing inappropriate behaviors
		Help client distinguish between grandiose ideas and own abilities	To provide information about his illness
To comply with medication regimen	Takes medications as directed	Establish one-to-one relationship with consistent nurse	To establish trust, to promote compliance with medication regimen
	Understands importance of taking medications as directed	Monitor client taking medications	To ensure compliance

Other types of self-destructive behavior include overeating, smoking, reckless driving, participation in hazardous sports or hobbies, and substance abuse.

THEORETICAL APPROACHES

Psychoanalytical

According to Freud,[38] an individual's two significant instincts are *eros* (instinct for life) and *thanatos* (instinct for death). Thanatos is inherent in all persons and is engaged in a constant struggle with eros. This accounts for the ambivalence experienced by suicidal persons—they wish to live, and they wish to die. Freud explained that a stressful event evokes confusion, guilt, and shame, which activate the death wish. The person kills himself instead of the object that he wants to destroy. Freud's anger-turned-inward theory is discussed on p. 259.

Sociological

Durkheim[30] discussed suicide within a sociological context. He stated that the nature of a society predisposes its individual members to suicide and that suicide can be expected when certain conditions exist. He believed any condition that interfered with a stable socioeconomic status influences suicide. For example, consider the high suicide rate during the start of the Depression in 1929. His studies showed a direct relationship between social conditions and the incidence of suicide. Durkheim described the following four forms of suicide:
- Egoistic—The individual lacks group support, resulting in extreme individualism.

- Altruistic—The individual identifies strongly with a group and is willing to die for the group's ideas and purposes.
- Anomic—The individual is in a period of normlessness, as occurs when society undergoes changes and moral authority is weakened.
- Fatalistic—The individual receives excessive regulation, the opposite of anomie.

Farberow[33] emphasized sociocultural conditions associated with suicide. Sociocultural influences such as religion, legal sanctions, and philosophical beliefs determine the meaning and pattern of suicide in a society. According to Farberow, suicide cannot be studied without considering the impact of these influences on the suicidal person. Table 14-9 summarizes theories of suicide.

NURSING PROCESS

Assessment

Physical dimension Any person in poor physical health with chronic pain or a chronic or terminal illness may be considered at risk for suicide. Many persons who commit suicide have visited a physician for a variety of physical complaints within 6 months of their deaths. Common complaints include chest pain, insomnia, fatigue, gastrointestinal upsets, backaches, and anorexia. These symptoms may indicate depression, and the nurse needs to be aware of the potential for suicide among clients having these complaints.

Other persons considered at high risk for suicide include those abusing alcohol and drugs, those engaged in risk-

▼ **TABLE 14-9** **Theories of Suicide**

Theory	Theorist	Dynamics
Psychoanalytical	Freud	The death drive (thanatos), inherent in all persons, is in constant struggle with the instinct to live (eros). It is this struggle that accounts for the ambivalence seen in suicidal persons.
Sociological	Durkheim	The nature of a society (for example, unstable socioeconomic conditions) influences suicide.
	Farberow	Religion, legal sanctions, and philosophical beliefs determine the meaning and pattern of suicide in a society.

taking activities such as mountain climbing, hang gliding, and car racing, and those who are accident prone. Age is also a factor because adolescents and older white men have the highest rates of suicide.

It is important to inquire about arrests, motor vehicle accidents, and court involvements, because many persons attempt suicide after being jailed. Inquiring about previous suicide attempts is equally important. A person who has made a previous attempt is likely to make another.

Emotional dimension Any depressed person, particularly one with feelings of hopelessness, is considered at risk for suicide. Not all depressed persons are suicidal, but the nurse needs to be aware of the possibility. The nurse is alert to the high risk of suicide as clients emerge from severe depression and their energy levels increase. She assesses depressed clients carefully at this time. Persons with excessive guilt may also attempt suicide.

Intellectual dimension The suicidal person may be preoccupied with thoughts of self-harm or self-destruction. He may actively state his wish to die, or he may give out subtle clues, such as saying "Good-bye" or "You won't have to bother with me any more."

Based on psychoanalytical theory, ambivalence may be seen in the suicidal client. It is essential to assess this behavior so that emphasis can be placed on the person's will to live.

The person with disorganized, fragmented, and distorted thinking is considered a high risk for suicide. Because of his confusion and disorientation, he may be unable to reason effectively or control his behavior, and he may act impulsively. Persons with schizophrenia or psychoses have a high potential for suicide. The client may describe hallucinations with voices telling him to jump out a window or walk out in front of moving vehicles, or he may describe delusions of being Superman and attempt to fly off a roof.

Because the risk is great in these persons, the nurse thoroughly assesses judgment, thought content, and impulsiveness.

Social dimension Most people who commit suicide have experienced turmoil or losses in their interpersonal relationships. According to interpersonal theory, sudden changes in life situations, such as separation, divorce, or death, may have created what is perceived by the client as insurmountable problems. The nurse assesses the client's relationships with family and friends and his perception of supportive persons. Frequently, isolation and alienation from significant others is seen. He may reject any offers of help from supportive persons. Dependence brought on by illness or injury may generate feelings of hopelessness and helplessness, with suicide seen as the only choice since the client thinks that nothing can be done about the situation and that no one can help.

An assessment of the person's personal, family, school, and work history may provide significant information. Persons living alone, particularly older, single, divorced, or widowed men, are prone to suicide. Persons with a family history of a committed suicide or an attempt are considered a risk for suicide. It is important to ask whether anyone in the family has ever attempted suicide. Real or perceived failure at school as well as unemployment and job stress contribute to suicide. The nurse needs to be aware that the anniversary date of a lost loved one may precipitate a suicide attempt as grief is reawakened.

Additional clues that may be significant in assessing suicide risk include giving away possessions, arranging personal and business affairs, contacting friends and relatives, and writing a will.

The client's self-concept is assessed. Because of upheavals in relationships and loss of loved ones, the individual's esteem may be lowered. Feelings of inferiority, incompetence, inadequacy, and worthlessness are common. The individual's resources are also assessed, including family, friends, agencies, employment, and finances, so that support systems can be strengthened.

Spiritual dimension The nurse explores the client's religious affiliation. Most studies indicate that white Protestants in the United States have the highest rate of suicide. However, people of other races and religions also commit suicide.

A discussion of the client's beliefs about life and death provide data on the client's potential for suicide. For some, death may be seen as a punishment for guilt or a way to punish others for inflicting guilt and pain. Others may view life as having no meaning or purpose or may believe that there is no help or hope that life will ever be better. Others see death as a relief from pain and suffering and better for themselves, the family, and loved ones.

The nurse assesses the client's sense of value and worth as a person. Many who attempt suicide feel unimportant and insignificant, that their life or death makes little difference to anyone.

Analysis
Nursing diagnosis

The following list provides examples of NANDA-accepted nursing diagnoses that may relate to suicide:

1. High risk for violence: self-directed, related to threats of suicide
2. High risk for violence: self-directed, related to suicidal gestures
3. High risk for violence: self-directed, related to inability to realistically evaluate the problem
4. High risk for violence: self-directed related to inability to control behavior associated with suicide attempt

The following case example demonstrates the characteristics of the nursing diagnosis, potential for violence, self-directed.

▼ **Case Example**

Terry, age 15, attempted to kill herself by taking an overdose of a combination of medications including Valium, aspirin, Sominex, and Dalmane. She had had a fight with her boyfriend of 7 months and had been grounded by her father for talking on the telephone too long. She does not have a good relationship with her mother, who said she "never listens to her." On returning from school she became angry at her hopeless situation and searched the house for any medications she could find and swallowed them. Thirty minutes later her mother returned and, on learning what Terry had done, had her admitted to a psychiatric unit for adolescents.

▼ **TABLE 14-10   NURSING CARE PLAN**

GOALS	OUTCOME CRITERIA	NURSING INTERVENTIONS	RATIONALES
NURSING DIAGNOSIS: Potential for violence: self-directed related to depression			
LONG TERM			
To have no thoughts of self-harm	States no suicidal thoughts		
To have no signs or symptoms of depression	Demonstrates no signs or symptoms of depression		
SHORT TERM			
To have a reduced potential for harm to self	Verbalizes anger appropriately	Monitor client for anger (verbal and physical) against self	To determine level of anger; to prevent escalation
	States no thoughts of suicide, has a will to live	Monitor client for suicidal risk	To determine seriousness of client intent
		Assess availability of weapons, drugs	To determine lethality of intent
		Establish a no-suicide contract with client	To prevent impulsive suicidal actions
		Provide one-to-one supportive observation	For client's protection; availability of supportive person
	Demonstrates effective coping skills in dealing with stress and frustration	Teach client problem solving	To help client solve problems rationally
To have a reduced level of depression	Performs own self-care	Help with activities of daily living (ADLs) when client is unable to perform them	To promote esteem, respect, and general well-being
	Participates in group activities	Facilitate expression of feelings	To help client identify and acknowledge feelings
	Interacts with others	Promote social interactions	To establish support system; to have pleasure in relationships with others
	Experiences pleasures	Encourage active participation in group activities	To promote social interactions
			To provide pleasurable experiences
			To promote a sense of worth and belonging
	Asserts self	Encourage independence through assertive behaviors	To help client feel more in control of self

Planning

Assessment of clients who are suicidal frequently results in setting goals that are related to the following client needs:

1. Safety
2. Expression of anger, rage, guilt, hopelessness
3. Adaptive coping skills
4. A support system
5. A will to live

The nursing care plan (Table 14-10) lists examples of long-term and short-term goals, outcome criteria, interventions, and rationales related to the suicidal client. These serve as examples of the planning stage of the nursing process.

Implementation

Physical dimension Hospitalization is generally the treatment of choice when a client has attempted suicide or appears in imminent danger of harming himself. The suicidal client requires close supervision as his depression lifts, and he seems more animated and energetic. It is during this time that he has the energy to make decisions, and suicide may be one of them. Before this time, he may lack the energy to make or carry out a decision to commit suicide.

Most hospitals have written policies about the care of suicidal persons that include the following:

1. Removing potentially harmful items such as belts, socks, boot strings, matches, lighters, hairpicks, sharp objects, watches, glass cosmetic containers
2. Observing the client 24 hours a day on a one-to-one basis
3. Having client sleep in a dimly lit area for observation purposes
4. Having the client eat on the unit
5. Maintaining special awareness at times when suicide attempts are known to be likely: early morning, on arising, during busy routines, while shaving, when there is a shortage of staff or change of shift, when suddenly cheerful
6. Isolating, if progressing toward destruction, to decrease stimulation
7. Encouraging to participate in activities

The client is given antidepressant medications to elevate his mood and make him more amenable to treatment. Electroconvulsive therapy (ECT) is an additional treatment that has proved effective.

Because the risk of suicide is high after the diagnosis of a terminal illness, during a chronic illness, or after an arrest for a motor vehicle accident, the nurse alerts the client's significant others to the possibility of suicide when clues have been observed. Physical complaints are treated as prescribed to promote comfort and a caring attitude.

Emotional dimension Anguish, anger, depression, and hopelessness are the most common emotions expressed by clients who are suicidal. Nursing interventions for these feeling states are discussed in the depression section of this chapter.

Intellectual dimension Threats of suicide are taken seriously. Listening attentively conveys the attitude of caring so desperately needed by the suicidal person. The nurse helps the client expand his thinking to consider options with more favorable consequences for himself and others. When the suicide threat is a manipulative maneuver for controlling others, assisting the client to sort out the meaning underlying the suicide threat is more helpful than labeling him a "manipulative client."

No harm contracts are an effective treatment method. The client states in writing that he will not hurt or kill himself, and, if he has self-destructive feelings, he will talk with a staff member about them. Threatening delusions or hallucinations necessitates protection from impulsive actions. Close observation and medication may be necessary. Once the risk of suicide is lessened, the client can be taught new methods of coping. Problem solving, decision making, and assertiveness are used to reduce the impact of stress.

Social dimension A vital task in working with a suicidal client is helping him improve his self-concept. It is important to involve the client in activities to prevent preoccupation with self-destructive behavior and to provide opportunities for increasing self-esteem through accomplishing useful and worthwhile tasks. This involves him with others and lessens his isolation and alienation. Helping the client reestablish relationships with family and significant friends also reduces the isolation. Until contact with family is made, the nurse may be the significant person. Family, friends, and other supportive persons need to be involved in the treatment plans.

It is helpful to plan for a friend or family member to be with the client on the anniversary of the death of a loved one. This contact may prevent loneliness and help the client reintegrate positive relationships with others. Providing the telephone number of hotlines and the name of a contact person at crisis intervention center is an additional effective nursing action.

Spiritual dimension The suicidal client's perception of an intolerable life situation requires the greatest nursing expertise. Feelings of hopelessness, purposelessness, and meaninglessness are diminished by warmth, a caring, confident attitude, and by offering alternatives for solving problems. The relationship with the nurse may satisfy his need for relatedness so that he finds the strength to come to terms with life, gain confidence, value himself, and live an enriched life. See the accompanying box for key interventions for suicidal clients.

See Table 14-10 for a sample nursing care plan.

See the box on p. 282 for guidelines for primary and testing prevention.

KEY INTERVENTIONS FOR SUICIDAL CLIENTS

1. Provide close observation.
2. Remove potentially harmful items.
3. Demonstrate a confident, "take charge" attitude.
4. Form a no-harm contract.
5. Promote expression of thoughts and feelings.
6. Help client to think of other options for resolving the problem.
7. Mobilize a support system.
8. Increase self-esteem.

GUIDELINES FOR PRIMARY/TERTIARY PREVENTION

Hope-Hopelessness

Primary Prevention

Teach client to:
- Have pleasures, such as hobbies, interests, and sports
- Adapt to losses
- Adopt a positive attitude; focus on accomplishments
- Maintain high self-esteem
- Restore self-esteem when lowered
- Share sad feelings with a supportive person
- Manage sad feelings: exercise, treat self to a special favor, spend time with a friend
- Problem solve
- Identify signs and symptoms of early depression
- Obtain information about antidepressant medications: name, dosage, side effects
- Become more independent
- Develop assertiveness skills

Teach family ways to be supportive to depressed family member

Tertiary Prevention

Community resources, such as community mental health centers
Self-help groups, such as manic-depressive groups and suicide survivor groups

Evaluation

The evaluation process for clients who are depressed or demonstrate manic or suicidal behavior includes consideration of the effectiveness and the appropriateness of the treatment plans.

Effectiveness

Were the interventions effective for the client's recovery? For the depressed and suicidal client ask the following questions:
- Does he have fewer physical complaints?
- Is his mood more animated?
- Is he less preoccupied with himself?
- Has his negative thinking decreased?
- Does he initiate new friendships or reestablish old ones?
- Does he have pleasures in his life?
- Does he state that he no longer wants to harm himself?

For the manic client:
- Has his activity level lessened?
- Are his emotions more stable?
- Does he have a realistic perception of himself?
- Are his thought processes reality based?
- Does he have accurate knowledge about his illness?
- Is his social behavior appropriate?
- Does he comply with his medication regimen?

For depressed, suicidal, and manic clients:
- Does the client know about his diagnosis, medications, and treatment regimen?
- Was the family or a significant friend involved in the client's care?
- Does the family and significant friend have knowledge of the client's diagnosis, medications, and treatment regimen?

- Does the client use what he has learned to manage or prevent depression and manic or suicidal behavior?
- Does the client know community resources available to depressed and suicidal persons or those with manic behavior?

Appropriateness

Were the interventions appropriate and realistic for the client's life-style, cultural background, educational level, developmental stage, economic status, and religious affiliation?

Did the client participate in the decision for choice of treatment?

BRIEF REVIEW

Depression, manic behavior, and suicide describe behaviors along the hope-hopelessness continuum. Hope enables a person to accomplish a goal and is related to trust and the expectation that help from another person is forthcoming. Hopelessness is a component of depression, a pathological state. Manic behavior, an affective illness, is characterized by symptoms that are the opposite of depression; these include hyperactivity, elation, and excessive verbal activity. Suicidal behavior is the ultimate act of self-destruction and frequently accompanies depression.

Theoretical explanations for depression include displaced anger, loss of esteem as a result of failure to achieve developmental goals, heredity, biochemical imbalances, negative thinking, lack of positive reinforcement, learned helplessness, losses, or a combination of factors. Explanations for manic behavior include heredity, chemical excesses, defects in cell membranes, and losses. Theoretical explanations for suicide include the individual's innate death drive, the nature of society, and religious and legal sanctions.

The nursing process is a systematic and organized method of working with clients who have lost hope, who are depressed, suicidal, or having manic episodes. The increasing number of suicides, particularly among adolescents and the elderly, challenge the nurse to identify persons at risk for suicide, to intervene quickly to prevent suicide, and to strengthen the person's coping skills so that life becomes bearable and meaningful.

REFERENCES AND SUGGESTED READINGS

1. American Psychiatric Association: *Diagnostic and statistical manual of mental disorders* (DSM-III-R), Washington, DC, 1987, The Association.
2. Barker P: The nursing care of people experiencing affective disorder: a review of the literature, *Journal of Advanced Nursing* 14:618, 1989.
3. Beck A: *Depression: causes and treatment*, Philadelphia, 1967, University of Pennsylvania Press.
4. Beck A and others: Hopelessness and eventual suicide: a 10-year prospective study of patients with suicidal ideation. American Journal of Psychiatry 142(5):559, 1985.
5. Beck A, Weissman A: The measurement of depression: the hopelessness scale, *Journal of Counseling and Clinical Psychology* 42(6):861, 1974.
6. Becker F: *The revolution in psychiatry*, New York, 1964, The Free Press.
7. Beeber L: Enacting corrective interpersonal experiences with

the depressed client: an intervention model, *Archives of Psychiatric Nursing* 3(4):211, 1989.

8. Belmaker R, van Pragg H: *Mania: an evolving concept,* Jamaica, NY, 1980, Spectrum Publications.

9. Berk J: *The down comforter,* New York, 1980, Avon Books.

10. Bibring E: The mechanisms of depression. In Greenacre P, editor: *Affective disorders,* New York, 1953, International Universities Press.

11. Blazer D: *Depression in late life,* St Louis, 1982, Mosby—Year Book.

12. Bowers W: Treatment of depressed in-patients, *British Journal of Psychiatry* 156:73, 1990.

13. Bowlby J: Processes of mourning. *International Journal of Psychoanalysts* 42:317, 1961.

14. Burns D: *Feeling good,* New York, 1981, The New American Library.

15. Bruss C: Nursing diagnosis of hopelessness, *Journal of Psychosocial Nursing* 26(3):28, 1988.

16. Campbell L: Hopelessness: a concept analysis, *Journal of Psychosocial Nursing and Mental Health Services* 25(2):18, 1987.

17. Cappodanno A, Targum S: Assessment of suicide risk: some limitations in the prediction of infrequent events, *Journal of Psychosocial Nursing and Mental Health Services* 21(5):11, 1983.

18. Carroll B: The blood test for depression: how to use it, *Diagnosis* 3(9):71, 1981.

19. Ciaramitao B: *Help for depressed mothers,* ed 2, Edmunds, Washington, 1982, Charles Franklin Press.

20. Cochran CC: Change of mind about ECT, *American Journal of Nursing* 84(8):1004, 1984.

21. Cowley PN: An investigation of patient's attitudes toward ECT by means of a Q analysis, *Psychological Medicine* 15(1):131, 1985.

22. Crowe RR: Current concepts of electroconvulsive therapy: a current perspective, *New England Journal of Medicine* 311(3):163, 1984.

23. Davis T, Jenson L: Identifying depression in medical patients, *Image: Journal of Nursing Scholarship* 20(4):191, 1988.

24. Davis J, Maas J: *The affective disorders,* Washington, DC, 1985, The American Psychiatric Association.

25. Deakin J: *The biology of depression,* Washington, DC, 1986, The American Psychiatric Association.

26. *Depression/awareness, recognition, treatment (DART),* National Institute of Mental Health, 1986, US Department of Health and Human Services, US Government Printing Office.

27. DeRosis H, Pellegrino V: *The book of hope,* New York, 1981, Bantam Books.

28. Dixon D: Manic depression: an overview, *Journal of Psychosocial Nursing and Mental Health Services* 19:28, 1981.

29. Dufault K: Hope: its spheres and dimensions, *Nursing Clinics of North America* 20(2):379, 1985.

30. Durkheim E: *Suicide,* New York, 1951, The Free Press.

31. Erikson E: *Childhood and society,* ed 2, New York, 1964, WW Norton.

32. Erickson R, Post R, Paige A: Hope as a psychiatric variable, *Journal of Clinical Psychology* 31(2):324, 1975.

33. Farberow N: *Suicide in different cultures,* Baltimore, 1975, University Park Press.

34. Farberow N: Suicide prevention in the hospital, *Hospital and Community Psychiatry* 32:99, 1981.

35. Fieve R: *Mood swing: the third revolution,* New York, 1981, Bantam Books.

36. Fraser RM: *ECT: a clinical guide,* New York, 1982, John Wiley & Sons.

37. Fraser RM, Glass IB: Recovery from ECT in elderly patients, *British Journal of Psychiatry* 133:524, 1978.

38. Freud S: Mourning and melancholia. In *The complete psychological works of Sigmund Freud,* vol 14, London, 1957, Hogarth Press. (Translated from the German under the general editorship of J Strachey and A Tyson.)

39. Gordon V and others: A 3-year follow-up of a cognitive-behavioral therapy intervention, *Archives of Psychiatric Nursing* 2(4):218, 1988.

40. Gottschalk L: A hope scale applicable to verbal samples, *Archives of General Psychiatry* 30:279, 1974.

41. Harris E: The dexamethasone suppression test, *American Journal of Nursing* 82:784, 1982.

42. Harris E: Lithium: In a class by itself, *American Journal of Nursing* 89:190, 1989.

43. Hatton C, Valente S: *Suicide, assessment and intervention,* ed 2, Norwalk, Conn, 1984, Appleton-Century-Crofts.

44. Hume A and others: Manic depressive psychosis: an alternative therapeutic model of nursing, *Journal of Advanced Nursing* 13:93, 1988.

45. Jacobson A: Melancholy in the twentieth century: causes and prevention, *Journal of Psychiatric Nursing* 18(7):11, 1980.

46. Janicak P and others: ECT: an assessment of mental health professionals' knowledge and attitudes, *Journal of Clinical Psychiatry* 46(7):262, 1985.

47. Jourard S: Suicide: an invitation to die, *American Journal of Nursing* 70:269, 1970.

48. Kalinowsky LB: The convulsive therapies. In Freedman AM, Kaplan HI, editors: *Comprehensive textbook of psychiatry,* vol 2, ed 2, Baltimore, 1975, Williams & Wilkins.

49. Kaplen R, Kottler D, Francis A: Reliability and rationality in the prediction of suicide, *Hospital and Community Psychiatry* 33:212, 1982.

50. Karasu T: Toward a clinical model of psychotherapy for depression: systematic comparison of three psychotherapies, *American Journal of Psychiatry* 147(2):133, 1990.

51. Kerr N: Signs and symptoms of depression and principles of nursing care, *Perspectives in Psychiatric Care* 24(2):48, 1988.

52. Kim M, McFarland G, and McLane A: *Pocket guide to nursing diagnoses,* ed 4, St Louis, 1991, Mosby—Year Book.

53. Kline N: *From sad to glad,* New York, 1981, Ballantine Books.

54. Kovacs M: The efficacy of cognitive and behavior therapies for depression, *American Journal of Psychiatry* 137:1495, 1980.

55. Lattaye T: *How to win over depression,* New York, 1980, Bantam Books.

56. Lewinsohn P: A behavioral approach to depression. In Friedman R, Katz M, editors: *The psychology of depression: contemporary theory and research,* Washington, DC, 1974, VH Winston & Sons.

57. Lewis S, McDowell W, Gregory R: Saving the suicidal patient from himself, *RN,* December, 1986.

58. Major LG: Electroconvulsive therapy in the 1980's, *Psychiatric Clinics of North America* 7(3):613, 1984.

59. Manderino M, Bzdek V: Mobilizing depressed clients, *Journal of Psychosocial Nursing and Mental Health Services* 24(5):23, 1986.

60. McEnany G: Psychobiological indices of bipolar mood disorder: future trends in nursing care, *Archives of Psychiatric Nursing* 4(1):29, 1990.

61. Mejo S: The use of antidepressant medication: a guide for the primary care nurse practitioner, *Journal of the American Academy of Nurse Practitioners* 2(4):153, 1990.

62. Menninger K: Hope, *American Journal of Psychiatry* 116:481, 1959.

63. Merz B: Cell membrane defects in mental illness, *Journal of the American Medical Association* 248:633, 1982.

64. Miller J: Inspiring hope, *American Journal of Nursing* 85(1):22, 1985.

65. Miller J, Powers M: Development of an instrument to measure hope, *Nursing Research* 37(1):6, 1988.

66. Motto J, Heilbron D, Juster R: Development of a clinical instrument to estimate suicide risk, *American Journal of Psychiatry* 142(6):680, 1985.

67. Murphy S: Preventative intervention following accidental death of a child, *Image: Journal of Nursing Scholarship* 22(3):174, 1990.

68. Nolen-Itoeksema S: Sex differences in unipolar depression: evidence and theory, *Psychological Bulletin* 101(2):259, 1987.

69. Obayuwana A and others: Hope index scale: an instrument for the objective measurement of hope, *Journal of the National Medical Association* 74(8):761, 1982.

70. Parent C, Whall A: Are physical activity, self-esteem and depression related? *Journal of Gerontological Nursing* 10(3):8, 1984.

71. Plumlee A: Biological rhythms and affective illness, *Journal of Psychosocial Nursing and Mental Health Services* 24(3):12, 1986.

72. Richman J: *Family therapy for suicidal people,* New York, 1986, Springer.

73. Rifkin A: ECT versus tricyclic antidepressants in depression: a review of the evidence, *Journal of Clinical Psychiatry* 49(1):3, 1988.

74. Rippere V, Williams R: *Wounded healers: mental health workers' experiences with depression,* New York, 1985, John Wiley & Sons.

75. Rogers C, Ulsafer-van Lanen J: *Nursing interventions in depression,* Orlando, 1985, Grune & Stratton.

76. Roose S and others: Depression, delusions and suicide, *American Journal of Psychiatry* 140(9):1159, 1983.

77. Rosenbaum J: Depression: viewed from a transcultural nursing theoretical perspective, *Journal of Advanced Nursing* 14:7, 1989.

78. Roy A: Risk factors for suicide in psychiatric patients, *Archives of General Psychiatry* 39(9):1089, 1982.

79. Rush J, Altshuler K: *Depression—basic mechanisms, diagnosis and treatment,* New York, 1986, Guilford Press.

80. Rutter J, Izard C, Read P: *Depression in young people, developmental and clinical perspectives,* New York, 1986, Guilford Press.

81. Sands D and others: Understanding ECT, *Journal of Psychosocial Nursing* 25(8):27, 1987.

82. Sartorius L: *Depressive disorders in different cultures,* Geneva, 1983, World Health Organization.

83. Schmale A: A genetic view of affects with special reference to the genesis of helplessness and hopelessness. In Nagera H: *The psychoanalytic study of the child,* Monograph no 2, New York, 1964, International Universities Press.

84. Seligman M: Depression and learned helplessness. In Freidman R, Katzi M, editors: *The psychology of depression: contemporary theory and research,* Washington, DC, 1974, VH Winston & Sons.

85. Selmi P and others: Computer-administered cognitive-behavioral therapy for depression, *American Journal of Psychiatry* 147(1):51 1990..

86. Simmons-Alling S: Genetic implications for major affective disorders, *Archives of Psychiatric Nursing* 14(1):67, 1990.

87. Smith DM: Guided imagination as an intervention in hopelessness, *Journal of Psychosocial Nursing and Mental Health Services* 20(6):29, 1982.

88. Staats S: Hope: expected positive affect in an adult sample, *Journal of Genetic Psychology* 148(3):357, 1987.

89. Stotland E: *The psychology of hope,* San Francisco, 1969, Jossey-Bass.

90. Talbot K: ECT: exploring myths, examining attitudes, *Journal of Psychosocial Nursing and Mental Health Services* 24(3):6, 1986.

91. Thompson C and others: A comparison of normal, bipolar, and seasonal affective disorder subjects using the seasonal pattern assessment questionnaire, *Journal of Affective Disorders* 14:257, 1988.

92. Weissman M, Paykel E: *The depressed woman,* Chicago, 1974, University of Chicago Press.

93. Willner P: *Depression: a psychological synthesis,* New York, 1985, John Wiley & Sons.

94. Zorumski C, Rubin E, Burke W: Electroconvulsive therapy for the elderly: a review, *Hospital and Community Psychiatry* 39(6):643, 1988.

95. Zung W: A self-rating depression scale, *Archives of General Psychiatry* 12:63, 1965.

ANNOTATED BIBLIOGRAPHY

Beeber L: Enacting corrective interpersonal experiences with the depressed client: an intervention model, *Archives of Psychiatric Nursing* 3(4):211, 1989.

This article explains the behavior of depressed clients using Sullivan's and Peplau's theoretical models. A case example illustrates the processes.

McEnany G: Psychobiological indices of bipolar mood disorder: future trends in nursing care, *Archives of Psychiatric Nursing* 4(1):29, 1990.

This report focuses on constructs that form a basis for understanding bipolar disorders. Also addressed is the application of the nursing process to psychobiological aspects of bipolar mood disorders, specifically, circadian rhythm disturbances and dietary influences on neurotransmission.

Zorumski C, Rubin E, Burke W: Electroconvulsive therapy for the elderly: a review, *Hospital and Community Psychiatry* 39(6):643, 1988.

The authors review indications, complications, and precautions related to ECT for older clients. Special attention is given to cardiovascular factors and concurrent medications is emphasized.

CHAPTER

15 Flexibility-Rigidity

Cathleen M Shultz

After studying this chapter, the student will be able to:

- Define flexibility-rigidity
- Discuss historical perspectives of flexibility and rigidity
- Describe the theoretical development of flexibility and rigidity
- Discuss the psychopathology of compulsive personality disorders and disorders of impulse control as described in the DSM-III-R
- Use the nursing process to care for clients experiencing difficulties with flexible or rigid behaviors
- Identify research findings relevant to flexibility and rigidity

Change is inevitable in life, and adaptation is essential to healthy maturation. The capacity to respond to change easily is central to flexibility.

A client's response to change reveals his place on the flexibility-rigidity continuum (Figure 15-1). Cues are seen in the person's activities and interactions, which are formed by developmental stages, early experiences, culture, and personality. For example, a 4-year-old who must stack play items neatly in a row before going to bed each evening is displaying early signs of rigid ritualistic behavior that could be problematic in later years. The environment also contributes to the type of responses; if the child's parents reinforce this behavior by insisting on the toys being placed neatly before bedtime, the rigid behavior can become permanently linked with going to sleep. If the client perceives the environment as stressful, there is a greater tendency to respond rigidly; the behavior becomes firmly entrenched.

Flexibility means that the person responds and can be influenced to change. The flexible person has many responses and maintains an open mind. Adjectives such as *resilient, pliant, accommodating,* and *adaptable* describe the flexible client. A flexible client displays an openness to change and even welcomes variety knowing that change is a healthy part of being.

When unhealthy, the flexible individual resembles a chameleon, which cannot be clearly identified in its native environment. Readily adopting others' beliefs and values, the client demonstrates little consistency, predictability, separateness from others, or sense of commitment. No or minimal personal boundaries are present. Terms such as

wishy-washy, wimpy, weak, blows with the wind, just a carbon copy, and *mimicking others* may be used to describe this client.

Failure to adapt and alter one's behavior as conditions change characterizes *rigidity.* Rigid behaviors are rooted in fear. Rigid or repetitive behaviors are commonly seen in rituals, phobias, compulsive personality disorders, and disorders of impulse control. The rigid client may not acquire new behaviors or different responses. Remaining with the familiar, the rigid client seeks security by minimizing risks and avoiding the unknown. The rigid client is also characterized as being obstinate, unyielding, closed minded, unbending, or unwilling or unable to consider new information. Thought processes involving decision making, problem solving, and the quality of interpersonal relation-

---

▶ **DIAGNOSES Related to Flexibility-Rigidity**

MEDICAL DIAGNOSES	NURSING DIAGNOSES
Obsessive compulsive disorder	**NANDA**
Obsessive compulsive personality disorder	Fear
Pathological or compulsive gambling	**PMH**
Kleptomania	Altered feeling pattern: fear
Pyromania	

HISTORICAL OVERVIEW

DATES	EVENTS
1500s-1800s	Discussion of rigidity first appeared in the literature in the sixteenth century.
	Rigid behaviors were believed to be due to a religious melancholy or the devil's work; treatment involved a ritual of exorcism by witch doctors, mystics, or religious leaders.
1900s-1920s	Rigid behaviors were first identified as a medical concern by Freud in 1915; he conceptualized symptomatology as unconscious with psychosexual roots in the libido.
1930s-1940s	A neurophysiological cause for rigid behaviors was sought; researchers discovered that the personality's socialization influenced the degree of rigidity.
1950s-1960s	Attempts were made to link the process of socialization with personality characteristics. Adorno and others[1] documented the authoritarian personality and thus caused a shift from a neurophysiological to a socialization basis.
	Rubenowitz[73] confirmed the impact of socialization on the development of rigidity. He revealed that both flexibility and rigidity existed in adults and influenced their thinking, attitudes, and behavior.
1960s-1980s	Behavioral therapy began with the conditioning studies of Pavlov[64] in the Soviet Union and Thorndike[50] in the United States. Until the development of behavioral treatments, the prognosis for clients with obsessive-compulsive personalities was poor and nurses were involved only peripherally in treatment.
	Phobias have emerged as the second most common mental health problem, with at least one in nine Americans having some form of phobia; only alcoholism occurs more often.
1980s-1990s	The prevalence rate of obsessive-compulsive disorders is 2.8%, with the most prevalent form being checking followed by repeating, counting, collecting, and washing.[34]
	Rigid behaviors are considered the mental health problem of the 1980s and 1990s corresponding to an increasingly insecure and complex world.
Future	Nurses, especially those with counseling credentials, will be more directly involved with treatment using relaxation and exposure techniques such as imagery and desensitization.
	Some view obsessions and compulsions as part of normal mental life. A current challenge involves understanding the relationship between normal obsessions and compulsions and those that lead to interference and distress.[41]

ships are profoundly affected by the client's rigidity. Considerable interpersonal skills are needed to effectively relate to these clients.

In the past, rigidity has been linked exclusively with aging, but current research[2,22] suggests that rigid characteristics, such as the inability to be flexible, are frequently found in young children.[7,9,88]

The rigid person needs structure, consistent expectations, specific instructions, and clear lines of authority. Excessive rigidity restricts the range of healthy behaviors, especially in emotional, intellectual, and social dimensions. For example, the client may have a diminished capacity to initiate and maintain interpersonal relationships. Also, oc-

cupations requiring considerable flexibility can be devastating to rigid clients.

In some cases, rigid behaviors may actually aid an individual. Denial of feelings and predominantly rigid responses have enabled prisoners of war to withstand solitary confinement and torture; thus rigidity became a survival technique. Famous prisoners such as Victor Frankl (WWII) actually reframed his concentration camp experience by not centering on the hopelessness of the situation.[20] The rigid person also may cope better in a regimented society such as those ruled by dictators. Denying feelings makes an indifferent and hostile environment more tolerable, thus enabling some to survive difficult home situations and governmental suppression.[35]

Identifying clients' responses to change can assist the nurse in minimizing or preventing health problems related to flexibility and rigidity. Intervening during pertinent developmental stages may help those at-risk individuals whose creative potential and capacity for enjoying life is already compromised by problems of rigidity or flexibility.

Obsessions and compulsions exist along a broad spectrum that incorporates rigidity. The terms *rigidity, obses-*

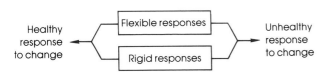

FIGURE 15-1 Flexibility-rigidity continuum of responses to change.

sions, and *compulsions* may be used interchangeably in health-related literature.

DSM-III-R DIAGNOSES

This chapter addresses disorders of impulse control: kleptomania, pyromania, pathological or compulsive gambling, obsessive-compulsive personality disorder, and obsessive-compulsive disorder. The discussion focuses on general information applicable to rigid personalities.

According to DSM-III-R criteria, impulse control disorders have these essential features in common:

1. Failure to resist an impulse, drive, or temptation to perform an act that is harmful to self or others. The act may or may not be resisted, premeditated, or planned
2. Increased tension/arousal before committing the act
3. Experience of pleasure, gratification, or release at the time the act is committed. Immediately after the act, there may be genuine regret, self-reproach, or guilt

Clients with kleptomania are unable to resist impulses to steal objects that they do not need for either personal use or monetary value. The theft is not premeditated and objects are either given away, discarded, returned quickly, or kept and hidden. No long-term theft planning occurs and others are not involved in the thefts. The disorder may be seen as early as childhood and is more common in females than males.

Deliberate and purposeful fire-setting on more than one occasion describes the client with pyromania. These people are fascinated with, curious about, or attracted to fire, details about fire, and associated characteristics of fire such as use, consequences, or exposure to fire. The fire is not set for monetary gain, to conceal criminal activity, to express anger or vengeance, to improve one's living circumstances, or in response to a delusion or hallucination. Usually the client spends considerable time and resources in preparing for the fire-setting and may leave obvious clues. They are often recognized as regular watchers at fires, frequently set off false alarms, and show interest in fire-fighting paraphernalia. Their fascination with fire leads some to seek employment or volunteer work in fire-fighting. They may be indifferent to the consequences of the fire for life or property, or they may get satisfaction from the resulting destruction. This disorder usually begins in childhood and is more common in males than females.

Clients who have a pathological gambling disorder have a chronic and progressive failure to resist impulses to gamble and gambling behavior that compromises, disrupts, or damages the person, family, or vocational pursuits. Characteristic problems include extensive indebtedness and consequent default on debts and other financial responsibilities, disrupted family relationships, inattention to work, and financially motivated illegal activities to pay for gambling. Persons with a pathological gambling disorder generally believe that money causes and is also the solution to all their problems. As gambling increases, the client usually lies to obtain money to continue gambling. There is no serious attempt to budget or save money. These clients are often overconfident, energetic, easily bored, and "big spenders," but there are times when they show obvious signs of personal stress, anxiety, and depression. About 2% to 3% of the population are affected, men more often than women.

The client with an obsessive-compulsive personality disorder (OCPD) displays a pervasive pattern of perfectionism and inflexibility beginning in early adulthood. The disorder is diagnosed more frequently in men than women. Clients strive for perfection, which interferes significantly with their functioning when their preoccupation with rules, trivia, procedures, or form decreases their ability to see the broad picture. These clients have trouble with time allocation and establishing priorities; work and productivity are prized to the exclusion of pleasure and interpersonal relationships. Often the person has a preoccupation with logic and intellect and an intolerance of affective behavior in others. Leisure activity is planned and pursued with diligence, and pleasurable activity may sometimes be postponed forever.

Decision making for the client with OCPD is avoided, postponed, or protracted often due to an inordinate fear of making a mistake. For example, assignments cannot be completed on time because the person is ruminating about priorities or wants to do the projects "just right." Clients with this disorder tend to be excessively conscientious, moralistic, scrupulous, and judgmental of themselves and others; they may be stingy with their emotions and material possessions. The disorder is often incapacitating, particularly in the client's work situation.

Obsessive-compulsive disorder (OCD) differs from OCPD. Clients with OCD have recurrent obsessions or compulsions with an awareness of the senselessness of the behavior, whereas clients with OCPD do not recognize the senselessness of the behavior. Clients can be affected with both disorders simultaneously.

OCDs are characterized by rigid behaviors, frequently treated on an outpatient basis. Obsessions and compulsions are time consuming and may interfere with relationships, social activities, or work. Preliminary data from a National Institute of Mental Health (NIMH) study suggest that OCDs may be far more prevalent than commonly believed.[74] The disorder has been identified in children, with the majority (68% to 87%) retaining the disorder into adulthood.[22,53] A genetic factor has also been suspected.[52] Repeated behaviors are numerous and can include rituals regarding eating (for example, if the client eats green beans, he will eat two at a time, or in multiples of 2, rather than eat without considering the amount on his fork) and drinking in 2s and 4s, handwashing, checking (for example, checking faucets for drips or making sure the stove is turned off before leaving the house), preoccupations with moral things, compulsion to talk, tapping, hoarding, preoccupations with numbers, being perfectionistic, repeating things until they are "right," counting, organizing, list making, demanding that others say certain words, and fear of contamination. For adults, the most prevalent form of obsessive-compulsive behavior is checking followed by repeating, counting, collecting, and washing.[34]

The prognosis of obsessional states is more severe than for other neurotic disorders. Thus the nurse is challenged to find and use effective interventions. Complete recovery is rare; however, complete disability is seen only in a minority of cases. Clients rarely report themselves symptom free at the completion of a treatment regimen, but all but the most severely affected continue to work.[22] Relapse is common among those clients who are only partially improved at the end of treatment.[45] However, successful treatment is possible, and the success rate is enhanced by the nurse's encouragement.

THEORETICAL APPROACHES

Psychoanalytical

Obsessions are intrusive recurring or persisting ideas, thoughts, images, or impulses that are unacceptable to the person, cause distress, and are *ego dystonic;* that is, the person does not consider them voluntarily produced or consistent with what the person desires to do. Frequently the obsession is repulsive, inane, or obscene to the client. Obsessional content usually centers around dirt and contamination, aggression, keeping things in strict order, sex, or religion. The client feels compelled to engage in these sometimes repugnant thoughts or fantasies.[57]

Continuous brooding or repetitive thinking about real situations, unpleasant possibilities, or difficult decisions is not considered obsessional thought because the individual is engaged in thinking in a meaningful way. Because the content is not ego dystonic, it is not a true obsession.[51]

Obsessional behaviors range from those that do not produce uncomfortable anxiety to those that pervade a person's life-style. If the behaviors are distressing or incapacitating, the syndrome is labeled *neurotic.* Between these extremes are obsessional traits that cluster into obsessional personality patterns, seen in a person with obvious anxiety (Figure 15-2). Traits are fixed, long lasting, and predictable. As long as clients remain productive, they are not neurotic even though they may be using rituals extensively.[76]

Rigid individuals have obsessive-compulsive patterns of behavior that are rooted in childhood. As the child passes through the phases of psychosexual development, the anxiety generated from socialization is manifested through various ego defenses. Later in life, a person's anxiety may cause him to become fixated or to regress to an earlier point because of conflicts that occurred during that stage. These fixations and regressions are examples of ego defenses that are part of normal development. In the neurotic person they become rigid. Even when they do not relieve anxiety they are repeated because they at least convey the illusion of control.[51] For example, Mary, who has considerable work-related anxiety, does not begin important paperwork; instead, she clears the top of her desk and countertops in her office until the activity consumes the time she allotted for the paperwork.

In the quest for total mastery, those with rigid personalities may use intelligence or magical thinking to diminish anxiety. Although phobias are covered in Chapter 10, they are briefly discussed here because they are also one of the control methods that those with rigid personalities use. Phobias permit a rigid client to avoid anything that threatens loss of control or is perceived as a potential danger. As

a response to fear, a phobia can occur about anything in the client's environment. Common phobias include fear of heights, cancer, leaving the home, snakes, and blood.

Obsessions and compulsions can occur simultaneously in an individual. Compulsions are repetitive acts regarded as excessive or exaggerated. The person does not achieve pleasure from completion of the activity. Although the behaviors are voluntary, the urge to do them is so strong that the person's volition seems diminished.

The dynamics for compulsions are similar to those for obsessions in that compulsions are obsessive thoughts that are acted out. The compulsion is not an end in itself, but is designed to neutralize or prevent discomfort or some dreaded event or situation. Compulsions may include handwashing, faucet checking, checking stoves and heaters, checking under the bed, repeatedly counting numbers in a sequence, or collecting soap samples from hotel rooms. Some compulsions take the form of repeated urges to act; although the thought recurs, the person resists overt action.

▼ **TABLE 15-1   Definitions of Terms from the Psychoanalytical Perspective**

Term	Definition
Obsessions	Intrusive recurring thoughts, images, or impulses unacceptable to client
Compulsions	Repetitive acts regarded as excessive or exaggerated
Phobias	Fears that are out of proportion to the demands of the situation and cannot be explained or reasoned away
Neuroses	Distressing or incapacitating symptoms that interfere with living
Obsessional personality	Obsessional traits in a person with obvious anxiety; not neurotic as long as the person remains productive
Obsessive-compulsive disorder (OCD)	Recurrent obsessions or compulsions without recognizing the behavior's senselessness; no pleasure is obtained from completing a compulsion or obsession
Obsessive-compulsive personality disorder (OCPD)	A pervasive pattern of inflexibility and perfectionism
Pathological gambling	Compulsive gambling to release anxiety; experiences pleasure, gratification, or release at the time the act is committed
Kleptomania	Compulsive stealing to release anxiety; experiences pleasure, gratification, or release at the time the act is committed
Pyromania	Compulsive setting of fires to release anxiety; experiences pleasure, gratification, or release at the time the act is committed

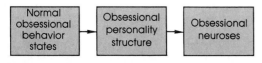

FIGURE 15-2 Obsessional behavior continuum.

The rigid personality has obsessive-compulsive patterns of perfection, *omnipotence,* and *omniscience,* with an overriding need for certainty and absolutes. Mounting anxiety may be released in a variety of syndromes, such as alcoholism, drug addiction, compulsive overeating or undereating (anorexia nervosa), compulsive masturbation, compulsive water drinking, compulsive gambling, compulsive stealing (kleptomania), or compulsive fire-setting (pyromania). In all these situations the person is driven to do the act, but pleasure does not accompany the behavior; only a diminishing of anxiety is felt. Table 15-1 summarizes definitions from the psychoanalytical perspective.

Rigidity mechanisms are defenses against powerlessness and helplessness. When these behavioral devices fail to serve their purpose, the client may experience a total breakdown of integrative capacities resulting in responses such as depression, schizophrenia, paranoia, or grandiose states.

Psychoanalytical theory proposes that conflicts in the anal phase are linked to obsessive symptom development. If the person unsuccessfully represses the anxiety attached to these conflicts and uses sublimation and reaction formation, obsessive and compulsive traits are likely to appear in later life but at a subclinical level.

When repression and sublimation fail, the defense mechanisms of *isolation,* undoing, reaction formation, and denial occur, in that order. With isolation the person separates feelings associated with a thought, as in the following case example.

▼ Case Example

Jay had repeated thoughts that his family was dead, but his reaction was unemotional. He effectively isolated the ordinary feelings that accompany such overwhelming loss. Unaware of the meaning behind such thoughts, he was annoyed with their intrusiveness and wished to be rid of them.[51] Jay will continue using isolation as long as his anxiety is minimized by its presence. When isolation fails, other defense mechanisms will replace it.

Rado[68] elaborated on Freud's theories regarding behavioral rigidity. He considered obsessions and compulsions to be overactive disorders. The person's emotions inflict damage rather than serve as emergency signals. Rado supported Freud's hypothesis that the cause of behavioral rigidity is the "battle of the chamber pot." The child responds to the demands for bowel training with enraged defiance and to the parent's punishments or threats with fearful obedience. Making the child feel guilty for not obeying becomes the parent's means of control.[51] This guilt creates a fearful conscience that demands perfection, repentance, or reparations known as expiratory behaviors (Figure 15-3) (see Chapter 12).

Biological

Increasingly, researchers have explored the relationship between rigid behaviors and biological causes and biochemical changes. For example, some theorists speculate that rigidity is associated with increased autonomic arousal. At this time whether the arousal is the cause or the result of rigid behaviors is difficult to ascertain.[8] Cases have been documented of obsessive-compulsive individuals who met DSM-III-R criteria who had elevated cerebrospinal fluid cor-

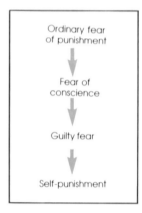

FIGURE 15-3 Steps in the development of expiratory behavior.

tisol levels.[85] Head injuries have also been identified as a probable contributor to the development of obsessive-compulsive neuroses.[59]

Rigid clients' diets have been studied. Hypoglycemia secondary to an inappropriate diet has been documented as causing obsessive behavior that cleared when a high-protein diet was administered.[70]

Blood type O may be associated with a decreased development of obsessive-compulsive symptomatology.[69] OCDs have been linked to neurological illness and depression. Electroencephalogram (EEG) changes have been consistent with temporal lobe epilepsy, indicating that this disorder may be associated with a brain disease. Specifically, a lesion in the limbic system has been theorized.[47]

Consideration has been given to genetic factors as a cause of obsessive-compulsive disorders. The results of a study of the relatives of children with obsessive-compulsive disorder showed a higher incidence of the disorder in the children's relatives (see research highlight on p. 290).

Interpersonal

Sullivan's concept of the self-system is relevant to rigid behaviors. The self-system encompasses all the energies and behaviors that an individual devotes to avoiding anxiety or increasing self-esteem and security. As the self-system forms, the person's emotional investment seems to be in maintaining that system, not in changing it. Security operations effectively steer the individual away from anxiety provoking situations, so the self-system becomes difficult to change. Three security operations are closely linked to rigidity: selective inattention, false personifications, and sublimation[51,81] (see Chapter 4).

Behavioral

Behavioral therapists focus on changing the observable behavior, ignoring the inner conflicts and motivations. The emotional reaction to danger is based on the person's appraisal of his own coping efforts. When confronted with anything perceived as a threat, rigid individuals are more upset than "normal" individuals. They believe that magical thinking will alter feared outcomes. Rather than confronting their anxiety feelings directly, they prefer to use rituals.

RESEARCH HIGHLIGHT

Psychiatric Disorders in First Degree Relatives of Children and Adolescents with Obsessive-Compulsive Disorder

- M Lenane, S Swedo, H Leonard, D Pauls, W Scery, and J Rapòport

PURPOSE

This study sought to determine the type and extent of psychiatric disorders in relatives of those with childhood obsessive-compulsive disorder (OCD).

SAMPLE

Forty-six consecutive admissions to the National Institutes of Mental Health's (NIMH) study of seven clients with primary childhood OCD were the subjects. Inclusion criteria were rituals and/or repetitive thoughts that were deemed unreasonable by the patients and experienced as distressful causing significant interferences at home, school or interpersonal functioning. Subjects ranged in age from 6 to 18 years (29 boys and 17 girls). The mean age of onset was 10.5, with a mean duration of 3.76 years. All parents but three fathers were interviewed and 98% of siblings aged 6 and older participated.

METHODOLOGY

Multiple instruments were used to diagnose possible disorders and symptoms. All are listed in this chapter's table of instruments (see Table 15-3).

Based on data from: *Journal of American Academy of Child and Adolescent Psychiatry* 29(3): 407, 1990.

FINDINGS

A higher incidence of psychiatric disorders was reported in relatives of clients with childhood OCD, thus suggesting a genetic factor in OCD. Fifteen of the 90 parents (17%) were diagnosed with OCD. Fathers were three times as likely as mothers to be affected. Subclinical OCD was comparable for fathers (13%) and mothers (13%). Three siblings (5%) met criteria for OCD and two (3%) for subclinical OCD. Twenty (45%) fathers and 30 (65%) mothers received a non-OCD Axis I diagnosis. The predominant non-OCD diagnoses were mood disorders, alcoholism, and anxiety disorder. Twenty-one (36%) siblings had non-OCD psychiatric diagnoses, which included affective disorder, conduct/oppositional disorder, attention deficit disorder, and an anxiety disorder. The largest afflicted OCD parent/OCD child combination was father/son, following the known male dominance of this disorder.

IMPLICATIONS

Once a client has been diagnosed with OCD, the nurse also takes a family history relative to OCD and other psychiatric disorders. Other family members are likely to have OCD and/or other emotional disorders.

Further, loss of control or uncertainty is intolerable and, therefore, feared and avoided. Rigid persons are not necessarily aware of the pattern of appraisal that they are using because the process may be preconscious and usually becomes automatic and intuitive. Figure 15-4 illustrates the rigid and normal patterns of danger appraisal and the likely outcomes.

Rigid disorders, like all other human behaviors, are responses that the individual has learned and selected or chosen to repeat. For example, the individual who compulsively counts has learned that counting fence posts somehow helps allay anxiety. Reinforcement (any event that increases the likelihood of a response being repeated) needs to occur for these behaviors to reappear. The ritualistic behavior relieves some of the anxiety and becomes a reinforcer, even though the relief may be momentary.

Anxiety provoking stimuli, such as unwanted thoughts or frightening situations, become paired with other stimuli. For example, John's sexual thoughts become paired with dirty hands, which leads to frequent hand washing; since the washing did not relieve all his anxiety, he repeats the procedure.

The behaviorists treatment of choice is exposure and response prevention.[89] A number of criticisms and objections have emerged.[44] For example, exposure techniques for fire setting may be dangerous to others. Also, these treatments are beyond the usual financial and people resources available to clients with the problem.

Cognitive

Cognitive structures (understanding, knowledge, or intelligence) designed to achieve equilibrium are organized mental activities. When a fear is perceived, the client organizes the fear response according to his past reactions to similar situations, and one of three results may occur:

1. The structure has responses similar to previous experiences if the fear is congruent with past situations.
2. If the fear has never been mentally processed, the individual does not assimilate it. Usually the response is avoidance or responding without understanding.
3. If conflict occurs between fear and the person's structure, change may result as the person strives to resolve the conflict and retain equilibrium. The change may or may not be healthy; for example, the fearful person may use compulsive rituals.

Working with the fearful individual requires using cognitive conflict therapeutically to produce the desired changes.[66]

Cognitive processes mediate any threat that creates anxiety. The person first evaluates the degree of danger and the available resources for coping with the danger. For example, if a person perceives someone in authority to be a threat, he decides how he is to behave in the presence of that person. When the individual has no idea what to do in the situation, the problem becomes frightening, whereas knowing what to do makes the problem manageable. Developing rigid responses helps the person maintain control and decrease his anxiety.

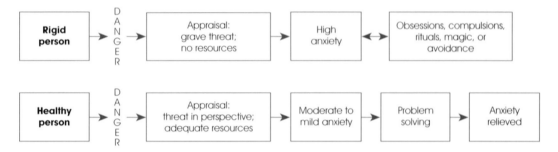

FIGURE 15-4 Paradigm of the rigid person's and the healthy person's appraisal of danger.

Piaget believes that rigid responses are selected and repeated by the client to minimize anxiety.[66] Critics assert that cognitive theories provide a rationale for treatment aimed at only symptom removal. They maintain that the problem is oversimplified.

Table 15-2 summarizes the theories and dynamics of flexibility-rigidity.

NURSING PROCESS

Assessment

Physical dimension The flexible person readily accommodates the ordinary changes that accompany maturation and aging. Daily routines are varied in response to unexpected schedule changes, illnesses, and the changing needs of family members or close friends. Body functions are accepted as natural phenomena and are not the object of undue concern. The flexible person is resilient in the face of adversity. Changes and some disorder are tolerated in the physical environment. A balance exists among concerns for the external world, the sensations and feelings generated within the person, and the more abstract inner thought processes of the person.[51]

The nurse assesses the ease with which the client accomplishes ordinary daily routines to determine how much the activities are bound to rituals. Many clients have lived with their rituals and obsessions for years as identified by behaviorists. Responses to certain key questions indicate whether the nurse needs to explore the responses further. For example, the nurse asks, "How long does it take you to get ready for work?" If the client responds, "Three hours,"

TABLE 15-2 Summary of Theories of Flexibility-Rigidity

Theory	Theorist	Dynamics
Psychoanalytical	Freud	Rigid behaviors result when an individual is fixated at or regresses to an early stage of psychosexual development. Behavior becomes rigid to convey an illusion of control. Defense mechanisms used include isolation, undoing, reaction formation, and denial. Rigidity mechanisms are defenses against powerlessness and helplessness. The rigid person functions effectively in most areas of living.
	Rado	Rigid behaviors are overreactive disorders that cause harm rather than convey that the individual has a problem. Behavioral rigidity begins with the "battle of the chamber pot."
Biological	Beech and Perrigault	Rigidity is associated with autonomic arousal.
	Lieberman	OCDs have been linked to neurological illness and depression.
	Traskman	Obsessive-compulsive people have elevated cerebrospinal fluid cortisol levels.
	Rippere	Hypoglycemia, secondary to an inappropriate diet, causes obsessive behavior.
	Rinieris	Blood type O may hinder the development of obsessive-compulsive personality.
	Jenike	A limbic system lesion has been theorized to cause obsessive-compulsive behavior. EEG changes indicate temporal lobe epilepsy in obsessive-compulsive clients.
Interpersonal	Sullivan	The individual's self-system uses energy and behavior to avoid anxiety or increase self-esteem or security. The rigid person's self-system seems to maintain the system, not change it. Three security operations are linked to rigidity; selective inattention, false personification, and sublimation.
Behavioral	Farkas	The focus is on changing the observable rigid behavior and ignoring inner conflicts and motivations. When confronted with anything perceived as a threat, the rigid person is more upset than "normal individuals."
Cognitive	Piaget	Rigid disorders are viewed as responses the persons selected or chose to repeat to decrease anxiety. The rigid individual's source of threats and anxiety is unacceptable ideas and feelings close to the person's conscious awareness. Cognitive processes assist in determining the severity of anxiety and fear as well as solutions.

this is the cue for further data collection. Most clients do not volunteer information about their obsessions and compulsions unless distressed or asked about them.[40] Even when confronted with the behavior, the client may not evaluate them negatively; this belief supports the maintenance of the disorders.[75]

In addition to questions, direct observation of routines or inquiry about the use of time is necessary to assess the extent of rituals or irrational fears. Rigid clients may repeat tasks such as hand washing or compulsive checking of water faucets or gas stoves and phobic avoidance.[89] Although rare, obsessive slowness can exist, such as taking an hour to brush one's teeth. Often the obsessions and compulsions occur in clusters involving washing, checking, thoughts of the past, and embarrassing behavior.[47] Even when the disability becomes more public, the client often has enough successful modes of functioning to maintain a job and prevent hospitalization. However, the quality of family life is often affected.

The person's health history reveals characteristic patterns of adapting to the shifting demands of life such as illnesses associated with stress and change. Some illnesses such as ulcerative colitis have been associated with the obsessional personality.[67] Repeated and exaggerated concerns about illness, such as cancer, AIDS, tuberculosis, or a cold, can prompt the person to seek unnecessary physical examinations and even multiple surgical treatments. Abuse of vitamins, herbal preparations, and over-the-counter medications can also occur. Medication histories including past and present use of drugs provide useful information about the rigid client's health behaviors.

Deficits in self-care may result from behavioral patterns that interfere with daily living. The obsessive-compulsive client is especially vulnerable to dietary deficiencies due to overeating or undereating.

Cleanliness can require hours and take priority over all activities. For example, a strange paradox exists in some rigid individuals who maintain scrupulous cleanliness in the bathroom, but who leave the remainder of the house in a chaotic mess with food encrusted on utensils in the kitchen and months of dust accumulated in other rooms. The person may manifest this same scrupulous behavior in his manner of dress.

According to behavioral theory, the rigid person develops rituals to diminish anxiety. The nurse observes and questions to determine the presence of rituals. The person may develop elaborate rituals around food preparation, paying mailed bills, eating, getting up, or preparing for bed. These activities, which need to be performed in a certain sequence, can consume nearly all of the client's waking hours. Any break in the routine usually means that the procedure is begun again until it is perfectly executed.[51]

The person feels inner resistance (rejects or disowns the impulse) and may even consider the act senseless but finds it necessary to complete. The most frequent forms of compulsions are cleaning (hand washing) and checking (making sure everything is turned off or locked). Males are more frequently checkers, and females are more frequently washers.[43]

When assessing the physical dimension of people with rigid behaviors, the nurse needs to consider the severity and type of dysfunctional behavior. Specific physical problems result from some stereotyped, rigid behaviors. Most frequently encountered in compulsive clients is dermatological problems. Repeated hand washing may lead to a skin surface breakdown. Chronic dry skin may occur from too frequent showering. Dermatitis, skin lesions, and chemical reactions to soap may be present. The client may also report physical problems such as fatigue, symptoms of anxiety, anorexia, nausea, diarrhea, sweating, paresthesia, and palpitations.

Normal eating and sleeping routines may be disrupted by phobias or premorbid obsessional thoughts. The dread of dying while asleep may cause insomnia. Wanting to maintain control may cause the client to have difficulty going to sleep.[42,84] From a cognitive perspective, the nurse assesses behaviors and thoughts the client uses to minimize anxiety.

The client's body language is revealing. The inflexible person often has a stiff body posture with muscle tightness. The arms are frequently crossed as if to shut out everyone. The facial expression is likely to reflect few emotions.

The nurse needs to be aware that rigid clients with problems of impulse control such as stealing, gambling, or fire setting may be a hazard to other clients during hospitalization. Precautions may be necessary to protect the rigid client and others. Assessment includes determining if the client has matches or other fire-setting paraphernalia and limiting access to items used as cigarettes or fuel. Agency policies on smoking, playing card games, and keeping personal items such as lighters may need to be reviewed and altered to ensure the safest possible environment.

Emotional dimension Using psychoanalytical theory, the nurse assesses the client's anxiety level and the presence of obsessions, compulsions, and phobias. Increasingly, these disorders are not seen in isolation. OCDs do occur in combination with other health problems such as mental retardation,[60] Tourette's syndrome,[71,86] catatonia,[36] post-abortion,[58] and panic.[12]

Problematic, rigid behaviors are often in close association with other emotional difficulties. Therefore the nurse assesses for the presence of associated emotional problems as well as rigid behaviors. To enhance success, associated problems, such as depression, need to be treated before the rigid behavior.[43]

Anxiety at the beginning of treatment has been related to the client's response to treatment. With mild anxiety the client is more likely to succeed. High anxiety needs to be reduced before the rigid behavior can be treated because extremely anxious clients are likely to fail.[43]

Severe fears of illness such as cancer or AIDS without any signs of disease and fears of dying when the person is actually in good health are also bases for psychiatric evaluation of obsessive-compulsive characteristics. Observations, examination, and laboratory tests are used to rule out the existence of any actual physical problem as psychiatric treatment is initiated.

Dominated by fears and anxiety that prompt them to seek absolute control over their emotions and environment, rigid persons use only a limited range of normal human potential according to psychoanalytical theory. Described as pseudoplacid (falsely calm), their emotional demeanor seems to be an unaffected, flattened emotional state unless they are confronted with one of their core concerns, as discussed in the following case example.

▼ Case Example

Sharon, an efficient keypunch operator, became upset when a new employee rearranged the office supplies. Sharon "blew up" and insisted that everything be returned to its original place so that she could inventory all supplies every morning and evening. Sharon's co-workers were surprised at Sharon's anger and puzzled that Sharon wanted to inventory supplies because it was not one of her assigned tasks. Her quiet, unassuming manner changed when she perceived that she lost control of her environment. Her co-workers had never seen her behave this way before, but neither had she ever had the amount of anxiety that she was experiencing in the work setting.

Many of the fears and repetitious thoughts that are a part of rigidity may be known to only the sufferer or the immediate family members. Clients are often embarrassed and disgusted by the irrational and senseless nature of their problems, as indicated in the following case example. The client's distress may be shared only after a trusting relationship has been established that clearly indicates unqualified acceptance of the client as a person.[51] These people typically intellectualize their feelings or do not mention them.

▼ Case Example

Although she held an important executive position, Lois recently experienced numerous personal changes and stressors that taxed her ability to adapt. The changes included a move, her son's hospitalization for asthma, her husband's job loss, and the theft of her jewelry. Her new job required that she hear employees' problems. While she was going through the motions of listening to the employees, she had irrational thoughts of "running away" from this work setting. After weeks of this pressure she sought counseling because her feelings frightened her.

When she was asked to describe herself and what frightened her she stated, "These people come to my office with difficult problems. After listening about 5 minutes I feel numb, like this is not real. If I touch my arm I can't feel it. The person is talking, but I can't hear all of it. I've managed to say the right thing and get them out of the office quickly. I'm frightened that someone will find that I feel like I'm falling apart and can't handle the job. I don't think anyone suspects that I feel this way. Please help me."

Intellectual dimension Assessing the client's response to change provides one of the major clues to flexibility. Change is a challenge that may trigger creativity and kindle enthusiasm in the flexible person, but it threatens the rigid individual, who is unable to accept it.

Similar to acceptance of change is the acceptance of differences. The flexible person accepts people with different values, skin color, language, or life-style. This acceptance carries with it a sensitivity to and appreciation of others' feelings based on trust and respect. The flexible person is comfortable with others and has a sense of self-worth and an optimistic outlook. Flexibility provides access to the entire range of human emotions, and this enables the person to express these feelings appropriately.[51] The inflexible person enjoys none of these responses.

Willingness to consider both sides of an issue, to change plans, and to be open to self-scrutiny demonstrates flexible thinking. The nurse assesses the client's thinking by getting answers to questions such as the following: How open is the person to new ideas? How able is the person to compromise or to see another's viewpoint?

The nurse assesses the client's interest in hobbies or civic activities, decision-making abilities, or abilities to prioritize or to determine the presence of rigid behaviors. Questions such as, "Do you have repeated thoughts or words that occupy your thinking?" or "Do you frequently forget?" can provide information that the nurse may need to explore further.

Rigid people appear to have a more restricted sphere of interest and knowledge than flexible people, and they are more concrete in their thinking and less introspective.[48] Kline and Cooper[49] found that rigid thinking and rigid personalities were not correlated. Other studies found evidence of concrete thinking when clients focus on the present rather than working toward a future goal. The extremely rigid person is too concerned with controlling the fears and anxieties of the moment to develop any action for the future. The isolation of feelings results in a limited capacity for introspection.[23,51] More frequently, rigid clients have associated cognitive problems such as dissociations,[72] information processing,[80] memory deficits,[79] and ruminations.[75]

Clients with problems of extreme rigidity are often above average in intellect. However, they may have a thinking deficit specific to topics they fear.[87] Clients may also believe that feared outcomes will definitely materialize if they do not protect themselves. They can be incapacitated by even trivial decisions. The need to always be correct and the reluctance to take any kind of risk render them ineffective at most administrative levels or positions requiring responsibility for decisions. If they are required to arrive at a decision, their solution includes finding a rule or policy to follow.

Rigid clients may appear preoccupied or have difficulty concentrating. They may be preoccupied with hoarding money or making lists like lists of everyone a client knows, what he has done each day, or to whom he has spoken. It is difficult for them to establish priorities. They may have doubt about their work and their decisions. Their thinking may be illogical. At home, work, or school, they may mismanage their time, especially if they have compulsive behaviors such as the woman who can't leave the driveway for work without going back into the house several times to check if the curling iron is off, "even though I know it is off." Some have reported resisting thinking by occupying their minds with counting real or imaginary items or being overcommitted to activities, projects, or unnecessary details such as the father who could not leave any store magazine rack without rearranging all the magazines in the rack.

Social dimension The nurse assesses the client's social networks and satisfaction with these relationships. A person's flexibility enables him to establish varied relationships with diverse degrees of closeness and to change the responses to these relationships over time. Success in establishing an intimate, lasting relationship suggests a certain amount of flexibility. Flexibility permits an individual to sustain a balance in dependent as well as independent relationships.

Another assessment area concerns the person's flexibility in social roles. This flexibility is important, as one's total identity can become submerged in one's primary role. Examples of types of inflexible persons can be the general, the scientist, the professor who responds to all situations as a professional, or the mother who responds to all situations as a mother, rather than as a person with a unique identity and who understands the differences in her many roles. Family members can provide information about the individual's flexibility in relating to others in varied situations.

Rigid individuals tend to have restricted social contacts, and their relationships are characterized by aloofness and superficial involvement. Their ruminations and morbid thoughts often lead to compulsive avoidance of others.[21] Assessing the individual's social network reveals few contacts, usually limited to family members and co-workers. Their social impairment covers all areas of their lives including involvement with others during their leisure time and activities. The person whose life is circumscribed by fears and repetitive behavior may devote all his energy to these symptoms, leaving no time for social contacts. When asked, these individuals deny that their rituals affect social functioning, but they may express loneliness in their relationships (see Chapter 21 for further information on loneliness). Recreational activities may be entirely missing or may be pursued ritualistically, suggesting that the goal is to achieve rather than to relax and enjoy. Even in recreation the obsessive individual is driven by the belief that one "should" relax as seen in the following case example.

▼ Case Example

Colby, a market analyst, has not taken a vacation in over 10 years. He is meticulous in his work and insists that employees do likewise. His children call him "stoneface"; rarely have they seen him display emotions such as fear or joy. His wife complains that no household repairs ever get done; he gets too bogged down in details.

The nurse assesses the individual's satisfaction with his sexual behavior. About one third of the obsessive compulsive individuals report obsessions related to sexual themes. Their symptomatology, such as obsessions about odors and bodily secretions interfered with their ability to relax and experience sexual satisfaction.[26]

Assessing the family is essential for quality care of a rigid individual. Frequently, the entire family is involved in maintaining the rituals because to do otherwise would precipitate unbearable anxiety in the afflicted member and create retribution and chaos within the family. Therefore knowing how the family functions and the role that each member plays in relation to the rigid person is important. Often the entire family is controlled by the member's idiosyncratic needs. A spouse can describe how the rigid person relates to her.

A *Samson's complex* has been identified where the client has compulsions to reenact betrayal and rage in close relationships. The person compulsively rages in response to others' behaviors.[50] Rigid people have a need to repeat trauma and victimization with significant others.[88] Major contributors to the development of OCDs are the unmet parental symbiotic needs of the child combined with perfectionistic family interaction styles.[39,51] Assessment includes obtaining information about the frequency and intensity of anger, themes of "poor me," and amount and resolution of the individual's crises.

In the work setting, compulsion or overachieving may be evident. Clients may complain of chronic job dissatisfaction or may fear success and unconsciously manifest behavior such as lateness or not meeting deadlines, which ensures that there will be no promotions.

Although some clients with rigid behaviors may be involved with antisocial behavior such as fire setting and shoplifting, they do not readily admit it. Even when caught they usually deny wrongdoing. In their minds, according to psychoanalytical theory, the act makes them feel better or helps someone else.

Cultural background needs to be assessed, since preliminary studies show ethnic groups such as the Irish are more likely to be obsessive. In addition, marital status and geographical location are influences: Bachelors and women living in rural areas without outside employment are more likely to be obsessional. The common factor among all three groups (the Irish; unemployed, rural women; bachelors) is their emotional or geographical isolation.

The nurse assesses the avoidance patterns used by people since those with rigid behaviors may abandon most of their friends and compromise personal aspirations. Even though they define their behaviors as self-defeating, they rationalize what they are doing as necessary and become skillful at inventing excuses so that others will not be aware of their fears. This tendency is illustrated in the following case example.

▼ Case Example

Even when her anxiety was minimal, Betty, an accountant, washed her hands 10 times before and after she ate. To hide this behavior, she did not date, did not invite people to her apartment, and did not eat with her co-workers. She believed she was effective at work and did not need to socialize with her colleagues to be good at her job.

Although Betty could do her job well she would probably be viewed more effectively and obtain more co-worker cooperation if she did not isolate herself. Her compulsions affected her social contacts as well as her overall job performance.

Spiritual dimension Assessment incorporates information about the client's religious beliefs; religious practices; creative outlets; and attitude toward self, others, and life in general. A flexible person develops a philosophy that guides conduct. His religious or philosophical convictions are personally satisfactory and can be used as a source of strength and self-renewal. Flexibility enables an unsatisfied person to search for a fulfilling faith.

Rigid people tend to profess faith in a supernatural power who is obeyed without thinking or questioning. This type of client seems to draw an imaginary box around his spiritual self and is intolerant if the lines are crossed. Religious principles are often accepted literally rather than investigated for philosophical or historical significance. Scrupulous moral standards or religious practices are very important and rigidly followed, often resulting in an unwillingness to recognize the validity of differing faiths.[51]

Similarities have been found between religious compulsions (such as compulsively attending church services or obsessively praying) and the obsessive-compulsive personality.[32,38]

Rigid adherence to religious and ethical beliefs creates guilt and feelings of inadequacy for many inflexible people. They set exceedingly high standards for themselves and for others; then, with failure, they are left guilty and disillusioned. Their need for perfection also makes it impossible for them to forgive themselves or others. (See Chapter 12 for further information about guilt.)

Thus in assessing the spiritual dimension the nurse needs to understand clients' meanings and perceptions of their faith. Are their beliefs a source of comfort or primarily a rigid demand for compliance? Does their faith offer hope and tolerance for others instead of judgmental attitudes? In what activities unrelated to compulsive behavior do they participate for spiritual fulfillment?[51]

Measurement tools

Numerous scales have been developed to determine varying facets of flexibility and rigidity. Table 15-3 summarizes the more common scales.

▼ **TABLE 15-3** **Instruments to Measure Flexibility-Rigidity**

Instruments	Measures
California F Scale[1]	Antisemitism and ethnocentrism (rigid thinking)
Gough-Sanford's Rigidity Scale[15]	Resistance to habit change and preference for order and detail
Obsessional Scales[55,57]	Self-reporting presence of obsessions
Gibb's Scale[29]	Degree of obsessive-compulsive traits
Sandler-Hazari Obsessionality Inventory[25]	Obsessional traits and symptoms in clinical and nonclinical populations
Hopkins Psychiatric Rating Scale[61]	Obsessive-compulsive judgments
Crown-Crisp Experimental Index[61]	Diagnostic information about obsessions
SCL-90-R Brief Symptom Inventory[61]	Obsessive-compulsive dimension
Leyton Obsessional Inventory[17,62]	Presence of obsessions in adults
Leyton Obsessional Inventory-Childhood Version[10]	Presence of obsessions in children
Yale-Brown Obsessive Compulsive Scale[30,31]	Severity of obsessive-compulsive symptoms that is not influenced by the type of obsessions or compulsions present; uses interview format
NIMH Clinical Global Obsessive Compulsive Scale[63]	Presence of obsessions and compulsions
Comprehensive Psychopathological Rating Scale, OCD Subscale[5]	Severity of obsessive-compulsive disorder symptoms including rituals and obsessions

Analysis
Nursing diagnosis

Fear is a nursing diagnosis approved by NANDA that applies to the rigid person. The defining characteristics of this nursing diagnosis are listed in the box below. The following case example illustrates the characteristics of the nursing diagnosis of fear.

▼ Case Example

Evelyn is a 30-year-old married administrative assistant. She sought a nurse counselor 1 month after her car was totalled. Her peace of mind was devastated, and she was preoccupied with the circumstances of the wreck. She was washing her hands "too many times to count" each day.

Although she had functioned successfully at work, her competence and job performance were decreasing due to the handwashing. She repeatedly told her co-workers that she was afraid to be in a car or any moving vehicle. Inwardly, she became frightened by her irrationality, and she became panicky as she feared the humiliation she would experience when others learned the truth. She had difficulty concentrating and recalling promises. When discussing her lack of concentration and poor recall, she appeared as if she were in control because she could identify that her problems were the result of her car wreck.

Evelyn also worried about her diminished activities as she forced herself to avoid cars. She lived 3 miles from her job and walking consumed considerable time.

▼ **FEAR**

DEFINITION

Feeling of dread related to an identifiable source that the person validates.

DEFINING CHARACTERISTICS

• **Physical dimension**

Wide-eyed
Attack behavior
Fight behavior-aggressive
Sympathetic stimulation-cardiovascular excitation, superficial vasoconstriction, pupil dilation

• **Emotional dimension**

Increased tension
Apprehension
Afraid
Scared
Terrified
Panicked
Frightened
Jittery

• **Intellectual dimension**

Impulsiveness
Increased alertness
Concentration on source
Focus on "it, out there"

• **Social dimension**

Decreased self-assurance
Flight behavior-withdrawal

Modified from Kim MI, McFarland GK, and McLane AM, *Pocket guide to nursing diagnosis,* ed 5, St Louis, 1993, Mosby–Year Book.

The following list provides examples of NANDA accepted nursing diagnoses with causative statements:

1. Ineffective individual coping: excessive handwashing related to anxiety
2. Ineffective individual coping: compulsive faucet checking related to loss of support secondary to recent death of spouse
3. Fear of contamination by germs related to guilt
4. Sleep pattern disturbance related to ruminating thoughts of dying in sleep
5. Ineffective family coping related to lack of ability to accommodate client's rigid behaviors
6. Noncompliance related to obsessive thinking
7. Altered thought processes: obsessive fear of death related to distorted perceptions about hospitalization
8. At risk for impairment in skin integrity: skin lesions related to frequent handwashing

Planning

See Table 15-4 for a nursing care plan with long-term and short-term goals, nursing interventions, outcome criteria, and rationales related to fear.

Implementation

Physical dimension Initially, the nurse needs to determine the length of time she may be working with the client to change rigid behaviors. Caution is urged if the time is short because working with the rigid client usually requires a long time. Change without appropriate support can cause this client's defenses to disintegrate. If the nurse does not have the time or the expertise, she needs to provide a supportive role rather than intervening directly.

The nurse reduces demands on the client when there is evidence of increasing tension such as agitation or escalation of ritualistic behavior. Medications may be ordered, especially during acute periods, when the client is near panic. Interventions include administering the medications as ordered and observing for side effects. Self-management techniques for controlling anxiety are preferable when possible. (See Chapter 10 for further information about anxiety.)

Antidepressant medications have been used with some success for depressed clients with obsessions, because depression appears to accelerate or maintain obsessive symptoms.[37,56] Antidepressants seem to have a primary effect of reducing the depression and a secondary effect of reducing obsessions. The nurse observes hospitalized clients for medication side effects and teaches outpatient clients to observe for side effects in their health regimens.

Numerous studies indicate that significant improvement in obsessive-compulsive symptoms may be seen with the use of clomipramine (Anafranil), even in nondepressed clients. The accompanying profile describes nursing care appropriate to the administration of clomipramine. Clients are told that the medication must be taken as ordered and that it may need to be taken for the rest of the client's life. Studies have reported that 35% to 42% of adults and 37% of children and adolescents improved while taking this drug.[*]

The nurse allows time for the hospitalized client to perform needed rituals. Some routine nursing activities can be

---

[*]References 19, 33, 37, 46, 64, 74.

▼ **TABLE 15-4   NURSING CARE PLAN**

GOALS	OUTCOME CRITERIA	INTERVENTIONS	RATIONALES
NURSING DIAGNOSIS: Fear of traveling in cars related to obsessive preoccupation with circumstances of recent car wreck			
LONG TERM			
To minimize fear of traveling in car	Voices fear associated with traveling in car	Encourage client to identify and discuss fears	Recognition and discussion will decrease anxiety
	Participates in desensitization therapy for 6 weeks	Refer for desensitization therapy	Desensitization will minimize or eliminate the thoughts
	Drives car by self in 6 weeks	Encourage client to drive	Driving the car will decrease fear and increase feeling of security
SHORT TERM			
To decrease preoccupation 1 month after beginning therapy	Verbalizes realistic aspects of the wreck	Assist to explore realistic aspects of wreck	Decreases irrational thinking
	Talks about car wreck less than twice a week	Teach to use thought-stopping techniques when unwanted thoughts occur	Helps limit preoccupation and increase feeling of control
	Substitutes relaxation as a response to obsessive thinking	Teach relaxation techniques; assist to imagine being free of obsessive thoughts	May motivate to change behavior
	Participates in social activities of interest	Encourage to become involved in social activities	Decreases time for obsessive thinking

CLOMIPRAMINE

(klom-ip′ra-meen)
Anafranil
Func. class.: Tricyclic
antidepressant
Chem. class.: Tertiary amine

Action: Not known. Potent inhibitor of serotonin uptake, also increases dopamine metabolism
Uses: Depression, dysphoria, phobias, anxiety, agoraphobia, obsessive-compulsive disorder
Dosage and routes:
Obsessive-compulsive disorder
▶ *Adult:* PO 25 mg hs and increase gradually over 4 wk to a dose of 75-300 mg/day in divided doses
▶ *Child (10-18 yr):* PO 50 mg/day gradually increased; not to exceed 200 mg/day
Depression
▶ *Adult:* PO 50-150 mg/day in a single or divided dose
Anxiety/agoraphobia
▶ *Adult:* PO 25-75 mg/day
Available forms include: Caps 25, 50, 75 mg
Side effects/adverse reactions:
HEMA: **Agranulocytosis, neutropenia, pancytopenia**
CV: Hypotension, tachycardia, **cardiac arrest**

CNS: Dizziness, tremors, mania, seizures, aggressiveness
ENDO: Galactorrhea, hyperprolactinemia
META: Hyponatremia
GI: Constipation, dry mouth
GU: Delayed ejaculation, anorgasmia, retention
INTEG: Diaphoresis
Contraindications: Pregnancy, hypersensitivity
Precautions: Seizures, suicidal patients
Pharmacokinetics: Extensively bound to tissue and plasma proteins, demethylated in liver (active metabolites), excreted in urine (metabolites); half-life: 21 hr parent compound, 36 hr metabolite
Interactions/incompatibilities:
—Hypotensive antagonism: bethanidine
—Toxicity: phenothiazines, cimetidine
—Ethanol reaction: disulfiram, guanadrel increased or decreased effects
—Increased or decreased effects of clomipramine: estrogens
—Delirium: ethchlorvynol
—Hypertensive crisis, convulsions, hypertensive episode: MAOIs

—Decreased seizure threshold: phenytoin, phenobarbital

NURSING CONSIDERATIONS
Assess:
—B/P (lying, standing), pulse q4h; if systolic B/P drops 20 mm Hg withhold drug, notify physician; take vital signs q4h in clients with cardiovascular disease
—Blood studies: CBC, leukocytes, differential, cardiac enzymes if patient is receiving long-term therapy
—Hepatic studies: AST, ALT, bilirubin, creatinine
Administer:
—Increased fluids, bulk in diet if constipation, urinary retention occur
—With food or milk for GI symptoms
—Gum, hard candy, or frequent sips of water for dry mouth
Perform/provide:
—Storage in tight container at room temperature, do not freeze
—Assistance with ambulation during beginning therapy since drowsiness/dizziness occurs
—Safety measures, including side rails, primarily in elderly
—Checking to see PO medication swallowed

Evaluate:
—Mental status: mood, sensorium, affect, suicidal tendencies; increase in psychiatric symptoms: depression, panic
—Urinary retention, constipation; constipation is more likely to occur in children
—Withdrawal symptoms: headache, nausea, vomiting, muscle pain, weakness; do not usually occur unless drug is discontinued abruptly
—Alcohol consumption; if alcohol is consumed, withhold dose until morning
Teach client/family:
—That the effects may take 2-3 wk
—To use caution in driving or other activities requiring alertness because of drowsiness, dizziness, blurred vision
—To avoid alcohol ingestion, other CNS depressants
—Not to discontinue medication quickly after long-term use, may cause nausea, headache, malaise
Lab test interferences:
Increase: Prolactin, TBG
Decrease: Serum thyroid hormone
Treatment of overdose: ECG monitoring, induce emesis, lavage, activated charcoal, administer anticonvulsant

Italic indicates common side effects.
Bold italic indicates life-threatening reactions.

Modified from Skidmore-Roth L: *Mosby's nursing drug reference,* St. Louis, 1993, Mosby–Year Book.

modified to accommodate the client's needs. The extremely ritualistic person may require prompting to eat meals on time or to meet specific appointments. Patience and tolerance are required to relate to the client bound by fears or rigidity. Waiting for the completion of ritualistic and compulsive behavior can be frustrating. The person's need to control everything can cause the nurse to feel manipulated into responding to irrational demands.[51]

Clients who wash their hands or shower frequently may require skin protection. Lotions, topical medications, or gloves can provide some protection for hand washers; and clients may need reminders to use prescribed soaps and lotions. Harsh soaps are eliminated so that the client does not continue to irritate the vulnerable skin surface. The client needs to be reminded to thoroughly dry the wet skin, especially when irritation is present or in cold weather.

Obsessions may be somatic. For example, fear of contracting cancer or the obsession that cancer has developed is best dealt with by not focusing on it. After examination to ensure that no pathological condition is present, diversion to activities that interest the client or a matter-of-fact acceptance of the complaints is indicated.[51]

Emotional dimension Rigidity demands tolerance, understanding, and acceptance by the nurse and significant others. Pressuring clients to hurry or to make decisions creates anxiety that results in increased rigidity. Familiar routines provide a reassuring structure. Discussing the situations and the accompanying feelings while encouraging clients to confront the problems that have compromised their ability to function is reassuring and can decrease anxiety.[51]

Since theories of causation differ, therapy sessions also differ. Because psychoanalytical theorists believe that obsessive-compulsive problems occur as a result of unresolved conflicts in the anal stage of development, the nurse assesses childhood experiences. Using the cognitive model, the nurse focuses on the individual's evaluation or cognitive appraisal of the threatening ideas or feelings that are central to the major symptoms. Since the person's belief system can be elicited by the nurse's focusing on self-statements and beliefs about the problem area, treatment such as desensitization is shorter and more direct than the psychoanalytical approach.[78]

With the nurse's assistance, clients need to first learn to

recognize the existence of feelings such as anger, guilt, and loneliness before discovering the presence of and expressing appropriately their own feelings. For example, the client may not initially realize that anger is an appropriate response to criticism by a friend. In an effort to avoid conflict and maintain a "nice" image the client may deny his anger and not acknowledge the criticism. The client needs to know first that anger exists and then learn how to recognize its presence within himself before therapeutically working with the anger. By being available and supportive, especially during periods of anxiety or an escalation of ritualistic behavior, the nurse can encourage the client's expression of independent feelings and reward any initiative for dealing with feelings, as illustrated in the following case example.

▼ Case Example

Kevin was critical of everyone because he missed an occupational activity which he enjoyed. As his anger and anxiety increased, he began rubbing his hands together rapidly. This be-

havior had recently been extinguished. The nurse who was working with Kevin sat down and they discussed the situation together. Kevin was asked to describe his feelings. After some hesitancy he said he felt left out and that no one cared enough to tell him that he missed the activity. The nurse pointed out that Kevin's behaviors indicated anger and resentment. She told Kevin that these emotions were related to feeling rejected. The nurse also mentioned the progress he had made in describing his feelings. Within the hour his hand rubbing decreased and it was not present 5 hours later.

Kevin may need many experiences like the one described in the case example. With patience and understanding the nurse assists Kevin to verbalize his emotions. Rigid clients have spent many years unaware of their internal self. Self-awareness is the foundation of their behavioral changes.

Current treatment methods for obsessions and compulsions can be divided into two types: (1) exposure procedures designed to reduce the anxiety related to obsessions and (2) blocking or punishing procedures developed to

▼ TABLE 15-5 Definitions and Examples of Treatment Methods

Term	Definition	Example
Imaginal flooding	Repeatedly recalling situations in the mind precipitate undesired behavior	A client recalls an image in his mind of a high wall as he learns to conquer his fear of heights. He repeats the image, often combined with relaxation, until anxiety is minimized.
Satiation	Designed to decrease potency of a reinforcer	The compulsive eater is placed before a large table of food and must eat until the compulsive desire is gone. The schedule is repeated until he no longer acts out his compulsive behavior with eating.
Thought stopping	Self-induced technique to stop undesired thoughts	A client actively recalls an unwanted thought and commands himself to "stop" at the same time he relaxes. The procedure is repeated until he satisfactorily stops the undesired thought.
Aversion therapy	Use of stimuli designed to create repulsion following undesired behavior	Disulfiram (Antabuse) is given to an alcoholic client to induce nausea when he drinks alcohol.
Modeling	Imitation as a method of behavior change	The nurse demonstrates the desired social skill that the client wishes to adopt, for example, introducing someone in a social situation.
Behavioral rehearsal	A rehearsal situation that simulates role-playing; client rehearses new responses to problem situations after learning new adaptive responses portrayed through modeling	The client rehearses the social skill (for example, answering the phone) that causes an anxiety response. The client is taught by the nurse until he can do the skill without using the undesired behavior.
Social reinforcement	Positive reinforcement to new behavior; both behaviors occur in a social setting important to client	The client demonstrates the changed behavior (for example, answers the phone and talks coherently without stuttering) and is complimented for his ability to do this by those who knew he had difficulty with the behavior.
In vivo exposure	Placing client in an artificial situation that resembles the real situation causing problematic behavior	The client who fears bridges is shown a video that mimics going over a bridge in a car. The situation is combined with a method (for example, relaxation or thought stopping) designed to prevent the undesired behavior. The client can view this situation as safer and able to be controlled.
Flooding	Repeated exposure to a situation that causes the undesired behavior; client is not to stop the exposure scheduling	The client is repeatedly driven down a street that causes anxiety until he no longer fears the street. Usually this approach is combined with a relaxation method to assist the client in changing the undesired behavior.

decrease the frequency of either obsessive thoughts or compulsive behaviors. Exposure procedures use systematic desensitization (see Chapter 10) and prolonged exposure to feared cues. Blocking or punishing procedures consist of thought stopping, aversion therapy, and covert sensitization. The last two have proved the most successful. Table 15-5 gives further definitions and examples.

Using desensitization, the client outlines the behaviors associated with the feared event, such as fear of bridges. The process uses a combination of techniques including guided imagery, relaxation, positive self-talk, and other anxiety reducing techniques as needed. Either with the assistance of a counselor or using a self-help product, such as a book, workbook, or audiotape, the client outlines and rehearses each behavior, first verbally and then mentally. For example, the client imagines successfully completing each step of going over a nearby bridge in a car without any associated feelings of fear. If fear is felt during the mental rehearsal, the client is encouraged to use relaxation immediately. The rehearsal is repeated until relaxation is automatically used when the fear is felt.

The final desensitization occurs when the client applies the mentally rehearsed behavior. First, using a support person who serves as a coach, the activity is attempted at a time most likely to ensure success. For example, attempting to cross a bridge during peak traffic when there is a strong chance the car may creep or stop on the bridge would not be conducive to successful desensitization. Finally, the client performs the behavior without a significant other. Allowing time for repeated attempts and providing rewards important to the client during each phase of the process promotes the likelihood that the new behaviors will quickly become habit. The new positive behavior is then associated with the bridge crossing; the healthy response replaces the unhealthy response. The goal is to see the client freed from the incapacitating affects of the fears. Desensitization has been used quite successfully; it does take time, energy, commitment, and work. A hopeful attitude from the nurse encourages clients to use this relatively inexpensive treatment method.

Verbal support may help when the person becomes anxious, but modeling calmness and empathy provides a more meaningful message. Praise helps as the ritualistic behavior decreases. If possible, the nurse provides opportunities for the client to talk with someone who has been successful in overcoming similar problems. Often persons with fears believe they are the only ones who are so fearful.[51] Being in a support group with others who have ritualistic behavior minimizes their isolation.

Changing rigid behavior can take up to several months as the client struggles to move from an intellectual to an emotional understanding of behavior. Even though repetition may be tiring, the nurse repeats insights often and in different ways to assist the client therapeutically.

The client may be tempted to end therapy when some anxiety has diminished within the first few sessions. The nurse encourages the client to continue therapeutic sessions because he needs long-term counseling to experience permanent, beneficial changes.

Treatment for both fire setting and stealing can be similar. A newly developed technique of line graphing has been helpful in sequentially correlating external stress, behavior,

and feelings. For example, a child fire setter is requested to discuss his feelings and behavior before, during, and after a recent fire-setting episode. Feelings and behaviors are graphed with the child present to visually represent the situation; this assists the child to see the cause-and-effect relationship between feelings and behavior. The child is then given a choice of adaptive responses other than setting fires. Graphing helps the child observe his feelings and provides strategies to interrupt the fire-setting act before it occurs.[14]

Intellectual dimension Using a cognitive approach, the nurse can offer the client new ways to view the core problem. Alternative responses to the problem forms the basis for developing effective coping skills. For example, a client has obsessive thoughts that a co-worker is her enemy; the nurse helps her consider other possible ways to interpret the co-worker's behavior.

A time when the client's anxiety is low is the best opportunity for teaching new coping skills. When the person is receptive, the nurse provides only the information about emotional insights that can be assimilated.[51] If the client's anxiety escalates or the person is resistant, it is better not to press the issue. During the relationship, the nurse may also engage in a power struggle with the client. The nurse's own flexibility may be tested by the client's rigid demands and need for control.

Argument and persuasion contribute to a rigid viewpoint, whereas a matter-of-fact presentation of information is more acceptable to the client. Rigid clients are more apt to portray remarkable intellectual understanding of their situation and do not benefit from intellectualization during therapeutic sessions. In fact, intellectualizing only reinforces the behavior that contributes to their denial of internal feelings.

Reviewing the therapeutic session with the client after the session closes is essential for developing insight. The nurse also needs to highlight positive client behaviors. Interactions with the client need to contain both positive and negative statements about the client because the balance and presence of both are important to long-term involvement with a client manifesting rigid behaviors.

The nurse strives to help the client connect intellect and emotions by encouraging related homework between therapy sessions. The client's ruminations may be helpful because he will remember and ponder these assignments. This refocuses ritualistic thinking into a useful tool for the client to become more healthy. For example, the nurse may tell the client to think about the topic of the next session and ask the client to think about and discuss his reaction and feelings about the topic. These clients cannot acknowledge the presence of feelings until they understand that feelings exist in every situation.

A number of behavioral management techniques have been developed in recent years. For example, response prevention keeps the client from ritualistic behavior by distracting his attention, redirecting his activity, or cajoling.[91]

Self-help information relevant to problems of rigidity is available to the general public. One technique that can be self-taught is thought switching, which is briefly outlined in the accompanying box. Another useful technique, thought stopping, is found in Chapter 12.

▼ THOUGHT-SWITCHING TECHNIQUE

Aim: To replace fear-inducing self-instructions with competent self-instructions.

Thought switching involves replacing negative thoughts with positive ones until the positive ones, through practice, become so strong that they replace the anxiety-provoking negative ones. A series of positive thoughts are deliberately strengthened until they override unwanted ones.

The following are steps in thought switching:

1. Recall anxiety associated with the fearful stimuli. List all self-instructions used in the situation. (For example, "As I enter the elevator, people will stare," and "As I enter the elevator, the walls will collapse.") Include small detailed thoughts as well as overwhelming ones.

2. List an opposite set of coping self-instructions. (For example, "As I enter the elevator, I'll tell myself it doesn't matter if people stare," and "As I enter the elevator, I'll tell myself the walls will not collapse.")

3. Put each coping self-instruction on a separate card. Keep cards in a convenient place, such as in a purse, in a pocket, or by the telephone. Their sequence does not matter.

4. Identify a high-frequency activity carried out every day, such as using the telephone, combing hair, or drinking coffee. Each time before the activity is carried out, the top card is read.

5. Use the coping self-instructions in real-life situations.

6. If better self-instructions are developed, use them but do not switch too often. Practice each one frequently enough for it to be useful.

Modified from Fensterheim H, Baer J: *Stop running scared!* New York, 1977, Dell Publishing Co.

Reading materials are likely to be helpful to clients who are moderately dysfunctional. Some clients, however, may read compulsively to gain insight; unless behavior is changed, this is an activity which delays progress. Severely impaired individuals require assistance to implement self-help measures; the family or significant others need to be involved in this treatment.

When the client shows considerable insight into his behavior with manifested changes in living, treatment may stop. The end of therapy is approached with an organized plan, including the review of the client's problem behaviors, the insights achieved, and the remaining tasks.

Social dimension Establishing a significant relationship with a constricted and inflexible person is a challenge. It may not be personally rewarding because the client may expect perfection and voice criticism if the nurse is imperfect. These clients are often as critical of themselves as they are of others. After the nurse establishes a trusting relationship with the client, she encourages interpersonal relationships, for example, by giving the client assignments such as calling a friend or meeting one new person each week. The client may need social skills training to diminish anxiety before he is able to increase the quality or quantity of social contacts. For example, the client may need to role-play telephone skills with a nurse before actually phoning a friend.

When the client's anxiety is low, participation in small group activity is encouraged. Meaningful responsibilities such as committee work, volunteer efforts, or assisting with work at home help thrust the person into social participation. Membership in a self-help group composed of persons with similar problems or in a therapy group can help the client increase social skills.[51]

Family members often experience intense frustration, especially as clients become more socially or occupationally dysfunctional. Impatient to see results, the family may need the nurse's guidance to convey patience while assisting in treating symptoms. In addition, the family may have experienced years of dysfunctional communication patterns and years of protecting the client from anxiety provoking situations. For example, if the client has a time-consuming compulsion such as washing his hands 30 times before leaving the house, this activity is worked into the family's schedules to leave the house. The time problem is compounded if the client must wash his hands at a bathroom sink used by most other family members. If the client's progress is hindered by the home situation, therapeutic intervention such as hospitalization or family therapy may be necessary.

Family members are encouraged to continue contact with the client during hospitalization. The nurse provides contact with both after the client's discharge to promote continuity in care as the family conveys the effect of the client's behavior on their interaction patterns. By sharing with the family the plans and expectations for change, the nurse promotes the family's ongoing involvement in the client's treatment. The home will be the crucial test of the new behavioral changes and will determine whether they will be lifelong.

Encouraging and supporting mature family relationships that provide opportunities for the client to exercise autonomy and independence are useful strategies. Family members often are locked into a pattern in which they foster and maintain the client's dysfunctional behaviors and dependence. Both the client and the family need help to change these dysfunctional patterns.

Various family therapies have had moderate to good success in changing problematic family patterns.[18] In a group setting, family members can discuss decisions to be made, such as how money may be spent or where to go on vacation. The nurse's presence can help them feel freer to explore previously unavailable options. The nurse can interject comments or questions that promote thinking and diverse responses. When one ignores rigid behaviors and concentrates on healthier ones, rigid behaviors can decrease.

Because of societal stigmas associated with compulsive gamblers, kleptomaniacs, and pyromaniacs, clients with an impulse control problem may not be included in social activities. These clients and families may need to develop an individualized social network.

Pathological gamblers may need their economic and job status reviewed for specific interventions that will assure their return as a contributing member of society. Kleptomaniacs may have stolen items accumulated in their home; someone needs to accompany the client and inventory their possessions, returning items when possible. The nurse may work directly with store personnel to assist the client in returning stolen items or making a plan for restitution. The pyromaniac may have destroyed his living area by fire, so the nurse may help find available housing when the client is discharged or refer him to a social worker for further assistance.

Because clients with pyromania or kleptomania may have broken the law by destroying property, stealing, or harming people, the nurse may need to be supportive of these clients when facing legal charges or being sent to jail. The client may be hospitalized temporarily for a court-ordered evaluation. The client with pyromania is never to be taken lightly, as he may be dangerous to himself or others unfortunate enough to be in the buildings he is planning to burn. Valuables need to be secured when accessible to the client with kleptomania.

 Spiritual dimension Rigid clients frequently have a constricted life-style. Typically, they have unrealistic expectations for perfection and become entangled with the religious rules and not with the predominant concepts. Comfort and support is seldom felt by the client's religious practices.

Guilt may absorb the rigid client who is unable to adhere to religious beliefs. The nurse can encourage the client to discuss these superhuman ideals in a factual manner. She can also exhibit acceptance and unconditional regard as she moves the client toward self-acceptance. (See Chapter 12 for additional information about guilt.)

Referral to counselors, ministers, or religious leaders with counseling experience may be necessary to assist these clients in moving from "the letter of the law" practice to a more tolerant and kinder approach toward the self and others. Focusing the client on self-acceptance rather than on changing others' behaviors may require repeated reinforcement.

Obsessions and compulsions may be manifest with self-deprecating religious thoughts and compulsive practices. When the client is hospitalized, the nurse may need to facilitate the compulsive acts. For example, the client may use a rosary and finger the beads throughout a catheterization procedure. Removing the beads without an awareness of the compulsive need can heighten anxiety in the rigid client who requires some control in unfamiliar surround-

ings. Providing a quiet room away from those who may be disturbed by the religious practice will help the rigid client practice his beliefs until they can be altered.

The rigid client may need to relearn personal caretaking in the form of nurturing, especially in the spiritual dimension. Some may have experienced being shamed or "made fun of" when they shared their compulsions or obsessions with others. Once the rigid practices are gone, the clients need continual encouragement to think of their own spiritual needs and to continue actions that meet those needs. Exploring and initiating new choices can be rewarding for rigid clients.[13] See the boxes for key interventions related to flexibility-rigidity and guidelines for prevention.

INTERACTION WITH A COMPULSIVE CLIENT

Nurse: (Approaching hospitalized client who is repeatedly and rapidly washing her hands. It is time for the client's antianxiety medication.) Miss Clark, your medication is ready for you to take.

Client: Okay. (No attempt is offered to stop the activity.)

Nurse: I brought water for you to take with the pill. Here it is. (The medication and pill are handed to the client.)

Client: (The client takes the pill and hands the empty containers to the nurse.) Thanks.

Nurse: I'll be back in 15 minutes so we can talk.

The client is preoccupied with compulsive hand-washing. Compulsive behavior usually temporarily releases the rigid client's anxiety. Rather than interrupting the hand-washing activity and risking a further increase in the client's anxiety, the nurse focused on administering the antianxiety medication rather than directly stopping the hand-washing activity. This is not the time to engage the client in a discussion of her hand-washing ritual, nor does the client need censorship or berating. Usually, rigid clients are well aware of the absurdity of their behaviors; they need help in associating their feelings with their actions. The nurse wisely allows the medication some time to be effective before exploring with the client those thoughts or activities preceding the hand-washing act. In a matter-of-fact manner,

---

▼ **KEY INTERVENTIONS RELATED TO FLEXIBILITY-RIGIDITY**

Reduce demands on client in response to escalation of ritualistic behavior
Allow time for rituals
Monitor medication regimen
Encourage client to eat meals as scheduled
Allow some control in nurse-client relationship
Provide skin protection, if needed
Assist client to recognize and express feelings of anger
Use systematic desensitization to help client control feelings of fear
Teach effective coping skills
Teach client to connect intellectual and emotional experiences
Encourage constructive relationships
Encourage involvement of family in care
Support mature family interactions
Encourage client to discuss religious ideals

▼ **PRIMARY/TERTIARY PREVENTIONS**

Primary

Teach caregivers the importance of consistent expectations during child rearing
Teach caregivers ways to allow the child to experience some control during bowel training
Teach parents approaches to decreasing anxiety and increasing child's self-esteem

Tertiary

Community resources
Community mental health centers

Self-help groups

Obsessive-compulsive groups
Phobia groups

the nurse approaches the client, truly expecting the client to take the medicine. Adding the choice of when the client wanted the nurse to give the medicine might have further increased the amount of anxiety.

Evaluation

Successful treatment may lead to unscheduled time in the client's day as the obsessions and compulsions are diminished. Time previously devoted to the rituals becomes available for entertainment, relationships, or projects. Clients may need assistance in acquiring new skills and in planning social and occupational activities. Evaluation provides an excellent opportunity to determine new needs for nursing intervention.

Evaluation of the nursing process includes a review of data and the client's and/or family's report on progress made to alleviate obsessions and compulsions. Although the literature indicates that setbacks are common, the nurse conveys hopefulness toward minimizing and eliminating rigid behavior throughout the interactions.

The following essential criteria to evaluate the interventions provide a framework for the nurse:
1. *Adequacy:* Were the symptoms stopped or minimized? Can the client manage the rigid behaviors should they reoccur?
2. *Appropriateness:* Were the interventions specific to the rigid behavior, the client's resources, and the client's life-style? Did the interventions match the client's cognitive abilities? Were significant others involved in the treatment? Were the interventions realistic?
3. *Effectiveness:* Was the client or his family satisfied with the outcomes of the interventions? Can the client or his family handle future episodes of rigid behavior? Can the client now recognize events that may trigger rigid behavior development?
4. *Efficiency:* Were interventions initiated in a timely manner and using the most cost-effective method? Did the client or his family decrease their reliance on the nurse and increase their own abilities to handle rigid behaviors?

The nurse needs to involve the client and his family to maximize the success of interventions. As clients learn new ways to cope with their fears, they are challenged to make new life-style changes.

In working with these long-term clients, the nurse may easily become discouraged with her own interventions. Meaningful employment evaluations that measure achievements by the nurse's activities as well as the client's progress may help provide satisfaction for the nurse.

Measurable goals and outcomes provide data for evaluating the intensity of the rigid behavior, the client's growth in understanding the origins of rigidity, new ways to cope with the problems, and the diminishment or elimination of rigid behaviors.

BRIEF REVIEW

Flexibility and rigidity are reactions to change that can be functional or dysfunctional. Inflexible behaviors alter one's capacities for developing interpersonal relationships and managing daily living. Rigidity, repetition, anxiety, fear, and a driven quality characterize rigid disorders, including OCDs, impulse control disorders, and phobias.

Freud's theories on neuroses influenced psychiatrists to favor psychoanalytical treatment. Learning theories emphasizing cognitive change as a means for altering behaviors are gaining acceptance. A holistic approach to the nursing problems related to rigidity involves a comprehensive assessment of all dimensions of the client's life.

As rigid behaviors have become more prevalent, nurses have become more involved in their direct treatment. Treatment of rigid clients with behavioral interventions rather than psychoanalysis has facilitated this role change for nurses. The bulk of the therapeutic work involves translating the client's intellectual, often profound, insight into emotional understanding and a commitment to change. The future promises expansion of nursing practice into broader care of rigid clients as more is learned about this complex and often distressing problem.

Being aware of one's own feelings, especially anger or frustration, is essential because these emotions can increase the client's anxiety level and exacerbate the symptoms the nurse is working to diminish. Keeping expectations realistic is important because changing extremely rigid behaviors is a difficult and slow process that involves ongoing self-awareness.

REFERENCES AND SUGGESTED READINGS

1. Adorno W and others: *The authoritarian personality,* New York, 1950, Harper & Brothers.
2. Allsopp M, Verduyn C: Adolescents with obsessive-compulsive disorder: a case note review of consecutive patients referred to a provincial regional adolescent psychiatry unit, *Journal of Adolescence* 13(2):157, 1990.
3. American Psychiatric Association: *Diagnostic and statistical manual of mental disorders (DSM-III-R),* ed 3, Washington, DC, 1980, The Association.
4. Apter A and others: Severe obsessive compulsive disorder in adolescence: a report of 8 cases, *Journal of Adolescence* 7(4):349, 1984.
5. Asberg M and others: A comprehensive psychopathological rating scale, *Acta Psychiatrica Scandinavia* 271:5-27, 1978.
6. Ballerini A, Stanghellini G: Phenomelogical questions about obsession and delusion, *Psychopathology* 229(60):315, 1989.
7. Barron-Cohen S: Do autistic children have obsessions and compulsions? *British Journal of Clinical Psychology* 28(Pt 3):193-200, 1989.
8. Beech H, Perrigualt J: Toward a theory of obsessional disorder. In Beech H, editor: *Obsessional states,* London, 1974, Methuen & Co.
9. Berg C and others: Obsessive-compulsive disorder: a two-year prospective follow-up of a community sample, *Journal of American Academy of Child/Adolescent Psychiatry* 28(4):528, 1989.
10. Berg C, Rapaport J, Flament M: The Leyton obsessional inventory-child version, *Journal of American Academy of Child and Adolescent Psychiatry* 25:84, 1986.
11. Berntson G and others: Cardiac reactivity and adaptive behavior, *American Journal of Mental Deficiency* 89(4):415, 1985.
12. Bodkin J, White K: Clonazepam in the treatment of obsessive-compulsive disorder associated with panic disorder in one patient, *Journal of Clinical Psychiatry* 50(7):265, 1989.
13. Buhler R: *New choices, new boundaries,* Nashville, 1991, Thomas Nelson Publishers.

14. Bumpass E, Fagelman F, Brix R: Intervention with children who set fires, *American Journal of Psychotherapy* 37:328, 1983.

15. Buros D, editor: *The fifth mental measurement yearbook,* Highland Park, NJ, 1959, The Gryphon Press.

16. Cassano G and others: Derealization and panic attacks: a clinical evaluation of 150 patients with panic disorder/agoraphobia, *Comprehensive Psychiatry* 30(1):5, 1989.

17. Clark D, Bolton D: Obsessive-compulsive adolescents and their parents: a psychometric study, *Journal of Child Psychology and Psychiatry and Allied Disciplines* 26(2):267, 1985.

18. Dalton P: Family treatment of an obsessive-compulsive child: a case report, *Family Process* 22(1):99, 1983.

19. DeVeaugh-Geiss J and others: Clinical predictors of treatment response in obsessive compulsive disorder: exploratory analyses from multicenter trials of clomipramine, *Psychopharmacology Bulletin* 26(1):54, 1990.

20. Erikson E: *Childhood and society,* ed 2, New York, 1964, WW Norton.

21. Farkas G, Beck S: Exposure and response prevention of morbid ruminations and compulsive avoidance, *Behavior Research and Therapy* 19(3):257, 1981.

22. Flament M and others: Childhood obsessive-compulsive disorder: a prospective follow-up study, *Journal of Childhood Psychology and Psychiatry* 31(3):363, 1990.

23. Foa E: Phobias, how to keep your fears under control, *US News and World Report* 91:69, 1981.

24. Foa E and others: Deliberate blocking and exposure of OC rituals: immediate and long-term effects, *Behavior Therapy* 15(5):450, 1984.

25. Freud S: *The ego and the id.* In Strachey J, editor: New York, 1962, WW Norton.

26. Freund B, Steketee G: Sexual history, attitudes and functioning of obsessive-compulsive patients, *Journal of Sex and Marital Therapy* 15(1):31, 1989.

27. Gagan J: Imagery: an overview with suggested application for nursing, *Perspectives in Psychiatric Care* 22(1):20, 1984.

28. Gallagher A, Newton S: Obsessional compulsive disorder, *Nursing Standard* 3(51):35, 1989.

29. Gibb G and others: The measurement of the obsessive-compulsive personality, *Educational and Psychological Measurement* 43(4):1233, 1983.

30. Goodman W and others: The Yale-Brown Obsessive Compulsive Scale. I. Development, *Archives of General Psychiatry* 46(11):1006, 1989.

31. Goodman W and others: The Yale-Brown Obsessive Compulsive Scale. II. Validity, *Archives of General Psychiatry* 46(11):1012, 1989.

32. Greenburg D: Are religious compulsions religious or compulsive?: a phenomenological study, *American Journal of Psychotherapy* 38(4):524, October, 1984.

33. Griest J and others: Clomipramine and obsessive compulsive disorder: a placebo-controlled double-blind study of 32 patients, *Journal of Clinical Psychiatry* 51(7):292, 1990.

34. Henderson J Jr, Pollard C: Three types of obsessive compulsive disorder in a community sample, *Journal of Clinical Psychology* 44(5):747, 1988.

35. Henry P, Stephens P: *Stress, health, and the social environment,* New York, 1977, Springer Verlag.

36. Hermesh H and others: Catatonic signs in severe obsessive compulsive disorder, *Journal of Clinical Psychiatry* 50(8):303, 1989.

37. Hewlett W, Vinogradov S, Agras W: Clonazepam treatment of obsessions and compulsions, *Journal of Clinical Psychiatry* 51(4):158, 1990.

38. Hoffnung R and others: Religious compulsions and the spectrum concept of psychopathology, *Psychopathology* 22(2-3):141, 1989.

39. Hoover C, Insel T: Families of origin in obsessive-compulsive disorder, *Journal of Nervous and Mental Disease* 172(4):207, 1984.

40. Insel T: Obsessive-compulsive disorder: five clinical questions and a suggested approach, *Comprehensive Psychiatry* 23:241, 1982.

41. Insel T: Phenomenology of obsessive compulsive disorder, *Journal of Clinical Psychiatry* 51:4, 1990.

42. Insel T: The psychopharmacological treatment of obsessive compulsive disorder, *Journal of Clinical Psychopharmacology* 1:304, 1982.

43. Insel T: *New findings in obsessive-compulsive disorder,* Washington, DC, 1984, American Psychiatric Press.

44. Jakes I: Salkoviskis on obsessional-compulsive neurosis: a critique, *Behavior Research Therapy* 27(6):673, 1989.

45. Jenike M: Obsessive compulsive disorder: a question of a neurologic lesion, *Comprehensive Psychiatry* 25(3):298, 1984.

46. Kelly M, Myers C: Clomipramine: a tricyclic antidepressant effective in obsessive compulsive disorder, *Drug Intelligence and Clinical Pharmacy* 24(7-8):739, 1990.

47. Khanna S and others: Clusters of obsessive-compulsive phenomena in obsessive-compulsive disorder, *British Journal of Psychiatry* 156:51, 1990.

48. Khanna S, Channabasavanna S: Phenomenology of obsessions in obsessive-compulsive neurosis, *Psychopathology* 21(1):12, 1988.

49. Kline P, Cooper C: Rigid personality and rigid thinking, *British Journal of Educational Psychology* 55:24, 1985.

50. Kutz I: Samson's complex: the compulsion to re-enact betrayal and rage, *British Journal of Medical Psychology* 62(Pt 2):123, 1989.

51. Larson M: Flexibility-rigidity. In Beck C, Rawlins R, Williams S, editors: *Mental health-psychiatric nursing: a holistic life-cycle approach,* St Louis, 1984. Mosby—Year Book.

52. Lenane M and others: Psychiatric disorders in first degree relatives of children and adolescents with obsessive compulsive disorder, *Journal of American Academy of Child/Adolescent Psychiatry* 29(3):407, 1990.

53. Leonard H and others: Childhood rituals: normal development or obsessive-compulsive symptoms? *Journal of American Academy of Child/Adolescent Psychiatry* 29(1):17, 1990.

54. Leone C: Thought-induced change in phobic beliefs: sometimes it helps, sometimes it hurts, *Journal of Clinical Psychology* 40(1):68, 1984.

55. Lerner P: The development of a self-report inventory to assess obsessive compulsive behavior, *Dissertation Abstracts International* 43(0-B):30, 1983.

56. Levine R and others: Long-term fluoxetine treatment of a large number of obsessive-compulsive patients, *Journal of Clinical Psychopharmacology* 9(4):281, 1989.

57. Magaro P: The personality of clinical types; an empirically derived taxonomy *Journal of Clinical Psychology* 37(4):796, 1981.

58. McCraw R: Obsessive-compulsive disorder apparently related to abortion, *American Journal of Psychotherapy* 43(2):269, 1989.

59. McKeon J, McGuffin P, Robinson P: Obsessive-compulsive neurosis following head injury: a report of our cases, *British Journal of Psychiatry* 144:185, 1984.

60. McNally R, Calamari J: Obsessive-compulsive disorder in a mentally retarded woman, *British Journal of Psychiatry* 155:116, 1989.

61. Mitchell J, editor: *The ninth mental measurement yearbook,* Lincoln, Neb, 1985, University of Nebraska Press.

62. Mothersill K, Neufeld R: Probability learning and coping in dysphoria and obsessive-compulsive tendencies, *Journal of Research in Personality* 19(2):152, 1985.

63. Murphy D, Pickar D, Alterman I: Methods for the quantitative assessment of depression and manic behavior. In Burdock E, Sudilovsky A, Gershon S, editors: *The behavior of psychiatric patients,* New York, 1982, Marcel Dekker.

64. Pavlov I: *Experimental psychology and other essays,* New York, 1959, Philosophical Library, Inc.

65. Persons J, Foa E: Processing of fearful and neutral information by obsessive-compulsives, *Behavior Research and Therapy* 22(3):259, 1984.

66. Phillips J: *The origins of intellect: Piaget's theory,* San Francisco, 1975, WH Freeman.

67. Rabavilas A: Relation of obsessional traits to anxiety in patients with ulcerative colitis, *Psychotherapy and Psychosomatics* 33(3):155, 1980.

68. Rado S: *Adaptational psychodynamics: motivation and control,* New York, 1969, Science House, Inc.

69. Rinieris P, Stefanis C: Obsessional personality traits and ABO blood types, *Neuropsychobiology* 6(3):128, 1980.

70. Rippere V: Dietary treatment of chronic obsessional ruminations, *British Journal of Clinical Psychology* 22(4):314, 1983.

71. Robertson M, Trimble M, Lees A: The psychopathology of the Gilles de la Tourette syndrome, *British Journal of Psychiatry* 152:383, 1988.

72. Ross C, Anderson G: Phenomological overlap of multiple personality disorder and obsessive-compulsive disorder, *Journal of Nervous and Mental Disorders* 176(5):295, 1988.

73. Rubenowitz S: *Emotional flexibility-rigidity as a comprehensive dimension of the mind,* Stockholm, 1963, Almquist, Wiskell, & Forlag.

74. Runck B: Research is changing views on obsessive compulsive disorder, *Hospital Community Psychiatry* 34(7):597, 1983.

75. Salkoviskis P, Westbrook D: Behaviour therapy and obsessional ruminations: can failure be turned into success? *Behavioural Research Therapy* 27(2):149, 1989.

76. Salzman L: Psychotherapeutic managment of obsessive compulsive patients, *American Journal of Psychotherapy* 39(3):323, 1985.

77. Sanavio-Ezio A, Vidotto-Giulio D: The components of the Maudsley Obsessional Compulsive Questionnaire, *Behavior Research and Therapy* 23(6):659, 1985.

78. Scott A and others: Regional differences in obsessionality and obsessional neurosis, *Psychological Medicine* 12(1):131, 1982.

79. Sher K and others: Memory deficits in compulsive checkers: replication and extension in a clinical sample, *Behavior and Research Therapy* 27(1):65, 1989.

80. Silverman S: Correspondences and thought-transference during psychoanalysis, *Journal of American Academy of Psychoanalysts* 16(3):269.

81. Sullivan H: *The interpersonal theory of psychiatry,* New York, 1953, WW Norton.

82. Swedo S and others: Obsessive-compulsive disorder in children and adolescents: clinical phenomenology of 70 consecutive cases, *Archives of General Psychiatry* 46(4):335, 1989.

83. Swenson R: Response to tranylcypromine and thought stopping in obsessional disorder, *British Journal of Psychiatry* 144:425, 1984.

84. Tan T and others: Biopsychobehavioral correlates of insomnia, *American Journal of Psychiatry* 141(3):357, 1984.

85. Traskman L and others: Cortisol in the cerebral spinal fluid of depressed and suicidal patients, *Archives of General Psychiatry* 37(7):761, 1980.

86. Trimble M: Psychopathology and movement disorders: a new perspective on the Gilles de la Tourette syndrome, *Journal of Neurological and Neurosurgical Psychiatry* Suppl:90-5, 1989.

87. Turns D: Epidemiology of phobic and obsessive compulsive disorders among adults, *American Journal of Psychotherapy* 39(3):360, 1985.

88. van-der-Kolk B: The compulsion to repeat the trauma, *Psychiatric Clinics of North America* 12(2):289, 1989.

89. Veale D: Management of obsessive-compulsive disorder, *British Journal of Hospital Medicine* 43(4):278, 1990.

90. Vitiello B, Spreat S, Behar D: Obsessive-compulsive disorder in mentally retarded patients, *Journal of Nervous and Mental Disorders* 177(4):232, 1989.

91. Weiner M, White M: The use of a self psychology approach in treating a compulsive 84-year-old man, *Clinical Gerontologist* 3(4):64, 1985.

92. Whitley GG: Ritualistic behavior: breaking the cycle, *Journal of Psychosocial Nursing* 29(101):31, 1991.

ANNOTATED BIBLIOGRAPHY

Fernsterheim H, Baer J: *Stop running scared!* New York, 1977, Dell Publishing Co.

   This paperback for anyone with distressing fears is a compendium of information on phobias and how to control them. The authors discuss fear and fear-control training. Programs for mild obsessive-compulsive symptoms are provided. Appendices include examples of relaxation exercises and hierarchies for systematic desensitization.

Jermain D, Crismon M: Pharmacotherapy of obsessive-compulsive disorder, *Pharmacotherapy* 10(3):175, 1990.

   A comprehensive overview of medications used to treat OCD. Research studies and clinical trials are summarized for effectiveness with OCD. All aspects of medications are explored. A helpful current reference for nurses involved with OCD clients.

Kellerman J: *Helping the fearful child,* New York, 1981, Warner Books.

   The author discusses how the child learns to be afraid. Common childhood fears such as darkness and new situations are covered. Those who raise children are offered methods to deal with the child's fears in the home and how adults may cope with the fears. The authors suggest finding professional help if the book's advice is ineffective or requires professional reinforcement.

Rachman S, Hodgson R: *Obsessions and compulsions,* Englewood Cliffs, NJ, 1980, Prentice-Hall.

   This book presents detailed theoretical explanations for the development of obsessions and compulsions. Research findings to support treatment methods are included. Discussions cover both conventional treatment and psychological modification.

CHAPTER 16

Dependence-Independence

Cathleen M Shultz

After studying this chapter, the student will be able to:

- Distinguish among dependent, independent, interdependent, and related terms
- Describe the historical development of dependence-independence
- Identify theories of dependent, independent, and interdependent behaviors
- Discuss the psychopathology of dependent, histrionic, and avoidant personality disorders as described in the DSM-III-R

- Apply the nursing process to care for clients experiencing difficulties with dependent or independent behaviors
- Identify current research findings relevant to the care of clients experiencing dependence or independence

Dependence on others is a fundamental human need during normal growth and development and a healthy response to crises throughout life. As individuals mature, they move toward increasing independence, with the goal of becoming interdependent, a necessity for survival. All individuals are dependent to some degree; no person ever becomes entirely independent.

Western society values independence and generally views dependency as a weakness or inadequacy. Our culture contributes to these feelings by encouraging standards that are difficult to achieve. We are taught, propagandized, and influenced to believe that total independence is not only possible but must be attained at all cost. Because of this societal view, children are often prematurely pushed toward independence and dependent behavior in adults is often regarded as negative and maladaptive. Conflict in the form of anxiety and self-hate frequently arises from frustration caused by dependent and independent needs.

Dependent behavior may be considered adaptive or maladaptive. For example, a newborn is totally dependent on caregivers; this dependence is adaptive because the behavior contributes to the infant's survival. By the age of 3 years, the child displays some ability to care for himself. However, if this same child has a new sibling and reacts by reverting to demands to be bottle fed, the dependent behavior is maladaptive.

During illnesses, the nurse expects acutely ill clients to be dependent on professionals or significant others for care.

Healing is facilitated by dependent behaviors. The behavior becomes maladaptive if the client does not become increasingly independent and remains inappropriately dependent when his condition no longer requires total care.

The illusion of dependency, a characteristic of neurosis, is common and can be crippling if not confronted. Individuals with illusions of dependency seem to be dependent but may become extraordinarily competent when their illusions are destroyed. For example, Cecilia believed that she was dependent and incapable of functioning without her spouse who made all family decisions. After her divorce and subsequent psychotherapy, she finished an associate degree in nursing and much to her surprise found that she is capable of functioning as an effective, responsible decision maker. Persons with illusions of dependency often

▶ **DIAGNOSES Related to Dependence-Independence**

MEDICAL DIAGNOSES

Histrionic personality disorder
Avoidant personality disorder
Dependent personality disorder

NURSING DIAGNOSES

NANDA

Powerlessness

PMH

Impaired work
  Role-dependence

	DATES	EVENTS
HISTORICAL OVERVIEW	Preindustrial Age	The individual was dependent on nature and became more independent when tools and materials were developed.
	Industrial Age	Technology made interdependent behavior essential for survival.
	Post-Renaissance	The frontier woman was expected to be dependent, while cherishing the spirit of independence. This dichotomous expectation of women continues to some extent to the present. Western society came to view independence as a right, with dependent behavior being discouraged. The client was expected to assume a passive, dependent role.
	1952	World Health Organization recognized the individual's dependence on alcohol in their definition of alcoholism.
	1960s	Nurses were found to have higher dependency scores than women tested in other fields.[46]
	1970s	Holistic medicine emphasized independence with its belief that the individual is responsible for self-care. Men and women were more apt to work interdependently in fulfilling family responsibilities. Encouraging dependence on the health care system was found to increase societal costs.
	1980s	Independence was valued more by society as clients become more mobile and encouraged to spend more time in the work settings. The success-at-all-costs mentality was seen more frequently. The nurse's role in the care of persons dependent on substances increased as the numbers of clients experiencing these dependency problems increased dramatically.
	1990s	The economic crisis and unemployment have led to a sense of dependence and helplessness in many people who previously functioned independently. The stress caused by this change has created a need for intervention by psychiatric/mental health nurses to prevent the development of maladaptive dependence.
	Future	Future challenges include participation in prevention and treatment programs to stop the growing numbers of those with personality disorders.

mirror the desires of the people they wish to please; Cecilia would always do what her husband wished her to do. This pseudodependence masks much ability because only those who can tap areas of themselves can do this mirroring effectively. Pseudodependent people usually have a keen ability to manipulate others to fulfill their own needs, while truly dependent people can manipulate only at the most infantile level. The truly dependent person cannot read the behavior of those to whom he is relating.

Maladaptive dependence is of central significance in the psychopathology of personality disorders and in individuals with addictive behavior involving excessive food, work, sex, and chemical substances. Due to pain and stress, these people seek comfort through drugs, alcohol, food, work, and addictive relationships. The dependence creates unhealthy limitations such as being unable to function occupationally if the job requires any independence, working to avoid feelings or other responsibilities such as family, or limiting the social contacts to those on whom they are dependent. Their dependence becomes an inflexible way of life and causes considerable distress for clients and their

significant others. (See Chapter 18 for further information on addictive behavior.)

Independent behavior develops at a later stage than dependent behavior, but it too continues throughout the individual's life. Healthy children become increasingly independent as they mature, leaving the family and beginning relationships outside their family structure. Independence encouraged at too early an age can contribute to *codependent* behavior development, isolation from others and oneself, and difficulty in seeking assistance from others when support is needed. Some people may manifest pseudoindependent behavior and send mixed messages to others; instead of asking for assistance, they convey being totally self-reliant.

Nurses need to understand adaptive and maladaptive dependence and independence to assist clients in meeting their needs and in attaining and maintaining health. Recognizing and supporting appropriate dependent and independent behaviors during the healing process becomes a challenge for the nurse to incorporate into care. Fostering independence maximizes the individual's abilities and has

Term	Definition
Dependence	Reliance on another individual or object for support or aid; individual seeks healthy physical contact, attention, proximity, physical help, and approval and praise
Adaptive dependence	Created when the internal and external environments prevent autonomous functioning; includes acceptance of physical and emotional limitations
Maladaptive dependence	Inappropriate or unrealistic reliance on others or objects; can cause a physical or emotional illness
Pseudodependence	False dependence, which, when confronted and altered, reveals a capable individual
Independence	Behavior that is free from external support and comes from within the individual; individual takes the initiative, overcomes obstacles, remains persistent, wants to do something, and wants to do things by himself
Adaptive independence	Individual acts according to own judgment
Maladaptive independence	Behavior interferes with an individual's ability to attain health
Interdependence	Balance between dependence and independence; behavior is used appropriate to situation; requires problem-solving abilities and is not a patterned response to stimuli

the potential to ensure care that is more cost-effective.

Providing support for those with excessive dependency needs is a challenge. Nurses need to thoroughly understand the relevance of dependence, independence, and interdependence to the development of psychopathology and to working successfully with clients experiencing related personality disorders (see Table 16-1 for definitions). The health-illness continuum can be used as a framework to conceptualize adaptive and maladaptive dependence and independence. The individual who maintains adaptive coping behavior is on the healthy end of the continuum (Figure 16-1) and thus able to develop interdependence that enables coping optimally within his abilities.

DSM-III-R DIAGNOSES

Maladaptive dependence-independence can permeate various psychopathological conditions. Emotional prob-

lems with a dependence-independence component include depression, substance addictions such as chemical abuse, codependency, and some personality disorders. This chapter focuses on the DSM-III-R characteristics of histrionic, avoidant, and dependent personality disorders, which have unhealthy dependent-independent factors.

Personality traits are enduring patterns of perceiving, relating to, and thinking about the environment and oneself; they appear in a wide range of social and personal situations. When personality traits become inflexible and maladaptive, causing either considerable impairment or distress, they become personality disorders. *Personality disorders* refer to traits that characterize the client's recent (past year) and long-term behavior; they are not limited to isolated episodes of the individual's behavior. For example, the client who delivers a child by cesarean section needs to have others care for her for a few weeks after surgery; this is normal dependency. However, if she still has the same expectations of others for the same problem 12 months later, the nurse may refer her for counseling due to the unhealthy dependency needs that are suggestive of a personality disorder.

The manifestations of personality disorders are often evident by childhood and early adulthood. The client often expresses dissatisfaction with the effect his behavior has on others or with his inability to function adequately. Generally, the behaviors are difficult to alter without long-term behavioral changes supported with counseling and continued throughout most of the adult's life; they usually are less obvious or modify without treatment in middle or old age.

Clients with *histrionic personality disorder* are emotionally excessive and attention seeking. They demand reassurance, approval, or praise from others. Emotions are often inappropriately exaggerated, for example, being more sad or angry than is usually seen in the situation. Needing immediate gratification, their behavior is lively and dramatic. They also exaggerate interpersonal relations and frequently adopt the role of "victim" or "princess." Typically attractive and seductive, they crave novelty, stimulation, and excitement and quickly become bored with normal routines. They may constantly demand reassurance because of feelings of helplessness and dependency. In close relationships, they attempt to control the opposite sex or to enter into a dependent relationship. Creative and imaginative, they show little interest in intellectual achievement and frequently complain of poor health or feelings of depersonalization. They tend to be impressionable and easily influenced by others such as authority figures or by fads.

Clients with *avoidant personality disorder* experience social discomfort when near others due to concerns about how others view them; they are easily hurt by criticism and devastated by the slightest hint of disapproval. Seldom will they enter close relationships unless guaranteed uncritical acceptance even though they desire affection and acceptance. These people often appear dependent because once a relationship is formed, they tend to be clinging and fearful of losing others. Berating themselves for the inability to form relationships, a social phobia may be present; their social and job-related functioning may become impaired.

Clients with *dependent personality disorder* have a pervasive pattern of dependent and submissive behavior, fre-

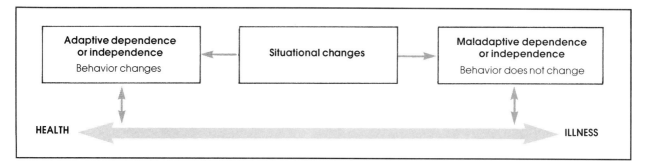

FIGURE 16-1 Dependence-independence on the health-illness continuum.

quently being unable to make everyday decisions without an excessive amount of advice and reassurance from others. Their excessive dependence on others prevents initiating projects or doing things on their own. They tend to feel uncomfortable or helpless when alone, are devastated when close relationships end, and are preoccupied with fears of being abandoned. They are easily hurt by criticism and disapproval and invariably lack self-confidence. They belittle their abilities and assets. Occupational functioning is impaired when independence is required, and they may avoid promotions that force them to make decisions.

THEORETICAL APPROACHES

Psychoanalytical

Freud[28] dealt with the development of dependence in the oral phase, which occurs during the first 2 years of life. During this phase the infant learns to depend on the parent or primary caregiver for both emotional and physical life support. The infant learns that dependency needs are met by the parent, and survival occurs only if minimal needs are satisfied.

According to Freud, if dependency needs are not met during the oral phase, the individual becomes fixated at this stage. This fixation results in the individual trying to meet his own dependence needs. Fixation at the oral stage can result in substance dependency, development of a dependent personality disorder, or other problems related to meeting dependent needs, such as eating disorders or smoking. The dependent individual relies on others to make his choices. The person's superego is inhibited by the demands and prohibitions of others. Use of chemical substances releases the inhibitions of the superego. The person is then able to be himself, talk more freely, and be more sociable. The individual's ego boundaries are loosened, and the person may act on id impulses that are ordinarily repressed. However, adaptive dependence occurs when the infant's dependence needs are adequately met, and he progresses successfully through the oral stage to the next stage of development.

Adaptive independence is learned at a later stage than adaptive dependence. According to Freud, during the anal stage the toddler begins to learn independent behavior. At this stage the child is able to move about somewhat without assistance, and the parent begins to expect certain things of the child, such as walking. The child learns that certain actions cause certain behaviors in others. For instance, when the toddler uses the toilet, the parent acts pleased; when the child wets the diaper, the parent shows disapproval. Parents start reinforcing independent behavior, and the child develops a need for achievement. This need activates internal pressure, which initiates a reponse from the child to relieve the pressure. Positive parental response to the child's beginning mastery over the environment rewards the child. Gradually, increasingly independent behavior is rewarded, and the toddler learns adaptive independence.

Erikson[22] called the first 18 months of life the trust versus mistrust period. The infant learns to trust himself and the environment by " asking" the parent for caring behavior. The asking behavior is repeated, and an effective response is expected. If the parent continues to deliver the necessary care, the baby learns trust and acceptance.

During the development of trust the infant begins to realize he is a separate entity. Parental behavior such as rejection or overprotection leads to dependent, attention-seeking behaviors. When rejected, the infant may hold his breath or stomp his feet to get attention. On the other hand, the overprotected child may be quiet and withdrawn so the caregiver will say, "What a good boy!" or "What a good girl!" Developing these dependent behaviors leads the infant to feel powerless and inadequate. As the dependent person gets older, he often finds the use or abuse of chemical substances or food allows him to feel better about himself. The person feels a false sense of control, more adequate, and more independent. While "high," he often feels he can accomplish anything.

Erikson labeled the beginning of adaptive independence as the autonomy versus shame and doubt stage. To progress successfully through this stage, the toddler needs to receive positive reinforcement for doing things for himself. At the same time the parents need to exert firm outer control. The toddler must be allowed to make decisions within his ability. During the next stage, initiative versus guilt, independent behavior is expanded. At the same time, the ability to communicate is enhanced. The child demonstrates independence by saying "no" to parental demands.

The most vital stage in the development of independent behavior is the industry versus inferiority stage. At this age the child wants to do things for himself, takes initiative, and works diligently to overcome obstacles. All of these are tasks of independence, and it is important for the parent to reinforce such independent behavior. Praise from the parents and others is an excellent positive reinforcement during this stage. Positive, consistent reinforcement needs to be given for both physical and emotional acts that reflect adaptive independent behavior.

Erikson dealt with independent behavior at all stages. The last stage of life, integrity versus despair, is an important stage for maintaining adaptive independence. Erikson described ego integrity as all previous phases coming together, whereas despair leaves the individual angry and filled with self-disgust. The aging individual with ego integrity is able to develop adaptive independence, which is the opposite of the adaptive dependence discussed earlier. The elderly person faces many changes. Along with increasing physical dependence, emotional independence is threatened by many losses that occur during the latter part of life. While the aging individual is attempting to cope with these losses, society says, "Independence is important" and "Worthwhile people work." The aging individual needs to receive positive reinforcement for realistic independent behavior to counteract the increased physical dependence and society's negative attitude. Rewards, such as positive statements and sincere praise, can be given for both adaptive dependent and adaptive independent behavior. During this phase, because of forced dependence in some areas, the client with interdependent coping skills is able to age more successfully.

Erikson described two stages in which interdependent behavior is developed, the identity stage and the intimacy stage. The identity stage occurs in adolescence. If the youth has accomplished the previous tasks adequately, developing interdependent behavior is easier. Having previously received positive reinforcement for adaptive dependent and adaptive independent behavior, the adolescent had already learned some interdependent behavior. The adolescent strives to be psychologically independent from the family and may express this independence by renouncing the parent's values and norms. However, the individual is extremely dependent on peers. The parents have the task of allowing the youth to make independent decisions and judgments when possible, while assuring the adolescent of continued family love and support. This period is often difficult for the parents and the adolescent. Frequently, it appears to the parents that the child who had excellent judgment 2 years earlier is now incapable of making any sound decisions at all. During this time the parent allows independent decisions while setting firm and consistent rules.

During the intimacy stage, adaptive coping behavior consists of the ability to move from a dependent to an independent position. Developing an independent coping style, the young adult then assumes a role that requires interdependence. If the individual has previously developed a realistic trust in others and is secure in his own identity, he is able to be self-disclosing and form an intimate relationship with another. This relationship fulfulls affiliation needs and achieves interdependence.

Bowlby emphasized the importance of bonding between the infant and the parental figure.[10] A bond or attachment phenomenon occurs between mother and infant at birth, and the newborn is soon conditioned to meet his dependence needs. Klaus and Kennell[42] expanded Bowlby's theory to include the newborn and both parents. The mother

and father need to see, touch, and cuddle the baby soon after birth. This time is critical in conditioning the parents to perform the role of parent. The sooner the bonding occurs, the more rapidly the parents receive positive reinforcement from the baby's touch, and the adaptive dependence needs of both the baby and parents are met.

Bowlby believed that independent behavior is fostered by parents who provide unfailing support along with consistent encouragement for the child to become independent. The parent gives unfailing support by allowing and encouraging the child to perform tasks that he can successfuly accomplish. At the same time, the parent needs to assist the child with tasks that are too difficult. While developing autonomy, the child needs to feel confident that the attachment figure will be available when needed. Development of independent behavior extends throughout childhood and adolescence; however, once the behavior is developed, it persists fairly consistently through life. Having had both dependent and independent needs met, the individual may use interdependent behavior.

According to Bowlby, the self-reliant person is not as independent as Western culture stereotypes project. Rather he is able to develop adaptive interdependent behavior. The well-adapted person and his attachment figure both give and receive support and love, are available when needed, and slowly build confidence in each other's availability.

Rubin[61] believes that children raised by significant others who have self-hate learn self-rejection, have diminished self-confidence, and feel that they cannot depend on themselves. Thus dependence on the parents becomes prolonged, which extends the children's exposure to this parental onslaught, completing a vicious cycle from which it is most difficult to remove themselves. As adults, they have many repressed feelings, which become exaggerated, develop an autonomy of their own, and when they emerge, bring on a conditioned pattern of self-hate, often in the form of personality disorders, addiction, abusive behavior, and depression. These reactions have an addictive quality, and, once used, are generally used again and again.

Mahler[47] considered the first few months of life as symbiotic months, which means that a union between the baby and the mother is essential for meeting adaptive dependence needs. During these months the baby learns to identify with the aspect of the baby's symbiotic self represented by the mother and responds mainly to the internal environment. For example, the baby internally identifies with the mother.

Maladaptive dependence is developed when the infant's dependence needs are not rewarded in a manner that allows the infant to progress from one stage to another. The infant who receives sufficient care for survival but does not receive loving care from the parental figure will not have his dependence needs met adequately. This infant develops maladaptive dependence. Equally harmful is the parental figure who has a smothering relationship with the infant, which results in maladaptive independence. In both cases the infant is taught a maladaptive mode of coping. Either the toddler tries harder to get dependence needs met or withdraws and develops maladaptive independence.

According to Mahler the development of independent behavior begins at 4 or 5 months, the peak of the symbiotic

▼ **TABLE 16-2** **Subphases of Mahler's Separation-Individuation Process**

Phase	Age	Description	Example
Differentiation	5-9 months	Becoming aware of being separate from mother. A powerful bond between mother and infant. Physical and psychological dependence on mother.	Smiles at sound of mother's voice and at sight of mother.
Practicing	9-14 months	Expanding independence. In latter part of phase learns to walk. Adaptive independence learned from games played with mother and other nurturing individuals. First notices inanimate objects in environment. Separation anxiety.	Plays game in which child runs away from mother and mother chases and catches child.
Rapprochement	14-24 months	Many conflicts need to be resolved. Increased awareness of external environment. Increased sense of physical separateness. Adaptive development depends on child resolving conflict related to wish to replace parent of same sex. Separation anxiety.	Shares achievements with mother.
Consolidation	24-36 months	Beginning of object constancy, which is the ability to hold a symbolic picture of loved object when object is absent. Child moves away from mother with less anxiety. Increased independence. Future mental health depends on the development of increased individuality and emotional object constancy.	Plays alone without physical presence of mother.

phase. At this time the infant begins the first subphase of *separation-individuation,* which are two separate but intertwined tasks. *Separation* is the development of the physical ability to move away from the mother, along with the mental awareness of being separate. *Individuation* is a cognitive, effective development that allows the infant to cope with the separateness. The subphases of the separation-individuation process are described in Table 16-2.

Interpersonal

Sullivan[65] considered infancy the "learning to count on others" phase. He stressed interpersonal relationships and socialization and contended that if dependent needs are met in infancy, the infant learns to trust himself with others. Through the interpersonal relationship with the mother, the baby's dependency needs are met and thus adaptive dependence occurs.

According to Sullivan, adaptive independence begins in the latter part of the infant stage, when the baby learns to satisfy some of his own needs independent of the mother. The growth of independence occurs during the second stage, childhood, which begins when articulate speech is learned. This stage occurs when the child develops a self-concept and recognizes himself as separate from others.

Sullivan's interpersonal relationship theory proposes that interdependent behavior is initiated during the juvenile stage. During this time the child learns both to cooperate and compete. The school-aged child learns to work and play with other children to attain established goals. At the same time they compete against those who are outside their own group. At this age children form clubs and gangs.

Internal control is strengthened, and external control is lessened somewhat.

The growth of interdependent behavior continues through the next two periods, preadolescence and adolescence. During preadolescence the child learns to form relationships requiring reciprocity and mutual sharing. By the end of adolescence the young adult has learned the rights and the responsibilities of living in society. The self-system is stabilized, and the individual is capable of forming indepth, interpersonal relationships.

Behavioral

The learning theories propose that maladaptive dependence occurs when positive reinforcement is not sufficient to meet the infant's needs. The baby learns to search for methods to meet these needs. As an adult, the individual may learn to rely inappropriately on others or objects such as food or chemicals to meet his needs. Overinvolvement with work, food, relationships, or chemical substances prevents one from dealing with painful issues and brings a temporary comfort or distraction from oneself. When the chemical action wears off or the relationship or work is not there, the good feelings are replaced by feelings of anxiety, guilt, inadequacy, and dependence, so the person uses the substances again to regain the good feelings. (See Chapter 18 for additional discussion of use of alcohol to meet needs.)

The psychodynamics of maladaptive independence are similar to those of maladaptive dependence. Maladaptive independence occurs at a later stage of development during early childhood. This mode of coping may be learned when

▼ **TABLE 16-3**   Development of Dependence, Independence, and Interdependence According to Various Theories

Theorist	Development of Dependence	Development of Independence	Development of Interdependence
Bowlby[10]	Birth—attachment	Childhood to adolescence—unfailing support	Adolescence—assurance of availability of attachment
Erikson[22]	Birth—trust	Age 2 to 3 years—autonomy Age 3 to 6 years—initiative	Age 13-18 years—identity Age 18 to 40 years—intimacy
Freud[28]	Birth to 2 years—oral phase	Age 2 to 3 years—anal phase	
Mahler[17]	Birth—symbiotic phase	Age 4 to 5 months—separation individuation Age 2 years—rapprochement	
Sullivan[65]	Birth—learning to count on others	Childhood—self-reliance	Age 6 to 9 years—looks to peers for a sense of companionship Age 9 to 12 years—forms an intense love relationship with person of same sex ("chum relationship") Age 13 to 18 years—able to establish relationships with persons of opposite sex; to be dependent, independent, and interdependent.

a child receives negative reinforcement for displaying adaptive dependent behavior. Rewarding inappropriate independent behavior can also result in maladaptive independent behavior. The individual who has developed a maladaptive independent coping style has difficulty accepting external control. When external control is necessary, the individual experiences a conflict between internal and external needs. Examples of this conflict are the elderly person who is confused at times and can no longer live alone and the alcoholic individual at a cocktail party. Both of these individuals want to pursue an independent course. The elderly person wants to live independently but is too confused to do so. An external control—living with someone else—is imposed. The alcoholic has an internal conflict. At cocktail parties the external control says, "Drink—it is the sociable thing to do." However, the alcoholic cannot drink socially without serious consequences.

In summary, the concepts of dependence, independence, and interdependence develop differently according to various theorists. Their ideas are included in Table 16-3. A summary of theories relating to independence and dependence is provided in Table 16-4.

NURSING PROCESS

Assessment

Physical dimension Assessing the physical dimension consists of determining the client's willingness and ability to perform tasks of daily living. According to Freud, the person with an interdependent coping style has achieved a balance between dependent and independent behavior that is appropriate to the situation. For example, an executive who is hospitalized for a possible myocardial infarction is able to accept the forced dependence and

allows others to perform his activities of daily living. He relies on health providers to bathe him, assist him in getting out of bed, and perform whatever other physical care is needed. However, as his condition improves, he performs self-care as appropriate. This client follows the regimen necessary to return to an optimal level of health. The nurse assesses the client's progress toward increasing independence throughout the healing process.

The client who exhibits predominantly maladaptive dependent behavior is reluctant to perform tasks of daily living. Interpersonal theories support that illness, for example, provides an excellent rationalization for being dependent. The hospitalized client is observed for behaviors such as refusing to take his own bath, not feeding himself, and not performing other hygienic care of which he is capable. This capable individual may actively refuse to care for himself or may wait passively for the nurse or family to provide the care.

Because the dependent client may demonstrate signs of poor physical health, the nurse assesses the client's total physical appearance and health status. Physical deterioration is more apparent in certain types of maladaptive dependent behavior than in others. An individual dependent on relationships, situations such as work, or substances such as cigarettes or coffee may neglect his physical needs as he relies more and more on work or other external means of comfort. The nurse may observe inadequate hygiene, inadequate nutrition, inactivity, weight loss, poor skin turgor or muscle tone, and unkempt appearance. Obtaining the addictive substances or circumstances such as work becomes the person's overriding objective, and the nurse needs to determine the significance of the dependence.

Distortion of an individual's body image may result from maladaptive dependence. Behaviorists believe that a person's body image can be distorted by low self-esteem, lack

▼ **TABLE 16-4** **Summary of Theories of Dependence-Interdependence**

Theory	Theorist	Dynamics
PSYCHOANALYTICAL		
Intrapsychic	Freud[28]	Maladaptive dependence results from the fixation of adaptive dependency needs that were not met during oral phase.
		Independent behavior is learned during anal phase in response to being allowed to exert appropriate control over actions. Becomes maladaptive when this need is frustrated.
	Erikson[22]	As the infant learns to trust his caregiver and himself, he learns adaptive dependence.
		Adaptive independence is learned during the stage of autonomy versus shame and doubt as the child receives positive reinforcement for doing things for himself. Both dependence and independence become maladaptive when the need is frustrated.
	Bowlby[11]	Adaptive dependence is learned during bonding between mother and infant.
		The child develops independent behavior when parent encourages him to perform realistic tasks for himself.
	Rubin[61]	Maladaptive dependence is learned from significant others who have self-hate.
		Self-hate behaviors are addictive and occur in the forms of personality disorders, abusive behavior, addictions and depression.
	Mahler[47]	The infant has a symbiotic dependent relationship with mother.
		Maladaptive dependence develops when child's dependence needs are not rewarded by mother.
Interpersonal	Sullivan[65]	Adaptive dependence learned during infancy when child learns he can count on others to meet his needs.
		Independent behavior begins in late infancy and continues into childhood in response to being rewarded for satisfying some needs independent of mother.
BEHAVIORAL		Dependence becomes maladaptive when positive reinforcement is not sufficient to meet infant's needs.
		Maladaptive dependence occurs when the child receives negative reinforcement for displaying adaptive dependent behavior.

of confidence, and helplessness, which are characteristics of a dependent person. Body image is also distorted by the individual who possesses a grandiose sense of self-importance and who is vain and self-indulgent, such as an individual with a narcissistic personality disorder.

Using behavioral theory as a framework, the nurse assesses the client for evidence of physical abuse, because the individual with maladaptive dependent behavior may accept many forms of physical abuse from significant others. They have high tolerance levels for abuse, especially if it was experienced during formative years. The client may have a number of bruises, small burns, or even human bites. Cues to assess include the client's wearing inappropriate clothing for the weather conditions or wearing clothing that covers large amounts of the body. For example, the client might wear long-sleeved shirts and long pants outside in 100°F temperatures or wear long-sleeved, high neck, and midcalf length dresses. When asked about the clothing, the client may ignore the questions or have difficulty talking about how the marks were incurred. The client may refuse a physical examination that requires removal of the clothing. The dependent person may find physical abuse less threatening than the fear of having to rely on himself.

The nurse assesses the client's general appearance because clients with a histrionic personality disorder are typically overly concerned with physical attractiveness, act seductive, appear flamboyant, and often complain of feeling bad or having poor health. For example, they frequently may complain of feeling weak, fatigued, or having a headache. Consider the following case example.

▼ **Case Example**

Kate, age 37 years, is a high school English teacher. She wears clothes similar to the young women she teaches. Consistently, she relates to male co-workers and students in a seductive manner. Her superintendent has spoken to her twice this semester about her classroom behavior. When confronted, she states that people are exaggerating and misjudging her intentions because she means nothing by it. She believes that she is just tired and feels so helpless that others misinterpret her intentions. The last episode has caused her superintendent to insist that she go to a counselor for diagnostic work and possible counseling. Her histrionic behavior is probably not in her awareness. If left unchecked, her seductiveness and inappropriateness could have serious employment consequences.

Determining disfigurements or the presence of chronic illnesses becomes important, as the former may predispose the client to an avoidant personality disorder and the latter may contribute to the development of a dependent personality disorder. Scars, birthmarks, limps, atrophied limbs, and fatigue suggest the need for further exploration by the nurse.

A characteristic of maladaptive independence is that the person needs to be in control of the external environment. One indicator of this behavior is performing tasks that are contraindicated by the person's physical or emotional status. For example, the individual insists on controlling his finances while he is emotionally too unstable to manage them.

 Emotional dimension The emotional dimension of an individual with a maladaptive dependent or independent coping style is believed by psychoanalytical theorists to be characterized by deep-seated resentment and anger, although the individual may not be aware of these feelings. The nurse observes for indications of anger and its expression. Because of the fear of abandonment, the client may not openly express the anger. Instead it may be manifested by loud, threatening outbursts, temper tantrums, threats of bodily harm to oneself or other, sullen withdrawal, or questions such as "Why did this happen to me?" The client may throw things or refuse medications or other necessary treatments. The dependent client has an underlying anger at himself because of his perceived inability to act and toward others because they reinforce but do not do enough for his dependence.

An individual who is extremely dependent may show signs of depression (see research highlight). Occasionally, helplessness and suicidal feelings are present. The nurse needs to look for signs and symptoms of helplessness, depression, and suicidal ideas. These feelings are especially pronounced during and after detoxification periods (see Chapter 18).

For those clients with a histrionic personality disorder, the nurse observes for rapidly shifting and shallow emotional expressions, attention-seeking behaviors, and depersonalization. On first impression, clients appear charming and appealing; they frequently lack genuineness. Their behavior is overly reactive and intensely expressed. For example, when seeing a childhood casual acquaintance pass by his hospital room, the client loudly calls the person's name and embraces him like a very close friend and sobs because they have not seen each other in such a long time; the client's reaction is inappropriate for the situation and warrants further assessment. The nurse assesses the client's reactions to others, the intensity of those reactions, and their need to be the center of attention in a variety of situations.

The individual with an avoidant personality disorder is crushed when criticized and constantly seeks approval. Maintaining routines, however boring, causes resistance to taking risks. Their reasons for avoiding changes are often exaggerated. For example, the client may cancel a needed return appointment to the physician's office because of a remote possibility that rain might make driving dangerous. Timidity is a predominant behavior. They fear being embarrassed by blushing, crying, or showing signs of anxiety before others.

Emotional abuse can be self-inflicted or received from others including those the client values most. The nurse assesses the dependent client for evidence of self-diminution (not recognizing or neglecting one's assets and possibilities), repression (pushing thoughts and feelings out of ready awareness), self-derision (derogatory statements such as "I'm ignorant," "I'm no good"), perfectionism (meeting impossible standards), destructive forms of relating to oneself (nightmares, panic and hypochondriacal attacks, and ruminations), accident proneness, and denying pleasure to oneself.

The nurse also explores the emotional quality of the

RESEARCH HIGHLIGHT

The Assessment of Personality Characteristics in Depressed and Dependent Psychiatric Inpatients
- J Overholser, R Kabakoff, and W Norman

PURPOSE

This study was designed to assess the personality characteristics of psychiatric inpatients according to their dependency and depression psychopathology.

SAMPLE

The convenience sample consisted of 106 psychiatric inpatients admitted to a private, university-affiliated hospital. All patients had been referred to the Psychological Consultation Program for assessment of personality functioning. All DSM-III-R diagnoses were established by the treating psychiatrists, who did not know the purpose of the research.

METHODOLOGY

Subjects were grouped into four categories based on a combination of the two variables of interest, depression and dependency. Subjects were given the Minnesota Multiphasic Personality Inventory (MMPI) and the Millon Clinical Multiaxial Inventory (MCMI), with results based on the MCMI Dependent subscale. The grouping procedures resulted in four subgroups: (1) depressed, (2) dependent, (3) depressed and dependent, and (4) nondepressed, nondependent control group.

Based on data from *Journal of Personality Assessment* 53(1):40, 1989.

FINDINGS

Although interpersonal dependency may be a part of the depressive episode, the findings showed that not all depressives display elevated levels of dependency. The presence or absence of dependency was associated with significant differences across demographic data, MMPI scores, and clinical variables. Dependent patients, regardless of their level of depression, were characterized by anxiety, self-doubts, and social insecurities. Depressed, dependent subjects were older and more likely to be women. Dependency was associated with reduced activity and energy levels, but only when seen in conjunction with depression.

IMPLICATIONS

Nurses may benefit from assessing dependency levels when working with depressed clients. Further testing may be of assistance in developing interventions specific to the depressed client's emotional pathology.

client's interactions. For example, a verbally abusive spouse may use strong, derogatory comments toward the submissive, dependent client with the nurse present. An abusive spouse could loudly say, "You're always late. You can't be counted on for anything. You'd think she never learned how to tell time," when his wife arrives 5 minutes after a scheduled appointment. The nurse maintains an awareness that public behaviors are less intense than what may be experienced in private. The client needs professional assistance to change abusive situations.

Intellectual dimension The interdependent individual is able to assess situations in a realistic way. Because his perception is not clouded by unmet dependent or independent needs, he can objectively evaluate each situation. When ill, the well-adapted or interdependent person listens to a health care provider and then decides on a course of action. The person neither blindly accepts the health care provider's word nor immediately rebels against any restrictions. This individual normally needs to have time to work through the emotional impact of any illness or trauma, whether emotional or physical, before being able to decide which course of action is best.

The intellectual dimension is affected by the degree of maladaptive dependent or independent behavior a person displays. The more severe the maladaptive behavior, the more rigid the client's functioning. From a psychoanalytical perspective, the nurse assesses the person's flexibility, ability to comprehend what is occurring, his knowledge base, and ability to analyze the relationships involved. The individual with maladaptive dependent behavior appears to accept any explanation of the problem or condition that the nurse or other authority figures offer, often displaying blind trust or overcompliance toward the suggestions of others.

The nurse assesses the client to determine the person's major coping styles. This assessment is best accomplished over time and includes the reactions of the client to both internal and external stimuli. Close attention is given to the subjective data that the client discloses. The nurse considers factors such as the individual's body posture and tone of voice. Especially pertinent is the congruency between the client's verbal and nonverbal messages. If the person states "Boy am I glad to see you!" then turns slightly away from the nurse or stands with tightly folded arms, the messages are incongruent.

Adaptive dependent and independent behavior enables the client to develop an interdependent coping style that allows movement back and forth from one coping style to the other as needed. Maladaptive coping patterns place the individual in a rigid response mode. Inability to move from one coping style to another interferes with attaining an optimal level of health.

The individual who uses a maladaptive independent coping style has difficulty accepting a dependent role. The client's internal message is "Be in control," but the external message is "You are not in control." Because there is a basic mistrust that anyone else can perform the task, any attempt to compel the client to accept external control is met by angry resistance. The nurse determines the client's response to newly created dependent roles, such as those which occur during hospitalization or during treatment for a newly diagnosed illness.

Lack of appropriate decision making characterizes the intellectual functioning of the maladaptive dependent person. The person does not know how to solve problems and cannot think beyond the moment or is unable to make decisions without continual reassurance. The nurse also observes limited impulse control; lack of concentration and insight; and faulty judgment, cognitive skills, and thought processes.

Delayed gratification and meeting goals are foreign to the client with a histrionic personality disorder, who must have immediate and complete gratification of his needs. Speech may be excessively impressionistic and lacking in detail. For example, when asked to describe her husband, the client answers, "He is a terrific person"; she is unable to elaborate beyond that response.

Decision making is difficult for the client with a dependent personality disorder. The nurse assesses clients for their abilities to initiate projects. She determines who makes the most important decisions in the client's life, such as where they live or what job they will take. She also observes for overcompliance and agreement with others' wishes. According to interpersonal theory, these people fear being rejected and will be motivated by the desire to have others like them and by their extreme fears of being abandoned. Determining their ability to follow suggested interventions becomes important to successful attainment of optimal health; they may comply simply because they desire being liked by the health care worker.

Denial is the defense mechanism most frequently used by the dependent person. The dependent person accepts society's belief that one "should" be independent; therefore the individual uses denial to prevent himself from experiencing pain and anxiety. The person who abuses chemical substances uses denial even more frequently than other dependent people. Part of the denial occurs because society considers chemical substance abuse not only a weakness but also a moral disgrace. This makes the role of the nurse extremely difficult because it is almost impossible to work with a client to change maladaptive behavior when the client denies the existence of the behavior.

Projection, another frequently used defense mechanism, allows the dependent person to place blame and responsibility on someone else. It demonstrates the person's lack of self-confidence and feelings of helplessness and powerlessness. The nurse assesses projection through words and speech patterns used by the client. For example, the use of projection is illustrated by the following statements: "I got drunk because my wife kept pushing me" and "I stole it because my dad said I was a coward. It is his fault."

Social dimension In the United States young children are taught to be competitive and to value independence; children are urged to leave home when they become young adults. Competition and independence can prevent having close relationships with others and with oneself. These values are not the same in some other cultures. The Japanese, Chinese, and Mexican cultures teach children to value interdependence. Families tend to stay close, and several generations may live together.

The person with maladaptive dependent behavior has a poor self-image, which leads to the firm belief that he is not capable of caring for himself. The individual also has a fear of being alone. These characteristics are often displayed by individuals with personality disorders, such as avoidant personality disorder and dependent personality disorder.

Awareness of individual and family developmental tasks is also important when assessing dependent and independent behavior. Is the client performing at the appropriate developmental level for his age and culture? It is usually considered appropriate for the 25-year-old to find a job and move away from home, but this behavior is not considered appropriate for most 14-year-olds. Is the family accomplishing its developmental tasks?

The nurse can assess interdependent behavior most easily in the social dimension. The interdependent person is able to function in both social and occupational settings. Some characteristics of interdependent behavior include developing meaningful relationships, being able to provide and accept nurturing care, and maintaining a good work record. In the occupational setting, interdependence allows the individual to accept authority when it is appropriate and to be the authority when needed. The interdependent person accepts the responsibility for his own actions.

Both maladaptive dependent and maladaptive independent behaviors have many social ramifications for the client and family. Manipulating others characterizes both styles. Manipulative behavior is used to "con" others into meeting the individual's needs (see Chapter 23).

The person who uses substances is often seen as a manipulative and exploitive client. Within the drug culture, manipulation is a way of life. The unhealthy payoff is in conning others into meeting the person's dependent needs at their own expense (see Chapter 18). The nurse may find such clients wanting special favors, wanting to bend the rules, and disregarding rules. Other behaviors such as seduction, helplessness, or interpersonal exploitation may be displayed. The manipulative client acts out his feelings rather than stating them verbally.

The client who uses helplessness tells the nurse how well the nurse is able to do things with remarks such as "I wish I were as competent as you," "I don't know how you manage everything so well," "I just can't seem to do it," or "I can't seem to do anything for myself. I am so dumb." Using knowledge of interpersonal theory, the nurse assesses conversations with the client to determine the client's manipulation.

The individual with maladaptive dependent behavior frequently has many social contacts. When left alone, even for a short time, however, this person becomes fearful and anxious. The spouse may miss work often because the dependent individual demands attention. When the client is ill and hospitalized, the family devotes full time to the client. Although there are many visitors, the social contacts do not reassure this individual, and as soon as he is alone, he becomes very demanding of the nursing staff. The nurse maintains an awareness of the number and quality of the client's relationships and the client's reaction to actual or anticipated alone times.

▼ Case Example

Alice is a 24-year-old homemaker with two children younger than 5 years. She came to the neighborhood, nurse-operated clinic for routine check-ups for her children. While in the waiting area, the nurse observes that she does not interact with the other women who also live in the same neighborhood. She appears withdrawn and rarely smiles, keeps to herself, and occupies her time slowly thumbing through a magazine while her children are running around the clinic waiting area. She seems ill at ease when other women try to draw her into their conversations.

When the nurse finishes examining the children, she focuses her attention on Alice. Assessing her social skills and feelings of control over her world would be part of the assessment with the whole group. Although the mother seems to be a dependent person, the nurse would further assess her behavior to determine the presence and extent of maladaptive dependence in her life.

The effects of maladaptive dependent behavior on interpersonal relationships depend on the type of behavior and the severity of the maladaption. Behavioral theory indicates that the client will demonstrate a range from suspiciousness and withdrawal from social contacts to overt acting out, such as lying or stealing to get attention. Characteristics to observe include clinging, having many acquaintances but no close friends, too much concern for the feelings of others, and jealousy. They tend to cling to whatever friends they have; this dependency often drives others away. There may be overt acting out, in which the individual engages in verbal or physical violence and aggression. In some cases the violence is self-directed.

The client may have legal problems caused by violent acts, thefts, illegal occupations, failure to honor debts, or reckless driving. These problems often occur in maladaptive people who use chemicals to meet their dependence needs.

Family assessment is essential because the family dynamics are related to the client's emotional problems. The nurse interviews the family to identify the family patterns and to investigate how the individual with the identified maladaptive dependence and independence is incorporated into the family dynamics.

The family may reinforce patterns of maladaptive dependence by doing for the client or insisting that the nursing staff do for him what he needs to do for himself. The nurse asks all family members how they see themselves and the other family members contributing to the problem. When talking with more than one family member, the nurse can observe the family's interactions with each other, including how they address each other, whether any one person is excluded from the conversation, and what tone of voice they use with each member of the family. The client can describe what role he believes the family plays in the present problem. Once the family dynamics are identified, the nurse can assess both the client's and the family's perception of the maladaptive dependent behaviors.

Family dynamics also play an important role in the development of the members' self-concepts and roles. Parents who are comfortable with themselves are able to portray this to their children, and they are also able to accept their children as they are. Through positive acceptance and appraisal from the parent, the children develop positive self-concepts and high self-esteem. The children are then able to make decisions when appropriate and thus experience beginning independence. Positive interactions with parents throughout the different developmental stages enable an individual to learn adaptive interdependence and self-acceptance.

The nurse assesses the effects of maladaptive dependent behavior on the client's social interactions. The degree of social impairment depends on the severity of the dependence needs. The individual who believes his dependence needs cannot be met feels pain; to allay this pain, the individual may display behavior such as whining or being very self-centered. The client tends to exclude the needs of others and gradually withdraws. As people withdraw from the client in response to his behavior, the client's behavior becomes more extreme. The behaviors become cyclical and the unmet dependency needs worsen.

Many persons with personality disorders demonstrate maladaptive dependence. Individuals with avoidant and dependent personality disorders have a need for uncritical acceptance by others. This need greatly interferes with social functioning. The individual's behavior estranges him from his family and other interpersonal relationships. The person then may experience loneliness and may seek excessive attention, or he may withdraw completely (see Chapter 21). The client may ask the nurse, "Why doesn't anyone like me?" or "Why am I always alone?" The client's response to this loneliness includes frequent touching, speaking loudly, asking for unnecessary help, soliciting praise for accomplishment, asking for approval of personal appearance, and other attention-seeking behavior.[8] This type of dependent behavior is self-defeating. Because the client is attempting to meet a basic need that was not met in infancy, the attention the client receives is never enough.

A client with a dependent personality disorder has a pervasive pattern of dependence, which can be incapacitating in relationships. Due to fears of being alone, they will go to great lengths to avoid being alone. Significant others frequently make the client's most important decisions, giving an illusion of closeness. Despite these dependency needs, the client usually has no close friends or confidants other than relatives. Clients avoid situations that increase social demands, and, when in social situations, they are reluctant to participate due to fear of saying something inappropriate or foolish or being unable to provide an answer to a question. The nurse assesses the type and amount of time spent in interpersonal situations and observes hospitalized clients as they make decisions and interact with others, especially if hospitalized for an emotional problem.

Clients with dependent personality disorders are also easily hurt by criticism and disapproval; they feel devastated when close relationships end. From interpersonal theory, the nurse understands that they will do things they dislike, that are unpleasant, or that are demeaning, believing that others will like them if they do these things. They lack self-confidence and frequently belittle their own abilities. They seek overprotection and dominance in others. The nurse assesses the clients' reactions to criticism, their satisfaction with their jobs and hobbies, their relationship with significant others, and their confidence levels. Being aware of the client's statements about himself assists in determining the value he places on himself. For example, statements such as "I'm so stupid," "I can never do anything right," or "I'm the world's clumsiest person" are devaluing and belittling statements that indicate low self-esteem.

Individuals with chemical dependence may cause family disintegration. The nurse assesses the family dynamics in terms of the effects the client's behavior has on the family as well as the family's needs that are met by his behavior. In the early stages of chemical dependence, the family may make excuses for the member's behavior. Later they may lie to relatives and friends in an attempt to conceal the problem. On the other hand, the family members may facilitate the dependence by obtaining prescriptions for him or creating and promoting situations that they know lead to the increased stress that results in drinking. The family may also use the dependent member as a scapegoat by focusing on his problem as the sole cause for the underlying family conflict. The family may become dysfunctional in a different way if the client recovers and the family does not deal with its addictive issues. However, the family problems increase as the client's chemical dependence increases, and sometimes the family unit dissolves, leaving the client alone. At other times the family stays together, continuing the same dynamics that perpetuate the problem. Recovery becomes extremely difficult.

Assessing the occupational history of the client with maladaptive dependent or independent behavior is important because the individual may have varying degrees of occupational impairment. The extent of occupational impairment varies with the amount of maladaptive dependence. Job-related behaviors to be assessed include increased absenteeism, absence from the job on Mondays, and prolonged breaks. The client who displays maladaptive independence to the extent of disregarding social norms has difficulty keeping a job. The behaviors that cause the individual to have legal problems also affect occupational functioning. The individual is impulsive, shows little or no responsibility, is late or does not show up, and often just walks off the job.

According to psychoanalytical theory, the maladaptive dependent individual placed in an unstructured work situation has difficulty structuring his work. The person also has difficulty with jobs that require independent decisions. Behaviors that interfere with the dependent person's occupational functioning include procrastination, stubbornness, indecisiveness, impulsiveness, depression, and frequent mood swings. The maladaptive independent individual usually appears to do well alone. The family dynamics are reversed from those of the dependent person's family. Often the family feels left out and not needed. In cases of extreme maladaptive independent coping behavior, the individual feels in total control of the external and internal environment. This interferes with social contacts, family, and occupational functioning.

Spiritual dimension Interdependence allows the individual to develop spiritually and to continue to strive for his full potential. By definition, interdependence permits one to be dependent on others (including a higher power) or to be dependent on self. Therefore the individual has the freedom to believe or not to believe in a higher power. The interdependent person does not have an excessive need for *affiliation*, which is a need to be very closely associated with an organization. Nor does the interdependent person have to feel totally in control of the internal and external environment.

Maladaptive dependent behavior makes it difficult to develop a realistic, meaningful philosophy. The extremely dependent person may avow a belief in a higher power; however, this belief is colored by the person's internal stimuli, which produces an excessive need for affiliation. These same stimuli influence the person to cling to family and friends. The dependent person does not allow enough self-growth to reach his full potential including creative endeavors. He may gravitate to cults because of a need to be told what to do. Superficial reliance on a higher power may occur, especially in the person with a dependent personality disorder who is easily influenced by authority figures and religious practices and who is unable to make one's own decisions.

Maladaptive independent coping behavior also interferes with spiritual needs. The person has difficulty forming a relatedness to a higher power or to other people because of a basic mistrust of himself and others. In severe cases, the individual may have no respect for the morals and values of others. This individual is not able to attain self-actualization.

Religious teachings and attendance at worship services may promote dependence on a higher power. These practices may be viewed as necessary for relating to a higher power. The nurse assesses the client's involvement by determining the amount of time spent in worship activities and the client's attitude toward these activities.

Measurement tools

Several tools have been developed to measure dependence, independence, and related concepts such as deference (to seek and sustain subordinate roles in relationships with others). Table 16-5 summarizes these scales.

Analysis
Nursing diagnosis

The NANDA nursing diagnosis related to dependence and independence is powerlessness. The defining characteristics of this diagnosis are summarized in the box.

The following case example illustrates characteristics of the nursing diagnosis of powerlessness.

▼ **TABLE 16-5** Instruments Used to Measure Dependence, Independence, and Related Concepts

Instruments	Measures
Bellar Checklist[5]	Changes in dependence and independence
D-1 Scale[12,19]	Dependence and independence
Minnesota Multiphasic Personality Inventory (MMPI)[56]	Dependence and independence
Millon Clinical Multiaxial Inventory[56]	Dependent subscale diagnoses dependent personality disorder
The Adjective Check List[44]	Subscale of deference is related to dependence
Edwards Personal Preference Schedule[5]	Three properties of dependency—reliance on others for approval, reliance on others for help, and conformity to the opinions and demands of others
Situational Test of Dependency[68]	Overt dependency

▼ **Case Example**

Paul, age 52, is an executive in a high-technology firm, where he has been employed for 26 years. Recently, the firm merged with an out-of-state firm. All the decisions are passed from headquarters without consulting anyone in the local office. Paul is a high achiever and had been in a control situation for more than 10 years. He now has an immense feeling of powerlessness. His opinion is no longer important.

Although he has drunk alcohol on social occasions since college, he always felt he was in control of his drinking. As his feelings of powerlessness have increased, so has his drinking. It has now reached a point where he is frequently late for work or misses work altogether. Although he quit a teen-age smoking habit 25 years ago, he has begun smoking again. He spends 12 to 16 hours a day at work, sometimes sitting at his desk staring straight ahead with a blank look on his face. His wife is worried about his changes and withdrawal from the family. He has agreed to see a counselor.

Paul's powerlessness is a reality, directly related to a sudden change in his work situation. He is unable to cope with his change. He denies and represses his feelings and turns to addictive behavior and social isolation for comfort. He has moved from an interdependent person with an independent view of his occupation to one of perceived and actual dependence. Much to his wife's dismay, he has turned

▼ **POWERLESSNESS**

DEFINITION
Perception that one's own action will not significantly affect an outcome; a perceived lack of control over a current situation or immediate happening

DEFINING CHARACTERISTICS
- **Physical dimension**

  Does not defend self-care practices when challenged

- **Emotional dimension**

  Depression over physical deterioration that occurs despite client compliance with regimens
  Apathy
  Expressions of dissatisfaction and frustration over inability to perform previous tasks and/or activities
  Reluctance to express true feelings, fearing alienation from caregivers

- **Intellectual dimension**

  Expressions of uncertainty about fluctuating energy levels
  Verbal expressions of having no control or influence over situation
  Verbal expressions of having no control or influence over outcome
  Verbal expressions of having no control over self-care
  Nonparticipation in care or decision making when opportunities are provided
  Does not monitor progress
  Inability to seek information regarding care

- **Social dimension**

  Dependence on others that may result in irritability, resentment, anger, and guilt
  Passivity

Modified from Kim MS, McFarland GK, McLane AM, editors: *Pocket guide to nursing diagnoses,* ed 5, St Louis, 1993, Mosby–Year Book.

▼ TABLE 16-6   NURSING CARE PLAN

GOALS	OUTCOME CRITERIA	INTERVENTIONS	RATIONALES
NURSING DIAGNOSIS: Impaired social interaction related to meeting dependency needs by manipulation			
LONG TERM To engage in effective social exchanges	Verbalizes awareness of factors that lead to difficulty in social interactions	Assist to identify factors that lead to unsuccessful social interactions	Knowledge about causes may contribute to changing the behavior
	Verbalizes desire to have positive social interactions	Give positive feedback for verbalizations	Positive feedback is an incentive to continue the behavior
	Demonstrates increased ability to have successful social interactions	Teach effective social skills	Client may never have learned to interact effectively
		Assist to identify people with whom client feels comfortable and encourage interaction with them	Provides opportunity for positive interaction without rejection and increases confidence in ability to have effective interactions
SHORT TERM To meet dependency needs without using manipulation	Verbalizes relationship between dependence and use of manipulation	Assist to explore relationship between dependence and use of manipulation	Client can learn that manipulation prevents direct expression of healthy dependence
	Expresses willingness to use constructive behavior to meet dependence needs	Assist to identify effective ways to meet dependency needs	Knowledge about effective ways to meet dependency needs serves as a foundation for changing behavior
	Demonstrates attempts to use nonmanipulative behavior to meet dependency needs	Give positive feedback when client uses nonmanipulative behavior	Positive feedback motivates client to continue behavior
			Conveys confidence in client's ability to use constructive ways to meet needs
		Role model constructive ways to meet dependency needs	Role modeling provides concrete example of desired behavior
NURSING DIAGNOSIS: Powerlessness related to perceived inability to make decisions.			
LONG TERM To experience increased sense of power and control in decision making	Verbalizes increased feeling of power in ability to make decisions	Assist to identify specific decision making situations in which he feels powerless	Recognition of what contributes to feeling of powerlessness Provides baseline data for plans to change behavior
		Provide opportunities for client to express feelings of control of decisions	Increases client's confidence in his abilities to be in control
	Engages in behavior to increase sense of power and control in decision making	Assist to identify decision making situations he can control	A sense of control is increased with knowledge
			Recognition that he can control some situations increases confidence in ability to assert himself with others
		Assist to develop coping strategies for situations he can realistically control	Availability of coping strategies and knowledge of what he can control reduces anxiety and increases confidence
		Role-play situations that involve control in decision making	Role-playing helps to try out behavior in a nonthreatening situation

▼ **TABLE 16-6   NURSING CARE PLAN** —cont'd

GOALS	OUTCOME CRITERIA	INTERVENTIONS	RATIONALES
SHORT TERM			
To experience increased ability to make decisions	Verbalizes willingness to make decisions	Assist client to examine behavior and arrive at reasons for inability to make decisions	Recognition of reason for behavior may motivate client to change behavior
		Review past experience with decision making	Provides frame of reference for examining present decision making behavior
		Teach client step-by-step process for making decisions	Client may be unaware of the process for making decisions
		Encourage client to defer fewer decisions to others	Making decisions increases confidence in ability to do so
			Contributes to independent functioning
		Support client's efforts in making decisions, even when not always successful	Reinforces independence in decision making
			Allows client to learn that he will not always be successful and to experience failure in a safe environment

to unhealthy behaviors for comfort rather than proactively solving the problem. Without intervention his behaviors will worsen and seriously affect his family and occupational situation. A nurse can use Paul's history of independence to assist him in reversing his destructive behaviors.

The following list provides examples of NANDA-accepted nursing diagnoses with causative statements related to maladaptive dependence and independence:
1. Ineffective individual coping related to maladaptive dependence on others.
2. Impaired social interaction related to inability to maintain close relationships with others.
3. Ineffective individual coping related to resistance to receiving help during an acute incapacitating illness.
4. Powerlessness related to inability to perform activities of daily living.
5. Powerlessness related to spouse making client's major decisions.

Planning

Table 16-6 provides a nursing care plan with some long-term and short-term goals, outcome criteria, nursing interventions, and rationales related to dependence-independence. These serve as examples of the planning stage in the nursing process.

Implementation

Physical dimension Once the nurse has ascertained the client's physical abilities, the nurse works with the client to develop a plan stating (1) the activities of daily living the client can execute independently, (2) the activities with which the client needs assistance, and (3) the

activities that the nurse needs to perform for the client. Using behavioral theory, the nurse may use positive reinforcement when the client demonstrates initiative in performing the activities of daily living as outlined. The positive reinforcement consists of simply praising the client for doing the tasks or, for hospitalized clients, of allowing the client extra privileges, such as a walk or other types of recreation. The nurse also uses the therapeutic relationship to work with the client who has difficulty either in taking the initiative in doing activities of daily living or in staying within the established limitations.

Initially, the nurse needs to meet the client's dependency needs. It may be necessary to assist the client in activities of daily living, help him in making decisions, and offer much praise and attention. In the client and his family's best interests, the nurse continually assists them toward increasing independence, realizing that setbacks may occur when a client is changing lifelong behaviors; considerable encouragement will be needed to alter his life-style.[62]

Once the client has discontinued using a chemical substance, the nurse needs to assist him to recognize and discuss that life without the substance is a major loss. The nurse's intervention needs to be directed toward helping the client grieve the loss of a significant aspect of his life-style (see Chapter 13).

Other interventions that the nurse may consider for the dependent client are weight control measures such as a weight reduction diet, an exercise regimen, and a balanced nutritional program. The nurse teaches the client stress management techniques and measures to alter any distortion of body image. The client with physical limitations due to trauma or arthritis may need assistive devices such as a cane, special eating utensils, or a wheelchair to attain more independence.

Emotional dimension Since a characteristic of dependent behavior is to allow significant others to physically or psychologically abuse them, the nurse needs to recognize signs of abuse and implement plans to change this behavior (see Chapter 34). Self-abuse can be altered by such interventions as thought-stopping techniques (see Chapter 12), participating in support groups, and encouragement to recognize and change the negative messages given by oneself.

The dependent person often has underlying anger. Once anger is identified, the nurse works with the client to express the anger using some of the interventions discussed in Chapter 11. One effective method for dealing with anger is learning how to be assertive. *Assertiveness* is the ability to express one's needs and desires directly to the appropriate person in an appropriate manner. Assertiveness, as opposed to aggressiveness, does not rely on sarcasm or belittling others. It involves assuming responsibility for one's self and one's emotions and not projecting these onto another individual. At the same time, the assertive person does not allow others to belittle him, nor does he accept responsibility for the other's behavior or emotions.

Assertive behavior is difficult for the dependent individual to learn, especially when he has been raised in an environment that gave no encouragement for this healthy behavior. An example of assertive behavior occurs when an alcoholic accuses his wife of being responsible for his drinking, and she informs him that he, not she, is responsible for his behavior. The nurse needs to work with the client to implement assertive behavior. Frequently, especially in the early stages of developing assertiveness, the client may display aggression, and the nurse assists the client to distinguish between the two behaviors and change aggression into assertion.

Assertiveness training is one method for reducing dependent, passive, and aggressive behavior and increasing assertive behavior. Nurses can conduct individual or group assertiveness training that can substantially alter a dependent client's life-style. Assertiveness training is a communication skill training that promotes more effective behaviors with respect to (1) firm, direct presentation of self; (2) active work orientation; (3) constructive work habits; (4) effectiveness in giving and taking criticism; (5) better control of anxiety or fear; and (6) satisfaction with performance.[16]

Assertiveness training typically involves people in a series of sessions that address various aspects of problem situations. Such problems may include managing aggression, getting needs met in a different way, speaking effectively, identifying intimidating factors, and enacting stress management techniques. The specific arrangement of content and sessions varies considerably, but assertiveness

---

RESEARCH HIGHLIGHT

The Effects of Assertiveness Training on Older Adults
• AW Franzke

PURPOSE

The purpose of this study was to determine whether assertiveness training is an effective intervention method for improving the quality of life for older adults.

SAMPLE

Eighty-four people (30 men and 54 women) over 65 years of age living in the San Antonio, Texas, area composed the sample. Forty-two people who were rated as upper class and were members of the American Association of Retired Persons (AARP) participated. Forty-two were lower or lower middle-class people from a nutrition center for the elderly. There were 21 people in each experimental and control group. The AARP members were volunteers recruited at a national meeting at which the researcher's offered a free assertiveness training class. The participants from the nutrition center were a convenience sample. Participants were chosen for the experimental and control groups after rating by the researcher on the Shevy and Bell Constructs of Social Rank allowing control for socioeconomic status. The participants were rated by preretirement occupation and educational level. The occupation of the husband was used for women who had not been employed outside the home.

METHODOLOGY

The experimental group was given a 6-week course in assertiveness training by the researcher; the control group was not given the training. Both groups were given pretests and posttests. Two self-report scales were administered: the Assertiveness Inventory and the Burger Scale for Expressed Acceptance of Self. For the assertiveness training, the experimental group was divided into four groups: two groups of AARP members and two groups from the nutrition center. The researcher taught six classes for all the groups.

FINDINGS

The assertiveness training had a significant effect on scores for assertiveness and self-concept. The upper-class experimental and control group (AARP) reported a more significant increase in positive self-concept than the lower classes (nutrition group). The difference between the pretest and posttest was significant for both groups on the assertiveness measure. There were no significant differences between men and women.

IMPLICATIONS

Nurses working with older clients can assist them to achieve a more productive and satisfying life by using an assertiveness training course as an intervention method. These participants learned and applied the assertiveness skills at a level that significantly improved their skills and self-concepts.

Based on data from *The Gerontologist* 27:13, 1987.

DRUG PROFILE

CLORAZEPATE DIPOTASSIUM
(klor-az'e-pate)
Tranxene
Func class: Antianxiety
Chem class: Benzodiazepine

Controlled Substance Schedule IV
Action: Depresses subcortical levels of CNS, including limbic system, reticular formation
Uses: Anxiety, acute alcohol withdrawal, adjunct in seizure disorders
Dosage and routes:
Anxiety
▶ *Adult:* PO 15-60 mg/day
Alcohol withdrawal
▶ *Adult:* PO 30 mg then 30-60 mg in divided doses; day 2, 45-90 mg in divided doses; day 3, 22.5-45 mg in divided doses; day 4, 15-30 mg in divided doses; then reduce daily dose to 7.5-15 mg
Seizure disorders
▶ *Adult and child >12 yr:* PO 7.5 mg tid, may increase by 7.5 mg/wk or less, not to exceed 90 mg/day
▶ *Child 9-12 yr:* PO 7.5 mg bid, may increase by 7.5 mg/wk or less, not to exceed 60 mg/day
Available forms include: Caps 3.75, 7.5, 15 mg; tabs 3.75, 7.5, 15 mg, single dose tab 11.25, 22.5 mg

Italic indicates common side effects.
Bold italic indicates life-threatening reactions.

Side effects/adverse reactions:
CNS: Dizziness, drowsiness, confusion, headache, anxiety, tremors, stimulation, fatigue, depression, insomnia, hallucinations
GI: Constipation, dry mouth, nausea, vomiting, anorexia, diarrhea
INTEG: Rash, dermatitis, itching
CV: Orthostatic hypotension, ***ECG changes, tachycardia,*** hypotension
EENT: Blurred vision, tinnitus, mydriasis
Contraindications: Hypersensitivity to benzodiazepines, narrow-angle glaucoma, psychosis, pregnancy (D), child <18 yr
Precautions: Elderly, debilitated, hepatic disease, renal disease
Pharmacokinetics:
PO: Onset 15 min, peak 1-2 hr, duration 4-6 hr, metabolized by liver, excreted by kidneys, crosses placenta, breast milk, half-life 30-100 hr
Interactions/incompatibilities:
—Decreased effects of clorazepate: valproic acid
—Increased effects of clorazepate: CNS depressants, alcohol, disulfiram, oral contraceptives, antidepressants, MAOIs

NURSING CONSIDERATIONS
Assess:
—B/P (lying, standing), pulse; if systolic B/P drops 20 mm Hg, hold drug, notify physician

—Blood studies: CBC during long-term therapy, blood dyscrasias have occurred rarely
—Hepatic studies: AST, ALT, bilirubin, creatinine, LDH, alk phosphatase
—I&O; may indicate renal dysfunction
Administer:
—With food or milk for GI symptoms
—Crushed if client is unable to swallow medication whole
—Sugarless gum, hard candy, frequent sips of water for dry mouth
Perform/provide:
—Assistance with ambulation during beginning therapy, since drowsiness/dizziness occurs
—Safety measures, including siderails
—Check to see PO medication has been swallowed
Evaluate:
—Therapeutic response: decreased anxiety, restlessness, insomnia
—Mental status: mood, sensorium, affect, sleeping pattern, drowsiness, dizziness

—Physical dependency, withdrawal symptoms: headache, nausea, vomiting, muscle pain, weakness after long-term use
—Suicidal tendencies
Teach client/family:
—That drug may be taken with food
—Not to be used for everyday stress or used longer than 4 mo, unless directed by physician; not to take more than prescribed amount, may be habit forming
—To avoid OTC preparations unless approved by physician
—To avoid driving, activities that require alertness; drowsiness may occur
—To avoid alcohol ingestion or other psychotropic medications, unless prescribed by physician
—Not to discontinue medication abruptly after long-term use
—To rise slowly or fainting may occur
—That drowsiness might worsen at beginning of treatment
Lab test interferences:
Increase: AST/ALT, serum bilirubin
Decrease: RAIU
False increase: 17-OHCS
Treatment of overdose: Lavage, VS, supportive care

Modified from Skidmore-Roth L: *Mosby's nursing drug reference,* St Louis, 1993, Mosby–Year Book.

programs consistently emphasize the development of new behaviors. In a comprehensive program, the client is taught new ways such as making simple requests, handling compliments and criticisms, diminishing the harmful effects of anger, building self-affirmations, and demonstrating caring and methods to reinforce and maintain assertive skills.

Training is usually limited to a number of weeks or a few months at most. Learning assertiveness in a shorter program without practice and constructive feedback can create significant problems in day-to-day living. When a client unexpectedly and abruptly becomes assertive in a situation in which he formerly was relatively passive, the new behavior often evokes anger rather than praise. Others have become comfortable with the person's lack of assertiveness and have developed their own roles around the client's role; the new behavior may evoke punishment rather than reward. Clients need to be taught to expect these reactions as they change their behaviors.

A second potential negative consequence of assertiveness training can occur. If the client's personality pattern and defenses depend on a passive stance, the seemingly simple change to more assertive behavior is likely to produce unexpected and intense anxiety and uncertainty. The nurse teaches the client to recognize these symptoms and seek appropriate assistance when the reactions become beyond the client's ability to alter. Clorazepate dipotassium (Tranxene) may be prescribed to help control anxiety. The accompanying profile describes nursing care appropriate to the administration of clorazepate. Mastering assertiveness requires a sizable investment of time and energy. Becoming skilled requires study and practice, trial and error sessions, and more study and practice.

For healthy people, assertiveness training may be another useful method for positive changes in behavior regardless of their age (see the research highlight on p. 320). However, for the person with subtle serious underlying mental health difficulties, in whom passivity is an integral part of the personality, the risk is significant; and the training is undertaken ideally only as a complement to ongoing counseling or psychotherapy.

◤ **Intellectual dimension** To help the client develop an interdependent coping style, the nurse encourages the client to generate solutions for his problems. She asks him to identify a simple problem and set easy, short-term goals to reach a solution. An example is a client who does not take care of his own hygiene. The nurse has the client identify the aspect of hygiene that would be easiest for him to initiate. The client then sets a short-term goal, such as "I will comb my hair by 9 AM daily without being reminded to do so." Using behavioral theory, the nurse compliments the client when he initiates the action on his own. The nurse thus can assist the client in making sound decisions and setting goals that he can accomplish. A positive approach is used, which involves the client without making him entirely responsible for making the decision. The environment can be structured so that the client can succeed in establishing and reaching goals.

Because denial is a defense mechanism used by the person with dependent behavior, especially one who abuses chemical substances or is involved in other addictive processes, sound nursing judgment is essential. The nurse does not attempt to force the client to eliminate using the denial mechanism. The client's long-term needs must be considered, and exploring the fears and anxieties underlying the denial is necessary. For instance, the person abusing a substance is more apt to be receptive to dealing with the problem when he is in a physical or emotional crisis; alleviating the crisis too soon may prevent seeking treatment. During this crisis time, denial is less pronounced, and the client is more willing to accept the reality of the problem and the need to take action. The nurse can now help the individual verbalize his feelings and perceptions about his problem. With verbalization, anxiety subsides and denial may not be necessary.

Instead of confronting the client about a dependency problem, the nurse may approach the situation by assisting the client in identifying the dependency behaviors. Once the client identifies the behaviors, the nurse can confront the client about the result of these behaviors. What is the impact on the client, the family, the client's job? While exploring these behaviors and their overall impact, the client may become conscious of the reality of dependency as a problem. Once this occurs, the client is able to begin accepting the treatment regimen. The dependent client's family also uses denial and needs to be supported to accept the reality of the situation and the client's maladaptive dependence and to help change the dependency.

The individual with a maladaptive independent coping style also uses denial to a degree that is detrimental to optimal health. In some cases, such as a client with diabetes mellitus or severe myocardial infarction, denial of the seriousness of the problem or denial of the need to change behavior can be life threatening. Because denial is usually based on a need to be independent, the nurse assists the client in identifying comfortable and uncomfortable dependent behaviors. She helps him accept comfortable dependent situations. She also allows the client as much control of the external environment as possible. For example, the client can make decisions such as when he will bathe or when he will meet with the nurse. The nurse needs to reinforce behaviors that indicate acceptance of the reality of dependent situations.

The individual with a dependent life-style, whether dependent on people or addictive substances and circumstances, needs to learn decision making skills. The client is taught how to make simple decisions and is supported throughout the process. First, he is taught to specify the problem and to gather data about it. Second, the client is taught to propose alternatives. Next, he discusses the pros and cons of the alternatives and then selects one of them. The client then applies the alternative and evaluates the result. By practicing these steps and making increasingly more complex decisions, he can learn how to make decisions unaided. Support from the nurse is essential in teaching the client how to problem solve throughout the process.

Social dimension From the outset of the relationship, the nurse sets limits on the amount and type of dependent behavior that will be tolerated and clearly communicates these limitations to the client. As the nurse begins the relationship with the client whose dependence is maladaptive, she meets and structures his social dependency needs and then gradually assists him to do more for himself. For example, as rapport increases, the client may want to talk longer and more frequently to the nurse. In the initial work with this client, the nurse could say, "Hi, I'm the nurse who will work with you. I'll want to talk with you for up to 10 minutes every day." The support and guidance to gradually increase self-care conveys recognition of the client as a responsible person.

The nurse can help the client feel more in control of the situation and less dependent by anticipating his dependency needs. Early in the relationship this approach helps to develop trust. Assisting the client in identifying ways he expresses his dependence as well as sources of the dependent behaviors is helpful. As he becomes aware of the dependent behavior, the client needs support to move toward greater independence. In the process of moving toward the goal of interdependence, the client may demonstrate exaggerated independent behavior. The nurse accepts this behavior and discusses possible motivations for the behavior with the client.

Behavior modification may be used for intervention in the client's attention-seeking behavior. Positive reinforcement involves giving consistent, positive rewards for identified desirable behavior. The nurse clearly communicates to the client and the health team members what is desirable behavior. She may positively reinforce the client's behavior by giving him attention at times other than when he asks for something. She praises him when he does not engage in the attention-seeking behavior. Negative reinforcement is achieved by consistently ignoring behavior that is clearly identified as undesirable. To implement this approach, the nurse ignores the client's attention-seeking behavior.

▼ Case Example

Max is a 27-year-old paraplegic hospitalized for reevaluation of his physical status. Each of the past four hospitalization days have been spent with his wife at his bedside from 7 AM to 9 PM. She leaves to stay with their 4-year-old son at night. As soon as she leaves, he operates the call light frequently for "small requests" such as a drink of water, pulling the pillow higher in bed, or obtaining a bed pan. Each request is separate, and the two evening and night shift nurses have a difficult time cordially meeting his requests with the other 34 clients on their unit. Finally, the night nurse realizes she has a fearful, dependent client who needs further assessment and interventions to diminish his fears and increase his independence in a situation that he views as frightening.

When a client like Max uses excessive attention-seeking behaviors, the nurse confronts the client about these behaviors and assists him in identifying them. The client is encouraged to talk about the feelings that the behaviors evoke. The nurse helps the client identify and establish mature types of behavior to meet his needs. For example, the nurse explores independent or interdependent behaviors that can replace the negative attention-seeking behaviors. The nurse helps the client identify behaviors that are comfortable for him and then sets stages for initiating this behavior. The client describes problems he encounters and rehearses more assertive responses with the nurse. The client may practice the comfortable behavior once a day and then increase it in small increments until the behavior is spontaneous and new skills such as assertion are learned. As the client changes to more interdependent behavior, the nurse gives the client positive reinforcement by praising him for displaying more adaptive behavior.

Maladaptive dependent behavior can lead to low self-esteem, resulting in numerous problems such as loneliness and physical and psychological abuse (see Chapters 21 and 34). The nurse uses a nonjudgmental approach, accepting the client's positive and negative attributes. The nurse sets attainable goals with the client so that he can achieve greater self-esteem. The nurse approaches the client in a consistent, accepting manner, thus indicating to the client that she considers him a person of value.

The first step in treatment of the abused client is to find out if the client recognizes the abusive treatment. The nurse can ask questions such as "Who abuses you?" "When does it occur?" and "What are your feelings about the abuse?" Developing increased self-esteem and encouraging the expression of feelings allows the abused client to recognize the abuse and the feelings it generates. These clients need support to treat themselves in a gentle and compassionate manner; often they have never experienced genuine caring for who they are as people. (See Chapter 34 for further discussion of abuse.)

The client with maladaptive dependence frequently feels lonely and needs to develop an interdependent behavior. Numerous interventions to increase socialization opportunities and skills for clients with personality disorders are detailed in Chapter 21. The nurse assists the client by first arranging to spend time with the client. It may be necessary just to sit with him. Once a therapeutic relationship with the nurse is established, the client may talk about his feelings of loneliness. The nurse then helps the client balance his needs for dependence with his needs for independence. As the client's maladaptive dependent behavior decreases and he is able to take initiative, the nurse explores ways of increasing contact with others. The nurse works with the client to change maladaptive behaviors to a socially acceptable mode.

Because the individual's maladaptive behaviors occur within the family, knowledge about how the family interacts is essential for successful treatment. Some substance abuse treatment centers use family intervention and milieu therapy in a family group situation. Community mental health agencies also work with the family. To ensure continuity of care, the community mental health nurse and the hospital-based nurse maintain open communication.

Twelve-step programs exist for almost every addiction

and abuse situation as Americans realize the epidemic proportions of these harmful problems and more openly address related problems such as codependency. Work settings also may offer counseling or support groups as employee benefits. These maladaptive dependencies and independencies create problems for the client, the family, the work setting, and society and require the attention and resources necessary to prevent and minimize their consequences.

The nurse is not usually involved with the client's legal problems which may result from addictive processes. However, the nurse explores the client's perception of the problem. What does the client see as the cause of the problem? The nurse identifies behaviors that have resulted in the legal problem and then explores with the client his responsibility for the problem.

Occupational impairment frequently occurs as a result of maladaptive dependent or independent behaviors. The nurse assists the client in realistically assessing personal capabilities and limitations by having the client list both strengths and weaknesses. The nurse expands the strengths and weaknesses that the client overlooks. The nurse also refers the client for job or educational counseling.

 Spiritual dimension To help the client meet his spiritual needs, the nurse encourages him to discuss his beliefs and values, to explore his own philosophy of life, and to identify whether his maladaptive dependent or independent coping has led him to develop values and behaviors that interfere with treatment. The nurse may need to encourage the client to seek spiritual guidance.

The maladaptive dependent client may meet spiritual needs through superficially developed ritualistic worship practice or be so dependent on others such as a parent that the creative self has never been discovered. Feelings of worthlessness may accompany dependency.

Clients with maladaptive independent behaviors may appear so busy or so self-reliant that time is never or only fleetingly taken to explore creative endeavors and relationships with a higher power, the self, and others. These clients

---

▼ KEY INTERVENTIONS RELATED TO DEPENDENCE-INDEPENDENCE

Determine range of client's need for assistance
Meet dependency needs initially
Assist with weight control measures
Allow for expression of anger
Teach assertiveness
Teach problem solving
Assist in indentifying dependency behaviors that are comfortable and those that are not
Teach decision making skills
Assist in identifying ways to get adaptive dependency needs met
Use behavior modification for attention-seeking behaviors
Explore independent and interdependent behavior to replace maladaptive dependence
Increase socialization opportunities and skills
Obtain knowledge about family's interaction patterns
Encourage to discuss religious beliefs and values related to dependence-independence

GUIDELINES FOR PRIMARY/TERTIARY PREVENTION

Primary Prevention

Identify risk factors that contribute to dependency
Teach parents about healthy child rearing practices such as bonding, need for development of autonomy
Teach parents decision-making/problem-solving skills

Tertiary Prevention
Community resources

Community mental health center
Advocates for battered women
Substance abuse treatment centers
Vocational counseling

Self-help groups

Codependents Anonymous
Emotions Anonymous
Alcoholics Anonymous
Narcotics Anonymous

may need to spend time and energy in activities that nurture the spiritual dimension.

Either extreme of the dependence-independence continuum creates problems with the client's spirituality. A healthy interdependent approach best helps the client mature, meet ongoing spiritual needs, and experience life to its fullest. See the box on p. 323 for key interventions for dependence-independence and the box above for guidelines for primary and tertiary prevention.

INTERACTION WITH A DEPENDENT CLIENT

Nurse: *(Enters the day room of the mental health center. Clients are involved in small group activities in clusters scattered around the room. Mr. Mitchell is being treated for depression; he has a flat affect, is recently widowed, and generally seems "lost." In this outpatient situation, he has paired with another male client, Mr. Coker, who frequently speaks for him, bosses him around, and makes decisions for him. They did not know each other before meeting at the center. She approaches both of them and interrupts their card game. Mr. Mitchell has an appointment with her in 5 minutes and then is scheduled to get his morning medication.)* Good morning Mr. Mitchell and Mr. Coker. I see you are busy playing cards again today. Mr. Mitchell, I just wanted to let you know that my office had a roof leak last night and we'll need to meet in the other nurse's office.

Client Mitchell: *Okay, I'll be right there. (He makes an effort to stand.)*

Client Coker: *Wait a minute. We're not done here and you promised to play gin rummy with me this morning. (He places his hand in a restraining manner on Mr. Mitchell's arm. Mr. Mitchell obeys and does not complete his standing effort.)*

Client Mitchell: *(Appears in conflict and anxious.) I'll come as soon as I finish. I've got to keep my promise to my friend.*

Nurse: *(Places her hand under his forearm and gently urges him to a standing position.) Mr. Mitchell, you'll be*

able to keep your promise to him after we talk. I'm sure Mr. Coker won't mind if you keep your promise to meet with me, too. You can play cards in between your treatment sessions. (Mr. Mitchell willingly stands and leaves with her.)

Underlying Mr. Mitchell's depression was maladaptive dependency. Such clients are vulnerable with people who may not have their best interest in mind when they develop relationships. Mr. Mitchell was unable to make a decision and would have acquiesced to the strongest personality in the interaction. This was not a time to teach him new behaviors; it was a time to act as an advocate and set limits for him. Limit setting and assertiveness training become part of a successful treatment regimen, ensuring his optimal recovery.

Evaluation

Treatment is considered successful when the client recognizes the maladaptive ways that he expresses his dependency needs and comfortably alternates between being dependent, independent, and interdependent. Evaluation centers on the client's ability to express satisfaction with his altered dependent or independent state, to reduce or eliminate the personality difficulties created by maladaptive dependence or independence, and to achieve awareness of these healthy alterations.

The individual with addictions and abuse shows success as he begins to attend the appropriate self-help group, admits his dependence on external substances and events, and develops new behaviors for meeting his needs. Recovery can take years and considerable effort. When constructive change does not occur, the nurse develops new goals and incorporates alternative strategies into the revised nursing care plan. The objective is to encourage the client toward healthy interdependence.

Criteria pertinent to determining the success of the treatment goals with the maladaptive dependent or independent client include the following:

1. *Adequacy*: Did the interventions alter the problems with dependency? Were the maladaptive behaviors changed and goals met? Were the interventions matched to the client's life-style? Were the behaviors altered over a long time?

2. *Appropriateness*: Was the intervention related to the severity of the symptoms? Were acute symptoms the focus of immediate attention? Did the recommended interventions consider the client's and family's personal abilities and resources including income?

3. *Effectiveness*: Did the client learn to manage maladaptive dependent or independent behaviors? Were the goals and interventions specific to dependence and independence problems? Did the client change behaviors to alleviate the harmful effects of dependence and independence?

4. *Efficiency*: Were interventions sufficient to prevent or minimize the negative consequences of maladaptive dependence and independence? Did the client and family experience relief from distress? Were resources helpful? Does the client have fewer unhealthy behaviors? Did the process move at a pace that considered the client's readiness and energy level?

Involving the client and family throughout the treatment program provides invaluable information about the effectiveness of the plan and can minimize or prevent relapses. Such involvement also enhances the likelihood of permanent change and the adoption of healthier behaviors. Reinforcing positive change encourages the client's receptiveness and adoption of new ways to relating to self, others, and circumstances. If the client reseeks the nurse's assistance after termination, the nurse needs to be accepting of the situation and willing to resume the relationship or refer the client for other help.

BRIEF REVIEW

The human infant begins life totally dependent on others for nurturing all facets of his person. If the infant's needs are adequately met in the dependent phase, the infant is able to move to the independent phase. Once the independent needs are met, the toddler is able to begin learning interdependent behavior.

The interdependent individual is capable of using both dependent and independent coping styles. Interdependent coping is the most adaptive mode of coping. However, everyone at times has difficulty accepting forced dependence or independence. This difficulty does not indicate an overall maladaptive coping style. However, when the individual predominantly uses one style to handle all situations, a maladaptive style exists. Such a rigid pattern is detrimental to attaining an optimal level of health.

Maladaptive behaviors related to dependence and independence include (1) doing more or less than one's physical capabilities allow: (2) seeking approval, praise, and proximity in a manipulative manner; (3) low self-esteem; (4) basic mistrust; (5) anger; (6) denial; (7) rationalization; (8) social isolation; (9) occupational impairment; (10) a rigid pattern of coping; and (11) a poorly defined philosophy of life, values, and mores. These behaviors are displayed by individuals with personality disorders and those who engage in addictive processes.

The nurse's role is to assess the client for dependent and independent coping behaviors, discussing any maladaptive behaviors with the client and working with him to change them. The goal is to move from maladaptive to adaptive coping styles that incorporate flexibility and interdependence so that clients have optimal health.

REFERENCES AND SUGGESTED READINGS

1. Aitken M: Self-concept and functional independence in the hospitalized elderly, *American Journal of Occupational Therapy* 36:243, 1982.
2. Angel G, Petronko D: *Developing the new assertive nurse: essentials for advancement*, New York, 1986, Basic Books.
3. Bartek J and others: Nurse-identified problems in the management of alcoholic patients, *Journal of Studies of Alcohol* 49(1):62, 1988.
4. Belenky M and others: *Women's ways of knowing; the development of self, voice, and mind*, New York, 1986, Basic Books.
5. Bellar E: Dependence and independence in your children, *Journal of Genetic Psychology* 87:25, 1955.
6. Bernardin A and others: A construct validation of the Edwards Personal Preference Schedule with respect to dependency, *Journal of Consulting Psychology* 21(1):63, 1957.
7. Blankfield A: The concept of dependence, *International Journal of Addiction* 22(11):1069, 1987.
8. Booth T: Institutional regimens and induced dependency in homes for the aged, *The Gerontologist* 26:418, 1986.
9. Bower S, Bower G: *Asserting your self*, Menlo Park, California, 1976, Addison-Wesley.
10. Bowlby J: *Attachment and loss,* vol I, New York, 1980, Basic Books.
11. Butler P: *Self-assertion for women*, New York, 1981, Harper and Row.
12. Carpenito L: *Nursing diagnosis: application to clinical practice*, Philadelphia, 1989, JB Lippincott.
13. Chang B and others: Adherence to health care regimens among elderly women, *Nursing Research* 34:27, 1985.
14. Chenevert M: STAT: *Special techniques in assertiveness training*, St Louis, 1983, The CV Mosby Co.
15. Chinn P: Debunking myths in nursing theory and research, *Image—The Journal of Nursing Scholarship* 17:45, 1985.
16. Clark C: *Assertiveness skills for nurses*, Wakefield, Mass, 1978, Nursing Resources.
17. Clark S: Nursing diagnosis: ineffective coping. II. Planning care, *Heart-Lung* 16(6):677, 1987.
18. Clough D, Derdiarian A: A behavioral checklist to measure dependence and independence, *Nursing Research* 29:55, 1980.
19. Derdiarian A, Clough D: Patient's dependence and independence levels on the prehospital-postdischarge continuum, *Nursing Research* 25:47, 1976.
20. Dracup K, Meleis A: Compliance: an interactionist approach, *Nursing Research* 31:31, 1982.
21. Eddins B: Chronic self-destructiveness as manifested by noncompliance behavior in hemodialysis patients, *Journal of Nephrology Nursing* 2:194, 1985.
22. Erikson E: *Childhood and society*, ed 2, New York, 1964, WW Norton.
23. Evers H: Old women's self-perceptions of dependency and some implications for service provision, *Journal of Epidemiological and Community Health* 38:306, 1984.
24. Faugier J: The changing concept of dependence in the drug and alcohol field, *Nurse Practitioner* 1:253, 1986.
25. Fisk N: Alcoholism: ineffective family coping, *American Journal of Nursing* 86(5):586, 1986.
26. Franklin D: Hooked, not hooked: why isn't everyone an addict?, *Industrial Health* 4(6):39, 1990.
27. Franzke A: The effects of assertiveness training on older adults, *The Gerontologist* 27:13, 1987.
28. Freud S: *An outline of psychoanalysis*, New York, 1969, WW Norton.
29. Goldin G and others: *Dependency and its implications for rehabilitation*, Lexington, Mass, 1972, Lexington Book Co.
30. Gorney-Lucerno M: Caring for yourself while caring for others: the issues of codependency, *Perspectives* 6(3):14, Summer, 1991.
31. Gough H: *The adjective check list*, Palo Alto, Calif, 1952, Consulting Psychologists Press.
32. Heller K, Goldstein A: Client dependency and therapist expectancy as relationship maintaining variables in psychotherapy, *Journal of Consulting Psychology* 25(5):370, 1961.
33. Herman S: *Becoming assertive: a guide for nurses*, New York, 1978, D Van Nostrand Co.
34. Higley R: Independence vs. dependence: whose decision? *ANNA Journal* 13:286, 1986.
35. Homer M, Leonard A, Taylor P: The burden of dependency, *Sociological Review* (Monograph)31:77, 1985.
36. Hutchings H, Colburn L: An assertiveness training program for nurses, *Nursing Outlook* 27:394, 1979.
37. Hutchinsen S: Chemically dependent nurses: trajectory toward self-annihilation, *Nursing Research* 35(4):196, 1986.

38. Jakubowski-Spector P: Facilitating the growth of women through assertive training, *Counseling Psychology* 4:75, 1973.

39. Kellner C, Best C, Roberts J and others: Self-destructive behavior in hospitalized medical and surgical patients, *Psychiatric Clinics of North America* 8:279, 1985.

40. Kilkus SP: Adding assertiveness to the nursing profession, *Nursing Success Today* 3:17, 1986.

41. Kilkus SP: Self-assertion and nurses: a different voice, *Nursing Outlook* 38(3):135, 143, 1990.

42. Klaus M, Kennell J: *Parent-infant bonding*, ed 2, St Louis, 1982, The Mosby—Year Book.

43. Lake A: Fostering dependency in the nurse-patient relationship, unpublished master's thesis, Atlanta, 1975, Emory University.

44. Leininger M: Caring: a central focus of nursing and health care services, *Nursing and Health Care* 2:135, 1980.

45. Lenters W: Sick love and sick religion: exposing our dependencies, *Journal of Christian Nursing* 3(1):7, 1986.

46. Levitt E, Bernard L, Zuckerman M: The student nurse, the college woman and the graduate nurse: a comparative study, *Nursing Research* 11(2):80, 1962.

47. Mahler M: *On human symbiosis and the vicissitudes of individuation*, New York, 1976, International Universities Press.

48. McCord M: Compliance: self-care or compromise? *Topics in Clinical Nursing* 1:1, 1986.

49. Milauskas J: Will nursing assert itself? *Nursing Administration Quarterly* 9:1, 1985.

50. Miller A: Nurse/patient dependency—a review of different approaches with particular reference to studies of the dependency of elderly patients, *Advances in Nursing Science* 9:479, 1984.

51. Miller A: Nurse/patient dependency—is it iatrogenic? *Advances in Nursing Science* 10:63, 1985.

52. Miller A: A study of the dependency of elderly patients inwards using different methods of nursing care, *Age and Aging* 14:132, 1985.

53. Mikulic M: Reinforcement of independent and dependent patient behaviors by nursing personnel: an exploratory study, *Nursing Research* 20(2):162, 1971.

54. Murphy R: Patient's advocate: when independence is good medicine, *RN* 47:25, 1984.

55. Numerof R: Assertiveness training for nurses in a general hospital, *Health and Social Work* 3:79, 1978.

56. Overholser J, Kabakoff R, Norman W: The assessment of personality characteristics in depressed and dependent psychiatric inpatients, *Journal of Personal Assessment* 53(1):40, 1989.

57. Padrick K: Compliance: myths and motivators, *Topics in Clinical Nursing* 7:17, 1986.

58. Reed P: An analysis of the concept of self-neglect, *Advances in Nursing Science* 12(1):39, 1989.

59. Reich J: Validity of criteria for DSM-III self-defeating personality disorder, *Psychiatry Research* 30(2):145, 1989.

60. Reid J: Medication compliance in the elderly: a review, *Journal of Clinical and Experimental Gerontology* 7:31, 1985.

61. Rubin T: *Compassion and self-hate: an alternative to despair*, New York, 1986, Macmillan.

62. Shultz C: Lifestyle assessment: a tool for practice, *Nursing Clinics of North America* 19:271, 1984.

63. Smith C: The relationship of nurse-client interaction frequency and duration to dependency scores of nurses and primipara clients in a public health setting, Unpublished master's thesis, Atlanta, 1976, Emory University.

64. Sprock J, Blashfield R, Smith B: Gender weighting of DSM-III-R personality disorder criteria, *American Journal of Psychiatry* 147(5):586, 1990.

65. Sullivan H: *The interpersonal theory of psychiatry*, New York, 1953, WW Norton.

66. Thomasma D: Freedom, dependency and the care of the very old, *Journal of the American Geriatrics Society* 32:906, 1984.

67. Watson J: *Nursing: the philosophy and science of caring*, Boston, 1979, Little, Brown.

68. Willis J: Simple scale for assessing level of dependency of patients in general practice, *British Medical Journal* (Clinical Research, Ed.) 292:1639, 1986.

69. Withers J: Background: why women are unassertive, *Nursing Digest* 6:68, 1978.

70. Zerwekh J, Michaels B: Co-dependency: assessment and recovery, *Nursing Clinics of North America* 24(1):109, 1989.

ANNOTATED BIBLIOGRAPHY

Hemfelt R, Minirth F, Meier P: *Love is a choice: recovery for co-dependent relationships*, Nashville, Tenn, 1989, Thomas Nelson Publishing.

This book summarizes important aspects of codependency in an easily understandable manner. Codependency is defined and causes are delineated. In addition factors that perpetuate the co-dependent cycle are explored. The authors relate the concept to interpersonal relationships surrounding the co-dependent personality. Offering encouragement to the reader, these noted counselors present the stages of recovery and challenge individuals to pursue breaking old, unhealthy ways of relating to others.

Rubin T: *Compassion and self-hate: an alternative to despair*, New York, 1986, Macmillan.

A self-help book emphasizing the development of self-hate. Direct and indirect forms of self-hate are described, and the reader is encouraged to confront and alter these behaviors such as addictions, negative thoughts, maladaptive dependence, illusions, and abuse. The author urges the reader to meet the painful challenge to change one's life. The answer rests with developing compassionate behavior toward oneself and practical "how-to" advice is offered. Change involves choice not compulsion and the reader is challenged to alter negative patterns and build a stronger sense of well-being and understanding.

Shramski T, Harvey D: Paradox of independence, *American Mental Health Counselors Association Journal* 3:4, 1981.

Independence emphasizing total self-reliance is an ideal often projected by mental health workers. To function in the community, however, an individual must adapt to interdependence. This paradox often leads to frustration for mental health counselors and their clients. To resolve the frustration, the goal of independence must be incorporated with the development of mutual support systems and group interactions. Goals need to assist the client in developing an interdependent coping style.

Thomasma D: Freedom, dependency, and the care of the very old, *Journal of the American Geriatrics Society*, 32:906-914, 1984.

Difficulties permeate treatment decisions for the very old and dependent client; these difficulties will increase with new treatments and more technology. Because aging is a process of becoming more dependent, the author proposes a dependency rule where greater responsibility for treatment decisions rests with caregivers. The article focuses on dependency in the aged and the role this plays, along with an increasing loss of personal autonomy, in quality of life judgments.

Waterman A: Individualism and interdependence, *American Psychologist* 36:762, 1981.

Waterman contends that to develop a truly synergistic society built on voluntary participation, individualism must be supported. Research indicates that individuals who are able to express personal beliefs are more able to develop identity, self-actualization, and moral reasoning. These characteristics enable one to function interdependently in society.

Zerwekh J: Co-dependency: assessment and recovery, *Nursing Clinics of North America* 24(1):109-120, 1989.

The author provides an overview of the development of co-dependency from a description of those who were emotionally involved with a chemically dependent person to the suggestion that it is a disease entity in itself. Co-dependency is discussed relative to process addictions (gambling, sex, religion, work, accumulating money, and worry) and substance addictions (alcohol, drugs, food, nicotine, and caffeine). The article broadly discusses codependency definitions, characteristics, stages, and recovery. A hopeful attitude is portrayed as the article gives practical advice on setting boundaries, recognizing shame and guilt, learning to reparent, and learning to give daily affirmations.

Sharon K Holmberg

After studying this chapter, the student will be able to:

- Define trust and mistrust
- Trace the historical perspectives of trust and mistrust
- Describe theories of schizophrenia and delusional (paranoid) disorders
- Discuss the psychopathology of schizophrenia; delusional (paranoid) disorders; and the personality disorders schizoid, paranoid, and schizotypal, as described in the DSM-III-R

- Use the nursing process in caring for clients who mistrust
- Identify current research findings related to mistrust

A mixture of trust and mistrust in a person's basic social attitudes is crucial in developing a health personality. At certain times, interactions clearly require caution. Naiveté or too little caution in adult life can make the individual feel vulnerable. On the other hand, with too much caution the individual will interact with immense wariness. Such extreme wariness puts the individual at risk for disturbed interactions with others. Ideally, the healthy person is able to strike a reasonable balance between these extremes of behavior.

A belief in the trustworthiness of others usually sets the tone for positive interactions. Doubts about trusting arise normally under certain circumstances, such as when promises go unfulfilled. These doubts, for most individuals, are temporary and circumscribed. However, inability to establish and maintain trusting relationships is a potential problem. When such circumstances prevail, pronounced distortions can occur in one's ability to relate to others. The individual may lose self-esteem, feel very unsure of himself, become highly anxious, and ultimately behave in a manner that is unusual or difficult to understand.

These responses may be accompanied by serious distortions in perception, cognitive abilities, and reality testing. When the perceptual and cognitive functioning includes the presence of delusions, hallucinations, disorganized behavior, marked loose associations, and emotional turmoil, the person is *psychotic*. Psychotic behaviors impair the individual's ability to think, respond, remember, communicate, interpret reality, behave appropriately, and meet the ordinary demands of life. These behaviors are seen in persons diagnosed with schizophrenia and paranoid disorders.

The development of the individual's ability to trust cannot be considered separately from the development of mistrust. Both can be viewed as a continuum (Figure 17-1). This section of the chapter focuses on normal aspects of trust and mistrust, followed by the evolution of pathological states in which mistrust appears to predominate. Many theoretical ideas are relevant to the psychotic disorders discussed in this chapter. They represent a variety of ideas

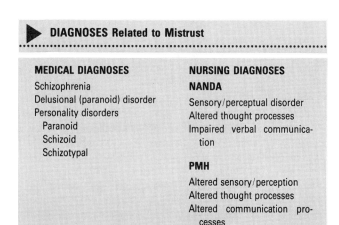

▶ **DIAGNOSES Related to Mistrust**

MEDICAL DIAGNOSES	NURSING DIAGNOSES
Schizophrenia	**NANDA**
Delusional (paranoid) disorder	Sensory/perceptual disorder
Personality disorders	Altered thought processes
Paranoid	Impaired verbal communication
Schizoid	
Schizotypal	
	PMH
	Altered sensory/perception
	Altered thought processes
	Altered communication processes

	DATES	EVENTS
HISTORICAL OVERVIEW	Primitive	Efforts are made to comprehend the environment, rendering it more manageable and trustworthy by ascribing magical qualities to natural forces such as the sun. People thank the "good gods" when economic conditions are good and harvests plentiful. The term *Vesania* or insanity is introduced by the Roman Cicero, who believed the art of healing the soul had been neglected.
	Third Century AD	A distinct separation between bodily causes of illness and other conditions caused by "passions of the soul" is a fairly well established idea.
	Tenth Century AD	Psychological problems have become so intertwined with theological ideas and monastic medicine that psychotic manifestations become known as diabolic possession.
	1700s	The nervous system is discovered. It is recognized that all parts of the body are connected by nerves. Psychiatric conditions are thought to be caused by diseases of the nerves.
	Late 1800s	Concerted efforts are made to classify serious mental disorders. A German, Kraepelin, creates a new category of disorder called *dementia praecox*. The establishment of major state psychiatric hospitals in the United States is in progress.
	1920s	Efforts are made to link psychoanalytical theories of Freud to the biological theories of Kraepelin with little success. Treatment is largely "custodial" and provided in large state hospitals.
	1930s and 1940s	There is an increase in the use of poorly understood biological treatments for severe mental disorders. Insulin therapy, electroconvulsive therapy, and psychosurgery are used to treat psychotic disorders, especially when accompanied by severe behavioral problems.
	1950s	Advances in treatment approaches, such as introduction of phenothiazines, allow for significant improvement of acute psychotic symptoms.
	1960s	With deinstitutionalization and the emphasis on shorter hospital stays followed by outpatient treatment and rehabilitation, the nurse needs to be prepared to work with mistrusting clients both in the hospital and in the community.
	1980s	Contemporary society demonstrates its vulnerability and lack of trust by the use of fences, walls, and security systems.
	1990s	The increase in the use of weapons, especially guns, is a graphic demonstration of the increase in the general level of social mistrust, but there is more discussion of gun control.
	Future	Research on the effectiveness of the therapeutic nurse–client relationship may provide additional understanding of the mistrusting client and lead to new approaches for nursing interventions.

with respect to causes, from biological to psychological and social.

Trust is necessary to interact successfully with others. It requires the individual to have an idea of what meaning to attribute to the words and behavior of another person. The trusting person accepts the fact that others can be relied on. Trust of another person is related to an expectation of a consistent response from the other individual in a given circumstance. Consistency and reliability allow the individual to develop a trust that similar actions, when repeated, produce a similar outcome each time. Thus, trust is reinforced.

When an expected outcome does not happen, the trusting person feels disappointed but is able to cope. The situation is carefully reevaluated. The trusting person is capable of evaluating both his own and the other person's verbal exchanges and behaviors. He may seek help from others in reviewing a particular puzzling or disappointing situation. In doing so, the individual will most likely test the reality of his perceptions and understand more fully what he misunderstood. Trust, then, is related not only to the expectation of similar outcomes in similar circumstances but also to the willingness and ability to analyze objectively deviations from these expected outcomes to realistically understand and explain the outcome.

People who are able to trust others can depend on others. The trusting person expects help from others in time of need and to receive it in a reasonably straightforward way. Trusting persons are able to outline what they need and assume that any negotiations for meeting these needs will take place in an atmosphere of mutual respect and honesty.

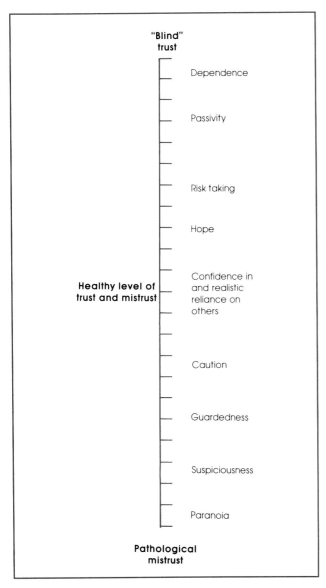

FIGURE 17-1 Trust-mistrust continuum.

Trust is related to faith in the good will of the human race. This philosophical approach assumes that people are basically kind and considerate. Too much trust, however, can have a devastating impact on an individual. Blind trust may evolve from an individual's fantasy that "all of my needs will be fulfilled." Blind trust can lead to easy and repeated psychological injury, resulting in a reluctance to trust at all.[50]

Mistrust is a mental state in which basic assumptions are fraught with suspicions about being able to understand and predict potential outcomes. When an individual perceives that a response from another is incompatible with factual data, it is difficult to comprehend the response or feel safe about arriving at a mutual understanding with the other person. Interactions become increasingly difficult when the outcome of an exchange cannot be anticipated or validated. Individuals who lack trust approach others with an assumption that they will not be accepted, understood, or

valued. Consequently, productive interaction is not possible. A certain amount of judicious mistrust is normal in relationships and is desirable in certain situations. If individuals develop the ability to make judgments and discriminations about factual data, mistrust, when it occurs, is based on sound reasoning. When judgment is impaired, as in mental illness, mistrust and suspiciousness may dominate interactions.

Pathological mistrust arises when feelings of mistrust are generalized indiscriminately, without sufficient regard to the nature of the relationship and its context. This pathological mistrust leads to a number of psychological responses. Fear of the unknown and the unpredictable, as when similar situations repeatedly result in dissimilar responses, can generate mistrust. Feelings of having little control combined with a fear of the unknown often leads to suspiciousness and withdrawal. The environment seems threatening and unpredictable. Withdrawal can reflect the individual's feeling of helplessness, or it may reflect the fear that any action will have catastrophic consequences. The person may feel very alienated. Alienation, withdrawal, and even an individual sense of nonexistence are means of coping with extreme mistrust.

Certain individuals are wary of others' motivations throughout life. The ability to exchange ideas and express feelings or to fully articulate one's own wishes is considered fruitless. Paranoia is an extreme form of this suspiciousness. Paranoid thinking is based on the expectation that others have devious, if not evil, intentions. A feeling that the world is basically good is lost. The world is viewed as evil, and others are perceived as attempting to thwart individual survival needs.

Pathological mistrust can be seen in numerous clinical syndromes. It is a dominant characteristic of paranoid disorders and may be a predominant characteristic in schizophrenic disorders. Considerable debate continues with respect to understanding how and why such symptoms develop. Psychological theories intended to describe and explain the development of personality are often applied to explain these pathological syndromes predominated by mistrusting behaviors. Others strongly argue that schizophrenic and paranoid disorders are largely due to an abnormal physiological state.

Recent theoretical approaches have viewed these psychiatric conditions as resulting from a complex interplay of many genetic, physical, psychological, social, and environmental conditions. (Table 17-1). Another important consideration is that these conditions may be thought of as a group of disorders that have yet to be differentiated. If this group of disorders (schizophrenia and paranoia) is ever differentiated, the primary and secondary cause of each condition could vary in importance in a given group of conditions. Several theoretical approaches to explain schizophrenia and paranoid disorders are briefly examined. At present, strong research emphasis is placed on biological considerations.

Several psychiatric diagnoses are discussed in relationship to the concept of trust-mistrust. These diagnoses include schizophrenia; delusional (paranoid) disorders; and three personality disorders schizoid, paranoid, and schizotypal.

In this chapter, trust-mistrust is seen as a continuum.

▼ **TABLE 17-1** **Summary of Theories of Mistrust**

Theory	Theorist	Dynamics
Biological		
Genetic		Genetic tendencies are linked with pathological mistrust.
Biochemical		Imbalances in chemistry of nervous system related to pathological mistrust, decreased prolactin secretions, and lowered MAO activity. Brain structure abnormalities and left hemisphere dysfunction may also contribute to pathological mistrust.
Psychoanalytical	Freud	The incompletely developed, weakened, or impaired ego contributes to distorted interactions. The individual has difficulty comprehending his experiences and becomes increasingly suspicious as his anxiety increases.
	Erikson	Inconsistency or failure to meet infant's basic needs results in infant being less able to develop trust.
Interpersonal	Sullivan	The "not me" aspect of personality accompanied with anxiety and confusion contributes to lack of trust.
Object relations	Mahler	When child's separation tasks are not fully accomplished, the person lacks a strong sense of self and is threatened, insecure, and mistrustful when interacting with others.
Cognitive	Piaget	Cognitive development between ages 4 and 9 months results in infant's recognition that his actions initiate reactions that may contribute to development of a sense of trust or mistrust.
Family interaction	Lidz et al	Overt marital conflict and parental characteristics of overprotective mother and passive father may lead to mistrust of others.
Communication	Bateson	Double-bind communication promotes insecurity and mistrust.
Stress vulnerability	Neuchterlin, Dawson	A developmental model that attempts to integrate the biological, social, and psychological aspects of many theories into an overall model. Factors that increase individual vulnerability are proposed. An individual's learned skills of coping are helpful in preventing illness unless stressors become too great, especially during adolescence or early adulthood.

Persons who have trouble trusting tend to be suspicious of others. Thus, suspiciousness falls on the mistrust end of the continuum (see Figure 17-1). Suspiciousness often leads to fear of others, which in turn causes the person to withdraw and become isolated. In general, persons with the previously mentioned disorders are characteristically suspicious and withdrawn. This chapter addresses these two behaviors in detail.

DSM-III-R DIAGNOSES

Schizophrenia

The onset of schizophrenic disorders most often occurs during adolescence or young adulthood. Only occasionally is someone diagnosed with this disorder after 30 years of age.

The essential features of schizophrenia are the presence of psychotic symptoms during the active phase of the illness and a decrease in the level of functioning. Other characteristics commonly seen include delusions and hallucinations, disturbances in affect and thought content, and impaired interpersonal functioning.

Several types of schizophrenia are defined based on the predominant clinical picture. The accompanying box describes the types of schizophrenia. This diagnostic category is further divided into categories of acute, chronic, in remission, or acute exacerbation of symptoms in a previously remitted or chronic state. Thus it is important to identify the type and severity of psychiatric symptoms as well as

the time perspective. Before making a diagnosis of schizophrenia, others causes of the symptoms such as organic mental disease should be ruled out. The symptoms of illness must have been present for at least 6 months before this diagnosis is made.

If these criteria are not met, other diagnoses, such as those listed as psychotic disorders not elsewhere classified, are considered. This category includes diagnoses that do

▼ **TYPES OF SCHIZOPHRENIA**

CATATONIC
Marked psychomotor disturbance including stupor, negativism, rigidity, excitement, or posturing

DISORGANIZED
Incoherence, loosening of associations, grossly disorganized behavior, flat or inappropriate affect

PARANOID
Preoccupation with systemized delusions or with auditory hallucinations related to a single theme

UNDIFFERENTIATED
Prominent psychotic symptoms (delusions, hallucinations, incoherence, disorganized behavior) that cannot be classified in any other category

RESIDUAL
At least one previous episode of schizophrenia; no psychotic symptoms, but signs of illness persist, such as emotional blunting, social withdrawal, eccentric behavior, illogical thinking, and loose associations

not fit the temporal characteristics necessary for schizophrenia, such as schizophreniform disorder or brief reactive psychosis. The diagnosis of schizoaffective disorder is unique because it is applied to persons who have had both schizophrenic symptoms and symptoms of a mood disturbance during the course of the disorder. The diagnostic manual should be consulted for additional information on all diagnoses.

Delusional (Paranoid) Disorder

Delusional (paranoid) disorder is characterized by the presence of a persistent delusion. The delusion usually involves any one of several themes and can be quite intricate and involved. These themes are discussed in the chapter. Other psychotic symptoms and unusual behaviors are limited in scope and intensity, although social functioning may be seriously limited. Auditory or visual hallucinations may be present but are not a prominent feature of the condition. The onset of the disorder is much more common in middle and late adulthood.

Personality Disorders: Paranoid, Schizoid, Schizotypal

The diagnosis of personality disorder is based on the individual's personality characteristics, which are typical of a person's recent past and long-term functioning and are relatively enduring traits. If psychotic processes are present, an Axis I diagnosis is made. A decision then is made whether to establish an Axis II diagnosis. The major traits associated with paranoid personality disorder include a tendency to expect exploitation by others, doubting trustworthiness of friends, bearing grudges, being easily slighted, and quick to anger. Characteristics associated with schizoid personality disorder are an inability to enjoy close relationships, a preference for being alone, a lack of strong emotions, indifference to opinions of others, a lack of close friends, and an inability to express feelings. Schizotypal personality disorder can be recognized by the presence of odd or eccentric behavior, beliefs and speech; constricted emotional expression; no close friends; unusual perceptual experiences; ideas of reference and paranoia; and excessive social anxiety. These conditions are more specifically defined in the diagnostic manual.[1]

THEORETICAL APPROACHES

Biological

Genetic

The genetic potential for developing schizophrenic syndromes is strongly supported by research. Twin and family studies indicate that schizophrenia occurs more frequently in the children of schizophrenic parents than those with nonschizophrenic parents.[8] However, there is incomplete expression of genetic predisposition in many mental disorders, including these. The expression of a particular genotype as mental illness may correlate with environmental and social conditions and the timing of stressful events in one's life.

Biochemical

The major groups of biochemical theories related to schizophrenia have been developed from attempts to understand the actions of psychotropic drugs. Studying the nervous system and the cause of *extrapyramidal symptoms* and *tardive dyskinesia* has led to a better understanding of the mechanisms of action of psychoactive drugs. These studies suggest the likelihood of imbalances in dopamine, serotonin, and norepinephrine in the neurotransmission process. The antipsychotic action of neuroleptic drugs probably results from the blockage of dopamine receptors. Related studies have focused on the possible dysfunction of the endocrine glands. Prolactin and growth hormone secretion from the pituitary gland have been studied, as the secretion of both may be controlled by the same neurotransmitter that is implicated in the cause of schizophrenia. Drugs that decrease dopaminergic activity, such as the neuroleptic drugs, increase serum prolactin levels.[27]

Another focus of biochemical research is the study of monoamine oxidase (MAO) activity.[25] MAO is an enzyme crucial to the metabolism of biogenic amines, and its activity is largely genetically determined. Different levels of MAO activity are found in acute and chronic schizophrenia. Generally MAO activity is lower in persons diagnosed as having chronic schizophrenia. Persons with acute schizophrenia, however, have normal or near normal MAO activity.

The search for physiological factors in schizophrenic illness is being pursued in other areas as well. The development of computed tomography (CT) and pneumoencephalography has allowed study of structural deviations of the brain. Recent evidence suggests that persons with schizophrenia may exhibit structural abnormalities.[60] Reasons for these abnormalities are as yet unknown. Some theories propose that conditions for structural abnormalities develop during pregnancy. The second trimester is a critical time for development of brain structures and neural migration. Minor congenital physical anomalies that occur in the second trimester may influence later brain development. One cause of the disruption may be genetics. Evidence suggests that alcohol abuse during pregnancy may be linked to the development of mental dysfunction in a child. Certain other events during pregnancy may cause minor disruptions in fetal neural development that later become problematic. Some of these events include the use of even small amounts of some drugs, exposure to radiation or other noxious environmental conditions, or the development of a common cold or flu virus at crucial times in fetal development.

The prominence of cognitive and language difficulties in schizophrenia may suggest abnormalities in brain hemisphere functioning, especially the left hemisphere, which is specialized for language and analytical processing. Tests for eye dominance, handedness, and lateral eye movements have been used to evaluate the possible existence of left hemispheric dysfunction. Another approach to examining psychological influences has been the study of attention and perceptual disorders. Many schizophrenic clients experience a deficit in selective attention and the ability to sustain attention. Research studies have documented the inability of clients to filter out extraneous noise from meaningful sensory input. The ability to integrate new information with previous knowledge may also be defective. The process by which the ability to focus attention and combine new knowledge with existing memories is poorly understood. This process may be related to an individual's emotional responses. When emotional responses are distorted or suppressed, the ability to remember and to make cognitive links is disturbed.

But one could ask the following question: "What are the causes of suppressed and/or distorted emotional responses?" A partial response to such a question would involve a discussion of the balance among dopamine, serotonin, norepinephrine, and the neurotransmission process, which is not well understood. At present, a well-integrated biological theory that can adequately explain the neurochemical interactions and relationships is lacking. This is an area of relatively intense basic science research.

Psychoanalytical

The intrapsychic theory proposed by Freud[19] is based on assumed mental mechanisms that govern cognitive and emotional processes. This theory suggests that mistrusting behaviors result from the failure of the ego to mediate between innate drives and reality. The ego functions that maintain contact with reality may be incompletely developed, weakened, or impaired; primitive modes of thinking and feeling predominate. Communication with others becomes distorted. The individual cannot comprehend his experiences and becomes more suspicious as the level of anxiety increases.

Erikson[17] described the first emotional developmental stage as basic trust versus basic mistrust. He stated that the way in which body needs are met has a direct bearing on the establishment of emotional trust. Consistency and the mother's ability to accept the baby's biological needs and functions influence the degree of self-acceptance and social trust an infant ultimately develops (see Chapter 4).

Interpersonal

Sullivan[55] suggested that feedback from significant others influences the development of trust. The child gradually incorporates experiences with others into images of "good me," "bad me," and "not me." "Good me" concepts develop from positive and rewarding experiences with significant others, usually parenting figures. The child views himself in a positive way and the environment as caring, responsive, trustworthy (Figure 17-2). Most children develop parts of the self that are "good me" and parts that are "bad me." These patterns of self-understanding stabilize during the first 3 years of life.

Mahler[38] and Sullivan[55] also developed concepts that help understand mistrusting behaviors. Mahler[38] described the development of emotional object constancy and individuality. When these separation tasks are not fully accomplished, the person lacks a strong sense of self and feels more vulnerable and threatened when interacting with others. This causes a decrease in the level of trust in both himself and others. Sullivan[55] described a similar process in the development of self-concept. In his terminology the

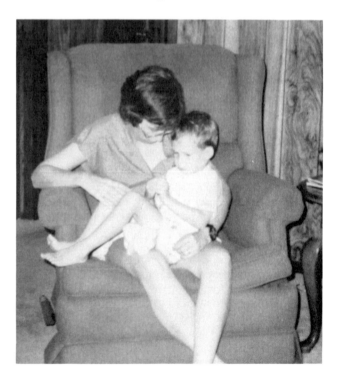

FIGURE 17-2 This child is receiving comfort and caring after shutting his fingers in a door and a positive lesson in trust.

"not me" is that aspect of personality accompanied by anxiety, confusion, and lack of trust.

Cognitive

Piaget and Inhelder,[45] in conceptualizing the cognitive development of the child, state that between the fourth and ninth months the child first begins to recognize that his actions result in reactions. He then slowly realizes that he is an integral part of the sequence of events. From this understanding, he begins to establish a sense of self-trust. During this same time, the infant begins to give up spontaneous smiling in favor of more selective responses. When seeing strangers, the child's reaction appears to be fear or anxiety.[52] Recent research indicates that this change in response is a result of cognitive development. The earlier egocentrism of the infant gives way to a more objective perception of reality. The infant has the cognitive ability to realize that things can act on their own and may be unpredictable or even alarming.

As the child recognizes the existence of causes that are independent of his own action, he can establish his own separateness and experience a sense of trust and confidence in others. Development of this cognitive mode of thinking is a necessary prerequisite and a preparation for physical separation from the mother, requiring the child to trust that his mother will not disappear during the separation. Without this cognitive evaluation of situations that involve separation, the child's emotional adjustment is thought to be more difficult.

The foundations of trust are tested with each developmental phase of life. These foundations can be reestablished and renewed or modified with each crisis and conflict. At any time during the remaining developmental phases, the individual may confront situations that seriously challenge his ability to trust. When basic trust cannot be restored through interactions with the environment and persons in it, the individual may experience a serious undermining of his previous concept of self and may develop distorted modes of relating to others.

Information processing as a cognitive dysfunction is seen in persons with pathological mistrust. Persons in a psychotic state such as schizophrenia may have difficulty making correct associations. Ideas and perceptions seem to develop without logical thought processes and are reflected in cognitive, linguistic, and perceptual deviations. Reasons for these association disorders are poorly understood, but may be a consequence of the individual's difficulty with attention. Zubin[64] has conceptualized three dimensions of attention: (1) selecting a focus, (2) maintaining a focus, and (3) shifting a focus. Most people can select relevant stimuli in the environment, direct their attention toward it, and become almost totally unaware of other stimuli. For example, a person wishing to read will focus on the book and disregard the radio playing, fluorescent lamp's buzz, other people's talking, flashing headlights through the window, and any other environmental noise. Persons who are unable to maintain a focus or who constantly shift their focus soon become confused, distracted, and unable to decipher relevant stimuli requiring a response. Such responses may be the result of impairment of the cognitive-perceptual filtering mechanism and may result in a mistrust of others.

Family Interaction

Initial theory about family relationships as a cause of mental illness seemed to have developed from the antagonistic views toward family members that clients expressed in therapy. For several decades, parents, especially the mother, were viewed as causing schizophrenia and the label *schizophrenogenic mother* was applied. Two versions of pathological family interaction was described by Lidz and others.[37] One version was of an outwardly harmonious family, termed *skewed,* which is characterized by a mother who is exceedingly intrusive into her child's life and overprotective, feeling that the child cannot exist without her supervision. The theory suggests that the child realizes that his mother opposes movements toward autonomy and becomes fearful of engulfment or incorporation, but on some level believes that neither he nor his mother can get along without the other. Fathers in this family structure are described as passive and feeling excluded from the family, based on the intensity of the relationship between mother and child.

The second version of family interactional dynamics is the *schismatic* family. In these families, overt conflict predominates between the spouses, who compete for the loyalty of the children. A child may feel caught in a bind, trying to please both parents and ultimately accepts the role of family *scapegoat* and behaves in ways that seem to cause parental conflicts. Family communication patterns become confusing, distorted, and even irrational. Overprotection undermines the child's ability to develop basic trust in his

world and his abilities. The child represses his feelings and needs in an effort to fit into the parents' requirements.

Generally, research that supports this theory has been strongly challenged by the fact that families were studied after an ill member had been identified. Therefore, assuming that pathological patterns of interaction actually exist, it was not possible to determine if they existed before the illness occurred or if the family was responding to having a person in the family with severe psychiatric disorder. It is recognized that families have communication problems and individual family members may have problems with alcohol abuse and/or expression of excessive violence toward other family members. However, there is no clearly established evidence that family interactions are considered the root cause of schizophrenic or paranoid behaviors. Many healthy adults have grown up in dysfunctional families.

In general, the role of the family in society and in facilitating the personality development of offspring occurs through the following family organizational elements: nurturance functions in caring for children, the dynamic family organization, and family social system that teaches role functions and the family's transmission of cultural values and expectations (see research highlight).

Communication

Distorted patterns of communication with inconsistent verbal and nonverbal messages can severely undermine trusting relationships. The individual sending a message gives one kind of signal on a verbal level and another, emotionally conflicting message, on the nonverbal level. This pattern of *double-bind* communication may be relatively common in social relationships but becomes problematic when there is no opportunity for clarification of conflicting messages. When this pattern of interactions is repetitive, it prevents a clear understanding or resolution of the inconsistencies in levels of communication and causes confusion and mistrust between all participants (see the following case example).

▼ Case Example

A nurse was attempting to establish a therapeutic alliance with Jerome whose history indicated that he was paranoid, trusted no one, and usually stopped therapy after one or two sessions. After several therapy sessions, Jerome telephoned the nurse and said to her, "Let's run off to Paris and get married." This serious verbal communication was accompanied by Jerome's laughter, and a radio was playing very loud disco music in the background. Jerome's message was unclear. He seemed to be indicating that the relationship should be greatly intensified (that is, marriage), but he was also laughing. The messages were conflicting, but a double-bind communication did not occur because no emotional prohibition in this relationship prevented discussion of the messages. It was possible to discuss the conflict in messages so the nurse initiated communication about the message. She responded to him by saying, "You know, I am your nurse, not your girlfriend. It's not clear what you mean when you're laughing and at the same time suggesting something serious." This communication allowed for clarification of the meaning of the message and relationship between the nurse and Jerome.

Double-bind interactions rather commonly occur in nor-

RESEARCH HIGHLIGHT

A Comparison of Short-Term Psychoeducational and Support Groups for Relatives Coping with Chronic Schizophrenia

- CF Kane, E DiMartino, and M Kimenez

PURPOSE

The overall purpose of this study was to compare the efficacy of two group programs offered to family members of state hospital inpatients diagnosed with schizophrenia. The two approaches that were compared were short-term psychoeducational groups and short-term multiple family support groups.

SAMPLE

After contacting 66 families, 37 families agreed to attend the group meetings held at the hospital. Families were assigned to one of the two groups. Forty-nine family members participated. Most participants were mothers, but fathers and siblings were also included. The majority of families were white and approximately half were in the higher socioeconomic levels.

METHODOLOGY

This study was a quasiexperimental design, with families assigned to whichever interventions (support group or education group) that was started next. Both interventions consisted of four group meetings. The support group was based primarily on a lay self-help group model, except for the group leaders who were professionals. The sessions were nonstructured discussions. The educational program consisted of a structured teaching program including information on the diagnosis, medications, managing negative feelings, and reducing stress. The measurement questionnaires were completed before the series of group sessions started and at the end of the set of four sessions.

FINDINGS

Both groups improved significantly on the knowledge measure over time. Family members whose pretest scores indicated clinical depression scored lower on posttest depression measures if they had participated in the educational program. There was no change in scores of those family members with high depression scores who participated in the support group. Family members in the educational group were more willing to recommend the group to others than were participants in the support group. This is one measure of family member satisfaction.

IMPLICATIONS

In this comparison, the psychoeducational group appears to be more effective in reducing depression in family members and providing a more satisfactory group experience than the support group model. These findings must be interpreted cautiously. Both groups were short term. A support group may be as effective as the educational group if extended over a longer period of time. The long-term effects of either group were not examined.

Based on data from *Archives of Psychiatric Nursing* 4(6):343, 1990.

---

mal human interactions, both within and outside the family. When caught in a double bind, a healthy individual may respond defensively because the nature of the expected response is not clear. The individual experiences discomfort, but corrective interactions and the nonrepetitive nature of the exchange prevent a pathological state.

Stress-Vulnerability Model

This model attempts to integrate the psychological, social, and biological information addressed earlier into a comprehensive theory that may be useful in clinical practice.[42] It is considered tentative because it is based on many assumptions that have not yet been firmly established as valid. However, there has been some examination of these ideas from a research perspective (see research highlight). This developmental model emphasizes that multiple factors contribute to the development of the illness over time. Characteristics of an individual that indicate vulnerability to the illness include (1) deficits in social competence and coping, (2) autonomic hyperactivity toward aversive stimuli, and (3) a reduction in information processing capacity. These characteristics may be a result of genetic influences and early social and environmental stresses. The degree of vulnerability to disease may depend on the extent of the problem with genetic, intrauterine, and early social and environmental influences. Learning coping skills and developing competence in various aspects of life help protect the individual and decrease vulnerability. Depending on the nature and severity of stressors later in life, however, illness may develop. Adolescence and early adulthood is an exceptionally stressful developmental period when the individual is attempting to accomplish developmental tasks of independence. Stressors such as use of street drugs, development of a physical illness, family conflicts, or inability to manage conflicts with peers may be sufficient to create psychotic symptoms. Such stressful life events or tensions in interpersonal relationships overwhelm coping skills. Onset of illness is often gradual so that early behavioral changes may not be recognized as symptoms of a potentially serious illness. Table 17-1 (p. 331) summarizes the major theories.

NURSING PROCESS
....

Assessment

Physical dimension A pathologically suspicious individual may appear strikingly different from the normal person. She may wear makeup abnormally, or her eyebrows

RESEARCH HIGHLIGHT

A Prospective Study of Stressful Life Events and Schizophrenic Relapse
• J Ventura, KH Nuechterlein, D Lukoff, and JP Hardesty

PURPOSE

Both vulnerability and stressful life events have been proposed as contributors to the onset of schizophrenia and are thought to contribute to its course. This study was designed to examine whether stressful life events increased in patients' lives before rehospitalization. It was hypothesized that persons who were rehospitalized would have more stress in their lives before rehospitalization than those patients who were not rehospitalized over the course of a year.

SAMPLE

The sample was comprised of 30 schizophrenic outpatients who had been treated in an outpatient clinic for approximately 1 year. Twenty-two men and eight women were in the sample. The mean age of the group was 23 years, and all patients had been diagnosed with psychosis within 2 years of their entry into the study. Persons with organic mental disorders, extensive habitual drug or alcohol abuse in the previous 6 months, mental retardation, and impaired vision were excluded from the study.

METHODOLOGY

Subjects continued in their usual treatment program. The subject was interviewed every month by a researcher, using a Life Events Interview, which examined 111 relatively independent life events. The interview also included open-ended questions, to find out about events that happened to subjects that were not on the interview schedule. The therapist filled out a Brief Psychiatric Rating Scale on each patient in the study every 2 weeks. At the end of the year, the social stressors of patients who had been rehospitalized were contrasted with those who had not been rehospitalized.

Based on data from *Journal of Abnormal Psychology* 98(4):407, 1989.

FINDINGS

The frequency of all life events, total negative events, and other events that were significant enough to be considered life changes were compared in several ways between those subjects that were rehospitalized and those that were not. Subjects who relapsed had a greater total number of life events over the year, a higher number of events in the month before relapse, and a greater number of life change events in the month before relapse than did those who did not relapse. Sixty-seven percent of relapsed patients who were without psychotic symptoms in the month before readmission experienced at least one independent life event during that month before they were rehospitalized. For patients who had persistent psychotic symptoms, only 20% experienced a life event in the month before readmission.

IMPLICATIONS

The results of the study are consistent with the heuristic vulnerability/stress model of schizophrenic episodes. The assumption is that there are predispositional factors, such as genetics, which contribute to vulnerability. In this study, it was clear that there was an increase in environmental stress in the month before hospitalization for those who relapsed. Experiencing a major life change event did not necessarily lead to hospitalization since 55% of relapsing patients did not have a major life event in the month before rehospitalization. Psychotic relapses may be triggered by social stressors, environmental stressors, such as drug abuse, and even by internal stressors (such as negative thinking) in those persons who are most vulnerable, as evidenced by the high return to hospital rate in persons who were chronically psychotic. Stress and life change events were less related to rehospitalization in this group.

---

may be arched too much. His plaid jacket of blue, green, and brown may seem strange when combined with plaid pants of bold red and purple that are three sizes too large. The client may appear disheveled, unkept, or even dirty and have a body odor. Sometimes the unusual manner of dress reflects the individual's distorted body image. The client who considers his body physically changed will report, for example, that a body part is no longer in proportion, or that his skull has become flat, or that he is falling apart at the joints. Body image distortions can be so severe that some individuals cannot recognize photographs of themselves or even identify their own body parts. Distortions may involve confusion of sexual identity and a feeling that some body parts are of the opposite sex or that they lack body parts. Homosexual or promiscuous behavior may be efforts to clarify sexual identity.

Preoccupation with somatic complaints is common for the person with a distorted body image. The body feels strange. The client who has become exceedingly self-fo-

cused may also be much more aware of normal body functions (for example, breathing, heartbeat, and peristaltic movements of the bowel) and consider them abnormal. Physical assessment needs to include attention to these physical complaints to separate realistic physical problems from hypochondriacal complaints. Equally important to assess are the client's diet and sleep patterns. Some clients may neglect necessary health care such as eating, dressing properly, elimination, and sleeping. Thus these fears can become a serious threat to survival.

The suspicious client may be unable to look directly at others. Often the suspicious person wears sunglasses to protect himself from eye contact. Other techniques to avoid eye contact include staring out the window, keeping eyes down toward the floor, or wandering about the room.

Motor activity for schizophrenic clients may be within the normal range or may be either of two extremes: too little or too much. Those with too little motor activity, *catatonic* clients, show marked withdrawal, sometimes to the point of being totally immobilized and unable to respond to commands. They may move themselves into unusual, seemingly uncomfortable positions and remain there for hours. *Waxy flexibility* is the term applied when a client's limbs can be placed in a given position that the individual makes no effort to change, sometimes for hours. At times, movements will be repetitive and stereotyped, such as plucking at the skin or pulling out hair. Other unusual or bizarre movements may also be seen, such as facial grimacing or sucking movements of the mouth. Some bizarre movements can result from psychotropic medications (see Chapter 24).

An increase rate of motor activity in suspicious clients is usually demonstrated by agitation, pacing, inability to sleep, loss of appetite, and weight loss. Increased motor activity may be accompanied by emotional lability, flight of ideas, and impulsiveness. When an individual is unable to exert the usual, socially expected controls, impulsive behavior may result. This behavior appears to be sudden, unpredictable, unmotivated, and illogical. The client may become verbally destructive, aggressive, or even violent. Persons who have been withdrawn and quiet for considerable periods may also demonstrate impulsive behavior. It is particularly important to recognize that such impulsive behavior can include serious suicide attempts.

Obtaining a thorough history as part of the assessment has two purposes: (1) to establish if any other family members have been treated for serious psychiatric disturbances, as some research supports a genetic predisposition to schizophrenia; and (2) to clarify where and how the client's symptoms began. Acute drug intoxication, especially amphetamines, hallucinogenic drugs of various types, and sometimes alcoholic hallucinosis may produce symptoms similar to those of schizophrenia. Laboratory studies of blood and urine may show toxic levels of some of these substances. Neurological conditions such as Huntington's chorea, Gilles de la Tourette's disease, tertiary syphilis, some forms of epilepsy (especially temporal lobe epilepsy), and brain tumors may manifest themselves with extreme suspiciousness in addition to psychotic components. Thus a thorough physical examination is essential to rule out physical causes of the behavior.

Emotional dimension The trusting person is able to express his own feelings relatively freely, in an honest and forthright manner, and expects the same from others. Emotions can be shown in an acceptable manner, accurately reflecting how the individual feels in a given situation. Facial expressions are a key to how one feels. Other behaviors, such as body movements and posture, are consistent with the person's facial expressions.

For the suspicious individual, feelings may not be easily interpreted. Because the individual experiences the world as threatening and unsafe, feeling comfortable, relaxed, and free to express himself is almost impossible. The person may be uncertain of his own feelings or may not realize what his behavior is saying. The client can appear angry and threatening or withdrawn and suspicious, or it may be difficult to interpret his mood at all. Characteristic feelings are negativism, helplessness, decreased self-esteem, anxiety, fear, anger, guilt, depression, and ambivalence. These feelings may not always coincide with what seems to be the dominant mood of the client.

Distortions in feelings may make it exceedingly difficult to interpret what is being communicated. The client usually is unaware of the distortions because he may find nothing unusual in his expression of feelings. Emotional lability is a common characteristic. For example, a client may laugh hysterically while describing an experience. A few moments later, he may burst into tears, with little having occurred to precipitate such an extreme change. When questioned, the client is not always able to explain this shift in expressed mood and may or may not be aware of its having occurred. Generally, the shift in mood is extreme, with the expression of feeling being an overreaction to what would normally be expected to accompany the content of the discussion. The client may explain the shift in mood as a response to other stimuli, such as hallucinations; thus the change, from the client's perspective, seems perfectly comprehensible.

The opposite of overreaction is *emotional blunting*, a decreased intensity of emotion from that normally expected from the specific situation. Such clients frequently seem to be apathetic, minimally responsive, or indifferent to the environment or events that happen to them. Another somewhat similar but more severe emotional response, known as *flat affect,* is demonstrated when a client does not communicate any feelings in his verbal and nonverbal responses. For instance, a client, in describing having been raped a few days ago, may talk of the event as if she had read it in a newspaper, showing no personal feelings or reactions. It is extremely difficult to understand emotional reactions of such clients or perceive how they are feeling.

Equally difficult to interpret are inappropriate affects. An inappropriate expression of emotion is seen when the content of a thought or an idea differs significantly from the emotional tone being expressed. For example, a client may laugh as he describes having threatened his wife with a knife during an argument.

Feelings experienced by the suspicious person can be potent despite the possible difficulties in interpreting them. The individual who has become uncertain of his identity also has difficulty understanding his environment. One likely outcome is a sense of overwhelming anxiety accompanied by feelings of impending doom. For example, a young woman was brought into the emergency room almost in shock after having collapsed in exhaustion. She had been running for 4 hours in an effort to escape unknown "pursuers" whom she believed were wishing to kill her, but there was no evidence that any pursuers existed. The client may be unrealistically convinced that death is almost certain but chooses to struggle against it. Such a reaction to overwhelming anxiety yields expression of fear or anger that may be difficult to differentiate from each other. The client who reacts in this manner to overwhelming anxiety can be volatile, threatening, and aggressive. The suspicious person is particularly sensitive to feeling trapped or closed in. Small rooms, limited access to exits, close physical proximity, and emotional intensity may cause the client to express his fear by fleeing or by explosive behavior. The client is generally more able to express anger than to acknowledge anxiety and fear. Clients may express their fear through paranoid ideas as in the preceding example. The nurse, then, is alert for behavioral cues that indicate anger (e.g., irritation, attention seeking, or restlessness).

Emotionally, the individual may experience depersonalization, a feeling of strangeness or unreality concerning the self. The client may feel a loss of identity or different, changed, or empty. Clients who experience depersonalization are likely to make statements such as the following:

My body is like a pillar of salt. Chips fall when I move. I can't look in a mirror because it isn't me anymore. Who is it?

A closely related experience, *derealization,* addresses the feeling of strangeness or unreality with respect to the environment, as if the environment has changed. Following are examples of statements that reflect this experience:

I've been walking around in a dream for days. Something has happened to the world. It's become evil and red.

A second means of expresssing confusion in self-identity and response to overwhelming anxiety may be withdrawal from the environment. The client becomes passive and unresponsive and withdrawn and may feel and act helpless. Severely withdrawn behavior, as in catatonia, can occur; but a more common response is the client's gradual or partial withdrawal from relationships. The client feels depressed and lonely. Feelings of guilt may arise from a sense of having failed himself and others. The experience of being unable to cope with self and others adequately (low self-esteem) accompanied by the discomfort (mistrust) felt in relating to others can further reinforce the passivity.

Ambivalence (the coexistence of contradictory emotions, attitudes, ideas, or desires about a particular person, object, or situation) may be a temporary feeling for most people. The healthy individual recognizes the contradictory feelings but can choose the option expected to be most satisfactory. When excessively ambivalent feelings are experienced, an alternative cannot be chosen. The highly suspicious individual may continually alternate between choices, feeling and expressing a wish to do one and then the other. For example, a client may repeatedly state that he wants to call his mother on the telephone but is constantly sidetracked by other activities on the way to the telephone. Ambivalent feelings can seriously disrupt the individual's ability to function and may produce any of the following behaviors: (1) compulsive rituals, (2) negativism, or (3) overcompliance (Table 17-2). The constant indecision of the ambivalent person most likely indicates that motivation to accomplish a task is missing or ability to concentrate and maintain attention is lacking. When independent positive volition is lacking, the individual may believe that whatever action he chooses will be wrong; he will feel guilty, hurt someone, or increase the seriousness of his own predicament. Committing to a specific action or feeling means that the individual may be held accountable for the choice, producing an intolerable situation for the person already feeling vulnerable.

Intellectual dimension One of the major characteristics of pathological mistrust is multiple difficulties in the process and character of thought. One hypothesis is that increasing stress accompanied by anxiety or fear reduces the ability to think clearly and logically. The person's thinking regresses to a more primitive level. As indicated by the stress/vulnerability model, increase in stress may influence biological processes in the brain, which might create further distortions in reality. Everyone is susceptible to some degree of impairment in thinking when under extreme stress. Persons with extreme difficulty in trusting relationships are more vulnerable to developing psychotic thought processes. Problems with thinking clearly or abstractly, communicating, and accurately perceiving the environment can develop.

The cognitive mechanisms used to arrive at conclusions do not follow the rules of ordinary logic used by adults. They follow some other process so that the conclusions reached are different from those ordinarily considered acceptable. This illogical process of arriving at conclusions may be experienced normally in dreams, when the connection between two events seem logical and obvious. This dreaming thought process in the awake adult is called *primary process thinking* (regressed thinking) and is an infantile form of cognition. It involves the use of mental images of objects and is supposedly controlled by id forces that seek instant gratification. The mental images that are created may relieve tension and allay anxiety, at least temporarily. As the level of anxiety increases, thinking may become increasingly distorted. To explore these interrelated cognitive distortions more fully, they are described

---

▼ **TABLE 17-2   Some Behavioral Manifestations of Ambivalence**

Behavior	Description	Example
Compulsive rituals	Attempts to solve conflicting feelings by constant, repetitive activity that may be stereotyped or seem meaningless	John has difficulty leaving his room. He gets up from the chair, takes three steps forward then three steps backward, sits again, touches the bed, stands up, taps the window, sits down, taps his knee three times, and then gets up and begins to walk forward again.
Negativism	Attempts to avoid opposing feelings by refusing, either verbally or nonverbally, to participate	Elizabeth's response to any request is always no. She refuses to get out of bed in the morning or participate in any ward activities. Once engaged in a given activity, the effort to have her change the activity is equally problematic.
Overcompliance	Attempts to deny responsibility for any action by doing only what another exactly instructs	Harold agrees to play checkers but will not move the pieces unless someone sits beside him to tell him exactly which way to move them and where to place them.

in the following categories: (1) disturbances in thought processes, (2) perceptual difficulties, (3) disturbances in language usage and communication, and (4) other intellectual disturbances.

Disturbances in thought processes

Three major disturbances in thought processes that commonly occur in highly suspicious clients are fragmented thinking, autistic thinking, and delusional thinking.

Fragmentation of the thought process occurs either by thoughts splitting off so the individual will "lose track of" thoughts or by the individual's blocking of thoughts. Thought blocking can be observed when an individual suddenly stops or abruptly changes the topic in the midst of a discussion. When fragmented thinking predominates, thoughts usually do not seem to occur logically. Consequently, the listener experiences the ideas being expressed as only slightly related to each other, or the transition between topics cannot be deciphered. The listener may find the interaction confusing or impossible to follow. For example, a client asked about his bus ride to the clinic responded, "The bus was late and warm; my bed was warm and comfortable; comfort for tears and sadness like my mother, when she was home yesterday."

Autistic thinking in the adult can be viewed as similar to the typical, normal childhood thought processes that occur before the child has sufficient intellectual and emotional maturity to perceive the environment in other than a self-centered way. This thought process is marked by a minimal distinction between self and others and an inability to distinguish between internal and external stimuli. For instance, the client may think "I want a glass of water," and then believe that others know his wish. The client's reality may be based on fantasy or wishes rather than on objective observations. Events or interactions may take on special, personal meanings for anxious, suspicious individuals. These meanings may not be understood or universally accepted by others.

With *magical thinking*, a form of autistic thinking, the individual equates thinking with doing. The logical link missing is that the client does not grasp the real relationship between cause and effect but believes he has secret powers or influences that "cause" other things to happen. For example, a client who lived near an air force base believed he controlled the taking off and landing of airplanes because the planes would fly in search of him when he was having "bad thoughts."

Concrete thinking is another type of autistic thinking. Concrete thinking reflects an inability to conceptualize meaning in words or thoughts. Therefore the ability to process information accurately may be lost. Understanding based on the context of words and nuances of meaning is lost. For example, *pare, pair,* and *pear* may seem to be the same, confusing the client because the client does not grasp the context of use and is therefore unable to determine which word is meant. The ability to classify in logical categories or abstract common qualities may fail; for example, when asked to explain the similarity between a car and a truck, the client may respond "They are both big," emphasizing a concrete quality. The client may be unable to associate other, more abstract qualities, such as that both are means of transportation. Concrete thinking does not allow the client to organize facts logically. Misinterpretations of casual remarks or jokes are common. The individual may not understand the subtleties of a joke and can only interpret proverbs concretely. For example, the proverb "People who live in glass houses should not throw stones" will be understood to mean that if a person in a glass house throws a stone, it will break a window.

The third major disturbance in thought processes is the *delusion,* or belief system, that is not validated or tested against reality (Table 17-3). Delusions are firmly maintained, even in the face of contradictory information or obvious proof to the contrary. Delusions usually reflect the client's denial of his own physical traits or feelings that he considers unacceptable. The delusional thought process begins to develop when the individual feels threatened by others or experiences anxiety related to a real or imagined trait of his own. As a protective measure, the individual projects outward these assumed negative qualities and may ascribe them to other persons, which can be accomplished by misinterpreting impressions of events and things. Thus

▼ **TABLE 17-3 Types of Delusions**

Term	Definition	Example
Ideas of reference	Belief that certain occurrences are directly related to oneself	An elderly woman, convinced she had a bad body odor, believed she caused others around her to rub their noses or sneeze.
Delusions of grandeur	An exaggerated sense of self-importance	A young woman who delivered a baby a few weeks earlier was brought to a psychiatric hospital because she was convinced she had given birth to the baby Jesus.
Somatic delusions	Belief that the body is changing or responding in an unusual way	A 22-year-old woman refused to wash her face, apply makeup, or look in a mirror because she believed that she had "turned into an old woman" as a result of being unfaithful to her husband.
Delusions of persecution	Belief that one is in danger, under investigation, persecuted, or at the mercy of some powerful force	A 52-year-old policeman under a great deal of job-related stress began to think his co-workers were against him. He was convinced they would harm him and refused to socialize with them.

for the individual, unacceptable thoughts, feelings, actions, and wishes come from outside rather than inside himself. For example, a person who considers himself lazy may develop the idea that others are talking about his laziness. Each time he sees people talking, he is certain they are talking about him.

The individual may also attribute to others his own unacceptable traits. Delusions develop essentially by reversing the usual deductive reasoning process. Usual logical thought processes move from description to conclusion. For the person with delusional thoughts, however, the conclusion is already clear. Evidence is mobilized and events are interpreted to support the conclusion. As the individual continues to use this false reasoning system, it can take on more organization, meaning, and complexity. Delusions may become systematized. That is, the delusional beliefs become more organized and the facts of events become changed in the individual's memory to be logical. Then the delusional beliefs can become integrated into the rest of the individual's life without seeming so discordant. When the person becomes utterly convinced of his false belief and all evidence to the contrary is ignored, a fixed delusion has developed. Table 17-3 defines common delusions.

Perceptual difficulties

The five senses facilitate one's accurate perception of the environment. Normal perceptions can be consensually validated by other individuals in the environment. For example, if a school cafeteria is serving fish on a particular day, most persons who walk by the cafeteria will receive some olfactory stimulation, and there will most likely be general agreement that the smell is one of fish cooking. As this example shows, perception involves a two-step process; recognition of the stimulus and an understanding or interpretation of the stimulus. Difficulties with perception may occur with either of these steps. The client may inaccurately perceive the nature of the stimulus or misinter-

pret it. Interpretation of and reaction to the stimulus are based on emotional associations with the stimulus. Regardless of previous experiences of the same or similar stimuli, however, the suspicious client may misinterpret or produce seemingly dissonant reactions to the current stimulus.

Perceptual distortions are common but usually transitory. Almost every person has experienced a situation such as waking up suddenly to misperceive an object in the room as an unknown person or catch a glimpse of an object out of the corner of his eye, such as a ball, and interpret it as an airplane. These distortions, known as *illusions*, are misrepresentations or misinterpretations of reality. They are usually brief, transitory experiences that may be accompanied by an equally temporary emotional reaction such as surprise or fear. Much more profound perceptual difficulties occur commonly in conjunction with distortions in body image. Depersonalization and identity confusion are examples of distortions in body image.

Other profound distortions in perception are *hallucinations* (Table 17-4). Hallucinations are perceptions of objects, sensations, or images that have no basis in reality. No stimulus exists; yet the individual perceives a stimulus and acts on it.

Hallucinations are frequently experienced as real sensations, or they may have an uncanny quality whereby the individual acknowledges their nonexistence to others but claims "they are real to me." For example, the client may be able to talk about the voices in his head and objectively describe what is being said, can sometimes identify who is talking, and will sometimes engage in a conversation with the voices. Most likely, hallucinations are a response to severe anxiety. As anxiety increases, dissociated components of the self-system begin to seem real and can meet needs such as improving or decreasing self-esteem and providing control or communications that are not being supplied in reality.

Four phases in the development of hallucinations have

▼ **TABLE 17-4   Types of Hallucinations**

Sense	Definition	Example
Auditory	Voices or sounds that have no basis in reality are heard. Voices may be a projection of inner thoughts, which can be comforting, derogatory, threatening, or commanding.	A young woman, very frightened of interaction with other people, hears a voice telling her what to do and how to act each time she leaves home.
Visual	Visual images of figures, objects, or events are experienced in the absence of external stimuli.	A middle-aged woman repeatedly sees glimpses of herself handcuffed and tied to a chair.
Gustatory	Tastes are experienced as distorted, or the client may experience taste without a stimulus.	A client who is concerned that some unknown person wants him dead experiences a bitter taste when he eats food in a restaurant.
Olfactory	Nonexistent odors that may arise from a specific or unknown place are smelled.	An adolescent girl, shortly after beginning menstruation, says her body smells bad. Repeated washing does not remove the odor.
Tactile	Strange body sensations are felt. Tactile hallucinations may be associated with distortions in body image. This hallucination frequently occurs with alcohol toxicity.	A young psychotic man repeatedly reports that he is unable to sleep because his penis is being massaged throughout the night by an unknown force.

been described. First, in response to anxiety, stress, or loneliness, daydreaming increases and focuses on comforting thoughts to relieve the discomfort. The client remains reality based and can still identify the thoughts as part of himself. In the second phase, however, as anxiety continues to increase, perceptual awareness becomes more intense and the client develops a "listening state" to hear the sensations, which are not dissociated from the self and are only vague, muffled sounds or whispers. The client, with ever increasing anxiety, wishes to put distance between himself and the developing hallucination by projecting the experience outward; thus it may seem to be coming from some place other than the self. In the third phase, the hallucination develops more prominence. The client adjusts and may find that the hallucination provides a sense of temporary security or comfort. Finally, the hallucination may lose its quality of comfort and become commanding, threatening, or disparaging. The client may feel controlled by the hallucination and become so involved with the experience that the possibility of outside interaction diminishes significantly. In this phase, hallucinations can powerfully influence the client's behavior. The client may act on hallucinations that command him to hurt himself or others.

The most common hallucinatory experiences are auditory or visual. Olfactory, tactile, and gustatory hallucinations are occasionally experienced by the psychotic individual but occur more commonly with persons who have an organic condition or are in alcohol or drug toxicity. When hallucinations are present, the nurse assesses their type and time of occurrence.

Disturbances in language usage and communication

Satisfactory interaction with others is based on the ability to adequately exchange ideas and thoughts, to share perceptions, and to express feelings. Disorders in language usage prevent this exchange from occurring. The resulting effect is a serious constriction or even total failure to establish a relationship.

When the individual experiences serious disruption in abstract thought patterns, speech patterns are likely to reflect the degree of chaos and fragmentation that the client experiences. Communication disorders can occur either because the individual is unable to organize his language properly or because a private language has developed. Inability to organize language can result from an association disorder or the loss of logical thought processes that occurs as autistic thinking develops. For example, a client who had begun to experience more symptoms told the nurse that he had begun to read normal words, such as *China*, as *C-hina*. He could not explain further. The individual fails to use conceptually based language patterns and may break speech into segments or fragments. As the breakdown of ideas and their expression continues, a single word or phrase may come to represent a whole meaning to the person. The person may feel he has communicated adequately but fails to be understood by the listener. Table 17-5 describes the most common language disorders.

Other intellectual disturbances

In addition to assessing thought processes, perceptual difficulties, and communication disorders in the suspicious client, evaluating other aspects of intellectual functioning is also important. Clients with a low level of intellectual ability may never have developed intellectually beyond the primitive thinking characterized by concreteness and magical thinking, and such thought processes in these persons may be normal.

Orientation disorders can have an organic or psychological basis. Orientation to person, place, and time is the normal state but is influenced by multiple factors. For example, a client who is suspicious and withdrawn, socially isolated, and preoccupied with hallucinatory experiences may know who he is and where he is but have no clear idea about the month or year.

A disturbance in the client's level of consciousness and ability to remember, particularly an abrupt change in these

---

▼ **TABLE 17-5   Language Disorders**

Language Change	Definition	Example
Asyndesis	A language disorder manifested by a juxtaposition of elements or meanings without adequate linkage	A client, when asked the name of the president, responds, "White House."
Metonymy	The use of imprecise terms or words with approximate meaning	"I have eaten three meals" becomes "I have eaten three menus."
Echolalia	The purposeless repetition of a word or phrase just stated by another individual	The nurse says, "Turn on the lights," and the client responds, "The lights, the lights, the lights, the lights."
Neologisms	A private word or phrase coined by the speaker that has special meaning to the speaker and cannot be understood by others	A client responds to a question by saying, "Ethuel, tanigram."
Clang associations	The repetition of words or phrases that have a similar sound but no other relationship	The nurse says, "What would you like to eat?" The client's response is "Eat, feet, meet, beat."
Word salad	The linking of ordinary words and phrases in a meaningless, illogical, disconnected manner	A client, pacing the hallway, says, "Vanilla reason lopsided can go left and right he is."

functions, may indicate a primary organic disease rather than a schizophrenic delusional disorder. Further neurological evaluation may be indicated.

When clients demonstrate severe impairment in attention span or ability to concentrate, they are experiencing severe anxiety and may be delusional, with hallucinations or other disturbances in the thinking process.

Social dimension Persons who trust readily show a willingness to meet others, feel relaxed and comfortable in making approaches, know that they have something of value to offer, and demonstrate some enthusiasm for doing so by displaying expressions of interest in another's feelings and reactions.

Social adjustment must be assessed by exploring specific details of the individual's life. For example, clients who have very few social contacts may respond to questions with "Oh, I don't do anything," or ultimately by admitting, "Oh, I watch the afternoon soaps." These comments can be explored further by assessing the level of involvement that the client can maintain. Assessment includes evaluating both the client's current and premorbid adjustment. Previous levels of adjustment can predict, to some degree, the client's potential. A positive change in social adjustment skills may indicate that the client is able to cope with the expansion of his social network. He may be receptive to socialization or job training programs that he previously refused. A client's withdrawal or refusal to participate may be viewed as one means of coping with an environment that seems overwhelming. Assessing the client's apparent "readiness" for rehabilitation programs is essential to successfully engaging the client at the appropriate time. Equally important is to recognize the value social and work programs can have in the overall improvement of the client's health.

Interpersonal trust plays a significant role in the successful establishment and maintenance of a social network. The nurse assesses the client's social network: his contacts with relatives, friends, and neighbors, through which he maintains a social identity, receives emotional support, material aid, services, information, and develops new social contacts.[40] Establishing and maintaining a social network is closely related to the ability to trust. For individuals who experience pathological mistrust, a simple interaction such as purchasing gasoline may be impossible.

One's concept of self is partially defined by responses from others. When early childhood relationships create much anxiety, the socialization process is disrupted, leading to inadequate social development. Socially inadequate development, resulting in the person's being unable to maintain communication with others can lead to private thinking, unique ways of experiencing the world, and a loss of the emotional meaning of social experiences. Socially accepted attitudes and roles may never be learned or can become distorted and are experienced by the client as loneliness, social isolation, mistrust of others, withdrawal, and dependence. The disordered interpersonal and object relations of the client do not result in a total rejection of social relatedness but are often characterized by an intense wish for, and an equally intense fear of, close relationships with other people, a need-fear dilemma.

Spiritual dimension The healthy, trusting individual may recognize spirituality as a natural part of his ex-

istence, providing a sense of meaning to life. For the trusting individual, reaffirmation of relatedness to a higher being comes from interaction and communication with others. Through relationships, the individual is able to maintain the sense of identity and inner strength necessary to cope with the stressors of normal development and the demands of human existence. When stresses become severe, a healthy person often seeks spiritual connectedness for support and guidance. Crises may produce opportunities for spiritual growth.

Individuals experiencing pathological mistrust are cut off from opportunities to reestablish a sense of being connected to a larger universe. The individual has lost a feeling of connectedness with significant others in his environment, so he no longer has access to resources critical for maintaining trust. When mistrust is severe, the individual loses the meaning to life. This loss can lead to despair, hopelessness, and withdrawal to the point of "feeling dead."

The individual who begins to experience disintegration of self-image, and with it a loss of the personal meaning to life, will usually struggle against the powerful feelings of potential doom and despair. The effort to maintain self-identity often occurs in the prepsychotic phase of illness. The person may not be clearly aware of the subtle changes that occur in thinking processes, emotional experiences, and modes of interaction. Some individuals may begin to seek religious groups and organizations to "shore up" the self-concept, to cope with a sense of impending doom, and to remain connected with a purpose to life. Experiences directly related to losing touch with reality, such as uncanny feelings or *deja vu* experiences, need to be explored. In an effort to find rational explanations for these experiences, the mistrusting client may place them in a religious context. The individual may suddenly begin to express increased interest in spiritual, religious, and philosophical questions, hoping to relieve the intense discomfort. It is not unusual for the client to change his religious affiliation, disclaim former beliefs, and insist that finally he has "found the truth"; no other approach is right, and he has been misled, fooled, or deceived by significant others.

The first task is gaining some understanding of a client's long-standing religious beliefs and values, as contrasted with beliefs that have developed as a consequence of personality disintegration. The client may have developed a complex system of beliefs, well supported by biblical teaching, or may have adopted philosophical positions that have been taken out of context.

An assessment of the client's religious background and the family's traditions and values about religious activities provide a rich source of information for understanding the client's religious beliefs and values.

The nurse also needs to be aware of the potential for suicide in clients who suffer a profound sense of isolation and meaninglessness of life. Suicidal behavior in such clients are likely to be successful, as motivation for suicide is rarely directed toward efforts to reestablish a connectedness to others but more toward acknowledging the feelings of "being dead." Because suicidal behavior may be impulsive, it may be difficult to recognize the danger signs (see Chapter 14). The reader is referred to the holistic assessment tool in Chapter 8 as a guide for a comprehensive assessment of the client who is mistrusting and suspicious.

TABLE 17-6   Instruments to Measure Trust

Instrument	Measures
The Interpersonal Trust Scale	Measures general trust expectancies
Trust Scale for Nurses[59]	Measures the nurse's trust of clients and the nurse's trust of other nurses

MEASUREMENT TOOLS

Table 17-6 summarizes the more common scales for measuring trust.

Analysis
Nursing diagnosis

The following list provides examples of NANDA-accepted nursing diagnoses[23] with causative statements:
1. Noncompliance with prescribed medication regimen related to thinking the medication is poisoned
2. Self-esteem disturbance related to distorted body image
3. High risk for violence related to hallucinatory voices
4. Noncompliance related to impotence associated with antipsychotic medications
5. Sleep pattern disturbance related to fears associated with delusions
6. Altered thought processes related to delusions
7. Sensory/perceptual alterations: hallucinations related to anxiety associated with multiple stressors
8. Impaired verbal communication related to loose associations
9. Ineffective individual coping: hostile behavior related to fear of others
10. Social isolation related to extreme suspiciousness

Impaired verbal communication, sensory/perceptual alterations, and altered thought processes are three nursing diagnoses approved by NANDA that apply to a person who mistrusts. The defining characteristics of the nursing diagnoses are listed in the accompanying boxes (pp. 343-344). The analysis stage also includes examining the defining characteristics of the medical diagnosis to understand how the client is expressing the diagnosis.

The following three case examples illustrates characteristics of the nursing diagnosis of impaired verbal communication, sensory-perceptual alterations, and alteration in thought processes, respectively.

▼ Case Example

Alan was brought to the hospital by the police. He had been found hiding in the underbrush in a restricted area near the airport. Alan was dirty and unshaven and wore torn clothing. In the hospital admitting office, Alan sat rigidly in one corner watching everyone in the room, his eyes reflecting sometimes fear and sometimes sadness. When asked questions, Alan made some mumbling, unintelligible sounds. It was later discovered that Alan had been

▼ IMPAIRED VERBAL COMMUNICATION

DEFINITION
A state in which an individual experiences a decreased or absent ability to use or understand language in human interaction.

DEFINING CHARACTERISTICS
- **Physical dimension**

  Physical impairment of sensory end organs, cerebral cortex, or afferent and efferent nerves
  Hypervigilance or hypovigilance to stimuli
  Speech impediments

- **Emotional dimension**

  Absence of, unrestricted, or inappropriate expression of feeling

- **Intellectual dimension**

  Disparate verbal and nonverbal messages
  Inappropriate selection of words
  Unable to speak dominant language
  Inability or refusal to speak
  Message does not coincide with context
  Verbosity
  Ill-timed message
  Illogical speech
  Speaking out of turn
  Disagreement on punctuation of communication
  Absent, irrelevant, or untimely feedback
  Unresponsive to feedback
  Disorientation
  Distorted, imaginary, or false perception

- **Social dimension**

  Withdrawal from interaction

Modified from McFarland G, McFarlane E: *Nursing diagnosis and intervention: planning for patient care,* ed 2, St Louis, 1993, Mosby—Year Book.

missing from home for 2 days. Before abruptly leaving home, Alan had spent the previous 3 weeks sitting alone in his room. He had refused food and would talk to no one.

▼ Case Example

Peter, a 29-year-old computer programmer, has worked alone in an office in the basement of a large manufacturing firm for the past 7 years. When the firm was bought by another company, Peter was told he could move to Baltimore, the new company headquarters, or he would be given compensatory pay for 6 months, allowing him time to find another job. Having to make such a difficult decision so disturbed Peter that he became unable to concentrate at work and believed the new company president was talking to him through the ventilators and sometimes followed him home. Peter became very tense on the walk home and would turn around to look for the new president and believed he saw a glimpse of a shirt sleeve or hat disappearing around the corner. One evening Peter believed he saw the company president sitting at the kitchen table talking. Peter yelled and screamed in anger and could not be calmed down.

▼ SENSORY/PERCEPTUAL ALTERATIONS

DEFINITION

State in which an individual experiences a change in the amount or patterning of incoming stimuli accompanied by a diminished, exaggerated, distorted, or impaired response to such stimuli.

DEFINING CHARACTERISTICS

- **Physical dimension**

  Diminished or distorted visual, auditory, tactile, gustatory, olfactory, and kinesthetic capabilities
  Motor incoordination
  Alteration in posture
  Changes in muscular tension
  Increased or decreased response to stimuli
  Altered sleep patterns
  Restlessness

- **Emotional dimension**

  Exaggerated emotional responses
  Rapid mood swings
  Anxiety
  Fear
  Apathy
  Flattened affect
  Anger
  Irritability

- **Intellectual dimension**

  Disorientation in time, place, or person
  Altered abstraction or conceptualization
  Bizarre thinking
  Decreased problem solving ability
  Disordered thought sequencing
  Hallucinations
  Illusions
  Daydreaming
  Altered communication patterns

- **Social dimension**

  Boredom

Modified from McFarland G, McFarlane E: *Nursing diagnosis and intervention: planning for patient care*, ed 2, St Louis, 1993, Mosby–Year Book.

▼ Case Example

Ellen, a 20-year-old unemployed woman, lives with her mother. She has been unable to finish high school and has never worked. In the first session with her nurse she says, "Can you give me feelings? I have no feelings. I am empty." She goes on to describe in a very disorganized manner that she is more than one Ellen. One Ellen is a famous movie actress; another is a bad evil person, maybe the devil; and the third is the Ellen sitting in the room. She insists that she knows this because it was reported in a national magazine and furthermore demands that the nurse arrange a television appearance for her so that "the whole world will know."

Planning

Examples of short- and long-term goals, outcome criteria, interventions, and rationales related to mistrust are

▼ ALTERED THOUGHT PROCESSES

DEFINITION

A state in which an individual experiences a disruption in cognitive operations and activities.

DEFINING CHARACTERISTICS

- **Physical dimension**

  Altered sleep pattern
  Hyperactivity

- **Emotional dimension**

  Inappropriate/labile affect

- **Intellectual dimension**

  Altered states of consciousness
  Disorientation to time, place, person
  Impaired memory
  Confabulation
  Distractability
  Disturbed thought flow (circumstantial, tangential, neologism, flight of ideas, word salad, blocking)
  Disturbed thought content (delusions, obsessions, preoccupations, phobias)
  Impaired problem solving
  Impaired judgment
  Perceptual alterations (hallucinations, illusions)
  Cognitive dissonance
  Suicidal/homicidal ideation
  Attention deficit
  Egocentricity
  Inappropriate/nonreality-based thinking

Modified from McFarland G, McFarlane E: *Nursing diagnosis and intervention: planning for patient care*, ed 2, St Louis, 1993, Mosby–Year Book.

presented. These examples illustrate how the nurse develops a client-specific plan for each client in the planning stage of the nursing process.

Implementation

Physical dimension The client's physical and safety needs are considered first. Clients who have experienced severe symptoms for a long time without receiving care may be suffering from malnutrition, dehydration, infections, and other phsyical disorders. Treating these physical problems is the first priority. Physical illnesses in conjunction with a psychiatric disorder can produce a synergistic effect of increasing the symptoms of either illness. For example, a mistrusting client who is also diabetic may refuse to eat because she believes her intestines have turned to stone. The resulting physiological imbalances created by her refusal to eat may further stimulate other distortions in body image as specific symptoms of hypoglycemia begin to occur. Prompt interventions to ensure adequate nutritional intake are necessary to maintain physical balance. Specific psychological interventions for the disturbance can be initiated after the life-threatening physical illness is controlled.

Occasionally, the nurse meets clients who have devel-

DRUG PROFILE

CHLORPROMAZINE HCl

(klor-proe'ma-zeen)
Chlor-Promanyl, Chlorpromanyl,* Largactil, Promaz, Thorazine
Func class: Antipsychotic/neuroleptic
Chem class: Phenothiazine-aliphatic

Action: Depresses cerebral cortex, hypothalamus, limbic system, which control activity aggression; blocks neurotransmission produced by dopamine at synapse; exhibits a strong α-adrenergic, anticholinergic blocking action; mechanism for antipsychotic effects is unclear
Uses: Psychotic disorders, mania, schizophrenia, anxiety, intractable hiccups, nausea, vomiting, preoperatively for relaxation, and acute intermittent porphyria, behavioral problems in children
Dosage and routes:
Psychiatry
▶ *Adult:* PO 10-50 mg ql-4h initially, then increase up to 2000 mg/day if necessary
▶ *Adult:* IM 10-50 mg q1-4h
▶ *Child:* PO 0.25 mg/lb q4-6h or 0.5 mg/kg
▶ *Child:* IM 0.25 mg/lb q6-8h or 0.5 mg/kg
▶ *Child:* REC 0.5 mg/lb q6-8h or 1 mg/kg
Nausea and vomiting
▶ *Adult:* PO 10-25 mg q4-6h prn; IM 25-50 mg q3h prn; REC 50-100 mg q6-8h prn, not to exceed 400 mg/day
▶ *Child:* PO 0.25 mg/lb q4-6h prn, IM 0.25 mg/lb q6-8h prn not to exceed 40 mg/day (<5 yr) or 75 mg/day (5-12 yr); REC 0.5 mg/lb q6-8h prn
▶ *Adult:* IV 25-50 mg qd-qid
▶ *Child:* IV 0.55 mg/kg q6-8h
Intractable hiccups
▶ *Adult:* PO 25-50 mg tid-qid; IM 25-50 mg (used only if PO dose does not work); IV 25-50 mg in 500-1000 ml saline (only for severe hiccups)
Available forms include: Tabs 10, 25, 50, 100, 200 mg; time-release caps 30, 75, 150, 200, 300 mg; syr 10 mg/5 ml; conc 30, 100 mg/ml; supp 25, 100 mg; inj IM, IV 25 mg/ml
Side effects/adverse reactions:
*RESP: **Laryngospasm**, dyspnea, **respiratory depression***

* Available in Canada only.
Italic indicates common side effects.
Bold italic indicates life-threatening reactions.

CNS: Extrapyramidal symptoms; pseudoparkinsonism, akathisia, dystonia, tardive dyskinesia, seizures, *headache*
HEMA: Anemia, ***leukopenia, leukocytosis, agranulocytosis***
INTEG: Rash, photosensitivity, dermatitis
EENT: Blurred vision, glaucoma
GI: Dry mouth, nausea, vomiting, anorexia, constipation, diarrhea, jaundice, weight gain
GU: Urinary retention, urinary frequency, enuresis, impotence, amenorrhea, gynecomastia, breast engorgement
CV: Orthostatic hypotension, hypertension, ***cardiac arrest***, ECG changes, ***tachycardia***
Contraindications: Hypersensitivity, circulatory collapse, liver damage, cerebral arteriosclerosis, coronary disease, severe hypertension/hypotension, blood dyscrasias, coma, child <2 years, brain damage, bone marrow depression, alcohol and barbiturate withdrawal states
Precautions: Pregnancy (C), lactation, seizure disorders, hypertension, hepatic disease, cardiac disease
Pharmacokinetics:
PO: Onset erratic, peak 2-4 hr, duration may be detected for up to 6 mo after last dose
IM: Onset 15-30 min, peak 15-20 min, duration may be detected for up to 6 mo after last dose
IV: Onset 5 min, peak 10 min, duration may be detected for up to 6 mo after last dose
REC: Onset erratic, peak 3 hr
Metabolized by liver, excreted in urine (metabolites), crosses placenta, enters breast milk; 95% bound to plasma proteins; elimination half-life 10-30 hr
Interactions/incompatibilities:
—Oversedation: other CNS depressants, alcohol, barbiturate anesthetics
—Toxicity: epinephrine
—Decreased absorption: aluminum hydroxide or magnesium hydroxide antacids
—Decreased effects of: levodopa
—Decreased serum chlorpromazine: lithium
—Increased effects of both drugs: β-adrenergic blockers, alcohol

—Increased anticholinergic effects: anticholinergics

NURSING CONSIDERATIONS
Assess:
—Swallowing of PO medication; check for hoarding or giving of medication to other clients
—I&O ratio; palpate bladder if low urinary output occurs
—Bilirubin, CBC, liver function studies monthly
—Urinalysis is recommended before, during prolonged therapy
Administer:
—IV after diluting 1 mg/1 ml with normal saline, give 1 mg/2 min; may be further diluted in 500-1000 ml of compatible sol
—Antiparkinsonian agent, to be used if extrapyramidal symptoms occur
—Drug in liquid form mixed in glass of juice or cola, if hoarding is suspected
Perform/provide:
—Decreased stimuli by dimming lights, avoiding loud noises
—Supervised ambulation until stabilized on medication; do not involve in strenuous exercise program because fainting is possible; client should not stand still for long periods of time
—Increased fluids to prevent constipation
—Sips of water, candy, gum for dry mouth
—Storage in tight, light-resistant container, oral solutions in amber bottles
Evaluate:
—Decrease in: emotional excitement, hallucinations, delusions, paranoia, reorganization of patterns of thought, speech
—Affect, orientation, LOC, reflexes, gait, coordination, sleep pattern disturbances
—B/P standing and lying; take pulse and respirations q4h during initial treatment; establish baseline before starting treatment; report drops of 30 mm Hg
—Dizziness, faintness, palpitations, tachycardia on rising
—For neuroleptic malignant syndrome: hyperpyrexia, muscle rigidity, increased CPK, altered mental status

—Extrapyramidal symptoms including akathisia (inability to sit still, no pattern to movements), tardive dyskinesia (bizarre movements of the jaw, mouth, tongue, extremities), pseudoparkinsonism (rigidity, tremors, pill rolling, shuffling gait)
—Skin turgor daily
—Constipation, urinary retention daily; if these occur, increase bulk, water in diet
Teach client/family:
—That orthostatic hypotension occurs often, and to rise from sitting or lying position gradually
—To remain lying down after IM injection for at least 30 min
—To avoid hot tubs, hot showers, or tub baths since hypotension may occur
—To avoid abrupt withdrawal of this drug or extrapyramidal symptoms may result; drug should be withdrawn slowly
—To avoid OTC preparations (cough, hayfever, cold) unless approved by physician since serious drug interactions may occur; avoid use with alcohol or CNS depressants; increased drowsiness may occur
—To use a sunscreen and sunglasses during sun exposure to prevent burns
—Regarding compliance with drug regimen
—About extrapyramidal symptoms and necessity for meticulous oral hygiene since oral candidiasis may occur
—To report sore throat, malaise, fever, bleeding, mouth sores; if these occur, CBC should be drawn and drug discontinued
—In hot weather that heat stroke may occur; take extra precautions to stay cool
Lab test interferences:
Increase: Liver function tests, cardiac enzymes, cholesterol, blood glucose, prolactin, bilirubin, PBI, cholinesterase, [131]I
Decrease: Hormones (blood and urine)
False positive: Pregnancy tests, PKU
False negative: Urinary steroids, 17-OHCS
Treatment of overdose: Lavage, if orally ingested, provide an airway; *do not induce vomiting or use epinephrine*

Modified from Skidmore-Roth L: *Mosby's nursing drug reference*, St Louis, 1993, Mosby—Year Book.

oped bizarre or socially unacceptable means of meeting basic needs, for example, eating with their fingers when using a fork is appropriate. These behaviors are sometimes a result of desocialization, which can happen in the hospital or at home, especially when the individual has little contact with or feedback from others about his behavior. The nurse may wish to implement a program to change these behaviors, which can be as simple as reminding the client of alternatives. The change may require more intensive behavior modification programs, with a reinforcement system to encourage systematic behavioral change.

In the hospital, several measures are taken to prevent self-destructive behavior, including checking the client's personal belongings for any instruments that can be used to inflict physical harm, such as razors, matches and cigarettes, and even forks and knives, as well as ensuring that the length of electrical cords on lamps are as short as possible, using unbreakable glass in the windows or mirrors, and keeping furniture in excellent repair to eliminate sharp or broken edges. If the client is treated in an outpatient setting, continual awareness of the client's ability to meet self-care needs is relevant to maintaining the living situation. Self-destructive behaviors in an outpatient or community setting may be more subtle and nonspecific but require an equal amount of attention. For instance, a client who repeatedly exposes himself to harsh weather without proper clothing or who walks alone for hours at night may be passively self-destructive rather than actively suicidal. Attention to these behaviors and appropriate intervention, such as facilitating a change in the treatment setting, may be necessary.

Suspicious clients are often unable to maintain proper sleeping and eating patterns. For the acutely psychotic individual, sleep may be disrupted by nightmares or severe anxiety, so that the individual cannot fall asleep, or the person may feel more comfortable in a less stimulating environment. Reversals of the sleep-wake pattern may be seen. Sleeping too much may be a way for the individual to manage difficulties in relating to others. The nurse must understand the precise cause of the client's difficulties. It is usually advisable not to encourage the use of medication for sleep but to provide whatever intervention is necessary in response to the cause of the sleeping problem. An active program during the day that keeps the client involved and prevents daytime naps can also facilitate normal sleep patterns, as can physical exercise based on the client's health status. In a hospital or day treatment program, these activities can be part of the overall treatment program. Referral to rehabilitation programs, job training programs, sheltered workshops, or volunteer activities may be necessary for clients out of the hospital to maintain a daily life structure that enables more normal sleeping habits.

Body image distortions and identity confusion are best managed by helping the client describe his perception as concretely as possible. Once the distortions are understood, the nurse can suggest alternate ways for the client to understand his experiences. For instance, the nurse observed a 20-year-old client's acne but had not discussed it with her. When the client explains that her face is rotting away the nurse can express doubt about her perception of present reality. The client's separate sense of self can be maintained by using proper pronouns to clarify a given situation. For instance, "I am Jean Johnson, your nurse, and I have come to help you, George, prepare for breakfast" encourages a recognition and reinforcement of separateness.

It is important to continually remind the client who is around him and what activities are in progress. Specific information, given in anticipation of activities or changes at the time of the event, can help the client maintain a sense of control and self-identity. Orientation to surroundings is helpful for clients who experience identity confusion; for example, "You and I are going to walk down this long hallway to the very end to my office." Anticipatory guidance, as in this example, can facilitate the client's ability to cope with events that seem distorted and unreal. Realizing the degree of body image distortion may require the nurse to make inferences from observed behaviors, as the client may not realize or be able to articulate his difficulty. Seeing the client in inappropriate clothing may lead to a discussion of how the client views himself. Sexual identity problems are often not addressed openly or directly by clients. A client's fear of being homosexual may be one way to indicate his concerns about sexuality. Providing information about normal sexual functions and behavior or discussions with the client about normal body and sexual functions can be exceedingly important.

Antipsychotic medications are a common intervention for coping with distortions. Antiparkinson medications are given to reduce the side effects of the antipsychotic medications (Table 17-7). Chapter 24 provides more specific information about medications. The accompanying profiles for chlorpromazine (Thorazine) (p. 345), fluphenazine (Prolixin) (p. 347), clozapine (Clozaril) (p. 349), and trihexyphenidyl (Artane) (p. 351) describe nursing care appropriate to their administration.

Emotional dimension The mistrusting individual may be totally out of touch with any feelings and thus cannot express them accurately. Or he may be so fearful of his own or the other's reactions that he relies on a number of mechanisms to hide, distort, or miscommunicate feelings. Interventions in the emotional dimension are directed toward understanding the client's emotional reactions and facilitating his interpretation of them by recognizing and acknowledging them. The client's goal is to accurately communicate his emotions in a culturally acceptable manner. To assist the client, the nurse needs to address factors that inhibit full expression of feelings, such as poor social skills, lack of self-confidence, a fear of rejection or punishment, the need to protect the self from emotional hurt, and memories of past unpleasant emotional experiences.

Nonverbal communication takes on a profound meaning: Body postures, degree of eye contact, physical proximity, and the degree of apparent tension in the nonverbal exchange are all measures of how the relationship is progressing. The nurse maintains an emotional posture of accessibility, respect, and interest. She concentrates on stimulating interest in the client and not filling in silences with chatter or talking about herself as a way of managing her own feelings of discomfort in the silence. The client easily recognizes these ploys and may respond with increased withdrawal. The nurse may be able to strengthen the relationship by using nonverbal methods of relating to the client, such as looking at magazines, playing games, or going

FLUPHENAZINE DECANOATE/ FLUPHENAZINE ENANTHATE/ FLUPHENAZINE HCl

(floo-fen'a-zeen)
Modecate Decanoate,* Prolixin Decanoate/Moditen Enanthate,* Prolixin Enanthate/Moditen HCl,* Permitil HCl, Prolixin HCl
Func class: Antipsychotic/ neuroleptic
Chem class: Phenothiazine, piperazine

Action: Depresses cerebral cortex, hypothalamus, limbic system, which control activity and aggression; blocks neurotransmission produced by dopamine at synapse; exhibits strong α-adrenergic and anticholinergic blocking action; mechanism for antipsychotic effects is unclear
Uses: Psychotic disorders, schizophrenia
Dosage and routes:
Enanthate, decanoate
▶ *Adult and child >12 yr:* SC 12.5-25 mg q1-3wk
HCl
▶ *Adult:* PO 2.5-10 mg, in divided doses q6-8h, not to exceed 20 mg qd; IM initially 1.25 mg then 2.5-10 mg in divided doses q6-8h
Available forms include: HCl Tabs 1, 2.5, 5, 10 mg; elix 2.5 mg/5 ml; conc 5 mg/ml; inj IM 10 mg/ml, enanthate, decanoate, inj SC, IM 25 mg/ml
Side effects/adverse reactions:
RESP: Laryngospasm, dyspnea, *respiratory depression*
CNS: Extrapyramidal symptoms: pseudoparkinsonism, akathisia, dystonia, tardive dyskinesia, drowsiness, headache, seizures, *neuroleptic malignant syndrome*
HEMA: Anemia, *leukopenia, leukocytosis, agranulocytosis*
INTEG: Rash, photosensitivity, dermatitis

EENT: Blurred vision, glaucoma
GI: Dry mouth, nausea, vomiting, anorexia, constipation, diarrhea, jaundice, weight gain
GU: Urinary retention, urinary frequency, enuresis, impotence, amenorrhea, gynecomastia
CV: Orthostatic hypotension, hypertension, *cardiac arrest,* ECG changes, *tachycardia*
Contraindications: Hypersensitivity, circulatory collapse, liver damage, cerebral arteriosclerosis, coronary disease, severe hypertension/hypotension, blood dyscrasias, coma, child <12 yr, brain damage, bone marrow depression, alcohol and barbiturate withdrawal states
Precautions: Pregnancy (C), lactation, seizure disorders, hypertension, hepatic disease, cardiac disease
Pharmacokinetics:
PO/IM (HCl): Onset 1 hr, peak 2-4 hr, duration 6-8 hr
SC (enanthate): Onset 1-2 days, peak 2-3 days, duration 1-3 wk, half-life 3.5-4 days; decanoate: onset 1-3 days, peak 1-2 days, duration over 4 wk, half-life (single dose) 6.8-9.6 days, (multiple dose) 14.3 days
Metabolized by liver, excreted in urine (metabolites), crosses placenta, enters breast milk
Interactions/incompatibilities:
—Oversedation: other CNS depressants, alcohol, barbiturate anesthetics
—Toxicity: epinephrine
—Decreased effects of: levodopa, lithium
—Increased effects of both drugs: β-adrenergic blockers, alcohol
—Increased anticholinergic effects: anticholinergics

NURSING CONSIDERATIONS

Assess:
—Swallowing of PO medication; check for hoarding or giving of medication to other clients
—I&O ratio; palpate bladder if low urinary output occurs
—Bilirubin, CBC, liver function studies monthly
—Urinalysis is recommended before and during prolonged therapy

Administer:
—Concentrate with juice, milk or uncaffeinated drinks
—Antiparkinsonian agent, to be used if extrapyramidal symptoms occur
—IM injection into large muscle mass, to minimize postural hypotension give injection with patient seated or recumbent
—Use dry needle or solution will become cloudy; use No. 21 G or larger due to viscosity
Perform/provide:
—Decreased noise input by dimming lights, avoiding loud noises
—Supervised ambulation until stabilized on medication; do not involve in strenuous exercise program because fainting is possible; patient should not stand still for long periods of time
—Increased fluids to prevent constipation
—Sips of water, candy, gum for dry mouth
—Storage in tight, light-resistant container in cool environment
Evaluate:
—Therapeutic response: decrease in emotional excitement, hallucinations, delusions, paranoia, reorganization of patterns of thought, speech
—Affect, orientation, LOC, reflexes, gait, coordination, sleep pattern disturbances
—B/P standing and lying; take pulse and respirations q4h during initial treatment; establish baseline before starting treatment; report drops of 30 mm Hg
—Dizziness, faintness, palpitations, tachycardia on rising
—Extrapyramidal symptoms including akathisia (inability to sit still, no pattern to movements), tardive dyskinesia (bizarre movements of jaw, mouth, tongue, extremities), pseudoparkinsonism (rigidity, tremors, pill rolling, shuffling gait)
—Skin turgor daily
—Constipation, urinary retention daily; if these occur, increase bulk, water in diet

Teach client/family:
—That orthostatic hypotension occurs often, to rise from sitting or lying position gradually
—To avoid hot tubs, hot showers, or tub baths since hypotension may occur
—To avoid abrupt withdrawal of this drug or extrapyramidal symptoms may result; drug should be withdrawn slowly
—To avoid OTC preparations (cough, hayfever, cold) unless approved by physician since serious drug interactions may occur; avoid use with alcohol or CNS depressants; increased drowsiness may occur
—To use a sunscreen during sun exposure to prevent burns
—Regarding compliance with drug regimen
—About extrapyramidal symptoms and necessity for meticulous oral hygiene since oral candidiasis may occur
—To report sore throat, malaise, fever, bleeding, mouth sores; if these occur, CBC should be drawn and drug discontinued
—In hot weather heat stroke may occur; take extra precautions to stay cool
Lab test interferences:
Increase: Liver function tests, cardiac enzymes, cholesterol, blood glucose, prolactin, bilirubin, PBI, cholinesterase, ^{131}I
Decrease: Hormones (blood and urine)
False positive: Pregnancy tests, PKU
False negative: Urinary steroids, 17-OHCS
Treatment of overdose: Lavage, if orally injested, provide an airway; *do not induce vomiting*

---

*Available in Canada only.
Italic indicates common side effects.
Bold italic indicates life-threatening reactions.

Modified from Skidmore-Roth L: *Mosby's nursing drug reference,* St Louis, 1993, Mosby–Year Book.

▼ **TABLE 17-7**   **Antipsychotic and Antiparkinson Medications**

Generic Name	Trade Name	Daily Dosage Range (mg)
ANTIPSYCHOTIC MEDICATIONS		
Chlorpromazine	Thorazine	30-800
Promazine	Sparine	40-1200
Mesoridazine	Serentil	30-400
Thioridazine	Mellaril	150-800
Fluphenazine	Prolixin	0.5-40
Perphenazine	Trilafon	12-64
Trifluoperazine	Stelazine	2-40
Haloperidol	Haldol	1-15
Chlorprothixene	Taractan	75-600
Thiothixene	Navane	8-30
Clozapine	Clozaril	300-900
ANTIPARKINSON MEDICATIONS		
Trihexyphenidyl	Artane	6-10
Benztropine	Cogentin	4-6
Biperiden	Akineton	2-6
Diphenhydramine	Benadryl	75-200

for a walk. The manner in which questions are phrased is important. Using open-ended questions or comments, such as "Tell me about your day's activities," followed by a pause to communicate interest and expectation of an answer is usually more productive than direct questioning. The client plays a key role in the pace of closeness that develops. The nurse may need to help facilitate the expression of feelings by noticing subtle changes in expression.

As the client is able to relate more comfortably to the nurse in an individual setting, the behavior can be generalized to other interactions. The client may be more accepting of the perspectives of others and can gradually identify his own feelings more accurately and express them to others. Self-identity is then strengthened, which initiates a cycle of increasingly healthy expression of feelings. As the client gains confidence in his ability to accurately reflect his feelings, he is rewarded by accurate responses from others.

Clients who express emotional reactions with ambivalence, flat affect, or inappropriate affect are using these means to keep their emotional reactions hidden, distorted, unclear, vauge, or diffused. Behaviors such as compulsive rituals, negativism, and overcompliance can create serious restrictions on the client's ability to perform activities of daily living. When this reaction occurs, the nurse may be required to intervene to ensure task accomplishment. Firm limit setting, with a focus on reality and recognition that certain tasks need to be accomplished, can be adequate intervention. At times, the nurse may have to provide specific, detailed, step-by-step directions or to actually do the task for the client. When a client's feelings and thoughts are exceedingly disorganized, the ability to make decisions is severely impaired. The client cannot decide which of the massive number of inputs requires a response. Under such circumstances, the nurse needs to limit choices. As the client becomes increasingly organized, the choices can be expanded. Gradually, with increasing integration of feelings

and thoughts, the client becomes more capable of self-care and will be able to choose for himself.

Principles to keep in mind when interacting with clients who have difficulty with expression of feelings are listed here.

1. The angry client is rarely angry at the nurse personally but may be projecting feelings from another relationship. It may be safer for the client to express anger at the nurse rather than the individual who actually generated the anger. If the nurse becomes angry with the client, she tells him so in a matter-of-fact way without making him feel guilty or depriving him of care.
2. The nurse does not encourage the client to express feelings unless she is comfortable with the client's feelings and can be available to listen.
3. Expression of feelings may not always be therapeutic. Catharsis may be good in certain situations, but expression of the same feelings over and over can serve as a constant focus on the feeling, becoming merely ruminations.
4. Too much focus on negative feelings may reinforce them or bring them to the point that the client feels a need to act out destructively rather than to cope with intense feelings.
5. Emotional expression and experiencing intense feelings can be painful, even for the client who seems out of contact with reality.
6. Clients may experience shame or embarrassment from expressing feelings. The nurse needs to be aware of these reactions and provide appropriate interventions, such as providing privacy to discuss significant feelings in a quiet and comfortable atmosphere and offering emotional support and sensitivity.

◣ **Intellectual dimension** Sometimes clarification is difficult because the client's ability to communicate is severely limited. The nurse needs to express clearly but gently that she does not understand, without emotionally

CLOZAPINE
(kloz-a′pin)
Clozaril
Func class: Antipsychotic
Chem class: Tricyclic
dibenzodiazepine derivative

Action: Interferes with binding of dopamine at D_1 and D_2 receptors with lack of extrapyramidal symptoms, also acts as an adrenergic, cholinergic, histaminergic, serotonergic antagonist

Uses: Management of psychotic symptoms in schizophrenic patients for whom other antipsychotics have failed

Dosage and routes:
▶ *Adult:* PO 25 mg qd or bid, may increase by 25-50 mg/day, normal range 300-450 mg/day after 2 wk, do not increase dose more than 2 × /wk, do not exceed 900 mg/day, use lowest dose to control symptoms

Available forms include: Tabs 25, 100 mg

Side effects/adverse reactions:
CNS: Sedation, salivation, dizziness, headache, tremors, sleep problems, akinesia, fever, seizures, sweating, akathisia, confusion, fatigue, insomnia, depression, slurred speech, anxiety

GI: Dry mouth, constipation, nausea, abdominal discomfort, vomiting, diarrhea, anorexia

MS: Weakness; pain in back, neck, legs; spasm

CV: Tachycardia, hypotension, hypertension, chest pain, ECG changes

---

Italic indicates common side effects.
Bold italic indicates life-threatening reactions.

GU: Urinary abnormalities, incontinence, ejaculation dysfunction, frequency, urgency, retention
RESP: Dyspnea, nasal congestion, throat discomfort
HEMA: **Leukopenia, neutropenia, agranulocytosis, eosinophilia**

Contraindications: Hypersensitivity, myeloproliferative disorders, severe granulocytopenia, CNS depression, coma

Precautions: Pregnancy (B), lactation, children <16, hepatic, renal, cardiac disease, seizures

Pharmacokinetics:
Steady state 2.5 hr, 95% protein bound, completely metabolized by the liver, excreted in urine and feces (metabolites), half-life 8-12 hr

Interactions/incompatibilities:
—Increased anticholinergic effects: anticholinergics
—Increased hypotension: antihypertensives
—Increased CNS depression: CNS drugs
—Increased bone marrow suppression: antineoplastics, other drugs suppressing bone marrow
—Increased plasma concentrations: warfarin, digoxin, other highly protein bound drugs

NURSING CONSIDERATIONS

Assess:
—Swallowing of PO medication; check for hoarding or giving of medication to other clients
—I&O ratio; palpate bladder if low urinary output occurs
—Bilirubin, CBC, liver function studies monthly
—Urinalysis is recommended before, during prolonged therapy

Administer:
—Antiparkinsonian agent, to be used if extrapyramidal symptoms occur

Perform/provide:
—Decreased noise input by dimming lights, avoiding loud noises
—Supervised ambulation until stabilized on medication; do not involve in strenuous exercise program because fainting is possible; client should not stand still for long periods of time
—Increased fluids to prevent constipation
—Sips of water, candy, gum for dry mouth
—Storage in tight, light-resistant container

Evaluate:
—Decrease in: emotional excitement, hallucinations, delusions, paranoia, reorganization of patterns of thought, speech
—Affect, orientation, LOC, reflexes, gait, coordination, sleep pattern disturbances
—B/P standing and lying; take pulse and respirations q4h during initial treatment; establish baseline before starting treatment; report drops of 30 mm Hg
—Dizziness, faintness, palpitations, tachycardia on rising
—EPS including akathisia (inability to sit still, no pattern to movements), tardive dyskinesia (bizarre movements of the jaw, mouth, tongue, extremities), pseudoparkinsonism (rigidity, tremors, pill rolling, shuffling gait)
—Skin turgor daily
—Constipation, urinary retention daily, if these occur, increase bulk, water in diet

Teach client/family:
—That orthostatic hypotension occurs often, and to rise from sitting or lying position gradually
—To avoid hot tubs, hot showers, or tub baths since hypotension may occur
—To avoid abrupt withdrawal of this drug or EPS may result; drug should be withdrawn slowly
—To avoid OTC preparations (cough, hayfever, cold) unless approved by physician since serious drug interactions may occur; avoid use with alcohol or CNS depressants; increased drowsiness may occur
—Regarding compliance with drug regimen
—About EPS and necessity for meticulous oral hygiene since oral candidiasis may occur
—To report sore throat, malaise, fever, bleeding, mouth sores, if these occur, CBC should be drawn and drug discontinued
—In hot weather, that heat stroke may occur; take extra precautions to stay cool
—To avoid driving or other hazardous activities; seizures may occur

Lab test interferences:
Increase: Liver function tests, cardiac enzymes, cholesterol, blood glucose, bilirubin, PBI, cholinesterase, ^{131}I
False positive: Pregnancy tests, PKU
False negative: Urinary steroids, 17-OHCS
Treatment of overdose: Lavage, activated charcoal, provide an airway; do not induce vomiting

Modified from Skidmore-Roth L: *Mosby's nursing drug reference,* St Louis, 1993, Mosby—Year Book.

---

rejecting the client as an individual. Both the client and nurse will need to continue trying to communicate. Sometimes the communication is similar to understanding a foreign language—a portion is comprehensible, but the whole does not fall together into a sensible meaning. The nurse needs to listen carefully and then share what is understood. The accuracy of understanding is checked with the client. If the content of the communication remains unclear, the feelings may be more obvious than the verbal message. Recognizing and acknowledging the feelings the client expresses can help explain the message.

Hallucinations are particularly disturbing experiences for the client. They may be related to especially strong feelings about something or may be an unconscious effort to control anxiety. Hallucinations may be a way to express feelings that are otherwise unacceptable to the client. Such experiences are often frightening and ultimately probably do not allay anxiety but can lead to increased anxiety and further distortions of reality. If, when clients describe hallucinations, the nurse is judgmental or attempts to argue with the client, the result may be a further decrease in trust and confidence. On the other hand, if the nurse encourages the client to share his perceptions, the client can begin to build a trusting relationship with the nurse. The nurse can aid reality testing for the client by acknowledging that, although the perceptions are real to the client, they are not shared by others. With sufficient observation and interaction, the nurse may be able to recognize the precipitants of the client's increased anxiety resulting in hallucinations. Once a pattern is identified, the nurse can discuss the precipitants and encourage the client to express whatever feelings were being experienced. Eventually, the client may be able to realize the relationship between the hallucination and particular strong feelings. The nurse can cast doubt on the hallucination as being a representation of reality without directly challenging the client.

Some clients readily recognize hallucinations as "out of reality" and will describe this experience. Even so, the client may feel out of control. Severe hallucinations, such as command auditory hallucinations, can cause the client to lose control of his behavior. Usually the nurse can recognize this behavior and can intervene before the client loses control by setting firm limits or moving the client to a quieter place. Setting up competing stimuli such as whistling or humming can interrupt the hallucination. Engaging in conversation, a game, or going for a walk can help divert the client's attention to something else. These interventions are particularly useful during the early phases of the development of hallucinations as described on p. 340.

From the client's perspective, delusional thoughts are real and seem absolutely true, regardless of how far-fetched the ideas. Arguing with the client about the reality of the delusions will only reinforce his wish to convince others of the belief and can help solidify the delusional system. A delusional system develops as a defense to protect the client from formidable feelings. With time the nurse can learn what symbolic meaning the delusion probably contains for the client and may be able to respond to the underlying theme. For example, a client who had become convinced that out-of-state cars followed him and were after him may actually have been expressing the wish for his family, who lived out of state, to pay more attention to him and not reject him. When this client begins to discuss the idea that cars were following him, the nurse, understanding the meaning, could refocus the discussion to his feelings of loneliness and rejection. Although his interpretation of reality seems right, the client needs to know that others have arrived at a different conclusion. The nurse shares that she interprets information in a different way and may make suggestions that cast doubt on the validity of the delusional thought process without directly challenging it.

Clients with paranoid delusions are generally suspicious and will promptly reject any questioning of their thought processes. They may consider anyone who challenges them to be dangerous. Communication with the very suspicious and delusional person needs to be direct, clear, and concrete. Providing accurate data as straightforwardly as possible is essential, as is being clear about boundaries. The nurse's use of "I" and "you" helps such clients differentiate themselves from the surroundings that seem so dangerous. The extremely paranoid client also needs to maintain a sense of being in control. Clear messages about what is expected, what are "rules," and what the individual has a choice about letting the paranoid person know exactly what he can and cannot do. This communication helps prevent the client's feeling that he has somehow been wronged by the staff or the nurse. For example, a paranoid client, upset that his primary nurse had been ill, asked her if he could be transferred to another unit. He, of course, knew that this was possible. The nurse responded to the situation by agreeing that, if he wished, he could be transferred; but she did not think it would be a good idea because he knew people on this unit and she felt that they had been working well together, despite her illness and 2-day absence. The nurse suggested that the client think about it for a while and they could talk more about it later. Later in the day the nurse approached the client, who said to her, "Oh, you are right. I guess I had better stay here."

Misinterpreting reality as a consequence of disorders in thought processes can result in impulsive or autistic behaviors. The client may not be able to stop autistic behavior, even at the request of the nurse; impulsive behaviors are, by definition, unpredictable. An example of autistic behavior is the client who sits in a corner and rocks back and forth in his chair. Impulsive behaviors can be more problematic, especially when they involve threatening others or aggressive acting out. Clients rarely refuse to comply, not because of obstinacy but because they cannot comply due to their own perceptions of reality. If the behavior is not harmful to the client or others nearby, it may not be helpful to persist in attempting to have the client stop. A person will not do something he absolutely does not want to do unless physical force is used. The nurse can be prepared to decide whether the behavior is destructive enough to require physical force. If the nurse decides that the client is not harming himself or others, she will not pressure the client to the point where he responds by lashing out. The nurse attends to the behavioral cues (for example, negativism, belligerence, irritation) that indicate that the client is unwilling to cooperate and tries again later. As a last

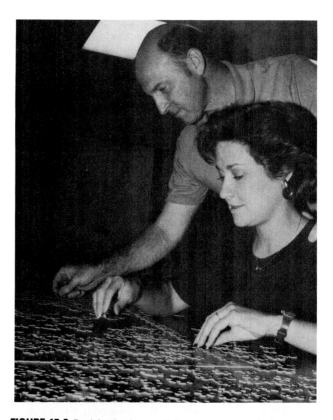

FIGURE 17-3 Participating in an activity on a one-to-one basis promotes interactions and helps to build trust.

TRIHEXYPHENIDYL HCI

(trye-hex-ee-fen'i-dill)
Aparkane,* Aphen, Artane, Hexaphen, Novohexidyl,* T.H.P., Trihexane, Trihexidyl, Trihexy
Func class: Cholinergic blocker
Chem class: Synthetic tertiary amine

Action: Blocks central muscarinic receptors, which decreases involuntary movements
Uses: Parkinson symptoms
Dosage and routes:
Parkinson symptoms
▶ *Adult:* PO 1 mg, increased by 2 mg q3-5 days to a total of 6-10 mg/day
Drug-induced extrapyramidal symptoms
▶ *Adult:* PO 1 mg/day; usual dose 5-15 mg/day
Available forms include: Tabs 2, 5 mg; caps sus-rel 5 mg; elix 2 mg/5 ml
Side effects/adverse reactions:
CNS: Confusion, anxiety, restlessness, irritability, delusions, hallucinations, headache, sedation, depression, incoherence, dizziness, flushing, weakness

---

Italic indicates common side effects.
Bold italic indicates life-threatening reactions.

EENT: Blurred vision, photophobia, dilated pupils, difficulty swallowing
CV: Palpitations, tachycardia, postural hypotension
INTEG: Urticaria, rash
MISC: Suppression of lactation, nasal congestion, decreased sweating, increased temperature
MS: Weakness, cramping
GI: Dryness of mouth, constipation, nausea, vomiting, abdominal distress, ***paralytic ileus***
GU: Hesitancy, retention
Contraindications: Hypersensitivity, narrow-angle glaucoma, myasthenia gravis, GI/GU obstruction, tachycardia, myocardial ischemia, unstable CV disease
Precautions: Pregnancy (C), elderly, lactation, tachycardia, prostatic hypertrophy, abdominal obstruction, infection, children, gastric ulcer

Pharmacokinetics:
PO: Onset 1 hr, peak 2-3 hr, duration 6-12 hr, excreted in urine
Interactions/incompatibilities:
—Increased anticholinergic effects: antihistamines, phenothiazines, amantadine

NURSING CONSIDERATIONS
Assess:
—I&O ratio; retention commonly causes decreased urinary output
—B/P, pulse frequently while dose is being determined
Administer:
—With or after meals for GI upset; may give with fluids other than water
—At hs to avoid daytime drowsiness in client with parkinsonism
Perform/provide:
—Storage at room temperature in light resistant containers
—Hard candy, frequent drinks, sugarless gum to relieve dry mouth

Evaluate:
—Parkinsonism: shuffling gait, muscle rigidity, involuntary movements
—Urinary hesitancy, retention; palpate bladder if retention occurs
—Constipation; increase fluids, bulk, exercise if this occurs
—For tolerance over long-term therapy; dose may need to be increased or changed
—Mental status: affect, mood, CNS depression, worsening of mental symptoms during early therapy
Teach client/family:
—Not to discontinue this drug abruptly; to taper off over 1 wk
—To avoid driving or other hazardous activities; drowsiness may occur
—To avoid OTC medications: cough, cold preparations with alcohol, antihistamines unless directed by physician
—To avoid sudden position changes
—To avoid hot climates, overheating may occur

Modified from Skidmore-Roth L: *Mosby's nursing drug reference,* St Louis, 1993, Mosby—Year Book.

---

resort, it may occasionally be necessary to restrain a client for his own or others' protection.

As the client's thought disorder begins to disappear, the nurse adopts a plan of care that further builds on the changes in behavior. More opportunities for task mastery can be provided. Gradually, the client becomes able to accomplish increasingly complex tasks and can build positive feelings about himself from experiences such as occupational therapy or tasks such as keeping his own room in order. These interventions can rebuild self-esteem and help the client obtain personal satisfaction. These therapeutic interventions also provide the nurse with opportunities to observe the client's strengths and weaknesses in areas such as manual skill, concentration and attention, and ability to follow directions. Information of this nature is exceedingly valuable in making realistic plans for rehabilitation and can provide data to determine the client's readiness for alternative opportunities to develop skills. Sometimes previously unknown organic deficits may be recognized, a special talent observed, or a specific limitation in ability to relate to others noted. Observations can be discussed with the client to enhance understanding. Knowing a client's limitations is important to ensure that the client

is not frustrated by being asked to perform tasks he cannot do.

Social dimension Initial efforts are directed toward reestablishing interpersonal contact on a one-to-one basis (Figure 17-3). Consistent, repeated, brief approaches to initiate social participation and aid communication may be necessary. Gradually, the client's relationships with others can be expanded.

When a pathological family pattern of interaction and communication emerges, treatment of the whole family may be indicated, with efforts toward repatterning the communication and role relationships (see Chapter 29). It is not unusual for the family to experience self-blame, guilt, anger, frustration, and disappointment with the ill member. The nurse needs to recognize, acknowledge, and explore these feelings. Families who blame themselves for the client's difficulty are particularly sensitive to comments that may implicate them as responsible for the client's behavior. The nurse needs to be aware of this possibility and approach the family with sensitivity to the difficulties they have experienced in their relationships with the mistrusting client.

Krauss and Slavinsky[33] point out the importance of establishing a working alliance with the family, especially the family of the client with a long-term disorder, to exchange information, provide guidance and support, relieve the family of guilt and responsibility, and prevent further deterioration of the family unit. Families of mistrusting clients often are isolated and do not have an adequate system of support, as a result of having to cope with the client's unusual behaviors. The financial burdens of providing treatment can become overwhelming for the family as well as decrease the resources available for social interaction with others. Interventions may be necessary to help the family reestablish previous network ties or to develop new ones. Families may profit from referral to self-help groups or family support groups. Providing families with information about the illness and helping them develop skills to manage daily activities are beneficial.

Clients may need help establishing themselves in the community after discharge from the hospital. Planning for community living includes attention to the basic minimal requirements: some form of economic support, including sufficient resources for food; a safe place to live; and referral to some form of follow-up treatment, including a means of obtaining medications. The nurse can be involved in initiating or providing any of these aspects of outpatient treatment. Ideally, the client is also taught about the purpose of his medications and when to take them. Other self-care skills may also need to be taught. The nurse's referral is made to other nurses and other professionals who will be providing further treatment. Assessment of the client's daily living skills and any special techniques that have helped accomplish self-care tasks are included on the referral.

Nurses who work with clients in the community focus their attention on helping the client build a social network. Often the client's social network is very small, including perhaps a visit to the therapist in an outpatient clinic and occasionally interacting with a family member. Expanding the client's social network can be a slow process, but it proceeds gradually and consistently from interactions with one to two persons to small groups. Clients who have demonstrated vulnerability to the stress of change are encouraged to make no more than one major life change at a time. Abrupt changes may exacerbate symptoms. Careful monitoring and timing affect the interventions. Some clients need firm expectations and specific goals to expand their social network.

Support for establishing a social network is often maintained in a concrete and specific way in the group or individual therapy provided in outpatient settings. Often the client and the nurse fail to recognize the importance of integration into and support from the community to enhance coping mechanisms. A structured daily life is an important way to prevent regression. The nurse who works with clients living in the community needs to monitor daily activities.

An individual's job is central to his definition of self. Even retired or unemployed persons think of themselves as "a retired shoemaker" or say, "I was a steel worker before the plant closed." Work not only provides a source of income but also can be a major source of social interaction, a means of self-satisfaction, and a way to contribute to society. Many clients who experience symptoms such as hallucinations or some other thought disorder can, despite these difficulties, maintain productive employment. Those

who cannot hold a job may need referral to rehabilitation programs or sheltered work environments. The nurse facilitates appropriate referral and also supports communication between the various service providers and aspects of treatment.

Spiritual dimension Work with the mistrusting client in the spiritual dimension is directed toward providing a sense of relatedness and meaning to life. This work often begins by establishing a sense of connectedness in a trusting relationship. Helping the client indirectly express feelings through creative arts, poetry, or music is a positive way for the nurse to make contact with a deeply disturbed client.

Religion may be overemphasized or religious teachings distorted by the client who is making a concerted effort to maintain cognitive and emotional stability. Previous religious beliefs can become distorted. The client may suddenly change beliefs, join a cult, or declare himself to be the son of God. The nurse, in her effort to differentiate between the client's psychotic processes and long-standing religious beliefs, needs to have some general knowledge of various religious denominations. Her own philosophy of life and religious beliefs may be challenged by the client. The nurse recognizes that maintaining a personal connection with the client is more therapeutic than debating specific beliefs. The nurse may openly acknowledge differences in religious teachings without presenting this difference as a barrier to a therapeutic relationship.

The client's interpersonal relationships may be lost or change dramatically as a consequence of pathological mistrust. Once having regained a reality base, clients may be ashamed or embarrassed by the behaviors they demonstrated and may need help understanding the impact of these behaviors on others. The client may also experience feelings of loss and grief when he is more realistically able to articulate his own strengths and limitations. The nurse will need to facilitate the client's grieving process while helping the client establish realistic life goals for himself. See Table 17-8 for a sample nursing care plan. See the boxes on p. 354 for key interventions.

INTERACTION WITH A MISTRUSTING CLIENT

Nurse: (In medication room, about to give fluphenazine hydrochloride [Prolixin Decanoate] injection) Mr. Evans, this is your usual medication. The amount you will get is what you have had before.

Client: I've been wondering, is there a way that someone can be killed with no trace of what caused it afterward?

Nurse: What are you referring to, Mr. Evans—this medication?

Client: Well. . . (pause) I was just wondering about, you know, my father died. . .

Nurse: I don't know of any way to kill someone without leaving evidence of what caused the person's death. I am giving you the medicine to help you, not to hurt you. What about your father?

Client: Well, he was a good man and yet he died at such a young age. The Mafia must know something. He was such a good man. God would not punish him.

Nurse: As we've talked about before, Mr. Evans, your father died from a heart attack. How long ago was that?

Client: Twenty years.

▼ **TABLE 17-8 NURSING CARE PLAN**

GOALS	OUTCOME CRITERIA	INTERVENTIONS	RATIONALES
NURSING DIAGNOSIS: Sensory-perceptual alteration: auditory hallucinations related to anxiety associated with multiple stressors			
LONG TERM			
To manage anxiety without hallucinations	Uses effective methods for managing anxiety		
	Demonstrates fewer (or no) hallucinations		
SHORT TERM			
To extinguish hallucinations	Takes medications as prescribed	Give medications as prescribed	Antipsychotic medications diminish psychotic symptoms
	Stays in contact with reality	Monitor for side effects of medications	Clients may stop taking medications when side effects are uncomfortable
		Present reality	To focus on reality and avoid belief that hallucinations are real
To interact with others	Interacts with others individually and in small groups	Teach social skills	Interpersonal contacts increase anxiety; competence in social skills builds self-esteem and decreases anxiety
		Provide group activities	To increase social interactions
		Provide group therapy, reality orientation	To receive feedback from others, to learn about hallucinations and ways to deal with them, to share feelings with others
To reduce anxiety	Verbalizes fears and feelings of anxiety	Facilitate expression of fears feelings of anxiety	Hallucinations often follow anxious feelings
	Identifies signs and symptoms of anxiety	Help client to identify signs symptoms of anxiety	Becoming consciously aware of bodily changes associated with anxiety helps client to recognize them and manage them effectively
	Seeks others when fearful or anxious		
	Uses effective stress reducing methods		
		Teach stress reduction: exercise, relaxation, talk to someone	Increases clients repertoirs of coping skills

Nurse: The anniversary of his death is next week, isn't it?
Client: Yes, I always dedicate that day to him. I go to his grave and say a prayer.
Nurse: I guess you must feel it was unfair that he died so young.
Client: Yes, I do. Can I call you if I want to talk some more?

This client demonstrates his lack of trust and severe paranoia by indicating indirectly that he does not feel safe with the nurse who has been giving him the same medication for several months. His delusion soon becomes quite apparent, although he does not say very much about what he believes regarding "the mafia."

The nurse approaches the situation through clear, direct questions that facilitate a better understanding of what the client is thinking. The nurse responds specifically and directly to the client's concerns. It is important to assure him of his safety and to emphasize the present reality. By stating facts in a nonargumentative tone and focusing on obtaining more information from the client, the nurse is better able to give accurate feedback. Sometimes the client's delusional thoughts confuse past memories, present activity, and thoughts about future plans. Here, the nurse has helped the client put each in proper perspective.

Ultimately, the nurse helps the client identify some of the feelings associated with the discussion that may have contributed to the delusional ideas. Over time, the client can better understand the relationship between his feeling state and thought process, and he may eventually draw conclusions that include both the real facts and the real feelings. See the box on p. 354 for guidelines for primary/tertiary prevention.

KEY INTERVENTIONS FOR MISTRUST/ SUSPICIOUSNESS

Meet physical and safety needs
Provide a busy day schedule of activities to enable client to maintain normal sleep habits
Present reality
Reduce anxiety
Strengthen self-image and self-identity
Set firm limits to enable task accomplishment
Use clarification when communication is not understandable
Encourage sharing of perceptions
Intervene when hallucinating
Cast doubt on delusions
State requests in brief, clear, simple words
Reestablish relationships, one-on-one initially, then with others
Include family in treatment and teaching
Help client plan for community living

KEY INTERVENTIONS FOR HALLUCINATIONS

Be alert to cues that client is hallucinating
Interrupt hallucination by calling client by name or other distraction
Avoid touching without first telling client
Ask what voices are saying and whose voice it is. Avoid further discussion of hallucination to prevent reinforcing inappropriate behavior
Present reality
Help client learn that he can dismiss hallucinations by humming or whistling or saying, "Go away or be quiet."

GUIDELINES FOR PRIMARY/TERTIARY PREVENTION

Mistrust

Primary Prevention

Teach person to maintain high self-esteem
    to resotre self-esteem, when lowered, with positive self-talk
    to reduce anxiety
    to manage stress
    to share suspicious feelings with a supportive person for validation
    to identify signs and symptoms of developing psychosis (when thoughts become disorganized)
    information about antipsychotic medications; name, dosage, side effects and about antiparkinson medications that relieve extrapyramidal side effects
Teach family signs and symptoms of developing psychosis, need for medication and/or hospitalization

Tertiary Prevention
Community resources

Community mental health centers
Day treatment centers
Crisis homes
Boarding homes

Self-help groups

National Alliance for the Mentally III

KEY INTERVENTIONS FOR DELUSIONS

Develop a trusting relationship to lessen anxiety and need for delusions
Identify the underlying feelings being expressed in the delusion, then refocus discussion on the feeling (e.g., loneliness, rejection)
Cast doubt on the validity of the delusional thought, e.g., "I know these thoughts are real to you, but I do not see them as real."
Avoid supporting/reinforcing delusions
Provide accurate information
Be alert to behavioral cues that client may act on the delusion
Provide opportunities for task mastery to increase self-esteem and personal satisfaction
Provide a busy schedule of activities to prevent alone time
Help client learn that if he cannot control delusions, he can learn to talk about them only with significant others or in therapy

Evaluation

In acute treatment settings, the mistrusting client may demonstrate dramatic behavioral changes, including a significant increase in reality orientation, increased ability to articulate feelings with appropriate affect, improved decision-making ability, and increased ability to tolerate interpersonal relationships. The client may be unable to acknowledge or directly articulate changes in a specific manner but will clearly demonstrate more healthy behaviors.

BRIEF REVIEW

Trust and mistrust influence personality structure and relationships. The ability to trust is strongly influenced by early parent-child relationships, family relationships, and inherited traits. Trust develops from consistent, reliable interpersonal exchanges in which the individual feels accepted, understood, and valued. Trusting relationships are maintained by a willingness to evaluate one's own behavior, the behavior of others, and the circumstances of the interaction in an objective and realistic manner. The individual's ability to trust may change or be modified in response to significant or traumatic events in adulthood. Healthy individuals establish relationships, assuming others are basically trustworthy, but are able to discriminate rationally and evaluate during the process of interaction.

Mistrust can develop into a pathological state in which interaction with others is characterized by suspiciousness of others, withdrawal, and difficulty in interpersonal relationships. Mistrust is seen in doubts about one's ability to communicate accurately, to understand others, and to predict the potential outcome of interactions. Multiple theoretical approaches have been applied to understanding the pathological states, such as schizophrenic and paranoid disorders, in which mistrust is a predominant characteristic. No single theoretical approach fully explains the multiple clinical syndromes marked by a defective interpretation or loss of contact with reality.

The nurse approaches work with mistrusting clients in a systematic, goal-oriented manner, facilitating the client's growth toward increasing healthy behaviors. As the nurse makes an assessment and begins to plan and implement treatment, she can relate her knowledge of the client to theories of behavior. Evaluation of care includes reviewing the client's movement toward health and planning for further treatment, as indicated.

REFERENCES AND SUGGESTED READINGS

1. American Psychiatric Association: *Diagnostic and statistical manual of mental disorders*, ed 3, Washington, DC, 1987, The Association.

2. Andreasen NC: *The broken brain: the biological revolution in psychiatry*, New York, 1984, Harper & Row.

3. Andreasen NC and others: Hemispheric asymmetries and schizophrenia, *American Journal of Psychiatry* 139: 427, 1982.

4. Andreasen N and others: Structural abnormalities in the frontal system in schizoprenia, *Archives of General Psychiatry* 43: 31, 1986.

5. Baxter D, Melnechuk T: *Perspectives in schizophrenia research*, New York, 1980, Raven Press.

6. Beard MT: Trust, life events, and risk factors among adults, *Advances in Nursing Science* 4(4): 26, 1982.

7. Bernstein A: Orienting response research in schizophrenia: where we have come and where we might go, *Schizophrenia Bulletin* 13(4): 623, 1987.

8. Bellack A: *Schizophrenia: treatment, management and rehabilitation*, Orlando, Fla, 1984, Grune & Stratton.

9. Bellack A: *Disorders of the schizophrenic syndrome*, New York, 1979, Basic Books.

10. Cohen R, Sample W, Gross M: Positron emission tomography, *Psychiatric Clinics in North America* 9(1): 63, 1986.

11. Callaway E, Naghdi S: An information processing model of schizophrenia, *Archives of General Psychiatry* 39: 339, 1982.

12. Caton D: *Management of chronic schizophrenia*, New York, 1984, Oxford University Press.

13. Chesla CA: Parents' illness models of schizophrenia, *Archives of Psychiatric Nursing* 3(4): 218, 1989.

14. Colliton MA: The spiritual dimension of nursing. In Beland I, Passos J: *Clinical nursing*, ed 4, New York, 1981, Macmillan.

15. D'Arcy C, Siddique CM: Social support and mental health among mothers of preschool and school aged children, *Social Psychiatry* 19: 155, 1984.

16. Erikson EH: *Childhood and society*, ed 2, New York, 1964, WW Norton.

17. Erikson EH: *Identity and the life cycle: selected papers*, New York, 1959, International Universities Press.

18. Fox J: Etiological factors and information processing deficits associated with schizophrenia: a review of findings. In *Conference proceedings: sttae of the art and science of psychiatric nursing*, 1990, National Institute of Mental Health.

19. Freud S: Analysis: terminable and interminable. In Freud S: *Collected papers*, vol 5, London, 1950, The Hogarth Press, Ltd.

20. Fromm-Reichmann F: Psychotherapy of schizophrenia, *American Journal of Psychiatry* 111: 410, 1954.

21. Gerace L: Schizophrenia and the family: nursing implications, *Archives of Psychiatric Nursing* 2(3): 141, 1988.

22. Glazer W and others: Chronic schizophrenics in the community: are they able to report their social adjustment? *American Journal of Orthopsychiatry* 52: 116, 1982.

23. Gordon M: *Nursing diagnosis: process and application*, ed 2, New York, 1987, Mosby–Year Book.

24. Gottesman I, Bertelsen A: Confirming unexpressed genotypes for schizophrenia, *Archives of General Psychiatry* 46: 867, 1989.

25. Gruen R and others: Platelet MAO activity and schizophrenic prognosis, *American Journal of Psychiatry* 139: 240, 1982.

26. Gur RE and others: Brain function in psychiatric disorders. III. Regional cerebral blood flow in unmedicated schizophrenics, *Archives of General Psychiatry* 42: 329, 1985.

27. Hemmings G: *Biochemistry of schizophrenia and addiction: in search of common ground*, Baltimore, 1980, University Park Press.

28. Houseman C: The paranoid person: a biopsychosocial perspective, *Archives of Psychiatric Nursing* 4(3): 176, 1990.

29. Kane D, DiMartino E, Jimenex M: A comparison of short-term psychoeducational and support groups for relatives coping with chronic schizophrenia, *Archives of Psychiatric Nursing* 4(6): 342, 1990.

30. Kim MJ, Moritz DA, editors: *Classified of nursing diagnoses: proceedings of the third and fourth national conferences*, New York, 1982, McGraw-Hill.

31. Klein M: *Love, guilt and reparation*, New York, 1975, The Melanie Klein Trust.

32. Korner A and others: The relation between neonatal and later activity and temperament, *Child Development* 56: 38, 1985.

33. Krauss JB, Slavinsky AT: *The chronic psychiatric patient and the community*, Oxford, England, 1982, Blackwell Scientific Publications.

34. Lantos P: The neuropathology of schizophrenia and a critical review of recent work. In Bobbington P, McGuffin P, editors: *Schizophrenia: the major issues*, Oxford, England, 1988, Heinemann.

35. Leff J: *Expressed emotion in families*, New York, 1985, Guilford Press.

36. Lettieri-Marks D: Research in short-term inpatient group therapy: a critical review, *Archives of Psychiatric Nursing* 1(6): 407, 1987.

37. Lidz T, Fleck S, Cornelison A: *Schizophrenia and the family*, New York, 1965, International Universities Press.

38. Mahler MS: A study in the separation-individuation process, *Psychoanalytic Studies of the Child* 26: 403, 1971.

39. Malone J: Schizophrenia research update: implications for nursing, *Journal of Psychosocial Nursing* 28(8): 4, 1990.

40. McKinlay JB: Social network influences on morbid episodes and the career of help seeking. In Eisenber L, Kleinman A, editors: *The relevance of social science for medicine*, New York, 1980, D Reide Publishing Co.

41. Millen T: *Disorders of personality*, New York, 1981, John Wiley & Sons.

42. Neuchterlin KH, Dawson MW: A heuristic vulnerability street model of schizophrenic episodes, *Schizophrenia Bulletin* 10: 300, 1984.

43. Neuchterlin KH, Dawson MW: Information processing and attentional functioning in the developmental course of schizophrenic disorders, *Schizophrenia Bulletin* 10: 160, 1984.

44. Northouse PG: Interpersonal trust and empathy in nurse-nurse relationships, *Nursing Research* 28: 365, 1979.

45. Piaget J, Inhelder B: *The psychology of the child*, New York, 1969, Basic Books.

46. Platt S: Social adjustment as a criterion of treatment success: just what are we measuring, *Psychiatry* 44(5): 95, 1981.

47. Ritzler BA: Paranoia—prognosis and treatment: a review, *Schizophrenia Bulletin* 7: 710, 1981.

48. Rotter JB: A new scale for the measurement of interpersonal trust, *Journal of Personality* 35: 651, 1967.

49. Rosenthal T, McGuiness T: Dealing with delusional patients: discovering the distorted truth, *Issues in Mental Health Nursing* 8: 143, 1986.

50. Ruditis SE: Developing trust in nursing interpersonal relationships, *Journal of Psychiatric Nursing and Mental Health Services* 17(4): 20, 1979.

51. Seiver LL and others: Smooth pursuit eye tracking impairment, *Archives of General Psychiatry* 39: 1001, 1982.

52. Spitz RA, Wolf KM: The smiling response and contribution to the otogenesis of social relations, *Genetic Psychology Monographs* 34: 59, 1946.

53. Strauss, J, Carpenter W: *Schizophrenia*, New York, 1981, Plenum Medical Books.

54. Strauss J: Subjective experiences in schizophrenia: toward a new dynamic psychiatry, II, *Schizophrenia Bulletin* 15: 197, 1989.

55. Sullivan HS: *The interpersonal theory of psychiatry*, New York, 1953, WW Norton.

56. Torrey EF: *Surviving schizophrenia: a family manual*, New York, 1988, Harper Collins.

57. Ulin P: Measuring adjustment in chronically ill clients in community mental health care, *Nursing Research* 30: 229, 1981.

58. Ventura J and others: A prospective study of stressful life events and schizophrenic relapse, *Journal of Abnormal Psychiatry* 98(4):407, 1989.

59. Wallston KA, Wallston BS, Gore S: Development of a scale to measure nurse's trust of patients, *Nursing Research* 22: 232, 1973.

60. Wasow M: *Coping with schizophrenia*, Palo Alto, Calif, 1982, Science and Behavior Books.

61. Weinberger D and others: Poor premorbid adjustment and CT scan abnormalities in chronic schizophrenia, *American Journal of Psychiatry* 137: 1410, 1980.

62. Weinberger DR: Implications of normal brain development for the pathogenesis of schizophrenia, *Archives of General Psychiatry* 44: 660, 1987.

63. Wright TL, Palmer ML: An unobtrusive study of interpersonal trust, *Journal of Personality and Social Psychology* 32: 446, 1975.

64. Zubin J: Problems of attention in schizophrenics. In Kietzman JL, Sutton S, Zubin J, editors: *Experimental approaches to psychopathology*, New York, 1975, Academic Press.

ANNOTATED BIBLIOGRAPHY

Cantor S: *Childhood schizophrenia*, New York, 1988, Guilford Press.

Recommended for readers especially interested in severe mental disorders of children. A good source of information about the early development of schizophrenia, this book contributes to a broader understanding of the disorder and the various understandings about causes, symptoms, and treatment.

Hatfield AD, Lefley HP: *Families of the mentally ill: coping and adaptation*, New York, 1988, Guilford Press.

The authors recommend that professionals view family members of psychotic patients as essential social supports for the patient. Parents are often integral to the patient's ability to manage successful community living. Family members usually provide the bulk of community care. Organized into three sections: (1) overview of the family's experience, (2) coping and adaptation theory, and (3) what families think they need for assistance.

North CS: *Welcome silence: my triumph over schizophrenia*, New York, 1989, Avon.

A personal narrative of a person with severe mental illness who describes her experiences attempting to manage schizophrenic symptoms and the personal work of recovery. Provides a view of the illness as experienced by the patient, which can facilitate development of a more supportive perspective towards persons with schizophrenia.

CHAPTER
18 Addictive Behavior

Laina M Gerace

After studying this chapter, the student will be able to:

- Identify addictive behaviors
- Discuss historical perspectives on addiction
- Discuss diagnostic criteria of psychoactive substance use disorders as described in the DSM-III-R
- List common substances of addiction and their effects
- Describe theories explaining various aspects of addictive behaviors

- Apply the nursing process to care for clients with addictive behaviors
- Identify selected current research findings relevant to addiction and client care
- Describe professional issues related to alcohol and other drug abuse

---

The need for gratification is common in all human beings. Particularly important is feeling physically satisfied. Physical satisfaction leads to general feelings of well-being and helps the person deal more effectively with the demands of life. Therefore gratification is often associated with eating and drinking.

Also important for gratification are psychosocial experiences such as being connected in relationships, satisfying work, and meaningful activities. Eating a wonderful meal and drinking pleasurable beverages in the company of good friends exemplify a gratifying experience. Enthusiastic devotion towards one's religion, earnest commitment for one's work, or zest for a chosen sport are further examples.

Although there are cultural variations, in our society the use of certain substances such as coffee or alcohol to feel better is common. Alcoholic beverages are often served at social gatherings and the 15-minute coffee break is an American tradition. Substances are also used for medical reasons to alleviate pain, alter mood, suppress appetite, or relieve anxiety. Moderate, controlled use of substances is considered acceptable. However, when use of substances gets out of control and continues regardless of adverse consequences, addictive behavior results.

Addictive behavior can be thought of as unrestrained searching for gratification. What once was experienced as pleasurable now becomes obsessive, compulsive, and uncontrolled. The object of gratification—alcohol, prescription drugs, illegal substances, a combination of substances, or even food—becomes so central in the person's life that

it continues to be sought despite harm to mental and physical health, family, and society. Instead of using substances and experiences in a mentally healthy way for normal coping, they are progressively used to avoid the demands of life. Paradoxically, although it continues to be sought, the substance of addiction no longer really satisfies, and life in general, seems out of control.

ADDICTION AS A DISEASE

The disease model of addiction holds that substance abuse, whether drugs, alcohol, or nicotine, has a characteristic symptomatology and a progressive and predictable course. Jellinek[18] first proposed that, as with any other

> ### DIAGNOSES Related to Addictive Behavior

MEDICAL DIAGNOSES
Psychoactive substance dependence
Psychoactive substance abuse

NURSING DIAGNOSES
NANDA
Ineffective individual coping
Defensive coping
Ineffective denial

PMH
Aggression/violence toward
    self: substance abuse

DATES	EVENTS
1600s	Tobacco a major export from American colonies to England.
1700s	Luxury tax placed on smokeless tobacco (snuff).
1800s	Virtually no laws governing drug sales and use. Chinese laborers introduced opium smoking to Americans. Heroin placed on the market as a "nonaddicting substitute" for codeine. Temperance movement led to increased beer production. The Prohibition movement led to prohibition of alcohol in various states.
1906	Pure Food and Drug Act prohibited interstate commerce of adulterated or mislabeled foods and drugs. The act specifically referred to alcohol, morphine, opium, cocaine, heroin, and marijuana.
1914	Harrison Narcotics Act was passed as result of an international agreement to control trade and sale of opium, morphine, and cocaine. Dealers and dispensers of opiates and cocaine had to register annually, pay a fee, and use special order forms provided by the government. Smuggling of drugs was a crime.
1920-1933	The Eighteenth Amendment for national prohibition of alcohol was passed. Illegal production of alcohol became profitable, organized crime grew. Concern about widespread disrespect for the law led to repeal. Increased clinical use of barbiturates.
1930-1940s	Major effects of amphetamines were discovered and used to treat narcolepsy and activity in hyperactive children. Appetite suppressive effect became a major clinical use of amphetamines. Later amphetamines were used by soldiers to promote alertness and manual dexterity.
1940-1970	Increasing crime due to critical shortage of heroin, which led to increased prices. Drug experimentation increased during 1960s "hippy" phase and Vietnam War.
1980-1990s	Emphasis on health lead to decreased use of nicotine and marijuana; however, use is still common. Decriminalization of marijuana debated but not resolved, whereas punishment for possession has decreased. Increase in polysubstance abuse.
Future	Polysubstance abuse will become a major problem and complicate assessment and treatment. A major problem will result from the development of illicit drugs that are easily available, cheaper, and rapidly addictive.

HISTORICAL OVERVIEW

chronic disease, alcoholism is characterized by distinct, progressive phases. Beginning with social drinking and use of alcohol to reduce stress and tension, the disease progresses to gradual increase in alcohol tolerance, blackouts (chemically induced periods of amnesia), and loss of control over drinking to the point where the person needs help to stop. In both alcohol and drug addiction, denial is an integral part of the disease and a major obstacle to recovery. Adverse medical consequences are common, especially when addiction progresses over a long time.

Addiction is a complex problem. Addictive behavior is increasingly viewed as a biopsychosocial problem in which genetics, neurochemistry, pharmacology, behavior, and social environment interact to produce the illness.[36] The accompanying box lists some terms used to describe addictive behavior related to alcohol and drugs and their definitions.

DSM-III-R DIAGNOSES

The DSM-III-R refers to addictive behaviors as psychoactive substance use disorders and distinguishes between substance dependence and abuse. *Psychoactive substance de-*

pendence is defined as impaired control of one or more substances that continues despite adverse consequences. According to the DSM-III-R, the symptoms of the psychoactive substance dependence include physiological symptoms of tolerance and withdrawal. At least three of the following patterns must be present: (1) more of the substance is taken than intended; (2) an unsuccessful attempt is made to reduce the amount; (3) preoccupation with the substance, including obtaining, using, and recuperating from the effects of the substance; (4) frequent intoxication so that it interferes with role obligations, family life, and psychological, and physical health; (5) important social, occupational, or recreational activities are stopped because of substance use; (6) the substance continues to be used despite knowledge of having persistent or recurrent social, psychological, or physical problems; (7) increased tolerance develops, which causes the person to take more and more of the substance; (8) withdrawal symptoms develop with continued use; and (9) continued use of the substance to avoid withdrawal symptoms.

Psychoactive substance abuse refers to a maladaptive pattern of substance use, such as using the substance despite resulting social, work, or personal problems that are

▼
COMMONLY USED TERMS RELATED TO ADDICTION

Misuse	Used for purposes other than those for which intended, or used incorrectly as prescribed
Abuse	Excessive use of a substance that differs from accepted social practice
Craving	Persistent psychological or physiological hunger or need for a substance
Dependence	Compulsion to take a substance either on a continuous or periodic basis to experience its effects and to avoid discomfort of its absence
Tolerance	The need for increasing amounts of a substance to achieve the same effects
Withdrawal	Characteristic physiological signs that occur when the addictive substance is reduced or stopped; sometimes called abstinence syndrome
Cross-dependence	Condition in which one substance can prevent withdrawal symptoms caused by a different substance in the same pharmacological class
Cross-tolerance	Condition in which tolerance to one substance results in reduced response to another, resulting in tolerance to both substances
Dual diagnosis	Alcohol and/or drug dependence occurring simultaneously with mental illness
Polyaddiction	Dependence on several substances, not necessarily similar in effect, such as alcohol, cocaine, and cigarettes
Relapse	Reestablishment of addiction after a period of abstinence
Codependency	Stress-related preoccupation with the addicted person's life, leading to extreme dependence on that person.

created with such use or using the substance repeatedly in situations when use is physically dangerous. Examples of substance abuse include drunk driving, using cocaine on weekends and then missing a major midterm examination, and drinking despite being diagnosed with an ulcer. Symptoms include at least one of the following patterns: (1) continued use despite knowledge of having a persistent or recurrent social, occupational, psychological, or physical problem that is caused or exacerbated by use; and (2) recurrent use of the substance in situations in which use is physically hazardous. These symptoms must have persisted for at least 1 month or have occurred repeatedly over a longer time.

THEORETICAL APPROACHES

There is no consensus about how and why addiction occurs. Most likely, many factors play a role in the addiction process. For example, family history seems to predispose people to addictive behavior, but not all persons with family histories of addiction become addicted. Why is it that some individuals can drink moderately or use cocaine occasionally whereas others cannot stop? Why is it that some individuals who are addicted can stop, either on their own or with the help of treatment, but others repeatedly relapse and eventually die from the consequences of addiction? Do these differences occur because of the person's physiological make-up, personality traits, or psychosocial needs or because of what they learned about substance use in the family and society? How does culture and substance availability contribute to substance abuse?

Because addictive behavior is a complex phenomenon, no single theory can fully explain the problem of addiction. Addiction most likely results because of an interplay among genetic disposition, biological factors, and environmental influences.[35] The theoretical perspectives that follow address various aspects of addictive behavior.

Psychoanalytical

The psychoanalytical perspective conceptualizes addictive behavior as extreme psychological dependence. This idea is reflected in the often used term *chemical depen-*

dency. Human beings start life in a completely dependent state. A baby must be nurtured and cared for in a consistent manner to survive. This first phase of development is known as the oral phase. The baby is extremely dependent on the primary caregiver and only gradually adjusts to being away from the mother. According to Freud, if dependence needs are not adequately met during the oral phase of infant development a fixation develops. The individual has difficulty moving beyond the oral phase of development and constantly seeks oral gratification. According to this way of thinking, substance use, eating, and smoking are ways to fill oral dependency needs. Extreme dependency needs result in a compulsion toward the object, activity, or experience. Despite recognition that the substance is harmful and attempts to change this drive for the addictive substance, there is an overwhelming urge to continue seeking it.

Underlying personality traits

Early psychoanalytical thinking viewed addictive behavior as symptomatic of underlying psychopathology rather than as a primary disease. Alcoholism, for example, was seen and treated as a problem secondary to personality disorders, depression, or maladaptive coping. Psychoanalytical thinking about addiction differs from the Alcoholics Anonymous approach, which is based on the assumption that addictive behavior is a primary disease for which recovery, but not cure, is possible. It is true that psychiatric disorders occur more frequently in addicted persons and vice versa. What is not known is whether certain personality factors predispose an individual to addiction.[33]

Research into the role of personality traits in addiction focuses on the question: Is there an "addictive personality?" This question grew out of the observation that drug addicts seem to manifest antisocial personality patterns. One problem in answering this question is that addicts are studied *after* they have been addicted, not before, making it difficult to determine whether the personality traits were a cause or result of the addiction. Another problem is that studies on personality traits were conducted mostly on hospitalized heroin addicts and cannot be generalized to other addictions.

The current viewpoint is that personality traits such as

low self-esteem, tendency to break rules, or frequent depressed mood may be predisposing factors.[25] For example, individuals with antisocial and borderline personality traits are at greater risk for developing alcohol or drug abuse. Likewise, individuals with major mental illnesses are more likely to develop substance abuse problems. However, research has not yet demonstrated that a consistent personality profile typifies someone with addictive behavior, whether the substance of addiction is alcohol or drugs. Many types of persons can become addicted.

Behavioral

Alcohol, drugs, and food are powerful reinforcers. From the behavioral viewpoint, a *reinforcer* is anything that increases the likelihood that a behavior will recur. Reinforcers work in a variety of ways. A *positive reinforcer* works by rewarding the behavior; a *negative reinforcer* works by removing an aversive stimulus. In the case of narcotics, for example, positive reinforcement consists of the pleasant, euphoric feelings that result when the substance is taken. The negative reinforcement consists of the uncomfortable or aversive effects (pain, anxiety, or withdrawal symptoms) the addicted person experiences without the substance. In other words, the addicted person continues the abused substance to avoid the negative effects, which reinforce desire for the substance. Similarly, aversive techniques may sometimes be used in treatment. For example, if an alcoholic is given an agent that creates unpleasant reactions when he drinks alcohol, the aversive reaction is a negative reinforcer, and alcohol may subsequently be avoided.

Once a pattern of substance abuse is established, objects, events, and persons associated with the pleasant effects also serve as secondary reinforcers. *Secondary reinforcers* are events or conditions that are associated with or supplemental to positive reinforcers. For example, repeated good feelings from alcohol use cause the presence of drinks, a bar, and "drinking buddies" to become secondary learned reinforcers.

Secondary reinforcers are important factors in the persistence of addictive behavior. Their presence continues to trigger the desire to use the addictive substance even after the addicted individual has been abstinent for long periods. This problem is well known in relation to illicit drug addiction. If the drug addict returns to the community and is again exposed to situations where drugs are present, it will be difficult to resist using drugs again.[25]

Sociocultural

Addictive behavior takes place in a social context. Understanding some of the social factors that influence the addiction process provides insight into how complex the problem of addiction really is in our society. Sociocultural theory considers factors such as (1) prevalence, (2) economics, (3) substance availability, and (4) cultural attitudes. Even though they are discussed separately, these factors are highly interrelated.

Prevalence

Addictive behavior is a health problem of increasing concern as the health, social, and financial costs of drug and alcohol abuse reach an all time high. Population surveys show that over 14 million Americans had used an illegal drug in the month before the survey and that 6.5 million were dependent on cocaine, heroin, and amphetamines. Similarly, about 10.5 million adults are alcohol dependent.[28] Consequences such as health effects, family distress and violence, serious and fatal accidents, and fetal alcohol syndrome create a ripple effect, involving others, not just the addicted person. It is also estimated that 20% to 50% of all illnesses requiring hospitalizations are alcohol and drug related.[35]

The prevalence of concurrent (use in same time period) and simultaneous (taking substances together at one time) use of alcohol and sedatives is increasing. A recent survey showed that a greater percentage of males, especially young adult men, than female drinkers used sedatives or tranquilizers.[14]

The prevalence of substance abuse varies in special populations.[20] Three special populations are of concern. One is the *elderly.* Prevalence of alcohol abuse and dependence is thought to be at about 2.2% in those over 65 years of age. A major concern in this population is prescription and over-the-counter drug misuse or abuse. Typical patterns of abuse involve *polypharmacy:* the use of many different medications prescribed by more than one physician and dispensed by more than one pharmacy. Memory deficits and poor vision can also lead to overuse or improper use of prescribed medications. Patterns of abuse may develop due to the stress and losses inherent in aging.[5,8] Nonprescription drugs most often misused by the elderly include analgesics, antacids, laxatives, and sedatives. Prescription drugs misused or abused include anxiolytics, sedatives, hypnotics, and analgesics.

A second special population of concern is the *adolescent.* Substance abuse among teenagers is often part of risk-taking behavior consistent with wanting to be independent, to separate from parents, and to explore new roles.[22] Alcohol is the most widely used and abused substance among young people, with prevalence of use reported anywhere between 60% and 80%. Use of other illicit drugs ranges from 3% to 20% depending on the substance.[32]

A third special population of concern is the *pregnant woman and her developing fetus.* Alcohol abuse is a serious problem in childbearing women and their infants. Prevalence in this population varies greatly with geographical region and ethnicity.

Fetal alcohol syndrome has been estimated at between 0.3 to 0.9/10,000 births nationwide. Estimates in lower socioeconomic areas is higher: 2.6 per 1000 births. Risk for fetal alcohol syndrome for blacks is about sevenfold higher than that for whites. While higher than in other groups, incidence varies among different cultures of Native Americans. Health units serving mainly Navajo and Pueblo tribes report prevalence similar to that for the overall US population, whereas, for Southwest Plains Indians, a much higher prevalence was reported (1 case/102 live births). Several factors, such as cultural influences, patterns of alcohol consumption, nutrition, and metabolical differences, have been suggested to play a role in this difference.[27]

Cocaine and crack abuse is another serious problem affecting the health of pregnant women and their infants. Again, prevalence varies with geographical region. A recent study by the National Association for Perinatal Addiction Research and Education surveyed 36 hospitals around the country and found that at least 11% of women in the hospitals had used illegal drugs during pregnancy. Specific medical effects of prenatal cocaine use includes increased rates of spontaneous abortion, premature detachment of the placenta, fetal growth retardation, and increased risk for cerebrovascular accidents in the infant.[21,29]

Economics

Measuring economic cost of an illness is one way to assess the overall impact of that illness on society. Research indicates that alcohol and other drug abuse costs society many billions of dollars each year in lost productivity, expenses related to medical consequences of substance abuse, and the loss to society from premature deaths due to substance abuse. These economic costs give an indication of the magnitude of substance abuse in our society.

Substance availability

To a great extent, the presence of a substance determines its use. For example, if freshly baked brownies are in the house, they will be eaten. Likewise, when there is an "open" bar at a big wedding, more liquor will be consumed.

Availability is a key factor in addiction. If alcohol or drugs are not available, abuse cannot occur; however, availability of a substance is not enough to cause addiction. Many people can obtain drugs if they want to, but do not. Therefore availability is a necessary condition for substance abuse, but it is not a cause.

Throughout history alcoholic beverages have often been subject to extra taxation and various legal controls. Behind controlling availability is the idea that reducing overall consumption is the best way to reduce alcohol abuse. However, controlling alcohol availability does not provide a simple solution to alcohol abuse. For example, prohibition in countries such as India, Russia, Sweden, and the United States led to illicit production and distribution. The only groups in which prohibition seems to work well are those for whom abstinence is a social norm as part of their religious beliefs. Cross-national studies show that increasing the price and tax on alcoholic beverages decreases consumption among moderate users, but heavy drinkers will make financial sacrifices to continue drinking the same amounts.[15]

Currently, the government has put great emphasis on drug-free work environments. Most places of employment, including hospitals and other health care agencies, have policies prohibiting alcohol, drugs, and cigarettes in the work place. The impact of these policies on use and abuse remains to be determined.

Cultural attitudes

Culture plays a major role in shaping human behavior. What is appropriate in one group may be quite different in another. Drinking patterns, especially, have been studied across cultures. It is difficult to make general statements about cultures because substance use varies widely even within a culture. Many factors, including cultural traditions, family patterns, and genetics probably play a role in why some cultures seem to have higher rates of substance abuse than others. The Italian and Irish cultures illustrate how culture plays a role in substance use.

In the Italian culture, drinking rates are high, but alcohol-related problems are low. Italians associate drinking with food and family. Children are introduced early to drinking small amounts of wine mixed with water at family mealtimes. Drinking becomes associated with daily life in the context of eating, not with the purposes of relaxation, relieving stress, or becoming drunk and engaging in risk-taking behaviors. As a result, alcoholics in the Italian culture have less overt "drunk" behavior (fighting, drinking with buddies at the bar) than alcoholics in the United States, but cirrhosis of the liver is high because alcoholism is kept in the family and not referred for treatment.[15]

In the Irish culture, drinking rates are high and alcohol-related problems, such as fighting, family disruption, and accidents, are also high. Excessive drinking among men is not unusual and is thought to relate to the tight social controls that exist, such as strict rules about birth control, premarital sex, marital roles, and family relationships. Drinking, therefore, is associated with stress relief and getting away from social controls.[4]

Family

Systems theory provides a framework for understanding how addiction affects the structure, roles, and functions of a family. A family carries out its functions through the subsystems, which are a part of its structure and guide its communication patterns.[36] It is important to recognize that addictive behavior is not necessarily an outcome of a dysfunctional family. Many times the opposite is true: Addiction creates so much stress in the family system that dysfunctional family patterns may result. Addictive behavior affects the entire family.[31]

For healthy family functioning, the boundaries of the family subsystems are clear. Parents form a special subsystem when they guide and direct the growth and development of their children. Spouses form a marital subsystem as they meet each other's need for support and intimacy. Likewise, siblings form a subsystem in which they learn to negotiate peer competition and relationships. Addiction can severely disrupt family subsystems and boundaries. For example, if a parent is addicted to a drug or alcohol, that parent is no longer dependable and available to the children. Parental boundaries are weakened. Family rules are unclear and a level of chaos develops in the family structure.

Family roles are also affected by addiction. As boundaries are altered, children may fill in parental roles by taking care of younger siblings and even the addicted parent. A female child, in particular, may take an *overachiever* role in which she assumes responsibility for family management. Other coping roles children may assume when parents are addicted are (1) *hero,* the child who provides self-esteem for the family by being successful; (2) *scapegoat,* the child who takes the focus off the addicted parent by seeking negative attention; (3) *mascot,* the child who relieves family tension by being endearing and funny; and (4) *lost child,* the child who withdraws from the family and feels lonely and unimportant.[6]

Codependency

The idea of codependency grew out of clinical observations that family members who live with an addicted member are significantly affected by that person's use of alcohol or mood-altering substances. *Codependency* is defined as stress-induced preoccupation with the addicted person's life, leading to extreme dependence and excessive concern with the dysfunctionally addicted person.[6] The family member may take on the same coping style (rationalization, denial) as the addicted person. The behaviors resulting from codependency are referred to as *enabling,* behaviors of the nonaddicted person that tend to help maintain the addiction. Enabling behaviors support the denial of addiction. For example, a supervisor ignores signs of alcoholism in an employee and "covers" for that employee by giving others heavier assignments.

Codependency is a popularized concept that tends to encompass a broad spectrum of meanings and implications. The concept is receiving some criticism because it tends to include a wide range of common behaviors. However, understanding codependency helps those who have relationships with addicted persons develop awareness of how their behaviors shield an addicted person from experiencing the impact of the consequences of addiction. The following case example demonstrates codependency.

▼ Case Example

Juan, a husband and father, routinely abuses alcohol on the weekends, having difficulty getting up and going to work on Monday mornings due to a hangover. Marissa, his wife, goes to great extremes to cover for him by calling his boss to say that her husband is sick. If her husband forgets his keys and locks himself out of the house on Sunday night, she waits up for him. If he vomits on the bathroom floor, she cleans up after him and the children are told that "Daddy was sick to his stomach last night." When empty beer bottles are left around the house, she quickly disposes of them. Juan's drinking is not mentioned. Even the children become so preoccupied with taking care of their addicted father and their distressed mother that they restrict their relationships with friends. As a result, Juan's addictive behavior is a family secret. The family's enabling behaviors actually help to maintain his addiction.

Consider how differently things might be in the case example if Marissa does not deny the problem or hide it from Juan's place of work or from the children. If Juan fails to show up for work on Monday morning, he alone has to answer to his boss. If he locks himself out, he has to create a disturbance to wake someone up to let him in. If he vomits on the floor, it remains there until he cleans it up himself. If empty beer bottles remain, evidence is provided for father and children to see how much he is actually drinking. If the consequences of his behavior are visible, he may begin to recognize and feel responsibility for his alcoholism.

It is not surprising that a spouse engages in enabling behaviors. Living with an addicted person in a society that avoids dealing with the problem can be very confusing. Not only does the addicted person disrupt normal family functions by being unpredictable and unreliable, but also society fails to acknowledge the scope of the problem. Many people still do not understand that addiction is a disease in which excessive denial is part of the problem. If the addicted family member is vital to the family's

---

RESEARCH HIGHLIGHT

Nursing Students with Alcoholic Fathers: Alcohol Consumption and Depressive Symptoms
- MR Haack and TC Harford

PURPOSE

The study examined the relationship between positive family history for alcoholism and the prevalence of alcohol consumption and depressive symptoms in a sample of undergraduate nursing students.

SAMPLE

Sample consisted of 179 student nurses in a large midwestern university. Response rate for data on family drinking history was 93%. Sample composition was 80% white, 13% Asian American, 4.2% black. Most were women under 25 years of age.

METHODOLOGY

The study relied on longitudinal data on drinking and drug use, depression, and burnout. On the last data collection cycle, students were asked if any of their relatives had been alcoholics or problem drinkers at any time of their lives. On the basis of this information students were classified into the following categories: (1) family history positive for alcoholic father and mother, (2) family history positive for other alcoholic relatives, and (3) family history negative for alcoholic relatives. Data gathered on students included measures on drinking patterns and depression (CES-D Depression Scale). Analysis of variance was used to explore the relationship between family history and the students' drinking patterns and depression scores.

FINDINGS

This sample of nursing students did not report a greater prevalence of parental alcoholism than other college students. Data indicated that students who are daughters of alcoholic fathers report higher levels of alcohol consumption when compared to either families with alcoholic relative other than father or nonalcoholic families. No relationship was shown between family history and the students' scores on the depression instrument.

IMPLICATIONS

A positive history for alcoholism or alcohol problems in the family may increase student nurses' risk for developing drinking-related problems. It is important for developing professionals to examine their own use of alcohol and other substances. Self-care is a vital component in a professional's life.

Based on data from *Issues in Mental Health Nursing* 9:181, 1988.

security, it is not surprising that a wife, and mother of young children, is reluctant to do anything to upset the family system.[12]

Biological

Current emphasis on the biological dimension of addiction focuses on research for risk factors related to deficiencies in various neurochemicals that have important functions in the brain. For example, noradrenergic neurotransmission has been linked to relapse in alcoholism.[36] Another area of research concerns the metabolism of acetaldehyde. Alcohol is oxidized in the liver to acetaldehyde and, mediated by aldehyde dehydrogenase (ALDH), is broken down further before it is eliminated from the body. Acetaldehyde seems to be mainly responsible for symptoms of alcohol-related sensitivity such as facial flushing, hot feeling in stomach, palpitation, tachycardia, dizziness/hangover, and muscle weakness. Many Asians experience these aversive "flushing" symptoms after a drink of alcohol. Their inability to metabolize acetaldehyde quickly and effectively is thought to be due to deficient amounts of ALDH needed to mediate the breakdown of acetaldehyde. Research shows that persons manifesting the "flushing" response tend to consume fewer alcoholic drinks in their daily life. The biologically based alcohol intolerance may protect Asians from alcoholism.[11]

The massive denial often occurring with the disease of addiction may be due, in part, to biochemical effects leading to a phenomenon called *euphoric recall.* Euphoric recall refers to the client's tendency to remember the good feelings about being under the biochemical influence of the addictive substance, but not the embarrassing or dysfunctional behaviors associated with it. An example is the drunk driver who feels jovial and confident while he weaves dangerously down the road. Later, he remembers only the good feelings, not the impaired driving. It is almost as if a delusional system develops in addictive behavior because reality is not perceived accurately. These symptoms create barriers to treatment for the addicted client.

Genetics

Alcoholism tends to run in families, but is that due to environmental influence (children drink because parents drink), or is it due to a genetic tendency? By studying identical twins and adopted children, it is possible to infer genetic patterns of transmission. If, for example, twins show considerably higher concordance rates for alcoholism than do regular siblings, a genetic factor may be present. Likewise, if children of alcoholic parents adopted into nonalcoholic homes develop a higher incidence of alcoholism, a genetic factor probably exists.

Evidence is convincing that children of alcoholics are more vulnerable to alcoholism, whether raised by their alcoholic parents or by nonalcoholic foster parents[7] (see research highlight). Very little is known about this genetic vulnerability. Especially important would be understanding the role of environmental influence with the genetic vulnerability. At this time, twin studies are inconclusive.[23] Genetic influence seems to be present for two types of alcoholism in men. Type I alcoholics have a later onset of the disease, and little or no criminality; type II have earlier

onset, considerable criminal behavior, and a higher risk for developing alcoholism than type I.[15]

NURSING PROCESS: ALCOHOLISM

Assessment

Physical dimension Areas assessed include (1) patterns of use, (2) physical indications, (3) negative consequences, and (4) risk factors.

Assessment of patterns of use includes the quantity, frequency, and the circumstances in which drinking takes place. The three areas taken together can determine the extent of alcohol abuse. For example, heavy drinking can include excessive drinking on the weekends (binge drinking), or a pattern of drinking four or more drinks (wine, beer, or hard liquor) per day. For women, heavy drinking is two or more per day because of body weight and different metabolism.

Clients feel ashamed about their inability to control drinking and use denial about the extent of their problem. Heavy drinkers have a tendency to underreport the amount of their drinking. The nurse needs to feel comfortable in conducting the assessment interview because of the sensitive nature of the data. Framing questions in a caring, collaborative, nonjudgmental manner improves client response. Strategies for interviewing alcohol-addicted clients can be learned from experienced nurses and other health care providers.

The kinds of questions used to assess patterns of use address quantity, frequency, and circumstances of use. For example: When was the last time you had any alcoholic beverages? What beverages (wine, beer, mixed drinks) did you drink? How many drinks did you have? How many times per week do you drink? How many drinks (glasses, cans, shots) do you typically drink each time? Where do you usually drink and with whom?

Assessment of physical indications may not yield obvious signs in the early stages of the disease. Early physical symptoms may include shakiness and nervousness due to the need for a drink. *Blackouts* (chemically induced periods of amnesia) are highly indicative of alcoholism. Later physical symptoms may include shakiness when not drinking, tolerance, and physical problems such as abdominal pain, nausea, and vomiting related to pancreatitis or gastritis. Symptoms of myopathy and peripheral neuritis may eventually develop. Table 18-1 lists early and late signs and symptoms of alcoholism.

Laboratory tests can aid in the assessment of alcohol abuse or dependence. Blood alcohol levels measure the concentration of alcohol in the blood. Levels are expressed in the number of milligrams of alcohol per milliliter of blood (mg %). Typically, the legal limit of blood alcohol is 100 mg/dl or 0.1%. The blood alcohol level is used mainly for medical and legal purposes, such as to determine whether a person was drunk when an accident occurred or whether a comatose person brought to the emergency room is drunk. To reach the legal limit, a 160-pound man would have to consume about five cans of beer in 1 hour.[10] The blood alcohol level indicates the current state of drunkenness (alcohol abuse), not whether the disease of alcoholism is present.

▼ **TABLE 18-1**   Alcohol

Early Signs and Symptoms		Later Signs and Symptoms	
Physical	**Behavioral**	**Physical**	**Behavioral**
Red eyes	Daily or binge drinking	Shakes when not drinking	Continuous drinking despite harmful effects
Headaches (i.e., hangovers)	Preparty drinking	Tolerance: needing more to get drunk	Excessive sleeping
Lack of coordination	Sneaking drinks	Physical illness: liver and cardiac damage	Fights/arguments
Unsteady gait	Work absences		Legal difficulties
Drowsiness			Family difficulties
Alcohol on breath			Dropping of nondrinking friends
Blackouts (periods of memory loss)			Loss of job
Slurred speech			Falls
			Burns
			Bruises
			Lack of control; saying unexpected things

COMMON MEDICAL COMPLICATIONS OF ALCOHOLISM

Alcohol and the Digestive System
Esophagus (varices, Mallory-Weiss syndrome, cancer)
Mouth (cancer)
Stomach (gastritis, ulcers)
Pancreas (pancreatitis)

Alcohol and the Liver
Cirrhosis

Alcohol and the Heart
High blood pressure
Cardiac dysrhythmias
Alcoholic cardiomyopathy

Alcohol and Pulmonary Disease
Pneumonia

Alcohol and Blood Disorders
Anemia

Alcohol and the Endocrine System
Gonadal and adrenal effects (decreased libido, impotence)

Alcohol and the Brain
Peripheral neuropathy
Wernicke-Korsakoff syndrome
Dementia
Seizures

Alcohol and the Fetus
Fetal alcohol syndrome

Liver function and other blood tests can be used as indicators of alcoholism, although other reasons for elevation of liver function and other tests would have to be ruled out. The accompanying box shows common medical complications of alcoholism.

Assessment of negative consequences includes family problems, job problems, and other problems, such as drunk driving arrests. A family member's complaints about the client's drinking is a reliable indicator of a drinking problem. A pattern of job "shrinkage," such as assuming fewer responsibilities, showing up late, calling in sick, is a common negative consequence. Accidents and injuries, such as falls, car accidents, leaving the stove on, and falling asleep with a lit cigarette, are other examples.

Assessment of risk factors includes a family history of alcoholism or medical complications of alcoholism. Other risk factors include a history of excessive drinking with peer group and using alcohol to relieve stress. Coming home from a hectic work day and using two or three drinks to "unwind" is an example of using alcohol to relieve stress.

Emotional dimension In the emotional dimension, the nurse is aware of her own values, attitudes, and feelings about alcoholism. Especially important are the nurse's past experiences with addictive behavior. Perhaps the nurse comes from an alcoholic home and has never resolved personal issues left over from these experiences. The nurse's religious orientation may forbid alcohol use and the nurse may believe that such use is "wrong" and that addicted persons are "bad." Recognizing one's own emotional feelings is an important part of being able to work effectively with alcoholic clients.

The client with alcoholism experiences a variety of emotional reactions, such as anxiety, anger, guilt, and depression. He may feel deeply embarrassed and ashamed about being addicted. Once in treatment and no longer drinking, the client may seem emotionally shallow and flat. Being under the prolonged influence of alcohol has blocked the experience of emotional feelings. Yet the client may express anger and belligerence. The prospect of life without alcohol constitutes a major adjustment. The client may feel angry because others have forced him to face up to the problem. Another emotion is grief. The chemical of abuse has been experienced as a "friend" that is now taken away. The addict craves for and feels sad about the lost substance.

Intellectual dimension *Denial,* part of the disease of alcoholism, prevents the client from acknowledging the reality of the addictive behavior and its effects, thus avoiding emotional pain.[5] Denial is present when the client minimizes the addictive behavior, saying things such as, "I only drink a little beer." Other examples of denial include statements such as, "I can cut down if I want to," or "I know I have a problem, but I don't think treatment is going to help me."

Another defense used to guard against emotional pain is *rationalization,* which consists of making excuses for one's behavior. For example, an alcoholic client might say, "If my boss wasn't so mean I wouldn't drink."

Alcohol can impair intellectual functioning such as thinking processes and accurate perceptions of reality. Acute, transient impairment results from intoxication. The nurse is likely to encounter intoxicated clients in the emergency room setting in connection with injuries or accidents. According to the client's unique response patterns, he may show paranoid ideas, confusion, grandiosity, or sedation. The client may be belligerent, silly, inaccessible, or unpredictable.

Long-term, chronic impairment occurs in chronic alcoholism. Severe and chronic alcoholics often have specific deficits in problem solving, abstract thinking, concept shifting, psychomotor performance, and memory. In some clients, brain damage from long-term alcohol use includes conditions such as alcohol amnestic disorders (Wernicke's and Korsakoff's syndromes). Wernicke's syndrome is related to nutritional deficiencies, especially thiamine (vitamin B_1). This disorder is characterized by apathetic behavior and, if not treated, progresses to a permanent amnestic syndrome known as Korsakoff's syndrome. In the latter, chronic, fixed memory deficits are present. Alcoholic de-

mentia related to cerebellar degeneration is another type of intellectual impairment occurring late in severe alcoholism. Alcoholic dementia is a general state of intellectual deterioration and personality change, often leading to the need for institutionalization.

Intellectual impairment is also a concern for the fetus of a mother who abuses or is dependent on alcohol. Even moderate use may affect the fetus. In severe cases, alcoholism can cause permanent damage to the growing fetus. Fetal alcohol syndrome consists of physical and mental defects including growth deficiency, mental retardation, learning problems, and other physical symptoms such as heart defects, malformed facial features, low birth weight, and hyperactivity.

What the client knows and does not know about his particular addiction needs to be assessed carefully. Many clients lack knowledge and understanding about addictive behavior. They lack knowledge about the addictive nature of the substances and about the process of addiction. Some of the misunderstandings about addiction reflect societal myths (see the accompanying box).

Social dimension Addictive behavior takes place in a social context. Society puts great emphasis on alcohol and drugs and these substances are readily available. It is important to assess the social context of the client's addictive behavior. Does the client's social system consist mainly of addicted friends? Is anyone else in the family addicted? It is important to gather information about how the client got into treatment. Was social pressure (such as pressure from family or work) used to motivate the client?

The family is a key factor in the social dimension. Family members have been affected by alcoholism. Having their addicted family member in treatment has an impact on the family system, subsystems, and boundaries. The whole family undergoes readjustment. Often counseling is necessary to help the family understand patterns of codependency and to deal with changes. Their support significant affects the client's treatment outcome.

Spiritual dimension In the face of life's difficulties, alcohol is often used to relieve stress and experience physical pleasure and good feelings. Once addiction sets in, however, the client begins to indulge not for the sake of pleasure but often to alleviate guilt and remorse about the harm done to others through the addiction. Often this harm is very real, yet the addicted person fails to assume responsibility for it because continued use of alcohol dulls awareness and distorts reality. The nurse assesses the client's perception of his moral responsibility as he progresses in treatment. In many programs, a chaplain is an integral part of the spiritual aspect of assessment and care.

As part of the spiritual dimension, the nurse needs to consider the detrimental effects of the *moral model* of addiction. The moral model views addictive behavior as a lack of will power and holds the individual wholly responsible for the addiction. Addiction is seen as sinful or bad. The message is that the individual should be able to control his drinking. Even greater moral stigma is attached to women who drink excessively; they are viewed as sexually "loose."[16] It is important that nurses use the disease approach rather than the moral model when working with addicted clients.

▼
COMMON MYTHS ABOUT SUBSTANCE ABUSE

Myth: Drinking beer or wine is not as serious as drinking "hard liquor."
Fact: One beer, 4 oz of wine, and one shot of whiskey all have the same alcohol content.
Myth: Stopping alcohol or drug use for 3 days proves that the person is not addicted.
Fact: Trying to cut down and stop is a typical pattern of addiction. The fact that the person resumes drinking indicates that addiction exists.
Myth: You have to "hit bottom" to accept treatment.
Fact: The addiction process can be interrupted at any point. Awareness of early symptoms of addiction is the key to early intervention.
Myth: Addicts have a lack of discipline and self-control.
Fact: Anyone with a predisposition for addictive behavior can become addicted in a society where alcohol and drugs are readily available and promoted.

▼
CAGE SCREENING TEST

C   Have you ever felt the need to **C**ut down on your drinking (drug use)?

A   Have you ever been **A**nnoyed at criticism of your drinking (drug use)?

G   Have you ever felt **G**uilty about something you've done when you have been drinking (high from drugs)?

E   Have you ever had a morning **E**ye opener (taken drugs) first thing in the morning to get going (avoid withdrawal symptoms)?

Measurement Tools

Because of their extensive contact with clients in a variety of clinical settings, nurses are in an excellent position to screen for alcohol and other drug problems. Screening is used to identify clients who are potentially abusing alcohol or drugs. If clients screen positive, further assessment is required to determine the exact nature of the substance abuse problem. Although several tools are available, the 4-question CAGE is a common screening test.[24] The instrument can effectively detect a problem with substance abuse. It can be easily incorporated into any clinical setting, including prenatal clinics, medical-surgical units, emergency rooms, and primary health care clinics. A positive response to two of these questions are strongly indicative of alcoholism or drug abuse. The CAGE questions are listed in the box.

The best way to introduce screening questions is to give the client a general introduction to the content and purpose of the questions. For example, the nurse says, "Because alcohol and drug use can interfere with health and medi-

cations, we need to ask you some general questions about your substance use." A good lead-in to the CAGE is: "Do you drink now and then?" A "yes" response indicates the need to administer the test. Then the test should be administered to screen for drugs.

Analysis

Nursing diagnosis

Following are the NANDA-accepted nursing diagnoses related to clients with alcoholism:

Coping, Ineffective individual
 Defensive coping
 Ineffective denial

The defining characteristics of these diagnoses are summarized in the accompanying boxes.

Other diagnoses apply as well because these clients present with complex problems, both physical and psychological. These other diagnoses include the following:

1. Powerlessness related to loss of control over alcohol use
2. Altered role performance related to effects of alcoholism
3. Self-esteem disturbance related to loss of control over alcohol use
4. Sexual dysfunction related to chronic use of alcohol
5. Sleep pattern disturbance related to alcohol use
6. Impaired social interaction related to alcohol use
7. Spiritual distress related to loss of control over alcohol use

▼
DEFENSIVE COPING

DEFINITION

The state in which an individual experiences falsely positive self-evaluation based on a self-protective pattern that defends against underlying perceived threats to positive self-regard

DEFINING CHARACTERISTICS

- **Emotional dimension**

  Hostile laughter or ridicule of others

- **Intellectual dimension**

  Denial of obvious problem or weakness
  Projection of blame/responsibility
  Rationalizes failure
  Defensiveness (hypersensitive to criticism)
  Superior attitude toward others
  Difficulty in reality testing of perceptions
  Lack of follow through or participation in treatment or therapy

- **Social dimension**

  Difficulty establishing/maintaining relationships

Modified from Kim MJ, McFarland GK, McLane AM, editors: *Pocket guide to nursing diagnoses*, ed 5, St Louis, 1993, Mosby–Year Book.

▼
INEFFECTIVE DENIAL

DEFINITION

A conscious or unconscious attempt to disavow the knowledge or meaning of an event to reduce anxiety/fear to the detriment of health.

DEFINING CHARACTERISTICS

- **Physical dimension**

  Delays seeking or refuses medical attention to the detriment of health
  Uses home remedies (self-treatment to relieve symptoms)

- **Emotional dimension**

  Displays inappropriate affect

- **Intellectual dimension**

  Does not perceive personal relevance of symptoms or danger
  Minimizes symptoms
  Displaces source of symptoms to other organs
  Unable to admit impact of disease on life pattern
  Makes dismissive gestures or comments when speaking of distressing events
  Displaces fear of impact of condition

- **Spiritual dimension**

  Does not admit fear of death or invalidism

Modified from Kim MJ, McFarland GK, McLane AM, editors: *Pocket guide to nursing diagnoses*, ed 5, St Louis, 1993, Mosby–Year Book.

▼ **TABLE 18-2 NURSING CARE PLAN**

GOALS	OUTCOME CRITERIA	INTERVENTIONS	RATIONALES
NURSING DIAGNOSIS: Coping, ineffective individual related to denial of alcohol dependence			
LONG TERM			
To acknowledge inability to control alcohol intake	Recognizes that alcoholism is a disease that needs treatment	Assess patterns of alcohol intake with client	Reviewing actual drinking patterns and giving feedback about adverse effects helps client work through denial
		Give client feedback about adverse effects and loss of control over drinking	
		Convey disease approach to alcoholism and explain recovery process	Conveying disease approach reduces stigma
			Explaining recovery process supplies hope
To abstain from alcohol	Makes commitment to abstinent life-style by using available support such as AA and 12-step approach	Encourage commitment to recovery	Recovery is a lifelong process and requires commitment on the part of the client
SHORT TERM			
To listen to feedback from others about adverse effects of alcohol intake	Agrees to listen and participate in a structured intervention* session in which others give feedback about drinking and its effects	Collaborate with certified alcohol counselor or other experienced person to plan a structured intervention*	Use of resources will increase likelihood of effectiveness and success of intervention
		Use family and employment as "leverage" to encourage client to participate in the intervention	Because denial is pervasive, external social pressure is often needed to motivate client into a structured intervention session
		Provide feedback to client in a caring, supportive manner	Objective feedback will penetrate denial; support will convey caring and maintain respect
		Present treatment as a reasonable alternative to client's pattern of alcoholism	Presenting treatment as a choice will foster commitment to sobriety
To agree to enter a treatment program	Selects a treatment program and makes appointment to enter	Provide information about treatment options	Providing information about treatment and helping client take the first step provides support
		Assist client to make appointment to enter a treatment program	
	Is compliant with treatment and follow-up care	Devise with client a plan for compliance with follow-up care	Keeping appointment indicates behaviorally that client is committed to the treatment plan

*A structured intervention is a session in which persons close to an addicted client meet to give feedback about that person's substance abuse and the effect of that abuse on work performance, responsibilities, and family relationships.

The following case example demonstrates the characteristics of a client with a nursing diagnosis of ineffective denial. (See the box on p. 366 for defining characteristics of ineffective denial.)

▼ Case Example

Lyonel is a 33-year-old construction worker who had an accident at the construction site because he failed to use required safety precautions. As a result he is hospitalized with a broken hip. At the time of admission to the Emergency Department, his blood alcohol level was 0.16, well over the legal limit for intoxication. While recovering from hip surgery, Lyonel becomes very shaky, agitated, and nervous, showing signs of alcohol withdrawal. His girlfriend tells the nurse that Lyonel "drinks a six-pack of beer every day," and that she has delayed their marriage because she is concerned about his drinking. The physician prescribes Valium for several days to facilitate alcohol withdrawal. The liaison nurse who has special expertise in substance abuse counseling is called in to talk with Lyonel about his alcohol problem. Even when Lyonel is presented with factual information about his drinking, he refuses to acknowledge that a problem exists, stating: "I don't drink any more than the rest of the guys. My girlfriend is just a worrier. Besides, if she would marry me I wouldn't drink as much."

Planning

See Table 18-2 for a nursing care plan with examples of long-term and short-term goals, outcome criteria, interventions, and rationales related to defensive coping and ineffective denial. These are examples of the planning stage in the nursing process for an alcohol-addicted client.

Implementation

Physical dimension When a client is brought into treatment for alcoholism, the alcohol is abruptly stopped and other drug agents are temporarily substituted. Withdrawal from alcohol may range from mild to severe in terms of the symptoms experienced by the client. The accompanying box summarizes the three stages of alcohol withdrawal. Although assessment data about drinking patterns will provide baseline information about the severity of the alcoholism, it is often not possible to determine in advance which clients will develop delirium tremens. Therefore it is important to monitor each client during the withdrawal phase.

A wide variety of medications will minimize symptoms in milder forms of alcohol withdrawal. Especially useful are medications that show cross-dependence with alcohol, for example, benzodiazepines such as oxazepam (Serax). The drug profile on p. 369 describes nursing care appropriate to its administration. If withdrawal is more severe or signs of delirium tremens (severe tremulousness, agitation, delirium, visual hallucinations) develop, more aggressive interventions include medications such as pentobarbital, chloral hydrate, or chlordiazepoxide.[17] In addition to medications, clients with poor nutritional status require fluid and electrolyte supplements during withdrawal. Thiamine is administered to prevent Wernicke's syndrome.[2] The nurse administers medications and monitors the client's responses. Mainly, she provides support, comfort, and encouragement during this phase of care.

▼
·········
STAGES OF ALCOHOL WITHDRAWAL

Stage I	Psychomotor agitation, tremors, hyperactivity, hypertension, tachycardia, diaphoresis, anorexia, insomnia, and illusions. This stage is usually self-limiting and lasts from a few hours to 2 days.
Stage II	Stage II consists of stage I symptoms plus hallucinations: auditory, visual, tactile and olfactory (rare), and paranoid ideation and behavior. The hallucinations may be transient and intermittent.
Stage III	This stage is called delirium tremens. Stage III consists of stage I and stage II symptoms with the addition of disorientation, delusions, and delirium. There may be seizure activity. There is an increased incidence of death at this stage.

Modified from Knott DH, Fink RD, Morgan JC: Intoxication and the alcohol abstinence syndrome. In Schwartz, GR and others, editors: *Principles and practices of emergency medicine*, Philadelphia, 1978, WB Saunders.

In all stages of withdrawal, the client needs to be carefully observed and monitored. The client is protected from physical injury. Addictive substances are not left within the client's reach, nor are any medications with an alcohol base, such as cough syrup and shaving lotion, which may be used to meet the craving for alcohol.

Although relatively less common, withdrawal delirium may occur in stage II and needs careful monitoring. Stage III, delirium tremens, is a medical emergency. Onset is 3 to 5 days after cessation of drinking and lasts about 72 hours. In delirium tremens, the client experiences illusions and hallucinations, is disoriented, and may develop seizures, in addition to becoming belligerent and difficult to manage. Sedation and physical restraints may be required. The client is carefully monitored and attended. Some of the same strategies used with violent clients may need to be initiated. After the symptoms abate, the client falls into a deep, prolonged sleep that may last 24 hours.[2]

Most patients who undergo alcohol withdrawal do not progress to these extreme stages. However, the nurse may encounter these problems in medical-surgical settings when alcoholism has not been identified and diagnosed. Lack of proper substance abuse screening can lead to difficult, unplanned situations in postoperative and other clients.

Once the client is successfully withdrawn from alcohol, the rehabilitation phase of care begins. This phase may occur in either an inpatient or outpatient setting, depending on the best approach for the particular client. During the rehabilitation phase, a holistic approach to physical health is important for the client. Often there are nutritional deficiencies and vitamins are sometimes administered. In addition, exercise, regular sleeping patterns, and a general healthy life-style are emphasized. Many modern inpatient treatment programs have a fully equipped exercise room and prescribe an exercise regimen for clients. Fresh fruits and vegetables are routinely included in the diet. No junk food is kept in the refrigerator. These are important details of a comprehensive treatment program. It takes time and practice for clients to alter longstanding, unhealthy practices.

Some clients are treated with disulfiram (Antabuse), a

OXAZEPAM

(ox-a′ze-pam)
Apo-Oxazepam,* Novoxapam,*
Serax
Func class: Antianxiety
Chem class: Benzodiazepine

Controlled Substance Schedule IV
Action: Depresses subcortical levels of CNS, including limbic system and reticular formation
Uses: Anxiety, alcohol withdrawal
Dosage and routes:
Anxiety
▶ *Adult:* PO 10-30 mg tid-qid
Alcohol withdrawal
▶ *Adult:* PO 15-30 mg tid-qid
Available forms include: Caps 10, 15, 30 mg, tabs 15 mg
Side effects/adverse reactions:
CNS: Dizziness, drowsiness, confusion, headache, anxiety, tremors, fatigue, depression, insomnia, hallucinations, paradoxical excitement, transient amnesia
GI: Nausea, vomiting, anorexia
INTEG: Rash, dermatitis, itching
CV: Orthostatic hypotension, **ECG changes, tachycardia,** hypotension

---

*Available in Canada only.
Italic indicates common side effects.
Bold italic indicates life-threat-

EENT: Blurred vision, tinnitus, mydriasis
Contraindications: Hypersensitivity to benzodiazepines, narrow-angle glaucoma, psychosis, pregnancy (D), child <12 yr
Precautions: Elderly, debilitated, hepatic disease, renal disease
Pharmacokinetics:
PO: Peak 2-4 hr, metabolized by liver, excreted by kidneys, half-life 5-15 hr
Interactions/incompatibilities:
—Decreased effects of oxazepam: oral contraceptives, valproic acid
—Increased effects of oxazepam: CNS depressants, alcohol, disulfiram, oral contraceptives

NURSING CONSIDERATIONS
Assess:
—B/P (lying, standing), pulse; if systolic B/P drops 20 mm Hg, hold drug, notify physician; respirations q5-15 min if given IV
—Blood studies: CBC during long-term therapy, blood dyscrasias have occurred rarely
—Hepatic studies: AST, ALT, bilirubin, creatinine, LDH, alk phosphatase

Administer:
—With food or milk for GI symptoms
—Sugarless gum, hard candy, frequent sips of water for dry mouth
Perform/provide:
—Assistance with ambulation during beginning therapy; drowsiness/dizziness occurs
—Safety measures, including side rails
—Check to see PO medication has been swallowed
Evaluate:
—Therapeutic response: decreased anxiety, restlessness, insomnia
—Mental status: mood, sensorium, affect, sleeping pattern, drowsiness, dizziness
—Physical dependency, withdrawal symptoms: headache, nausea, vomiting, muscle pain, weakness, tremors, **convulsions** after long-term use
—Suicidal tendencies

Teach client/family:
—That drug may be taken with food
—Not to be used for everyday stress or used longer than 4 mo, unless directed by physician; not to take more than prescribed dose, may be habit forming
—To avoid OTC preparations (cough, cold, hay fever) unless approved by physician
—To avoid driving, activities that require alertness, since drowsiness may occur
—To avoid alcohol ingestion or other psychotropic medications unless prescribed by physician
—Not to discontinue medication abruptly after long-term use
—To rise slowly or fainting may occur
—That drowsiness might worsen at beginning of treatment
Lab test interferences:
Increase: AST/ALT, serum bilirubin
Decrease: RAIU
False increase: 17-OHCS
Treatment of overdose: Lavage, VS, supportive care

Modified from Skidmore-Roth L: *Mosby's nursing drug reference,* St Louis, 1993, Mosby–Year Book.

---

prescribed medication that, when ingested with alcohol, creates nausea, vomiting, flushing, hypotension, anxiety, and palpitations within minutes. Based on the behavioral principle of stimulus-response, this approach creates an aversive response when alcohol is taken. The client takes disulfiram on a regular basis, then, if drinking (stimulus) does take place, instead of the usual pleasant reaction, a very unpleasant reaction (response) occurs. The unpleasant reaction serves as a deterrent (negative reinforcer) to alcohol use. The person stops drinking to avoid the unpleasant effects experienced due to the disulfiram. However, this treatment approach only works if the client is compliant with the disulfiram. It should be combined with other rehabilitation strategies. The drug profile on p. 371 describes additional nursing care appropriate to its administration.

Emotional dimension Once the client is withdrawn from alcohol, many emotions are experienced. One predominant emotion may be anger. The client may feel angry because, now that alcohol is removed and the disease is being confronted, he is no longer able to completely deny the reality of alcoholism. Other feelings are anxiety and guilt. The nurse allows expression of feelings realizing that for a period of time such feelings were covered with the depressant effects of alcohol. Setting limits on the expres-

sion of anger is also appropriate. The nurse need not be the target for verbal abuse. An example of limit setting is, "Mr. Jones, I understand that you have been through a lot, and it is okay for you to feel angry. But it is not okay for you to shout at me and call me names."

Another common feeling the client deals with is grieving the loss of alcohol. The substance of addiction was a central part of the person's life. When that is taken away, feelings of loss and emptiness are experienced. This is a normal part of the recovery process and can be long and difficult to work through. It is helpful for the nurse to discuss this period of grieving with the client. Techniques used to facilitate grieving the loss of alcohol include writing a "letter of good-bye" to alcohol because alcohol was like a "friend." Such letters can be shared with a small group of similar clients under the nurse's guidance. Gradually, the client learns to substitute healthier activities and relationships in the place of the lost substance.

The family of the alcoholic client also experience a range of emotions. They often feel angry toward the client for the pain and disruption that the alcoholism has caused. When the client begins to assume more responsibility within the family, family members often feel upset by the changes they must make to accommodate their recovering family member. It is important for families to participate in the recovery process. For example, they need to be educated about the disease of addiction and learn about the roles they have assumed in the process of addiction. They may need guidance to reorganize their roles as the addicted family member recovers and takes on more responsibility within the family. It is important for family members to attend special family meetings and other planned programs offered through the treatment program.

Intellectual dimension Denial and rationalization are two ineffective coping mechanisms often seen in the alcoholic client. The nurse intervenes in the denial and rationalization by gently and persistently helping the client recognize his alcoholism. It is important to gauge interventions so as not to overwhelm and demoralize the client, recognizing that alcoholism occurs in all types of individuals, and not everyone benefits from the same approach. Confrontation, when needed, is not punitive or brutal. It is important to temper confrontation with respect and empathy. For example, the nurse may say in a direct manner, "In looking at your patterns of behavior, it seems to me that alcohol is interfering with your family life and job performance. You need help to stop drinking."

Intoxicated clients are often treated in the Emergency Department for injuries or accidents. Blood alcohol readings can confirm alcohol intoxication. Health care providers in the Emergency Department may become frustrated with intoxicated clients, seeking to discharge them as rapidly as possible. However, it is important to provide some intervention in relation to the alcohol problem. Once the acute intoxication has passed, the client is given feedback that may raise awareness of the alcohol problem. For example, the client can be given written information about alcohol abuse or can be referred to a treatment program or be given an Alcoholics Anonymous telephone number before being discharged. If transferred to a medical-surgical unit, information about drinking patterns is recorded in the admission note for later follow-up.

One of the most important interventions the nurse can provide is knowledge about the adverse effects of alcohol and alcoholism as a disease. Such information can be given in any health care setting. For example, nurses in prenatal care clinics provide information to pregnant women about the potential harm of alcohol on fetal development. School nurses should be involved in preventing alcohol abuse and drunk driving among teenagers.

Most alcohol treatment programs, whether inpatient or outpatient, provide structured educational programs that emphasize the disease process of alcoholism. Nurses are part of the team providing educational interventions. Clients are taught about the disease model of addiction (see discussion under Biological Theory), about the recovery process, craving, and relapse. As part of recovery, they are taught how to live in a world where alcohol is promoted at most social functions.

Social dimension Social pressure often is applied as an initial intervention to bring the client into treatment. In the area of substance abuse, the term *intervention* has a special meaning. It means confronting the addicted person with the facts about his addiction in a caring manner.[19] The following case example demonstrates such an initial intervention.

▼ Case Example

Jeanine works in an automobile plant. In the past few months, her supervisor notices alcohol on Jeanine's breath after lunch and observes a decline in her work productivity. Jeanine calls in sick more often than previously and no longer volunteers for extra tasks. Fellow workers notice that Jeanine drinks too much. After first covering for her job shrinkage, they decide to talk to the supervisor. The supervisor consults with the employee assistance counselor at the plant. Together they decide to meet with Jeanine and confront her in a nonjudgmental manner with specific incidents that provide evidence that her job performance is impaired by alcohol. Evidence they provide include dates and times that slurred speech and the smell of alcohol was noticed on her breath, specific data about her shrinking job performance, a record of her Monday morning absences, and comments about her co-workers' concerns. Jeanine is surprised by the feedback, but is able to acknowledge that she has been drinking at lunch time, as well as evenings and weekends because she "gets shaky and nervous." The employee assistance counselor and the supervisor offer Jeanine the option of going into treatment (the employee assistance counselor has a specific program for the referral) rather than losing her job. Jeanine decides to go into treatment. The counselor helps her make the telephone call to the treatment agency.

Once in treatment, interventions occur in a social milieu setting. Being in a group with other recovering persons strengthens the treatment program by providing support and feedback from others with similar problems. The client feels less alone and is provided with honest feedback from peers. Nurses working in treatment settings often conduct various groups as part of the treatment program. These groups include educational sessions, such as learning about the addiction process. In addition, there may be groups on special topics such as sexuality, interpersonal relations, and relapse prevention.

▼ THE TWELVE STEPS OF ALCOHOLICS ANONYMOUS

1. We admitted we were powerless over alcohol—that our lives had become unmanageable.
2. Came to believe that a Power greater than ourselves could restore us to sanity.
3. Made a decision to turn our will and our lives to the care of God as we understood Him.
4. Made a searching and fearless moral inventory of ourselves.
5. Admitted to God, to ourselves, and to another human being the exact nature of our wrongs.
6. Were entirely ready to have God remove all these defects of character.
7. Humbly asked Him to remove our shortcomings.
8. Made a list of the persons we had harmed, and became willing to make amends to them all.
9. Made direct amends to such people whenever possible, except when to do so would injure them or others.
10. Continued to take a personal inventory and when we were wrong, promptly admitted it.
11. Sought through prayer and meditation to improve our conscious contact with God as we understand Him, praying only for knowledge of His will for us and the power to carry that out.
12. Having had a spiritual experience as a result of these steps, we tried to carry this message to alcoholics, and to practice these principles in all our affairs.

DISULFIRAM

(dye-sul'fi-ram)
Antabuse, Cronetal, Ro-Sulfiram
Func class: Alcohol
deterrent
Chem class: Aldehyde
dehydrogenase inhibitor

Action: Blocks oxidation of alcohol at acetaldehyde stage; accumulation of acetaldehyde produces the disulfiram-alcohol reaction
Uses: Chronic alcoholism (as adjunct)
Dosage and routes:
▸ *Adult:* PO 250-500 mg qd × 1-2 wk, then 125-500 mg qd until fully socially recovered
Available forms include: Tabs 250, 500 mg
Side effects/adverse reactions:
CNS: Headache, drowsiness, restlessness, dizziness, fatigue, tremors, psychosis, neuritis, sweating, **convulsions, death,** peripheral neuropathy

Italic indicates common side effects.
Bold italic indicates life-threatening reactions.

GI: Nausea, vomiting, anorexia, severe thirst, ***hepatotoxicity,*** metallic, garliclike aftertaste
INTEG: Rash, dermatitis, urticaria
RESP: **Respiratory depression,** hyperventilation
CV: Tachycardia, chest pain, hypotension, ***dysrhythmias***
Disulfiram: Alcohol reaction: flushing, throbbing, headache, respiratory difficulty, nausea, vomiting, sweating, thirst, chest pain, palpitations, dyspnea, hyperventilation, tachycardia, confusion, CV collapse, MI, CHF, convulsions, death
Contraindications: Hypersensitivity, alcohol intoxication, psychoses, CV disease, pregnancy (X)
Precautions: Hypothyroidism, hepatic disease, diabetes mellitus, seizure disorders, nephritis
Pharmacokinetics:
PO: Onset 12 hr, oxidized by liver, excreted unchanged in feces
Interactions/incompatibilities:
—Increased effects of: tricyclic antidepressants, diazepam, oral anticoagulants, paraldehyde, phenytoin, chloriazepoxide, isoniazid, caffeine

—Disulfiram reaction: alcohol
—Psychosis: metronidazole

NURSING CONSIDERATIONS
Assess:
—Liver function studies q2 wk during therapy: AST, ALT
—CBC, SMA q3-6 mo to detect any abnormality including increased cholesterol
Administer:
—Only with patient's knowledge; do not give to intoxicated individuals
—Vitamin B₆ to decrease cholesterol levels, which often increase with this drug
—Once per day in the AM or hs if drowsiness occurs
—Only after patient has not been drinking for >12 hr
Evaluate:
—Mental status: affect, mood, drug history, ability to follow treatment, abstain from alcohol
—For signs of hepatotoxicity: jaundice, dark urine, clay-colored stools, abdominal pain

Teach client/family:
—Effect of this drug if alcohol is taken; written consent for disulfiram therapy should be obtained
—That shaving lotions, creams, lotin, cough preparations, skin products must be checked for alcohol content; even in small amount, alcohol can produce a reaction
—That tolerance will not develop if treatment is prolonged
—That reaction may occur for 2 wk after last dose
—That tablets can be crushed, mixed with beverage
—To carry ID listing disulfiram therapy
—To avoid driving or hazardous tasks if drowsiness occurs
—That disulfiram reaction can be fatal, occurs 15 min after drinking
Lab test interferences:
Increase: Cholesterol
Decrease: ¹³¹I uptake, PBI, VMA
Treatment of overdose: IV vitamin C, ephedrine sulfate, antihistamines, O₂

Modified from Skidmore-Roth L: *Mosby's nursing drug reference,* St Louis, 1993, Mosby–Year Book.

As part of the rehabilitation, most alcoholic clients are referred to Alcoholics Anonymous (AA), a well known self-help organization based on the idea that people can help each other in the recovery process. It is the largest self-help group in existence and is considered so vital in recovery that most treatment programs refer clients to it while they are still in the treatment program. Run by recovering volunteers, AA provides a 12-step program that emphasizes a structured, progression toward recovery. The steps start with personal recognition of alcoholism, acknowledgment of loss of control over one's life to the group, progress to a commitment to sobriety, and restitution to others for past harm due to alcoholism. See the accompanying box for the 12 steps of AA. Other self-help groups include Al-Anon for spouse, adult relatives, and friends of alcoholics and Alateen (for Children of Alcoholics). Local telephone directories list these groups.

Spiritual dimension The client may experience overwhelming feelings of guilt about the loss of control inherent in being addicted. The feeling that addiction is immoral is still commonly held by society, as well as by the individual who is addicted. In addition, the client becomes aware of the hurt and harm that was done as a consequence of the addiction. Spirituality addresses both the loss of control and the harm that may have been done to others as a result of the addiction. Part of therapy is for the client to accept responsibility for past transgressions and harm done to others through careless behaviors while under the influence of alcohol.

In the AA 12-step program, spirituality is emphasized. The need for a higher being addresses the loss of control experienced by the addicted person. Sometimes the reference to a higher being creates problems for clients who are atheists. However, spirituality can be interpreted in a nonreligious way (that is, there are life forces higher than we are), and AA is not a religious organization. The issue about harm done to others is addressed in the 12 steps of AA. See the box on p. 372 for key interventions for alcohol abuse.

Evaluation

In working with clients with alcoholism, the nurse needs to be flexible in evaluating the success of the nursing care plan. The nursing care is part of an overall interdisciplinary treatment program in which the client is a partner. Much depends on where the client is in terms of working through denial and being motivated for recovery. Rehabilitation and maintaining an alcohol-free life-style is difficult and typically consists of multiple relapses. It is easy to feel critical of clients when they relapse, but the nurse need only think about how difficult it would be to forever give up a favorite

▼ **KEY INTERVENTIONS FOR ALCOHOL ABUSE**

Monitor alcohol withdrawal
Administer medications to minimize withdrawal symptoms
Provide support, comfort, and encouragement
Provide safety measures in severe withdrawal
Promote holistic health (nutrition, exercise, sleep)
Promote the concept of recovery as a lifetime commitment

Recognize own feelings about addictive behavior
Allow expression of client's feelings
Set limits on verbal (or physical) abuse
Facilitate grieving of the "lost substance"
Assist family members to express feelings

Help client to recognize own addiction
Use confrontation and give feedback in a caring manner
Provide education about addiction and recovery
Promote attendance at educational groups and programs
Teach client how to deal with craving

Use structured intervention (social pressure) to work through denial
    about addictive behavior
Promote peer interaction and feedback
Encourage attending Alcoholics Anonymous
Encourage attending Alateen, Adult Children of Alcoholics, and Al-Anon
    by family members

Recognize that client may feel overwhelming guilt about addiction
Help client recognize own responsibility for hurt and damage caused
    by addictive behavior
Use chaplain if client desires

food such as desserts, ice cream or cookies, or coffee or pop, while these are available and promoted in virtually every social setting. Giving these up is very difficult. Giving up alcohol is even more difficult because some of the reasons for addiction are physiological. The craving for alcohol often remains even in those clients who stay "dry" for years.

Adequacy of the care depends on how reasonable the goals are and whether the client is able to work through some of the denial associated with alcoholism. Appropriateness of the interventions is evaluated through feedback and discussion with the interdisciplinary team. Nursing interventions should be coordinated with those of the primary physician, the social worker, and other therapists or counselors.

Effectiveness of care is evaluated through observing changes in the client's behaviors. Is the client beginning to acknowledge realistically the extent of his addiction? Is the client becoming educated on the disease process of alcoholism by participating in the structured program? Is the client adjusting to the treatment program and relating effectively with other clients and staff? Can the client identify ways to deal with relapse, family issues, the work setting?

Treatment outcomes include measures such as length of time before relapse, relapse rates, social readjustment, and job reentry. It is not yet clear what kind of treatment program (inpatient, outpatient, length of program, type of therapeutic interventions) works best for each particular type of client.

NURSING PROCESS: DRUG ADDICTION

Assessment

Physical dimension Assessment for drug use may be even more complex than assessment for alcohol use for several reasons. First, because drugs are illegal, persons using them may try to hide or greatly minimize use. Second, drug use results in a wide variety of effects because of the many types of illicit drugs that are available. Effects of drug use include effects of the drugs themselves, effects of overdose, and signs and symptoms of withdrawal. To complicate things even further, polydrug use leads to mixed signs and symptoms. Table 18-3 provides an overview of information about commonly abused substances, their uses, and effects.

Assessment in the physical dimension addresses three main areas: (1) patterns of use, (2) signs and symptoms of withdrawal, and (3) signs of medical complications. Effects of overdose is typically assessed in the Emergency Department.

Assessment of patterns of use begins with a series of questions concerning specific drugs, starting with those considered more acceptable, such as marijuana and cocaine, and moving on to those considered to be hard drugs, such as heroin. Assessment of drug use includes quantity, frequency, and situations in which drug use takes place. Assessment includes drug of choice or substance primarily used, possible interactions of polysubstance use, past drug history and experience with withdrawal, and time last dose of drug was taken before assessment interview.

Assessment of signs and symptoms of withdrawal requires knowledge of withdrawal syndromes of the drugs typically abused. Withdrawal syndromes vary with the *half-life* of the substance being used. For example, heroin and morphine withdrawal signs start in 10 to 12 hours; amphetamines, 4 to 6 hours. Generally speaking, withdrawal symptoms tend to be opposite from the drug's effects. Withdrawal from a stimulant, for example, will result in depression and lethargy; withdrawal from a narcotic will result in irritability. However, withdrawal from any class of drug tends to result in anxiety and prolonged anhedonia, an uncomfortable state of extreme pleasurelessness and depression. Severity of withdrawal relates to length of use, degree of tolerance established, and individual patterns of use. Table 18-3, lists specific withdrawal syndromes for each major drug classification.

Assessment of medical complications of drug abuse may help identify a drug user. Drug abuse may present with physical signs such as track marks and other evidence of intravenous drug use. The client may present with some medical complication of drug abuse. The accompanying box lists common complications. Runny nose or engorged nasal mucosa, chronic cough, and dilated pupils are other physical signs. Screening for specific drugs can be conducted with urine toxicology tests; however, false positive results may occur with certain foods (e.g., poppy seeds) and medications (e.g., decongestants). Some drugs may be detectable for only a short time (as little as 12 hours: cocaine, LSD); others are not detectable in urine (inhalants). Drug screening is also used to monitor recovery. See Table 18-4 for drug detection periods.

Emotional dimension As with the alcohol-addicted client the drug-addicted client experiences anxiety,

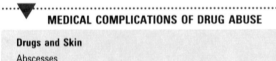

MEDICAL COMPLICATIONS OF DRUG ABUSE

Drugs and Skin
Abscesses
Cellulitis
Thrombophlebitis

Drugs and the Heart
Endocarditis

Drugs and the Lungs
Pneumonia
Abscess
Tuberculosis
Adult respiratory distress syndrome

Drugs and the Liver
Hepatitis

Drugs and the Brain
Meningitis
Abscesses

Drugs and the Fetus
Addicted infant, drug withdrawal
Developmental problems

Miscellaneous
Acquired immunodeficiency syndrome (AIDS) from needle sharing and unsafe sex
Nasal deterioration from cocaine sniffing

anger, guilt, and despair. These emotions are painful and often result in defensive behaviors, such as rationalization, projection, and denial, which makes it difficult for others to comprehend the emotional pain experienced by the addicted person.

Emotional maturity is another area to assess. Due to prolonged drug use, clients may lack maturity and show inability to accept responsibility.

Intellectual dimension Just as is true in alcohol addiction, defense mechanisms of denial and rationalization can be observed in the drug addicted client. Manipulative behavior, especially in relation to drug seeking, is often observed in treatment settings. For example, the drug-addicted client may have family members or friends sneak in drugs during hospitalization.

Prolonged drug use often disturbs intellectual functioning. Memory impairment can result in prolonged cocaine use. Paranoid thinking can result from prolonged cocaine, amphetamine, and barbiturate use.

Social dimension As was discussed under behavioral theory, drugs have an ability to reinforce the behaviors that lead a person to continue taking drugs. Part of the reinforcement system is the social context in which drug addiction takes place. Often the addict's main social contacts are other drug users. Family ties may not be as strong as they once were. If the addict remains in the drug culture where pleasant experiences associated with drug taking occurred it will be extremely difficult, if not impossible, for that person to stay off drugs. Therefore assessing the client's social system is important.

Spiritual dimension Experiencing powerlessness and loss of control over drug use leads to loss of hope and spiritual well-being. In addition, the client may have been involved in illegal activities around drug procurement. The client may have been forced into treatment by the judicial system. These factors contribute to feelings of low self-worth and dehumanization.

Analysis
Nursing diagnosis

Nursing diagnoses that apply to clients with drug abuse or dependence are found in the discussion of alcohol abuse.

The following case example demonstrates the characteristics of a client with a nursing diagnosis of defensive coping who abuses drugs. (See the box on p. 366 for defining characteristics of defensive coping.)

▼ Case Example

Sandra is a single 25-year-old woman admitted to a drug rehabilitation program for chronic polydrug abuse (prescription drugs, cocaine, heroin). Over the past 3 years she has been involved in prostitution to support her drug habit. Before admission she was incarcerated for 2 months and detoxified. Admission to the rehabilitation program was part of a diversion arrangement with the court system. Sandra told the court that she is "sick of being on the streets and on drugs" and "wants to make changes" in her life. Once admitted to the program, Sandra seems anxious about being there. She tends to avoid others, stating she doesn't need to participate in group sessions because she already knows what her problems are. Her low self-esteem and defensive coping are reflected in her lack of follow-through.

Planning

See Table 18-5 for a nursing care plan with some long- and short-term goals, outcome criteria, interventions, and rationales related to defensive coping.

Implementation

Physical dimension Withdrawal from drugs varies according to the nature of the drugs the client was taking. It is not uncommon for clients to abuse several classes of drugs at the same time. The general principle in facilitating withdrawal is that the client is given sufficient quantities of whatever prescribed medications are necessary to suppress severe withdrawal symptoms, and the doses of these medications are then gradually reduced.[17] The purpose of pharmacotherapy is also to control or relieve the severe anhedonia that persons experience during drug withdrawal. Anhedonia, in conjunction with physical discomfort, tends to make the client inaccessible to therapeutic interventions.[34] Prescribed medications are not a substitute for the abused substance; rather, they are a treatment for physiologically induced withdrawal effects.

The nurse's role is to administer medications that facilitate withdrawal and to monitor the client's responses. Withdrawal from opiates (heroin, morphine, meperidine) can be achieved with methadone, a substitute for these agents. Methadone doses are gradually reduced over about a 10-day period. Some clients may be enrolled in metha-

Text continued on p. 378.

▼ **TABLE 18-3** **Controlled Substances: Uses and Effects**

Drugs	Trade or Other Names	Medical Uses	Physical Dependence	Psychological Dependence
NARCOTICS				
Opium	Dover's Powder, Pantopan, Paregoric, Parepectolin, Deodorized Tincture of Opium	Analgesic, antidiarrheal	High	High
Morphine	Morphine, MS Coutin, Pectoral Syrup	Analgesic, antitussive		
Codeine	Codeine, Empirin w/Codeine, Robitussin A-C, Tylenol w/Codeine, many cough syrups	Analgesic, antitussive	Moderate	Moderate
Heroin	Diacetylmorphine, Horse, Smack	Under investigation	High	High
Hydromorphone	Dilaudid	Analgesic		
Meperidine (Pethidine)	Demerol, Pethadol	Analgesic		
Methadone	Dolophine, Methadone, Methadose	Analgesic, heroin substitute		
Other Narcotics	Darvon, Fentanyl, LAAM, Levo-Dromoran, Lomotil, Numorphan, Percocet, Percodan, Talwin, Tussionex	Analgesic, antidiarrheal, antitussive	High-Low	High-Low
DEPRESSANTS				
Choral Hydrate	Noctec	Hypnotic	Moderate	Moderate
Barbiturates	Alurate, Amobarbital, Butisol, Florinal, Gemonil, Lotusate, Mebaral, Nembutal, Phenobarbital, Phenoxbarbital, Secobarbital, Tuinal	Anesthetic, anticonvulsant, sedative, hypnotic	High-Moderate	High-Moderate
Glutethimide	Doriden	Sedative, hypnotic	High	High
Benzodiazepines	Ativan, Azene, Centrax, Clonopin, Dalmane, Diazepam, Halcion, Librium, Paxipam, Restoril, Serax, Tranxene, Valium, Versed, Verstran, Xanax	Anti-anxiety, anticonvulsant, sedative, hypnotic	Low	Low variable
Other Depressants	Equanil, Miltown, Noludar Placidyl, Paral, Valmid	Antianxiety, sedative, hypnotic	Moderate	Moderate
STIMULANTS				
Cocaine	Coke, Flake, Snow	Local anesthetic	Possible	High
Amphetamines	Biphetamine, Delcobese, Desoxyn, Dexedrine, Mediatric	Hyperkinesis, narcolepsy, weight control		
Phenmetrazine	Preludin			
Methylphenidate	Ritalin			
Other Stimulants	Adipex, Bacarate, Cylert, Didrex, Ionamin, Plegine, Pre-Sate, Sanorex, Tenuate, Tepanil, Voranil			
HALLUCINOGENS				
LSD	Acid, Microdot	None	None	Degree unknown
Mescaline and Peyote	Mesc. Buttons, Cactus	None	None	Degree unknown
Amphetamine Variants	2,5-DMA, PMA, STP, MDA, MMDA, TMA, DOM, DOB		Unknown	Degree unknown
Phencyclidine	PCP, Angel Dust, Hog	Veterinary anesthetic	Degree unknown	High
Phencyclidine Analogs	PCE, PCPy, TCP	None	Degree unknown	Degree unknown
Other Hallucinogens	Bufotenine, Ibogaine, DMT, DET, Psilocybin, Psilocyn	None	None	Degree unknown

National Institute of Drug Abuse.

Tolerance	Duration of Effects (in hours)	Usual Methods of Administration	Possible Effects	Effects of Overdose	Withdrawal Syndrome
Yes	3-6	Oral, smoked	Euphoria, drowsiness, respiratory depression, constricted pupils, nausea	Slow and shallow breathing, clammy skin, convulsions, coma, possible death	Watery eyes, runny nose, yawning, loss of appetite, irritability, tremors, panic, chills and sweating, cramps, nausea
		Oral, injected, smoked			
		Oral, injected			
		Injected, sniffed, smoked			
	12-24	Oral, injected			
	Variable				
Possible	5-8	Oral	Slurred speech, disorientation, drunken behavior without odor of alcohol	Shallow respiration, cold and clammy skin, dilated pupils, weak and rapid pulse, coma, possible death	Anxiety, insomnia, tremors, delirium, convulsions, possible death
Yes	1-16	Oral, injected			
	4-8				
Possible	1-2	Sniffed, injected, smoked	Increased alertness, excitation, euphoria, increased pulse rate and blood pressure, insomnia, loss of appetite	Agitation, increase in body temperature, hallucinations, convulsions, possible death	Apathy, long periods of sleep, irritability, depression, disorientation
Yes	2-4	Oral, injected, smoked			
		Oral			
Yes	8-12	Oral	Illustrations and hallucinations, poor perception of time and distance	Longer, more intense "trip" episodes, psychosis, possible death	Withdrawal syndrome not reported
		Oral, injected			
	Up to days				
	Variable	Smoked, oral, injected			
Possible		Oral, injected, smoked, sniffed			

Continued.

▼ **TABLE 18-3   Controlled Substances: Uses and Effects—cont'd**

Drugs	Trade or Other Names	Medical Uses	Physical Dependence	Pyscological Dependence
CANNABIS				
Marijuana	Pot, Acapulco Gold, Grass, Reefer, Sinsemilla, Thai Sticks	Under investigation		
Tetrahydrocan-nabinol	Cesamet, Marinol, THC	Control nausea and vomiting for cancer chemotherapy	Degree unknown	Moderate
Hashish	Hash	None		
Hashish Oil	Hash Oil			

▼ **TABLE 18-4   Drug Detection Periods**

Drug	Category	Detection Period*
AMPHETAMINES	Stimulants	
Amphetamine		2-4 days
Methamphetamine		2-4 days
BARBITURATES	Sedative hypnotics	
Amobarbital		2-4 days
Butalbital		2-4 days
Pentobarbital		2-4 days
Phenobarbital		Up to 30 days
Secobarbital		2-4 days
BENZODIAZEPINES	Sedative hypnotics	
Diazepam (Valium)		Up to 30 days
Chlordiazepoxide (Librium)		Up to 30 days
COCAINE	Stimulants	
Benzoylecgonine		12-72 hours
CANNABINOIDS (MARIJUANA)	Euphoriants	
Casual use		2-7 days
Chronic use		Up to 30 days
ETHANOL	Sedative hypnotics	Very short†
METHADONE	Narcotic analgesics	2-4 days
METHAQUALONE (QUAALUDE)	Sedative hypnotics	2-4 days
OPIATES	Narcotic analgesics	
Codeine		2-4 days
Hydromorphone (Dilaudid)		2-4 days
Morphine (for Heroin)		2-4 days
PHENCYCLIDINE (PCP)	Hallucinogens	
Casual use		2-7 days
Chronic use		Up to 30 days

*Detection periods vary; rates of metabolism and excretion are different for each drug and user. Detection periods should be viewed as estimates. Cases can always be found to contradict these approximations.

†Detection period depends on amount consumed. Alcohol is excreted at the rate of approximately 1 oz/hr.

Tolerance	Duration of Effects (in hours)	Usual Methods of Administration	Possible Effects	Effects of Overdose	Withdrawal Syndrome
Yes	2-4	Smoked, oral	Euphoria, relaxed inhibitions, increased appetite, disoriented behavior	Fatigue, paranoia, possible psychosis	Insomnia, hyperactivity, and decreased appetite occasionally reported

▼ **TABLE 18-5   NURSING CARE PLAN**

GOALS	OUTCOME CRITERIA	INTERVENTIONS	RATIONALES
NURSING DIAGNOSIS: Defensive coping, related to failure to participate in treatment program.			
LONG TERM To demonstrate commitment to recovery and rehabilitation	Keeps appointments	Establish trust and rapport	Client needs to feel accepted and respected
	Verbalizes a sense of purpose and hope in daily living activities	Assist client to talk about resistance to participate Assist client to relate to other clients in unit	Verbalizing resistance will help client make better choices Meeting others with similar problems fosters help
	Makes appropriate future plans	Provide feedback to client about effect of substance abuse on health and relationships	Feedback is necessary to help client work through denial about the scope of problem
SHORT TERM To verbally indicate that treatment is important for recovery from addiction	Acknowledges loss of control over substance use	Encourage client to acknowledge loss of control over substance use	Acknowledging loss of control over substance use is necessary before treatment
To participate in planned treatment program	Understands various components of the treatment program	Explore with client various components offered by the treatment program	Understanding the treatment program helps client make informed choices
	Feels safe and supported within first 3 days	Orient client to treatment unit, schedules, etc	Orientation to the setting fosters a sense of belonging
	Accepts feedback from staff and other clients	Provide feedback in a support environment	Confrontation and feedback is more effective in an atmosphere of support
	Demonstrates increased self-esteem and confidence	Convey respect Allow the client to make choices about care Acknowledge client's difficulties and successes as these occur	Respect and an atmosphere where choices are allowed raise self-esteem and confidence Providing feedback about difficulties and success of client provides support and conveys respect

done maintenance program as ongoing treatment. Methadone inhibits craving for illicit narcotics in carefully selected clients who are unable to maintain a drug-free lifestyle. Withdrawal from barbiturates, benzodiazepines, and related drugs is carefully managed because seizures and fatal reactions can occur if withdrawal is abrupt. Withdrawal is managed by tapering benzodiazepine use gradually or administering a general depressant such as phenobarbital, gradually reducing the dose over a period of 10 days to 3 weeks. Careful observation is necessary. If insomnia, tremulousness, irritability, and orthostatic hypotension occur, further withdrawal is suspended until these symptoms disappear. Monitoring drug metabolite levels is advisable in cases of severe, longstanding addiction.

During the rehabilitation stage, the nurse facilitates an approach to physical health that encourages the client to exercise, eat nutritious foods, and develop regular sleeping patterns. A comprehensive treatment unit has the facilities and programs to facilitate a general healthy life-style.

Emotional dimension It is not uncommon for clients who are addicted to drugs to seem emotionally immature and manipulative. Although not all drug-addicted clients are alike, many appear demanding and in need of immediate gratification. Much of this behavior may be driven by drug craving. The client was accustomed to the good feelings of being under drug influence. The intensive desire to have the drug can lead to sneaking drugs into the treatment unit. Wanting immediate gratification to requests can lead to staff splitting. For example, a client may ask one nurse for a privilege, such as preparing a snack in the kitchen. The nurse says, "No, you cannot do this now because you are supposed to be in your group meeting." The client then finds another nurse who is new on the unit and tearfully repeats the request. The new nurse does not realize that the client is supposed to be in a treatment meeting and goes with the client to the kitchen. The client thanks the new nurse for "being so nice when some other nurses are so mean." Such behaviors give rise to divisive feelings among staff, sometimes pitting one staff group against another. It is best for nurses and other health care providers to work closely together in setting firm limits on manipulative behavior (see Chapter 23).

Drug-addicted clients often have difficulty identifying their own emotions and may express them through somatic concerns. They may focus on bodily functions and complain of headaches, backaches, and the like. Once physical disturbances have been ruled out, it is best to minimize vague somatic complaints and refocus on the goals of the treatment program. Holding clients responsible for their behaviors, rather than focusing on vague symptoms and undefined feelings, is a better overall strategy of intervention.

Intellectual dimension Drug-addicted clients have defenses similar to clients with alcoholism: denial and rationalization. Being confronted with their addiction and the effects of addiction on their own and others' lives is a painful experience. It has often been found to be more effective if recovering drug addicts are part of the treatment team. They "have been there" and can speak frankly to another addict about addiction.

The drug-addicted client also participates in structured educational sessions to learn about drug addiction. Educational sessions address the disease model of addiction,

---

▼ **KEY INTERVENTIONS FOR DRUG ABUSE AND ADDICTION**

Monitor client's response to withdrawal
Recognize that withdrawal symptoms vary according to substance(s) used
Acknowledge difficulty client will have with feelings of anhedonia
Promote physical health (exercise, nutrition, sleep)
Set limits on drug-seeking behavior
Work closely with other staff to minimize manipulative behaviors
Minimize vague somatic complaints
Hold client responsible for behavior
Use recovering addicts to help confront client with addiction
Provide education about drug addiction, craving, and relapse
Help client recognize social reinforcers that help maintain addictive behavior
Promote supportive relationships with other recovering addicts
Recognize own feelings in relation to working with addicted clients
Help client acknowledge loss of control over behavior
Help client acknowledge responsibility for hurt and damage caused to others through addictive behavior

---

craving and relapse, grieving the lost chemical, and other aspects of rehabilitation.

Social dimension In addition to learning about addiction, clients are also taught about primary and secondary reinforcers (see section on Behavioral Theory). Clients must restructure their social lives so that they do not return to the life-style associated with taking drugs. This process is difficult for many clients. Recovering drug addicts are often helpful to each other in providing confrontation, support, and resources. The nurse needs to be supportive as well. Especially important is not to become overwhelmed by the client's problems and the potential for relapse. The nurse provides professional care within the context of a comprehensive team approach and uses the team to process the nurse's own feelings in relation to giving care to addicted clients. See the accompanying boxes for key interventions for drug abuse and addiction and for guidelines for primary and tertiary prevention.

Spiritual dimension The drug-addicted client experiences a sense of fear and failure. The client's life may be in shambles, and he may have lied, cheated, or stolen to support his drug habit. As the client recovers and becomes aware of the hurt and harm done to others as a result of addiction, the guilt and shame can be overwhelming. Similar to AA, the Narcotics Anonymous (NA) 12-step program approaches recovery as a spiritual process, and reliance on a higher power is emphasized. The issue about harm done to others is addressed in a concrete step-by-step manner. For example, the client makes an inventory of positive and negative personal characteristics. He makes a list of all persons harmed and, when possible, makes amends for harm done. These, as well as other NA steps, foster a sense of integrity and responsibility that are crucial to a wholistic recovery.

It is important for the nurse to support the philosophy of a 12-step program. The nurse should encourage the client to participate in and follow through with NA activities.

▼

Evaluation

Evaluation has been discussed under the section in nursing process for the client with alcoholism. The same points apply for the care plan for drug-addicted clients. The nurse needs to be flexible about the progress of these clients, realizing that addiction, although a common problem, is difficult to treat. It is important to understand that relapses are part of the recovery process. Relapses are common in many illnesses; for example, diabetes, arthritis, multiple sclerosis, mental illnesses. There are also many variations in how clients recover. There may be times when the client is drug free, or the client may return to a life-style where drug behavior is modified. Some clients "burn out" on drugs as they get older. Other clients go back to the same addictive behaviors.

It is helpful to recognize the limitations to what a health care professional can do for any client. The nurse cannot force a client to be drug free anymore than the nurse can enforce a low cholesterol diet for someone with heart disease or a calorie reduction diet for an obese person. It is the nurse's responsibility to educate clients about alcohol and drugs and to give nursing care to addicted clients according to standards of excellence. Although the nurse is responsible for giving safe and effective care, the ultimate responsibility for changing addictive behavior and the accompanying life-style lies with the client.

PROFESSIONAL ISSUES

The Impaired Nurse

Professional organizations and societies have begun to develop policies, procedures, and programs for helping nurses deal with addictive behavior. The American Nurses' Association passed a formal resolution declaring that the profession needs to address misuse of alcohol and other drugs and emotional and psychological dysfunction in its own members.[1] This resolution calls for ongoing collection and dissemination of infomation, including educational and research activities related to the impaired nurse.

The idea that nurses can become addicted seems somehow unthinkable to many. Nevertheless, nurses are as vulnerable as everyone else to substance abuse. Being a professional does not necessarily protect someone from becoming addicted. In fact, health care professionals may be at increased risk because of work stress and drug availability. The policies and procedures developed through the ANA and implemented at the state level through peer assistance networks have been helpful in facilitating identification and treatment for addicted colleagues. Many states have instituted collaborative relationships between the state licensing department and the state nurses' association to protect the impaired nurse's license while she is in recovery. The nurse needs to be familiar with the policies and procedures for the impaired nurse in her own state. Addressing the problem of professional impairment is a positive step for the profession.

Addiction Nursing Specialty

Addiction nursing is a specialty with nursing organizations of its own. The American Nurses' Association in conjunction with the National Nurses Society on Addictions and the Drug and Alcohol Nursing Association have developed standards of practice.[1] Certification is also available. Some schools of nursing have developed addiction nursing specialties in their graduate programs.[26]

Nursing Education

In 1989 and in 1990, the National Institute of Alcoholism and Alcohol Abuse (NIAAA) and the National Institute of Drug Abuse (NIDA) funded 10 schools of nursing across the nation to develop faculty and curriculum in substance abuse. The focus of these 3-year programs is to prepare faculty in various practice areas so that the teaching of substance abuse nursing can be improved. Substance abuse content and clinical skills are integrated throughout undergraduate and graduate nursing curricula so that every practicing nurse is able to screen, assess, and provide intervention and referral for clients with substance abuse problems. These funded programs are part of a national effort to improve substance abuse education for all health care professionals, including nurses, physicians, social workers, and psychologists. It is encouraging to document nursing's progress in this vital area of health care.

BRIEF REVIEW

Addictive behavior is viewed as a biopsychosocial problem in which genetics, neurochemistry, pharmacology, behavior, and social environment interact to produce the disease of addiction. The main features of addiction include loss of control over, and preoccupation with, substance use.

Denial leads to continued use despite persistent social, psychological, or physical problems.

Because addictive behavior is a complex phenomenon, no single theory can fully explain the problem. Theoretical perspectives address various aspects of addictive behavior. Psychoanalytical theory explains addictive behavior as resulting from extreme dependency needs leading to a compulsion for the substance. Although no certain type of personality profile typifies someone with addictive behavior, personality traits of low self-esteem, tendency to break rules, or frequent depressed mood add to the risk for substance abuse. Behavioral theory explains addiction in terms of reinforcers. Once a person is addicted, reinforcers such as pleasant effects and associations will increase the likelihood that addictive behavior will recur.

Sociocultural theory considers factors such as prevalence, economics, substance availability, and cultural attitudes. These factors explain variability of addiction in different cultures and age groups. Populations of special concern are the elderly, adolescents, and pregnant women. Family theory provides a framework for understanding how addiction affects the structure, roles, and functions of the family. Codependency leads to enabling behaviors in families of a dysfunctionally addicted person. Biological and genetic research provide evidence of physiological factors contributing to addiction.

The nursing process for both alcohol and drug addiction includes assessment of patterns of use, physical indications of use, negative consequences, and risk factors. Because denial is a crucial factor in addiction, social pressure is often applied in a structured intervention to facilitate client entry into treatment. Withdrawal is managed with medications, comfort measures, and monitoring. Recovery includes client and family teaching about addiction, craving, relapse prevention, a healthy life-style, and stress reduction without substance use. The spiritual dimension plays an important role in recovery.

A variety of activities within the nursing profession make important contributions to the field of addiction. Nursing has addressed addiction in its own members by developing policies and procedures through the American Nurses' Association. Addiction nursing is a specialty with its own nursing organizations and certification examinations. Nursing education programs across the nation are making special efforts to integrate substance abuse education as part of every basic nursing curriculum.

REFERENCES AND SUGGESTED READINGS

1. American Nurses' Association: *Standards of addictions nursing practice with selected diagnoses and criteria,* Kansas City, 1988, The Association.
2. Alpert MA: Modern management of delirium tremens, *Hospital Medicine* 125:111, 1990.
3. Amodeo M: Treating the late life alcoholic: guidelines for working through denial, integrating individual, family and group approaches, *Journal of Geriatric Psychiatry* 23(2):91, 1990.
4. Bennett LA: Family, alcohol, and culture. In Galanter M, editor: *Recent developments in alcoholism: treatment research,* vol 7, New York, 1989, Plenum Press.
5. Caaroselli-Darinja M: Drug abuse and the elderly, *Journal of Psychosocial Nursing and Mental Health Services* 23 (6):25, 1985.
6. Carruth B, Mendenhall W: *Co-dependency: issues in treatment and recovery,* New York, 1989, Haworth Press.
7. Dinwiddie SH, Cloninger CR: Family and adoption studies of alcoholism. In Goedde HW, Agarwal DP, editors: *Alcoholism: biomedical and genetic aspects,* New York, 1989, Pergamon Press.
8. Ellor JK, Kurz DJ: Misuse and abuse of prescription drugs by the elderly, *Nursing Clinics of North America* 17: 319, 1982.
9. Ewing JA: Detecting alcoholism: the CAGE questionnaire, *Journal American Medical Association* 252:1905, 1984.
10. Fell JC: Drinking and driving in America: disturbing facts—encouraging reductions. *Alcohol Health and Research World* 14: 18, 1990.
11. Goedde HW, Agarwal DP: *Alcoholism: biomedical and genetic aspects,* New York, 1989, Pergamon Press.
12. Gomberg ES, Neson BW, Hatchett BF: Women, alcoholism, and family therapy, *Family and Community Health* 13 (4):61, 1991.
13. Goodwin DW: Genetic determinants of alcoholism. In Mendelson JH, Mello NK, editors: *The diagnosis and treatment of alcoholism,* New York, 1985, McGraw-Hill.
14. Grant BF, Harford TC: Concurrent and simultaneous use of alcohol with sedatives and with tranquilizers: results of a national survey, *Journal of Substance Abuse* 2 (1):1, 1990.
15. Heath DB: Environmental factors in alcohol use and its outcomes. In Goedde HW, Agarwar DP, editors: *Alcoholism: Biomedical and genetic aspects.* New York, 1989, Pergamon Press, 312-332.
16. Hughes TL: Models and perspective of addiction: implication for treatment, *Nursing Clinics of North America* 24: 1, 1989.
17. Jaffe JH: Drug addiction and drug abuse. In Goodman LS, Gilman A, editors: *The pharmacological basis of therapeutics,* New York, 1990, Macmillan.
18. Jellinek EM: *The disease concept of alcoholism,* New Haven, 1960, Hillhouse Press.
19. Johnson VE: *Intervention: how to help someone who doesn't want help,* Minneapolis, 1986, Johnson Institute Books.
20. Lex BW: Alcohol problems in special populations. In Mendelson JH, Mello NK, editors: *The diagnosis and treatment of alcoholism,* New York, 1985, McGraw-Hill.
21. Lindenberg CS and others: Review of the literature on cocaine abuse in pregnancy, *Nursing Research* 40 (2):69, 1991.
22. Logan BN: Adolescent substance abuse prevention: an overview of the literature, *Family and Community Health* 13:25, 1991.
23. Marshall EJ, Murray RM: The contribution of twin studies to alcoholism research. In Goedde HW, Agarwar DP, editors: *Alcoholism: biomedical and genetic aspects,* New York, 1989, Pergamon Press.
24. Mayfield J, McLeod G, Hall P: The CAGE questionnaire: validation of a new alcoholism screening instrument, *American Journal of Psychiatry* 131: 1121, 1974.
25. Milby JB: *Addictive behavior and its treatment,* New York, 1981, Springer.
26. Murphy SA: Addiction nursing: an agenda for the 1990's, *Issues in Mental Health Nursing* 9:115, 1988.
27. National Institute on Alcohol Abuse and Alcoholism: Fetal alcohol syndrome, *Alcohol Alert* DHHS PH 297, 1991.
28. National Institute on Drug Abuse: National household survey on drug abuse: Population estimates. DHHS Publication No 1 89-1636, 1989.
29. Schneider JW, Griffith DR, Chasnoff IJ: Infants exposed to cocaine in utero: implications for developmental assessment and intervention, *Infants and Young Children* 2 (1): 25, 1989.
30. Schuckit MA: *Drug and alcohol abuse: a clinical guide to diagnosis and treatment,* New York, 1984, Plenum Press.

31. Silva LY, Liepman MR: Family behavior loop mapping enhances treatment of alcoholism, *Family and Community Health* 13 (4): 72, 1991.
32. Smart RG, Jansen VA: Youth substance abuse. In Annis HM, Davis CS, editors: *Drug use by adolescents: identification, assessment and intervention,* Toronto, 1991, Alcoholism and Drug Addiction Research Foundation.
33. Solomon J: Alcoholism and psychiatric disorders. In Goedde HW, Agarwal DP, editors: *Alcoholism: biomedical and genetic aspects,* New York, 1989, Pergamon Press.
34. Taylor WA, Gold MS: Pharmacologic approaches to the treatment of cocaine dependence, *Western Journal of Medicine* 152: 573, 1990.
35. Tweed SH: Identifying the alcoholic client, *Nursing Clinics of North America* 24: 13, 1989.
36. Wallace J: The new disease model of alcoholism, *Western Journal of Medicine* 152:502, 1990.
37. Wright LM, Leahy M: *Nurses and families: a guide to family assessment and intervention,* Philadelphia, 1984, FA Davis.

ANNOTATED BIBLIOGRAPHY

Estes NF, Heinemann ME, editors: *Alcoholism: development, consequences, and interventions,* St Louis, 1986, Mosby−Year Book.
Edited by two nurses who are leaders in the field of substance abuse, this book provides a broad spectrum of topics related to alcoholism. Timely content on substance abuse in nurses and the elderly is included.

Hughes TL, Gerace LM, editors: *Family and community health: current topics in substance abuse,* Gaithersburg, Md, 1991, Aspen Publishers.
Alcohol and drug abuse are addressed within the broad social and cultural contexts in which it takes place. This special journal issue, edited by two nurses, covers a wide range of current topics. Included are issues related to ethnicity, adolescence, women, the elderly, and the family.

Jack L, editor: *Nursing care planning with the addicted client,* Skokie, Ill, 1990, National Nurses Society on Addictions.
Issued by the NNSA, this manual provides an excellent update on nursing care for addicted clients with complex problems. Material is presented through case studies reflecting various types of addictive behaviors. Included are clients with polysubstance abuse and AIDS, as well as the older alcoholic, a pregnant woman who drinks alcohol, and a homeless schizophrenic.

Kinney J: *Clinical manual of substance abuse,* St Louis, 1991, Mosby−Year Book.
Emphasizing the skills necessary for effective treatment of substance abuse, this manual features a wealth of information on the scope of the problem, screening, assessment, treatment modalities, and roles of the nurse.

Ray O, Ksir C: *Drugs, society and human behavior,* St Louis, 1990, Mosby−Year Book.
This comprehensive, readable book provides information on commonly abused drugs. The social context in which drug use takes place is examined.

CHAPTER
19 Somatization

Sharon K Holmberg

After studying this chapter, the student will be able to:

- Define somatization
- Discuss the historical development of theory related to the interaction of psychological and biological states
- Define and describe the most common psychiatric diagnoses related to somatization as described in the DSM-III-R

- Describe the most common physical conditions in which mood states and responses to stressors may contribute to illness
- Discuss theory related to somatization disorders
- Apply the nursing process in the care of clients with somatization disorders
- Identify current research findings related to somatization

In Western medicine, labeling the cause of a specific disease is complete when the reason for a diseased organ can be attributed to a physiological cause, such as bacterial growth, atherosclerosis, abnormal cells, or some other biological change. Increasingly, however, emphasis is being placed on the role of an individual's life-style—the psychological, social, and environmental factors—on health. In fact, for some persons, a common way to express psychological distress and social anxieties is through physical complaints. This is commonly known as *somatization.* In this chapter, two general categories of somatic disorder will be discussed: (1) those in which there is a known, documented, physiological change that is thought to have resulted, at least partially, from psychosocial and environmental influences; and (2) disorders in which the documentation of biological changes is scant or nonexistent, although symptoms expressed are largely biological and clients are convinced that they are physically ill.

Somatization disorders are health problems that result from influences of both the mind and body. This term expresses the idea that emotional aspects of a person influence the functioning of various body organs and functioning of the body organs may influence emotions. Broadly speaking, somatization is considered a process by which psychological distress becomes physical symptoms. Another term, *psychosomatic,* meaning mind and body, is used to describe emotional symptoms, such as phobias, obsessions, insomnia,[19] and other expressions of physical complaints for which a biological cause may or may not be found. A closely related term, *psychobiological,* suggests that specific psy-

chological conflicts from early life are triggered by later life experiences and produce diseases such as peptic ulcer, rheumatoid arthritis, bronchial asthma, migraine, essential hypertension, ulcerative colitis, and dermatitis. This term evolved from applying psychoanalytical thinking to physical conditions, but these ideas have not been well substantiated so the term is now less commonly used.

The terms *somatization* and *psychosomatic* may sometimes be used interchangeably, although the term psychosomatic has a longer history of use in the health sciences. The use of these terms is further complicated by the application of both terms to some psychiatric diagnoses in which the client experiences physical symptoms but no disturbances of physiology can be found. These psychiatric diagnoses are known as somatoform disorders. For the sake of clarity in this chapter, the term *somatization* will be considered a broad, general term that includes illnesses

---

▶ **DIAGNOSES Related to Somatization**

MEDICAL DIAGNOSES	NURSING DIAGNOSES
Somatiform disorders	**NANDA**
Conversion disorder	Ineffective individual coping
Somatization disorder	
Hypochondriasis	**PMH**
	Ineffective individual coping

HISTORICAL OVERVIEW

DATES	EVENTS
Ancient	Hippocrates describes the unity of the individual in the environment, recognizing how health is affected.
	The Greek philsopher, Aristotle, observed that afflictions of the soul, such as passion, pity, joy, loving, and hating, have corresponding afflictions of the body.
1600s	Descartes reasons that the human is divided conceptually into body and mind, a description of Western, dualistic thought.
1700s	Some writings suggest the interaction of the mind and the body by describing verbal suggestions that can produce physiological changes.
1800s	The term psychosomatic is introduced, referring to emotional symptoms such as phobias, obsessions, and insomnia.
1900s	Freud publishes his first papers describing the psychodynamics of anxiety and conversion hysteria.
1920s	Psychoanalytical formulations are further developed. Somatic symptoms are interpreted as hysterical and viewed as symbolic expressions of unconscious instinctual urges.
1930s	The research of Cannon[9] in physiology leads to the concept of homeostasis.
	Pavlov's research with dogs, which demonstrate stimulus-response feedback mechanisms, is published.[46]
	von Bertalaniffy[85] describes new approaches to biological research, which are later developed into general systems theory.
1940s	Constructs are developed by Wolff and Wolff[88] and Dunbar[20] that attempt to link a specific personality pattern or conflict situation to specific diseases such as migraine, diarrhea, or ulcerative colitis. Specificity theory, developed by Alexander, French, and Pollock,[2] suggests that every emotion has a somatic concomitant; certain kinds of conflicts have affinities for certain organ systems.
1950s	Psychosomatic research includes the cause of duodenal ulcer, the relationship of separation and depression to illness, and the psychological stress of surgical patients.
	Selye[73] publishes a seminal work defining stress as the nonspecific response of the body to any demand made on it. This response leads to increased damage in the organism, predisposing the individual to disease.
	Friedman and Rosenman[28] identify a cluster of behavior traits (type A personality) that is correlated with coronary atherosclerosis.
1960s	Sources of environmental stress are identified and described, including noise, job stress, environmental hazards, and sensory deprivation.
	Holmes and Rahe[41] develop a stress scale in an effort to standardize the extent of stress experienced by a person and relate it to the disease process.
	Lazarus[48] publishes the first phases of research emphasizing cognitive processes and adaptive mechanisms in stress. The role of major life changes and disruption in social networks is related to increased episodes of physical illness.
	Type A and B behaviors are further related to the predisposition to coronary heart disease.
1970s	Newly discovered hypothalamic factors and hormones demonstrate the connection between the brain and neuroendocrine axis.
	Complex models of stress and illness are proposed and tested. These examine stimulus characteristics, response characteristics, and attempt to describe a "lack of fit" between person and environment.
	Psychiatric nursing programs that integrate biological and psychological studies in the curriculum are developed.
	Roy[70] and Rogers[68] propose theories of nursing based on an integrated, holistic concept of humans.

Continued.

DATES	EVENTS
1980s	Links between anxiety and the immunological system are established in animal research. The discovery of hormones secreted by the brain, such as endorphins, open new avenues for research and demonstrates the complexity of biochemistry associated with behavior.
	Psychiatric–medical units are developed in general hospitals that recognize the need for a holistic nursing approach.
1990s	Stressful life events, such as test anxiety during final examinations, are found to suppress the immune functioning in people. This research establishes the link between psychological stress and illness.
Future	With emphasis on the biological bases of illness, nurses will be more active in managing psychophysiological disorders in direct and indirect roles.

with and without biological changes. The term *psychosomatic* will apply to conditions in which there are documented biological changes, and the term *somatoform* disorders will be used to refer to conditions in which biological change had not been documented.

Understanding how the body and the mind function together in health and illness is a relatively new and rapidly expanding field. The idea that it is impossible for the mind to suffer without the body becoming sick[5] is at least two centuries old. However, the complex, synergistic action of biological, psychological, social, and environmental factors is just beginning to be understood (see historical overview). Basic research, especially in neuroendocrinology, immunology, and neurobiology, and the study of psychological adaptation processes have developed an expanding scientific base for analysis and treatment of somatization disorders.

Psychosocial stressors can affect most body systems or the whole person. Psychological factors are believed to have significant influence on the following systems and physical conditions: the gastrointestinal tract (peptic ulcer, nausea and vomiting, ulcerative colitis, irritable bowel syndrome), the cardiovascular system (hypertension, dysrhythmia, tachycardia, angina pectoris), musculoskeletal system (tension headaches, rheumatoid arthritis), genitourinary tract (painful menstruation, urinary frequency, impotence), and the respiratory system (asthma). Other illnesses, such as obesity, anorexia nervosa, some skin conditions, and migraine headaches, are also referred to as psychosomatic or somatization. It is apparent from this list that some of these are symptoms and others are actual signs of a documentable physical change. As scientific knowledge expands, growing evidence supports theories about the probable impact of stress in the development or exacerbation of biological diseases such as diabetes, hyperthyroidism, hypothyroidism, cancer, myocardial infarction, and kidney disease.

Because somatization disorders can become serious and even life-threatening, appropriate medical treatment is essential. Control of life-threatening symptoms may be the first phase of a comprehensive treatment program. Such treatment usually occurs in the general hospital. Increasingly, psychiatric–medical units are emerging in general hospitals.[23,40] The psychiatric liaison nurse may also contribute significantly to the care of these clients in a general hospital setting, by either providing direct services or consulting with the nusing staff. Psychotherapy and pharmacotherapy extend beyond the phase of acute illness to treatment in psychiatric hospitals, outpatient clinics, and private offices. Approaches to therapy need to be client specific because the illness reflects the individual's particular difficulty in coping with his own life situation in a way tolerable to the physiological system.

DSM-III-R DIAGNOSIS

Somatoform disorders are the psychiatric diagnostic categories associated with the combination of physical and psychiatric symptoms. The essential feature of this category of psychiatric diagnoses is that physical symptoms being described by the client cannot be associated with pathological changes at the cellular or organ level, yet the client does not attribute the sensations to any psychological factors. The client does not deliberately produce these physical symptoms; rather they occur as an expression of emotional conflict. Somatization disorders, conversion disorder, and hypochondriasis are subcategories of somatoform disorders.

Somatization disorder is characterized by recurrent, multiple physical complaints affecting various body systems. The symptoms may be vague or presented in an exaggerated manner. Despite repeated efforts to obtain medical attention, no physical pathology is diagnosed. Most persons with this disorder develop symptoms before the age of 30 and continue to experience somatic symptoms to a greater or lesser degree throughout their lives. Persons with a somatization disorder usually experience a high level of anxiety, depression, and irritability.

Conversion disorder is diagnosed when symptoms such as sudden onset of paralysis, blindness, aphonia, seizures, or other neurological disorders occur and an appropriate investigation finds no physical causes to which the symptoms can be attributed. Conversion symptoms may be expressed by the autonomic and endocrine system and include vomiting and *pseudocyesis*. These symptoms are not intentional or consciously produced but are thought to be a means to resolution of unconscious conflicts.

Hypochondriasis is a preoccupation or belief that one has a serious disease based on his interpretation of certain symptoms, in spite of reassurances to the contrary. Additional details of diagnostic criteria can be obtained from the diagnostic manual.[1]

THEORETICAL APPROACHES

Psychoanalytical

An early concept of Freud's description of hysteria or hysterical neurosis was that certain physical symptoms such as paralysis, tics, and nervous coughs, were related to early psychological trauma. Physical symptoms would occur when incomplete repression had taken place. The most common physical symptoms were conversion symptoms.

More specifically, the process involves the occurrence of several related, highly unpleasant, psychological events in an individual's childhood that are put out of mind, or repressed. *Repression,* the involuntary exclusion of painful or conflictual thoughts, impulses, or memories from awareness is the primary defense of the ego. By this mechanism, the individual "forgets" early memories or traumas. These memories, however, can be brought near the surface of consciousness and almost remembered under certain conditions. These conditions are specific to the individual and are in some way related to the early emotional traumas. For example, a person who, as a child, was very frightened by being placed in a big bathtub by an unkind and cruel baby-sitter might become very upset by working in the enclosed space of a manhole after a flood. A man with these "forgotten" memories may experience rapidly escalating anxiety and rush to get out of the manhole, bumping his arm on the ladder and falling into the water in the process.

Conversion symptoms occur only in instances when the mental mechanism of repression fails or is incomplete. The repressed impulse, thought, or idea continues to exist in the unconscious. If the impulse is expressed in a disguised or unrecognizable form, such as paralysis, the feelings associated with the impulse become centered in this physical symptom. Returning to the preceding example, this individual is unlikely to be able to associate his anxiety with those early memories. Instead, the person experiences a feeling of fear but cannot understand the intensity of the feeling or why it is occurring in this situation. By removing himself from the situation immediately, he again may gradually feel fine. If the supervisor insists that he reenter the manhole to continue working, however, he may develop a paralysis in the arm that was bumped when he fell during the earlier effort to escape. This paralysis could have a sudden or more gradual onset, occurring over a few days. Examination by health care personnel may reveal bruising but no reason for paralysis. Thus psychological trauma of years ago becomes converted into an active, current physical symptom, precipitated by events that influence the individual's inability to maintain complete repression.

In psychoanalytical terms, the mechanisms associated with conversion symptoms are considered to be that of primary gain, in which there is a temporal relationship between the psychological conflict and the physical symptom. The individual obtains a partial solution to the underlying psychological conflict. Another mechanism proposed is that of secondary gain, in which the individual avoids a particular upsetting activity through the symptom. These mental mechanisms are not deliberate or conscious but occur totally out of the individual's conscious control. They are often seen in persons with the medical diagnoses of conversion disorder.

An extension of the psychoanalytical theory that early psychological trauma is converted into physical symptoms has been applied to psychosomatic conditions. Known as the specificity theory, it states that various parts of the body are associated with certain developmental phases as outlined by psychoanalytical theory (see Chapter 4). Anxiety or psychological maladjustment during a certain development phase may lead to illness in the body site associated with that developmental phase. For example, psychological maladjustment during the oral phase of development (associated with eating) may lead to later development of peptic ulcer. Psychological maladjustment in the anal phase (associated with elimination) may be the root of lower bowel disease, such as ulcerative colitis. This theory was well accepted in the 1950s and somewhat after that, but research examining the proposed relationships did not strongly support the theory. The specific theory of body organs corresponding to psychological developmental phases has essentially been replaced by more general theories regarding effects of stressors and anxiety on the body.

General Systems

The foundations of general systems theory are outlined in Chapter 4. Systems theory was an outcome of new scientific doctrines of wholeness, dynamic interaction, and organization. As such, it provided the possibility of an integrated concept of mental disorder. Biological factors (physical appearance, endocrine balance, intellectual endowment, sex, and age) and life experiences (family relationships, interpersonal relationships, education, social status, and cultural factors) were viewed as interacting together with the environment. These interactions create unique individualistic responses.

In this framework, *mental health* was viewed as a state in the interrelationship of the individual and the environment in which the personality structure is relatively stable and the environmental stressors are within an absorptive capacity.[48] Therefore mental illness exists on a continuum that extends from the well-integrated (healthy) personality to the poorly balanced personality structure that can tolerate few internal or external demands. Constitutional factors such as genetic endowment, physical and intellectual functioning, body size, and traits of temperament function together as an interacting substance, molding and being molded by environmental influences. Disturbances in any of the systems influence the individual. For example, an overlying stressful job that produces prolonged emotional imbalance is likely to produce physical symptoms or biological changes.

Somatization is an expression of the interactions among

biological traits, life experiences, and the environment. This group of disorders represents an exaggerated physiological response to prolonged stress and can occur in all human beings. Reasons for the psychosomatic reaction or the development of somatic symptoms severe enough to meet diagnostic criteria for a psychiatric condition rather than other neurotic reactions are specific to the individual, probably based on previous life experiences or learned behavior. Systems theory, as an interactional theory, also addresses the nature of the many interactions and reactions taking place.

Stress

The basic concepts of stress described by Selye are discussed in Chapter 4. Stress theory applies to somatization as it clearly demonstrates the interrelationship of the mind and body. Selye defined stress as a set of bodily defenses against any form of noxious stimuli, a universal physiological set of reactions and processes,[50] created by an environmental demand. In this framework, stress is the individual's physiological response and the stressor is an environmental condition. A variety of environmental conditions, such as natural disasters, war, imprisonment, and forced relocation, may produce a stress response in almost anyone. More mundane daily life events can also be stress producing. The stress response is individualistic. What one person finds stress producing may be pleasurable for another, such as being at a large, noisy, active family gathering. *Psychological stress* occurs when a particular relationship between the person and the environment occurs that the individual views as threatening or exceeding personal resources.

Psychological stress can produce the physiological changes described by Selye. For example, depending on an individual's relationship with a particular family member, the death of that family member, usually a stressor, may vary greatly in intensity. If the individual perceives the death of a family member as a stressor, the stress response may lead to illness. Levi and Kagan[53] suggest that psychosocial stimuli can cause physical disease. Their thesis is that most life changes evoke physiological stress responses intended for the physical activity of coping. The nature and extent of the stressor and its interaction with the individual's genetic and psychosocial responses may trigger precursors to disease that can lead to disease itself. The stress-illness response for psychological stress that leads to physical illness is complex. One must consider the following factors: (1) the nature and extent of environmental stressors; (2) the individual's characteristics, usually genetic and physical; (3) the individual's perception of, or the meaning given to, the event, called *cognitive appraisal,* and (4) the individual's coping abilities.

Environmental stressors

Both quantitative and qualitative differences affect psychological stress. For instance, in the preceding example, the death of a family member, how could a quantitative difference in stress be evaluated? First, consider the death of a mother who was the primary source of financial and emotional support for two preadolescent children. Her death resulted in the children being moved to foster homes, changing schools, giving up friendships, and adapting to different expectations. Second, consider a married man in his 50s whose mother dies while in a nursing home, where she has been living for the past 3 years. The adjustment of the children in the first example is extensive compared with that of the man in the second because the objective change in the lives of the children is greater. This addresses *quantitative* demand for change that imposes on an individual from an environmental stressor.

The *qualitative* demand may vary, depending on the individual's ability to anticipate or control an environmental stressor and the degree of positive or negative feelings associated with the stressor. For example, the man who can anticipate his mother's death because of an extended illness is likely to experience it differently than if she died suddenly in her home from a heart attack. The children in the preceding example would be likely to experience a high degree of qualitative demand as they have very minimal control of their environment and may not even understand the situation. Emotional maturity, including the ability to work out a successful positive relationship, will also lessen the emotional response to a stressor.

Another suggested way to categorize stressors is based on *duration.* Four broad and somewhat overlapping categories have been defined[21]:
1. Acute, time-limited stressors, such as arriving late to work or falling out of a canoe.
2. Stressor sequences, which involve a series of events over time but which occur as the result of one event, such as losing a job.
3. Chronic, intermittent stressors, such as disliked in-laws coming to dinner, which may occur regularly but are not constant stressors.
4. Chronic stressors, such as coping with a long-term physical illness or long-term job stress, in which there is no clear initiating factor but the stress is continuous and long lasting.

These general categories are intended to help one think about stressors. The crucial test is how the individual responds. For example, disliked in-laws coming to dinner could be a chronic stressor for the individual who is frequently preoccupied by the problem relationship.

Stressors can also include environmental characteristics, such as heat, humidity, cold, altitude, noise, and amount of light. Overexposure or underexposure to any of these may cause serious physical illness or minor changes in physiological functions or mood. For example, studies have shown two effects of noise: (1) it damages hearing, and (2) it has a "stress" effect, changing mood, intellectual and motor performance, general behavior, and general body physiological state. Some people exposed to high noise levels for several years develop hypertension. Environmental pollutants are another source of stress gaining increasing recognition. Some of these, such as ionizing radiation, are severe enough to produce immediate illness. Other stressors, such as repeating the same hand movements for several hours, are sources of chronic stress that gradually change physiological functioning.

Individual characteristics

The individual has obvious traits (for example, sex, age, physical appearance) and less obvious traits (for example, endocrine balance, genetic makeup, functioning of the immune and autonomic nervous systems). When these traits are combined with personality characteristics, the available coping abilities and techniques of the individual emerge and develop.

The physical properties and chemical composition of body tissues tend to be reasonably constant. When there is too much variation, such as with elevated body temperature, the individual is considered ill. More understanding of physical systems, however, has led to new theories about the importance of subtle variations and the extent of system interdependence. For example, some persons may be more prone genetically to develop cancer, so the physiological changes due to psychological stress may be reflected through this illness. Stress can ultimately produce observable changes in various body systems. Reactions of physical systems, that is, the internal environment, depend on the person's emotional and social responses, activity, and the external environment. For instance, the person with a childhood back injury, later employed in a job that puts physical strain on the back, is probably more likely to develop back pain than many others, particularly if the individual is in an unhappy marriage and is chronically tense and irritable. Some of the physical systems associated with stress responses are summarized in Table 19-1.

Figure 19-1 demonstrates the complex interactions of the brain and neurological system on modifying and interpreting stimuli from the internal environment and the external environment. Documentation of the interactions between the neurological, endocrine, and immune systems has gradually expanded. The relationship between life changes or stressful life events and the likelihood of developing an illness was substantiated in the 1960s. The reasons for these relationships were unknown. Recent research confirms that many stressful life events, even commonplace events such as school examinations, may depress the level of response protection of the body that is provided by the immune system (see the research highlight on p. 389). The mechanism of interaction between these systems is poorly understood but is presently an active focus of research. Connections between psychological distress produced by life event and biological change as measured by immune responses is the first specific evidence that challenges the traditional mind/body separation of Western health care practices. This research may suggest that practices such as meditation, relaxation techniques, and others, can have a positive influence on health.

Cognitive appraisal

Cognitive appraisal, a process that probably occurs in the cerebral cortex, intervenes between the environmental stimulus and the person's reaction. It is the mental activity of judgment, discrimination, and choice before action, an analysis based on past experience. Thus the degree and type of reaction to the same event can vary considerably from person to person. Consider, for example, two women, each of whom is sitting alone in her house late at night. Both women hear a weird, indiscriminate noise from the upstairs bedroom. Woman A has a recent history of being assaulted and robbed. Her response is immediate panic: her pulse rate and respirations increase, and her pupils dilate; she jumps from the chair to telephone a friend, fearing grave danger. Woman B feels a slight chill run up her spine but rapidly concludes that it is a windy evening and the bedroom door has swung shut. When a crisis or threatening situation occurs, these physical and mental processes seem to occur instantaneously and intuitively. Clearly, there is an instant arousal response in which the autonomic nervous system responds but can be rapidly modified by cognitive appraisal. Usually the appraisal process considers (1) risks and consequences ("What will happen if I don't change?"), (2) resources ("Am I strong enough to tolerate this? Who [or what] would help?"), and (3) imminence ("Do I have time to search, to think more?").

Lazarus and Folkman[50] describe three types of stress appraisals: harm/loss, threat, and challenge. When some damage has already been done to the individual, *harm/loss* appraisals primarily evaluate the degree of loss. *Threat* appraisals concern the anticipation of harm/loss and include anticipation of future problems resulting from the harm/loss already incurred. Both have primarily negative emotional implications, such as fear, grief, or anger. *Challenge* appraisals involve the potential for harm/loss or for gain and growth. Thus pleasurable emotions of eagerness or excitement are associated with challenge appraisals.

Cognitive appraisal is subjective. How a specific environmental event, especially an ambiguous one, is perceived does not necessarily relate to objective reality. Personality factors can influence or distort perceptions. For example,

....

▼ **TABLE 19-1** **Examples of Physical Systems and Their Role in Stress Responses**

Physical System	Role in Stress Response
Brain	Interprets and evaluates stressors Provides memories of past emotional experiences Controls feelings, emotions, and behaviors that ensure survival and perhaps sociability and sexuality
Autonomic nervous system	
Sympathetic	Reacts to acute demands made on the body, such as in acute anxiety or the fight or flight response
Parasympathetic	Directs functioning of physiological processes, such as digestion and body fluids
Endocrine system	Stressful environmental events change neurochemical and hormonal levels in the body, which prevents illness and facilitates adaptation, but can also cause illness
Immune system	Stress has an immunosuppressant effect that can increase vulnerability to certain diseases Major life changes, such as bereavement, increase the risk of illness, probably by suppression of the immune system

....

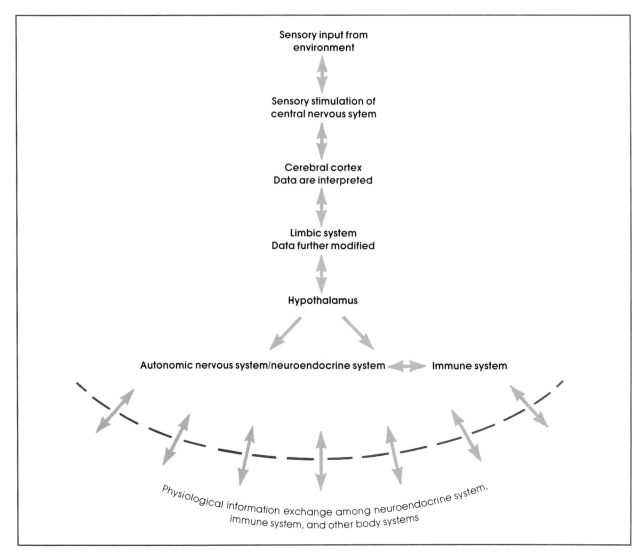

FIGURE 19-1 The path of information exchange between sensory inputs and body organs.

a person judges a new situation on past similar experiences. Timing of the event may also influence perception. Events that occur at an unexpected life phase (for example, a teenager whose parents die) or several stressful events together may influence the person's overall interpretation of those events. It has been suggested that the individual who tends to perceive things negatively or who expects fear, harm, or danger will more likely interpret new situations from that perspective. Cognitive responses can probably be changed or influenced by a variety of factors, such as psychotherapy, advice from family or friends, or a change in one's physical health. The individual's philosophy, beliefs, and sense of control also influence cognitive appraisals.

Coping

Coping addresses the active process of using personal, social, and environmental resources to manage stress. Three coping models are discussed here. The first model views coping as a stress-control mechanism by which

arousal is minimized through learned behaviors. The second, the ego psychology model, considers coping to be the most effective approach to managing person-environment relationships. The third model suggest that coping does not necessarily imply control over noxious stimuli but implies making an effort to minimize their effects. It is unclear how one's coping style develops. One important factor is temperamental style, which is thought to be partially a genetic trait. Other factors relevant to coping style relate to biological and socially learned differences in the individual's sensitivity to noxious stimuli as well as patterns of behavior learned from other family members, especially parents or significant others.

The first model states an individual's particular set of psychological adaptive mechanisms remain relatively constant throughout life. This theory proposes that one can define personality styles and associate them to illness. An individual's coping style can presumably be described and future responses predicted from studying the person's reactions in a few specific situations. If specific sets of coping

RESEARCH HIGHLIGHT

Stress, Loneliness, and Changes in Herpesvirus Latency
• R Glaser, JK Kiecolt-Glaser, CE Speicher, and JE Holliday

PURPOSE

A growing body of evidence suggests that major life changes can influence the incidence and course of illness by modifying the body's immune response. Stressful life events and loneliness may also affect the immune response. In this study, the goal was to examine the possible responsiveness of the immune system to these psychosocial influences.

SAMPLE

The initial sample consisted of 76 first-year medical students; 49 subjects could be used in the study. Twenty-one subjects were excluded from the study because there was insufficient plasma collected or the subject did not have antibody to the herpesvirus, which was to be used for evaluating the immune response. The final sample consisted of 16 women and 33 men, with an average age of 23 years.

METHODOLOGY

Three blood samples were drawn at the following time periods: 1 month before final examination, the first day of final examinations, and just after subjects had returned from summer vacation. Blood was analyzed to determine the level of herpes virus antigens in each of the three samples. Some other assays were also performed. Self-report questionnaires were filled out byt he subjects at the time that blood was drawn. These questionnaires consisted of the brief symptom inventory, which was administered at all three time periods, and UCLA loneliness scale, which was administered only once, at the first data collection point. The subjects were grouped into two groups of high and low loneliness. Data were analyzed using a 2×3 ANOVA design to test the effects of the different time periods and level of loneliness. The number and type of physical symptoms were examined in relationship to the three data collection periods.

Based on data from *Journal of Behavioral Medicine* 8(3):249, 1985.

FINDINGS

Self-reported symptoms were different at the three sample points. The greatest number of physical symptoms were reported on the day of final examinations, followed by the time period 1 month before examinations and the fewest symptoms were reported after summer vacation. The high loneliness subjects had significantly higher antibody titers across all of the three sample points when one assay method was used. Using another measure of antibody titer, a similar finding was reported, although the level of difference did not reach statistical significance. The combined factors of loneliness and time were not statistically significant.

IMPLICATIONS

This study documented significant and measurable changes in cellular immune response due to commonplace stressors in healthy adults. Elevation of antibody titers at the first data collection period and an even greater compromise in cellular immunity at the higher stress level of the examination period were reported. This study, along with others previously reported, consistently demonstrate the effects of loneliness on suppression of the immune system. The consistency of these findings across several studies lends strong support to theories about the importance of interpersonal relationships in influencing health-related outcomes. This study is consistent with a growing body of research demonstrating the importance of psychosocial variables as modifiers of immunocompetence, which is mediated through multiple pathways.

---

styles can be observed and documented, the relationships between these and the development of specific illnesses can be studied. To date, the only personality style that has been fairly well established in relationship to a specific disease is type A personality and coronary artery disease. Type A personality represents one coping style. These coping traits are having a strong desire to control situations, receiving personal gratification from achievements, setting very demanding work standards, and having a great sense of urgency. Failure in any of these personal standards leads to despair, anxiety, and frustration, which is dealt with by a redoubled effort to achieve, creating coronary-prone behavior. Efforts to associate other personality styles with illnesses have been inconclusive, although examination of these relationships continues.

An alternative, the *ego psychology* model, considers coping as a process between the individual and a constantly changing environment. This model views cognitive appraisal as essential to the determination of a behavioral response. Shontz[75] examined individuals' responses to being told of a serious physical illness and suggested that various stages may occur in the coping response. The first is shock, followed by encounter, then retreat, and gradually reality testing. These cycles repeat as the coping process continues, leading eventually to psychological growth.

Lazarus and Folkman[50] describe a third model of the coping process which is an interactive model. The emphasis in this model is on the individual's process of thinking through and evaluating the situation. It includes *problem-focused coping*, which means intellectually evaluating a situation and then selecting one or more alternative actions, and *emotion-focused coping*, a cognitive process in which the meaning of the stressful transaction is changed by rethinking a situation. The effect of emotional responses on

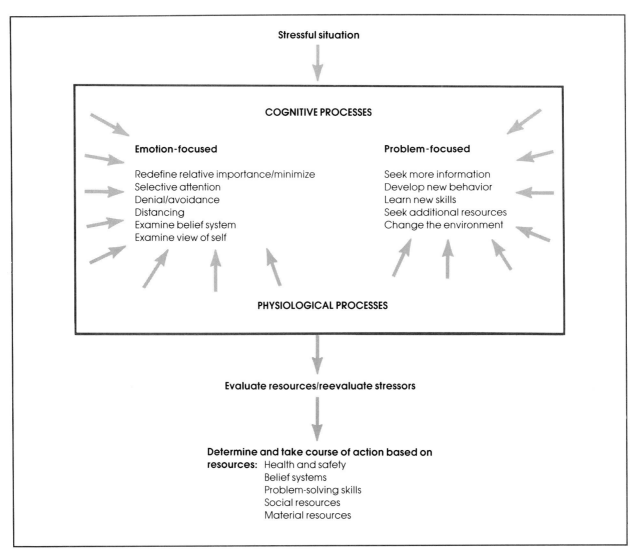

FIGURE 19-2 Interactional mode of coping.

Theory	Theorist	Dynamics
Psychoanalytical	Freud	Through the mechanism of repression early traumatic events are "forgotten." Later in life, specific events may trigger the possible resurfacing of painful memories. Somatic symptoms emerge when the mechanism of repression is only partially successful.
General systems		Dynamic interaction occurs between various parts of the individual's physical, social, psychological systems. Any disturbance in any of the systems influences the individual as a whole.
Stress	Selye	The nature and extent of the stressor and its interactions with the individual's genetic and psychosocial responses may lead to disease.
Cognitive model	Lazarus and Folkman	The process of cognitive evaluation of the stressor, then assessing personal, social, and environmental resources to determine the most effective means to manage, followed by action, then cognitive reassessment.

bodily systems and on the cognitive processes of making an evaluation is not particularly clear or well defined in this model. According to this theory, however, the person takes a selected action directed toward coping, then reevaluates the situation to determine the effectiveness of the coping actions. The person then decides what, if any, further action is necessary. How an individual responds depends on how the stressor is evaluated and what resources are available and accessible. In this coping model, to understand behavior one must understand the individual's process of analysis. Figure 19-2 illustrates this model. Emphasis is on the thought processes and reevaluation of the situation with little description of the impact of physiological processes and feedback mechanisms.

Table 19-2 provides a summary of theoretical approaches relevant to somatization disorder.

NURSING PROCESS

Assessment

Physical dimension Assessment of a client with a somatization disorder may reveal symptoms in only one body system, symptoms in several body systems, or responses that include the whole individual. Consequently, this discussion presents a general overview of physical assessment and then focuses on the assessment of specific body systems. Persons with physical health problems induced or exacerbated by stress are likely to have specific physical complaints that correspond to physical changes documented by laboratory studies and other diagnostic tests. The physical complaints described by persons with one of the somatoform disorders may be inconsistent and physical pathology, if found, will probably be incongruent with what is expected, based on knowledge of anatomy and physiology.

Assessment generally includes a complete physical examination and general laboratory tests. When gathering the health history, the nurse might inquire about a family history of disorders such as diabetes, cancer, hypertension, various cardiovascular disorders, and genetic diseases. The nurse obtains specific information about use of prescription and nonprescription drugs. The health inventory includes information about risk factors such as smoking, use of illegal drugs or alcohol, caffeine intake, and exposure to environmental contaminants such as chemicals, pesticides, radiation, and automotive exhaust. If relevant, the nurse explores with the client the nature of contaminants in the work place such as frequent contact with specific chemicals, high levels of noise, or strenuous physical activity. The nurse also assesses the client's life-style, including general activity level, diet, and eating patterns. It is important to inquire about the use of dietary supplements such as vitamins, which are known to cause health problems with insufficient or excessive intake.

Cardiovascular system

Distinctly pleasant or unpleasant stimuli usually evoke cardiovascular responses such as changes in heart rate, heart rhythm, blood pressure, and stroke volume. Research has indicated that cognitive work, such as mental arithmetic or public speaking and psychological stresses or intra-

psychic conflicts, can produce tachycardia and increase levels of norepinephrine and free fatty acids in the blood. The atherosclerotic process, which occurs in children as young as 15 years of age, is thought to result from several interacting variables, including lack of exercise, high fat diet, genetics, obesity, and central nervous system functions.

Physical assessment includes checking pulse, respirations, weight, and blood pressure and performing specific tests (see Table 19-3) that may be diagnostic if a particular condition is suspected. The nurse asks the client specific questions about episodes of tachycardia and any other related physical symptoms. Most diseases of the cardiovascular system develop subtly and slowly. They are not likely to be discovered until there is recurrent chest pain or a dramatic manifestation of acute illness such as myocardial infarction. In addition to those illnesses presented in Table 19-3, other conditions, such as cardiac dysrhythmias or sudden death (see the following case example), may also be partially attributed to psychological factors.

▼ Case Example

Sam, 27 years old and single, walked into the psychiatric emergency room one morning and asked to be seen. He complained of severe anxiety and a sense of impending doom. During the examination Sam stated that he was living in a somewhat unhappy situation with his mother after having broken up with his girlfriend approximately 4 months ago. He also acknowledged that he occasionally used some drugs, primarily marijuana and cocaine. Occasionally, he sold drugs to get money because he did not have a steady job. The mental status examination revealed an acutely paranoid, very guarded, and highly anxious man. All other cognitive and mental functions were normal. His blood pressure was 170/90. Sam reported that he had been seen in a local health clinic about 2 weeks earlier, where he had been told that he had mild hypertension.

Sam remained in the emergency room for several hours for observation, during which time the paranoid and anxious symptoms abated and he requested to leave, stating that he felt much better. He was released after signing permission for medical records to be obtained from the health clinic and accepting an appointment at the mental health clinic for the next day. That evening's local news reported a "crackdown" on local drug dealers; seven people had been arrested in Sam's neighborhood. The following morning the emergency room staff learned that Sam had been found dead at home at approximately 9 PM the previous night. Several weeks later the coroner's report indicated that the most probable cause of death was cardiac arrest, but the reason for cardiac arrest was never determined.

Severe cardiovascular disease may also produce circulatory difficulty severe enough to create other organic conditions. One of the most serious is delirium and other organic mental disorders associated with cerebral anoxia (see Chapter 33). Another psychogenic cardiovascular disorder causes the person to experience and describe symptoms of a cardiac condition when there are no physiologically measurable changes, such as can be measured by ECG or serum enzymes.

Gastrointestinal system

An emotional response is accompanied by a variety of gastrointestinal changes. Some are clearly physiological, and many have been individually learned from repeated

Text continued on p. 398.

► **TABLE 19-3** Common Psychophysiological Illnesses

Body System Affected	Illness	Significant Physical Signs and Symptoms	Associated Emotional Components	Associated Social or Environmental Conditions
Cardiovascular system	Coronary artery disease	Episodic chest pain usually on exertion, in cold weather, or in emotionally charged situations Characterized by dull, aching sensation in middle sternum Pain may radiate to left shoulder or arm and lasts approximately 5 minutes Diagnosed by ECG, cardiac catheterization May be accompanied by complaints of fatigue, irritability, insomnia	May be accompanied by depression, anxiety, chronic poor self-image, decreased energy, lowered ambition May exhibit overt anxiety, emotional lability in response to stress Elation, excitement, or frightening dreams can precipitate attacks	Smoking Employment demands related to deadlines, intense desire for achievement, work overload, job conflicts Frustration and discontent of persons with little education and low economic status; hard work not associated with success Diets rich in saturated fats or calories
	Myocardial infarction	Damage and death of cardiac muscles Characterized by severe, prolonged chest pain described as crushing and radiating to left arm and shoulder Frequently occurs during rest Accompanied by ashen color; cold sweats; tachycardia or dysrhythmias; nausea and vomiting; rapid, shallow breathing Diagnosed by ECG, elevated serum enzymes	Initial response of fear and apprehension followed by minimization or denial During hospitalization, feelings of anxiety and depression Severe emotional response possibly leading to inability to return to work Generally repression of emotions	As for coronary artery disease Also increased work responsibility, loss of spouse by death or divorce, social isolation Increased anxiety or depression, business or domestic problems possibly precedes myocardial infarction
	Essential hypertension	Blood pressure over 140/90 can indicate development of disease; may increase with age Occurs more often in black population May be accompanied by morning headaches, shortness of breath, chest pain, intermittent claudication in legs, and vascular changes in retina Hypertensive encephalopathy: serious risk of death	Theory of personality or intrapsychic conflicts between passive-dependent and aggressive impulses; repressed anger, resentment, or hostility not proved Positive association between anxiety, anger, and elevated blood pressure Stress from broad environmental conditions leading to fear, anger, or frustration Elevated blood pressure: noted, for example, after disasters or loss of job and in air traffic controllers	Contributing factors: rapid sociocultural change, urbanization, socioeconomic mobility, high-stress job, natural disasters

Headaches	Mild to severe, bilateral, throbbing or nonthrobbing; pain lasting a few hours to several days May be accompanied by nausea and vomiting or neurological symptoms No organic cause such as brain tumor May be associated with trigger factors, such as premenses or allergic response	Emotional conflicts dealt with ineffectively Response to anxiety or worry	Trigger factors possibly environmental, such as specific foods, glare, weather changes, alcohol, odors, hunger
Gastrointestinal system Irritable bowel syndrome	Motility disorder that can affect both large and small bowel Episodic abdominal pain and change in bowel habits, including diarrhea, constipation, passing of mucus No abnormal physical or laboratory findings Symptoms: possible nausea, vomiting, abdominal distention, headaches, insomnia, dizziness, appetite and weight loss	Conscious reports of a distressing event, nervous symptoms Possibly represents struggle over controlling and letting go of aggressive impulses Alternative suggestion: constipation associated with stubborn active striving and diarrhea associated with inadequate and helpless feelings	Precipitated by obviously stressful life events such as illness of family member, financial loss, job loss, increase in work hours
Ulcerative colitis	Inflammation of colon mucosa, primarily in rectum and sigmoid colon Can occur in ileum Onset may be acute and can be lethal in severe cases Symptoms: rectal bleeding, diarrhea, weight loss, fever, abdominal tenderness Diagnosed by proctoscopic examination or biopsy More common in whites and Jews May be genetic predisposition or autoimmune disorder Anal fissures, fistulas, perirectal abscesses possible Associated with high incidence of colon cancer	Personality type described as "primitive personally organization," characterized by neatness, oversensitivity, egocentrism, grandiose self-concept, and excessive need for love, sympathy, affection Naive concept of love and overattachment to mother Inability to be aware of or express feelings and fantasy Exceedingly sensitive to interpersonal loss but also maintains ambivalent object attachments	May be precipitated by separation, bereavement, or situations in which individual feels unable to cope or has failed

Continued.

TABLE 19-3   Common Psychophysiological Illnesses — cont'd

Body System Affected	Illness	Significant Physical Signs and Symptoms	Associated Emotional Components	Associated Social or Environmental Conditions
Gastrointestinal system— cont'd	Crohn's disease (regional enteritis)	Inflammation of small bowel and sometimes colon Similar to ulcerative colitis except abscess, fissures, ulceration, and perforation of bowel more common Cause thought to be genetic, immunological, or slow virus	Very similar to ulcerative colitis Early ego deficits resulting in compulsive or paranoid traits, excessive dependence, demanding or explosive manipulation Regression, helplessness, hopelessness possible	Symptoms may be precipitated by object loss, loss of self-esteem, interpersonal struggles
	Peptic and duodenal ulcer	Chronic ulceration of digestive mucosa in esophagus, stomach, or duodenum Onset acute, possibly accompanied by tarry stools depressed hemoglobin and erythrocyte counts, vomiting, epigastric pain Hemorrhage or perforation: medical emergency Less acutely, pain may be relieved by food or antacids Diagnosed by x-ray examination or endoscopy May be genetic predisposition since members of blood group O more likely to develop the illness	No reliable personality factors May be associated with oral conflict and frustration, accompanied by physical predisposition Personality factors in men described as assertively independent and in women as overly dependent	Situations where personal defeat is imminent but individual blocks this awareness May be associated with being single or alcoholic Higher frequency of ulcers in concentration camp survivor Associated with high-stress jobs
Respiratory system	Bronchial asthma	Recurrent bronchoconstriction, edema, excessive secretions in response to varied stimuli Wheezing that is mild or severe, episodic or paroxysmal Respirations may increase in frequency, accompanied by coughing, increased perspiration More common in boys than girls in childhood but approximately equal frequency in adults	Psychological profile confounded by inability to determine if certain factors cause disease or develop in response to it Relevant psychological factors: strong wish for protection, especially by mother Separation may precipitate attack, or intense conflict associated with separation may be relieved by being apart and other symptoms decrease Other causes: sexual excitement, fear, angry outbursts, disappointment, jealousy May be poorly attuned to environment, with immature coping mechanisms, dependence, tendency to become depressed and helpless unless given much support from others	Allergens, cold air, odors, and physical exercise can precipitate attacks Increased frequency of attacks at night and during weather changes

Hyperventilation syndrome	Breathing rapidly and deeply for a few minutes; produces vertigo, giddiness, buzzing in the ears, fainting, blurred vision, dry mouth, uncontrolled laughter or crying May be followed by apnea Can include increased heart rate, lowered blood pressure, nausea, increased perspiration	Responses to fear, anxiety, pain, anger, or situations with special meaning to person	Exercise, such as climbing stairs or running
Dermatological			
Generalized pruritus	Abnormal sensation in itching not caused by insect bites, dermatitis, diabetes, nephritis, liver disease, leukemia, or other diseases associated with itching May also be localized to specific areas of body such as anus or vulvae May lead to an itch/scratch such that individual produces severe, self-inflicted wounds	Anxiety and tension possibly producing a misinterpretation of cutaneous sensations May be a means to express repressed anger Possible exceptional need for affection	Lack of sexual partner or sexual outlets
Atopic dermatitis	Also known as neurodermatitis Dry, flaky skin with redness, papules, scaly hyperkeratosis, exudation of clear serum, crusting Typically on the face, knees, elbows Occurs intermittently May be allergic response	Related to lack of physical contact early in life Precipitated by emotionally disturbing situations, loss of or longing for love	Reaction to loss of significant person
Psoriasis	Large red plaques covered with thick white scales, usually on elbows and knees May involve deformity of nails May be genetic predisposition	Response to worry or stress Person with symptoms likely to feel repulsive May reflect desire for security	Systemic infection, excess or insufficient sunlight, dampness, cold weather
Acne vulgaris	Common at puberty; related to androgen-estrogen imbalance and overproduction of androgens Sebaceous glands overactive	Emotional stress or sexual difficulty may aggravate condition Sebaceous secretions may increase with anger	Diets rich in fats and carbohydrates may aggravate condition

Continued.

▶ **TABLE 19-3** Common Psychophysiological Illnesses — cont'd

Body System Affected	Illness	Significant Physical Signs and Symptoms	Associated Emotional Components	Associated Social or Environmental Conditions
Musculoskeletal system	Rheumatoid arthritis	Symmetrical joint swelling and deformity accompanied by morning stiffness and tenderness or pain on motion of joint Other systemic symptoms: fatigue, loss of appetite and weight, occasional fever Most frequently involves joints in knees, hands, feet Subcutaneous nodules and ocular lesions possible Diagnosed by x-ray examination of joints Rheumatoid factor and anemia may be found in laboratory report	Personality: self-sacrificing, conforming, inhibited or shy, perfectionistic, masochistic Varied patterns of controlling anger, hostility, and aggression but tendency for experiencing conflict over expression of anger Personality traits possibly caused by pain, distress, and treatment of illness rather than by preillness traits May be chronic depression	Many life changes in year preceding onset of symptoms; major life conflicts, sexual difficulty, marital problems likely High incidence of family members with psychiatric disturbance
Endocrine system	Thyrotoxicosis	Excess thyroid hormone Symptoms: palpitations, heat intolerance, increased appetite with weight loss, increased sweating, generalized weakness, insomnia, fine tremor of hands, elevated temperature, tachycardia, exophthalmos Diagnosed by protein-bound iodine, basal metabolic rate, iodine-131 uptake	Tension, excitability, and possible emotional lability, temper outbursts, crying spells, distractibility, short attention span, impaired recent memory; severe symptoms may include overt psychosis Disease possibly precipitated by acute emotional trauma or extreme fright	
	Hypothyroidism	Insufficient thyroid hormone Symptoms: peripheral neuropathy; hearing loss; headaches; skin pale, yellow, thickened; husky voice Accompanied by cold intolerance, aching muscles, irregular menstrual periods, weight gain, lowered body temperature Diagnosed by thyroid hormone level, iodine-131 uptake	Predominant depression, sometimes dementia, complaints of fatigue, lethargy, decreased initiative, impaired recent memory May include paranoid suspicions and auditory hallucinations	

Addison's disease	Decrease in corticosteroid caused by adrenal insufficiency Symptoms: weakness, fatigability, anorexia, weight loss, hypotension	Poverty of thought, apathy, fatigue, psychomotor retardation, depression May be frank psychosis, stupor, coma	
Cushing's syndrome	Excess of circulatory cortisol leading to increased appetite, truncal and facial obesity, frail skin, weakness, hypertension, muscle wasting, lowered glucose tolerance, impotence, amenorrhea	Depression with high risk of suicide, acute anxiety, emotional lability, irritability, insomnia Confusion and disorientation similar to organic mental disorders	
Diabetes	Disordered glucose metabolism caused by insufficient insulin Genetically transmitted Symptoms: polydipsia, polyuria, increased appetite with weight loss, fatigue	Produces psychological stress and may provide means to meet needs for attention, caring, affection	Need for insulin possibly altered by life changes, such as loss of interpersonal relationships
Hypopituitarism	Lack of pituitary hormone caused by lesions in gland, such as infections, head injury, tumors, myxedema, loss of pigmentation of breast areolae, inability to tan in the sun, loss of body hair, weight loss In children: dwarfism Severe symptoms: hypothermia, delirium, hypertension, stupor, coma, ultimately death	Mental disturbance typical and includes apathy, indifference, fatigue, drowsiness, depression, dependence, cognitive deficits, delusions, loss of libido	

training. Consider, for example, the learning process established by a mother who always feeds her crying infant, regardless of the cause of the crying. A person who has been fed as treatment for discomfort as a child, may be more likely to overeat as an adult, whenever discomfort or anxiety arises. The nurse, then, assesses the client's eating patterns.

Some persons respond to stress with serious or life-threatening conditions involving massive changes in gastrointestinal mucosa. These changes occur in conditions such as ulcerative colitis, irritable bowel syndrome, Crohn's disease (regional enteritis), and peptic or duodenal ulcers. In addition to psychological factors, persons who develop these conditions are thought to have a genetic predisposition. They also may tend to develop the illness because of some other cause, such as a change in neuroendocrine function, a metabolic dysfunction, an immunological disorder, or a slow virus. Sometimes these other causes can be documented but more often the reason for onset of symptoms is not clear.

Respiratory system

Many factors influence the normal functioning of the respiratory system. Exercise increases rate and depth of breathing. Severely obese people may have shallow breathing because of restricted movement of the diaphragm. Drugs such as morphine and codeine suppress respirations, whereas others such as salicylates are likely to increase them. The respiratory system can also be controlled voluntarily. Physical disorders that affect the respiratory system and result in difficult breathing include lung cancer, emphysema, congestive heart failure, and tuberculosis. The nurse looks for disorders that produce psychological responses, primarily fear and axiety, that further increase respiratory difficulty.

Bronchial asthma has multiple predisposing and interacting factors, including (1) possible genetic factors, (2) exposure to viruses or bacteria that results in infection, (3) exposure to allergens, (4) a tendency to bronchoconstriction, (5) a family history of allergy, and (6) psychological components. Physical symptoms are produced by a combination of events that lead to partial obstruction of bronchial passages because of constriction and edema. Acute asthma attacks are apparent, with audible wheezing, diaphoresis, increased respirations, and the use of accessory muscles to aid ventilation and forced expiration.

The nurse may note hyperventilation in persons who report repeated episodes of losing consciousness but who do not have epilepsy or other physical disorders that can cause loss of consciousness. Rapid breathing can be observed when the individual is under emotional stress.

Dermatological conditions

An itch, a tickle, and a pain are all conducted by the same nerve fibers. The individual may interpret the same sensation differently. The skin and its sensations are a major source of environmental stimuli. Responses to pain, temperature, and touch are essential for maintaining body integrity, protecting the body, and providing a means of interaction with the environment. The sexual function of skin has been demonstrated by Freud's descriptions of libidinal erogenous zones. Touch is also important to normal physical and psychological development.

Abnormal skin sensations and manifestations can occur as a result of allergies, damage (for example, burns, nerve trauma), infections, and emotions. Exaggerated responses such as blushing with embarrassment or pallor with fear are relatively common. In addition to those disorders listed in Table 19-3, several other primarily physical skin responses to emotional states include the following:

1. Hyperhidrosis: excessive sweat secretion, especially of the palms, soles of feet, and axillae, which may lead to rashes, blisters, or infections
2. Rosacea: a vascularity with papule formation, usually occurring on the face or upper chest
3. Alopecia areata: sudden patchy hair loss more common in children and young adults and usually occurring about 2 weeks after a significant emotional event

Musculoskeletal system

Rheumatoid arthritis affects primarily the musculoskeletal system, but it is considered a systemic disorder with an unknown cause. Onset of the disease most often occurs in the fourth decade of life but can occur at any age, including childhood. Several causes have been suggested, but most data point to multifactorial influences, including (1) genetic predisposition; (2) disordered immune mechanisms, especially cell-mediated ones; (3) a slow virus; and (4) psychosomatic mechanisms that influence several hormones, such as growth hormones, thyroxin, androgens, estrogens, and adrenocorticosteroids. Hypothalamic regulation of the immune response, especially in relation to corticosteroid production, may ultimately reveal an autoimmune response as responsible for rheumatoid arthritis symptoms.

The illness is usually not life threatening but can lead to chronic pain and disability. An acute onset is characterized by high fever, extensive polyarticular inflammation, and rapid development of joint deformities. (See Table 19-3 for other symptoms.) After the initial onset most persons will improve, and about one fifth will recover completely. Despite remissions and exacerbations, most persons continue to work and function in daily activities to some degree.

Endocrine system

The endocrine system is ultimately involved in mediating mind-body interactions, although the exact mechanisms of hormonal influence on mood, cognitive functions, and response to psychological and social factors are poorly understood. Disorders of the endocrine system, as with the disorders already described, may result from psychosocial stress and therefore may be considered psychosomatic. However, it is acknowledged that endocrine disorders may also be somatopsychic. That is, the hormonal imbalance caused by glandular dysfunction may produce mental symptoms, sometimes severe and difficult to differentiate from depression or psychosis.

The major endocrine disorders are listed in Table 19-3. In addition, gonadal dysfunctions, such as decreased androgen production in men and decreased estrogen secretion in women, are known to result both normally and from psychological causes. For instance, acute physical or psychological stress may lead to decreased testosterone production in men, which leads to decreased beard growth. Menopause is a normal reduction in estrogen secretion for women. It may produce significant changes in calcium and lipid metabolism that are associated with coronary atherosclerosis and osteoporosis. Menopause also causes changes in skin and mucosal surfaces, hot flashes, and insomnia. Most of these symptoms are biologically generated due to the internal change in estrogen levels. Some symptoms, such as hot flashes, can be quite distressing, resulting in increased stress. Amenorrhea may occur in premenopausal women as a result of certain drugs, such as reserpine and phenothiazines, extreme obesity, or excessive physical exercise.

Multiple systems responses

Several disorders involve responses to combined physical and psychological factors. Eating disorders, for example, are common, complex, serious, and involve an interrelationship of physical and psychological factors (see Chapter 31). Pain responses can also be considered partly psychosomatic. Headaches are a typical cause of pain, which may be transitory or severe and disabling. "Tension" headaches, usually mild and self-limiting, represent one end of the scale. Migraine headaches can be severe, lasting for days and accompanied by other symptoms, such as flashes of color or wavy lines in the visual field. Migraine headaches are usually thought to be caused by increased vasomotor activity, and tension headaches by contraction of skeletal muscles. Both causes coexist in some persons with headaches (Table 19-3).

The general category of somatoform disorders incudes the recognition that clients may experience a single symptom or many complex somatic symptoms. When physical assessment reveals a single symptom, the medical diagnosis of conversion disorder is usually applied. A common symptom is the relatively sudden onset of the temporary loss of functioning of a body part. This symptom often occurs in conjunction with a psychologically traumatic event. Such clients are more often seen in emergency rooms or physicians' offices. Physical assessment includes the diagnostic workup appropriate for evaluating the complaints of the client. If no organic cause can be found to explain the symptoms, referral to a psychiatric clinic or other outpatient service for evaluation may be indicated.

In clients who have multiple complaints in various organ systems, the diagnosis of somatoform disorder is complicated. The nurse is alert to the possibility of a psychiatric diagnosis of somatoform disorder when the client's medical history includes multiple surgical procedures, contact with a number of primary care physicians all of whom the client believes to have been unhelpful, and frequent referral to a variety of medical specialists. Such a client will often describe a history of poor health from childhood, and the family history is likely to be positive for many family members having illnesses that were disabling. These clients are much more likely to have been evaluated in medical and surgical settings rather than in psychiatric settings because they focus on physical health problems, may refuse to consider psychological or social factors, and are likely to be offended by the suggestion that some aspects of their condition may have psychological cause. Somatoform disorders are associated with other psychiatric conditions such as major depression, anxiety disorders, substance abuse, phobic disorders, antisocial personality, and schizophrenia. Thus it is important for the psychiatric nurse to be alert to clients' somatic complaints and understand how to obtain treatment for them.

Emotional dimension The range of emotional expression in persons who somatize is broad. The nurse works with clients who have the ability to be consciously aware of their feelings and emotional responses and with those persons who are far removed from realizing, understanding, or accurately expressing their feelings. The client's present symptoms may evolve from the individual's current life-style or be related to very early traumatic experiences that the client has suppressed (see the research highlight on p. 400). Therefore it is important both to listen to the client's description of feelings and to observe the expression of feelings. Conflicting data may give important clues to appropriate intervention.

One of the client's most significant problems is learning how to identify and develop more effective modes of coping with generalized anxiety. Generalized anxiety is reflected by physiological measures such as elevated blood pressure, tense muscles, and exaggerated reflex responses to environmental stimuli. Anxiety can also be expressed indirectly through anger, irritability, and frustration. Persons with significant disabling symptoms over time also may respond with depression, grief, and despair (see Chapter 14).

The major emotions associated with most somatization disorders are negative, such as anger and anxiety. Observing the client in a variety of situations helps to determine what causes these feelings. Listening to descriptions of the client's daily activities and relationships is another source of data. The client may be overcommitted or responsible for too many others, believe that others do not care, or long for more attention or affection. These feelings may be expressed through hostile or sarcastic humor rather than directly.

Table 19-3 lists some of the common feelings and personality traits associated with specific psychosomatic disorders. Much of the available data indicate that emotional expressions related to any one disorder can range from seriously distorted to quite normal, and there is considerable debate about whether the emotional difficulties of the client existed before the onset of the physical health condition or whether they resulted from the physical health condition itself. Psychosomatic disorders may be chronic, painful, debilitating, and socially restricting, such as is the case for rheumatoid arthritis. These factors alone can contribute to distorted emotional responses, for example, overreation or hostility. Therefore if a client has been ill for an extended period, it may be useful to consider and even discuss with the client and family members, the emotional impact and changes since the first onset of symptoms.

It is critical to recognize that certain of the conditions described in Table 19-3 should be considered *somatopsychic* conditions rather than psychosomatic. For example, thyroid disorders can result from several different causes, including viruses; that is, the condition results from a somatic illness. In these cases, there may be clear changes

RESEARCH HIGHLIGHT

Childhood Sexual Histories of Women With Somatization Disorder

• J Morrison

PURPOSE

The purpose of this research was to determine whether the childhood sexual experiences of women with somatization disorder was different from persons without this disorder. Women with somatization disorder have a high rate of sexual dysfunction and unhappy marriages.

SAMPLE

Ninety-one subjects participated in the study. Sixty subjects with somatization disorder were recruited from a psychiatric practice. Another 31 women diagnosed with primary affective disorders were used as a comparison group. The subjects were matched on the basis of race, age, and level of education.

METHODOLOGY

All subjects were first interviewed by the researcher. A second, structured interview was then conducted by a female research assistant. This interview was detailed and structured to obtain all data needed to establish a psychiatric diagnosis. Student's T-test and Fisher's exact test were used to evaluate differences between groups.

Based on data from *American Journal of Psychiatry* 146(2):239, 1989.

FINDINGS

Comparison between the two groups indicated that subjects with somatization disorder began sexual activity somewhat earlier than those with affective disorders. Both groups experienced menarche and learned about sex at about the same age and had similar sources of sex education. A history of unwarranted sexual contact during childhood, with or without intercourse, was found significantly more often in somatization disorder subjects. The average age at the time of sexual molestation was 10. Over 25% of subjects with somatization disorder had been sexually abused by more than one person. Subjects with somatization disorder were much less likely to report the ability to reach climax with intercourse in their present adult sexual relationships.

IMPLICATIONS

This research concurs with the few other existing studies that also reported a higher rate of sexual abuse in persons with somatization disorder. Childhood sexual abuse is also found in other diagnostic groups such as multiple personality disorder, chronic psychosis, post-traumatic stress disorder, and borderline personality disorder. Further study is needed to determine the specific ways in which childhood sexual abuse influences later emotional problems.

---

in emotional responses and sometimes evidence of organic mental changes. Many of the symptoms of psychiatric disorder dissipate when appropriate physical treatment is initiated. However, some personality changes may remain for many months or sometimes result in permanent personality changes.

Self-expectations for controlling emotions may be high. The individual may experience jealousy or anger but consider it weak to express such feelings, and if expressed, there is an accompanying sense of guilt. Both the holding in of emotions and the feeling of guilt for expressing feelings can lead to psychological distress that is ultimately expressed through body symptoms. Another manifestation of high self-expectations is excessive competitiveness. Friends and family members may describe the individual as a perfectionist, unwilling to accept anything that is not done perfectly. The person's usual emotional expressions, such as angry outbursts, crying, or admitting disappointment, are thought to be not only irrational but also personal failures. This can lead to a high level of generalized anxiety, which is expressed through the body. Social norms dictate what is within the realm of appropriate emotional behavior. Clients will need assistance to find the balance that is healthy for them and within that which is considered acceptable.

One of the common emotional responses to chronic physical discomfort and somatic symptoms is depression.

The client may use self-derogatory comments to discuss feelings of sadness and helplessness. The belief that one is unable to cope, expressed directly or indirectly, is often another sign of acute or chronic depression, which must be treated in conjunction with other illnesses. Assessment of the degree of depression and potential for suicide is essential (see Chapter 14).

◤ **Intellectual dimension** Psychophysiological illnesses usually do not have a direct impact on the individual's intellectual capacity or cognitive abilities. Occasionally, however, cognitive functions are compromised by an acute medical crisis or a chronic degenerative process. Symptoms then are similar to organic mental disorders (see Chapter 33), or the person may develop psychotic symptoms; and sometimes, with more severe brain damage, coma ensues. In addition to determining the medical and organic processes, the most significant aspects of the intellectual dimension to be assessed are the client's:

1. Knowledge about the disorder
2. Understanding of the disorder
3. Decision-making processes
4. Cognitive processes used in coping

Knowledge about the disorder refers to the client's information about the illness, that is, what changes may occur or have already taken place in the body and the potential or real limitations these impose. It is helpful to discuss the long-term implications of the specific health condition with the individual, allowing opportunity for discussion of alternatives and options. Clients with somatoform disorders may strongly persist with the belief that the condition is purely physical, which greatly complicates working with them on an intellectual level, thus helping these clients understand the complicated psychological and biological interactions may be time-consuming and require considerable repetition. These clients may also become very angry and rejecting of care providers. They imply or franky state dissatisfaction with the medical system and the care provided.

Understanding of the disorder involves what the client believes to be the cause or causes. Typically, the client has some basic knowledge about the effect of the disease process on the body. Assessment determines the advisability of providing more information to the client. For some persons, this increases their anxiety and use of defense mechanisms; for others, it facilitates their interest in managing the disease and contributes to self-care practices. It is probably helpful to give the client limited amounts of information at any given time to gradually increase their knowledge and then provide opportunities for review of information on a regular basis.

Clients' understanding of the disorder is influenced by their individual decision-making approaches and the cognitive processes used in coping. Clients with psychosomatic disorders typically are constant worriers. They may put off important life-style changes, or they may selectively exclude data that do not fit into the client's coping plan. For example, the client may use rationalization or denial to ignore, minimize, or dispute data suggesting that emotional responses are in any way related to physical symptoms, especially if admitting such data means drastically altering one's self-concept or learning a new way to relate to one's environment is implied. Understanding the client's intellectual style and cognitive processes helps the nurse develop a more effective teaching plan.

Denial is common, especially if the psychophysiological condition is not observable but either requires making major life changes or influences the person's view of self. For instance, denial can be readily recognized in the person who has had a myocardial infarction who does not follow the prescribed treatment and acts as if nothing has changed. Other clients are directly confronted with the physical realities of an illness, such as immobility of joints or learning to manage a colostomy. In spite of the very real nature of these physical changes, clients may still successfully deny that these events have taken place and develop rationalizations for why they cannot continue as they have in the past. Such rationalizations may include refusal to learn the necessary self-care skills for independent functioning.

Social dimension Assessing the social dimension with the client establishes what aspects of work life, family life, friends, and community involvement are creating stress sufficient to cause illness. Interpersonal relationships are usually the most significant aspects, both for creating stress and for healing. Establishing what life-style changes are necessary is also an important goal.

How an individual's personality interacts with employment demands can be an essential element in stress. Significant assessment questions to ask include the following:
1. Does the client consider reasonable the demands, expectations, and workload?
2. Is there a possibility of loss of job?
3. Are job responsibilities and expectations in keeping with the client's skills and intellectual capacity?
4. Are there conflicts with a supervisor or manager that prove difficult for the client?
5. What, if any, satisfaction is obtained from employment?
6. Are financial rewards reasonable, and do they meet client's needs and expectations?

Other sources of interpersonal stress in the work place may come from sexual harassment, ridicule, or other forms of abusive behavior. Support, understanding, and friendship from co-workers may be essential to job satisfaction for some individuals. For instance, one young woman began to complain that her job in a factory had become "too stressful," ostensibly because a procedure on the assembly line had been changed. Further exploration revealed that an older employee had resigned. This worker had been a significant buffer, protecting the young woman from intimidation by other co-workers. Without her, the job was no longer satisfying to the young woman, as relationships with other employees deteriorated.

Some clients may have been unemployed for an extended period of time. As a result social contacts, a sense of self-worth, and fulfillment all may have diminished. Furthermore, financial problems are almost always a concern of the unemployed. A drastic change in life-style frequently accompanies long periods of unemployment. Due to lack of money, the individual may have to change or give up social activities, such as regular aerobics classes, playing golf, or bowling. Each of these changes multiplies and further destabilizes the individual's interpersonal environment.

Disturbed interpersonal relationships may contribute to the client's maintenance of symptoms once they are established. The nurse can assess these relationships through discussions with the client, but discussions with family members and close friends may be necessary as well. Sometimes significant others are more able than the individual client to describe changes over time. A family evaluation, during which the client and family members are interviewed together, may be required to determine troublesome patterns of interaction. Family and marital assessment, as described in Chapters 29 and 30, is applicable to this client group.

Finding a satisfying balance of interdependence with others can be a source of unconscious conflict, especially for persons with somatoform disorders. The wish for dependency cannot be acknowledged, but the consequence of having chronic medical complaints is the socially acceptable opportunity to ask someone to be interested and give care. However, these wishes are unconscious and are usually denied if the topic is broached. The conflict of striving for independence, accompanied by the wish to be dependent, can be "acted out" through the development of a real physical illness. Being sick allows the adult to be cared for in a socially acceptable way, but the person may still express anger and resentment for needing the care.

Table 19-3 describes some of the social and environmental conditions relevant for specific diseases. One of the more common themes for persons who become ill is the impact of losses, especially the loss of significant others in the year preceding illness. The assessment of loss includes exploring the meaning of losing intimacy, such as affection, concern, touching, and sexual intercourse, as well as losing practical supports, such as fixing the car, paying the bills, doing the dishes, or cooking the meals.

Community involvement can be stressful if it is either too much or too little. Some persons become so overinvolved in church, civic, and social clubs that these activities, intended as a source of pleasure, become liabilities. Illness becomes a way to lessen the involvement. At the opposite extreme are other clients who are totally isolated from developing friends or participating in community life, which may be a personality style or a consequence of the debilitating symptoms. Determining the cause of social isolation will provide data about possible solutions. It is most important to determine how the individual views his involvement with the community and consider these relationships as part of the overall picture in making an adjustment.

The nature of the community may be a significant factor in psychophysiological illnesses. Neighborhoods with a high incidence of crime or much traffic or noise can be stressful, although those living there do not realize it. The nurse also examines factors such as the frequency of moves from community to community, a change in socioeconomic status, or the client's wish to modify his life-style. These factors may influence the stability of the client's social network, create unexpected problems with adaptation, and require making new friends.

The client's life-style and habits arising from personal interests and the social network may contribute to a psychophysiological illness. Excessive use of alcohol, smoking, or use of illegal drugs negatively influence health. Assessing the client's use of leisure time will yield important data about the degree of physical activity, the need for competitive interactions, and the ease of adjusting to new environmental demands and making new friends.

Spiritual dimension Personal beliefs and values contribute to the individual's understanding of the environment and help give life meaning. They contribute in conscious and unconscious ways to establishing a life-style, determining a hierarchy of importance for life demands, and providing the guiding principles on which to make choices. Existential beliefs, such as faith in God, fate, or some other higher authority, contribute to maintaining hope and giving meaning to life. Although these personal beliefs usually are helpful, they can become a source of stress when clients cannot reconcile their behaviors with their belief system or when others' expectations and demands are contrary to clients' interpretation of right and wrong.

Assessment of the client's values and value conflicts may best be completed indirectly. Often clients are aware of feeling stressed but do not relate this directly to their beliefs. Acting contrary to the belief system may lead to feelings of guilt, personal condemnation, or even hopelessness. Sometimes careful listening to details of a client's problem with strategically placed questions from the nurse helps clients become aware of and begin to understand these conflicts. Clients may realize they are questioning the validity of beliefs and values they previously took for granted. Resolution of these value conflicts may contribute significantly to improved physical health.

When others' expectations and demands do not fit into the client's view of proper behavior and actions, he may be faced with giving up long-held beliefs, learning to live with the conflicts, or modifying the source of unacceptable expectations and demands (for example, changing jobs, moving to another community, becoming divorced). Sometimes the client is unaware of the source of the conflict or ways to resolve it and responds with hopelessness, powerlessness, and despair.

These situations can trigger a spiritual crisis. Assessing these conflicts and determining how the client usually fulfills his spiritual needs can be valuable to planning the client's care.

The use of nonmedical healing techniques has become increasingly common as the traditional view of the mind/body dichotomy is challenged and as the success of high technology techniques fail to cure chronic diseases such as most somatization disorders. According to McGuire,[55] at least four forms of healing rely on an alternative understanding of the nature and etiology of illness: Christian healing, Eastern meditation or human potential groups, traditional metaphysical groups, and psychic and occult groups. Clients may already be involved with one of these forms of healing, which focus on a more holistic philosophy of human beings, relying on various ways to make meaning out of physical symptoms and suffering. Many of these forms of healing have been considered quackery by medical practitioners, so clients may be hesitant to discuss their beliefs. It is becoming more common for some persons to use both the technical advances of Western medicine in conjunction with another form of therapy, such as prayer groups, meditation, or yoga. Assessing the client's actual beliefs about causes, methods of diagnosis, and effective treatments is essential for a collaborative and successful working relationship.

Analysis
Nursing diagnosis

Ineffective individual coping is an example of a nursing diagnosis approved by NANDA,[61] which applies to clients with somatization disorders. The defining characteristics of this nursing diagnosis are listed in the box. Several other diagnoses could also apply, depending on the client's unique problems. Some examples include pain, disturbance in self-esteem, impaired social interaction, self-care deficit, dysfunctional grieving, and impaired physical mobility.

The following case example demonstrates the characteristics of the nursing diagnosis of ineffective individual coping.

▼ Case Example

Elaine, a 31-year-old single woman, was brought to the emergency department yesterday by ambulance. She had severe epigastric pain, vomited "a brown liquid," and had been having "black, soft stools for several days." Endoscopy revealed a gastric ulcer, and she was admitted for further treatment.

Elaine had lost her job as a typist about 5 months ago after missing many days because of severe headache, allergies, and "premenstrual tension" that involved irritability, crying, abdominal cramps and swelling, fatigue, and back pain. She had seen three physicians in the past year and had undergone many tests to de-

DEFINITION

The impairment of adaptive behaviors and problem-solving abilities of a person in meeting life's demands and roles.

DEFINING CHARACTERISTICS

- **Physical dimension**

  Nonperformance of activities of daily living
  Hypervigilance pattern
  Unconflicted inertia pattern
  Unconflicted change pattern

- **Emotional dimension**

  Unhappiness
  Hopelessness

- **Intellectual dimension**

  Lack of future orientation
  Self-absorption
  Inflexibility
  Clear and frequent expressions of pessimism
  Excessive use of denial

- **Social dimension**

  Overdependence on significant others, on professional help, or on institutions
  Nonproductive life-style
  Lack of functioning in usual social roles
  Continuance of escape-avoidance behavior
  Defense avoidance pattern
  Unconcerned and detached from usual social supports
  Refusal or rejection of help
  Noncompliance

- **Spiritual dimension**

  Purposelessness
  Quality of life not acceptable to person

Modified from McFarland G, McFarlane E: *Nursing diagnosis and intervention: planning for patient care,* ed 2, St Louis, 1993, Mosby–Year Book.

termine the cause of the allergic reaction and find an explanation for her "premenstrual tension." Outcomes of the tests revealed that she was allergic to house dust. The results of a 24-hour urine test showed mildly elevated corticosteroid levels, consistent with ovarian cysts. Oral estrogens were prescribed, but according to Elaine, "they did not help." She is angry with the physicians for not helping her feel better.

In addition, Elaine's 73-year-old mother had fallen and broken a hip about 2 months ago and was recently placed in a nursing home. Elaine and her mother cannot afford the nursing home, but Elaine is unable to decide if she can care for her mother at home. Today she said to the nurse, "I can't cope with all of these problems, I don't know what to do."

The following list provides examples of NANDA-accepted nursing diagnoses with causative statements for this case:

1. High risk for self-esteem disturbances related to role change

2. Dysfunctional grieving related to altered relationship with mother

3. Anxiety related to fear of living alone

4. Ineffective individual coping related to excessive uncontrolled internal anger

Planning

The planning phase of the nursing process for clients with psychosomatic and somatoform disorders is unique for each individual since the expression of health problems is very individually based and the expression of the health problems can vary greatly. Planning for care emerges directly from the nursing assessment. The medical diagnoses of the physical and psychiatric conditions are also considered in developing a nursing care plan during the planning phase. The nursing care plan (Table 19-4) provides examples of long- and short-term goals, outcome criteria, interventions, and rationales related to somatization. These serve as examples of the planning stage of the nursing process.

Implementation

Physical dimension The first intervention for clients with somatization disorders is to evaluate and treat the physical symptoms. Many clients are seen in an acute or even life-threatening state, so diagnosis and determining an initial plan of care are carried out quickly. A thorough physical examination with routine laboratory studies provides the initial basis for decisions. Specific procedures such as x-ray films, cardiac catheterizations, endoscopy, and proctoscopy may be necessary. The nurse explains these procedures to the client, telling him what to anticipate, why the test is being performed, and what may be learned from it. Such explanations facilitate the client's understanding and decrease anxiety and fear. The nurse needs to be available to respond to the client's questions and uses these opportunities to discover how much the client knows about the condition.

Some psychosomatic disorders require surgical procedures. Certain conditions require urgent surgery, but more often surgery is anticipated and planned in advance. This time with the client can be used for preoperative teaching and to prepare the client physically and psychologically. The aspect of care usually occurs in the general hospital, where the psychiatric nurse may be consulted. However, the inpatient or outpatient psychiatric nurse often discusses these issues with the client before general hospital admission.

As a result of the surgical procedure or the disease process, the client needs assistance to cope with changes in body image. For example, the client with rheumatoid arthritis notes changes in body size and shape accompanied by pain and loss of function. The nurse assists clients to examine realistically the meaning and impact of such changes. Some clients prefer to deny these changes and persist with attempts to do tasks that can cause further harm. A gentle approach aimed at helping the client gradually understand the reality of the limitations allows the client to make a psychological adjustment while learning new behaviors. At the other extreme, inadequate adjust-

▼ **TABLE 19-4** **NURSING CARE PLAN**

GOALS	OUTCOME CRITERIA	INTERVENTIONS	RATIONALES
NURSING DIAGNOSIS: Ineffective individual coping related to inability to deal effectively with conflicts as evidenced in multiple physical complaints			
LONG TERM			
To cope with conflicts with fewer symptoms	Verbalizes relationship between conflict and symptoms		
	Demonstrates appropriate coping skills in response to conflict		
SHORT TERM			
To express fewer symptoms	Has fewer symptoms	Acknowledge symptoms without undue emphasis	To show empathy for client's discomfort with focus on person, not symptoms
To use new coping skills for handling conflict	Uses new coping skills effectively	Teach new coping skills; assertiveness, relaxation, exercise, talking with supportive person	To promote healthy ways to handle conflicts that do not cause behavioral symptoms
To gain an understanding of relationship between conflict and physical symptoms	States relationship of physical symptoms to psychological conflict	Help client express feelings about conflicts	To identify feelings and gather data about factors that may contribute to symptoms

ment to a change in self-image is also seen in the client who refuses to participate in any aspects of self-care. Such clients need assistance to discuss their reactions. A behavioral approach that reinforces the client in gradually taking over a self-care activity may be effective.

Another concern for the client is how significant others will react to the physical changes, especially if the client's body is obviously distorted. Clients with alterations in some body areas or physical functions that are considered sensitive in most cultures, such as persons with colostomies and ileostomies, may also be greatly concerned and have serious difficulty adjusting. The client must adapt to these changes and learn new procedures to manage elimination. Persons intimately involved with the client must adjust to the changes as well.

Sexual problems may develop as a result of body changes. The client and significant others may feel embarrassment and shame because they cannot adapt to body alterations. Other reasons for sexual problems may be related to a lack of desire because of generalized pain, chronic discomfort, or restrictions of flexibility and ease of movement. Treatment of the underlying cause, such as the use of analgesics for pain, is a helpful first step. If problems are not resolved, however, further evaluation may necessitate referral to sex therapy or marital counseling.

A common medical intervention is the prescription of one or more medications specific to disease symptoms. The nurse needs to be familiar with the medication regimen and sufficiently knowledgeable to assess the expected effects. The nurse identifies side effects; allergic or other untoward effects, medication and food interactions; and the combined effects of several medications, alcohol, and food. Teaching the client about the medication regimen, including the schedule, effects, and precautions, is an important nursing responsibility that provides an opportunity to educate the client, perhaps improve compliance, and obtain data for other interventions. Some physical interventions will have little immediate impact and require more time before changes are apparent. The nurse encourages the client to stay with the treatment. Another problem that may be encountered with some clients is addiction to medications (for example, Librium) that have been used for pain management. The accompanying profile for chlordiazepoxide (Librium) describes nursing care appropriate to its administration. Psychological techniques for management of addictive behaviors (see Chapter 18) and teaching alternatives to pain management (see Chapter 20) are then implemented.

Certain physiological problems, such as insomnia or discomfort, may not be related to the specific disease process. Rather, they may be responses to factors such as the physical environment, generalized anxiety, or fear of the unknown. The client is encouraged to discuss the responses before alternative measures are implemented, as this discussion may be sufficient to resolve the problem. Pawlick and Heitkemper[63] have described behavioral approaches to

CHLORDIAZEPOXIDE HCl

(klor-dye-az-e-pox'ide)
A-poxide, Libritabs, Librium, Medilium,* Novopoxide,* Relaxil, Solium,* Lipoxide, SK-Lygen
Func class: Antianxiety
Chem class: Benzodiazepine

Controlled Substance Schedule IV
Action: Depresses subcortical levels of CNS, including limbic system, reticular formation
Uses: Short-term management of anxiety, acute alcohol withdrawal, preoperatively for relaxation
Dosage and routes:
Mild anxiety
▶ *Adult:* PO 5-10 mg tid-qid
▶ *Child >6 yr:* 5 mg bid-qid, not to exceed 10 mg bid-tid
Severe anxiety
▶ *Adult:* PO 20-25 mg tid-qid
Preoperatively
▶ *Adult:* PO 5-10 mg tid-qid on day before surgery; IM 50-100 mg 1 hr before surgery
Alcohol withdrawal
▶ *Adult:* PO/IM/IV 50-100 mg, not to exceed 300 mg/day
Available forms include: Caps 5, 10, 25 mg; tabs 5, 10, 25 mg; powder for IM inj 100 mg

Side effects/adverse reactions:
CNS: Dizziness, drowsiness, confusion, headache, anxiety, tremors, stimulation, fatigue, depression, insomnia, hallucinations
GI: Constipation, dry mouth, nausea, vomiting, anorexia, diarrhea
INTEG: Rash, dermatitis, itching
CV: Orthostatic hypotension, **ECG changes, tachycardia,** hypotension
EENT: Blurred vision, tinnitus, mydriasis
Contraindications: Hypersensitivity to benzodiazepines, narrow-angle glaucoma, psychosis, pregnancy (D), child <18 yr
Precautions: Elderly, debilitated, hepatic disease, renal disease
Pharmacokinetics:
PO: Onset 30 min, peak ½ hr, duration 4-6 hr, metabolized by liver, excreted by kidneys, crosses placenta, breast milk, half-life 5-30 hr
Interactions/incompatibilities:
—Decreased effects of chlordiazepoxide: oral contraceptives, rifampin, valproic acid
—Increased effects of chlordiazepoxide: CNS depressants, alcohol, cimetidine, disulfiram, oral contraceptives

NURSING CONSIDERATIONS

Assess:
—B/P (lying, standing), pulse; if systolic B/P drops 20 mm Hg, hold drug, notify physician

—Blood studies: CBC during long-term therapy; blood dyscrasias have occurred rarely
—Hepatic studies: AST, ALT, bilirubin, creatinine, LDH, alk phosphatase
—I&O; may indicate renal dysfunction
—For ataxia, oversedation in elderly, debilitated clients
Administer:
—By IV 5 ml saline 100 mg/powder, agitate ampule gently; do not use IM diluent for IV use
—With food or milk for GI symptoms
—Crushed if client is unable to swallow medication whole
—Sugarless gum, hard candy, frequent sips of water for dry mouth
Perform/provide:
—Assistance with ambulation during beginning therapy, since drowsiness/dizziness occurs
—Safety measure, including side rails
—Check to see PO medication has been swallowed
Evaluate:
—Therapeutic response: decreased anxiety, restlessness, sleeplessness
—Mental status: mood, sensorium, affect, sleeping pattern, drowsiness, dizziness

—Physical dependency, withdrawal symptoms: headache, nausea, vomiting, muscle pain, weakness after long-term use
—Suicidal tendencies, paradoxical reactions such as excitement, stimulation, and acute rage
Teach client/family:
—That drug may be taken with food
—Not to be used for everyday stress or used longer than 4 mo, unless directed by physician
—Not to take more than prescribed amount, may be habit-forming
—To avoid OTC preparations unless approved by physician
—To avoid driving, activities that require alertness; drowsiness may occur
—To avoid alcohol ingestion or other psychotropic medications, unless prescribed by physician
—Not to discontinue medication abruptly after long-term use, may precipitate convulsions
—To rise slowly or fainting may occur
—That drowsiness might worsen at beginning of treatment
Lab test interferences:
Increase: AST/ALT, serum bilirubin
False increase: 17-OHCS
Decrease: RAIU
Treatment of overdose: Lavage, VS, supportive care

*Available in Canada only.
Italic indicates common side effects.
Bold italic indicates life-threatening reactions.

Modified from Skidmore-Roth L: *Mosby's nursing drug reference,* St Louis, 1993, Mosby–Year Book.

---

the management of insomnia. These approaches include keeping a diary of sleep patterns, eliminating sleep outside of normal nocturnal patterns, going to bed and getting up at the same time each day, increasing physical exercise, and reducing caffeine intake.

Emotional dimension Clients need help to identify their unique emotional responses. The nurse can facilitate this process through careful listening and reflection. Identifying and exploring sensitive issues may help clients consider the interrelationships between feeling states and physical symptoms. Until clients accept that emotional states can be related to physical symptoms, they will probably give little credence to important techniques of stress management and evaluating factors that lead to psychological discomfort.

The nurse can teach the client several stress management techniques that will help control severe anxiety. Relaxation techniques and guided imagery encourage positive thinking, support the client's use of self-control measures, and modify the neuroendocrine response system. These techniques, once learned, are readily available to the client in any environment. Other relaxation techniques, such as various forms of meditation and biofeedback, are helpful for some persons. The nurse can explain the essential elements of these techniques and help interested clients seek the necessary resources. Special training or specialized equipment may limit the availability of these resources. Nonmedical interventions such as physical exercise, yoga, massage, and meditation are helpful to some individuals. Some evidence suggests that combining the emotional and cognitive aspects of a program of treatment with skill development of the various techniques may be more helpful than providing only one aspect alone (see the research highlight on p. 406).

Attempts to study the personality profile of persons with specific psychosomatic disorders suggest that certain emo-

RESEARCH HIGHLIGHT

A Study of the Effectiveness of Two Group Behavioral Medicine Interventions for Patients With Psychosomatic Complaints

• CJC Hellman, M Budd, J Borysenko, DC McCelland, and H Benson

PURPOSE

The study was designed to compare the effectiveness of three group treatments. Two similar versions of behavioral medicine interventions that included teaching mind/body relationships, relaxation-response training, awareness training, and cognitive restructuring were compared with a group that focused exclusively on information about stress.

SAMPLE

Subjects were adult (age range from 20 to 73) patients at a Health Maintenance Organization (HMO) referred for psychological treatment because the primary care provider believed psychosocial factors played an important role in generating the presenting symptoms. Of 116 patients called, 80 patients participated in the research study, but only 63 were part of the final data analysis due to missing data and dropouts. The researchers considered subjects to be typical of high users of primary care services at the HMO.

METHODOLOGY

Subjects were randomly assigned to one of three treatment groups. Treatment interventions consisted of the behavioral medicine groups that met 1 and ½ hours weekly for 6 weeks and the education group that met 1 and ½ hours for 2 times, separated by a 2-week interval. Pretreatment and posttreatment measures were the following: num-

ber of physical symptoms, level of psychological distress, and number of visits to the HMO. Posttreatment measures were taken 6 months after the intervention. Analysis of variance and covariance was used to examine the data.

FINDINGS

Generally, there was a greater reduction in physical symptoms, level of psychological distress, and number of visits to the HMO in the behavioral medicine groups than in the education-only group. The greatest reduction in health care visits occurred in subjects who had a reduction in physical symptoms as a response to the intervention. More than half of subjects not experiencing a reduction in physical symptoms did not reduce the number of visits for health care. In contrast, less psychological distress did not lead to a reduction in health care visits.

IMPLICATIONS

This study suggests that including interventions in which the subject has the opportunity to practice various techniques can help the individual to learn to decrease physiological arousal through the use of relaxation techniques. Addressing the relationships among thoughts, behaviors, and symptoms may be more beneficial than providing education alone.

Based on data from *Behavioral Medicine* 16(4): 165, 1990.

---

tional expressions may be responses to the illness and long periods of disabling symptoms rather than the result of preexisting character traits. Nevertheless, responses such as depression, guilt, and despair interfere with adequate coping. These symptoms may become severe enough to be identified as primary problems requiring specific interventions. The treatment often involves long-term psychotherapy, which could be individual, group, or family therapy, depending on problem behaviors. Psychotherapy can help clients learn to understand psychological traumas that occurred earlier in life. It is a useful intervention for somatoform disorders, especially conversion disorder. Supportive group interventions encourage the expression of troublesome emotions in an accepting environment. This type of intervention can be valuable for clients who fear rejection or lack of understanding from their family and friends. Some individuals find supportive groups through self-help movements, such as ostomy groups or arthritis groups, or through religion.

Intellectual dimension Because the client's intellectual and cognitive functions are essentially intact, the nurse usually focuses on assessing knowledge deficits and implementing appropriate teaching plans. Teaching plans are developed to address the client's specific needs. Besides intellectual capacity, the nurse considers the client's physical and emotional state. High levels of anxiety, for example,

are known to decrease retention of information. The most effective teaching plans support the individual's active involvement in the recovery and rehabilitation process. The nurse provides specific information and at the same time addresses the emotional and social components related to the factual data. The timing of interventions to match the client's interest or curiosity also facilitates learning.

The etiology of most somatization disorders is complex, and the specific mechanisms leading to particular symptoms are often poorly understood by both medical professionals and clients alike. Therefore the nurse does not overwhelm the client with too much information or discussion of complex and confusing theories. A simple and clear explanation is best. It may be helpful to let the client know that some things are poorly understood. The nurse can develop interesting ways to raise the client's interest in the health and illness process and then gradually present information as the client's knowledge base expands. The ultimate aim is to help the client realize that heredity, diet, life-style, stressful events, emotional responses, and social interactions can affect health states. With this knowledge, clients may begin to formulate their own care plan and strategies to reduce or resolve stressors.

The need for medical regimens such as exercise programs, dietary restrictions, or medication schedules makes more sense to clients if they understand the disease process.

Because the client may view some medical regimens (for example, hypertension medications) as more troublesome than helpful—that is, they are associated with more problems than positive gains—understanding the rationale may enhance compliance. As the complexity of the interventions increases, the more important it becomes for clients to understand the rationale for the interventions.

The nurse can choose from a broad range of behavioral and educational approaches to complement physical interventions. Some techniques of stress management can be taught effectively (see Chapter 10). Combining psychotherapy with other methods of stress reduction may be the most beneficial (see research highlight, p. 406). Other methods, such as relaxation techniques, can be taught by the nurse on an individual basis. The nurse can make specific referrals for the client interested in biofeedback, meditation, or acupuncture. The nurse explains to the client that, although these techniques can be helpful, they are not always effective; and not everyone is willing or able to fit them into daily activities. However, effectiveness may depend on the client's attitude and willingness to try different approaches. The nurse may need to assist the client in developing a plan that includes these interventions as a way to modify certain life-style factors.

Understanding the client's use of defense mechanisms in coping with emotional responses facilitates reinforcing effective ones and modifying unhelpful ones. The nurse determines how to modify the client's cognitive appraisal (subjective interpretation) of situations and events. The nurse may offer alternative interpretations to a client's description of events that may not be as anxiety producing. Offering alternatives helps the client develop new patterns of assessing situations without directly confronting ineffective coping behavior. Directly confronting clients' style of coping can further escalate their anxiety responses by leaving them vulnerable and psychologically unable to defend themselves.

Social dimension Interpersonal relationships can provide personal fulfillment or be a source of great stress. The nurse first identifies the client's social network and the significant positive or troublesome relationships. Then the nurse and client can begin to evaluate what changes are needed. Whenever possible, the nurse encourages the client to make decisions regarding treatment by providing information and allowing the client to choose a course of action.

Conflicts from interpersonal relationships may evolve from the person's view of self. To relate well to others, persons must have self-worth and believe they have positive traits and characteristics. Clients, particularly those with long-term disabling symptoms, may have little self-worth. The nurse can work with the client to identify the positive interpersonal traits and styles of relating, such as a sense of humor, thoughtfulness, or interest in another's ideas. Observing the client with significant others followed by a discussion with the client can help the nurse identify how the client distorts or misperceives the relationship. Comments from the nurse describing the positive qualities observed may initiate the client's redefinition of self. Often a negative sense of self arises from problems in early childhood relationships. In-depth exploration of these is best managed by long-term individual psychotherapy.

If the locus of control remains with the client, it provides some independence, even while the client is dependent in other respects. The nurse and the client discuss the realistic aspects of dependence. For instance, the person severely crippled by rheumatoid arthritis realistically may not be able to get to the bathroom alone, but resulting angry and resentful feelings only increase relationship tensions and the stress level. Behavioral approaches may help the client intellectually determine which dependence issues are "worthy" of the response and which are not. The nurse then supports the client's implementation of these decisions (see Chapter 16).

Symptoms of physical illness tend to gradually narrow or change the client's cultural roles and network of social supports. The client's central support network and role identity may slowly shift away from work and family into illness roles and reliance on health professionals for support. The nurse is actively involved with the client and family to help them maintain normal role behavior. Serious interpersonal problems in the client's family life may require resolution, which may involve terminating or drastically changing significant relationships. In addition to family or marital therapy, the nurse can encourage the client to develop new support systems when necessary by joining church groups, adult education classes, community activity groups, or special interest groups.

Sources of stress in the work place include environmental factors, difficult interpersonal relationships, or the type of work. Once the sources of stress and anxiety have been identified, the client may want assistance in determining a plan of action. For example, if the stress results from unavoidable environmental pollutants, the client may need to decide between continuing exposure to the health risks and finding another job. The nurse encourages the client to resolve these questions through discussion with significant others. The client's family and friends are often the most important source of assistance in alleviating stress from the work itself. The nurse teaches the client that certain life-style changes can help reduce stress by exploring with the client areas of stress and ways to reduce or alleviate them.

Maintaining social contacts away from work, developing hobbies or learning new skills, and following an exercise program divert the client's preoccupation with work problems. Assertiveness training may help the client cope better with difficult workplace relationships, especially if these relationships are the only problem area. More generalized interpersonal problems usually require psychotherapy.

The nurse also should consider self-help groups and other supportive group approaches for clients with somatization disorders. Specific support groups such as ostomy clubs allow members to share feelings, advice, and practical ways of coping. Discovering that others share similar problems reduces loneliness and the feelings of alienation while providing emotional support to cope with the problems. For example, Levitt and others[52] describe a support group for women with premenstrual syndrome, which focuses on helping clients increase their self-control. Self-help or support groups may be available in the community or at local mental health facilities or hospitals. The nurse who identifies a need but cannot find a specific group for a specific client may consider developing one.

▼ **KEY INTERVENTIONS**

Treat the physical symptoms without undue emphasis

Focus on the person, not the symptoms

Help client express feelings about sensitive issues

Teach stress management

Provide psychotherapy, group therapy

Provide information on the disease process, ways one's life-style and responses to stress effect health and illness

Offer alternative interpretations to client's description of events

Identify troublesome relationships at home, at work

Divert client's preoccupation with symptoms by developing new skills, hobbies

Reduce secondary gains of "sick role"

Refer to supportive self-help groups

Spiritual dimension Clients may be confused about their belief system, or they may recognize inconsistencies between behavior and their beliefs or values. Identifying this stress may be a key in determining an overall treatment program. Discussion of the client's beliefs and values does not necessarily involve the client's religious affiliation. Sick persons often ponder existential questions about the meaning of life or one's responsibility for behaviors, actions, and physical condition. These questions intensify if the individual begins to consider the possibility that a person has some control over physical symptoms. Thus helping the client understand that he can choose feelings and behavior is an essential intervention.

Troublesome spiritual conflicts are usually unconscious and difficult to verbalize, as many beliefs and values developed early in life from unquestioned social and cultural influences. Life experiences can expose the client to unfamiliar ways of thinking and behaving that challenge previously learned beliefs. Sometimes clarifying the conflict is sufficient to resolve it.

Illness as punishment for misbehavior is a common theme; the client may feel guilt for known or unknown misbehaviors. Beyond this, the client may ask, "Why me?," "Why now?," or "What value is my life?" This may reflect confusion about the validity of long-held beliefs and values, and the client may be ready to change his basic approach to life. For example, the client may begin to consider that an intimate relationship is more valuable than earning a lot of money or that good health should be highly valued. Patterns such as constant striving for power or control may be modified. The client may realize the mental and physical "expense" of these wishes when compared to satisfying needs through less demanding alternatives.

The nurse provides a stable, open-minded approach to the client's examination of these questions. Providing feedback, the nurse helps clients draw their own conclusions and make decisions according to their own beliefs and values. The nurse's major task is to assist the client to attain peace of mind. See Table 19-4 for a sample nursing care plan and the accompanying boxes for key interventions and guidelines for primary and tertiary prevention.

Evaluation

Evaluation of nursing care is ongoing throughout the treatment process. The specific aspects of care evaluated

▼ **GUIDELINES FOR PRIMARY/TERTIARY PREVENTIONS**

Primary Prevention

Teach person to identify feelings experienced, positive and negative ways feelings are expressed; verbally, nonverbally, in physical symptoms

to understand he has choices in ways to respond to stress/conflicts

to adopt a healthy life-style with a balance among working, playing, and loving

to identify interactions among mind, body, and the environment and their effects on health and illness

to strengthen independent functioning

stress management/relation techniques

conflict resolution

problem solving

to have hobbies/interests and join in group activities that are stimulating and interesting

Teach family to prevent client's secondary gains from "sick" role

Tertiary Prevention
Community resources

Community mental health centers

Self-help groups

Ostomy groups

Headache groups

varies depending on client needs. Four general guidelines to consider when evaluating care are adequacy, appropriateness, effectiveness, and efficiency. To evaluate adequacy, one should consider whether symptoms were relieved and if the deterioration in physical status was sufficiently interrupted, which is especially important in the acute phase. During the recuperative phase, adequacy of care includes determining if the client has developed the self-care skills to manage the illness.

Appropriateness of care in some ways reflects the importance of timing. Were the necessary acute interventions performed immediately and well? Were measures instituted to explain procedures to the client and begin involvement in care at the initial stages? Were interventions targeted to the client's level of understanding and ability to participate?

Effectiveness of care addresses the degree to which presenting problems have been modified, based on the assessment and the initial plan of care, which should be realistic and specifically targeted to meet the most troublesome of the client's physical and psychological problems. One of the essential measures of effectiveness relates to the progress clients are able to make relative to understanding ways to identify and control stress levels.

Evaluating the efficiency of care relates to effective coordination of resources. For example, the nurse should discuss referral to a community support group (such as an ostomy club, Alcoholics Anonymous) as part of preparation for discharge rather than considering referral just before the client is to leave.

BRIEF REVIEW

Somatization is the manifestation of physical illness or physical symptoms in one or more major organ systems with or without physical pathology. A major factor in symptom development is the client's response to stress. This stress could be events in one's current life or may be based on psychologically and physically traumatic events that occurred earlier in life. How the illness manifests itself depends on genetic traits, personality, and the particular pattern of environmental stressors.

Possible mechanisms for somatization disorders have been studied for the past 60 years, but they have been the focus of concern and debate since antiquity. Freud described the process of repression and some of the possible outcomes of incomplete or failed repression of early childhood traumas. Other theories expanded and modified the psychoanalytical theories. Some theories proposed that the parts of the body affected later in life would be those relating to the specific developmental phase in which the psychological trauma occurred. Another theory suggested that a certain personality profile resulted in the development of specific disorders. Later approaches were represented by general systems theory, which recognized the interrelationships of body systems. New understanding about the neuroendocrine system and cognitive mechanisms in the cerebral cortex has led to complex theories about person-environment interactions.

The nurse uses these theoretical ideas in the assessment and management of clients with stress-related disorders. The nurse assesses symptoms and evaluates the client's emotional, social, intellectual, and spiritual components regarding conflicts and demands from sources of stress. Environmental factors are also assessed. The assessment leads to individualized interventions directed toward maximizing the client's effective coping potential. Establishing new coping patterns may require psychotherapy, behavioral techniques, education, and environmental changes.

The overall therapeutic goal is to minimize the client's stress response through changes in the environment and within the client. The physical environment or interpersonal relationships may be changed to decrease conflicts that have resulted in stress. The nurse also helps the client learn new ways of thinking, new approaches to problems, and techniques that influence biological responses to stress-producing events.

REFERENCES AND SUGGESTED READINGS

1. American Psychiatric Association: *Diagnostic and statistical manual of mental disorders (DSM-III-R)*, Washington, DC, 1987, The Association.
2. Alexander F, French TM, Pollock G: *Psychosomatic specificity: vol I, experimental study and results*, Chicago, vol 1, 1968, University of Chicago Press.
3. Axen DM: Chronic factitious disorders: helping those who hurt themselves, *Journal of Psychosocial Nursing* 23(3):19, 1986.
4. Baker G: On the affections of the mind and the diseases arising from them. In Hunter R, MacAlpine I, editors: *Three hundred years of psychiatry: 1535-1860,* New York, 1963, Oxford University Press.
5. Baker GHB: Life events before the onset of rheumatoid arthritis, *Psychotherapy and Psychosomatics* 38:173, 1982.
6. Besedovsky H and others: Hypothalamic changes during the immune response, *European Journal of Immunology* 7:323, 1977.
7. Burchfield SF, editor: *Stress: psychological and physiological interactions*, Washington, DC, 1985, Hemisphere Publishing Corp.
8. Campbell C: *Nursing diagnosis and intervention in nursing practice,* New York, 1978, John Wiley & Sons.
9. Cannon WB: *Bodily changes in pain, hunger, fear and rage,* ed 2, Boston, 1953, Charles T Branford Co.
10. Carroll-Johnson RM, editor: *Classification of nursing diagnoses; proceedings of the eighth conference,* Philadelphia, 1989, JB Lippincott.
11. Chess S, Thomas A: *Origins and evolution of behavior disorders,* New York, 1984, Brunner/Mazel Publishers.
12. Chess S, Thomas A: *Temperament in clinical practice,* New York, 1986, The Guilford Press.
13. Choi M, Steptoe A: Instructed heart rate control in the presence and absence of a distracting task: the effects of biofeedback training, *Biofeedback and Self-Regulation* 7(3):257, 1982.
14. Cohen S: Benzodiazepines in therapy, *Current Psychiatric Therapy* 22:111, 1983.
15. Cox T: *Stress,* Baltimore, 1979, University Park Press.
16. Daines B, Holdsworth AV: Impotence, *Nursing Times,* 78(18):763, 1982.
17. D'Arcy C: Unemployment and health: data and implications, *Canadian Journal of Public Health* 77 (suppl 1):124, 1986.
18. Doenges ME, Jeffries MF, Moorhouse MF: *Nursing care plans: guidelines for planning patient care,* ed 2, Philadelphia, 1989, FA Davis.
19. Dorfman W, Cristofar I, editors: *Psychosomatic illness review,* New York, 1985, Macmillan.
20. Dunbar F: *Emotions and bodily changes,* ed 4, New York, 1954, Columbia University Press.
21. Elliott GR, Ensdorfer C: *Stress and human health,* New York, 1982, Springer.
22. Field H: Psychosomatic illness: semantic and theoretical evolution. In Gallon RI, editor: *The psychosomatic approach to illness,* New York, 1982, Elsevier Biomedical Publications.
23. Fogel B: A psychiatric unit becomes a psychiatric-medical unit, *General Hospital Psychiatry* 7(1):26, 1985.
24. Fontaine R, Roisvert D: Psychophysiological disorders in anxious patients: hypertension and hypotension, *Psychotherapy and Psychosomatics* 38:165, 1982.
25. Ford CV: *The somatizing disorders: illness as a way of life,* New York, 1983, Elsevier Biomedical Publications.
26. Ford MR and others: Quieting response training: treatment of psychophysiological disorders in psychiatric in-patients, *Biofeedback and Self-Regulation* 7(3):331, 1982.
27. Frederickson RCA and others: *Neuroregulation of autonomic, endocrine and immune systems,* Boston, 1986, Martinus Nijhoff.
28. Friedman M, Rosenman RH: *Type A behavior and your heart,* New York, 1974, Alfred A. Knopf.
29. Frese M: Stress at work and psychosomatic complaints: a causal interpretation. *Journal of Applied Psychology* 70(2):314, 1985.
30. Gadlin W: Psychiatric consultation to the medical ward: a group analytic and general systems theory point of view, *International Journal of Group Psychotherapy* 35(2):263, 1985.
31. Gagan JM: Imagery: an overview with suggested application for nursing, *Perspectives in Psychiatric Care* 22(1):20, 1984.
32. Gallon RL, editor: *The psychosomatic approach to illness,* New York, 1982, Elsevier Biomedical Publications.
33. Ganong WF: The neuroendocrine system. In Frederickson, RCA and others, editors: *Neuroregulation of autonomic, endocrine and immune systems,* Boston, 1986, Martinus Nijhoff Publishing.
34. Goldsmith S: Strategic psychotherapy in psychiatric consultations, *American Journal of Psychotherapy* 37(2):279, 1983.
35. Gould D: The myth of menopause, *Nursing Mirror* 160(23):25, 1985.
36. Glaser R and others: Stress, loneliness, and changes in her-

pesvirus latency, *Journal of Behavioral Medicine* 8(3):249, 1985.

37. Gunderson EKE, Rahe RH, editors: *Life stress and illness,* Springfield, Ill, 1974, Charles C Thomas.

38. Hebert DJ: Psychophysiological reactions as a function of life stress and behavior rigidity, *Journal of Psychiatric Nursing and Mental Health Services* 14(51):23, 1976.

39. Hellman CJC: A study of the effectiveness of two group behavioral medicine interventions of patients with psychosomatic complaints, *Behavioral Medicine* 16(4):165, 1990.

40. Hoffman RS: Operation of a medical-psychiatric unit in a general hospital setting, *General Hospital Psychiatry* 6(2):93, 1984.

41. Holmes TH, Rahe RH: The social readjustment scale, *Journal of Psychosomatic Research* 11:213, 1967.

42. Hopping M: Psychic seizures, *Bulletin of the Menninger Clinic* 48(5):401, 1984.

43. House A, Andrews HB: The psychiatric and social characteristics of patients with functional dysphonia, *Journal of Psychosomatic Research* 31(4):483, 1987.

44. Iyer PW, Taptich BJ, Bernocchi-Losey D: *Nursing process and nursing diagnosis,* Philadelphia, 1986, WB Saunders.

45. Kaplan HI, Freedman AM, Sadock BJ, editors: *Comprehensive textbook of psychiatry,* vols 1 to 3, ed 3, Baltimore, 1980, Williams & Wilkins.

46. Kaplan M: *Essential works of Pavlov,* New York, 1966, Bantam Books.

47. Kiecolt-Glaser J, Glaser R: Psychological influences in immunity: making sense of the relationship between stressful life events and health, *Advances in Experimental Medicine and Biology* 245:237, 1988.

48. Lazarus RS: *Psychological stress and the coping process,* New York, 1966, McGraw-Hill.

49. Lazarus RS, Monat A, editors: *Stress and coping,* ed 2, New York, 1984, Columbia University Press.

50. Lazarus RS, Folkman S: *Stress, appraisal and coping,* New York, 1984, Springer Publishing Co.

51. Lesse S: Masked depression, *Current Psychiatric Therapies* 22:81, 1983.

52. Levitt DB and others: Group support in the treatment of PMS, *Journal of Psychosocial Nursing* 26(1):23, 1986.

53. Levi L, Kagan A: Adaptations of the psychosocial environment to man's abilities and needs, In Levi L, editor: *Society, stress and disease,* vol 1, London, 1971, Oxford University Press.

54. Lilliston L, Brown P, Schliebe HP: Perceptions of religious solutions to personal problems, *Journal of Clinical Psychology* 39(3):546, 1982.

55. McGuire MB: *Ritual healing in suburban America,* New Brunswick, NJ, 1988, Rutgers University Press.

56. Marmor J, Pumpian-Mindlin E: Towards an integrative conception of mental disorder. In Gray W, Duhl FJ, Rizzo ND, editors: *General systems theory and psychiatry,* Boston, 1969, Little, Brown.

57. Meichenbaum D, Jaremko ME, editors: *Stress reduction and prevention,* New York, 1983, Plenum Press.

58. Mendelson G: Psychosocial factors and the management of physical illness: a contribution to the cost-containment of medical care, *Australian and New Zealand Journal of Psychiatry* 18:211, 1984.

59. Miller D and others: A pseudo-AIDS syndrome following from fear of AIDS, *British Journal of Psychiatry* 146:550, 1985.

60. Mitchell WD, Thompson TL: Some methodological issues in consultation-liaison psychiatry research, *General Hospital Psychiatry* 7:66, 1985.

61. North American Nursing Diagnosis Association: *Taxonomy I; with official nursing diagnoses,* St Louis, 1990, The Association.

62. Pasnau RO: Psychiatric considerations in coronary artery disease, *Bulletin of the Menninger Clinic* 48(31):209, 1984.

63. Pawlick RE, Heitkemper T: Behavioral management of insomnia, *Journal of Psychosocial Nursing* 23(7):14, 1985.

64. Peplau H: *Interpersonal relations in nursing,* New York, 1952, GP Putnam's Sons.

65. Philippopoulos GS, Lucas X: Dynamics in art group psychotherapy with psychosomatic patients, *Psychotherapy and Psychosomatics* 40(1/4):74, 1983.

66. Purilo DT, Hallgren HM, Uris EJ: Depressed maternal lymphocyte response to phytohaemagglutinin in human pregnancy, *Lancet* 1:769, 1972.

67. Redd WH: Behavioral analysis and control of psychosomatic symptoms of patients receiving intensive cancer treatment, *British Journal of Clinical Psychology* 21:351, 1982.

68. Rogers M: *An introduction to the theoretical basis of nursing,* Philadelphia, 1970, FA Davis.

69. Rogers MP, Dubrey D, Reich P: The influence of the psyche and the brain on immunity and disease susceptibility: a critical review, *Psychosomatic Medicine* 41:147, 1979.

70. Roy SC: Adaptation: a conceptual framework for nursing, *Nursing Outlook* 18(3):43, 1970.

71. Sarti MG, Cossidente A: Therapy in psychosomatic dermatology, *Clinical Dermatology* 2(4):255, 1984.

72. Schwartz GE: Testing the biopsychosocial model: the ultimate challenge facing behavioral medicine? *Journal of Consulting and Clinical Psychology* 50(6):1040, 1982.

73. Selye H: *The stress of life,* New York, 1976, McGraw-Hill.

74. Selye H, Neufield RWJ: *Psychological stress and psychopathology,* New York, 1982, McGraw-Hill.

75. Shontz FC: *The psychological aspects of physical illness and disability,* New York, 1975, Macmillan.

76. Sifness PE: Short-term dynamic psychotherapy for patients with physical symptomatology, *Psychotherapy and Psychosomatics* 42(1/4):48, 1984.

77. Smith GR, Brown FW: Screening indexes in DSM-III-R somatization disorder, *General Hospital Psychiatry* 12:148, 1990.

78. Smith GR, McDaniel SM: Psychologically mediated effect on delayed hypersensitivity reaction to tuberculin in humans, *Psychosomatic Medicine* 45(11):65, 1983.

79. Smith GR, Monson RA, Ray DC: Patients with multiple unexplained symptoms: their characteristics, functional health, and health care utilization, *Archives of Internal Medicine* 146(1):69, 1986.

80. Stefanek ME, Hodes RL: Expectancy effects on relaxation instructions: physiological and self-report indices, *Biofeedback and Self-Regulation* 11(1):21, 1986.

81. Svedlund J, Sjodin I: A psychosomatic approach to treatment in the irritable bowel syndrome and peptic ulcer disease with aspects of the design of clinical trials, *Scandinavian Journal of Gastroenterology* (suppl) 109:147, 1985.

82. Takashima H: *Humanistic psychosomatic medicine,* Berkeley, Calif, 1984, Institute of Logotherapy Press.

83. Throll DA: Transcendental meditation and progressive relaxation: their physiological effects, *Journal of Clinical Psychology* 38(3):522, 1982.

84. Viney LI and others: The effect of hospital-based counseling service on the physical recovery of surgical and medical patients, *General Hospital Psychiatry* 7(4):294, 1985.

85. von Bertalaniffy L: *General systems theory,* New York, 1968, George Braziller.

86. Ward SE and others: Repression revisited: tactics used in coping with a severe health threat, *Personality and Social Psychology Bulletin* 14(4):735, 1988.

87. Weiner H, Hoffer MA, Stunkard AJ: *Brain, behavior and bodily disease,* New York, 1981, Raven Press.

88. Wolff GA Jr, Wolff HG: Studies on the nature of certain symptoms associated with cardiovascular disorders, *Psychosomatic Medicine* 8:293, 1946.

89. Wong ID: The interface between medicine and psychiatry, *Bulletin of the Menninger Clinic* 48(3):193, 1984.

90. Young ID, Harsch HH: An inpatient unit for combined physical and psychiatric disorders, *Psychosomatics* 27(1):53, 1986.
91. Zales MR, editor: *Stress in health and disease,* New York, 1985, Brunner/Mazel Publishers.
92. Zenmore R: Systematic desensitization as a method of teaching a general anxiety-reducing skill, *Journal of Consulting and Clinical Psychology* 43:157, 1975.

ANNOTATED BIBLIOGRAPHY

McGuire MB: *Ritual healing in suburban America,* New Brunswick, NJ, 1988, Rutgers University Press.

This text provides an excellent resource for understanding the basic categories of healing groups used by large numbers of middle-class suburbanites. The diverse ideas about health and illness, causes of illness, diagnostic approaches, healing practices, and attitudes toward therapeutic failure and death are described for each category of nonmedical healing group. The author provides data to indicate that these rituals provide an important source of empowerment to ill persons. Most persons use physicians' services in addition to participation in alternative healing. For most practitioners of alternative healing, all aspects of life are connected so the approach to healing must reach beyond the "secularized" institutions and include consideration of and the interaction of the spiritual, biological, mental, emotional, and social aspects of life. It provides a good overview of nonmedical healing practices.

Smith GR: *Somatization disorder in the medical setting,* Washington, DC, 1991, The American Psychiatric Press.

An excellent review of somatoform disorders from the perspective of primary care practitioners. A brief historical review of these psychiatric conditions is provided. Clear descriptions of the presentation of this illness, differential diagnosis, and management of such conditions in the primary care setting are given. The text provides guidelines regarding how to determine whether specialized psychiatric services are needed. Case examples illustrate various points throughout the text, and typical reactions and possible negative responses of the caregiver are addressed. Written for physicians, the text also provides essential evaluation information for all professionals, especially those working in primary health care delivery systems.

Sharon K Holmberg

After studying this chapter, the student will be able to:

- Define and describe the differences between acute and chronic pain
- Discuss the historical development of pain and pain management
- Describe theories of pain

- Use the nursing process to care for clients with pain
- Identify current research findings related to the pain syndrome

Pain is a universal human experience. In the broadest definition, pain is a personal, private sensation of hurt. This defines pain in the subjective realm, implying that the individual experiencing pain is the true expert on the sensation. Other definitions of pain suggest its usefulness to the human organism. For example, pain has been defined as the experience of harmful stimuli that warns of current or impending tissue damage and as a pattern of responses used to protect the person from harm.

Pain is the most common symptom of disease or injury that precipitates entry into the health care system. It was once thought to emanate from the heart, but gradual understanding of the nervous system has modified this view. Acute pain usually triggers self-protective behaviors that prevent the person from further harm, such as withdrawing one's hand from a hot stove or supporting behaviors that encourage healing, such as immobilizing a twisted ankle. Acute pain is usually time limited and likely to disappear once the precipitating cause has been resolved and healing has taken place. On the other hand, chronic pain may or may not be associated with pathological findings, can lose its specific meaning in relationship to disease processes, and may actually be a hindrance to the individual's health and well-being. Such pain may be experienced by some persons without demonstrated pathological findings. Persistent pain, either with or without pathological findings, may become a health problem in its own right, affecting all aspects of the individual's life.

Chronic pain is the most frequent cause of disability in the United States. In one survey[45] internists estimated that approximately 13% of their clients could be classified as chronic pain sufferers. Estimates of the economic cost of this syndrome through the loss of work productivity, the

cost of workers' compensation payments, health care costs, and related expenses are as high as $60 billion annually. These numbers relate to economic expenditures and do not begin to address the emotional cost to the individual experiencing pain, who comes to view the suffering as endless, purposeless, and unavoidable.

Because pain is a common symptom of a wide range of disorders, there is no universally accepted method of classifying pain. Pain taxonomies have been developed based on the duration of pain and various aspects of pathological findings and assumed cause. Generally, pain of less than 6 months' duration is considered acute, whereas chronic pain lasts for more than 6 months. Agnew, Crue, and Pinsky[1] classified pain as follows:

1. Acute pain, with a duration of a few days, can be mild to severe. As a symptom of an underlying physical problem, it will abate once the pathological condition is treated. An example is postoperative pain.

▶ **DIAGNOSES Related to Pain**

MEDICAL DIAGNOSES	NURSING DIAGNOSES
Somatoform pain disorder	**NANDA**
Factitious disorders	
Conversion disorder	Pain
Hypochondriasis	Chronic pain
	PMH
	Altered comfort patterns
	Pain: Acute
	Chronic

2. Subacute pain, which has a somewhat longer duration, can be either mild or severe, is caused by known pathological conditions, and involves a prolonged period of healing. An example is the pain experienced by someone with a bone fracture.
3. Chronic malignant pain is defined as pain caused by uncontrolled neoplastic disease. Metastatic cancers can cause severe pain in various parts of the body, depending on the disease process and the organ systems involved.
4. Chronic benign pain has persisted for more than 6 months. It may have an unknown or a known cause other than neoplastic disease. The client demonstrates an adequate ability to cope. A client with rheumatoid arthritis may experience this type of pain.
5. Chronic intractable benign pain is the same as chronic benign pain except that the client demonstrates inadequate coping mechanisms. Pain then becomes a primary diagnosis.

Pain is also described as limited, intermittent, or persistent. Limited pain, similar to acute and subacute pain, relates directly to the presence of a pathological condition. It ends once the healing process is complete. Intermittent and persistent pain, not recognized in the preceding classification, may or may not be caused by an identifiable physical lesion. Persistent pain is often considered resistant to treatment and may cause individuals to seek out many different resources in an effort to find relief. This pain is what is usually meant by a *pain syndrome.*

Chronic pain conditions that are treated in psychiatric settings can arise from many different circumstances. The chronic condition may begin with an acute episode of painful physical illness. Curative treatments, accidents, and the like, leading to amputations or other major surgery, can produce residual damage that causes chronic pain. Another cause of pain may be due to a slow, insidious disease with progressive deterioration of both physical and psychological health. Failure to cope can lead to psychiatric treatment. Clients who make multiple, unsuccessful efforts to find a physical cause for their pain by consulting numerous specialists may also be referred to psychiatric treatment settings.

A number of psychogenic and sociological factors contribute to the development and continuation of pain syndromes. This chapter addresses current theoretical constructs of the interaction between physical and biological systems in the development of pain syndromes, discusses various ways of describing and understanding pain phenomena, and uses the nursing process to address nursing's responsibilities in treatment of persons with pain syndromes.

Nurses, as the professionals with the most direct contact with clients experiencing pain, require knowledge of pain assessment and management. The most common pain experiences related to emotional distress and occasionally experienced by most people are headaches, muscle aches, or low back pain. These symptoms may or may not be associated with a physical health condition. If the pain becomes severe or chronic or if the person is no longer able to cope, specific treatment for pain may be indicated. The overall goal is to minimize significantly both the pain experience and the effect of pain on the client's life.

Helping clients cope with pain is a familiar task of the nurse in both medical and psychiatric settings. Current theories of how pain develops address both physiological processes and psychological processes. In all cases, each physiological explanation of pain includes an emotional component. Experiencing pain is a combination of the stimulation of neural receptors with a substrate of past experience, anxiety, cultural learning, and meaning of the illness. The term *somatogenic* refers to pain that occurs as a consequence of some identifiable physiological process *Psychogenic* is applied to pain that occurs without a clearly identifiable physiological lesion being present. Thus it is assumed that this pain originates in the mind.

Psychogenic pain is not necessarily experienced any differently than pain with an obvious physical cause. Qualities of pain, such as severity and intensity, are influenced by psychological factors in both somatogenic pain and psychogenic pain. Psychogenic pain can be distressing in exactly the same ways as somatogenic pain. Identifying pain as psychogenic implies only that adequate physical explanations for the pain experience cannot be given but that psychological explanations better clarify the cause.

DSM-III-R DIAGNOSES

Certain psychiatric disorders may be expressed through pain syndromes. Hysterical pain may be brought on by a specific, highly charged emotional event that is related to earlier unconscious emotional conflicts. Known as a *conversion disorder,* it is similar to other hysterical physiological symptoms, such as blindness (see Chapter 19). A related term, *hypchondriacal pain,* describes persons who have a constant preoccupation with their bodies, fear disease or body malfunction, and also experience pain. A hallucination of pain is relatively rare but may be experienced by the psychotic individual and is likely to be accompanied by body delusions such as the body changing size. A third psychiatric diagnosis applied to persons with pain that cannot be explained on the basis of physical lesions is known as *somatoform pain disorder.* It is characterized by pain symptoms that are inconsistent with the anatomical distribution of the nervous system. The cause of pain cannot be adequately accounted for by organic pathology after an extensive medical workup, and no other known pathophysiological mechanism can explain the pain symptoms. In addition, the symptoms of pain must have been present for at least 6 months.

Munchausen's syndrome, a type of *factitious disorder* described in the DSM-III-R,[3] is applied to persons who repeatedly come to acute care settings with convincing but false symptoms of almost any illness or injury, at times accompanied by falsified documents that support evidence of the disease. Self-mutilation (e.g., dislocating one's shoulder) or self-infliction (e.g., lupuslike syndromes) of a disease may also occur. This syndrome may extend to children through their parents, as cases have been reported of parents deliberately and repeatedly infecting their children with various illnesses.[2] These situations and this disorder are considered relatively rare. Making an appropriate diagnosis is complicated because clients often use many different sources to obtain care so evidence to support the diagnosis may be difficult and time-consuming.

THEORETICAL APPROACHES

Biological

At present, the most widely accepted, comprehensive theory of pain is the gate control theory, which suggests that pain is modulated by a gating mechanism located in the spinal cord, as well as by activities in the higher central nervous system. Therefore other central nervous system activities, such as memories and emotions, can influence the perception of pain. Sensations are transmitted from nerve receptors into the spinal cord and then to the brain; but these impulses can be modulated or altered in the spinal cord, brain stem, or cerebral cortex.

The nerve fibers transmit impulses to the spinal cord. At the dorsal horn of the spinal cord the impulses encounter a "gate," which may be open, partially open, or closed. The gate is thought to be the substantia gelantinosa, consisting of highly specialized cells throughout the length of the spinal cord that can modulate the transmission of nerve impulses.

If this gate is open or partially open, the pain impulses stimulate T cells (transmission or trigger cells), allowing the pain sensation to proceed through the spinal cord to the brain. If the gate is closed, pain impulses are blocked. As the pain impulses ascend to the brain, activity in the brain stem, thalamus, or cerebral cortex—all of which influence or control emotions, memory, and attention—influence the individual's perception of pain (Figure 20-1).

Cerebral processes descending from the brain may also have an impact on the gating mechanism. Melzack and Wall,[48] who originally developed this theory, have proposed three types of cerebral processes: (1) sensory-discriminative, which relays information about time, space, location, and intensity; (2) motivational-affective, which provides information about the presence of unpleasantness or discomfort, resulting in action that decreases noxious stimuli; and (3) central control processing, the cognitive aspect of the brain, which analyzes the meaning of pain as well as past experiences and probable outcomes. Together this cerebral processing defines the pain experiences, determines motivation for alternative responses, and projects possible outcomes, thus interacting to influence the perception of and response to pain. In this way cerebral processing influences the physiological processes of the gating mechanism.

Psychological

Pain may occur primarily in conjunction with psychological factors. For example, a person uninjured in an automobile accident may express the pain of having destroyed his car or having a friend injured in the accident by developing severe pain in some part of the body. Also, persistent somatogenic pain may lead to psychological distress, which can be expressed as depression, anxiety, anger, and feelings of loss of control. In these cases the psychiatric disorder is a secondary consequence of pain but may take on primary importance in the treatment.

PAIN PATHWAYS

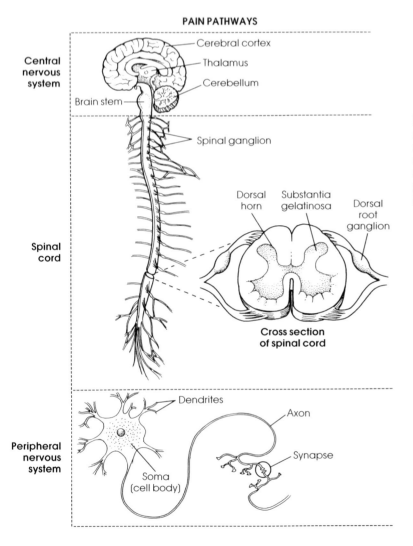

FIGURE 20-1 Pain pathways. The peripheral nervous system, made up of millions of neurons, transmits pain and other sensations by chemical exchange at the synapse into the dorsal horn of the spinal cord and then up through the substantia gelatinosa into the central nervous system. Pain perception is the outcome of multiple chemical exchanges in this complex pathway.

Psychoanalytical

Early psychoanalytical theoretical writings discuss pain primarily in the context of the pleasure-pain principle (see Chapter 4), but little is written about physical pain. In describing her observation of infants during the first year of life, Anna Freud[21] believed that "any tension, need or frustration is probably felt as 'pain' because the infant is not yet mature enough to separate bodily events from emotional events."

Szasz[68] formulated a general psychoanalytical theory of pain by articulating some basic assumptions. First, the ego system relates to the body as an object, just as the ego system relates to other persons as objects. Second, anxiety is an emotional state that occurs as a signal of danger to the ego. For an adult, danger could be the threat of losing a needed object, such as another person who is important. Third, according to Szasz, pain is an emotional state (affect) that has to do with the relationship of the ego to the body. As such, pain warns the ego of the potential loss (or damage) of a part (or the whole) of the body.

Szasz noted that the terms *organic* and *psychogenic* as applied to pain only locate it in an area of the body, rather than differentiate the experience. A parallel is drawn be-

tween these terms and the psychoanalytical application of *objective fear* and *neurotic anxiety.* Just as the source of objective fear can be validated by others (for example being stopped with drugs in the car by police), the source of organic pain can be validated (for example, a fractured leg). In this case, pain is a symptom. The source of neurotic anxiety is not validated by others because it is not objectively dangerous (for example, fear of cats) but represents something specific to the individual. Similarly, psychogenic pain cannot be validated by objective tests (for example, most headaches) but is nonetheless experienced by the individual as pain. In this case, pain becomes a form of communication, a means of soliciting help.

Every small child experiences pain. Pain signals to the child that something is wrong, a message that is likely to be communicated to others in a variety of ways. The response depends on a multitude of factors in the child, the situation, and significant others. The cause of the pain, either physical or emotional, the perceived seriousness of the cause, and whether these perceptions are mutually shared influence the response. Also important to determine the response are factors in significant others, such as how the child's message is interpreted; the child's own personal expectations; and the cultural expectations, values, and attitudes of significant others. Through a series of experiences beginning in earliest life, each person develops a set of assumptions about expressing pain and what the correct response should be. Certain established response patterns may be repeated later in life (see the following case example).

▼ Case Example

As an infant, Sarah had a particularly sensitive gastrointestinal tract. She frequently developed colicky symptoms an hour or so after being fed. These symptoms usually coincided with her mother leaving for work. Sarah's mother, anxious to arrive at work on time, was frequently impatient with her irritable, crying child and rushed to dress Sarah and drop her off at a babysitter. Sarah, now 10 years old, sometimes gets a "stomachache" before school in the morning and was unable to attend a 3-day sleep-over camp last summer because she developed abdominal pain, nausea, and vomiting the day before camp started.

The experience of acute pain is usually accompanied by fear, anxiety, or both: fear related to the loss or injury of a body part and anxiety about the response of significant others. A small child's response to acute pain includes looking to others for relief. If the wished-for response is not soon forthcoming, anxiety may increase as the child becomes concerned about a real or threatened separation or loss of love from an important person. This is one of the psychological processes that can associate anxiety with pain in the individual's emotional life. Another is an injury or hurt induced by significant others, as in receiving punishment. Pain is directly linked to the withdrawal of love. Not only is the physical pain accompanied by anxiety, but also anxiety and fear can recur if the individual believes that punishment is anticipated or deserved.

Anticipatory anxiety has a role in the psychological mechanisms related to chronic pain. When what is feared (that is, loss of something important) actually does or seems to have come to pass, the individual's response may be to feel grief and anger or disappointment, to feel punished, or to expect punishment. These dynamic psychological processes are similar to those that occur in depression. Instead of depression, however, pain becomes the predominant manner used to express the sense of loss, anger, hostility, and feelings of being responsible and guilty. This theory of anger turned inward and repressed hostility has been used to describe the *pain-prone person*. A history of physical abuse as a child, with pain used as a means of discipline, and parents who are attentive only when the child is sick or hurt are thought to be common experiences of the pain-prone person.

Given certain circumstances, individuals with certain character traits, such as being somewhat demanding and complaining, are more likely to develop chronic pain. It has also been suggested that having a limited formal education, a manual or routine job, and a lack of environmental supports may contribute to developing chronic pain. Many clients may express emotional distress through physical

---

RESEARCH HIGHLIGHT

Chronic Pain: Lifetime Psychiatric Diagnoses and Family History
• W Katon, K Eagan, and D Miller

PURPOSE

This study was conducted to develop more information about the relationship between chronic pain and psychiatric disorders. Specifically, the lifetime psychiatric diagnoses and family history of both psychiatric illness and chronic pain were examined in a group of people with chronic pain.

SAMPLE

From a pool of all persons admitted to an inpatient chronic pain treatment program over 8 months, 37 persons (two of every three) agreed to participate in the study. There were 20 women and 17 men ranging in age from 24 to 70 years. Subjects had experienced chronic pain severe enough to cause substantial impairment of at least 1 year, and a medical cause had been ruled out. Excluded were persons with a history of severe abuse or dependence on narcotic analgesics and those with an extensive psychiatric treatment history.

METHODOLOGY

Subjects were interviewed using the NIMH Diagnostic Interview Schedule. A family history of mental illness and chronic pain was obtained in the interview. Subjects also filled out an extensive packet of psychological tests. Among the scales used for this report were the Beck Depression Inventory, the Sarason Social Support Questionnaire, and the Beck Hopelessness Scale.

FINDINGS

The most common psychiatric diagnoses were either current or past depressive episodes or both (56.8%) and current or past alcohol abuse (40.5%). Twenty-four subjects (64.9%) had a past diagnosis of either alcohol abuse or major depression or both. Nineteen (51.4%) had an onset of these problems before developing chronic pain. A total of 54.4% of subjects had family histories of alcoholism, depression, or both.

IMPLICATIONS

This study demonstrates the association of chronic pain symptoms with either a past or present diagnosis of depression, alcohol abuse, or both. A strong association between a past history of alcohol abuse and the future development of chronic pain is shown. Since more than half of subjects experienced depressive episodes or alcohol abuse before the onset of chronic pain, the pain may be an expression of chronic psychiatric illness.

Based on data from *American Journal of Psychiatry* 142:10, 1985.

language because their vocabulary is not adequate to explain the emotional concepts that lead to pain. Somatic symptoms may be used as a defense against intolerable feelings. For example, a person who has learned that expressing anger is unacceptable may experience and describe his feeling of anger as physical pain. It is thought that some persons with chronic pain use that symptom as as emotional defense against a core conflict or a psychotic process. Without the symptoms of chronic pain such individuals may become acutely psychotic.

The individual who develops chronic pain related to physical illness or injury may experience both psychological losses and real losses, among which may be loss of mobility, loss of job, loss of independence, or significant changes in appearance. These losses can then lead to depression. The depression and pain, accompanied by feelings of being punished (perhaps unfairly), perpetuate and complicate the problem. According to Sternbach[67] chronic pain and depression seem almost interchangeable: Chronic pain usually leads to reactive depression, and reactive depression is frequently accompanied by complaints of pain. Recent research supports the interrelationship of depression and chronic pain (see the research highlight).

NURSING PROCESS

Assessment

Physical dimension The physical expressions of pain vary depending on the conditions causing pain. Therefore the physical assessment of the client should begin with an understanding of the client's medical history and any documented medical conditions. The nurse then familiarizes herself with the pain patterns usually associated with the documented condition. This knowledge helps the nurse develop precise and clear questions for discussion with the client.

The extent to which pain is evaluated can vary considerably. For acute pain, when the cause of pain is clearly evident, an extensive evaluation of pain is not usually indicated. When the individual is suffering from chronic pain, which is likely to be caused by numerous complex factors, the physical assessment of pain may need to be quite complex and detailed. The following list provides questions and topics for discussion relevant to physical assessment:

1. Where is the pain? Ask the client to point to specific painful areas of his body or to draw painful areas on a diagram of the front and back of the human body (Figure 20-2). A drawing is advantageous as a way to determine if and how the client's pain changes in response to situations or over time.
2. When did the pain start? Details of the client's first experience of this pain and its cause can be significant to the treatment.
3. Is the pain continuous or episodic?
4. Do you recognize patterns of occurrences associated with time of day, mood, emotional stress, or work demands?
5. How would you describe the quality of the pain? Is it well localized or dull, diffuse pain (see the box on p. 418).
6. How intense is the pain? The use of rating scales helps to objectify intensity and provides a standard measure

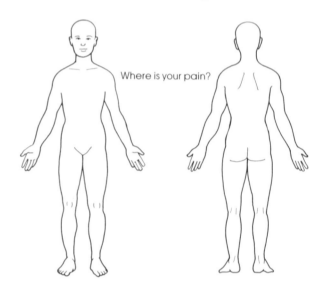

FIGURE 20-2 Identification of pain sites. Instruct the client as follows: Please mark, on the drawings, the areas where you feel pain. Put E if external, or I if internal, near the areas which you mark. Put EI if both external and internal. (From Jacox A: Pain: *A source book for nurses and other health professionals,* Boston, 1977, Little, Brown & Co.)

for the client and the nurse to measure changes (see the box on p. 418).
7. Does the description of pain change over time? Such changes may reflect an actual change in the client's physical status.
8. Discuss physical and environmental factors that influence the severity of pain (see the box on p. 419). Body functions such as eating, coughing, or defecating may influence pain experiences, as does body posture, weather, room temperature, and noise.

The physiological processes that change as a consequence of pain are related to the autonomic nervous system and are common with experiences of acute pain but may be totally absent in clients with chronic pain. The nurse looks for elevated blood pressure, elevated pulse and respirations, pupil dilation, skin color changes (pallor or flushing), and diaphoresis. Acute pain may also lead to nausea, vomiting, or diarrhea. Because clients with chronic pain may have few if any observable physiological changes, these are not necessarily reliable indicators of the presence of pain. Chronic pain may affect other physiological processes, such as decreased appetite, sleep disturbances, and the lack of sexual desire.

Most clients with pain do not describe significant changes in perception of the body's shape, size, or appearance except when these changes are based on reality. For example, an individual with chronic pain as a result of severe arthritis or a person who had lost a limb in an accident will have significant, obvious changes. Such changes will influence the person's perception of his body and require significant emotional adjustment. Other individuals who experience pain as one aspect of another psychiatric disorder, especially psychotic disorders, may believe that the body has actually changed dimensions or is distorted.

▼ **WHAT DOES YOUR PAIN FEEL LIKE?**

Some of the words below describe your *present* pain. Circle *ONLY* those words that best describe it. Leave out any category that is not suitable. Use only a single word in each appropriate category—the one that applies best.

1	2	3	4	5
Flickering	Jumping	Pricking	Sharp	Pinching
Quivering	Flashing	Boring	Cutting	Pressing
Pulsing	Shooting	Drilling	Lacerating	Gnawing
Throbbing		Stabbing		Cramping
Beating		Lancinating		Crushing

6	7	8	9	10
Tugging	Hot	Tingling	Dull	Tender
Pulling	Burning	Itchy	Sore	Taut
Wrenching	Scalding	Smarting	Hurting	Rasping
	Searing	Stinging	Aching	Splitting
			Heavy	

11	12	13	14	15
Tiring	Sickening	Fearful	Punishing	Wretched
Exhausting	Suffocating	Frightful	Grueling	Blinding
		Terrifying	Cruel	
			Vicious	
			Killing	

16	17	18	19	20
Annoying	Spreading	Tight	Cool	Nagging
Troublesome	Radiating	Numb	Cold	Nauseating
Miserable	Penetrating	Drawing	Freezing	Agonizing
Intense	Piercing	Squeezing		Dreadful
Unbearable		Tearing		Torturing

Modified from Jacox A: *Pain: a source book for nurses and other health professionals,* Boston, 1977, Little, Brown & Co.

▼ **HOW INTENSE IS YOUR PAIN?**

People agree that the following five words represent pain of increasing intensity.

1	2	3	4	5
Mild	Discomforting	Distressing	Horrible	Excruciating

To answer each question below, write the number of the most appropriate word in the space beside the question.

1. Which word describes your pain right now?   _____
2. Which word describes it at its worst?   _____
3. Which word describes it when it is the least?   _____
4. Which word describes the worst toothache you ever had?   _____
5. Which word describes the worst headache you ever had?   _____
6. Which word describes the worst stomachache you ever had?   _____

Modified from Jacox A: *Pain: a source book for nurses and other health professionals,* Boston, 1977, Little, Brown & Co.

Other physical signs of pain include body posture and facial expression. The body part with pain may be held stiffly or immobile. Limps or paralysis can also occur. The person with acute pain sometimes moans or grimaces. The facial expression of chronic pain sufferers reflects tension or anxiety.

Emotional dimension Emotions associated with chronic pain are complex. Over time the pain experience may have taken on a variety of meanings and be attached to emotional experiences that have little to do with the original causes of pain. Pain begins to develop a symbolic meaning. Living with chronic pain produces significant real and emotional changes in the person's life and may mean adopting a totally new life-style. Once the person has accepted the notion that the pain cannot be cured, loss is the most common feature of the emotional experience. Anger, frustration, and resentment may be the first expressions of loss. These feelings can be directed outward toward others who are blamed for the situation. The health care team is especially vulnerable to receive the blame and anger because the client expected them to cure the problem. When anger is directed inward, the client may feel both guilt and the wish for or expectation of punishment. Self-destructive behaviors in the form of noncompliance or not caring for self are expressions of guilt and punishment. Guilt is also associated with self-blame. The individual may express this by stating "I have brought this on myself" and also feels responsible for disrupting the lives of others. Anhedonia is a prevalent emotional tone. The client feels there is little opportunity to experience job and happiness.

When discussing the client's pain, the nurse should not only listen to the content of what the person says about the location of, intensity of, changes in, and type of pain, but also should listen for the emotions expressed at the same time. The emotional experience of pain has three phases: anticipation, the sensation itself, and the aftermath. These phases occur in sequence, especially with acute pain, but vary in length and intensity depending on the nature of the pain. For example, in acute pain, anticipation may be short, whereas for the person with intermittent pain, it may be a common, almost continuous, emotional state. The individual with continuous pain may experience all three phases but may not be able to distinguish them clearly because he perceives that he is in continuous pain at varying levels of severity.

Persons with acute pain are most likely to feel anxiety about causes and consequences. Anticipating the pain that accompanies diagnostic procedures or surgery raises the individual's anxiety. When the onset of pain is sudden, unanticipated, and unexplained, anxiety is related to a lack of understanding. This anxiety is expressed by agitation, restlessness, irritability, and demanding behavior (see Chapter 10). The client may seem pressured and may demand time,

attention, and explanations. As the individual obtains more information about the cause of the acute pain and its meaning relative to body injury or illness, the anxiety may change to fear or relief. Fear about the meaning of the illness or injury and worry about long-term consequences may lead to further anxiety.

Depending on the location of the pain, clients may feel embarrassed to discuss it, particularly when pain is located in the groin, genitals, or rectum. Shame is another common emotion associated with pain, particularly for those referred to psychiatric treatment or specialty clinics for chronic pain treatment. Others may have been told repeatedly that "it's all in your head" with the implicit message being that the individual is simply complaining, has control over the pain, and should "make it go away." Discussion of pain has become associated with humiliation. Persons reluctant to describe their pain are asked how others have responded to them in the past.

Grief and depression over the significant losses that accompany major physical illness or injury are appropriate and necessary for the individual's emotional adaptation to chronic pain and adjustment to a changed life. These emotional responses are expected as one aspect of the recovery process and require the nurse's attention.

On the other hand, pain may be a symptom of intolerable stress. In these cases, physical pain is a secondary consequence and a means of coping with pain in other aspects of life. Depression, anger, guilt, or frustration may be expressed as physical pain. This pain may mask serious emotional disturbances or be an expression of childhood abuse, neglect, or other negative experiences that are expressed bodily. The research highlight on p. 420 indicates that several factors likely occur together to produce psychogenic pain symptoms, including a history of abuse, certain ways of thinking, and psychosocial stressors in the present. Clients are likely to be less resentful of the physical sensation of pain and more willing to talk about the pain than about any other emotions or feelings. The emotions of such clients are assessed slowly and carefully to avoid precipitating severe depression or a psychotic state.

Finally, the emotional pain felt by the mentally ill client himself needs to be acknowledged and addressed. The frustrations and anguish resulting from mental disabilities such as confusion; intense fears; racing, illogical, or uncompleted thoughts; and deep despair, which may not have existed previously, affect the client in ways difficult to comprehend. Likewise, family and friends share the anguish of their loved one as they strive to understand and help him. The sensitive and caring nurse is aware of this anguish and emotional pain in both the client and family and seeks ways to demonstrate her caring.

◤ **Intellectual dimension** A state of hyperresponsiveness to sensations may accompany pain and is an essential aspect of pain assessment. The client is more sensitive to noxious stimuli and may negatively interpret interactions with others in the environment. The irritability that accompanies discomfort can lead to a negative interpretation of verbal exchanges. The client can easily misinterpret the meaning of comments and may take offense or view neutral comments in a negative light. For example, in responding to a request for assistance, the nurse may say, "Can I help you?" only to receive an angry or sarcastic reply from the

RESEARCH HIGHLIGHT

Psychogenic Abdominal Pain

• PLG Jenkins

PURPOSE

In this study of persons with nonspecific abdominal pain, a comparison was made between persons referred for psychiatric consultation and those that were not referred. The intent was to determine differences between the groups in pain experience, life events associated with the pain, and treatment recommendations. If there were differences, how could these be characterized?

SAMPLE

Twenty-five persons with abdominal pain for which no organic cause had been found were referred for psychiatric consultation. The subjects consisted of an experimental group and a consultation group. From a consecutive series of 1000 surgical admissions in another institution, 24%, or 51 cases were for nonspecific abdominal pain. From this unselected prospectively obtained group, 21 persons were matched with the consultation group, based on sex and age; and four additional subjects were added, making up the comparison group of 25 subjects. The majority of subjects were women, with a mean age of 44 years.

METHODOLOGY

Individuals in the experimental group were seen by the author as part of the work on an inpatient liaison service over a 2-year period. A full psychiatric interview was conducted with special attention to life events associated with pain. Length of time with pain and treatment recommendations were obtained from chart review. It is not clear how information was obtained from the comparison group,

Based on data from *General Hospital Psychiatry* 13:27, 1991.

except that they were sent a follow-up questionnaire. It is also not clear how this group differed in clinical symptoms from the consultation group.

FINDINGS

The consultation group had a mean duration of pain of 8.47 years, in contrast to the comparison group, which had a mean duration of pain of 5.56 years. In the consultation group, a psychiatric diagnosis was made in 20 of the 25 cases, whereas 12 psychiatric diagnoses were made in the comparison group. A history of childhood abuse and the subject's having a symptom model for pain were also associated with those persons who received psychiatric consultation. In the consultation group, 21 subjects reported one or more severe life events associated with the development of abdominal pain. From the questionnaire sent to the control patients, seven of eleven responses indicated no significant life event in the 6 months before admission.

IMPLICATIONS

Results of this study seem to support that female sex, duration of pain, and the three screening questions of psychiatric morbidity, childhood abuse, and the client having a symptom model are associated with psychogenic abdominal pain. Stressful life events also seem to be associated with the development of psychogenic abdominal pain. The most common psychiatric diagnoses were major depression, anxiety disorder, psychogenic pain, and conversion disorder. Study design problems and a small sample size indicate that these conclusions are tentative.

---

client such as, "I didn't mean to interrupt your busy day." Perception may also be heightened. The client may interpret the weight of a blanket or the smell of a cigarette, for example, as an exceedingly noxious stimulus, whereas these same sensations experienced without pain are not troublesome. A diminished response to sensations and lack of perception occur frequently when the individual is both depressed and in pain, sometimes resulting in a minimal reaction to others and the environment.

The client's attention span and concentration are likely to be disturbed by acute pain. The pain and attempts to manage the pain may so absorb thinking and cognition that he cannot attend to other matters. Clients with intermittent or chronic pain may ruminate about previous pain experiences, relating them to the current sensations. These cognitive processes can intensify pain sensations.

Social dimension The impact of pain affects all aspects of the individual's social role and requires careful assessment. Perception of self changes, as well as close relationships with family and friends. The ability to function adequately in previously established work roles can be severely curtailed, thus significantly influencing one's income, social status, and life-style, ultimately reinforcing a negative view of self.

The nurse assesses a person's self-esteem or self-worth. These aspects of self may change negatively as a result of real physical damage due to illness or injury. Persons who experience major physical changes may alter their emotional concept of self to include these real changes. The degree of change in self-worth is likely to be associated with the person's meaning of pain and the responses of others in the individual's social network. Persons who are adaptable and flexible with a secure sense of self are likely to require a period of adjustment to accommodate the change but then think of themselves in a changed but relatively positive way. Less adaptable persons will require a greater period of adjustment or may experience long periods of poor adjustment. Chronic pain is frequently associated with depression, one aspect of which is low self-regard. This low self-regard may have been a personality trait before the experience of pain or may develop as a consequence of the meaning given to chronic pain, as well as the stress of coping with it. To assess a person's change in self-perception, self-reports and data from significant others need to be obtained.

A positive sense of self is related to feelings of independence, the ability to maintain control of one's body and feelings, and having some influence on the environment.

These abilities are sometimes lost or reliquished. For example, in most health care facilities, the client is required to give control of medications to the nursing staff, resulting in the need to rely on others for pain control. This situation leads to dependence, similar to childhood, and will bring up memories or emotional conflicts about child-parent interactions. Although comforting for some persons and threatening for others, the fact of dependence produces more regressive behaviors. The client may begin to complain as much about trivial matters as about important ones. Other clients will express nothing, assuming that others do not care about their problems or discomforts, including pain. Assessment of dependence or independence includes the environment's expectation of dependent behavior as well as the client's reaction to increased dependence. Clients who develop pain syndromes as an unconscious wish to withdraw from social and environmental demands may actually receive some secondary gain from the dependent position.

The nurse assesses the client's coping abilities. Coping with pain can take considerable emotional energy. Clients feel too exhausted or depressed to maintain social contacts and slowly withdraw from their social networks, which eventually leads to loneliness and isolation. The person loses interest in others, including the desire for intimacy and sexual relations with a significant other. Friends and family members are likely to withdraw from the person in pain, not wishing to face their own emotional trauma caused by seeing someone close to them suffer. These significant others both identify with the suffering and feel helpless to intervene. Family members, in an effort to protect the person in pain, sometimes decide to withhold certain information or do not express their concerns to the client. Rather than discuss the stresses of daily living, family members attempt to project a happy, if superficial, image, further isolating the individual through emotional distance, lack of knowledge, and lack of shared experiences. Other family members attempt to pick up the tasks of the person in pain, changing the expectation of who is to fulfill any given family role.

Loss of employment is common for the individual with chronic pain. Physical disability, with or without chronic pain, may make a return to previous employment impossible. Job retraining may be possible, but it is accompanied by lost earning time and the cost related to retraining. Beyond the real expenses entailed, however, is the question of whether the person with chronic pain is able to and desires either to return to a former job or to be retrained. According to Unikel[70] people who display symptoms of pain and sickness learn, either through their own experience or from observations, that pain has three consequences: obtaining increased attention from others, avoidance of stressful situations, and economic advantage. Assessment of how these three factors influence the individual's pain experience is important.

The relationship between chronic pain and economic support is significant to treatment planning. Factors to consider in the assessment process are success or failure at the job, ability to cope with work-related stress, positive or negative feedback from others, a sense of control or powerlessness, and general job satisfaction. Some persons receive disability payments or workers' compensation payments roughly equivalent to their previously earned income, producing an unconscious incentive for continued uncontrolled pain, especially if the job was stressful and the person finds relief in avoiding stressful situations. Only rarely does the individual consciously and deliberately avoid employment by developing symptomatic behavior. However, individuals experiencing a real illness or injury may discover that their needs continue to be met, perhaps with less personal effort. The individual may feel more gratification from the role of sick person than from a job. These emotional factors reinforce the illness.

The client's present experience and expression of pain are strongly influenced by early experiences with pain and associated memories. Cultural factors, especially the means of reacting to and expressing pain within the family, influence behavior. These subtle but strong influences are usually difficult for the client to verbalize because they are based on early, preverbal, learned behaviors. For example, in general, women have been found to have a lower maximum tolerance for pain than men, although individual variations are great.[55] These variations are thought to be culturally determined, especially in Western cultures, as men are not supposed to cry out in pain as quickly as women. In summary, an assessment of pain includes its effect on one's perception of self, friends and family relationships, social and work roles, feelings of dependence or independence, degree of withdrawal from social contacts, employment status, economic support, and cultural factors.

Spiritual dimension An important aspect of the assessment process is to understand what meaning the client gives to the experience of pain. The person may or may not express, but probably often thinks about, the following questions: "Is pain associated with death? Will it be permanent? Do I deserve to suffer? Am I devalued as an individual because of pain and infirmity?"

Feelings of decreased value and worthlessness develop with persistent pain, especially when accompanied by physical incapacitation. Life may not seem worth living because the pain is sometimes unbearable. The individual feels that the pain represents punishment for being bad or unworthy or that life with physical incapacitation and pain is too difficult. Persons may also feel they are a burden for the family. The risk of suicide can be great at these times and needs to be carefully assessed.

The client's philosophy of life, religious beliefs, and spiritual ideas may be seriously challenged by living with pain. The values, beliefs, morals, and ethics that have held meaning for the individual in the past, such as "God is good," may seem to be a mockery given present experiences. The client who attempts to think through questions related to the "why" of pain will at least confront, if not modify, his philosophy to fit the present situation. The person with no meaningful philosophy of life may be overwhelmed by the experience of pain and lack a belief system that provides solace and aids with coping.

Assessment is made of the person's belief system, which is more than determining the individual's religion. The nurse inquires about the client's religious beliefs, but it will also be necessary to gradually understand how the client's belief system fits the present experience. For example, the client who believes pain is a punishment for wrongdoing may spend considerable time and energy mentally searching for those things that may be deemed "bad enough" to deserve the level of pain being experienced. Such persons are also likely to be consumed with feelings of guilt. Clients may express this belief by wishing to "do over" some aspect of their life, continually regretting having failed, and becoming preoccupied with the extent of their "punishment." Doubts about either the existence of or the fairness of a deity may be expressed. Assessing the strength of the client's belief system is important in understanding the client's perspective.

Another common reaction to pain is for the client to view the experience as a test of commitment to his religious beliefs. The client with this perspective can be reticent to complain of discomfort or ask for medication to relieve the pain. Pain becomes something to be endured as a means of proving worthiness. Proving that one can meet these religious challenges can mean unnecessary suffering, and ultimately the client will probably express anger and frustration or even question whether the effort to endure has any benefit. The individual may express hopelessness. When the nurse notices that a client seems to be in pain but says nothing, exploring his belief system may provide some understanding of how the client hopes to cope with pain or whether he has abandoned all hope.

The assessment includes an understanding of how the client in pain views prayer and meditation. Some questions to consider include the following:

1. Has the use of prayer or meditation alleviated pain in the past?
2. Does the client receive relief from pain from these activities?
3. Under what circumstances do these activities relieve pain?
4. Do they produce relaxation, improve self-control, or facilitate a more positive sense of self that facilitates pain management?
5. Is the client sufficiently knowledgeable about any of the relaxation or meditation techniques that may help reduce pain, such as transcendental meditation or self-hypnosis?

Measurement Tools

Measurement tools are useful to assist the nurse in systematically assessing the client's subjective experience of pain. One of the most common measurement tools is a simple descriptive scale, sometimes called a pain ruler, that asks the client to select a place on the scale that most accurately reflects the level of pain experienced. One end of the scale indicates no pain and the other end indicates severe pain (Figure 20-3).

The McGill-Melzack Pain Questionnaire is a specific, detailed measurement tool, which is most often used to collect research data, but it can be useful in clinical settings to elicit specific information about a client's pain. It is designed to measure the strength (severity) of pain and to delineate pain location. In addition, the client is asked to choose from lists of word descriptors that specify different aspects of the pain experience. The words are categorized into three major classes:

1. Words that describe the sensory qualities of the experience
2. Words that describe the affective qualities of the experience
3. Evaluative words that describe the intensity of the pain experience

The advantage of this measurement tool is its sensitivity to the subtle changes in aspects of the pain sensation that would not be reflected in more general questioning or by other, less specific measurement tools.

Analysis
Nursing diagnosis

The following list provides examples of NANDA-accepted diagnoses,[54] with causative statements related to pain:

1. Impaired physical mobility related to pain secondary to paraplegia
2. Sleep pattern disturbance related to pain
3. Self-care deficit requiring assistance with dressing and grooming secondary to low back pain

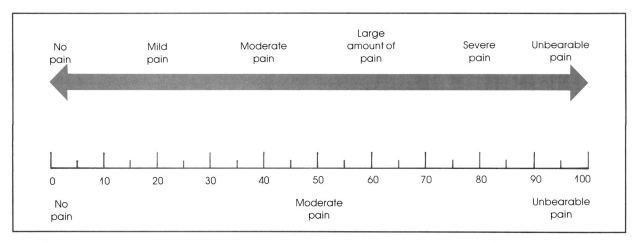

FIGURE 20-3 Pain rulers.

4. Powerlessness related to intolerable pain

The two nursing diagnosis approved by NANDA that apply to persons with pain are *pain* and *chronic pain*. The defining characteristics of these nursing diagnoses are listed in the accompanying boxes.

The following case example is a description of an individual who meets criteria for a nursing diagnosis of chronic pain.

▼ Case Example

Frank, a 47-year-old former employee of a public works department, received an on-the-job injury to his left eye, chest, and arm 14 months ago. He had been working in a park cleaning up brush and tree branches after a major storm. In the process of throwing tree limbs on a dump truck, one bounced back from the top of the truck, hitting Frank on the left side. The most immediate, serious, and obvious injury was to the left eye, requiring ambulance transport to a local emergency room. Other injuries included severe bruises to the left arm and two fractured ribs. The eye injury was of serious concern and the physician expressed concern that Frank may lose vision in the eye or actually lose his eye. Frank's wife or other family member had to take him to the ophthalmologist daily for approximately 3 weeks. The eye healed well with little loss of vision and no physical deformity. Frank, increasingly anxious, began to develop severe headaches and paralysis in his left arm and side, which persisted even after the eye and the fractured ribs were fully healed (at least in terms of what could be discovered by eye examinations and x-ray studies of the chest). He has seen four other physicians who can find no physical cause for the persistent headaches. Neurological examination of Frank's left arm finds no nerve damage that fits the pattern of numbness he describes. Frank, now at home and unemployed, needs assistance with dressing because the arm remains painful and paralyzed. He sometimes spends the whole day in bed due to a headache. He has filed for workers' compensation and feels very angry that no one has been able to find out what is wrong with his arm and tell him how to cure it.

The following case example describes a psychiatric diagnosis of somatization disorder and a nursing diagnosis of chronic pain.

▼ Case Example

Paula, 37 years old, was referred to a pain treatment program after all physical and neurological studies failed to show organic cause for her severe headaches, tingling on the scalp, and the sensation that her head was swelling up at night, symptoms that

---

▼ PAIN

DEFINITION

A state in which an individual experiences and reports the presence of severe discomfort or an uncomfortable sensation.

DEFINING CHARACTERISTICS

- **Physical dimension**

  Protective, guarding behavior
  Altered time perception
  Distraction behaviors (e.g., moaning, whimpering, crying, rubbing, pacing)
  Agitation
  Restlessness
  Facial mask of pain (e.g., beaten look, pinched features, tightened jaw muscles, clenched teeth, lackluster eyes, widely open or tightly shut eyes, knotted brows)
  Unusual posture
  Blood pressure and pulse change
  Increased or decreased respiratory rate
  Dilated pupils
  Diaphoresis
  Increased muscle tension

- **Emotional dimension**

  Irritability

- **Intellectual dimension**

  Verbal report of intense, limited pain experience
  Self-focusing
  Narrow focus
  Impaired thought process

- **Social dimension**

  Withdrawal from social contact

Modified from McFarland G, McFarlane E: *Nursing diagnosis and interventions: planning for patient care,* ed 2, St Louis, 1993, Mosby–Year Book.

▼ CHRONIC PAIN

DEFINITION

Pain: State in which the individual experiences and reports the presence of severe discomfort or an uncomfortable sensation.
Chronic Pain: State in which the individual experiences pain that continues for more than 6 months.

DEFINING CHARACTERISTICS

- **Physical dimension**

  Protective guarded behaviors
  Changes in sleep pattern
  Restlessness
  Facial mask of pain (beaten look, lackluster eyes, knotted brows)
  Altered ability to continue previous activities
  Weight changes

- **Emotional dimension**

  Irritability
  Depression

- **Intellectual dimension**

  Verbal report of pain for more than 6 months
  Self-focusing

- **Social dimension**

  Disruption of family and social relationships

Modified from McFarland G, McFarlane E: *Nursing diagnosis and interventions: planning for patient care,* ed 2, St Louis, 1993, Mosby–Year Book.

have increased in frequency and severity for the past several months. Paula quit her job 4 years ago due to persistent headaches brought on by conflict with her boss. She has been living with her parents, providing company for her mother who experiences chronic leg pain secondary to diabetic neuropathy. Six months ago, Paula's father retired and is now home every day caring for his wife. With a reduced family income, there are financial pressures. Paula resents her father's presence, admits that she sometimes feels "in the way" now, and says she should consider finding a job to help the financial situation but cannot do so because of her medical problems. After coping with the pain that keeps her awake all night, Paula has no energy left for a job.

Planning

When planning, the physical health problems and psychiatric diagnoses must be taken into account as well as the information gained on the nursing assessment. The physical health status and medical conditions of the client are particularly important to consider, as these have an impact on determining what goals can be accomplished with a given client. The other critical information to consider is how much the client is willing to accept the idea that the condition is related to psychological factors, rather than being strictly a physical condition. Table 20-1 provides

examples of goals, outcome criteria, interventions, and rationales related to pain, which are examples of the planning stage of the nursing process.

Implementation

Physical dimension Pain may be treated in a variety of settings. Clients with pain syndromes are usually seen first in medical clinics or hospitals because the client believes the cause is physiological. When no definable physiological causes are determined or the pain experience becomes further complicated by emotional factors, the client is likely to be referred to a psychiatric treatment setting or a specialty clinic for chronic pain sufferers. Clients with pain from emotional causes rarely seek psychiatric treatment initially and may be unwilling to acknowledge an emotional component. Moreover, members of the health care team may have a number of misconceptions and prejudices that interfere with adequate and accurate treatment. Chief among them are personal notions that prevent the nurse from accurately interpreting behavior. If the nurse understands her own attitudes and feelings related to pain behaviors, she can more objectively analyze discrepancies between her own expectations of behavior and the real

▼ TABLE 20-1 NURSING CARE PLAN

GOALS	OUTCOME CRITERIA	NURSING INTERVENTIONS	RATIONALES
NURSING DIAGNOSIS: Chronic pain (low back) related to auto accident 1 year ago			
LONG TERM			
To achieve optimal control of pain	Uses pain management techniques that control pain effectively		
SHORT TERM			
To describe pain control measures that reduce or eliminate pain	Describes pain control measures that reduce or eliminate pain	Assess pain level	To determine a baseline for progress or lack of progress in controlling pain
		Assess characteristics of pain	To determine a baseline for progress or lack of progress in controlling pain
		Discuss past measures for controlling pain; pharmacological and nonpharmacological	To find out what helps and what does not
		Describe methods for pain relief; biofeedback, hypnosis, physical therapy, TENS, relaxation, guided imagery, desensitization	To provide options to client for managing pain
To use pain control measures to manage pain	Uses measures that reduce or eliminate pain	Guide and support patient in deciding on method of pain control	To increase self-esteem by participating in the decision making, to promote self-responsibility
To state resources available in the community for help with pain control	Names resources available in community for help	Provide information about community resources	Providing information relieves anxiety that may exacerbate pain

behaviors of the client. Clients sometimes feel their responses to pain are negatively judged, that they cannot measure up to the expectations of others, or that they are ashamed of their behavior. Comparing one client's pain response to another's or comparing a client's response to what the nurse considers ideal is not fair to the individual. Discussions with clients about the meaning of their physical expressions of pain can facilitate the acceptance of behavioral responses and arrive at mutually agreeable, acceptable, and individualized understanding of the efficacy of treatment. Implementing pain treatment involves a combination of approaches.

Specific interventions for pain include medications, nerve blocks, and occasionally surgical interventions. Other possible interventions more frequently used in physical care settings and less often in psychiatric settings include massage and application of heat or cold. The use of *transcutaneous electrical nerve stimulation (TENS)* or acupuncture has become more common in recent years. Each of these interventions is discussed here.

Medications used to treat chronic pain range from analgesics to antidepressants and may also include placebos. A placebo is any medical or nursing measure that works because of its implicit or explicit therapeutic intent instead of its specific chemical or physical properties. It may be a pill containing lactose, an injection of saline, or even a surgical procedure. Contrary to popular belief, the use of placebos does not differentiate "real" pain from psychogenic pain. Placebos can and do relieve pain, both psychogenic pain and pain caused from obvious physical stimuli. They may work by reducing anxiety or by the classical conditioning response. Because taking a pill or receiving an injection is expected to relieve pain, it does. There may also be a biochemical response. Some researchers theorize that the cognitive expectation of a response actually stimulates a physiological response that produces more of the body's natural pain-relieving substances, endorphins.

Using sedatives and narcotic analgesics to treat acute pain is a standard practice. In the treatment of chronic pain, however, these drugs may be more problematic. The possibility for developing tolerance, dependence, or addiction is always present when these drugs are used. The nurse monitors and documents the effects of pain medications. In general, physical tolerance (but not necessarily addiction) develops after continuous use of narcotics for 2 weeks or longer but can be quickly reversed when the drug is no longer needed for pain relief.

Neurosurgical techniques are sometimes used to treat intractable pain.[69] All neurosurgical techniques cause permanent lesions of the nervous system and thus are used cautiously. There has been debate about the usefulness of these procedures and which clients are appropriate candidates for surgery. Some reports suggest that the procedures have not been considered highly successful in the long-term treatment of pain, whereas others express the view that neurosurgical techniques are usually used for those with severe, intractable pain and have been helpful (see research highlight on p. 426).

Nerve blocks are one neurological technique intended to interrupt pain pathways in the peripheral nervous system. Nerve blocks may be temporary, of the type dentists use to block pain or the spinal blocks used in labor and delivery. A temporary block is used diagnostically to investigate the anatomical pain pathways. It may also be used prognostically so that the client can experience the probable effect before a permanent procedure is undertaken. The nurse needs to be aware of possible complications, such as severe systemic reactions to the anesthetics that could require emergency interventions such as intubation and cardiopulmonary resuscitation during the procedure.

TENS consists of electrodes powered by a battery-operated generator that send a mild electrical current into the body at or near the pain site and can be used to control both acute and chronic pain. TENS is the most common peripheral stimulation technique. Others, such as vibratory stimulation and acupuncture, have come into use over the past 10 years and are effective for some clients and some types of pain. Just why TENS and other stimulation techniques are effective is unknown, but theories are that (1) blood flow is increased near the electrodes, increasing muscle relaxation and healing; (2) the body may be stimulated to release endorphins, increasing natural pain relief; or (3) electrical stimulation closes the neurological "gate" to pain impulse transmission. Some clients who benefit from TENS will use these units continuously and need to be taught correct application of electrodes and other important aspects of how the unit functions so they can use it at home. The nurse observes for possible complications, such as skin irritation or electrical burns from the electrodes. Therapeutic controversies about acupuncture, another form of peripheral stimulation, are far from resolved but research shows possible benefit in 60% to 75% of clients with chronic pain,[43] at least for a short time.

Two of the most traditional, effective, and universal nursing measures for pain control are the use of massage and the application of heat and cold. Not only does massage facilitate relaxation and help to relieve anxiety, but the action of massage stimulates large-fiber nerve impulses, according to the gate control theory, and thus closes off the reception of pain impulses. Massage can be performed lightly or deeply. Back massage can be used to reduce pain regardless of the site, although the specific pain site can sometimes be massaged.

The application of heat increases blood flow to injured tissues and thereby reduces inflammation. It is especially useful for bruises, muscle spasms, and arthritis. Heat also has a stimulating effect on large nerve fibers similar to that of massage, thus reducing the small fiber pain sensations. Applying heat will not relieve some types of pain, such as that caused by pressure on a nerve. Superficial dry heat is applied by heating pads or heat lamps. Moist heat is applied by hot-water bottles or hot baths. The nurse needs to be particularly cautious and alert to avoid burns. Occasionally, deep heat from an ultrasound device may be administered for specific types of pain, such as back pain. Cold therapy is more effective for acute pain than for chronic pain and is especially useful for burns or sprains.

Emotional dimension For the client with acute pain, the most common emotional experiences are anxiety and fear. Interventions from the nurse are directed toward reducing anxiety (see Chapter 10). The nurse needs to respond to the demands of the client; provide accurate, clear, and simple explanations of procedures and treatments; and respond to the client's questions. Verbal interaction and

RESEARCH HIGHLIGHT

Spinal Cord Stimulation and the Relief of Pain
- TH Koeze, AC Williams, and S Reiman

PURPOSE

In previous studies the outcome of spinal cord stimulation has been reported as equivocal. Subjects have been persons with several other possibly complicating diagnoses and the study designs were considered inadequate. This study was designed to overcome some of these research problems. The authors examined the amount of pain relief obtained from spinal cord stimulation in a group of patients who did not have other complicating factors that might influence perception of pain. The factors excluded were subjects with drug abuse, those involved in litigation regarding the pain or disability, those with overt psychosis, and those seen in special follow-up clinics.

SAMPLE

Ten women and 16 men patients who were using spinal cord stimulation for pain control were subjects in this study. The median age of the sample was 65 years. Twelve subjects experienced pain due to traumatic causes and 14 experienced pain due to nontraumatic conditions or unknown causes. Subjects had previously used several other treatments for pain control such as ultrasound, TENS, vibration, nerve blocks, nerve root section, cordotomy, and the like. A variety of analgesics including narcotics had also been used in attempts to control pain. Electrodes were implanted epidurally under general anesthesia, and each subject had an individualized schedule for spiral cord stimulation, which varied from continuous to intermittent stimulation weekly.

METHODOLOGY

All subjects were interviewed by one of two psychologists who had not met the subject previously or been involved in their treatment. A videotaped structured psychiatric interview was used for data collection as was the adjective check list of the Melzack pain questionnaire. Subjects evaluated their pain relief on a visual analog scale. For 16 subjects, a relative or close friend was also interviewed

Based on data from *Journal of Neurology, Neurosurgery and Psychiatry* 50:1424, 1987.

and rated the subject's pain. The treating clinician was also asked to rate the subject's pain.

FINDINGS

Estimates of the subject's pain by the subject, the relative, and the clinician were highly correlated (between 0.71 and 0.74, $P = 0.001$). Using the mean of these three scores obtained from the visual analog scale, pain relief was calculated for each subject. Thirteen of the 26 subjects had a pain relief estimate of 50% or more. However, there were five subjects whose estimate was less than 10% relief and four subjects whose estimate was over 90% relief. The amount of pain relief was not associated with age or sex. Outcomes suggested that the "trauma" subjects had better outcomes than did the "nontrauma" subjects and there seemed to be a tendency for subjects who had used this method for 1 to 2 years to report more positive outcomes than those who had used this method for 5 to 10 years. Subjects with pain relief increased domestic activity but not work or leisure activity. Fifteen subjects decreased analgesic drug use and only two subjects increased their use of analgesic drugs.

IMPLICATIONS

There was a general reduction in drug use for all drugs except antidepressants and the degree of pain relief was correlated with a shorter time using the stimulator. Given that most subjects were using this technique as a "last resort" the results should not be considered disappointing. These authors believe that other methods of pain control would also fail if equally stringent criteria for evaluation were used. Nine of the 13 subjects with less than 50% pain relief considered this method to be valuable, in spite of the large number of complications reported by these authors (which have been reported in other studies, too). More research should be directed toward determining what characteristics predict which individuals are most likely to benefit from this procedure.

---

the presence of others help reduce the client's anxiety. It is important that the nurse control her own responses to situations such as severe injury or uncomfortable procedures. Because the client may be able to see the nurse's face but not the site of the injury or procedure, his emotional response may be guided by what is reflected on her face.

The nurse keeps in mind that no pain, from the slightest to the most severe, is purely physical or purely emotional. Seeing the client as a whole person can facilitate the development of an effective supportive relationship. Establishing a positive alliance is essential. An initial positive relationship with a client can be established by conveying to the client that you know "it hurts." Frequently, the

client's behavior does not invite an empathic or positive response. The client is likely to be angry and resentful or depressed, sullen, and withdrawn. Referral to a psychiatric treatment setting may be viewed as just another way for others to communicate that the pain is not "real" and the psychiatric treatment is viewed as just another treatment attempt doomed to failure. The nurse takes into account the impact that previous negative reactions have had on the client and works toward building trust (see Chapter 7). The client needs to trust the nurse to believe in his pain.

Equally important is the nurse's respect for the client's response to pain. The client and the nurse may have different attitudes about appropriate behavior with regard to reporting pain and the verbal and nonverbal expressions of pain. Because of the differences in cultural expectations, values, beliefs, previous experiences, and memories of pain, there may be significant communication gaps between the nurse and the client. Sometimes it may be difficult for the nurse to acknowledge the patient's pain.

Clients with chronic pain present complicated emotional features. Some of the most common psychotherapeutic interventions are psychotherapy (see Chapter 7), group therapy (see Chapter 28), and couples therapy (see Chapter 30). Because the phenomenon of pain arises from physiological, emotional, and social factors, multimodel therapy is likely to be more effective than any single approach.

The major goal of psychotherapy is to help the client with chronic pain reduce helpless and hopeless attitudes by gaining control of the symptoms. This goal can be achieved by identifying and reducing anxiety states; identifying irrational cognitions, thinking, and personal beliefs; and then helping the client make modifications.

Intellectual dimension Theories related to pain mechanisms show that the individual can influence experiences of pain by thought processes. Clients can be taught to block pain sensations at the cortical level by a number of cognitive strategies, including distraction, relaxation, guided imagery, biofeedback, and hypnosis. The major advantage of these approaches is that the client is given a participatory role in pain relief and thus can develop a sense of control. Effective teaching from the nurse allows the client to use several of the cognitive approaches without assistance and on an as-needed basis. Working with the client to modify cognitive processing has the added advantage of requiring little technical equipment, except for biofeedback training, which requires monitoring equipment to provide feedback to the client. The nurse must have knowledge of these techniques, which are taught in educational programs or are available through seminars that vary in length from one day to several weeks of theoretical teaching and observed practice. Another important element in these techniques is that the nurse is confident of the helpfulness of the technique, can project this attitude to the client, and has been able to establish an alliance that facilitates the teaching process.

Reality testing and teaching the client to identify patterns of response that cause pain and to develop new response patterns are helpful interventions. Many clients with chronic pain need assistance to identify and express their emotional responses rather than respond with an expression of physical pain. On the inpatient unit, the nurse is responsible for designing and implementing a carefully conceived milieu, which encourages clients to problem solve, to develop better communication skills, and to understand the relationship between emotional stress and pain. A therapeutic milieu is an ideal environment for clients to develop an understanding of their emotional responses to daily life stresses.

Nurses use distraction, often without awareness of it as a treatment approach. Pain is relieved by focusing one's attention on something other than pain. When concentrating on a book, a television program, or a conversation with another person, pain is no longer at the client's center of attention and will be felt less intensively. This short-term relief technique may be especially helpful for managing periods of more acute pain, but it does not generally provide a long-term solution. Effective distracters are those involving the client's sense of hearing, sight, or touch. Information about the client's hobbies or interests helps the nurse select an appropriate distraction. Rhythm and repetition facilitate these techniques, so the use of headphones to listen to favorite music, rhythmic breathing exercises, frequent repetition of a word or phrase, poetry, singing, or tapping the foot or hand is encouraged. Another approach is to give the client a picture and ask him to describe it in detail or ask him questions about it. On an inpatient unit, encouraging visitors or the client's interaction with others can also serve as an effective distraction. The client needs to be taught these techniques, which can be used at will once the benefits are experienced.

Guided imagery and relaxation exercises are related techniques for pain control. Guided imagery uses the client's ability to create mental images of pleasant places or experiences based on previous events. It resembles a form of self-hypnosis. A comfortable environment with minimal noise and interruptions facilitates the exercise. Relaxation exercises may be used before guided imagery exercises to help induce a relaxed state. Initially, guided imagery involves the nurse, who helps the client create a relaxed, comfortable mental image by encouraging and asking questions that stimulate the client to create the imagined scene. Once the client has learned techniques of relaxation or imagery, client-specific cassette tapes can be made. The tape can be used by the client to recreate the imagery and induce a relaxed state; 15 to 20 minutes is usually long enough to be helpful. Imagery uses the mind's ability to create physiological responses. Just as watching a frightening scene in a movie can increase an individual's pulse rate, other imagery can facilitate the body's ability to relax. Clients often experience drowsiness after using this technique.

When used properly, hypnosis can alleviate severe pain. *Hypnosis* is an altered state of consciousness where distraction is minimized and concentration is heightened. Pain signals may be processed by the brain at an unconscious level but are not felt consciously. In responsive subjects all pain can be removed for controlled periods of time by the use of hypnotic suggestion. It can also be used selectively to block or partially block pain in certain regions of the body. It has been suggested that all pain should not be blocked, especially when it accompanies some organic conditions, as a change in the course of a clinical condition needs to be detectable by the clinical signs and symptoms of pain. Important diagnostic clues can be missed with a total block of pain sensation. The length of time that hypnotic analgesia is effective varies from a few hours to several days or weeks. With repeated hypnotic suggestion, pain relief can be reinforced and the effective time extended. Clients can be taught self-hypnosis, effectively gaining control over their pain.

Biofeedback provides the client with information about specific body functions such as skin temperature, pulse rate, blood pressure, or muscle tension by using equipment that measures these functions and provides feedback information to the client with visual and auditory signals. Its major use in chronic pain is to help the client control muscle tension, anxiety, and some autonomic nervous system functions, thereby influencing the physiology of the body and aiding in pain control.

 Social dimension It is important to stress that certain pain behaviors can be learned and unlearned. Once pain behaviors begin to occur, they can be influenced by factors outside the person and may be controlled by various environmental factors. Reported intensity of pain by clients is systematically influenced by social reinforcers. Treatment manages excess disability from pain by focusing on the actions of clients and their families to determine what pain behaviors are reinforced and how they are reinforced. The theoretical approach is based on learning theory. A behavior is learned by being reinforced from others' responses, but the behavior can be unlearned or modified by changing those factors that reinforce it (see Chapter 4).

Family and social roles can be changed significantly when the individual develops a serious medical condition accompanied by pain. Most often these changes are initially protective, intended to allow the individual time and opportunity for recovery. Any individual recovering from an extended illness will be faced with giving up a sick role and returning to a more functional, productive role. This task is more difficult when symptoms of the illness, such as pain, persist. Identifying variables that reinforce and maintain sick role behavior is important in implementing behavior modification techniques. Clear limit setting and consistent responses are necessary for a positive outcome.

Clients who have been unemployed for long periods, and especially those who receive monetary compensation, such as workers' compensation, are particularly difficult to rehabilitate. The longer an individual stays away from work, the less likely he is to eventually return to work. Behavioral techniques that address the client's low level of motivation and stimulate emotional insight have been successful. Behavioral therapy focuses on increasing the client's physical abilities, such as increasing activity levels, reducing the amount of pain medications used, and a specific program designed to reinforce nonpain behaviors. Behavioral therapy is almost always combined with several other therapeutic approaches. Special rehabilitation clinics have been developed to centrally locate rehabilitation services, including physical therapy, and intensify the effects of a well-coordinated team approach.

A self-help organization for persons with chronic pain was founded about 10 years ago.[13] It is intended to provide a support system for those suffering from chronic pain by encouraging positive attitudes and enhancing the perception of self-control. It is one possible source of information for clients who wish to learn relaxation techniques, communication skills, physical exercise, increase knowledge about nutrition and sleep aids, as well as discuss with others the impact that chronic pain can have in families. Some printed materials and video educational information can be obtained that are designed to assist persons to develop a better understanding of the effects of chronic pain. A professional organization for clinicians and researchers is the American Pain Society.

Spiritual dimension Some clients need or ask for spiritual guidance specific to their beliefs that is best provided by clergy. This guidance may be especially helpful for those who feel unfairly punished by their God and find their religious beliefs challenged. Some beliefs and religious ideas may interfere with treatments, such as occurs when a client has lost hope and the will to live. Discussions with the client concerning these beliefs help the client reestablish the will to participate in treatment programs.

Some specific treatments use the client's belief system in the treatment process. The aim is for the client to gain existential knowledge about himself through introspection and meditation. Especially relevant are yoga and transcendental meditation. A passive attitude, relaxation, and focused concentration are particularly helpful aspects of meditation for the person in pain. See the accompanying boxes for key interventions and for guidelines for primary/tertiary prevention. See Table 20-1 for a sample nursing care plan.

▼ **GUIDELINES FOR PRIMARY/TERTIARY PREVENTION**

Primary Prevention

Teach person to "think safety", for example, when lifting heavy objects, by wearing seat belts or crash helmets

- to identify signs and symptoms of anxiety that lead to increased pain
- to reduce anxiety and stressors
- to function as independently as possible in spite of pain
- to become aware of gains and benefits from pain
- to identify noninvasive methods for relieving pain
- to develop a sense of control by managing own pain with distractions such as music, imagery, massage, heat or cold applications, or biofeedback
- to identify relationship between emotional stress and pain
- to modify beliefs about pain so that hope and a will to participate in treatment is established
- to use community resources for help with pain management, for example, group therapy

Teach family to avoid reinforcing clients' pain behaviors

- to help client assume responsibility for own pain management regimen

Tertiary Prevention
Community Resources

Mental health centers for group and behavioral therapy
Pain management clinics
Rehabilitation clinics for physical therapy

Self-help groups

Chronic pain management groups

▼ **KEY INTERVENTIONS FOR PAIN**

Monitor effects of medications
Provide massage
Apply heat (to increase blood flow) or cold (for relief of pain)
Reduce anxiety and fears
Respect clients response to pain if different from one's own
Promote distraction: music, reading, singing
Teach relaxation, meditation
Use guided imagery, biofeedback, hypnosis
Provide psychotherapy, behavior modification
Prevent "sick role"
Refer to self-help groups for pain management

INTERACTION WITH A CLIENT IN PAIN

Client: (Partially sitting in bed with eyes downcast.) Don't trouble me this morning with breakfast or anything else. This has been the worst night.

Nurse: What has made it the worst night?

Client: Oh, the pain in my back was just awful. I couldn't sleep.

Nurse: What was it like?

Client: It went down my leg and then . . . . oh, never mind.

Nurse: Mr. B., I am interested in hearing how you describe the pain. It will help us work together on this problem.

Client: I don't think it can be solved.

Nurse: Are you feeling more hopeless after the bad night you had?

Client: I don't see how being in this hospital is going to help.

Nurse: Right now you sound discouraged. First, I'd like to help you get into a more comfortable position. Then we can talk to get a better understanding of what the pain is like.

This client and nurse are establishing a working alliance. The client with chronic pain may have learned that others do not wish to hear about his pain, depression, and hopelessness. Such expectations can produce initial rejection of the nurse.

The nurse responds with a direct question that indicates her interest in the client's experience. The tone of voice is nonjudgmental, reflecting concern and interest. She does not become frustrated by his initial hesitance to explain but rather indicates the need for a shared understanding of the problem. The nurse has begun the process of involving the client in the process of finding solutions to his pain and has conveyed a willingness to further engage the client in the pain assessment.

The nurse also has introduced the idea that the client's mood is relevant to the experience of pain and includes it in a discussion of pain. She does not pursue further discussion of mood at this time because the client, in this phase of the alliance, has defined the problem as pain and is unlikely to understand the interrelationship. There is a general acknowledgment and acceptance of the client's feeling state.

Ultimately, the intervention suggested by the nurse implies that she does not believe the situation is hopeless. The client's expectation of rejection has been derailed by the nurse's offer to further explore the situation with him.

Evaluation

Evaluation of the nursing interactions for the client with pain is based on both what the client says about the level of pain and behavioral cues the client demonstrates. It is important for the nurse to review with the client accomplishments toward the established treatment plan, as well as those areas of minimal improvement. Positive changes are reinforced, which, when discussed, contributes to the client's positive sense of self. Anxiety about maintaining the improvement is a common concern of the client that will need to be addressed. More difficult, but necessary, is a realistic discussion of treatment goals not completed and an evaluation of what else may be possible.

In general, successful outcome is indicated when the client is able to describe a decrease in the severity or frequency of pain. For those clients with chronic pain, it is important to consider what techniques for pain management have been learned successfully and to ensure that the client understands them. When used successfully, the client may describe feeling more in control of himself, may be better able to function in daily activities, and will demonstrate improved self-confidence. Family interventions may result in changed family dynamics that encourage the client to perform in expected roles. Some clients with chronic pain can have sufficient return of their functions so that they return to work or consider participation in retraining programs. Since pain treatment requires many different levels of expertise, participation from a number of health care providers is usually necessary. Evaluation should consider the coordination of care with regard to effectiveness, efficiency, and the ability to work as a well-integrated team. Evaluation also considers which treatment intervention programs are most successful.

BRIEF REVIEW

Pain is an abstract concept whose presence is indicated by the client's expression of the feeling and by his behaviors. As a syndrome, pain continues to be an economically and emotionally costly problem for both the individual and society. In part because of the economic and emotional burden, the problem of pain in health care has received much more attention during the past 20 years. New theoretical constructs have facilitated interest and research related to pain management.

Pain involves not only physiological mechanisms, but also emotional, intellectual, social, and spiritual components. The interaction of all factors determines the client's experience and expression of pain. There are several classifications of pain, based on cause and time factors. Persistent pain with no known physiological cause is known as psychogenic pain. The most commonly accepted theory of pain is the gate control theory first described by Melzack and Wall in 1965.

The nurse has a significant responsibility in working with clients experiencing pain. Chronic pain can be severely disabling. In addition to the discomfort of the client, social role functions are lost and the individual loses productivity and a positive sense of self. Together with the client, the nurse assesses severity, location, intensity, and duration of pain, as well as evaluating the contributing emotional, social, cultural, and spiritual factors. From the assessment, a plan of care is developed and implemented. The first intervention establishes a working relationship with the client; then goals can be developed. In addition to medications, several other effective interventions are available. The nurse becomes involved with teaching clients about their pain and about the techniques, such as guided imagery, that alleviate pain. Evaluation of progress is based on criteria established for the client to achieve.

REFERENCES AND SUGGESTED READINGS

1. Agnew D, Crue B, Pinsky J: A taxonomy for diagnosis and information storage for patients with chronic pain, *Bulletin of the Los Angeles Neurological Societies* 44:84, 1979.
2. Alexander R, Smith W, Stevenson R: Serial Munchausen syndrome by proxy, *Pediatrics* 86:581, 1990.
3. American Psychiatric Association: *Diagnostic and statistical manual of mental disorders (DSM-III-R)*, Washington, DC, 1987, The Association.

4. Barber J, Adrian C: *Psychological approaches to management of pain,* New York, 1982, Brunner/Mazel.

5. Beckman CE and others: Self-concept: an outcome of a program for spinal pain, *Pain* 22:59, 1985.

6. Blazer DG: Narcissism and the development of chronic pain, *International Journal of Psychiatry in Medicine* 10(1):69, 1980.

7. Blessing D: *Free yourself from pain,* New York, 1981, Simon & Schuster.

8. Brenz SF, Chapman SL: *Management of patients with chronic pain,* New York, 1983, Spectrum Medical and Scientific Books.

9. Bromm B, editor: *Pain measurement in man: neurophysiological correlates of pain,* New York, 1984, Elsevier Press.

10. Brown JM: Imagery coping strategies in the treatment of migraine, *Pain* 18:157, 1984.

11. Carroll-Johnson RM, editor: *Classification of nursing diagnoses; proceedings of the eighth conference,* Philadelphia, 1989, JB Lippincott.

12. Catchlove R, Cohen K: Effects of a directive to work approach in the treatment of workmen's compensation patients with chronic pain, *Pain* 14:181, 1982.

13. Cowan P, Lovasik DA: American Chronic Pain Association: strategies for surviving chronic pain, *Orthopaedic Nursing* 9:47, 1990.

14. Crook J, Rideout E, Brown G: The prevalence of pain complaints in a general population, *Pain* 18:299, 1984.

15. Davitz JR, Davitz LL: *Inferences of patient's pain and psychological distress: studies of nursing behaviors,* New York, 1981, Springer Publishing Co.

16. Dudley SR, Holm K: Assessment of the pain experience in relation to selected nurse characteristics, *Pain* 18:179, 1984.

17. Fordyce WE and others: Pain measurement and pain behavior, *Pain* 18:53, 1984.

18. Fordyce WE, Roberts AH, Sternbach RA: The behavioral management of chronic pain: a response to critics, *Pain* 22:113, 1985.

19. France RD, Houpt JL: Chronic pain: update from Duke Medical Center, *General Hospital Psychiatry* 6:37, 1984.

20. France RD, Houpt JL, Ellinwood EH: Therapeutic effects of antidepressants in chronic pain, *General Hospital Psychiatry* 6:55, 1984.

21. Freud A: The role of bodily illness in the mental life of children. In *The psychoanalytic study of the child,* New York, 1952, International Universities Press.

22. Geach G: Pain and coping, *Image* 19(1):12, 1987.

23. Geracioti TD and others: The onset of Munchausen's syndrome, *General Hospital Psychiatry* 9:405, 1987.

24. Graffam S, Johnson A: A comparison of two relaxation strategies for the relief of pain and its distress, *Journal of Pain and Symptom Management* 2:292, 1987.

25. Grainger S: No cause, no cure . . . but he's still in pain, *RN* 50:43, 1987.

26. Gruber M, Beavers F, Amodeo DJ: Trying to care for the great pretender, Nursing grand rounds, *Nursing* 17:76, 1987.

27. Hendler N: *Diagnosis and nonsurgical management of chronic pain,* New York, 1981, Raven Press.

28. Hendler NH, Long DM, Wise TN: *Diagnosis and treatment of chronic pain,* Boston, 1982, John Wright, P.S.B., Inc.

29. Houpt JL, Keefe FJ, Snipes MT: The clinical specialty unit: the use of the psychiatric inpatient unit to treat chronic pain syndromes, *General Hospital Psychiatry* 6:65, 1984.

30. Jacox A: *Pain: a source book for nurses and other health professionals,* Boston, 1977, Little, Brown.

31. Jacox A, Stewart M: *Psychosocial contingencies of the pain experience,* Ames, Iowa, 1973, University of Iowa Press.

32. Jenkins PLG: Psychogenic abdominal pain, *General Hospital Psychiatry* 13:27, 1991.

33. Jamison RN, Sbrocco R, Parris WCV: The influence of physical and psychosocial factors on accuracy of memory for pain in chronic pain patients, *Pain* 37:289, 1989.

34. Katon W, Eugan K, Miller D: Chronic pain: lifetime psychiatric diagnoses and family history, *American Journal of Psychiatry* 142:10, 1985.

35. Keefe FJ, Bradley LA: Behavioral and psychological approaches to the assessment and treatment of chronic pain, *General Hospital Psychiatry* 6:49, 1984.

36. Kerr FWL: *The pain book,* Englewood Cliffs, NJ, 1981, Prentice-Hall.

37. Khatami M, Rush JA: A one year follow-up of the multi-model treatment for chronic pain, *Pain* 14:45, 1982.

38. Kramlinger KG, Swanson DW, Maruta T: Are patients with chronic pain depressed? *American Journal of Psychiatry* 140:6, 1983.

39. Koeze TH, Williams A, Reiman S: Spinal cord stimulation and the relief of chronic pain, *Journal of Neurology, Neurosurgery and Psychiatry* 50:1424, 1987.

40. Kores RC and others: Predicting outcome of chronic pain treatment via a modified self-efficacy scale, *Behavior Research and Therapy* 28:165, 1990.

41. Kumar K, Wyant GM, Nath R: Deep brain stimulation for control of intractable pain in humans, present and future: a ten-year follow-up, *Neurosurgery* 26:774, 1990.

42. Levitan S, Berkowitz H: *New developments in pain research and treatment,* Washington, DC, 1985, American Psychiatric Association.

43. Lewith GT, Machin D: On the evaluation of the clinical effects of acupuncture, *Pain* 16:111, 1983.

44. Lipton S, Miles J, editors: *Persistent pain: modern methods of treatment,* vol 5, New York, 1985, Grune & Stratton.

45. Margolis RB and others: Internists and the chronic pain patient, *Pain* 20:151, 1984.

46. Meinhart NT, McCaffery M: *Pain: a nursing approach to assessment and analysis,* Norwalk, Conn, 1983, Appleton-Century-Crofts.

47. Melzack R, editor: *Pain measurement and assessment,* New York, 1983, Raven Press.

48. Melzack R, Wall P: *The challenge of pain,* New York, 1983, Basic Books.

49. Melzack R, Wall PD: Pain mechanisms: a new theory, *Science* 150:971, 1965.

50. Melzack R, Wall PD: Psychophysiology of pain. In Jacox A, editor: *Pain: a source book for nurses and other health professionals,* Boston, 1977, Little, Brown.

51. Miller TW, Kraus RF: An overview of chronic pain, *Hospital and Community Psychiatry* 41:433, 1990.

52. Mittal B and others: Dorsal column stimulation (DCS) in chronic pain: report of 31 cases, *Annals of the Royal College of Surgeons of England* 69:104, 1987.

53. Nigl AJ: Biofeedback and behavioral strategies in pain treatment, New York, 1984, *Spectrum Medical and Scientific Books.*

54. North American Nursing Diagnosis Association: *Taxonomy I: with official nursing diagnoses,* St Louis, 1990, The Association.

55. Notermans SLH, Tophoff MMWA: Sex differences in pain tolerance and pain appreciation. In Weisenberg M, editor: *Pain: clinical and experimental perspectives,* St Louis, 1975, Mosby—Year Book.

56. Nursing Now: *Pain: nurse 85 books,* Springhouse, Pa, 1985, Springhouse Corporation.

57. Pilowski I, Barrow CG: A controlled study of psychotherapy and amitriptyline used individually and in combination in the treatment of chronic intractable psychogenic pain, *Pain* 40:3, 1990.

58. Ramamurthy S and others: Long thorasic nerve block, *Anesthesia and Analgesia* 71:197, 1990.

59. Reich J, Tupin JP, Abramowitz SI: Psychiatric diagnosis of chronic pain patients, *American Journal of Psychiatry* 140:11, 1983.

60. Schaffer CB, Donlon RT, Bittle RM: Chronic pain and depression: a clinical and family history survey, *American Journal of Psychiatry* 137:1, 1980.

61. Schwartz DP and others: A chronic emergency room visitor with chest pain: successful treatment by stress management training and biofeedback, *Pain* 18:315, 1984.

62. Shacham S, Dar R, Cleeland CS: The relationships of mood state to the severity of clinical pain, *Pain* 18:187, 1984.

63. Sherman RA and others: Phantom pain: a lesson in the necessity for careful clinical research on chronic pain problems, *Journal of Rehabilitation Research and Development* 25:vii, 1988.

64. Skevington SM: Chronic pain and depression: universal or personal helplessness? *Pain* 15:309, 1983.

65. Steger JC, Fordyce WE: Behavioral health care in the management of chronic pain. In Milton T, Green C, Meagher R, editors: *Handbook of clinical health psychology*, New York, 1982, Plenum Press.

66. Swerdlow M, editor: *Relief of intractable pain*, ed 3, New York, 1983, Elsevier Science Publishers.

67. Sternbach RA: *Pain patients: traits and treatment*, New York, 1974, Academic Press.

68. Szasz T: *Pain and pleasure: a study of bodily feelings*, ed 2, New York, 1975, Basic Books.

69. Thomas DG: Surgical management of benign intractable pain, *International Disabilities Studies* 9:27, 1987.

70. Unikel IP: How we learn chronic pain and sickness. In Brena SF, editor: *Chronic pain: America's hidden epidemic*, New York, 1978, Atheneum/SMI.

71. Urban BJ: Treatment of chronic pain with nerve blocks and stimulation, *General Hospital Psychiatry* 6:43, 1984.

72. Urban BJ, Keefe FJ, France RD: A study of psychophysical scaling in chronic pain patients, *Pain* 20:157, 1984.

73. Wain HJ, Devaris DP, editors: *The treatment of pain*, New York, 1982, Jason Aronson.

74. Weh-Hsein W, editor: *Pain management, assessment, and treatment of chronic and acute syndromes*, New York, 1987, Human Sciences Press.

75. Wood DP, Wiesner MG, Reiter RC: Psychogenic chronic pelvic pain: diagnosis and management, *Clinical Obstetrics and Gynecology* 33:179, 1990.

76. Wynn P, Girgis F: The assessment and management of the failed back, Part II, *International Disabilities Studies* 10:25, 1988.

ANNOTATED BIBLIOGRAPHY

McCaffery M, Beebe A: *Pain: clinical manual for nursing practice*, Philadelphia, 1989, Mosby–Year Book.

Covers a significant portion of what the nurse can do with or for clients on a one-to-one basis. Strategies that require nursing judgment and are used independently are a central focus of the text. A number of noninvasive techniques for pain relief are discussed such as cutaneous stimulation, relaxation, and imagery. There are excellent chapters on chronic nonmalignant pain, problems of pain in children, and the elderly. The text is easy to read, well indexed, designed to find information quickly, and presents the essential information needed to guide care of patients in clinical settings.

McGrath PA: *Pain in children: nature, assessment and treatment*, New York, 1990, The Guilford Press.

The unique tasks of understanding and responding to children in pain are described clearly and sensitively. This very current information on assessment and control of acute, recurrent, and chronic pain from a multidimensional perspective make this book particularly useful in both general hospital pediatric settings and child psychiatric hospitals. Also included is a brief history of the study of pain and an excellent discussion of the neurology and physiological mechanisms of pain.

Roy R, Tunks E, editors: *Chronic pain: psychosocial factors in rehabilitation*, Baltimore, 1982, Williams & Wilkins.

Emphasis is on how sociocultural and environmental factors influence chronic pain. Of most value are chapters describing various methods of psychotherapy (family, marital, group, individual) with the chronic pain patient. Case examples illustrate the application of these techniques to persons with pain.

Cathleen M Shultz

After studying this chapter, the student will be able to:

- Define loneliness
- Discuss historical perspectives of loneliness
- Describe theories of loneliness

- Apply the nursing process to care for clients experiencing loneliness
- Identify current research findings relevant to loneliness and client care

Loneliness usually is defined as the absence of anticipated relationships. Thus individual perceptions, learned behavior, social skills, and social network have considerable effect on whether a person acknowledges loneliness. Nurses usually describe loneliness as a negative feeling that is chronic and a source of potential harm to health.

Loneliness is caused by the lack of certain kinds of social contact. In the everyday world, clients may use different words to describe loneliness, but they can easily report its presence or absence. Usually the person feels that something is missing because relationship expectations have not been realized.

Loneliness is a dynamic, cyclical process that can create, as well as result from, numerous health problems. In other words, loneliness can cause illness and illness can cause loneliness. Scholars agree on three important points: (1) loneliness results from deficiencies in a person's social relationships, it is subjective and often not directly related to social isolation, and it causes unpleasant feelings; (2) loneliness affects not only the individual who fails to benefit from personal contacts but also the health of a society and the quality of its human relationships; and (3) loneliness is so prevalent in the United States that a whole industry of national "telephone-a-friend" numbers and tapes has sprung up in an attempt to meet and capitalize on the nation's loneliness needs. The best estimates of incidence indicate that between 50 and 60 million Americans, or one fourth of the population, are lonely at some time during any given month.[40] Loneliness appears to be age related. Data from many studies suggest that loneliness is a major social problem among adolescents. As many as 10% to 15% are labeled as seriously lonely.[10] Loneliness peaks at adolescence. The incidence of loneliness declines with increasing age, and its occurrence becomes relatively constant at about age 70.[57]

Adaptive loneliness is healthy because it helps the client gather strength from internal resources. At these times loneliness is a normal reaction to life's circumstances rather than a problem that needs nursing intervention. Ending a friendship, beginning a new job, moving, and changing marital status are common occurrences that may cause loneliness. Loneliness does not automatically cause damage; it can provide time to develop creative potential in poetry, art, and music.

DSM-III-R DIAGNOSES

Loneliness can cause psychopathological conditions; it also can mask them. Loneliness is a component of many of the DSM-III-R diagnoses discussed elsewhere in the book. For example, loneliness has been linked to schizoid and schizotypal personality disorders. See Chapters 14 and 18 for further information on these topics.

> ▶ **DIAGNOSES Related to Loneliness**
>
> **NURSING DIAGNOSES**
> **NANDA**
> Impaired social interaction
> Social isolation
>
> **PMH**
> Loneliness

HISTORICAL OVERVIEW

DATES	EVENTS
Ancient Times	Historical accounts of the Jews and Christians acknowledged man's loneliness as the impetus for Eve's creation. Strong leaders such as David and Solomon sought people and God to reduce their loneliness. Numerous religions and other social groups urged frequent contacts among members to continue the groups' beliefs and maintain a social network.
Before 1960	In 1955 Hildegard E. Peplau, a nurse, was among the first to write about loneliness as a concept.[48] Only 12 publications about loneliness existed in English, including works by Sullivan[64] and Fromm-Reichmann.[23]
1970-1975	Written material on loneliness, including research, grew rapidly during this time. Weiss,[67] the father of the concept of loneliness, wrote his classic book entitled *Loneliness: The Experience of Emotional and Social Isolation.*
1975-1980s	Loneliness has obtained major attention by those involved in health care. Dramatic changes in relationships occurred in Western culture increasing social isolation. In the nursing literature loneliness is interwoven with commonly occurring events such as hospitalization, institutionalization of elderly individuals, bereavement, and suicide. Published information evolves from descriptions of loneliness and the behavior of lonely people to loneliness intervention programs. A loneliness prevention industry emerges and is thriving via self-help books, support groups, video dating clubs, national telephone numbers, and video and cassette tapes.
1990s	Increased attention is given to experiences of loneliness in special populations such as adolescents, widowed, pregnant teenagers, clients with medical problems.
Future	With the development of an increasingly high technology–low touch society, it is probable that the incidence of loneliness will become greater and consequences will be more problematic to both the individual and society. Public awareness of loneliness will increase and nurses will be challenged to include loneliness prevention and treatment interventions in all health care settings, including school systems, to reach more people in their formative years.

THEORETICAL APPROACHES

Psychoanalytical

Psychoanalytical theorists who wrote about loneliness obtained their data in clinical situations with emotionally troubled individuals. Thus they viewed loneliness as harmful and negative.

Zilboorg[71] distinguished between the terms *lonesome* and *lonely*. Lonesomeness is transient and normal; loneliness is a consuming, negative experience with underlying hostility and narcissism. The lonely person has childish, self-centered feelings. Loneliness has roots in infancy when the child learns (1) the pleasure of being cared for and loved and (2) the dismay associated with unmet needs.

Sullivan[64] claimed that loneliness appears first in childhood because of a need for human intimacy. From the infant's initial desire for human contact to the preadolescent's desire for a friend, everyone needs relationships. Yet faulty parent or peer interactions can result in failure to gain social skills. Later this lack can lead to adult loneliness.

Fromm-Reichmann[23] agreed with Sullivan that loneliness was unpleasant and originated in childhood. In extreme cases, loneliness could lead to psychosis.

Cognitive

Cognitive theorists such as Perlman and Peplau[50] suggest that loneliness results from inconsistencies between actual and perceived levels of social contact. Causes for this discrepancy vary and include character and situational factors, as well as past and present influences. Loneliness is one end point of the social interaction continuum (Figure 21-1). Everyone has an optimal level of social interaction: too little results in loneliness; too much creates a sense of crowding or feeling that one's privacy is invaded.

Sociocultural

For sociologists the cause of loneliness is created by factors outside the individual, that is, society. Social learning theorists Reisman, Glazer and Denney[51] believe lonely behavior begins in childhood, is reinforced in adolescence, and continues in adult life. In modern society three sociological forces create increased loneliness: (1) a decrease in meaningful group relationships, (2) an increase in geographical mobility, and (3) an increase in social mobility.

Loneliness can be divided into three categories: tran-

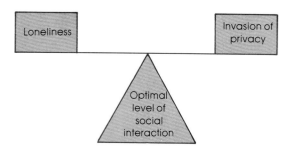

FIGURE 21-1 Social interaction continuum.

sient, situational, and chronic (Table 21-1). *Transient lone-liness* is temporary. It is not recognized as a problem that requires professional intervention. Clients either relieve their own loneliness by seeking the companionship of others, or the unpleasant feeling subsides with time.

Situational loneliness is triggered by a specific life event. Common events that cause situational loneliness include moving, going away to college, divorce, death of a family member or friend, changing jobs, and losing friends who move away or withdraw their friendship. The client's reactions are beyond just the feeling of being lonely. Additional reactions include headaches, depression, sleep disturbances, anxiety, and physical complaints. Clients with situational loneliness are more likely to seek professional assistance than are those who experience transient loneliness.

When loneliness lasts longer than 2 years with no apparent traumatic event, it is considered *chronic loneliness*. Loneliness becomes a way of life. Even when social opportunities arise, established patterns prevent healthy interactions with others. Intimacy is minimal or nonexistent. Those who suffer from chronic loneliness tend to have only superficial relationships because of their difficulty in establishing intimate contact.

Like so many negative emotions, destructive or maladaptive loneliness creates other problems. Persons who are chronically lonely blame themselves and feel hopeless about changing their circumstances. Because they believe that they lack the power to change their life, they expect others to shun their company. Thus they become even more lonely. In addition, their general state of health may suffer because of continuing physical symptoms.

Some professionals view the lonely client's main problem as a lack of social reinforcement. That is, each person needs social relationships that are uniquely satisfying in type and number. Some need many close friends, whereas others need only one close confidant. If the person's perceived optimal level decreases, loneliness results.

Two sociological positions predominate in explaining loneliness: the other-directed position[51] and the individualism position.[62] When people become other-directed and desire to please, they become conformists, alienated from their inner beings, including their feelings and goals. These traits are shaped by significant others and the mass media. Consequently, diffuse anxiety results because the need to please others motivates behavior and is rarely completely satisfied. The members of the other-directed society form what Reisman and others[51] call "the lonely crowd."

 TABLE 21-1 **Types of Loneliness**

Types	Characteristics
Transient	Duration: few minutes or hours; loneliness relieved by client
Situational	Precipitated by a life event of significance to the client; severe reactions, possibly lasting up to 1 year
Chronic	Extends beyond temporary circumstances to become a way of life; faulty interaction patterns; minimal or nonexistent intimacy

Slater[62] believes individualism is the cause of loneliness in America. Basically, people desire community and other people. The American pursuit of individualism (need to control one's behavior and to be self-directed) contradicts the basic nature of human beings, which is to be with others. The result is loneliness.

In terms of either position, loneliness is normal and is a common experience. The nature of loneliness is affected by sociological forces and is shaped by both the past and the present.

Not all individuals who are alone are lonely. Although the terms frequently are used interchangeably, aloneness, solitude, and boredom are not synonymous with loneliness (Table 21-2). People can be by themselves for a long time and not feel lonely because of their attitude. That is, they perceive themselves as having friends, neighbors, or a higher being to whom they can turn for comfort and company. Being bored is not the same as being lonely. Some individuals have a strong social network but still experience *boredom* or a lack of something to do.

Humanistic

In his theory of personality, Rogers[54] proposed that there is a discrepancy between one's inner self and the self seen by others. He believed that clients are pressured by society

TABLE 21-2 **Definitions of Loneliness and Related Terms**

Term	Definition
Loneliness	A negative experience caused by lack of contact; feeling that something is missing
Aloneness	An observable deficiency in social contacts; may or may not lead to loneliness
Solitude	Voluntary withdrawal from interpersonal relationships
Boredom	Lack of something to do

to behave in certain ways and that loneliness is a natural outcome of performing expected roles. As the individual performs these various roles, an empty existence emerges.

People remain "locked in their loneliness" because they believe their real inner selves are unlovable. Fearing rejection prevents them from truly exposing their real selves. Thus people continue to perform their social roles despite the accompanying feelings of emptiness; consequently, they can expect to experience loneliness. The cause lies within the client and is shaped more by current experiences than by childhood experiences.

Existential

Moustakas[15] differentiates between "loneliness anxiety" and "real," or "existential," loneliness. The former contributes to loneliness; the latter is loneliness. Loneliness anxiety results from a discrepancy between what one is and what one pretends to be. The resulting anxiety causes the use of defense mechanisms that prevent people from examining themselves and, frequently, from seeking activity with others. Facing genuine life experiences and realizing one's aloneness cause real or existential loneliness. Almost exclusively, Moustakas regards this kind of loneliness as an essentially positive experience.

Interactionist

Weiss[67] regards the cause of loneliness as the interaction between personality and situational factors. On the basis of his clinical work, he has described two types of loneliness. *Emotional loneliness* occurs when close intimacy is lacking; *social loneliness* happens when meaningful friendships or a sense of community is lacking. Emotionally lonely individuals feel restless and empty, whereas socially lonely people are bored and feel socially inadequate. Interactionists also view loneliness as normal. Table 21-3 summarizes the theoretical approaches.

▼ **TABLE 21-3**   **Summary of Theories of Loneliness**

Theory	Theorist	Dynamics
Psychoanalytical	Zilboorg	Loneliness has roots in infancy. The lonely person has infantile, omnipotent feelings.
		Lonesome is transient and normal; loneliness is a consuming, negative experience.
	Sullivan	Loneliness first appears in childhood with a need for human intimacy. Failing to gain social skills can lead to adult loneliness.
	Fromm-Reichman	Loneliness originates in childhood, can be unpleasant, and can lead to psychoses.
Cognitive	Perlman and Peplau	Loneliness results from discrepancies between actual and perceived levels of social contact.
		Loneliness is one end point of a social interaction continuum.
Sociocultural	Reisman, Glazer, and Denney	Loneliness is shaped by society, originates in childhood, and is reinforced in adulthood.
	Slater	Loneliness results from a pursuit of individualism that contradicts the human desire to be with others.
		Loneliness is normal and commonly experienced.
Humanistic outcome	Rogers	Loneliness is a natural consequence of performing one's societal roles.
		People are "locked in their loneliness" because they believe that their inner selves are unlovable.
		The cause of loneliness is within and is shaped more by current experiences than by childhood experiences.
Existential	Moustakas	Loneliness is viewed as a positive experience.
		Real loneliness and loneliness anxiety are different entities.
Interactionist	Weiss	Loneliness is caused by the interaction between personality and situational factors.
		Two types of loneliness exist: social loneliness and emotional loneliness.

NURSING PROCESS

Assessment

 Physical dimension Loneliness places the client at risk for serious health problems, and physical health problems can cause loneliness. A comprehensive life-style assessment provides clues for the nurse to identify not only potential physical problems and chronic illnesses but also risks for development of loneliness in the future.[61] The accompanying box lists possible health problems that have a loneliness component. Some physical problems necessarily lead to loneliness because human contact is minimized. Some diseases and physical problems carry a social stigma, causing others to avoid people with those medical diagnoses.

Loneliness can develop in clients with various physical disorders that affect not only them but also their families or support systems (see the research highlight on p. 437). Decreasing intimacy or quality and quantity of supportive relationships can cause loneliness. A client's loneliness can

▼ **HEALTH CONDITIONS THAT INCREASE THE RISK FOR DEVELOPING LONELINESS**

Cardiovascular Conditions

Myocardial infarction
Congestive heart failure
Coronary thrombosis
Ventricular fibrillation
Hypertension

Body Image Conditions

Overweight or underweight
Limb amputation
Scars
Facial deformities
Mastectomy
Colostomy

Conditions with a Social Stigma

Cancer
Tuberculosis
Alcoholism in self or family member
Acquired immunodeficiency syndrome (AIDS)

Communication Disorders

Dyslexia
Stuttering

Sleep Disturbances

Hypersomnolence
Hyperactivity

Conditions Altering Social Relationships

Chronic disease
Malnutrition
Chronic pain
Somatic illnesses

Congenital Malformations

Achondroplasia
Craniofacial defects
Amelia or hypomelia

Dermatological Conditions

Port-wine stains
Acne
Ichthyosis
Scleroderma
Visible skin cancers

Conditions Usually Requiring Limited People Contact

Hemophilia
Osteogenesis imperfecta
Immunodeficiencies
Leukemia

Altered Activity Levels

Cushing's disease
Paraplegia
Quadriplegia
Gait disturbances

Conditions Altering Sexual Activity

Impotence
Premature ejaculation
Frigidity
Sexual deviance
Genitourinary surgery
Herpes zoster or shingles
Surgeries
Colostomy
Hysterectomy
Foul body odors

a family member's health problem. For example, the child with an alcoholic parent may have limited social contacts because of the family's denial of the problem. Thus assessment takes into consideration the physical health status of both clients and their family members.

The nurse correlates various components of treatment, such as the type of hospitalization, with loneliness. Hospitalization that requires isolation and a limited number of visitors, recovery from an acute illness, or being in the final stages of an illness that leaves the client too weak for socializing, can all create temporary loneliness. In these situations temporary loneliness is inevitable. Both social isolation and feelings of loneliness occur among hospitalized and dying clients, especially those in acute-care, cure-focused settings.[19,33] Consider the lonely state of Mary Beth in the following case example.

▼ Case Example

Mary Beth is a 25-year-old artist with a traumatic injury to her right arm that resulted in a below-elbow amputation. She was right handed. She has been hospitalized 8 days and has been out of the intensive care unit for 2 days.

Because of his job, Mary Beth's husband can visit only briefly and infrequently. Mary Beth has not seen her children, 4 months old and 5 years old, since her hospitalization on the day of the accident. She cries frequently, snaps at hospital personnel when answering their questions, has been unable to sleep easily at night, and claims she is useless to everybody.

She will not look at staff members when they try to engage her in conversation; she tells them she wants to be alone. She has asked to see her parents and children, but visits have not been possible because of distance from the hospital, lack of funds, and her parents' lack of desire to visit. She has no interest in television or reading.

The staff learned that Mary Beth operates her own craft business from a building near her home. Mary Beth sells her oil paintings and gives art lessons at her business establishment. A friend has agreed to operate the business while she recuperates.

Assessment of Mary Beth's health included information contributing to loneliness. Once the nurse assessed the significance of her contacts with family, friends, and staff and determined the relevance of diversionary activities, Mary Beth can assist the nurse to develop goals and interventions to relieve or minimize loneliness and enhance her recovery. The nurse, using sociocultural theory, continues to assess her social relationships throughout the hospitalization and discharge to prevent the development of chronic loneliness as Mary Beth's healing progresses. Humanistic theory guides the nurse's assessment of Mary Beth's adjustment to the traumatic amputation and later to the prosthesis.

The nurse determines the medications the client is taking because they can contribute to the development of loneliness. Drugs such as antipsychotics and strong sedatives alter the client's thinking. Medications can cause communication disorders or neurological dysfunctions. Long-term cortisone therapy alters the client's physical appearance and activity level. These in turn can affect the client's ability to relate to others and the desire of others to be with the client.

Other health-related factors such as sleep patterns, socially unacceptable diseases, aesthetics, nutritional state,

RESEARCH HIGHLIGHT

Loneliness of Chronically Ill Adults and Their Spouses

• MJ Foxall and JY Ekberg

PURPOSES

This study determined the presence of and significant differences in frequency of loneliness between chronically ill adults and their spouses. It also examined the relationship between loneliness and sociodemographic, disease-related, sociological, and psychological characteristics. The data were part of a study on the adjustment of couples to chronic illness.

SAMPLE

Subjects were 80 nonhospitalized chronically ill persons and their 80 spouses purposively selected from sources such as self-help groups, clinics, and volunteers. Although they represented a variety of chronic illnesses, the majority of conditions were arthritis, chronic obstructive pulmonary disease, and peripheral vascular disease. Criteria for selection included age 25 years and older, husband and wife living together, either husband or wife but not both with at least one diagnosis of chronic illness (self-defined) for at least 6 months duration before the date of the interview, and the ability to respond appropriately in an interview.

Ill subjects were 47 men and 33 women, ranging in age from 26 to 85 years. The number of chronic illnesses ranged from 1 to 8 ($M = 2.78$; $SD = 1.65$) and the duration of illness ranged from 1 to 42 years ($M = 10.15$; $SD = 10.03$). Twenty-nine percent reported complete disability and 49% reported partial disability. Spouses ranged in age from 25 to 82 years ($M = 54.81$; $SD = 11.10$), and marriage length ranged from 2 to 63 years ($M = 30.79$; $SD = 13.10$). The majority were high school graduates, with a median annual income between $20,000 and $29,999.

METHODOLOGY

Loneliness of both groups was assessed using a single dichotomous item from the Oars Multidimensional Functional Assessment Questionnaire. Data on selected characteristics were collected using four instruments: subscales from the Oars, Disability Classification Index, Social Role Rating Scale, and Life Satisfaction Index-Z Scale. The instruments were administered separately to each member of the couple in their home by two nurse researchers.

Based on data from *Issues in Mental Health Nursing* 10(2):149, 1989.

FINDINGS

When subjects were asked whether they were lonely, 31% of the ill persons and 41% of the spouses reported "Yes." There was no significant difference between the two groups ($Z = 1.30$; $P = 0.19$). For both groups, women were more lonely than men; this difference was significant for the ill group ($P < 0.001$).

The highest correlation between loneliness and sociodemographical characteristics was the need for financial assistance for ill respondents and inability to afford luxuries for spouses; between lonely and disease-related characteristics, the highest correlation was the number of chronic illnesses for the ill and disability of the ill partner for spouses; between lonely and sociological characteristics, the highest correlation was decrease in the homemaker role for the ill and decrease in the leisure role for spouses. For both groups, loneliness was significantly related to lower life satisfaction and unrelated to mental health.

IMPLICATIONS

Differences found in the two groups indicate a need for alternative approaches in nursing interventions for lonely ill adults and their spouses. The nurse needs to encourage couples to recognize and clarify loneliness and develop realistic expectations to alleviate loneliness needs related to changes brought about by a chronic disease state.

Because women tended to express more loneliness and to be more socially responsive, the nurse can encourage their use of support systems within both family and community. For caretaking spouses who are socially isolated, the nurse needs to suggest methods for them to gain some personal time. These activities can occur with meaningful others if the ill spouse is unable to participate. Short-duration activities include physical exercise, walking, shopping, playing cards, and eating with friends. Longer-duration activities can be a weekend away from the home for the caretaker or a few days of respite care in a skilled nursing facility for the ill spouse. Together, the nurse and the couple can develop meaningful ways to alleviate loneliness.

---

illness treatments, and pain tolerance have been linked to loneliness and warrant assessment. Loneliness can cause sleep disturbances, and sleep disturbances can cause loneliness. Lonely clients often manifest sleep disturbances similar to those of depressed clients.

Visible congenital defects, inherited diseases, and aesthetic problems can diminish the desire of others to be with the client. Offensive odors, chronic nausea, vomiting or diarrhea, incontinence of stool or urine, and mutilating surgery need to be addressed as possible barriers to socialization and intimacy.

Poor nutrition among elderly persons often is due to

loneliness rather than to food or money. Women who have cooked for family or friends and who ate with them are especially vulnerable to loneliness at mealtimes when these significant others are gone. The client avoids meals to prevent feelings of loneliness.

Chronic diseases that require numerous treatments, such as renal dialysis, and chronic pain limit the client's quality of social activities. Social activities often become secondary to treatment of the client's health problem.

Lonely people have reported lower pain tolerance levels. Some require higher doses of pain relief medication; others may have somatic complaints. The astute nurse assesses the loneliness needs of clients who request frequent pain relief or higher doses of pain relief medication. The nurse explores the client's needs for the presence of other persons to relieve loneliness.

Emotional dimension There is no one simple way to describe how lonely clients feel. Their expression of loneliness may be similar to the following responses by clients who were asked to describe what it was like to be lonely:

"I felt so empty inside."

"I was totally unlikable."

"I did not know what to do with myself. Nothing I did was satisfying, and I felt so aimless."

"I was depressed and felt unwanted. I was leprous and unclean."

"Nothing meant anything to me. I had no one to share my life with . . . everyone was gone."

"I'm afraid to be with people. I never feel good enough or pretty enough around them."

"I feel so isolated. No one wants to be around me."

These statements indicate the complexity of the client's feelings. They express a variety of reactions from depression, insecurity, anger, despair, sadness, boredom, aloneness, self-pity, self-deprecation, shame, and hopelessness to phobic behavior (see accompanying box). The nurse needs to explore the intensity of the client's loneliness, the reasons behind the loneliness, the times or days when loneliness occurs, the length of time that loneliness has been present, and measures used to relieve loneliness.

Loneliness is seldom seen in isolation. Using psychoanalytical theory, the nurse assesses the client for the presence of other emotional pathology such as depression, hopelessness, and personality disorders. Hopelessness has been found to be a significant prediction of loneliness in women and men (see research highlight on p. 439). The accompanying behaviors can prevent the development and continuation of meaningful relationships. This theory supports obtaining a history of early childhood, as loneliness has its roots in infancy.

A client can feel afraid to express feelings toward others when faced with difficult circumstances. Unless feelings are expressed, however, he can feel alienated. Encouraging the expression of feelings in a safe environment and conveying acceptance of those feelings clarify the client's perspective on the situation.

Intellectual dimension When needs for relationships are met, people can be more creative, rational, and logical. Problem solving is easier. The nurse assesses problem-solving abilities, use of defense mechanisms such as rationalization and intellectualization, reality orientation, and perceptions and beliefs about the client's health. Extreme loneliness can lead to altered perceptions and ultimately suicidal thoughts and actions.

From the interactionist perspective, the nurse assesses the client's involvement with meaningful relationships and the community. Assessing involvement via organizations that require interacting with others and creative thinking provides important information to determine intervention strategies.

Sensory stimulation provides data for the client's thoughts. If the senses such as sight and hearing are malfunctioning, the client cannot receive accurate cues. Logical thinking may be altered, creating loneliness. Consider the following case example.

▼ CLIENT FEELINGS WHEN LONELY

Category 1: Desperation
Desperate
Panicked
Helpless
Afraid
Without hope
Abandoned
Vulnerable

Category 3: Impatience, Boredom
Anxious
Not attentive
Desirous to be elsewhere
Uneasy
Angry
Unable to concentrate

Category 2: Depression
Sad
Depressed
Empty
Isolated
Self-pitying
Melancholy
Alienated
Longing to be with one special person

Category 4: Self-deprecation
Unattractive
Down on self
Stupid
Ashamed
Insecure

▼ Case Example

Auda, 75 years old, has numerous lifelong friends. She is widowed and lives alone in a rural community where friendships are the essence of living. Two years ago she developed a hearing loss. Surgery to restore hearing was unsuccessful, a hearing aid will not be beneficial.

Several friends came by to wish her a happy birthday. She has difficulty hearing when there is considerable background noise. The kitchen is humming with activity. Two of her friends, Exie and Darlene, are laughing and talking to each other; Darlene says "That Auda is such a darling." Auda barely catches the conversation. She heard "That Auda is such a . . . " and completes the sentence with the word " . . . bother."

Moments later Auda is found crying in her bedroom. She is inconsolable. The party atmosphere vanishes.

In this case example, the client's diminished hearing caused her to hear only part of the conversation. Her perceptions were based on inaccurate information. She may find herself increasingly lonely as her friends tire of her inability to relate to them as before. These situations are common among persons with impaired hearing. If family or friends cannot cope with the person's behavior changes or if the hearing loss is not corrected, hearing impaired-individuals soon experience a shrinking social network.

Assessing the client's attitude toward self and others can provide cues to loneliness that have been associated with cynicism, rejection of life and others, doubting, and pessimistic beliefs. The client feels an inability to control his destiny. Researchers have found that lonely people have a negative view of marriage and either see themselves as never marrying or report the likelihood of a marriage ending in divorce.[29,63] If clients actually believe that others are not worth knowing and that little can be done to change their relationships, they probably will not be motivated to change. Thus they will continue to isolate themselves.

RESEARCH HIGHLIGHT

Predictors of Loneliness in Older Women and Men
• C Beck, C Shultz, C Walton, and R Walls

PURPOSES

This pilot study explored how the predisposing and precipitating factors of loneliness differed between older women and men. The predisposing factors addressed included age; education; health status, including hearing; marital status; spiritual well-being; and hopelessness. The precipitating factors addressed included geographical location, living arrangements, mobility, presence of living children, adequate contacts, retirement, and stress.

SAMPLE

The nonprobability sample was one of convenience. The sample was obtained from older people who were attending classes offered by a private southern university during summer sessions. These formal and informal 1-week classes are conducted for older persons in colleges and universities throughout the United States.

Eighty-five subjects (52 women, 33 men) participated in this study and returned completed questionnaires. Although the majority of the subjects were from Arkansas, 17 other states were represented. Most of the subjects reported a religious affiliation. The subjects came from varied previous occupational backgrounds including the military, sales, teaching, medicine, farming, and bookbinding.

METHODOLOGY

Data were obtained using the subjects' answers on the Demographic Questionnaire, the Abbreviated Loneliness Scale, the Hopelessness Scale, the Social Readjustment Scale, and the Spiritual Well-Being Scale. One of the co-investigators attended one of the group's functions and presented an overview of the research before administering the instruments. Subjects were given 3 days to complete the instruments, which were returned to the co-investigator.

FINDINGS

Univariate comparisons on the study variables revealed no significant differences between women and men. Hopelessness was found to be a significant predictor of loneliness in both women and men. Spiritual well-being (existential) and education were less predictive for women than for men.

IMPLICATIONS

Results and their interpretation are considered exploratory. Until more studies are available on gender differences in loneliness, nurses assessing and treating loneliness in the older person should not assume that predisposing and precipitating factors are the same for women and men. Especially valuable would be developing specific interventions to prevent or diminish loneliness, for example, discovering how to increase an older woman's sense of spiritual well-being or how to decrease an older person's sense of hopelessness.

Based on data from *Journal of Women and Aging* 2(1):3, 1990.

Social dimension According to sociocultural theory, assessment of the social dimension of a client's loneliness includes determining the following factors: the number and type of social contacts in the social network, intimacy, recent moves, status of pets, desire for human contact, job status, relationship satisfaction, feelings such as shyness when with others, self-concept, times when loneliness occurs, number of people living in the client's home and their relationship to each other, marital status, income level, recent life or role changes, recent losses such as divorce or death, culture, economic factors, social skills, and the concept of trust. Cognitive theory also encourages the nurse to assess expected levels of social contact. Together these theories guide the obtainment of information that contributes to discovering if clients are at risk for developing loneliness and their coping strategies for relieving and preventing loneliness.

Social skills are necessary to form relationships and to meet the human being's need for companionship. Because lonely people seem to have problems relating to others, it is likely that their social skills are deficient. A lonely client may describe feeling awkward in social situations, may suffer from low self-esteem, or may feel alienated from family members or friends. Thus it is important to assess what

loneliness means to the indiviudal client so that interventions are based on the specific circumstances involved.

Typically, lonely people take fewer social risks. They tend to avoid meeting new friends, include fewer people in their social network, express less affection for others, and give only minimal self-disclosure. They have difficulty being close to others and letting others be close to them. Lonely people often report being shy, introverted, and self-conscious. They may have had poor role models regarding relationships in their formative years.

Slater's theory of individualism (need to control one's behavior and to be self-directed) indicates that some lonely people have increaesd self-focused attention that prevents them from being empathic and responsive to the needs and feelings of others.[62] Psychoanalytical theory also supports this view. Some are inhibited socially and shy and do not enjoy parties or the company of others. Lonely people are more likely to strongly influence others to meet their goals, which may prevent relationships from developing.

Loneliness is age related; its intensity is more prevalent among adolescents and older adults. Among older people, loneliness is more related to socioeconomic status than to age or health. Elderly persons may be unable to form new friendships as their social circle decreases because of death and disability. Fixed incomes alter their life-styles and ability to maintain friendships; for example, if they can no longer drive, it may become more difficult to visit family and friends. Loneliness is acutely painful and widespread among adolescents, particularly those who live in divorced families. Adolescent loneliness is more frequent on Fridays and Saturdays. Adolescents also are more likely to feel isolated from parents, teachers, and peers. Adolescents of the lowest social classes, regardless of culture or ethnic group, are more likely to be lonely in their search to belong. Social skill deficits have been found in adolescents who describe themselves as unpopular, shy, and passive. The most vulnerable group seems to be 13-year-old girls.[37] Williams[70] has linked delinquent behavior with loneliness.

An association has been found between loneliness and the absence of close personal relationships, that is, friends, dating partners, and mates. Some adults without mates experience more intense loneliness than those with mates. For college students the absence of dating partners and friends is closely related to the development of loneliness. Students who have never had steady dating partners are lonelier than those who have.

Economic factors also may relate to loneliness, especially as they affect the client's self-esteem. Particularly important is the link between low socioeconomic status and loneliness. Poor persons may view their status as inferior and consequently may not relate to others because they may be embarrassed about their clothing or housing.

Loneliness is not related to the total number of friends.[45] One friendship can meet the client's needs for relationships. Loneliness, then, according to cognitive theory is in the eye of the beholder. Consider the following case example.

▼ Case Example

Michelle, 35 years old, was widowed 3 years ago. She had had a close relationship with her husband, and all social activities had involved them as a couple. As a career woman she made the decision to remain near her friends rather than move close to her family, who lived more than 2000 miles away.

Grieving was intense as was the loneliness she felt over the next 2 years. She attended many social functions, dated often, and visited friends frequently. Despite these social activities and numerous friends, loneliness was prolonged and a severe depression occurred. Michelle felt hopeless and had suicidal thoughts. Her loneliness was unrelieved by social activity and professional involvement.

The nurse knows that experiencing a death, divorce, or loss of a lover places clients at risk for loneliness. Thus using humanistic theory, the nurse assesses Michelle's role changes and social dimension beyond the number of persons in her social network. Obviously the one close relationship had provided satisfaction; removing that relationship made the client vulnerable.

Satisfaction with relationships is more important than frequency or length of interactions. Many lonely people have reported frequent interactions with strangers and acquaintances and fewer interactions with family and friends. In other words, lonely people meet many individuals, but they remain lonely because these persons are not as important as family, friends, or work.

Not to be overlooked is the client's physical environ-

ment, for example, whether the client is housebound or lacks mobility. The nurse assesses the location of the home or apartment relative to meaningful social activities, resources to seek social activities (that is, car, money, or phone), the size of the home, the number of people in the home or rooms for privacy, the home's appearance and cleanliness, the presence of pets, and safety factors. Persons who live in urban areas and in communities with high crime rates are more vulnerable to loneliness because they fear venturing out or cannot afford transportation to social activities.

Employment factors may contribute to loneliness. Workers whose roles are primarily technical and those who perform repetitive tasks that require minimal thinking may not consider themselves valuable to the work setting. They may feel isolated even from their co-workers. On the other hand, the higher one rises in the organization and the more power one attains, the more likely that feelings of loneliness may develop. Too much work or the hours people work may limit the time clients can spend in social activities.

Time of day may affect the client's loneliness and is considered in the assessment of a hospitalized client. Specific times when hospitalized clients feel most lonely include late evening after visitors have left and before bedtime.[46] The nearness of meaningful holidays or anniversary dates heightens lonely feelings.

From an interactionist perspective, cultural factors that promote loneliness relate to moving. The move can be related either to a change in one's socioeconomic status or to moving to a different geographical region. Culture exclusion occurs when one cultural group does not accept another.[11] With the frequency of upward mobility and moves from one area of the country to another, people require time to learn a new group's values. Until then, loneliness may result. If for any reason a person does not attain full group membership, lonely feelings increase.

Typically, lonely people dislike not only themselves but others. Understanding the client's general attitude toward self and others may provide cues about the presence of loneliness. Lonely people express less interest in sustaining contact with people, perhaps to avoid the pain of rejection or possibly because of lack of positive social reinforcement.

▼
CLIENT-REPORTED REASONS FOR LONELINESS

Category 1: Being Unattached

Having no spouse
Having no sexual partner
Breaking up with spouse or lover

Category 2: Alienation

Feeling different
Being misunderstood
Not being needed
Having no close friends

Category 3: Being Alone

Coming home to an empty house
Having no social contacts

Category 4: Forced Isolation

Being housebound
Being hospitalized
Having no transportation

Category 5: Dislocation

Being far from home
Being in a new job or school
Moving too often
Traveling often

They can avoid or distance others by projecting their own inadequacies and expecting perfection in acquaintances and friends.

Reasons for being lonely are as diverse as the expressions of loneliness. Rubenstein and Shaver[57] placed reasons for being lonely into the five categories, which are summarized in the box on p. 440.

Spiritual dimension Feeling alone can be a painful experience. Determining the client's meaning of life and desire for relationships with others and a higher power provides an indicator of the extent of loneliness. Lonely clients may not have much hope of being liked or even tolerated by others. They often express feelings of alienation. Without a faith in themselves, others, or a higher power, they are unlikely to explore new relationships or to take risks with current relationships.

Most religious groups encourage the concept of companionship. In Western culture an ongoing relationship between individuals and a higher power and among individual persons is at the center of religious beliefs and practices. Thus assessment includes the client's focus of worship and concept of a higher being as well as the degree of support that is perceived as necessary.

Religious teachings include general principles of conduct. In many religions, people are reminded to love self and others and to actively express that love. Assessment includes determining the beliefs the client actively practices in relating to fellow human beings. The following questions deal with the client's spiritual dimension:

- How frequently are you with others? Alone?
- Do you view others as friendly or hostile?
- What does your religion believe about the need to be alone?
- When have you felt isolated from a higher being? From family and friends?
- What religious practices do you use to relieve loneliness?
- What are your creative abilities? Do you practice them alone or with others?

▼ TABLE 21-4   Instruments to Measure Loneliness

Instruments	Measures
UCLA Loneliness Scale	Presence and degree of loneliness
NYU Loneliness Scale	Long-term loneliness and its extent; directly measures feelings associated with loneliness
Revised UCLA Loneliness Scale	Presence and degree of loneliness; modified for middle-age and elderly populations; indirectly measures loneliness as it assesses relationships to people
Schedules for the Measurement of Loneliness and Cathectic Investment (SMLC Scale)	Presence of loneliness and cathexis (attaching significance to important persons and objects)
Abbreviated Loneliness Scale	Developed to improve the original UCLA Loneliness Scale

Measurement Tools

Two different approaches are available to measure loneliness. One approach is unidimensional and describes loneliness as a single experience with common themes. The second approach is multifaceted and views loneliness with multiple components. Table 21-4 summarizes the more common tools.

Analysis

Nursing diagnosis

The NANDA nursing diagnoses related to loneliness are impaired social interaction and social isolation.

The following case example illustrates characteristics of the nursing diagnosis of impaired social interaction.

▼ Case Example

Jason is a 14-year-old boy who has recently moved with his parents from a rural area of Arkansas to Atlanta, Georgia. The move occurred several months before his graduation from the school system he has attended for the last 8 years.

Jason's parents are concerned because after 3 months in his new school he continues to verbalize his inability to meet new friends. He complains every weekend about being lonely and not having anything to do. When his parents suggest that he call someone or go to school functions, he gets very angry and says that "the kids here don't like to do the same things I like to do."

He leaves home for school in time to arrive for his first class and comes home directly after school ends. He complained that some classmates have made fun of his accent; he often comes home in tears. One teacher recently called and talked to Jason's parents about Jason's difficulty concentrating in the classroom. His parents believe that he is depressed and have called the school counselor.

▼ IMPAIRED SOCIAL INTERACTION

DEFINITION

The state in which an individual participates in an insufficient or excessive quantity or ineffective quality of social exchange.

DEFINING CHARACTERISTICS

- **Intellectual dimension**

  Verbalized or observed inability to receive or communicate a satisfying sense of belonging, caring, interest, or shared history

  Family report of change in style or pattern of interaction

- **Social dimension**

  Verbalized or observed discomfort in social situations

  Observed use of unsuccessful social interaction behaviors

  Observed use of successful social interaction behaviors

  Dysfunctional interaction with peers, family, and/or others

Modified from Kim MJ, McFarland GK, McLane AM, editors: *Pocket guide to nursing diagnoses,* ed 5, St Louis, 1993, Mosby–Year Book.

▼ **SOCIAL ISOLATION**

DEFINITION

Aloneness experienced by an individual and perceived as imposed by others and as a negative or threatened state.

DEFINING CHARACTERISTICS

- **Physical dimension**

  Evidence of physical and/or mental handicap or altered state of wellness

- **Emotional dimension**

  Sad, dull affect
  Projects hostility in voice, behavior
  Expresses feeling of aloneness imposed by others
  Expresses feelings of rejection
  Experiences feelings of indifference of others

- **Intellectual dimension**

  Inappropriate or immature interests and activities for developmental age or stage
  Preoccupation with own thoughts; repetitive, meaningless actions
  Inability to meet expectations of others
  Expresses interests inappropriate to developmental age or stage

- **Social dimension**

  Absence of supportive significant other(s)—family, friends, group
  Seeks to be alone or exist in subculture
  Shows behavior unacceptable by dominant cultural group
  Insecurity in public
  Expresses values acceptable to subculture but is unable to accept values of dominant culture

- **Spiritual dimension**

  Inadequacy in or absence of significant purpose in life

Modified from Kim MJ, McFarland GK, McLane AM, editors: *Pocket guide to nursing diagnoses,* ed 5, St Louis, 1993, Mosby–Year Book.

The following case example illustrates characteristics of the nursing diagnosis of social isolation.

▼ Case Example

James, a 59-year-old Korean War veteran, is single and has been chemically dependent since spending several years of his military service in the Aleutian Islands. As a child, he was indulged by parents who rarely punished him, met his every need, and required no accountability from him. He had developed no intimate friend-ships and never learned how to relate to his classmates. He had no household chores and seldom stayed with one activity for long.

Today he leads a lonely existence in an unkempt trailer. A dog is his only companion. He never married and often talks about wanting to have female friends. He has hypertension, chronic obstructive pulmonary disease, and epilepsy. Receiving disability benefits, he holds no job and has no social ties other than occasionally visiting two aunts who live nearby. His parents died years ago and he continues to live in his childhood neighborhood. He is chronically depressed, makes no major decisions greater than grocery choices, and often sleeps 12 to 18 hours a day.

Last week one of his aunts died suddenly. As so often occurred in the past, James reacted to the crisis by turning to diazepam (Valium), meperidine (Demerol), and beer. The prescription drugs are provided for old war wounds and their complications. His chemically altered consciousness prevented his experiencing the immediate loss and subsequent loneliness. He did not attend the funeral telling relatives that he was "just too tired and had too much pain."

Emotional pain is intolerable to him to so he escaped via drugs and avoided the experience. Chemicals prevented feeling the loneliness by altering his awareness and thinking. He is a very lonely individual because of his early childhood and lifelong maturation experiences. His loneliness is chronic and typical of those individuals who did not receive interventions early in life. Unfortunately, loneliness was not widely recognized as a problem worthy of attention in his formative years.

The following list provides examples of NANDA-accepted diagnoses with causative statements:
1. Social isolation related to being raped.
2. Social isolation related to move to a new community.
3. Social isolation related to recent diagnosis of AIDS.
4. Impaired social interaction related to admission to a nursing home.
5. Impaired social interaction related to role changes due to husband's recent death.

Planning

Table 21-5 provides some long- and short-term goals, outcome criteria, nursing interventions, and rationales related to loneliness, which are examples of the planning stage of the nursing process.

Implementation

 Physical dimension Loneliness has been linked with alcoholism, suicide, and physical illness. Because loneliness has life-threatening consequences, the nurse uses the loneliness health-illness continuum model as a reference for client care (Figure 21-2). The nurse strives to prevent or minimize the detrimental effect of loneliness on health by recognizing indicators of loneliness and initiating interventions that increase the likelihood of successfully relating to others. Interventions need to be meaningful to the client and involve participating in activities with small or large numbers of people. Interventions also need to be directed toward developing social skills and promoting a positive attitude toward self.

Groups can be formed for at-risk persons. The nurse arranges programs in which clients share activities, eat together in restaurants, or share meals in each other's homes.

▼ **TABLE 21-5 NURSING CARE PLAN**

GOALS	OUTCOME CRITERIA	INTERVENTIONS	RATIONALES

NURSING DIAGNOSIS: Social isolation related to decreased social contacts while hospitalized in protective isolation

LONG TERM

GOALS	OUTCOME CRITERIA	INTERVENTIONS	RATIONALES
To use effective coping strategies to relieve feelings of loneliness	Use coping strategies that effectively relieve loneliness feelings as evidenced by:		
	• Listing coping strategies used to resolve previous episodes of loneliness	Assist client to recall and list previously used coping strategies.	Increases security by conveying to client he can cope; provides positive reinforcement.
	• Verbalizing loneliness feelings	Encourage client to verbalize feelings of loneliness.	Reduces anxiety.
	• Participating in daily activities that relieve loneliness (e.g., letter writing, phone calling)	Request family to provide material for activities and encourage client to participate.	Diversional activities decrease monotony and limits time client has to think about how lonely

SHORT TERM

GOALS	OUTCOME CRITERIA	INTERVENTIONS	RATIONALES
To maintain social relationships he perceives as positive	Initiates social relationships as energy level permits as evidenced by:		
	• Outlining a schedule to pace social contacts and activities throughout the day	Assist client in developing a daily schedule that allows for social contact and activities.	Helps to structure day and provides opportunity for social contacts.
	• Identifying activities that help keep the client busy, especially during times of high-risk loneliness (e.g., evening hours and weekends)	Encourage client to identify activities of interest.	Allows client to have available a list from which he can plan activities before loneliness becomes intense; increases self-responsibility for managing loneliness.
	• Identifying people the client positively views as desiring communication with while hospitalized.	Assist client to identify people he wants to visit him.	Planned interactions with others break up periods of isolation and minimizes episodes of loneliness.

Churches, neighborhood, and senior citizen groups have regular meetings that include meals; Sunday dinners for widowed individuals provide companionship at a vulnerable time of the week. Older adults who are able to participate in the following activities have found them extremely helpful[26,34]: hobbies; sports; reading; playing cards; watching television; praying; meditating; work such as housework, cooking, and gardening; and completing jigsaw or crossword puzzles.

Regular physical exercise (for example, using a stationary bike, weight lifting, walking, golfing, and swimming) not only improves physical health but also contributes to general emotional health because endorphins are produced, promoting a sense of well-being. Those who feel good about themselves are more likely to interact with others.

Relieving lonely feelings requires accepting an unalterable physical problem such as a congenital syndrome or altering a problem such as obesity. Changing the client's perceptions or his body image is paramount to developing relationships. Assisting clients to accept themselves noncritically may be handled with interventions such as thought-stopping techniques (see Chapter 12). More resistant problems may require referral to a counselor.

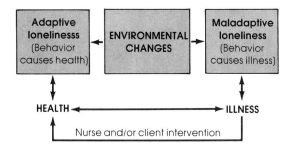

FIGURE 21-2 The client's response to loneliness on a health-illness continuum.

Correcting disfigurements that can be changed by cosmetic surgery may result in the client's desire to be with others. Persons with missing or nonfunctional body parts can be referred to organizations that provide support and guidance for obtaining and using prostheses. These organizations can assist the client to locate stores that sell clothing for persons who have had disfiguring surgeries.

When the problem is decreased mobility as a result of a fractured hip or paralysis, physical supports such as canes, walkers, and wheelchairs are available. These supports increase mobility, which in turn increase social interaction.

If sensory perceptions are altered and the problem is correctable, the nurse explores ways to obtain items such as glasses and hearing devices. Community organizations such as the Lions Club and Kiwanis Club assist in purchasing these items for low-income individuals. Support groups are available for hearing and visually impaired persons. The client may need to learn a new method of communication such as the Braille alphabet or sign language. Tutors and volunteers are available in most large communities. Attachments to amplify voices may be placed on the client's telephone and are usually available from an electronics store, the telephone company, or community service organizations.

If the client is homebound, visiting nurses from the private or public health sector are incorporated into discharge planning. The community nurse facilitates continuity of care into the home and works with clients to minimize social isolation. In some states social services provide transportation to buy groceries, keep health-related appointments, or ensure opportunities for social outings. Other communities may coordinate these services through volunteer efforts.

Odors can contribute to isolation. Simply improving personal hygiene may also eliminate the problem. In managing these aesthetic problems, professionals such as enterostomal therapists are available for consultation. Bowel and bladder training regimens, as well as odor eliminators, are identified in the nursing literature if specific instructions are needed.

Urban clients who live in unsafe neighborhoods are especially likely to be lonely. Moving may be impossible and may create more problems than it solves. Interventions are designed that consider the client's habits and habitat. For example, a lonely client living in a innercity can use community-supported transportation to receive health care in free neighborhood clinics; the client may need assistance

only in identifying transportation and the clinic location. Another challenge is presented by the client who lives in an isolated rural area or in a high-income area distant from neighbors. Neighborhood support groups, law enforcement officials, and community organizations may be used to develop an informal social network to check on these individuals periodically and assist in meeting their needs for social interaction.

Emotional dimension The nurse helps lonely clients by acknowledging their loneliness. Encouraging clients to describe what they feel may prevent avoidance or denial of loneliness. They may need assistance in expressing loss of power, diminished prestige, anger, and dependence.

The client's predominant feeling state, such as depression and anger, initially directs the nursing interventions. If the client is in an acute care setting, sometimes the nurse's availability and willingness to talk are all that are needed. The nurse thus provides support during hospitalization. Hospitalized clients with few visitors or with long spans of time between visitors have found visits by the nurse helpful. Short, frequent visits and expression of interest and concern minimize loneliness.[46]

The nurse's communication portrays hopefulness, concern, acceptance, and a willingness to spend time with the client. Many people believe the common myth that nothing can change the behavior of lonely persons. This myth has prevented lonely individuals from seeking help. The nurse cannot convince the lonely client to change unless she believes changes can occur. Without hope and encouragement from the nurse, the relationship may not progress beyond superficial interactions.

Several activities have been identified that individuals engage in to relieve the discomfort of loneliness.[57] These include crying, sleeping, thinking, doing nothing, overeating, taking tranquilizers, watching television, drinking or getting "stoned," studying or working, writing, listening to music, exercising, walking, working on a hobby, going to a movie, reading, playing music, spending money, calling a friend, and visiting someone. Some are therapeutic; others are not. The most commonly used activities were reading, listening to music, and calling a friend. At first glance they may appear to be overly simple. Yet clients have documented that these kinds of activities work for them. Thus nurses incorporate them into plans to relieve client loneliness.

Because loneliness is so prevalent and accompanies numerous disorders and situations, the psychiatric nurse can serve as a consultant for lonely clients and their families. The need to help staff members develop interventions or provide direct care through counseling in nonpsychiatric settings has increased considerably.

Intellectual dimension If the client has negative thoughts about himself and others that prevent him from developing relationships, the nurse directs him in using thought-stopping techniques discussed in Chapter 12. Converting negative thoughts to positive thoughts can break the self-deprecating cycle that many lonely people experience and prepare these clients for better relationships.

Scheduling diversional activities for evenings or weekends when loneliness is most likely to occur prevents the client from having time to think about how lonely he is.

These activities are based on the client's interests, physical functioning, and resources such as money and equipment or supplies needed to participate in the activity.

Therapeutic reminiscing has proved helpful for older clients who can share interesting events about their past. Previous successes and coping mechanisms prove to the client he is worthwhile and his life has meaning. By reflecting on skills used previously to solve socially related problems, clients can gain hope to face present problems that lead to loneliness.

Social dimension Interventions to enhance social skills and to increase the number and quality of relationships are firmly established in terms of what the client values. The client's need for autonomy affects the success of the intervention. For example, clients who value their independence will receive the greatest benefit from interventions that allow them to maintain control. For the lonely client, this means helping him develop his own plan to minimize loneliness.

The client needs continual encouragement to explore other relationships and test newly found social skills. As they build confidence in their social abilities, clients need frequent reminders that relationships are complicated and imperfect. Pain and hurt are inevitable, and the nurse needs to be sensitive to the negative aspects of trying new social behaviors. Nursing interventions involve teaching social skills to the client or altering the client's life-style to meet relationship needs. The time needed to learn new ways of relating depends on how quickly clients learn new behaviors and the number and quality of relationships needed to alleviate loneliness. The nurse uses this time to role model appropriate social skills and increasingly to expose the client to other clients using the group process. Additional clients could be added one by one to groups to gradually expand the number until the client is comfortably relating well to the total group.

With a motivated client, the nurse encourages learning new coping behaviors or assists the client to retain successful coping behaviors to attain an optimal health state. The client then adapts in a healthy way to the frequent encounters with situations that produce loneliness. For example, the client who has moved to a new city and knows no one may exhibit disturbed sleep patterns, such as waking in the early morning hours. Over time, exhaustion interferes with work productivity and health, even further reducing the client's ability to develop new friendships. The nurse helps the client alter this cycle and regain optimal health before the maladaptive behavior leads to permanent or destructive results.

Identifying tasks the client can perform during high-risk times prevents lonely feelings. Relatives and friends can be included in activities if the client desires. Holiday and anniversary celebrations are more meaningful if they follow the client's customary plans.

A social network plan involves evaluating the scope of a client's social contacts and enacting a plan to increase the quantity or quality of those contacts. Budget, geographical location, resources, transportation, likes and dislikes, availability of significant others, and health state are considerations in implementing a social network. Willing family members or friends are included in the treatment. The plan belongs to the client; the nurse is the facilitator. For those persons who no longer have an intimate relationship, the nurse gives encouragement while assessing and determining the need to "repeople" their world.

Day-care centers, garden clubs, foster grandparent programs, senior citizen groups, community coffee klatches, church groups, mixers, summer Elderhostel programs, and college classes open to handicapped or senior citizens create opportunities for various age groups to make new social contacts. The nurse gathers pertinent information about these activities to assist the client's decision making. Informing, discussing advantages and disadvantages, establishing priorities, and periodically checking the client's progress toward becoming part of these groups are important nursing interventions. The nurse may assist in forming these activities if none exist within the community.

If the client has diminished self-esteem, some situational changes can be considered. For example, a retired client may have recently moved to a retirement village. Esteem may be lessened if the person no longer views himself as contributing meaningfully to life. A niche usually can be found for the client's talents and abilities. Organizing parties, participating in community political campaigns, volunteering for hospital work, and visiting others in the same area who are temporarily housebound are activities that involve the client's ability to relate to others. Sharing past experiences as a volunteer consultant to those who may benefit from them is a method to develop work-related contacts. Retirement communities with planned activities provide additional options that increase socializing opportunities and the client's social network.

For those confined to prisons, loneliness may be a significant problem. The nurse serving these vulnerable populations may diminish the level of loneliness by encouraging visitors and the development of friendships, especially within the facility. Women are more receptive than men to these interventions.[17]

Sharing housing with someone who is compatible also prevents loneliness. Some individuals have successfully attempted communal living to provide companionship, share expenses, achieve safety, and give meaning to life.

Nursing of clients in long-term care settings such as nursing homes or mental hospitals requires that nurses teach unskilled workers how to meet companionship needs during routine care. Talking while ambulating clients, touching clients when entering their rooms, and allowing clients to talk during mealtimes offer opportunities to enhance the quality of institutional living while encouraging the client's reality orientation. Workers are given this information, but they also need to see nurses who provide models for caring behavior.

Pets can serve as people substitutes (see the research highlight on p. 446). Their companionship has been helpful to persons of all ages, most particularly to those with illnesses that leave them housebound or in nursing homes. As a source of comfort they offer meaning to clients who view their world as hopeless and void. If the client's life-style, resources, and desires permit, a pet not only offers companionship but occupies the client's time. Usually a veterinary medical association and a humane society have guidelines for placing animals in private dwellings and in nursing homes and for arranging pets to visit clients in mental hospitals. During periods of hospitalization the

RESEARCH HIGHLIGHT

Human-Pet Interaction and Loneliness: A Test of Concepts from Roy's Adaptation Model
• M Calvert

PURPOSE

The purpose of this study was to examine the extent to which interaction with an animal in the environment reduced loneliness in nursing home residents.

SAMPLE

The sample consisted of 65 residents from two county homes with resident pet programs and two nursing homes with visitation pet programs. All subjects voluntarily agreed to participate in the study and were able to pass a mental status screening using the Pfeiffer Short Portable Mental Status Questionnaire (SPMSQ).

The sample was divided into two groups depending on the level of interaction the participant rated himself as having with the animals in the pet program using a four-point scale. Thirty-two subjects were in the high pet interaction group and 33 were in the low pet interaction group.

Fifty-seven percent were from the county homes with resident programs. The majority of subjects were women (74%); the age range was 42 to 92 years with a mean age of 73.8 years. Both groups were comparable with regard to age and sex. The majority of subjects in both pet interaction groups (91% in high pet interaction and 97% in low pet interaction groups) were previous pet owners.

METHODOLOGY

Two instruments were used in this study. A researcher-designed demographical questionnaire was used to collect sample characteristics and measure human-pet interaction. The simplified version of the revised UCLA Loneliness Scale was used to measure loneliness.

Two resident pet programs and two visitation pet programs were in place for this study. In the resident pet programs, a dog is permitted to live in the facility and roam all areas except the dining rooms. The dog may also sleep or sit on the beds or chairs of the residents who allow this. The staff primarily grooms and feeds the dogs. Participants pet the animals as desired.

In the visitation pet programs, domestic animals such as puppies and kittens are taken by volunteers to the facilities for approximately 1 to 3 hours per visit. The residents are gathered in the hallways and allowed to interact as desired with the animals. The animals may be taken to the rooms and beds of selected residents as permitted by the nursing staff.

Based on data from *Nursing Science Quarterly* 2(4):194, 1989.

One resident program had been in effect for 2 years, the other for 6 years. The monthly visitation programs had existed for 3 months in one home and for 2 years in the other; the former had weekly pet visits for 2 weeks before the data collection.

After gaining permission from each participant, the researcher and two assistants conducted interviews with the subjects. After answering the SPMSQ items correctly, the subjects were interviewed according to the simplified version of the UCLA Loneliness Scale. Response cards written in large, bold print were used to assist the subjects in answering the questions.

FINDINGS

The loneliness scores ranged from 26 to 58, with a high and low pet interaction mean of 38.22 and 42.85, respectively. An independent two-tailed t-test was used to analyze the significance of differences between the mean loneliness scores of the two groups of pet interaction ($t = 2.24$; $P < 0.03$). The subjects in the high pet interaction group were statistically and significantly less lonely than those in the low pet interaction group. Also using an independent two-tailed t-test, the subjects from the homes with the resident pet programs were somewhat less lonely than those from the pet visitation programs ($P = 0.06$).

IMPLICATIONS

Findings were consistent with previous reports about the beneficial effects of human pet contact. Findings also support Roy's adaptation model of nursing, specifically that an individual's adaptive ability is influenced by the presence of environmental stimuli. The findings suggest that interaction with a pet is a positive contextual stimulus that reduces loneliness in nursing home residents, despite the negative factors to which they are exposed.

The study supports Roy's conceptualization of the interdependence mode of adaptation where interaction with a pet may be an important aspect of a person's interdependence mode of adaptation, especially for persons in settings where alienation is present. This study suggests that loneliness can be reduced as one gives attention and recognition to a pet.

---

client needs contact with the pet, either through the caregiver telling the client that his pet is being fed and cared for or through arranging a "visit" by the pet.[18]

Social skills can be developed by methods such as role playing. Imagery assists the client to view himself as successful in social situations. Big Brother, Big Sister, Adopt-A-Grandparent, and Adopt-A-Grandchild groups offer meaningful social outlets and also promote role development according to sociocultural theory.

Spiritual dimension Interventions depend on past practices clients have used to express their belief in a higher being. To clients who value and practice their beliefs, the inability to do so creates an all-consuming loneliness. Encouraging prayer and meditation helps bridge the feelings of alienation. Visits to the hospital or nursing home chapel offer an atmosphere conducive to interacting more meaningfully with their higher being.

When a client is doubting, suffering, lonely, or hurting,

prayer brings relief. When an individual feels alone, reaching out to others becomes a means to forget one's aloneness while fulfilling scriptural intent.

A client can be in conflict over his beliefs and feel alienated from his world. Verbalizing this conflict without fear of censure may relieve the tension and enable the client to solve the problem. In addition, reading favorite passages of the Bible or other inspirational books may provide comfort during times of loneliness.

The nurse fosters the client's own spiritual resources in coping with loneliness rather than imposing new, unfamiliar practices. If the nurse feels inadequate about discussing spiritual matters or cannot support the client's beliefs or

practices, arranging a visit from a chaplain, minister, or rabbi is a logical step.

Some churches have members or ministers who regularly check the religious status of persons admitted to hospitals. These groups schedule frequent visitation and offer services specific to the client's beliefs. Paid or voluntary hospital chaplains may provide the same services. For example, communion can be served at the client's bedside.

Depending on the religious group's outreach services, a member may expect numerous cards, assistance with caring for his family or home, regular visitation, and home care after discharge. Clients may spend years developing relationships with their church groups; the nurse fosters and incorporates this system into the client's interventions.

Clients who are alienated from others may need assistance from the nurse and family members. Encouraging activities involving nature, such as walking outdoors, or involvement with the community, such as volunteering one's services, may cause the client to be more creative and feel like a worthwhile, contributing, and valued member of society. See the accompanying boxes for key interventions for loneliness and guidelines for primary and tertiary prevention.

▼ **KEY INTERVENTIONS**

Arrange programs for clients to share activities such as eating together
Assist client to accept unalterable problems
Refer clients with missing or nonfunctioning body parts to organizations for support and guidance
Plan a regular physical exercise schedule
Relieve physical symptoms such as sleeplessness
Promote expression of lonely feelings
Plan meaningful diversional activities
Provide visits with friends
Acknowledge client's need for autonomy in interventions
Assist client to use thought-stopping techniques to decrease negative thoughts
Encourage therapeutic reminiscing for older, lonely clients
Design activities to enhance social skills
Develop a social network plan to "repeople" client's world
Encourage family to visit and to become involved in client's care
Offer a companion animal

▼ **GUIDELINES FOR PRIMARY/TERTIARY PREVENTION OF LONELINESS**

Primary Prevention

Identify high-risk groups, such as children from families that are isolated
Teach prospective parents about the need for human intimacy
Provide prenatal teaching about early development
Provide supportive follow-up during child's early developmental years
Teach healthy adolescents and elderly about causes of and ways to prevent loneliness

Tertiary Prevention
Community resources

Community mental health centers
Therapeutic group experiences for lonely elderly
Adult day care centers
Residential housing

Self-help groups

Groups for the widowed
Share-a-meal groups
Meditation groups

INTERACTION WITH A LONELY CLIENT

Nurse: *(Making afternoon rounds, entering the room of a hospitalized man who is several hundred miles from home; he is sitting in a chair, the television is on, and he is staring out a window.) Good afternoon, Mr. Graddy; how are you?*
Client: *(He offers no eye contact and continues staring out the window.) Okay.*
Nurse: *You're all alone.*
Client: *(Turning to face her.) Well, yes I am.*
Nurse: *(Indicating an empty chair near him and maintaining eye contact.) May I sit with you?*
Client: *(Nods affirmatively and pulls the chair closer to him so they are sitting across from each other.) Sure. I need some company.*
Nurse: *(Sitting down and placing her paperwork on the dresser nearby.) You seem to be deep in thought. (Pause)*
Client: *(Speaking slowly and with hesitation.) No... not really. I was just thinking about my kids and how much I miss them.*

The preceding conversation continued for about 5 minutes, and the nurse agreed to come by his room again later in the evening.

Mr. Graddy was lonely, and the nurse encouraged him to acknowledge how he felt. Her conversation prevented him from denying the presence of loneliness. By conveying acceptance and spending some time with Mr. Graddy, she provided a caring human contact. In this case, nursing intervention included offering an alternate support system by means of short, frequent visits during the client's hospitalization.

The nurse used verbal and nonverbal communication skills to convey interest, concern, acceptance, and caring. She was not discouraged by his initial lack of interest in her presence. She did not remain standing in a position of authority, and she put down her "professional equipment" to indicate this time was his. He easily responded to her cues, and this visit may become the basis for future positive nurse-client interactions.

Evaluation

Evaluation centers on the client's ability to express loneliness, to reduce or eliminate health problems caused by loneliness, and to achieve awareness of these changes. Generally, people cope with loneliness in one of three ways: (1) changing their relationships, (2) changing their social desires or needs, and (3) decreasing the importance of their relationships. When constructive change does not occur, the nurse develops new goals and incorporates more pertinent strategies into the nursing process. The objective is to replace maladaptive loneliness behavior with positive relationship patterns and effective social skills.

Criteria pertinent to determining the success of the nursing process with the lonely client include the following:

1. *Adequacy:* Did the interventions relieve the loneliness? Were the symptoms of loneliness relieved over time (for example, longer than 1 week)? Were the interventions matched to the client's life-style?

2. *Appropriateness:* Was the intervention related to the severity of the loneliness symptoms? Were acute symptoms the focus of immediate attention? Were the recommended interventions considerate of the client's personal abilities?

3. *Effectiveness:* Did the client learn to manage loneliness feelings? Were the goals and interventions specific to loneliness and related health problems? Did the client change relationship behaviors to alleviate loneliness?

4. *Efficiency:* Were interventions sufficient to prevent or minimize the feelings of loneliness? Was the client's distress relieved? Were resources helpful? Did the process move at a pace that considered the client's readiness and energy level?

Involving the client and family throughout the nursing process provides valuable information about the effectiveness of the plan. Such involvement also enhances the likelihood of permanent change and the adoption of healthier behaviors. Reinforcing positive change encourages the client's receptiveness and adoption of new ways of relating to others.

BRIEF REVIEW

Loneliness is a universal phenomenon that tends to be viewed as negative and unpleasant. About one fourth of the American population (60 million) experience loneliness during any given month. Caused by the inadequacy or lack of certain kinds of important contacts, loneliness has been linked to numerous health problems.

The study of loneliness is a recent development, and nurses such as Peplau have contributed to loneliness information and treatment. Heightened public awareness of the problem provides an excellent opportunity for nurses to assist lonely clients.

Loneliness theories have emerged from the psychological and sociological sciences. Most theorists believe loneliness is an unpleasant emotion that is linked to current situational factors.

Among the at-risk groups for loneliness are adolescents, those with chronic or socially unacceptable illnesses, those with body image problems, those who have lost significant relationships, those who have relocated geographically, and dying persons.

Loneliness and health problems are interrelated; each can cause the other. Health problems related to loneliness include cardiovascular diseases, body image problems, various chronic disorders, emotional disorders, and impaired learning. Situational factors such as divorce, death of significant others, moves, role changes, transportation, problems, lack of employment, and socioeconomic changes and spiritual difficulties contribute to the development of loneliness.

Nursing diagnoses for the lonely client center on social isolation and impaired social interaction. Interventions are designed by both the nurse and client. The goal is to help the client cope through change: change of social needs and relationships and the importance of those relationships. Strategies such as obtaining companion animals, determining transportation needs, altering social skills, and encouraging spiritual beliefs help prevent or minimize lonely feelings.

The nurse is unable to meet all the loneliness needs of her clients in their various development stages. However, she can offer a climate conducive for preventing or minimizing loneliness. This climate contains recognition, regard, respect, understanding, caring, and encouragement to enter relationships with others. In such a climate the client can express himself without fear, test new ways to handle his relationships, reevaluate his behavior, change negative attitudes toward himself and others, and grow toward becoming a more integrated and less lonely human being.

REFERENCES AND SUGGESTED READINGS

1. Anderson C, Arnoult L: Attributional style and everyday problems in living: depression, loneliness, and shyness, *Social Cognition* 3:16, 1989.

2. Anderson C, Harvey R: Discriminating between problems in living: an examination of measures of depression, loneliness, shyness, and social anxiety, *Journal of Social and Clinical Psychology* 6(3/4):482, 1988.

3. Anderson L: Narcissism and loneliness, *International Journal of Aging Human Development* 30(2):81, 1991.

4. Austin A: Becoming immune to loneliness: helping the elderly fill a void, *Journal of Gerontological Nursing* 15(9):25, 1989.

5. Austin B: Factorial structure of the ULCA Loneliness Scale, *Psychological Reports* 53:883, 1990.

6. Beal G: Helping men cope with divorce, *Journal of Psychosocial Nursing and Mental Health Services* 27(8):30, 1989.

7. Beck C and others: Predictors of loneliness in older women and men, *Journal of Women and Aging* 2(1):3, 1990.

8. Blai B: Health consequences of loneliness: a review of the literature, *Journal of the American Association of College Health Services* 37(4):162, 1989.

9. Brennan T: Loneliness at adolescence. In Peplau L, Perlman D, editors: *Loneliness: a sourcebook of current theory, research, and therapy,* New York, 1982, John Wiley & Sons.

10. Brennan T, Auslander N: *Adolescent loneliness: an exploratory study of social and psychological pre-dispositions and theory,* vol 1, National Institute of Mental Health, Juvenile Problems Div., Grant no. R01-MH 289 12-01, Behavioral Research Institute, Washington, DC, 1979.

11. Brody E: Cultural exclusion, character and illness, *American Journal of Psychiatry* 8:852, 1966.

12. Calvert M: Human-pet interaction and loneliness: a test of concepts from Roy's adaptation model, *Nursing Science Quarterly* 2(4):194, 1989.

13. Christian E: Sounds of silence: coping with hearing loss and loneliness, *Journal of Gerontological Nursing* 5(11):4, 1989.
14. Copel L: Loneliness: a conceptual model, *Journal of Psychosocial Nursing and Mental Health Services* 26(1):14, 1988.
15. Davies C: What Ruby really wanted, *Nursing* 20(2):97, 1990.
16. De la Cruz L: On loneliness and the elderly, *Journal of Gerontological Nursing* 12(11):22, 1986.
17. Desmond A: The relationship between loneliness and social interaction in women prisoners, *Journal of Psychosocial Nursing* 29(3):5, 1991.
18. Erickson R: Companion animals and the elderly, *Geriatric Nursing* 6(2):92, 1985.
19. Feifel H: The meaning of dying in American society. In Davis RH, editor: *Dealing with death*, San Diego, 1973, University of Southern California, Ethel Percy Andrus Gerontology Center.
20. Foxall M, Ekberg J: Loneliness of chronically ill adults and their spouses, *Issues in Mental Health Nursing* 10(2):149, 1989.
21. Francis G: Loneliness: measuring the abstract II: *International Journal of Nursing Studies* 17(2):127, 1980.
22. Francis G: Loneliness: the syndrome, *Issues in Mental Health Nursing* 3:1, 1981.
23. Fromm-Reichmann R: Loneliness, *Psychiatry* 22:1, 1959.
24. Gfellner B, Finlayson C: Loneliness, personality, and well-being in older widows, *Perceptual and Motor Skills* 67(1):143, 1988.
25. Hays R, DiMatteo M: A short form measure of loneliness, *Journal of Personality Assessment* 51:69, 1987.
26. Hood P: Perceived loneliness among the aged and associated factors, Unpublished master's thesis, Seattle, 1974, University of Washington.
27. Horowitz L, French R, Anderson C: The prototype of a lonely person. In Peplau L, Perlman D, editors: *Loneliness: a sourcebook of current theory, research and therapy*, New York, 1982, John Wiley & Sons.
28. Hoskins L and others: Nursing diagnosis in the chronically ill: methodology for clinical validation, *Advances in Nursing Science* 8(3):80, 1986.
29. Jones W, Hobbs S, Hockenberry D: Loneliness and social skill deficits, *Personality Processes and Individual Differences* 9(3):682, 1983.
30. Jourbert C: Relationship among self-esteem, psychological reactance, and other personality variables, *Psychological Report* 66(3 Pt 2):1147, 1990.
31. Kim M, McFarland G, McLane A, editors: *Pocket guide to nursing diagnoses*, ed 4, St Louis, 1991, Mosby–Year Book.
32. Knight R and others: Some normative, reliability, and factor analytic data for the Revised UCLA Loneliness Scale, *Journal of Clinical Psychology* 44:203, 1988.
33. Kübler-Ross E: *On death and dying*, New York, 1969, Macmillan.
34. Lopata H: Loneliness: forms and components, *Family* 35:2, 1971.
35. Lund D and others: Can pets help the bereaved? *Journal of Gerontological Nursing* 10:8, 1984.
36. Mahalski P, Jones R, Maxwell G: The value of cat ownership to elderly women living alone, *International Journal on Aging Human Development* 27(4):249, 1988.
37. Mahon N: The relationship of self-disclosure, interpersonal dependency, and life changes to loneliness in young adults, *Nursing Research* 31:343, 1982.
38. Mahon N, Yarcheski A: The dimensionality of the UCLA loneliness scale in early adolescents, *Research In Nursing & Health* 13:45-52, 1990.
39. Mahon N, Yarcheski A: Loneliness in early adolescents: an empirical test of alternate explanations, *Nursing Research* 37:330, 1988.
40. Meer J: Loneliness, *Psychology Today* 7:28, 1985.
41. Miller J: Assessment of loneliness and spiritual well-being in chronically ill and healthy adults, *Journal of Professional Nursing* 1(2):79, 1985.
42. Monk A: Aging, loneliness, and commnications, *American Behavioral Scientist* 31(5):532, 1988.
43. Moustakas C: *Loneliness*, Englewood Cliffs, NJ, 1961, Prentice Hall.
44. Mullins L, Dugan E: The influence of depression, and family and friendship relations, on residents' loneliness in congregate housing, *The Gerontologist* 30(3):337, 1990.
45. Norbeck J: Social support: a model for clinical research and application, *Advances in Nursing Science* 3:48, 1981.
46. O'Dell S: Someone is lonely, *Issues in Mental Health Nursing* 3:7, 1981.
47. Page R: Adolescent loneliness: a priority for school health education, *Health Education* 19(3):20, 1988.
48. Peplau H: Loneliness, *American Journal of Nursing* 55(12):244, 1955.
49. Peplau L, Perlman D, editors: *Loneliness: a sourcebook of current theory, research and therapy*, New York, 1982, John Wiley & Sons.
50. Perlman D, Peplau L: Theoretical approaches to loneliness. In Peplau L, Perlman D, editors: *Loneliness: a sourcebook of current theory, research and therapy*, New York, 1982, John Wiley & Sons.
51. Reisman D, Glazer N, Denney R: *The lonely crowd: a study of the changing American character*, New Haven, Conn, 1961, Yale University Press.
52. Ribeiro V: The forgotten generation: elderly women and loneliness, *Recent Advances in Nursing* 25:20, 1989.
53. Robb S and others: A wine bottle, plant and puppy: catalysts for social behavior, *Journal of Gerontological Nursing* 6:721, 1980.
54. Rogers B: Loneliness: easing the pain of the hospitalized elderly, *Journal of Gerontological Nursing* 15(8):16, 1990.
55. Rokach A: Surviving and coping with loneliness, *The Journal of Psychology* 124(1):39, 1990.
56. Roscoe B, Skomski G: Loneliness among late adolescents, *Adolescence* 24(96):947, 1989.
57. Rubenstein C, Shaver P: The experience of loneliness. In Peplau L, Perlman D, editors: *Loneliness: a sourcebook of current theory, research and therapy*, New York, 1982, John Wiley & Sons.
58. Rubin K, Mills R: The many faces of social isolation in childhood, *Journal of Consulting Clinical Psychology* 56(6):916, 1988.
59. Russell D and others: Social and emotional loneliness: an examination of Weiss's typology of loneliness, *Journal of Personality and Social Psychology* 46:1313, 1984.
60. Russell D, Peplau L, Ferguson M: Developing a measure for loneliness, *Journal of Personality Assessment* 42:290, 1978.
61. Shultz C: Lifestyle assessment: a tool for practice, *Nursing Clinics of North America* 19:271, 1984.
62. Slater P: *The pursuit of loneliness*, Boston, 1976, Beacon Press.
63. Solano C: Two measures of loneliness: a comparison, *Psychological Reports* 46:23, 1980.
64. Sullivan H: *The interpersonal theory of psychiatry*, New York, 1953, WW Norton.
65. Sullivan W, Poertner J: Social support and life stress: a mental health consumers perspective, *Community Mental Health Journal* 25(1):21, 1989.
66. Weeks D and others: The relation between loneliness and depression: a structural equation analysis, *Journal of Personality and Social Psychology* 39:1238, 1980.
67. Weiss R: *Loneliness: the experience of emotional and social isolation*, Cambridge, Mass, 1973, MIT Press.

68. Welt S: The developmental roots of loneliness, *Archives of Psychiatric Nursing* 1:25, 1987.
69. West D, Kellner R, Moore-West M: The effects of loneliness: a review of the literature, *Comprehensive Psychiatry* 27(4):351, 1986.
70. Williams E: Adolescent loneliness, *Adolescence* 18:51, 1983.
71. Zilboorg G: Loneliness, *Atlantic Monthly* 1:45, 1938.

ANNOTATED BIBLIOGRAPHY

Peplau H: Loneliness, *American Journal of Nursing,* 55:244, 1955.
In this classic article by a renowned nurse, the author shares insights about loneliness that remain helpful to contemporary nurses.

Peplau L, Perlman D, editors: *Loneliness: A sourcebook of current theory, research and therapy*, New York, 1982, John Wiley & Sons.
In this comprehensive overview of loneliness, knowledge and summaries of relevant research are combined into a practical sourcebook. Historical and current concepts are explored, including self-help practices of lonely people.

West D, Kellner R, Moore-West M: The effects of loneliness: a review of the literature, *Comprehensive Psychiatry* 4(27):351, 1986.
An excellent overview of research studies regarding loneliness and its prevalence, demographics, and relationship to psychiatric disorders and physical disease. This article explores loneliness among the aged. Loneliness was found to be a problem for a significant portion of the population and was reported more in the young and in women with the exception of older unmarried men. Studies that examine the relationship between loneliness, depression, alcoholism, child abuse, and bereavement are discussed. Succinct information is provided about correlates of loneliness in the elderly and future research suggestions for this group.

Carter L, Meier P, Minirth F: *Why be lonely?: a guide to meaningful relationships*, Grand Rapids, Mich, 1990, Baker Book House.
This book provides a positive view of treating loneliness. Written in a style that would appeal to the non health-care worker, the book would be useful as a reference to clients who benefit from reading about their problems and finding self-help strategies to ease their recovery. Discussion centers on three chapters that present a portrait of loneliness, the causes and consequences of loneliness, and overcoming loneliness.

Desmond A: The relationship between loneliness and social interaction in women prisoners, *Journal of Psychosocial Nursing and Mental Health Services* 29(30):5, 1991.
Loneliness is an inevitable factor in prison settings. This study measured loneliness of women prisoners as compared to the frequency of visits they received from family and friends. The results indicated that women prisoners were very lonely. The study did not support the relationship to visits, but did find a significant relationship to the presence or absence of a friend and the number of friends within the facility. These relationships were more significant to women prisoners than to men prisoners. This article would be especially helpful to nurses providing nursing services to the prison population.

Bernikow L: *Alone in America: the search for companionship*, Boston, 1987, Faber and Faber.
The author's years of work on loneliness is summarized in this book and presented in reference to societal issues, norms, and trends. Loneliness as related to individuals (adolescents, men, women, and widows and widowers), families, and communities is explored. The author reviews the meaning of having and being out of work and its effect on loneliness. The book contains many personal examples collected throughout America and provides thoughtful comments about the "number one cause of death" in America.

CHAPTER

22 Boredom

Cathleen M Shultz

After studying this chapter, the student will be able to:

- Discuss historical perspectives of boredom
- Describe theories of boredom
- Discuss the psychopathology of narcissistic personality disorder and borderline personality disorder as described in the DSM-III-R

- Apply the nursing process to care for clients experiencing boredom
- Identify current research findings relevant to the care of clients experiencing boredom

Boredom is an affective mental state primarily caused by prolonged exposure to dull, uninteresting, or monotonous stimuli. Boredom, a common phenomenon, can result in harmful stress that can lead to disease and accidents. Persons who are particularly vulnerable to experiencing the negative aspects of boredom include those who do repetitive tasks over a long time, those who are institutionalized or recuperating from a lengthy illness, those in prolonged isolation or solitary confinement, and those with certain personality disorders. Also at risk are persons who are retired, socially withdrawn, homebound, or institutionalized; adolescents; and those with handicaps that cause sensory deprivation. In at least one extreme case, a client who experimentally entered a cave and experienced months of boredom, isolation and no exposure to outside life developed permanent personality changes during the project. She later committed suicide.

Boredom frequently is confused with monotony, tedium, or apathy. These states are related to boredom and have common features as summarized in Table 22-1. Those who work in isolation or view their work as monotonous are less efficient and alert after only short work periods. Health problems such as accidents that cause injury and death are inevitable. People with monotonous jobs tend to be more neurotic and less mentally healthy than those in other jobs.[9,20]

Monotony alone, however, is not sufficient to cause boredom. Other factors include emotional lability, age, and satisfaction with personal life.[27,60,67,68] In addition, others believe that boredom results when an activity lacks meaning to the person or is perceived as boring.[13,41]

Nurses are expected to use specific interventions to minimize the effects of boredom. They also are challenged to gather empirical data that result in more effective care of the bored client. Limited success has been achieved in certain disorders using planned boredom as a treatment modality. Table 22-2 lists types of boredom and their causes.

DSM-III-R DIAGNOSES

Boredom is a problem experienced by many people with one or more personality disorders and is listed among their DSM-III-R characteristics. This chapter addresses two disorders with boredom as a component, narcissistic personality disorder and borderline personality disorder.

▶ **DIAGNOSES Related to Boredom**

DSM-III-R DIAGNOSES	NURSING DIAGNOSES
Borderline personality disorder	**NANDA**
Narcissistic personality disorder	Diversional activity deficit
	PMH
	Inadequate diversional activity

HISTORICAL OVERVIEW

DATES	EVENTS
1860	Florence Nightingale wrote that sick patients are adversely affected by seeing the same walls and ceiling while confined.
1913	Munsterberg recognized boredom in actual working situations.
1920s-1940s	A series of papers was published in England describing how boredom and monotony affect work.
1927	McDowall and Wells published an account of the genesis of boredom.
1930-1937	Earliest systematic psychoanalytical discussions of boredom were written by Fenichel,[12] Spitz, and Winterstein.
1953	Greenson[19] distinguished between an apathetic and an agitated boredom.
1972	First nursing article addressing boredom was published; the topic has since appeared in 10 publications with nurse authors.
1975	Bernstein[4] integrated psychoanalytical and sociological constructs to describe the recent increase in boredom. He proposed a dual taxonomy by differentiating responsive boredom from chronic boredom created by internal causes. Wangh[79] viewed boredom as an outcome of intrapsychic struggle.
1981	The first research on boredom conducted by nurses was published by Savitz and Friedman.[63] Smith's work indicated that only about 40 papers have been published on boredom since 1926.[68] Boredom is associated with narcissistic and borderline personality disorders.
1990s	Nurses are challenged to incorporate knowledge about boredom into practice as they learn to recognize boredom; distinguish it from related states of confusion, monotony, and adaptation; and develop and use interventions to help the client change the bored state.
Future	As the number of clients with borderline and narcissistic personality disorders increases, nurses will be more involved in treating these clients and providing prevention techniques and consultation services in schools, families, and work settings.

Personality traits can become personality disorders and the nurse must distinguish between them. According to the DSM-III-R *personality traits* are patterns of perceiving, relating to, and thinking about oneself and the environment; these traits are most frequently manifested in social and personal situations. When these traits become inflexible and maladaptive causing considerable impairment or distress, they become *personality disorders.* Usually evident in adolescence, the disorders continue throughout the adult's life and are often lessened by middle or old age without treatment. At this time, even with treatment, exacerbation of symptoms is common, especially in those with the borderline personality disorder.

The incidence of both disorders has increased during the past 10 years, perhaps due to their classification in the DSM-III-R and also due to more sophisticated diagnosing. These clients are usually treated on an outpatient basis and, depending on their symptom severity, can create considerable turmoil in group situations such as the home or work settings.

With the narcissistic personality disorder, the client has a pervasive grandiose (in fantasy or behavior) sense of self-importance and requires constant attention and admiration

such as "fishing for compliments" from co-workers, friends, and bosses. The client exaggerates his abilities and achievements, expecting to be inordinately noticed and recognized beyond his achievement level. Preoccupied with fantasies of unlimited success, power, brilliance, beauty, or ideal love, the client lacks empathy toward others and exploits them for personal gain. Hypersensitive to being evaluated, the client reacts to criticism with feelings of rage, shame, or humiliation even if the feelings are not verbally expressed. Believing that his problems are unique and can only be understood by special people, the client has a sense of entitlement, including an unreasonable expectation of especially favorable treatment. For example, he will superficially learn a physician's first name and as a result of this "friendship," expect to see the physician without an appointment. When others achieve or seem to "have more" or to "do more," the client is preoccupied with feelings of envy.

The client with a borderline personality disorder is unstable in several areas such as interpersonal relationships, moods, and self-image. Those closest to him at work or home cannot predict his reaction to a situation, creating a sense of hypervigilance and guardedness. He has a pattern

▼ **TABLE 22-1**   Definitions of Boredom and Related Terms

Term	Definition
Boredom	An affective mental state primarily caused by prolonged exposure to monotonous stimulation
Monotony	Tedious uniformity or lack of variety
Apathy	Lack of interest or concern
Emptiness	Lack of feeling
Sensory deprivation	Removal or minimization of sensory stimulation
Tedium	Disgust or weariness
Ennui	Feeling of mental weariness produced by lack of interest in surroundings.

▼ **TABLE 22-2**   Types of Boredom

Type	Cause
Apathetic	Repression of forbidden instincts and a decreased imagination
Agitated	Secondary state caused by failure of available activities to gratify wishes and fantasies
Responsive	Inevitable reaction to a monotonous task or life situation
Chronic	Unresolved inner struggle causing boredom to persist
Existential	Occurs from extraneous, multiple factors
Interpersonal	Occurs when other people are present

of unstable and intense interpersonal relationships vacillating between overidealizing and devaluing of the friend, family member, lover, or co-worker. Affectively, the client is unstable, experiencing mood shifts that last a few hours or days, alternating from depression, irritability, and anxiety to recurrent suicidal threats, gestures, or behaviors. The client has inappropriate or intense anger or cannot control his anger, displaying temper, rage, or actual fighting. The client is impulsive in at least two of the following areas, which are potentially self-damaging: spending, sex, substance use, shoplifting, reckless driving, and binge eating. He presents a marked and persistent identity disturbance with uncertainty in at least two of the following areas: self-image, sexual orientation, long-term goals or career choices, type of desired friends, and preferred values. The client has chronic feelings of emptiness and boredom. He often makes frantic, impulsive efforts to avoid real or imagined abandonment.

The nurse is challenged when working with clients who manifest borderline and narcissistic personality disorders. As with so many other new diagnoses, few long-term studies are available that demonstrate clearly effective treatments or prognoses with these disorders. Because clients with these personality disorders are becoming increasingly prevalent and contribute to dysfunctional homes and work settings, new information regarding cause and treatment methods including medications will likely emerge over the coming years.

THEORETICAL APPROACHES

Psychoanalytical

Information about boredom has emerged in bits and pieces through numerous psychoanalytical theories. In general, boredom is perceived as a complicated, internal, affective experience that results in the client's disinterest in the environment. This disinterest prevents a clash between desires and constraints. Thus the cause is internal and self-created.[79,80] For example, the school-aged child with a desire to fulfill a fantasy to play outdoors is unable to do so

because he is confined to his desk. To prevent intrapsychic conflict he may become bored.

Fenichel's classic work related boredom to depression, neurotic states, narcissistic needs, oral-sadistic needs, and diminished self-esteem.[12] Bored clients with narcissistic needs express vague complaints, including feelings of emptiness and lack of initiative.[37-39] Clients with oral-sadistic needs abuse substances and other items ingested with the mouth. These symptoms are linked to chronic boredom, and Fenichel believed that they relate originally to a lack of empathic mothering. He noted that people frequently relieved bored feelings by oral activities such as eating, drinking, and smoking.

Although Fenichel primarily focused on internally caused boredom, he believed that boredom can be caused externally. The best example is the assembly line worker whose many impulses conflict with his work; he resists acting out his impulse to briefly stop the work flow and talk with a co-worker because he will be fired. The work continues despite his boredom.

Hartocollis[24,25] studied boredom in certain mental health problems and believed boredom to be particularly characteristic of borderline personality disorders. He concluded that borderline and narcissistic clients are chronically bored. The behavior of borderline clients originates with problems in identity and intimacy. Erikson[11] believed that people who have successfully completed early adolescence have a sense of who they are and their likes, values, and important views. Clients with borderline personality disorder lack that sense of identity. Their relationships are fragmented and superficial.

Biological

Biological theories view boredom as a consequence of inattention which they relate to physical maturation. Biological theorists have linked cortical maturation to the development of the capacity to be attentive.[59] Myelination of certain nerve fibers may not be completed until 12 years of age, and measures such as electroencephalogram (EEG) and reaction time reflect the ability to be attentive.[21]

Some theorists link boredom to a decreased heart rate, while others report an association between boredom and an increased or erratic heart rate.[2,75,76] Hill and Perkins[28] believe this discrepancy to be caused by the attitude of the worker to the task rather than whether the task is identified as boring. Further study is needed before cardiac difficulties are definitely associated with boredom. Work continues on biological causes and results of boredom as it is studied in individuals' personal lives and occupations.

Behavioral

Behaviorists believe that boredom is caused by the client's environment. As the first to study boredom, McGill University researchers placed individuals on a bed with planned decreased stimulation, called "perceptual isolation." Their eyes were covered, they heard a constant buzzing noise through earphones, and their arms and hands were covered with cardboard cuffs. The experience became unpleasant within a few days, and diverse effects were found, including mood lability, visual and auditory hallucinations, EEG alterations, and an ability to be persuaded.[26] Later studies expanded the findings of the McGill researchers and other early studies.[14,56,59] Behaviorists then renamed perceptual isolation as *sensory deprivation.*

Boredom is recognized as a unique psychophysiological state that is best explained as an unusual emotional response to predictability. When individuals experience too much predictability, bordeom develops; too little predictability causes confusion.

When the client is bored, task performance becomes impaired and perceptions altered. The client is at risk for accidents and injuries, especially if operating heavy equipment or driving a car. The ideal aim then is an adaptive response with optimal predictability (Figure 22-1).

It must be remembered that some bored clients find a reward in boredom. When they are bored they focus on the past and the familiar. By choosing the known over the unknown, they avoid undesired emotions.

Cognitive

Cognitive theorists generally believe that lack of attention is a factor in the development of boredom. According to Hamilton,[20] attention is essential to learning and creative problem solving. Inattention leads to boredom. Perkins and Hill[56] found that boredom can develop subjectively in response to lack of interest in a task. They found that a person could initially be interested in the task only to become bored later because of his own perceptions and response to the situation.

Sociocultural

Generally, the sociological viewpoint is that individuals, groups, and society may become bored. Boredom is considered to be caused less by personality traits than by the various situations in which people find themsleves. This view is best illustrated by sociologist Robert Nisbet's warning in 1969 that the traditional power of society's authority was being undermined.[35] Nisbet believed that an increasing incidence of boredom and apathy began to occur during this time of social upheaval. Sociologists link boredom with physical disease, cruelty, and nihilism. Harlow Shapley even placed boredom as third in a list of five possible causes of world destruction.[35]

Orcutt[53] identifies two forms of boredom. Existential boredom occurs without the presence of other persons, whereas interpersonal boredom occurs when others are present. Both forms are internally felt and caused by lack of involvement with the self, others, or the environment. Studies reveal that younger and lower income persons are more likley to experience existential boredom than are older and more wealthy respondents. The latter groups report more interpersonal boredom.[54] The former group has more antisocial behavioral responses to boredom and are more likely to perform acts such as theft, gang attacks on another person, or substance abuse.

Table 22-3 summarizes the theoretical approaches.

NURSING PROCESS

Assessment

Physical dimension Assessment of the physical dimension includes obtaining a history of the client's work habits and productivity, sensory abilities such as hearing level, eating habits, physical surroundings, and activities to relieve boredom. The negative effects of boredom, especially in the work environment, adversely affect job performance, employee safety, morale, and eventually the actual work quality. The nurse assesses the individual's occupation, visits to company health clinics, and work-related accidents. Consider the following case example.

▼ Case Example

Herbert, age 58 years, works on a car assembly line. He mentions to the industrial nurse during a routine visit for a blood pressure check that he "really feels fatigued and has trouble staying alert on the job." A review of his records shows that he has been to the nurse three times in the past 6 months; two visits were for minor lacerations requiring stitches and one was for a stumbling accident resulting in a sprained ankle.

The nurse assesses the type of work Herbert does, the length of time doing his work, his reaction to his work, and sleep history to rule out other causes of fatigue. Accidents, however minor, are taken seriously, especially in a work setting concerned with employee safety and federal standards for employee work environments.

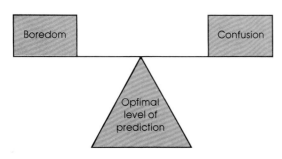

FIGURE 22-1 Response to human predictability.

▼ **TABLE 22-3** Summary of Theories of Boredom

Theory	Theorist	Dynamics
Psychoanalytical	Wangh[79]	Boredom results from conflicting internal forces.
	Greenson[19]	Boredom is due to repressing forbidden instincts causing conflict.
	Fenichel[12]	Boredom is associated with persons experiencing neuroses; it involves narcissistic needs, oral-sadistic needs, and diminished self-esteem.
	Erikson[11]	Clients with borderline personality disorders have problems in identity and intimacy. They lack a sense of identity.
Biological	Pribram[59]	Altered EEGs and decreased reaction time are among the physiological variables indicative of the presence of and reaction to boredom.
Behavioral	Herron[26]	Boredom results from sensory deprivation caused by the environment.
Cognitive	Perkins and Hill[56]	Boredom develops subjectively in response to lack of interest in a task.
	Hamilton[21]	Boredom occurs with inattention.
Sociocultural	Orcutt[53]	A society may experience boredom because of a perceived loss of authority; societal boredom is viewed as destructive.

Table 22-4 lists occupations and activities that place clients at risk for accidents and personal injury caused by boredom. Especially vulnerable are those whose jobs are characterized by fast, machine-paced work requiring heightened attention to avoid serious personal injury. Included in this category are forklift drivers and assemblers, whether or not their work is machined-paced. The machine-paced assemblers report somatic complaints, anxiety, depression, and frequent visits to the company's health clinic. The first survey of the physical consequences of occupation-related, severe boredom revealed a high incidence of psychosomatic diseases such as gastritis and peptic ulcers.[62] As one gets older, occupational boredom seems to diminish.[27,51,69] It is not known if this is due to adaptation to the work setting or to the possibility that bored, younger workers leave the setting.

The nurse assesses the individual's sensory functioning and physical environment. Boredom also may occur in seeing- or hearing-impaired persons; the physically restrained; clients in lengthy isolation; those in protected environments such as the laminar airflow rooms in which the client has little human contact; those recovering from drug or alcohol abuse; the alert but physically limited terminally ill; and those individuals institutionalized in rehabilitative facilities, mental health centers, and nursing homes.

The physical environment and circumstances can contribute to boredom, for example, drab hospital rooms or workrooms; visually unappealing food such as that often found in some prisons; and broken, dysfunctional, or inappropriate hearing aids or glasses. Dim or flickering lights, uncomfortable room temperatures, and annoying or humming noises may alter attentiveness, thus increasing the client's susceptibility to boredom. Assessment then includes notations of sensory deprivation and sensory impairment.

A myth prevails that only obese people eat more when bored. In actual studies obese persons ate significantly more food than normal persons, but boredom markedly increased food consumption for both obese and nonobese persons.[9] The nurse assesses the client's food intake and associated feelings for specified time intervals, (e.g., 24 hours).

The nurse and client as members of the health care team determine if boredom is related to personality disorders, fatigue, anger, grief, fear, avoidance, conflict, or loss of purpose. Changing the client's life-style depends on the client's motivation and resources, as well as on how long the client has been bored and how quickly he can make necessary changes.[67]

Occasionally, bored clients actively seek inappropriate stimuli to remove the feeling or prevent its recurrence because it is so uncomfortable. These are the excessively action-oriented, self-destructive thrill seekers, including those who abuse stimulant and depressant drugs. On psychological tests they will respond favorably to items such as "I would like to hunt lions in Africa" and "I would like to race motorcycles."

Adolescents and the elderly are at risk for development of boredom and its harmful consequences. The presence of boredom requires further assessment to determine what clients do to relieve feelings associated with bore-

▼ **TABLE 22-4** Occupations and Activities that Place Clients at Risk for Accidents and Personal Injury Caused by Boredom

Sample Occupation	Sample Activity
Lathe operator	Industrial inspection
Assembly workers	
Punch press operator	Machine punching
Drill operator	
Navy bomber pilot	Radar target detection
Military plane or ship navigator	Radar navigation
Air traffic controller	Television or screen surveillance
Train controller	
Airplane pilot	
Night watch person	
Security guard watching monitors	
Truck driver	Prolonged driving

dom. The nurse inquires about alcohol and drug consumption, since these substances may be used to relieve boredom.

The chronically bored client with borderline or narcissistic personality disorder also actively relieves boredom through reactions such as mood swings and intense anger. The narcissistic client is painfully self-conscious and preoccupied with activities involving grooming and remaining youthful. The nurse assesses the borderline client for evidence of physical fights and self-mutilation activity such as wrist slashing. These reactions are especially distressing to family members or co-workers.

Employee evaluation results may highlight difficulties in relating to others or clients hospitalized for emotional disorders may engage in fights with other inpatients to relieve bored feelings. Bored people may change jobs frequently or cause commotions in the school or work setting because they are bored and want to experience excitement.

Boring activities are associated with a high level of frustration and monotony (see the research highlight below).[56] Keen[34] believed the bored person has lost momentum and has a weak will. Nothing appears exciting to these people.

Emotional dimension The nurse assesses for the presence of boredom by inquiring about the individual's attitude toward life and how his time is managed. Initially, boredom seems to be a problem created by a lack of energy. The bored client has lost momentum and motivation, and nothing appears exciting. For some, boredom is a temporary result of a lack of adequate stimuli or a retreat from overstimulation. Clients' statements such as "I feel trapped," "I'm bored to death," "It's a blah day," "I've nothing to do,"

and "I just do not want to do that" reveal the characteristics of the boredom experience.

The nurse assesses the severity and significance of the problem by determining the intensity of boredom, the presence of related feeling states such as depression, and the client's need and desire to reduce the effects of boredom on his life. The nurse also assesses the client's ability to develop and incorporate successful coping mechanisms into his life-style. When bored feelings degenerate into chronic resignation, frustration, fear, resentment, apathy, depression, and hostility, the problem further challenges the client's and family's coping abilities.

From behavioral theory, sensory deprivation also can act as a stimulant that leads to a heightened awareness and readiness to act. The relationship is U-shaped; as arousal increases, performance first improves and then diminishes to the beginning performance level.[44] Particularly affected is the person's heightened ability after sensory deprivation to memorize lists and to recall previously learned material. Short periods of decreased stimuli with no people contact, no radio or television, minimal sound, closed eyelids, and lying down are helpful for those studying for tests that require memorization.[71,72] Thus the nurse assesses the frequency of times that individuals perform unstructured activities and their attitude during these times.

When boredom is present in someone with a borderline personality disorder, the person often displays anger or rage and may keep the work or home setting in turmoil to offset the distress experienced when feeling bored. This turmoil leads to ineffective social and occupational functioning. Consider the following case example.

RESEARCH HIGHLIGHT

Cognitive and Affective Aspects of Boredom
• RE Perkins and AB Hill

PURPOSE

This study investigated whether boredom is associated with subjective monotony and a high degree of frustration and whether it occurs when the stimuli lack personal meaning.

SAMPLE

Twenty-four undergraduates were chosen after responding to a set of eight questions about motorcycles. Their mean age was 21.6 years. Two groups were developed; each had six men and six women. One group would likely find the study task interesting (I); the other group would likely find it boring (B).

METHODOLOGY

Seven 6 × 8 inch color pictures of motorcycles were shown to each subject individually. The subject was given a list of constructs related to the quality and use of motorcycles and was asked to rate these constructs on a 7-point scale. At the end of the task, the subjects were asked to rate their degree of interest or boredom on a 6-point scale (slightly, reasonably, very interesting/boring).

Based on data from *British Journal of Psychology* 76:221, 1985.

Total discrepancy scores (TDS) were obtained for each elicited construct (TDSE) and for supplied constructs (TDSS). The higher the TDS, the more meaningful the stimuli or picture to the subject.

FINDINGS

Using a *t*-test of the TDS, means of the I group and B group indicated a significant difference. No evidence supported that boredom was associated with a lack of meaningful stimulation. In the second experiment, boredom was found to be associated with subjective monotony, and the third experiment provided strong support for previous speculations that boredom is associated with frustration.

IMPLICATIONS

The study presented more data to describe the cognitive and affective activity associated with monotony and boredom. Questions remain about the origins of boredom. The authors believe that subjective monotony may induce or represent boredom and that boredom occurs as a result of unknown processes. The field remains open for further investigation.

▼ Case Example

Linda, a 28-year-old former beauty queen with a master's degree, accepted a teaching position with no prior teaching experience. After her first year of employment, she announced her intention to become the school's assistant principal, a vacant position; she threw a temper tantrum when she was not selected. Her work history included frequent requests for special favors, requests to be placed in influential positions beyond her capabilities, and requests for prime office space. When such requests were denied, she reacted with rage and attempted to polarize the school's faculty and staff. Those who worked with her found that they did all the work while she openly took the credit for positive outcomes. She often sent her picture to the local newspaper to be included with articles concerning work mainly done by her colleagues. She joined influential community clubs outside the work setting. No one was her "friend" unless she benefited directly. She never understood why people disliked working with her; people frequently felt manipulated and used when around her. Close acquaintances were discarded when they no longer were able to assist her in her career goals. Co-workers who were aware of her negative contribution to the work environment stress were relieved to see her leave and the havoc diminish.

The nurse then assesses Linda's behavior toward her career goals and observes, where possible, her interactions with others. She will probably not be able to express what she values best about her co-workers.

Intellectual dimension Boredom can affect one's intellectual dimension both positively and negatively. When a person is bored, creativity comes to a halt. However, after lengthy boring experiences some persons have produced creative work such as painting and writing.

Splitting and *projective identification* are two defense mechanisms that frequently mask boredom. Splitting enables the client to view the world either as all bad or as all good. Projective identification allows the client to displace self-hatred and anger. Rather than admit that he has intense anger, the client who uses projective identification believes that someone else has the anger. The nurse probes beyond these reactions and assesses the intensity of the client's boredom and its relationship to the presence of defense mechanisms or personality disorders.

Psychoanalytical theorists believe that the clients with a borderline personality disorder commonly "splits" (primitive dissociation) their world into the two extremes of good and bad for fear of the results if the two were meshed; the bad could engulf and destroy the good. Their views of others and circumstances are labile and can change from moment to moment. The nurse assesses their sense of personal identity as in the following case example.

▼ Case Example

Kate had no idea what she wanted to do 5 or even 10 years from now. As an attractive 28-year-old single parent, she lived with her own parents who threatened to "kick me out of the house and take my child if I didn't get my act together. So I'm here to see you because they forced me." She had wanted to go to college for the last 3 years but had made no attempt to do so. Getting her to talk about herself was difficult and she could not name one thing about her life that she enjoyed; there was no substance to her conversation. The men in her life abused her physically and emotionally. Kate, with a borderline personality disorder, gave the nurse all the "right answers" because they were the ones she thought the nurse wanted to hear. She took on the values of those

around her like a chameleon. She had what Deutsch" calls the "as if" personality. It is "as if" they were like those to whom they relate most often.

The bored person may have more difficulty with long-term projects and situations requiring creative problem solving. When bored with a task, some persons may leave it incomplete or may mechanically complete it without giving attention to detail or quality. Moreover, the long-term project in itself may be boring.

Chronic physical problems that alter the mind's ability to function normally may contribute to boredom. Examples are post-traumatic head injury; cardiovascular accident; and emotional problems such as autism, psychoses, drug abuse, or drug treatment.

Determining the school progress of the student may be a clue to a decreased attention span and the presence of boredom. Learning is intense during primary and secondary school years. Yet, according to cognitive theory, the young child or adolescent may not be able to attend to learning that is accompanied by minimal stimulation or that requires long periods of intense attention. Generally educators agree that boredom inhibits learning.[15] The Boredom Confusion Adaptation Scale (BCAS) is an instrument designed to diagnose boredom in schoolchildren (see the research highlight on p. 458). Because boredom is inversely related to creativity,[66] the nurse assesses the client's creativity by asking about hobbies and work.

Social dimension Assessment of the social dimension includes determining if the client is an introvert or an extrovert. Extroverts are more likely to be bored, especially in a socially isolated situation.[61]

While assessing occupational status, the nurse also may determine the client's attitude toward the job or position. For those who are unemployed, the nurse can obtain sample schedules of their daily activities. This may provide information about how clients occupy their time. Busy and creative people seldom complain of boredom, especially over a prolonged time.

Boredom often has been called the culprit in "problem drinking" and other antisocial behavior. Numerous respondents to public surveys report that their excessive drinking was due to trying to kill time because there was nothing to do.[60] Other problems can result in legal problems as described in the following case example.

▼ Case Example

Greg is a 16-year-old who dropped out of high school because he was bored. He spends his time watching television and smoking marijuana. He lacks the social and occupational skills to get a job, and his friends are in school all day. His own efforts to fill the void are ineffective, and he looks to the outside world for needed stimulation. Stealing cars, racing, and speeding occupy his time until he is finally arrested. Boredom has resulted in serious consequences for Greg.

A client may perceive himself as bored from being in a job, friendship, or marriage too long. Or, a person may be bored if he is transferred to a new job, especially when the activity level decreases from that of his previous position. The nurse assesses whether a client is bored with an occupation, a relationship, or a change in the activity levels of a job.

RESEARCH HIGHLIGHT

Diagnosing Boredom, Confusion, and Adaptation in Schoolchildren
• SB Frick

PURPOSE

Using Friedman's rational theory as a framework, this study was designed to develop and test an instrument that could diagnose middle-school children's bored (B), confused (C), or adapted (A) states of mind.

SAMPLE

Subjects were from two middle schools in central South Carolina. One hundred fifty-four students in the seventh grade participated, with the median age being 11.9 years (range, 11 to 15). There were 90 boys and 64 girls. Ninety-six students were white, 28 were black, and 30 did not identify their race.

METHODOLOGY

Middle-school counselors, using definitions of B, C, and A, identified school situations specific to each construct. From the situations, declarative statements pertinent to B, C, and A were developed for the Boredom Confusion Adaptation Scale (BCAS) instrument, which then was independently reviewed and rated by five experts including Friedman. Only statements agreed on by all five experts remained. Sixty items, 20 for each construct, were retained and randomly arranged in the final instrument. Each statement was followed by two blanks that students could respond to with "like me" or "unlike me."

The BCAS was read aloud to each student who then checked his own responses. The researcher was not involved in this phase of data collection. Other information was obtained from school records including the Comprehensive Test of Basic Skills (CTBS) subscale and total skills scores; year-end grades received by students in mathematics, social studies, language arts, and reading; and total number of times tardy and absent. All data related to the school year in which the BCAS was given were collected.

Kuder Richardson 20 reliability estimates were obtained for each subscale (confusion = 0.77, and adaptation = 0.71). Other statistical correlations and factor analyses revealed 33 significant items (14 confusion, 12 bore-

dom, and 7 adaptation), which were included in the final form of the BCAS.

Pearson product moment correlation coefficients were calculated to obtain relationships between the BCAS subscales and the other data.

FINDINGS

The results revealed several significant findings, including support of assumed instrument reliability and validity. Generally scores and grades compared as follows:

SCALE SCORES	CTBS SCORES	TEACHER GRADES
Increase on the confusion score	Decreased	Decreased
Increase on the boredom score	Decreased	Decreased
Increase on the adaptation score	Increased	Increased

IMPLICATIONS

The BCAS score may be used diagnostically by school health professionals to determine boredom, confusion, or adaptation states. Interventions specific to the confused or bored state may be determined individually to achieve a more adaptive state in the learning environment. Bored students need varied assignments and teaching methodologies to enhance learning. Confused students benefit from simplification of assignments, increased structure such as an assignment calendar, more regulation at school, and a decreased amount of variety of classroom stimuli. These states are challenges for the teacher, especially when both types are in the same classroom.

Boredom and confusion are considered situation specific, so the measurement tool may differ in other settings. The development and determination of the effects of interventions to change the confused or bored state await further study.

Based on data from *Journal of School Health* 55:7, 1985.

Boredom can be especially devastating to a person planning to retire. The nurse assesses persons of retirement age for their preparedness. The following questions will provide the nurse with helpful information to guide her actions: "When does your retirement occur?" "What do you and your family plan to do following your retirement?" "What activities do you do regularly other than work?"

The homebound, nursing home, or hospitalized client may experience boredom without sufficient diversional activities. The assessment will include questions about the presence of a telephone, television set, or radio; the frequency and length of television or telephone use; and the frequency and purpose of visitors.

The client who is bored in social situations may withdraw. Bored clients do not attract people. Consequently, clients with few contacts with others may be more sus-

ceptible to boredom. Therefore assessment contains information about the client's comfort level in social settings or with groups, the number of new friends made in a recent time period (in the last 6 months, for example), and what the client does, feels, and thinks when bored.

With intimacy, approach-avoidance conflict is observed in clients with borderline personality disorder. Yearning for intimacy, they fear being subsumed by those closest to them and vice versa. Their desire and fear of intimacy create a history of stormy interpersonal relationships. Expressions of caring elicit opposite feelings of longing and rage. To put distance between the client and person "getting too close," the client openly devalues the other. The client alternates between idealization and devaluing to act out the conflict. The client may say that you are a wonderful boss, friend, or co-worker or later in the same day, say you are definitely the worst. These clients cannot accept contradictions in others, the good and the bad in those for whom they most care. They lack what psychoanalysts call "object constancy," which is the ability to have an overview of the other person's core personality. When others gratify them they are terrific; when they frustrate them they become the object of rage. Family members, to avoid the storms, will often gratify them rather than face the onslaught of rage.

These clients in an insatiable longing for love express projective identification. In other words, they hate anyone who stirs up these longings. They cannot tolerate both love and hate for the same person. Projecting the hate justifies abusing the hated person. They deliberately provoke, an action closely associated with projective identification. The nurse notes these behaviors when relating to the clients and obtaining descriptions of their relationships.

The client may often express feelings of depersonalization (feeling unreal) and derealization (feeling that the environment is unreal) because they abhor being alone. Due to their lack of personal identity, they need others to create the illusion of completeness. In the extreme, they can feel panic and participate in self-mutilation such as cutting the skin in an attempt to reassure themselves that they really do exist. Seeing blood and feeling pain assure them that they are alive.

Spiritual dimension The chronically bored, withdrawn client has difficulty relating to his world. Aimless and lacking purpose, this person is alienated from a higher being during periods of boredom. Assessing his attitude toward goals and his desire to relate to himself and others provides information about the extent of his boredom. Whether or not the client participates in creative activities can give the nurse information about the client's bored state relative to his spiritual dimension.

Characterized by *anhedonia*, the borderline personality disorder clients cannot enjoy life. Despite their intense involvement with activities, they feel little pleasure at their involvement with activities, others, or a higher being. Internal peace is difficult and they seem to be unable to put themselves in a calm state; constant activity such as finger tapping or rocking is typical. Any stress will disrupt their equilibrium. Actions are impulsive and distressing. The nurse finds little in this client's history that elicits personal contentment and serenity with self or others. The client will be unable to voice contentment, pleasure, goals, and inner peace during the assessment.

Measurement Tools

Tools to measure the presence and severity of boredom have emerged primarily from industry and from studies of vigilance, attention, and sensory deprivation. Nurses can use these tools in a variety of settings to determine boredom susceptibility, the presence of the types of boredom, and the client's ability to cope with boredom.

A summary of the tools to measure boredom is presented in Table 22-5.

Analysis
Nursing diagnosis

The defining chracteristics of the NANDA-accepted nursing diagnosis of diversional activity deficit are presented in the accompanying box. Other NANDA-accepted nursing diagnoses and causative statements for boredom include the following:

1. Diversional activity deficit related to boredom from lack of activities during an illness of 2 months.
2. High risk for diversional activity deficit related to monotonous environment in hospital isolation room.
3. Social isolation: boredom related to visitors limited by hospital isolation procedures.
4. Sensory-perceptual alteration: boredom related to need to immobilize hip joint for recent hip replacement surgery.
5. Ineffective individual coping: boredom related to unplanned use of time during occupational retirement.

The case example on p. 460 illustrates characteristics of the nursing diagnosis of diversional activity deficit.

▼ **TABLE 22-5**   **Tools to Measure Boredom**

Measurement Tool	Measures
Sensation Seeking Scale, Form V[14] (SSS-V)	Determines number and diversity of stimuli desired by individual; explores boredom susceptibility and need for stimulation
Boredom Coping[22] Scale (BCS)	Reflects how the person copes with boredom; measures person's ability to alter his perceptions of and ability to participate in boring activities
Orcutt's Scale[53]	Differentiates between interpersonal and existential boredom
Boredom Confusion Adaptation Scale[15] (BCAS)	Diagnoses the presence of boredom, confusion, or adaptation to predictable circumstances

▼ **DIVERSIONAL ACTIVITY DEFICIT**

DEFINITION

The state in which an individual experiences a decreased stimulation from or interest or engagement in recreational or leisure activities.

DEFINING CHARACTERISTICS

- **Physical dimension**
  Usual hobbies cannot be undertaken in hospital

- **Emotional dimension**
  Boredom

- **Intellectual dimension**
  Desire for something to do or read

Modified from Kim MJ, McFarland GK, McLane AM: *Pocket guide to nursing diagnoses,* ed 5, St Louis, 1993, Mosby–Year Book.

▼ Case Example

Virgil worked for 45 years as an engineer, always arriving at least an hour before the scheduled workday. He worked hard and received a good income, but his job was boring and he felt trapped. When he realized he would never attain the level in the company that he desired, he lost interest in his work and resigned himself to tolerate it until retirement.

Although Virgil was educated and bright, he had no outside interests other than his lawn work following his retirement. He and his wife had few friends and spent most of their time at home. With his work interest removed, he felt lonely and bored.

He quickly lost interest in anything new he attempted. Nothing needed the old skills he had used for decades. He wanted to help his wife, but he felt in the way. She had her own schedule and had not retired from her activities. Gradually he lost his appetite and interest in anything. He began waking at 4 AM. When his movements and speech slowed down, and he joked about ending it all, his wife arranged for him to see a counselor. Virgil's situation was serious and required attention because it was inherent in his depression and suicidal thoughts.

Planning

Table 22-6 provides a nursing care plan with long- and short-term goals, outcome criteria, nursing interventions, and rationales related to boredom. These serve as examples of the planning phase of the nursing process.

Implementation

Physical dimension Everyone experiences fleeting boredom, which is easily relieved by changing one's thoughts, engaging in an activity, or varying activities. How-

ever, boredom, with the potential for harmful consequences such as accidents or depression, usually is subtle and complex. It leaves the client unable to use his usual coping strategies. In addition, environmental constraints such as office rules may prevent an individual from using previously successful coping mechanisms to minimize boredom. For example, when bored while pounding nails in a new roof, the person can take a 5-minute break whenever needed. The same person on an assembly line can only leave at scheduled times or when a relief worker arrives.

The bored client needs a balance between routine activities and novel activities, as well as a change in the predictability of his situation. Placing readable calendars, clocks, newspapers, and television sets in clients' rooms or lounge areas is a simple but significant strategy to prevent confusion and boredom. In addition, changing the environment can positively influence client behaviors and feelings.[52] For example, moving the furniture to create a more pleasing atmosphere can enhance the quantity and content of conversation between caring staff members and clients.

The nurse also can have a positive effect on the sensory environment of the client by teaching those with impaired hearing and vision to periodically assess their hearing aids or glasses. Touch becomes essential for some isolated, institutionalized, or dying clients. The back rub may be a welcome contact for clients with decreased sensory stimulation. Sensory deprivation, long linked as causing boredom, has therapeutic value in treating clients with conditions such as stuttering, esophoria (one or both eyes turn toward the nose), infantile colic, snake phobia, narcotic addiction, compulsive overeating, smoking, alcoholism, hypertension, autism, and retardation. Increased short-term

---

▼ TABLE 22-6   NURSING CARE PLAN

GOALS	OUTCOME CRITERIA	INTERVENTIONS	RATIONALES
NURSING DIAGNOSIS: Diversional activity deficit: boredom related to postretirement inactivity			
LONG TERM			
To use effective coping strategies to relieve boredom during retirement	Uses strategies that worked in the past to relieve boredom	Assist to identify and examine coping strategies previously used	Feels secure to know he has used effective coping strategies
	Participates in activities of interest to relieve boredom (e.g., bowling, community activities, home or neighborhood repair project)	Assist to identify, establish priorities, and participate in hobbies and recreational activities and community agencies	Knowledge of activities from which to select gives client some degree of control in decision making
SHORT TERM			
To maintain positive social network following retirement	Initiates social relationship with retirees	Refer to community organizations with activities for retirees/senior citizens	Provides a pool of people with whom he can interact
	Participates in activities with preretirement friends at least once a week	Assist to identify those people with whom he wants to remain in contact	Incorporating these people encourages continuation of meaningful preretirement activities

TRAZODONE HCI

(tray′zoe-done)
Desyrel
Func class: Antidepressant—
tricyclic-like
Chem class: Triazolopyridine

Action: Selectively inhibits serotonin uptake by brain, potentiates behavioral changes
Uses: Depression
Dosage and routes:
▶ *Adult:* PO 150 mg/day in divided doses, may be increased by 50 mg/day q3-4d, not to exceed 600 mg/day
Available forms include: Tabs 50, 100, 150, 300 mg
Side effects/adverse reactions:
HEMA: **Agranulocytosis, thrombocytopenia, eosinophilia, leukopenia**
CNS: Dizziness, drowsiness, confusion, headache, anxiety, tremors, stimulation, weakness, insomnia, nightmares, EPS (elderly), increase in psychiatric symptoms
GI: Diarrhea, dry mouth, nausea, vomiting, **paralytic ileus,** increased appetite, cramps, epigastric distress, jaundice, **hepatitis,** stomatitis
GU: Retention, **acute renal failure, priapism**
INTEG: Rash, urticaria, sweating, pruritus, photosensitivity

Italic indicates common side effects.
Bold italic indicates life-threatening reactions.

CV: Orthostatic hypotension, ECG changes, tachycardia, **hypertension,** palpitations
EENT: Blurred vision, tinnitus, mydriasis
Contraindications: Hypersensitivity to tricyclic antidepressants, recovery phase of myocardial infarction, convulsive disorders, prostatic hypertrophy
Precautions: Suicidal patients, severe depression, increased intraocular pressure, narrow-angle glaucoma, urinary retention, cardiac disease, hepatic disease, hyperthyroidism, electroshock therapy, elective surgery, pregnancy (C)
Pharmacokinetics:
Metabolized by liver, excreted by kidneys, feces; half-life 4.4-7.5 hr
Interactions/incompatibilities:
—Decreased effects of: guanethidine, clonidine, indirect acting sympathomimetics (ephedrine)
—Increased effects of: direct acting sympathomimetics (epinephrine), alcohol, barbiturates, benzodiazepines, CNS depressants
—Hyperpyretic crisis, convulsions, hypertensive episode: MAOI (pargyline [Eutonyl])

NURSING COMSIDERATIONS
Assess:
—B/P (lying, standing), pulse q4h; if systolic B/P drops 20 mm Hg hold drug, notify physician; take vital signs q4h in patients with cardiovascular disease

—Blood studies: CBC, leukocytes, differential, cardiac enzymes if patient is receiving long-term therapy
—Hepatic studies: AST, ALT, bilirubin, creatinine
—Weight qwk, appetite may increase with drug
—ECG for flattening of T wave, bundle branch block, AV block, dysrhythmias in cardiac patients
Administer:
—Increased fluids, bulk in diet if constipation, urinary retention occur
—With food or milk for GI symptoms
—Dosage hs if over-sedation occurs during day; may take entire dose hs; elderly may not tolerate once/day dosing
—Gum, hard candy, or frequent sips of water for dry mouth
Perform/provide:
—Storage in tight, light-resistant container at room temperature
—Assistance with ambulation during beginning therapy since drowsiness/dizziness occurs
—Safety measures including side-rails, primarily in elderly
—Checking to see PO medication swallowed
Evaluate:
—EPS primarily in elderly: rigidity, dystonia, akathisia

—Mental status: mood, sensorium, affect, suicidal tendencies, increase in psychiatric symptoms: depression, panic
—Urinary retention, constipation; constipation is more likely to occur in children
—Withdrawal symptoms: headache, nausea, vomiting, muscle pain, weakness; do not usually occur unless drug was discontinued abruptly
—Alcohol consumption; if alcohol is consumed, hold dose until morning
Teach client/family:
—That therapeutic effects may take 2-3 wk
—To use caution in driving or other activities requiring alertness because of drowsiness, dizziness, blurred vision
—To avoid alcohol ingestion, other CNS depressants
—Not to discontinue medication quickly after long-term use, may cause nausea, headache, malaise
—To wear sunscreen or large hat since photosensitivity occurs
Lab test interferences:
Increase: Serum bilirubin, blood glucose, alk phosphatase
False increase: Urinary catecholamines
Decrease: VMA, 5-HIAA
Treatment of overdose: ECG monitoring, induce emesis, lavage, activated charcoal, administer anticonvulsant

Modified from Skidmore-Roth L: *Mosby's nursing drug reference,* St Louis, 1993, Mosby–Year Book.

---

memory, enhanced visual concentration, increased daydreams, and increased persuasiveness may follow periods of decreased boredom or stimulation.[72]

The boring work setting may or may not be alterable to diminish the causes of boredom. The nurse explores with the client what can be changed, such as the type of work and variety of tasks, the location of office equipment or lounges, and pictures on the wall. Reassignment of personnel may be needed to maintain productivity as well as to enhance creativity. The client may consider instituting small frequent breaks and varying activity. If these changes are not possible, the client may need to consider other employment, especially when safety or health is a concern.

Thrill seekers may require specific interventions to prevent physical harm to themselves and others. Increasing awareness of the destructive possibilities of their behavior is helpful. Because drug abuse may accompany their bored behavior, both the drug abuse and the boredom may need the nurse's attention simultaneously. The nurse determines

activities that prevent boredom and ultimately lead to drug abuse episodes.

Emotional dimension Clients may need assistance in acknowledging their boredom. Encouraging them to express their feelings based on psychoanalytical theory may be a new experience, especially for the chronically bored who believe that boredom is a way of life. Verbalization can occur directly with the nurse or during group therapy with those who have similar problems. Music therapy offers soothing sensory stimulation and may be scheduled before a group session to promote communication and relax the group members.

The bored client's predominant feeling states of frustration, restlessness, and apathy best respond to strategies used with the depressed or lonely client. Trazodone (Desyrel) may be used to treat the depression. The accompanying profile describes nursing care appropriate to the administration of Desyrel. See Chapters 14 and 21 for additional information on depression and loneliness. Countertransference also occurs particularly with bored clients.[40,50,74] The nurse is likely to become bored, lack energy, and be less motivated to interact with the boring client during the therapy sessions. Awareness that one can become bored with a chronically bored client is the first step in preventing one's own boredom.

The nurse strives to teach the client that alleviating boredom is a worthwhile goal. Expressing encouragement in these interactions assists the client in resolving difficulties caused by boredom. Attention to detail becomes necessary as the nurse asks for specific boredom examples and assists the client to explore these difficult situations in depth.

The nurse works with the client to clarify his boredom episodes. Questions such as "How frequently does boredom occur?," "How long does it last?," and "What prevents or alleviates the episode?" elicit the necessary information. Throughout the relationship the nurse encourages any sign of increased motivation to deal constructively with boredom. Support is necessary to assist the client in reversing his attitude toward his life and making changes. The nurse assists the client to risk greater unpredictability, which may be accompanied by fear. The client needs support to change his behavior.

Clients with borderline personality disorder can be exhausting as the nurse becomes the object of hatred and devaluation. The nurse monitors the caring that is expressed because too much can cause rage and destructive acting out. Clients learn from the nurse that love and hate can exist simultaneously in the same person and the nurse confronts projection of feelings. For example, if the client says that the nurse is deliberately trying to hurt him, the nurse states that she is not doing so, if that is true.

Using a psychoanalytical approach, these clients need long-term therapy to "heal the split." In therapy, the client learns "how to be"[58] and how the average person lives and receives encouragement that he can change. Using behavioral theory, the nurse focuses on behavioral change, goal attainment, and the client's ability to perceive events realistically. With the assurance of support, the client assumes more responsibility for his actions as he moves to decrease boredom. The client is encouraged to practice new learned behaviors daily.

Intellectual dimension Preventing boredom by means of intellectual processes may involve altering both the client's activity level and attitude. Dividing a complex task into simpler steps may help the client see it as achievable. Using behavioral theory as each step is successfully completed, the client can give himself positive rewards that are meaningful. For example, the client may have a large report due as part of his work. Because the topic is boring, he has difficulty completing the document. By breaking the report into smaller sections that take one day each to prepare, the client perceives the task as more manageable. After each section is finished, he treats himself to some time reading a book he has long wanted to finish. The success sustains his momentum, and he alternates a boring task with a pleasurable activity. Effective coping generally incorporates two strategies: changing one's habits to minimize what causes the boredom and changing one's attitude toward the activity associated with boredom.

Breaking down goals into measurable steps creates a sense of progress in these clients who are emotionally re-

moved from thoughts of the future. With each step, praise and encouragement are warranted.

Other choices may be presented, such as taking small frequent breaks or decreasing the total amount of time spent on a boring task during any workday. Intellectual stimulation, especially strategies to develop original responses, encourages creativity. For example, during therapy the nurse may give scenarios that motivate the client to use his imagination while problem solving. The idea is to produce a response that shows the client understood the scenario and found relevant solutions. For example, the nurse asks Sam, his client, what he would tell a fictitious friend, Toni, who wanted advice about how to handle his boring days now that he has lost his job. Toni has been anxious and is having trouble thinking. Theoretically, Sam's solution would show that he does have some understanding about how to deal with boredom in a healthy way. The nurse uses his response to build on possibilities to solve his own boredom problem.

Alleviating classroom boredom that inhibits learning requires teacher cooperation. The nurse may arrange meetings between student, parents, teachers, and guidance counselors to facilitate a team approach to problem solving.

Social dimension If the client is hospitalized for short-term, acute illnesses, the nurse plans socialization opportunities using sociocultural theory. Providing client lounge areas, ensuring that client rooms have adequate space and furniture for visitors, and promoting visiting hours that consider the schedules of visitors are strategies the nurse uses to alleviate boredom.

When clients do not have visitors, especially while in isolation, staff members need to periodically visit the client at times other than those for administration of medication or treatment. The personal touch and attention are meaningful. Those clients who are institutionalized either permanently or for a lengthy rehabilitation may benefit from planned as well as unplanned diversionary activities. The goal is to reach the client's optimum level of activity whether through singing, games of checkers, or walking field trips. Dining rooms for group eating are excellent places, not only to enjoy meals but also to break up the long day. Clients need encouragement to maintain communication by telephone calls, writing letters, or sending cards. It is essential to increase their social option whenever possible. The client's social skills also may need modification to produce more satisfying relationships and to prevent boredom.

Boredom can result from external pressures to conform.[66] When the client does not feel free to respond differently from his peer group and he chooses to remain with his peer group, then boredom may become a coping method. The client would rather be bored than become alienated from his peers. Thus the nurse encourages the client to have contacts outside one group and to decrease the amount of conformity exhibited when the client is with others.

Everyone needs to prepare for retirement to decrease the likelihood of boredom. Joint decision making with significant others to determine activities that prevent boredom can ensure a meaningful retirement period.

Initially, clients with borderline personality disorder may be charming. Manipulation will eventually become

▼
KEY INTERVENTIONS FOR BOREDOM

Balance schedule between routine and novel activities
Alter predictability of situations
Encourage participation in recreational activities
Use touch with clients experiencing sensory deprivation
Encourage small, frequent breaks during boring tasks
Vary activities where possible
Encourage verbalization of feelings associated with boredom
Teach value of alleviating boredom
Encourage use of music therapy and group therapy
Explore episodes of boredom
Reinforce motivation to deal constructively with boredom
Decrease complexity of tasks
Reward activity directed at decreasing boredom
Encourage to use creative approaches to problem solving
Arrange for visitors, a change in environment, and other activities to reduce boredom for the hospitalized client
Encourage client to maintain contact with other people via telephone calls, letters
Encourage prayer, meditation, and imagery
Encourage client to attend to relationship with self, others, and a higher being

▼
GUIDELINES FOR PRIMARY/TERTIARY PREVENTION

Primary Prevention

Identify at-risk groups
Teach importance of participating in diversional activities
Prepare for retirement
Maintain a circle of friends
Teach factors that lead to boredom

Tertiary Prevention
Community resources

Churches
Spas
Libraries
Community clubs

Self-help groups

Share-a-meal groups
Social skills groups
Meditation groups

part of the relationship. The nurse needs to minimize her response to their manipulative tactics such as suicidal gestures or threats.

Spiritual dimension A client may decrease boredom by concentrating on his relationship with himself, with others, or with a higher being. This process may require the nurse's support as the client changes his behavior. Encouraging prayer, meditation, imaging, and the development of meaningful goals also may help the client decrease boredom.

The emptiness due to lack of identity felt by the client with borderline personality disorder leaves a void difficult to minimize. As the client enters long-term therapy and begins the healing journey, all dimensions are affected. The client may need assistance in verbalizing spiritual needs and in implementing decisions that are spiritually uplifting.

Each client has unique spiritual resources that can be incorporated into the nursing care plan. Whether those resources are organized church groups, time alone, religious practices, or a search for a more meaningful existence, the nurse incorporates what the client values to help alleviate boredom. See the accompanying boxes for key interventions for boredom and guidelines for primary and tertiary prevention.

INTERACTION WITH A CLIENT EXPERIENCING BOREDOM

(Nurse enters room of hospitalized male client who is staring at walls as he sits in the lounge chair. His morning care is completed; no visitors are expected because his spouse and friends work during the day. He is 45 years old and has been admitted because of depression secondary to an adjustment to disability. He has not worked in 3 months. The nurse has been in the room twice this morning. She has interacted with him daily since his admission.)

Nurse: *Mr. Sayers, I see you glanced at the magazines your wife left. What did you find that was interesting?*

Client: *(Talking slowly and softly). Oh, one article on antique cars but I finished it.*
Nurse: *Oh, are you interested in old cars?*
Client: *Yes, but I'd rather be tinkering with one than reading about one. I like to keep busy at home.*
Nurse: *What are your plans for this morning? (The unit's activity schedule has already been discussed with him; a printed schedule is in his room and in the hall and lounge area.)*
Client: *None really. Time sure drags in here. I'm bored.*
Nurse: *(Sitting beside him and extending the printed schedule.) This morning some recreational activities are planned in the lounge. You mentioned yesterday that you liked classical music. Today a group is getting together to listen to Chopin. Afterward they talk about the artist and his music. It may interest you.*
Client: *(Indicates a little interest as he leans forward in his chair and gives her eye contact for the first time.) Well, yeah, it might... (Hesitates and pauses.)*
Nurse: *I would be glad to go with you to the area and introduce you to the people. (He nods affirmatively.) I've got to finish giving these medications; then I'll come back for you in about 20 minutes.*
Client: *(Smiles slightly.) Okay, I would like to do that.*

Even though Mr. Sayer's primary problem was depression, boredom became an integral component of his problem, his hospitalization, and his coping with a changed work status. The nurse entered the room with an awareness of all three components and attempted to focus on the first two.

Her visit provided stimuli in the form of a forced but friendly interruption. The visit prevented the client from dwelling on his own thoughts and encouraged him to do some constructive planning of his time. Without this interaction and attention to the unit's resources, Mr. Sayers may have spent the morning alone, more bored than ever.

The nurse focused the client's attention on unit activities. She encouraged him by linking the unit activities with knowledge she had gained during a previous nursing assessment. She supported him by offering to take him to the setting where the activity was scheduled and introducing him to unfamiliar people. By these actions she increased the likelihood of a successful intervention, which the client would incorporate into his hospital routine.

Although this interaction was brief, the nurse used a number of strategies to alleviate situational boredom. These strategies included maintaining trust, offering a suggestion, respecting the client's individuality, varying his hospital routine, displaying interest in him, using diversional activities, offering hope, providing support and encouragement, considering the client's interests, and promoting his independence. She does not let his lack of energy, insight, initiative, or attention to surroundings, such as the posted schedule, interfere with the possibility of his relating to others through a meaningful activity.

Nursing interventions in similar situations require a sensitive, creative nurse who is aware of the client as an individual and the practice setting's resources and capabilities. This nurse also plans to address the chronic boredom that contributed to the client's depression as she strengthens her relationship with him.

Evaluation

Evaluation includes examining the concrete data and the client's self-reporting on the success of the nursing process. Goals and outcomes concentrate on decreasing or alleviating boredom. Interventions are evaluated in terms of the intensity of boredom, the presence of related feeling states, the client's need and desire to reduce the effects of boredom on his life, the family's involvement, and the development of successful coping mechanisms that the client can eventually incorporate into his life-style.

The nurse hopes for a positive result: the alleviation of boredom or at least a decrease in its intensity. If neither occurs, new goals and more relevant strategies are implemented until new behaviors are evident.

The following criteria to evaluate the mutually developed interventions provide guidance for the nurse:
1. *Adequacy:* Were the symptoms of boredom stopped or diminished? Can the client self-manage his boredom?
2. *Appropriateness:* Were the interventions specific to the degree of boredom felt? As more acute symptoms appeared, did they receive prompt intervention (e.g., incapacitating anxiety, severe depression, the borderline personality disorder client's rage)?
3. *Effectiveness:* Was the client and/or his family satisfied with the effects of the interventions? Does the client have sufficient resources to handle similar future boredom situations?
4. *Efficiency:* Were interventions implemented in a timely manner and in the client's own environment where boredom is most often experienced? Was there a gradual decrease in reliance on the nurse's guidance and an increase in the client's ability to handle his own episodes of boredom?

Throughout the nursing process, the client and his family need to be involved. The nurse's sensitivity to this inclusion enhances the likelihood of the success of interventions and their use over long periods of time. Clients who learn using this methodology can make permanent life-style changes and prevent the harmful effects of untreated boredom.

BRIEF REVIEW

Boredom is a common experience that has received little attention by health professionals until recently. Because boredom is linked with predictability, researchers found that subjects functioned best when their stimulation level was moderate. If the subjects were overstimulated, they become confused; if they were understimulated, they become bored.

Boredom has been addressed by numerous theorists. All acknowledge boredom as a feeling state with diverse causes that can be generally categorized as internal, external, or a combination of the two. Initially believed to have only unpleasant consequences, boredom is now known to have numerous benefits for certain population groups. Among them are clients with stuttering problems, autism, mental retardation, alcoholism, hypertension, and compulsive overeating.

Adolescents; retired persons; those with monotonous occupations; the hearing and visually impaired; and those experiencing social isolation, depression, confinement, and restriction of movement are among the at-risk groups for developing boredom. Most persons in these groups experience some form of sensory deprivation, which creates too little stimulation with too much predictability.

The negative effects of boredom include altered job performance and work quality, missed work time, somatic complaints, anxiety, depression, and accidents that could possibly lead to death. In the work setting, the results have been costly in lost working hours and injuries and have included even death. Boredom is associated with decreased attention, gastritis, peptic ulcer, chronic resignation, frustration, apathy, hostility, thrill seeking, decreased creativity, altered learning, and alienation from self and others.

Boredom is also a characteristic of the narcissistic and borderline personality disorders. Relieving boredom impulsively in these clients causes inappropriate maladaptive responses such as rage and temper tantrums.

REFERENCES AND SUGGESTED READINGS

1. Aronson T: A critical review of psychotherapeutic treatments of the borderline personality: historical trends and future directions, *Journal of Nervous Mental Disorders* 177(9):511, 1989.
2. Bailey J and others: Boredom and arousal: comparison of tasks differing in visual complexity, *Perceptual and Motor Skills* 43:141, 1976.
3. Benson K and others: Sleep patterns in borderline personality disorder, *Journal of Affective Disorders* 18(4):267, 1990.
4. Bernstein H: Boredom and the ready-made life, *Social Research* 42:512, 1975.
5. Bloom H, Rosenbluth M: The use of contracts in the inpatient treatment of the borderline personality disorder, *Psychiatric Quarterly* 60(4):317, 1989.
6. Brockman R: Medication and transference in psychoanalytically oriented psychotherapy of the borderline patient, *Psychiatric Clinics of North America* 13(2):287, 1990.
7. Deering C: A review of the borderline diagnosis for children, *Issues in Mental Health Nursing* 11(3):255, 1990.
8. Deutsch H: Some forms of emotional disturbance and their relationship to schizophrenia, *Psychoanalysis Quarterly* 11:301, 1942.
9. Drory A: Individual differences in boredom proneness and task effectiveness at work, *Personnel Psychology* 35:141, 1982.

10. Eppel A: Inpatient and day hospital treatment of the borderline: an integrated approach, *Canadian Journal of Psychiatry* 33(5):360, 1988.
11. Erikson EH: *Childhood and society,* ed 2, New York, 1964, WW Norton.
12. Fenichel O: On the psychology of boredom. In Fenichel H, Rapaport D, editors: *The collected papers of Otto Fenichel: first series,* New York, 1953, WW Norton.
13. Fine M, Sansone R: Dilemmas in the management of suicidal behavior in individuals with borderline personality disorder, *American Journal of Psychotherapy* 44(2):160, 1990.
14. Fiske D: Effects of monotonous and restricted stimulation. In Fiske D, Maddi S, editors: *Functions of varied experience,* Homewood, Ill, 1961, Dorsey.
15. Frick S: Diagnosing boredom, confusion, and adaptation in school children, *Journal of School Health* 55:254, 1985.
16. Gallop R, Lancee W, Garfinkel P: How nursing staff respond to the label "borderline personality disorder," *Hospital and Community Psychiatry* 40(8):815, 1989.
17. Gibson D: Borderline personality disorder issues of etiology and gender, *Occupational Therapy Mental Health* 10(4):63, 1990.
18. Goldstein W: Beginning psychotherapy with the borderline patient, *American Journal of Psychotherapy* 42(4):561, 1988.
19. Greenson R: On boredom, *Journal of the American Psychoanalytic Association* 1:7, 1953.
20. Hamilton J: Attention, personality and the self-regulation of mood. In Maher BA, editor: *Progress in experimental personality research,* vol 10, New York, 1981, Academic Press.
21. Hamilton J: Development of interest and enjoyment in adolescence. II. Boredom and psychopathology, *Journal of Youth and Adolescence* 12(5):363, 1983.
22. Hamilton J, Haier R, Buchsbaum M: Intrinsic enjoyment and boredom coping scales: validation with personality, evoked potential and attention measures, *Personality and Individual Differences* 5(2):183, 1984.
23. Hartman D, Boerger M: Families of borderline clients: opening the door to therapeutic interaction, *Perspectives of Psychiatric Care* 25(3-4):15, 1990.
24. Hartocollis P: Affects in borderline disorders. In Hartocollis P, editor: *Borderline personality disorders: the concept, the syndrome, the patient,* New York, 1977, International Universities Press.
25. Hartocollis P: Affective disturbance in borderline and narcissistic patients, *Bulletin of the Menninger Clinic* 44:135, 1980.
26. Herron W: The pathology of boredom, *Scientific American* 52, 1957.
27. Hill A: Work variety and individual differences in occupational boredom, *Journal of Applied Psychology* 60:128, 1975.
28. Hill A, Perkins R: Towards a model of boredom, *British Journal of Psychology* 76:235, 1985.
29. Johansson G: Job demands add stress reactions in repetitive and uneventful monotony at work, *International Journal of Health Services* 19(2):365, 1989.
30. Johnson C: Recognizing borderline personality disorder in the primary care client, *Nurse Practitioner: American Journal of Primary Health Care* 13(8):11, 1988.
31. Kaplan C: The challenge of working with patients diagnosed as having a borderline personality disorder, *Nursing Clinics of North America* 21(3):429, 1986.
32. Katz S, Levendusky P: Cognitive-behavioral approaches to treating borderline and self-mutilating patients, *Bulletin of the Menninger Clinic* 54(3):398, 1990.
33. Kavoussi R and others: Structured interviews for borderline personality disorder, *American Journal of Psychiatry* 147(11):1522, 1990.
34. Keen S: Chasing the blahs away: boredom and how to beat it, *Psychology Today* 78, 1977.
35. Kelly G: *The psychology of personal constructs,* vol 1, New York, 1975, WW Norton.
36. Kernberg P: Resolved: borderline personality exists in children under twelve. Affirmative, *Journal of the American Academy of Child and Adolescent Psychiatry* 29(3):478, 1990.
37. Kohut H: *The analysis of self: a systematic approach to the psychoanalytic treatment of narcissistic personality disorders* (Psychoanalytic study of the child, monograph no 4), New York, 1971, International Universities Press.
38. Khout H: *The restoration of the self,* New York, 1977, International Universities Press.
39. Kohut H, Worf E: The disorders of the self and their treatment: an outline, *International Journal of Psychoanalysis* 59:413, 1978.
40. Kulick E: On countertransference boredom, *Bulletin of the Menninger Clinic* 49:95, 1985.
41. Landon P, Suedfeld P: Complex cognitive performance and sensory deprivation: completing the U-curve, *Perceptual and Motor Skills* 34:601, 1972.
42. Link P and others: The occurrence of borderline personality disorder in the families of borderline patients, *Journal of Personality Disorders* 2(1):14, 1988.
43. Ludolph P and others: The borderline diagnosis in adolescents: symptoms and developmental history, *American Journal of Psychiatry* 147(4):470, 1990.
44. Marsh J: The boredom of study: a study of boredom, *Management Education and Development* 14(2):120, 1983.
45. Masterson JF: Psychodynamic therapy with borderline patients, *American Journal of Psychiatry* 145(1):135, 1988.
46. McEnamy G, Tescher B: Contracting for cure: one nursing approach to the hospitalized borderline patient, *Journal of Psychosocial Nursing & Mental Health Services* 23(4):11, 1985.
47. McGlashan T, Heinssen R: Narcissistic, antisocial, and noncomorbid subgroups of borderline disorder: are they distinct entities by long-term clinical profile? *Psychiatric Clinics of North America* 12(3):653, 1989.
48. Mihalitsianou G, Soth N: Females with borderline personality disorder: personal and familial characteristics, *International Journal of Family Psychiatry* 9(2):169, 1988.
49. Miller L: The formal treatment contract in the inpatient management of borderline personality disorder, *Hospital and Community Psychiatry* 41(9):985, 1990.
50. Morrant J: Boredom in psychiatric practice, *Canadian Journal of Psychiatry* 19:431, 1984.
51. Nachreiner F: Experiments on the validity of vigilance experiments. In Mackie RR, editor: *Vigilance: theory, operational performance, and physiological correlates,* New York, 1977, Plenum Press.
52. Olsen R: The effect of the hospital environment: patient reactions to traditional versus progressive care settings, *Journal of Architectural and Planning Research* 1(2):121, 1984.
53. Orcutt J: Some social dimensions of boredom. Paper presented at the Annual Meeting of the American Sociological Association, Detroit, 1983.
54. Orcutt J: Contrasting effects of two kinds of boredom on alcohol use, *Journal of Drug Issues* 14:161, 1984.
55. Perkins R: The nature and origins of boredom, PhD thesis, Staffordshire, United Kingdom, 1981. University of Keele.
56. Perkins R, Hill A: Cognitive and affective aspects of boredom, *British Journal of Psychology* 76:221, 1985.
57. Plakun E: Narcissistic personality disorder. A validity study and comparison to borderline personality disorder, *Psychiatric Clinics of North America* 12(3):603, 1989.
58. Platt-Koch L: Borderline personality disorder: a therapeutic approach, *American Journal of Nursing* 83(12):1666, 1983.

59. Pribram K: *Languages of the brain,* Englewood Cliffs, NJ, 1971, Prentice Hall.
60. Robinson W: Boredom at school, *British Journal of Educational Psychology* 45:141, 1975.
61. Rosseel E. Fatigue and boredom resulting from reduced task motivation, *Psychologica Belgica* 14:67, 1974.
62. Samoilova A: Morbidity with temporary loss of working capacity of female workers engaged in monotonous work (Russian), *Sovetska Zdravookhranenie* 30:41, 1971.
63. Savitz J, Friedman M: Diagnosing boredom and confusion, *Nursing Research* 30:16, 1981.
64. Schaffer N: Maintaining a balanced treatment approach with the borderline patient, *British Journal of Medical Psychology* 63(Pt 1):11, 1990.
65. Schane M, Kovel V: Family therapy in severe borderline personality disorders, *International Journal of Family Psychiatry* 9(3):241, 1988.
66. Schubert D: Creativity and coping with boredom, *Psychiatric Annals* 8:46, 1978.
67. Shultz C: Lifestyle assessment: a tool for practice, *Nursing Clinics of North America* 19(2):271, 1984.
68. Smith R: Boredom: a review, *Human Factors* 23:329, 1981.
69. Stagner R: Boredom on the assembly line: age and personality variables, *Industrial Gerontology* 2:22, 1975.
70. Stone M: Long-term follow-up of narcissistic/borderline patients, *Psychiatric Clinics of North America* 12(3):621, 1989.
71. Suedfeld P: Changes in intellectual performance and in susceptibility to influence. In Zubek JP, editor: *Sensory deprivation: fifteen years of research,* New York, 1969, Appleton-Century-Crofts.
72. Suedfeld P: The benefits of boredom: sensory deprivation reconsidered, *American Scientist* 63:60, 1975.
73. Swenson C, Wood M: Issues involved in combining drugs with psychotherapy for the borderline inpatient, *Psychiatric Clinics of North America* 13(2):287, 1990.
74. Taylor G: Psychotherapy with the boring patient, *Canadian Journal of Psychiatry* 29:217, 1984.
75. Thackray R, Bailey J, Touchstone R: Physiological subjective and performance correlates of reported boredom and monotony while performing a simulated radar control task, *FAA Office of Aviation Medicine Reports* 8:9, 1975.
76. Thackray R, Jones K, Touchstone R: Personality and physiological correlates of performance decrement on a monotonous task requiring sustained attention, *British Journal of Psychology* 65:351, 1974.
77. Thompson J: Finding the borderline's border: can Martha Rogers help? *Perspectives in Psychiatric Care* 26(4):7, 1990.
78. Vaccani J: Borderline personality and alcohol abuse, *Archives of Psychiatric Nursing* 3(2):113, 1989.
79. Wangh M: Boredom in psychoanalytic perspective, *Social Research* 42:538, 1975.
80. Wangh M: Some psychoanalytic observations on boredom. *International Journal of Psychoanalysis* 60:515, 1979.
81. Wenning K: Borderline children: a closer look at diagnosis and treatment, *American Journal of Orthopsychiatry* 60(2):225, 1990.
82. Westen D and others: Object relations in borderline adolescents, *Journal of the American Academy of Child and Adolescent Psychiatry* 29(3):338, 1990.
83. Wester C: Managing the borderline personality, *Nursing Management* 20(2):49, 1989.
84. Wester J: Rethinking inpatient treatment of borderline clients, *Perspectives in Psychiatric Care* 27(2):17, 1991.

ANNOTATED BIBLIOGRAPHY

Braverman BG, Shook J: Spotting the borderline personality, *American Journal of Nursing* 87(2):200, 1987.

A case example is offered of team management of the borderline client who appears in the emergency room. Presenting symptoms and behaviors, including boredom as a component of the DSM-III characteristics, are presented. Specific nursing interventions such as limit setting, family involvement, safety measures, and need for psychiatric consultation are discussed.

Levy S: Psychoanalytic perspectives on emptiness, *Journal of the American Psychoanalytic Association* 32(2):387, 1984.

The author considers emptiness as a component of boredom. The article reviews emptiness from a psychoanalytical perspective and its treatment modalities. Suggestions are offered in the management of the complaint of emptiness.

Buhler R: *New choices: new boundaries,* Nashville, Tenn, 1991, Thomas Nelson Publishers.

From his nationally syndicated talk show, the author discusses the basics of spiritual nourishment. As a concept, he found that few people know much about nourishing themselves or others. He provides numerous examples of nourishing decisions people can make to enrich their lives in ways to prevent feelings such as boredom, loneliness, and self-pity. He discusses self-responsibility for nourishment, seeking multiple sources for nourishment, determining healthy choices, and identifying and overcoming obstacles to nourishment. He provides challenges to people to enrich their lives by making nourishing choices.

23 Manipulation

Elizabeth G Maguire
Nancy Kowal Ellis

After studying this chapter, the student will be able to:

- Discuss manipulation within a historical perspective
- Define manipulation
- Discuss the psychopathology of antisocial personality disorder, adult antisocial behavior, and malingering as described in the DSM-III-R
- Discuss theories of manipulation
- Use the nursing process to provide care for a manipulative client

Manipulation is behavior in which an individual tries to control others to fulfill his immediate desires. The manipulative person often feels satisfaction when he controls others. The terms *manipulative client* and *manipulator* usually evoke negative emotions because the recipient of the manipulation often feels victimized.

Although manipulation is commonly seen as destructive, virtually all interpersonal actions involve conscious or unconscious manipulation. The term *manipulative* has been misused to refer to any individual who tries to gain control or to become assertive.

In a therapeutic relationship, the nurse strives to encourage growth and independence. Achieving this goal is often difficult when the client is manipulative. The nurse must deal with the process as well as the content of the interaction.

Unfortunately, when a client manipulates as part of his pattern of interacting, the nurse has strong emotional responses and may neglect the process of the interaction. Understanding the dynamics of a client's manipulative behavior can help the nurse deal with her emotional response and further the client's growth and independence. The degree to which manipulative behavior is used also influences the nurse's and client's range of long- and short-term goals.

Destructive manipulation is a common pattern of relating for many clients with a psychiatric diagnosis, especially those with a personality disorder. Narcissistic personality disorder and antisocial personality disorder are two diagnoses where destructive manipulation is found in an extreme form. Narcissistic personality disorder is described in Chapter 22. This chapter describes the essential features and manifestations of the features of antisocial personality disorder, adult antisocial behavior, and malingering according to the DSM-III-R.

Destructive manipulation is used in each of the preceding disorders due to personality (ego) deficits. Destructive manipulation is a behavior learned in an environment that lacked the security for the client to have his needs met otherwise. Antisocial personality disorder is the more socially malignant of the disorders and appears to have the most severe consequences. For instance, it is common for a client with antisocial personality disorder to have been prosecuted by the legal system for conscienceless crimes and to have served time in prison.

DSM-III-R DIAGNOSES

According to DSM-III-R, the essential feature of antisocial personality disorder is a pattern of irresponsible and antisocial behavior beginning in childhood or early adolescence and continuing into adulthood. Common signs seen

 DIAGNOSES Related to Manipulation

MEDICAL DIAGNOSES
Antisocial personality disorder
Adult antisocial behavior
Malingering

DATES	EVENTS
1500s	Machiavelli published *The Prince,* which described manipulative strategies to succeed in politics. Power, not ethics, was stressed.
Early 1800s	The labels *morally deficient* and *morally insane due to genetic impairments* were introduced. They included individuals who showed obvious destructive manipulation.
Early 1900s	The label *psychodynamically impaired* replaced the moral labels. Destructive manipulative behavior was included in this category. The term *psychopath* was commonly used to describe individuals who functioned without regard to others' rights and outside of social rules and laws.
1930	Cleckley[4] replaced the term *psychopath* with *sociopath,* explaining that these individuals' destructive behaviors were directed toward society.
1952	The first DSM offered the diagnostic category *sociopathic personality,* which included manipulative behavior.
1963	Kumler,[17] a nurse, published an article on manipulation that recognized the impact of manipulation on the nurse-client relationship.
1968	DSM-III placed the diagnostic category *sociopath* under the general heading *personality disorders.* Wiley,[35] a nurse, published her conceptualization of manipulation.
1970s	Christie and Geis, researchers in Machiavellian behaviors, extensively studied manipulative individuals' abilities to exploit others, remain emotionally detached, and be continually opportunistic. They predicted that manipulative behaviors would increase in society, because these behaviors were reinforced by role models. Several popular books on succeeding through manipulation appeared.
1980	DSM-III altered the previous diagnostic category to *antisocial personality disorder.*
1986	An article by Chitty and Maynard[5] reflected renewed interest in managing manipulation.
1990	Johnson and Werstlein,[16] both nurses, published an article called "Reframing: a Strategy to Improve Care of Manipulative Patients."
Future	Manipulative behavior and personality disorders will be more easily recognized and managed as health care providers' awareness and understanding increase.

in childhood are physical cruelty, truancy, lying, stealing, running away from home, expulsion or suspension from school, and vandalism. The antisocial activities continue into adulthood and are reflected in behaviors such as failure to honor financial obligations, inability to sustain a job, disregard for honesty, and repeatedly performing antisocial acts that are grounds for arrest. There is generally no feelings of guilt or sorrow for the effects of their behaviors on others, and they often feel jusitifed for having injured or mistreated others.

Individuals with antisocial personality disorders are likely to get into physical fights, including physical abuse of spouse and children. Violation of legal norms is common and may be observed in activities such as driving while intoxicated and stealing. The individual is unable to have a meaningful relationship with others and typically never has a lasting monogamous relationship. The individuals tend to be promiscuous. Once the client is 30 years old,

the antisocial behavior, especially promiscuity, fighting and criminality are less pronounced. Males are more likely than females to have antisocial personality disorder.

The DSM-III-R contains a category termed *conditions not attributable to a mental disorder.* Adult antisocial behavior is in this category and is considered as a diagnosis when antisocial behavior occurs but does not meet the full criteria for antisocial personality disorder.

Malingering is another example of a diagnosis in this category in which destructive manipulation is an essential feature. The DSM-III-R describes malingering as an intentional production of false or grossly exaggerated physical or psychological symptoms motivated by external incentives such as avoiding work, obtaining financial compensation, evading criminal prosecution, obtaining drugs, or securing better living conditions.

Key factors in recognizing malingering is marked discrepancy between what the client reports as the stress or disability and the findings of a physical and mental assessment. Malingering may also be suspected when the client refuses to cooperate during the diagnostic evaluation and does not adhere to the prescribed treatment regimen. An individual with antisocial personality disorder is likely to use malingering. Malingering can be adaptive when a person consciously feigns an illness to protect himself, for example, while a prisoner during wartime.

Although the nurse may see extreme forms of manipulation in her practice, such as those described earlier, it is much more common to see subtle forms of destructive manipulation. This chapter describes ways for the nurse to assess and handle manipulation.

THEORETICAL APPROACHES

Psychoanalytical

Webster's defines *manipulation* as "skillful handling or operation, or artful management and control with the use of shrewd influence, especially in an unfair or fraudulent manner."

Psychoanalytical theory associates manipulation with the development of the superego. The superego emerges in an infant in response to rewards and punishments from significant others, most often parents. For this development to begin, the infant must be able to identify and internalize parental responses, demands, and prohibitions.

The infant's superego is reinforced when his self-esteem and fulfillment grow as he lives up to the standards of the superego. Failure to meet these standards results in guilt and shame. The development of primary morality therefore is directly linked to the morality of the significant others.

The child is also exposed to the standards of his peer group. As the child identifies with this peer group, he begins to adopt its morality. The internalized morals of early significant others and the peer socialization process contribute to the developing conscience. An individual's moral stance and feelings of guilt when being manipulative are influenced by both the conscience and the individual's perception of the values of his peer group or society.

The development of the superego and the conscience is influenced by various factors of early infancy and childhood. A child who has strong aggressive feelings and fears retaliation from his parents may turn his aggressive feelings inward. The result may be an overly severe superego and conscience. Such as individual would probably manipulate very little.

A child may develop a weak superego as a result of his inability to internalize social expectations. The parents may be inconsistent in their morality or demands, giving the child a false impression of their actions. The resultant weak superego gives the child a decreased sense of guilt and weak conscience.

A child who identifies strongly with his peer group may feel guilty when he himself manipulates. However, manipulation in collaboration with others may free him from guilt.

A person with a manipulative personality often uses manipulation as his primary goal. Punishment or reward has no effect because the gain is from the act itself. Psychoanalytical theorists view the manipulative individual as a fragile form of a *narcissistic personality*. The narcissistic individual manipulates in response to a wound that causes shame. The need to restore a sense of balance assumes primary importance, which involves restoring pride and decreasing the shame. Through manipulation the indivudal is relieved and exhilarated at pulling something over on someone and setting the balance right.

The narcissistic person views others as an extension of himself and uses them to mirror his grandiose self-image. The narcissistic manipulator cannot tolerate imperfection in others and therefore avoids all genuine intimate relationships. The individual with a manipulative personality puts his appearance before all his other aspects. Any threat to his appearance results in manipulative attempts to redeem his image, regardless of the impact on others or the violation of rights or rules. If the manipulative act is exposed, the manipulator pretends to be contrite to present the image that society expects. Remorse is acted out only because the individual with a manipulative personality has not developed a strong enough superego to truly experience this reaction.

Bursten,[3] in his psychoanalytical study of manipulation, emphasized the conscious nature of manipulation. The individual may not know the reason for his behavior, but he usually is aware that he is controlling another person to his own advantage. Bursten identified four essential components of manipulation[3]:
1. *Conflict of goal*—the manipulator must want something from the other person that he thinks the person does not want him to have.
2. *Intentionality*—the manipulator must intend to influence the other person. This component requires planning by the manipulator with an intent that is conscious or readily accessible to consciousness.
3. *Deception*—the manipulator knows his plan is to deceive the person.
4. *Sense of satisfaction*—the manipulator must feel a sense of satisfaction in deceiving the other person.

The four components are related; in some instances one may be more easily recognized, and in other situations another component may be more obvious. Bursten emphasized that all components must be observed or reasonably inferred for the behavior to be identified as manipulation.

Bursten[3] described three groups of manipulative situations. A person in group I uses manipulation only occasionally to achieve a goal or attain satisfaction and pleasure. For example, this person may manipulate to get a special privilege or to draw attention to himself. People in the second group may use manipulation to avoid danger and discomfort, as when a child does a special favor for a parent when he thinks punishment is forthcoming. Persons in both groups do not manipulate repeatedly or chronically. Their reason for manipulation usually becomes obvious and the advantages are at a conscious level.

People in the third group seem to manipulate for the sake of manipulating. Manipulation is the person's life-style; he has a manipulative personality. The manipulative behavior may be silly, involving pranks that may lead to repeated punishment. The basis for the manipulation is primarily a need to "pull something over" on another person. People in this group may be classified as having an antisocial personality disorder.

Interpersonal

Wiley[35] described two types of manipulation: constructive and destructive.

Constructive manipulation is using one's strengths to promote successful relationships. The constructive manipulator knows he is using manipulation and accepts responsibility for it.[35] Communication continues consciously and maturely. Both parties in the interaction know what is occurring and can decide whether to participate.

Destructive manipulation is using others for one's own purposes. This manipulator promotes difficulties in or destroys relationships, and personal growth is stunted. Communication is often at an unconscious level. The victim, however, responds negatively, often with anger and withdrawal. The manipulator may feel rejected, which increases his anxiety and need to manipulate.

Manipulative behavior is never eliminated (Shostrom[32]); all individuals use some degree of manipulation throughout their lives. This behavior can be viewed on a continuum from manipulative behavior to actualized behavior. (See Table 23-1 for the range of behaviors.) Most individuals fall between the two extremes. An individual in the actualized range may engage in manipulation but is aware of it and accepts responsibility for it.

The term *adaptive maneuvering* may be used to describe the manipulative responses of newborns (Kumler[17]). Adaptive maneuvering is an automatic behavioral pattern used to decrease anxiety without learning or interpersonal growth.[17] Newborns learn several adaptive maneuvers to fulfill basic needs. They influence or manipulate without regard for others' needs and without responsibility. Although this behavior is necessary for newborns, it is usually viewed as unacceptable in adults.

A child tests a variety of maneuvers to manipulate the environment. Significant others respond by setting limits. However, the child is allowed to test these limits and to occasionally fail. If the child's experimentation is met with consistent, clear limits and unconditional love and acceptance, he begins to develop self-control and self-esteem and to form a healthy identification with his parents. Gradually, the child replaces the adaptive maneuvers with independence and self-regulation. He learns to express his needs and to trust that they will be fulfilled.

▼ TABLE 23-1   Continuum of Manipulative Behavior

Manipulative Behavior	Actualized Behavior
Conceals sincere emotions	Trusts own emotions
Serves own desires	Openly communicates desires
Disregard for others	Aware and trusts himself and others
Deceives by playing role to create impression	Shows honest and genuine emotion
Constant need to control others	Free and spontaneous in interactions

A child may remain at the manipulative end of the continuum if his adaptive maneuvers do not get the ideal responses. This child's experimentation is met with inconsistent limits or no limits, conditional love, and nonacceptance. The child does not learn how to fulfill his needs or gain acceptance and love from others. He becomes insecure and submissive to external controls, lacking self-esteem.

As the manipulative individual grows, he becomes trapped in a vicious cycle: He has needs to be met, but he has learned to expect inconsistency and lack of fulfillment. Thus he becomes anxious when faced with his needs or fears and begins to disregard the needs and rights of others. Adaptive maneuvers learned in infancy—in this case manipulation—are repeated to gain fulfillment. If the individual gets a positive response and his needs are met, his anxiety temporarily decreases. However, his use of manipulation is reinforced. If he is met with a negative response and his needs remain unfilled, his fears, insecurities, and anxiety greatly increase; and he becomes angry and frustrated. His self-esteem diminishes and feelings of helplessness and insecurity grow. To fulfill his needs and control his anxiety, he again tries to manipulate. He attempts learned adaptive maneuvers for self-protection. His inability to trust others to respond to his needs and his frustration with the external world are reinforced, and his sense of worthlessness and helplessness increases.

This individual has learned that he cannot risk losing control or feeling vulnerable. His inability to take a risk makes a sincere relationship impossible. Lacking basic trust, he is trapped in attempts to gain and maintain control.

Table 23-2 summarizes the theoretical approaches.

NURSING PROCESS

Assessment

Physical dimension The nurse first assesses the client's perception of the threat to his physical security. Any threat may increase anxiety and cause regression to maladaptive coping mechanisms. Physical illness often results in a sense of loss of control and a fear of becoming helpless and dependent. Further, the health care system often strips a client of control. Within the health care system, a client often feels vulnerable and anxious and tries to manipulate the environment to increase his security. He may rely on manipulation to fulfill the phsyical needs that he has been able to meet independently in the past. The nurse assesses the client's stress level and past coping responses. Verbal and nonverbal behaviors tell the nurse that the client is feeling threatened or stressed.

The client's manipulations may interfere with his ability to express his physical needs. Depending on the nurse to meet physical needs makes the client vulnerable. The client may exaggerate a physical condition or need or withhold important information. For example, the client who exaggerates his pain to get extra medication ensures that his need (pain relief) will always be fulfilled and under his control. A client who wants to be discharged or to have special visiting privileges may also withhold information. To validate these clients' physical conditions, the nurse observes both verbal and nonverbal signals. Pain assess-

▼ **TABLE 23-2** **Summary of Theoretical Approaches**

Theory	Theorist	Dynamics
Psychoanalytical		Manipulation develops in response to a weak superego.
		The individual with a manipulative personality uses manipulation as a primary goal.
	Bursten	Manipulation operates on a conscious level.
		There are four essential, interrelated components of manipulation: conflict of goal, intentionality, deception, and sense of satisfaction.
		There are three groups of persons who manipulate—those who (1) manipulate occasionally to achieve a goal or satisfaction, (2) sometimes manipulate to avoid danger and discomfort, (3) manipulate as a life-style—for the sake of manipulation.
Interpersonal	Wiley	Constructive manipulation occurs on a conscious level.
		The person uses assets to promote successful interpersonal relationships.
		Destructive manipulation is unconscious and destroys relationships.
	Shostrom	All people use manipulation throughout their lives.
		The behavior can be placed on a continuum from manipulative behavior (conceals emotion and serves own needs) to actualized behavior (trusts own emotions and openly communicates needs).
	Kumler	Manipulative behavior of the newborn is adaptive maneuvering to meet his needs.
		Positive responses to adaptive maneuvering lead to independence and self-regulation.
		When adaptive maneuvering is not successful for getting needs met, the person remains manipulative.

ment, for example, includes both the client's perceptions of pain and observation of his appetite, sleeping pattern, ability to concentrate, and level of activity.

Emotional dimension The nurse tries to determine whether the client's manipulative behavior is a response to anxiety or an established, destructive pattern. A client who temporarily regresses may be aware of and disturbed by his behavior. This client may be able to discuss the fears or anxieties that triggered the behavior. Further exploration may reveal that manipulative behavior occurs only in response to high stress.

A client who manipulates destructively as a pattern, as described by Wiley,[35] may appear pleased when his manipulations are successful; he does not show sincere remorse or embarrassment. When the nurse explores the client's behavior, the client may respond with self-pity, anger, or frustration instead of accepting responsibility.

The destructive manipulator often shows superficial emotions; the expression of sincere anxiety, guilt, or fear makes the client vulnerable. The nurse may observe that the client can express hostility and anger only when he is anxious or fearful and frustration only when he feels guilty.

The nurse differentiates among assertive, aggressive, and manipulative behaviors. Many clients are encouraged to become assertively involved in their care and to question the health care providers. However, the system often remains rigid, and these attempts may be met with anger or power struggles. Clients may be negatively labeled because they have confronted the health care team or changed a routine. The nurse who is aware of the differences between assertive, aggressive, and manipulative behaviors can identify whether the behavior is constructive or destructive. (See Chapter 16 for a discussion of assertive and aggressive behavior.)

Intellectual dimension Manipulative behaviors are often learned as survival skills in childhood; therefore a client who is cognitively impaired may still be a skillful

manipulator. If the client has not learned to express his needs and to trust that they will be fulfilled, adaptive maneuvering may continue into a congitively impaired individual's adulthood. Attempts to get needs met show little regard for other's needs or personal responsibility. The manipulator often gives seemingly rational reasons for his behaviors and may present a sound defense when challenged. The client may continually express a conflict between his perceived needs and the needs of others. The nurse is likely to observe difficulties with roommates, conflicts with hospital routines and rules, and a resistance to limits set by the hospital staff. As the client's anxiety builds, complaints may involve several levels of hospital administration.

The client may use flattery to get people "on his side." He may request special privileges because of his "special circumstances." When staff do not respond positively to his manipulative behavior, the client may get angry and frustrated. He may think that staff members are resistant because, as in his other relationships, they are "against him." This behavior is an example of the vicious cycle manipulative clients perpetuate. When the client receives a negative response, his self-esteem diminishes and feelings of helplessness and insecurity increase. Manipulative behavior is repeated in search of fulfillment. If a positive response is received the manipulative behavior is reinforced.

The client who has been in the health care system for a long time may have learned several ways to gain control. He may use medical jargon, drop board members' names, or refer to physicians and nurses as personal friends. These behaviors often cause the health care team to feel threatened, to withdraw, and to try to placate the client.

The nurse assesses the client's motivation to change his behavior. She finds out how the client sees his behavior and whether his behavior has caused difficulties in the past. The nurse can ask directly whether he is willing to change his behavior.

Social dimension The nurse determines which of the three types of destructive manipulation the client is using[35]: (1) *Aggressive maneuvering,* exemplified by multiple demands, threats, requests for special consideration, and playing members of the health care team against each other; (2) *distracting maneuvering,* exemplified by changes of subject, flattery, expressions of helplessness, tearfulness, dawdling, and last minute stalling; and (3) *disparaging maneuvers,* exemplified by reprimands or self-pity.

The social life of a destructively manipulative client is often severely impaired and can be assessed by observing the client's present and past social interactions. A social history may reveal no sincere relationships. The client may also transfer frustrations and anger onto any significant social support that does remain. If family members are present, they may act ambivalent toward the client.

The client's job history may show an inconsistent work pattern, possibly resulting in financial instability. The client often speaks of a troubled past in which he has been victimized. A manipulative pattern may be evident since early childhood. A review of the client's childhood and adolescence may show periods of aggressiveness and early sexual behaviors. Drug or alcohol abuse may have started in childhood and continued into adulthood, possibly impairing work performance and parenting. The client may have shown lack of respect for social norms, values, and laws.

What may initially appear to be manipulative behavior may actually be the client's cultural pattern. For example, many cultures view women as submissive and allow men to make demands and to dominate. In such a case the nurse must be objective; an angry reaction can interfere with an accurate assessment. At times the nurse may have to use other staff to help assess a client's behaviors.

When involved with a destructively manipulative client, the health care team often becomes unable to work together harmoniously. The treatment plan is often debated because each team member perceives the client differently. Although the nurse expends a great deal of energy on the client, the client appears uninterested and uninvolved. As the nurse is manipulated, she may begin to give special privileges. According to Wiley,[35] the nurse commonly responds to destructive manipulation by feeling threatened or alienated or reinforces the behavior by pitying or mothering the client. These reactions, objectively identified, suggest that the client is manipulating.

Spiritual dimension A client's behavior can be influenced by religions that are manipulative rather than actualized.[32] *Manipulative religions* encourage helplessness by stressing the inability of individuals to trust their own nature. The nurse may observe overdependence on the religious community. The client may refuse to think through situations because he has learned to respond only as the religion demands. Such a client may resist helping himself, assuring the nurse that his religion will take care of him. He may rationalize that difficult events are God's will or the will of some higher power.

Actualized religions stress trust in one's own nature and encourage self-direction and growth. A client whose religion is actualized may rely on his religious community for support, guidance, and strength but accepts responsibility for his behavior and the direction of his future.

The nurse remains objective by assessing the client's perception of the meaning of religion in his life. The client may blame God or his religion for his situation or his dissatisfaction with life. Such a client may also attempt to use religion in a manipulative pattern.

The client's level of self-actualization and life satisfaction are typically low because he cannot fulfill his basic needs or form relationships. He may also have been involved in activities that are illegal, unethical, or outside social norms and values and may express pride in past violations of others' rights.

Analysis
Nursing diagnosis

Manipulative behavior is an example of a nursing diagnosis that applies to the behavior of clients discussed in this chapter. NANDA-accepted nursing diagnoses with causative statements appropriate for clients with manipulative behavior include the following:

1. Powerlessness related to altered ability to meet social responsibilities
2. Impaired social interaction related to inability to maintain enduring relationships
3. Ineffective individual coping related to disregard for social norms
4. Ineffective individual coping related to lack of impulse control.

The following case example illustrates the characteristics of manipulative behavior:

▼ Case Example

John, age 26 years, has lost his third job as a salesman. He blames his boss for "being against him" and his co-workers for "setting him up." He expresses a geat deal of anger at all his former co-workers for being jealous of him. John relates that his whole life has been this way. External circumstances consistently stand in the way of his fulfillment. At present John is hospitalized for elective surgery. He demands that his visiting hours be extended because he is expecting contacts for future employment. He is aware of his roommate's condition and need for sleep but sees this as just another obstacle in his way. John continues to enlist the assistance of other patients in violating the visiting hours and appears to enjoy deceiving the staff. When confronted, John immediately appears sorrowful and states that he breaks rules only because his life has been so difficult.

Planning

The nursing care plan gives examples of long- and short-term goals, outcome criteria, interventions, and rationales related to manipulation (Table 23-3). These serve as examples of the planning stage in the nursing process.

Implementation

Physical dimension The nurse providing physical care for the manipulative client ensures basic physical safety while holding the client responsible for his own behavior. The client may have a variety of basic unmet physical needs. A client who manipulates by making himself dependent is encouraged to assume responsibility for self-

▼ **TABLE 23-3   NURSING CARE PLAN**

GOALS	OUTCOME CRITERIA	INTERVENTIONS	RATIONALES
NURSING DIAGNOSIS: Manipulative behavior related to no sincere relationships			
LONG TERM			
To replace manipulative behaviors with more actualized, mature patterns of relating	Demonstrates mature behaviors role modeled by the health care team. Engages in long-term therapy as an outpatient to maintain support for new behaviors and patterns of relating.	Provide ongoing therapy sessions in which new behaviors and positive relating is practiced, role modeled and supported.	Mature patterns of relating can be learned with consistent and long-term treatment.
SHORT TERM			
To verbalize awareness of the use of manipulation and its effect on the ability to gain true fulfillment of one's needs and desires	Begins to identify own manipulative behavior. Explores what it feels like to be manipulated. Explores past uses of manipulation and assesses outcomes of those experiences.	Encourage open and honest discussion of (1) client's manipulative behaviors, (2) how it would feel to him if he were manipulated, and (3) analysis of the outcomes of past manipulations.	Gaining insight increases motivation and ability to change behavior.
To identify the stimuli that prompt the use of manipulative behaviors	Explores past situations that prompted the use of manipulation and identifies feelings experienced.	Encourage identification of feelings or situations that trigger manipulative behaviors.	Recognizing situations that trigger manipulative behavior promotes insight and ability to change behavior.
To use alternative, more actualized methods of identifying and meeting needs	Substitutes new methods of relating while hospitalized. Accepts feedback on new behaviors.	Role play situations in which client may practice actualized methods of relating. Provide feedback when client interacts without use of manipulation	Practicing new methods of mature relating will increase confidence and ability to use them long term. Acknowledgement reinforces the use of nonmanipulative behavior
To self-evaluate behaviors and identify when support is needed to avoid relying on old patterns of communication	Identifies when old, manipulative patterns of relating are used and begins to accept responsibility for them. Begins to request support when anxiety or stresses are high to avoid reliance on old patterns of relating.	Teach client to self-evaluate his behaviors and ask for support in a nonmanipulative way. Provide positive feedback when this behavior occurs. Encourage and reinforce client as he requests support when anxiety and stress are high	Self-evaluation and use of support will promote permanent use of new pattern of relating. Encouragement and reinforcement will motivate clients to continue to request support as needed

care. After assessing the client's perception of the threat to himself, the nurse can decrease that threat by allowing the client to assume as much control as possible. For example, a manipulative client may not ask the nurse to explain a procedure for fear of exposing this vulnerability. Carefully explaining the procedure without a request may lower the client's anxiety.

◢ **Emotional dimension** Anxiety often stimulates regression to maladaptive communication or destructive manipulation. A manipulative client feeling anxiety may camouflage his emotions and try to gain external control. The nurse looks beyond these maneuvers, discusses the client's perception of his anxiety, and explores his past patterns of coping with anxiety. Stripping such a client of his defenses is not useful.

The first intervention is to establish expectations, set limits, and communicate these to the client and the health care team. Limits are effective only if communicated consistenty and firmly. They are routinely reviewed to ensure they do not become punitive. The client's requests are objectively considered and not automatically opposed. The box on p. 475 given an approach to setting limits. Inappropriate limits may be set when the nurse becomes angry or exerts too much control. Limits must be reasonable and easily applied because, according to Kumler, the manipulative client has probably been exposed to inconsistent idle threats throughout his life. For example, the threat of not providing care if he does not cooperate cannot be carried out; it only perpetuates the cycle of maladaptive communication. The client's ability to set his own limits is assessed and encouraged. Encouraging self-control not only deters power struggles but also provides a model for a mature approach to relating.

Power struggles may result if the nurse phrases limits in a personal manner, beginning with "I want" or "you must." This sets up a struggle over control. Limit setting should be impersonal (for example, "Part of your treatment plan is that you attend one group today.") so that the client's anger does not focus on the nurse.

Davidhizar[6] stresses the importance of the nurse's personal self-awareness to effectively handle manipulative behavior. Inexperienced nurses should thoroughly investigate situations before taking action. Personal feelings of fear, guilt, responsibility, and obligation increase vulnerability to manipulation. She may choose to use more assertive body language and behavior to decrease susceptibility to manipulation.

Feelings of being used and powerlessness in the nurse may indicate that she is being manipulated. Alertness to and understanding of personal feelings can help the nurse recognize subtle manipulation.

The client will test limits and expectations. Consistent responses from the entire health care team are essential. As the client learns that the limits and expectations are firm and constant, he may begin to substitute one maladaptive behavior for another. Again, clear communication and consistency are necessary.

Although the entire health care team remains aware of expectations and limits, one primary nurse handles the client's requests. This approach lessens confusion and inconsistency, both of which a manipulative client can readily exploit. The primary care nursing system is ideal in this situation; requests for special privileges or changes in treatment are referred to one nurse who knows all aspects of the treatment.

The nurse can avoid power struggles by explaining to the client that confidentiality is maintained in the health care system. If the client asks a nurse to keep a secret or not share certain information, the nurse clearly and consistently avoids becoming engaged in any special relationship.

The nurse responds to the process or meaning of manipulative behavior to avoid unnecessary power struggles over content. This approach allows the nurse to respond to the client's maneuvers objectively. For example, if a client wants to slip out of the hospital for an hour, the nurse acknowledges that it must be hard to be hospitalized and unable to continue with normal routines. This acknowledgement allows the nurse and client to explore the client's actual need, instead of struggling over the content of the request. A manipulative client often responds to limits with anger. The nurse may acknowledge that the client is angry and that his situation is difficult. Such a response avoids punitive reactions or power struggles. If possible, the nurse discusses the process when the client's anxiety has decreased. The client's needs at the time limits were set and his ineffective communcation can be explored. More constructive patterns of coping and communicating are discussed if the client is receptive.

It is difficult to avoid reinforcing the cycle of manipulative behavior. For example, a client may angrily demand that his medications be given 30 minutes later than usual, and a busy nurse may comply to save time and avoid a conflict. However, this response reinforces the manipulative behavior. If a client's request is possible, he may be allowed the control he is seeking. By being a constructive role model, however, the nurse encourages learning by later exploring with the client his angry reaction and indirect request for control. Gratifying a client's manipulative requests without encouraging learning or growth only reinforces the behavior. Ignoring or neglecting the client also reinforces the behavior because the client expects that his needs will not be met.

Finally, the entire health care team's responses to the client should be explored continually. Conscious and unconscious anger, frustrations, and judgments are common. Putting the client's behaviors in perspective is helpful. The nurse reminds the team that the client's behavior results from a lifelong pattern of relating and is unrelated to any particular team member. For example, a client may cooperate with and complement the day nurse and resist the evening nurse, blaming her for his resistance. These nurses objectively assess their treatment of the client but remember that his reactions to them are most likely insincere. Rather, they are part of a pattern that somehow meets what the client perceives as his needs.

Intellectual dimension If manipulative behavior has been consistently reinforced, the client's motivation for change may be minimal, especially if stress is high and he is relying on previously successful coping mechanisms to control anxiety. Attempts to change the behavior of an unmotivated client may fail, but the nurse continues to be a constructive role model and avoids emotional responses that would reinforce manipulative behaviors. Again, responding to the process helps the nurse control her response. For example, the nurse may simply tell a client that a particular subject (such as another nurse's personal life) is inappropriate. She may then offer a more appropriate subject in its place.

Johnson and Werstlein[16] describe a therapeutic intervention in manipulation called reframing, which is defined as changing a person's interpretation of a given situation and therefore changing his behavioral response to it. For instance, the manipulative client's intention is usually to get attention or to gratify needs. If a client asks a nurse to hold his hand because of impending surgery, the request will usually be honored. If a client rings the call bell every 5 minutes because he is scared, many times the nurse will respond to the action, and not to the reason behind it. The nurse might initially see the client as demanding and bothersome, but then reframe her assessment to note the fear driving the behavior. If the nurse can use reframing in dealing with a manipulative client, she may help him meet his needs and decrease the maladaptive behavior. They can then work on developing adaptive and constructive patterns of relating.

The most effective intervention for a skillful manipulator is to explore the meaning of the behavior with him and the health care team. A client may be intelligent yet not be able to change behavior without therapy. Such a client may be able to identify and discuss his own maladaptive behavior, but he may be unable or unwilling to work at changing the behavior. The nurse may first explore with the client past actions that prevented him from meeting his needs. The client can then be encouraged to review past behavior to see how it was destructive. This information encourages the client to plan new methods for meeting his needs and provides positive reinforcement when these methods are tried.

 Social dimension The nurse gives the client the chance to see the destructive nature of past relating patterns and demonstrates constructive patterns. She encourages the client to explore his reactions to manipulation by others as a first step in realizing how his manipulative behavior affects others. The client is encouraged to identify manipulation in the past and to try out new communication techniques. The nurse encourages these new techniques only when the client's anxiety is low. Attempting a behavior change when anxiety is high sets up the client for frustration and failure. The nurse discusses past and present behaviors nonjudgmentally. The client and nurse explore the consequences of these behaviors, such as the client's failure to learn from past events. The nurse demonstrates to the family or significant others techniques that do not reinforce manipulation. These persons can also benefit from observing constructive communication and limit setting.

The client's strengths are supported to increase self-esteem. He needs encouragement and room to test new techniques; temporary regression is common. A structured setting is ideal for this testing period because it provides consistency, opportunities for learning, and safety. In such a setting the nurse can encourage the client's strengths and interactions with others, while the client remains independent. A structured environment can also support the nurse by holding the client responsible for his behavior.

In a group setting the manipulative client often emerges as a leader because of his need to control, and power struggles with the staff may develop, which can be difficult for the health care team. Nevertheless, the positive aspects of the client's behavior can be emphasized, as leadership ability is a strength.

Any change in the client's long-term pattern of relating should be reinforced after he leaves the health care system. Long-term psychotherapy can provide this reinforcement as well as an opportunity to learn to gain true fulfillment. Therapy can help the entire family learn constructive communication.

 Spiritual dimension The nurse remains aware of her values and of how they affect her perceptions of the client. Even if the client is involved in illegal or abnormal activities, objectivity remains necessary.

Some clients ask to include clergy in their care just to have another person to manipulate. Other clients may appear insincere in requesting religious support to cover their vulnerability and maintain control. Regardless of the rationale, the client's requests for religious assistance are supported. If the client involves a consistent religious representative, such as a hospital chaplain, this person should be regarded as part of the treatment team. The plan of care can be shared to keep communication open and to keep limits and expectations constant. The accompanying boxes describe key interventions for manipulation and guidelines for primary and tertiary prevention.

▼········
LIMIT SETTING

Expectations

Make expectations clear to client and other staff members.

Client-Centered Limits

Be sure that limits are in the best interest of the client and not punitive.

Communication

Avoid using personal statements, such as "I don't want you to drink alcohol while I'm on duty." Offer the true rationale: "Alcohol is not allowed in the hospital."

Consequences

When consequences are needed, avoid those that are absurd or cannot be enforced, such as "Put the alcohol away or I won't come into your room." Offer only enforceable consequences, such as "If you don't dispose of the alcohol, I will call security to dispose of it."

Testing

Remain firm and consistent as the client tests the limits that have been set.

Venting

Allow the client to vent feelings about limits, but do not engage in power struggles or attempt to rationalize (for example, "The hospital policy was written because things would get out of control if all clients could drink alcohol . . ."). Instead, verify the client's feelings and repeat the limit as necessary: "I hear that you are angry about this, but alcohol is not allowed."

Positive Reinforcement

Return to the client's room when the affect has subsided to demonstrate that you are not angry and have not withdrawn. Offer positive reinforcement for strengths.

Clarifications for Staff

Explain the expectations, limits, and consequences discussed with the client to all staff members to provide consistency and avoid confusion.

▼········
KEY INTERVENTIONS FOR MANIPULATION

Ensure physical safety
Encourage client to assume responsibility for self-care
Set consistent limits on manipulative behavior
Assist to identify manipulative behavior
Encourage self-control
Be consistent in approaches to client
Role model constructive pattern of coping/mature interaction
Explore meaning of manipulative behavior
Explore the consequences of manipulative behavior
Support strengths
Reinforce constructive use of leadership abilities
Demonstrate to family techniques that do not reinforce manipulation
Discuss client's perception of his anxiety
Respond consistently to testing behavior
Encourage client to try out new communication techniques
Support client's request for religious assistance
Allow client to assume as much control as possible
Channel requests to primary nurse

GUIDELINES FOR PRIMARY/TERTIARY PREVENTION

Primary Prevention
Identify high-risk groups through collaboration with community mental health nurse/school nurse

Initiate counseling with family of high-risk individuals

Provide education to parents regarding the importance of consistent child rearing practices

Teach family ways to strengthen their support system

Teach family effective and socially acceptable ways to communicate

Teach parents socially acceptable child-rearing practices

Tertiary Prevention
Community resources

Community mental health centers

Self-help groups

Groups for parental training, such as Parent Effectiveness Training

INTERACTION WITH A MANIPULATIVE CLIENT

Client: I want my medication at 9:30 AM. Any earlier than that is inhumane! You nurses are all worthless idiots anyway. Call my doctor. I'm leaving right now!

Nurse: John, it sounds like it has really been difficult for you to be in the hospital and on a hospital routine. I can discuss changing your medication time with your primary nurse and doctor.

Client: What's the matter? Can't you make a decision on your own? Or are you too new?

Nurse: A decision like this involves all of us. It is important that we make it together and then stick to it.

Client: Well, that could take time. When you're here, you can accommodate me. You're the nicest one, you know. You seem to understand more than those others.

Nurse: It sounds like it's difficult for you to work with a team of people. But we will meet and try to work it out.

Client: Please, do it for me just this one time. I promise I won't tell.

Nurse: The unit policy is that medications are given within 30 minutes of when they are ordered. But we will discuss it as a team with your doctor.

John tries to manipulate the nurse several times. First, he attempts to change her behavior through anger. The nurse responds to the process of the interaction (John's difficulty with being on a hospital schedule), not the anger. She also avoids a power struggle and remains objective by offering to discuss the client's request with team members. John again attempts to manipulate by trying to make her feel insecure, and then special. The nurse responds by consistently offering the same solution. The nurse reinforces the limit in an impersonal manner in her last statement. The unit policy, not she, sets the limits; thus she avoids being the focus of John's anger and power issues. The nurse also reinforces her solution consistently. The consistent and depersonalized limits set by the nurse will reinforce a mature communication pattern and maintain the consistency necessary among the health care team. If this pattern is reinforced, John can learn that his needs are met when appropriate, without the use of manipulation.

Evaluation

The evaluation of a change in a client's manipulative behaviors is based on the client's actions, not his words. Promises to change are respected, but they do not constitute change. Regression can be expected and is not considered failure.

The nurse can base an evaluation on small changes in a client's behavior; more obvious, long-term changes will most likely result only from long-term therapy. The nurse also evaluates her own expectations. The prognosis for the client with an antisocial personality disorder is often poor. In such cases, the long-term goal of the nurse is to be a role model of constructive behavior to help the client change. All evaluations are based on the long-term goal of learning from role modeling of mature behavior. The client is given the opportunity to learn and grow, and change is supported.

The evaluation of the manipulative client's care can be divided into four areas for a thorough and objective review.

Adequacy

- Was the client's behavior assessed objectively, or was he labeled negatively?
- Did the behavior meet the criteria for destructive manipulation, or was it a regression because of stress?
- Was a distinction made among aggressive, assertive, and manipulative behavior?
- Did the treatment plan encourage the client to learn?
- Were communication and limit setting clear and consistent, or was the cycle of manipulative behavior reinforced through inconsistency and anger?

Appropriateness

- Were consistent limits and plans established early and communicated to the entire health care team?
- Were interventions objective and punitive responses avoided?
- Were the client's needs considered and met when possible?
- Was the process of the client's interactions, not just their content, addressed?

Effectiveness

- Did the client's behavior change?
- Was the client able to see the need for learning and support?
- Was the client able to identify manipulative communication patterns when his anxiety was low?
- Were basic needs fulfilled by a supportive staff?

Efficiency

- Was the health care team's communication clear and open?
- Did members of the team support each other during the client's manipulative attempts?
- Was the health care team able to identify the dynamics involved in interactions with the client and with each other?
- Were limits and expectations consistent?
- Was the manipulative behavior identified early?
- Was information shared with all persons involved with the client?

- Has the health care team learned and grown from working with this client?

BRIEF REVIEW

An infant learns manipulative behavior to ensure that basic needs are met. Usually, as a child grows, manipulative behaviors are replaced with actualized behaviors. To some extent, all individuals use constructive or destructive manipulation. A child who receives inconsistent and conditional love often learns maladaptive relating and coping patterns and continues to manipulate. An individual falls into a manipulative cycle when needs are not met and anxiety increases because of negative past experiences. He disregards the needs of others and begins to manipulate to fulfill his needs. When the individual succeeds, the behavior is reinforced. When he fails, anxiety and frustration increase and often are manifested as hostility toward the persons he thinks are failing him. This reaction leads to further attempts to manipulate to decrease the anxiety.

Destructive manipulative behaviors are often associated with the DSM-III-R diagnostic categories of antisocial personality disorder and malingering. A client with these disorders may come into contact with the health care system for a number of related reasons. The long-term goal of the nurse is to be a role model of constructive behavior to help the client change. This approach may result in an initial behavioral change. The client is encouraged to pursue long-term change through long-term therapy.

Anger and frustration are common health care team reactions to manipulative behaviors. Open communication and consistency are essential for the staff to work together toward constructive role modeling. Early identification of manipulative behavior is essential. The nurse is often the first in identifying this behavior and mobilizing the health care team and other resources to coordinate the client's care. The nurse also plays a key role in helping the client become aware of the available long-term treatment. Major changes are rarely seen in the short term, but success can be evaluated on the basis of the health care team's offering of constructive role models and opportunity for growth.

REFERENCES AND SUGGESTED READINGS

1. American Psychiatric Association: Diagnostic and statistical manual of mental disorders (DSM-III-R), Washington, DC, 1987, The Association.
2. Bigler ED: Neuropsychology and malingering: comment on Faust, Hart, and Guilmette (1988), *Journal of Consulting and Clinical Psychology* 589(2):244, 1990.
3. Bursten B: *The manipulator: a psychoanalytic view,* New Haven, Conn, 1973, Yale University Press.
4. Cleckley H: *The mask of sanity,* St Louis, 1982, Mosby–Year Book.
5. Chitty KK, Maynard CK: Managing manipulation, *Journal of Psychosocial Nursing and Mental Health Services* 24(6):8, 1986.
6. Davidhizar R: Handling manipulation, *Health Care Supervisor* 8(3), 37, 1990.
7. Davidson GC, Neale JM: *Abnormal psychology: an experimental clinical approach,* ed 3, New York, 1982, John Wiley & Sons.
8. Faust D, Guilmette TJ: To say it's not so doesn't prove that it isn't: research on detection of malingering, *Journal of Consulting and Clinical Psychology* 58(2):248, 1990.
9. Finchy J: Nurse and mental health law: psychopaths—who are they? *Nursing Mirror* 119(4):24, 1984.
10. Groves JE: Taking care of the hateful patient, *New England Journal of Medicine* 298(16):883, 1978.
11. Hare RD: *Psychopathy: theory and research,* New York, 1970, John Wiley & Sons.
12. Hare RD, Schalling D: *Psychopathic behavior: approaches to research,* New York, 1978, John Wiley & Sons.
13. Hood M: New horizons: special units, the psychopathic patient, *Nursing Times* 81(12):53, 1985.
14. Holderby RA, McNulty EG: Feelings: how to make a rational response to emotional behavior, *Nursing 79* 9:39, 1979.
15. Hughes J: Manipulation: a negative element in care, *Journal of Advanced Nursing* 5:21, 1980.
16. Johnson GB, Werstlein PO: Reframing: a strategy to improve care of manipulative patients, *Issues in Mental Health Nursing* 11:(3):237, 1990.
17. Kumler FR: The interpersonal interpretation of manipulation. In Burd SF, Marshall MS, editors: *Some clinical approaches to psychiatric nursing,* New York, 1963, Macmillan.
18. Luetje V, Murray R: The person whose behavior is abusive. In Murray R, Huelskoether M: *Psychiatric mental health nursing: giving emotional care,* Englewood Cliffs, NJ, 1983, Prentice Hall.
19. Lyon GG: Limit setting as a therapeutic tool, *Journal of Psychiatric Nursing and Mental Health Services* 8(6):17, 1970.
20. MacMillan J, Kofued L: Sociobiology and antisocial personality: an alternative perspective, *Journal of Nervous and Mental Disease* 172:701, 1984.
21. McMorrow ME: The manipulative patient, *American Journal of Nursing* 81:1188, 1981.
22. Murphy GE, Guze SB: Setting limits: the management of the manipulative patient, *American Journal of Psychotherapy* 14:30, 1960.
23. Pasquali E and others: Mental health nursing: a holistic approach, St Louis, 1985, Mosby–Year Book.
24. Pelletier LR, Kane JJ: Strategies for handling manipulative patients, *Nursing* 19(5):82, 1989.
25. Reid WH: *The psychopath: a comprehensive study of antisocial disorders and behaviors,* New York, 1978, Brunner/Mazel.
26. Reid WH: *The treatment of antisocial syndromes,* New York, 1981, Van Nostrand Reinhold.
27. Reid WH: The antisocial personality: a review, *Hospital and Community Psychiatry* 36:831, 1985.
28. Richardson JI: The manipulative patient spells trouble, *Nursing* 11:48, 1981.
29. Ruesch J: Disturbed communication, New York, 1972, WW Norton.
30. Schultz JM, Dark SI: *Manual of psychiatric nursing care plans,* Boston, 1982, Little, Brown.
31. Self CA, Rogers RW: Coping with threats to health: effects of persuasive appeals on depressed, normal, and antisocial personalities, *Journal of Behavioral Medicine* 13(4):343, 1990.
32. Shostrom E: *Man the manipulator,* Nashville, 1967, Abingdon Press.
33. Smith RJ: *Personality and psychotherapy: a series of monographs, texts, and treatises,* New York, 1978, Academic Press.
34. Widiger TA, Frances A: Axis II personality disorders: diagnostic and treatment issues, *Hospital and Community Psychiatry* 36:619, 1985.
35. Wiley PI: Manipulation. In Zderad LT, Belchen HC, editors: *Developing behavioral concepts in nursing,* Atlanta, 1968, Southern Regional Education Board.

ANNOTATED BIBLIOGRAPHY

Davidhizar R: Handling manipulation, *Health Care Supervisor* 8(3), 37, 1990.

Davidhizar proposes that it is important for a nurse to be able to recognize manipulation and handle it to maintain an effective work relationship. She describes both manipulators and nurses susceptible to manipulation. Approaches are discussed for handling manipulation in others.

Johnson GB, Werstlein PO: Reframing: a strategy to improve care of manipulative patients, *Issues in Mental Health Nursing* 11:(3):237, 1990.

This article discusses the use of *reframing* as a means of increasing nurses' choices in their responses to manipulative patients and as a way of varying their perceptions. Reframing is a process of challenging the attitudes, values, and responses of a person to expand choices and provide improved patient care.

PART III

Therapeutic Modalities

Mental health–psychiatric difficulties may respond to a single treatment modality or a combined regimen. Part III addresses the most frequently used of these modalities. Each chapter lays a foundation for the nurse to develop strategies for maintaining mental health as well as for intervening in psychiatric illnesses. Following a general introduction, selected theoretical approaches are discussed for each treatment modality. Specific characteristics of each type of therapy are presented. In addition, the psychiatric nurse's role, goals for therapy, and qualifications for practice are described. Each chapter concludes with application of the five-step nursing process.

Part III begins with a discussion of psychotropic medications (Chapter 24) that are a vital aspect of the psychiatric nurse's responsibilities. Milieu therapy is presented in Chapter 25. Chapter 26 applies the nursing process to the community and to major community health problems, including homelessness and AIDS. Chapter 27 covers the use of crisis intervention. The focus of Chapter 28 is group therapy, one of the predominant types of therapy for clients of all age groups. Building on the foundations established in group therapy, the treatment modalities of family therapy and couples therapy are described in Chapters 29 and 30. Therapy directed toward the mental health–psychiatric nurse's role in caring for clients with eating disorders, chronic mental illnesses, dementia, and in abuse situations is presented in Chapters 31 to 34.

CHAPTER

24 Psychotropic Medications

Eleanor Gilliam Moon
Virginia Burke Karb

After studying this chapter, the student will be able to:

- Define the major categories of psychotropic medications
- Trace the historical development of psychotropic medications
- Discuss indications, usual dosage, common side effects, and nursing implications of psychotropic medications
- Describe psychotropic medication interactions with foods and other drugs
- Discuss tolerance and physical dependence
- Discuss the problem of noncompliance with medication regimens in the psychiatric client
- Identify current research findings related to psychotropic medications

A psychotropic medication is any medication that alters the mind. The major categories of psychotropic medications are the antipsychotic agents, antianxiety agents, antidepressant agents, and antimanic agents. Although these medications calm agitated, excited, and hyperactive clients, they are more than sedatives or tranquilizers, thus the term *tranquilizer* is a misnomer and is no longer used today. Antiparkinsonian medications are also discussed in this chapter because they lessen the side effects of many of the antipsychotics.

Medications can control violent, dangerous, or destructive behavior, improve the client's subjective feelings, shorten inpatient treatment time, and hasten the recovery of some clients. With medications, many clients who once required inpatient treatment can be treated at home, in the physician's office, or at the community mental health center.

As the use of psychotropic medications grows, so does the awareness that many of the agents can be abused, addictive, and attractive to those using illegal drugs. Researchers continue to look for the ideal psychotropic medications—those that alleviate symptoms, produce no side effects, have low abuse potential, do not cause dependence or addiction, are inexpensive, and do not interact with other medications.

When psychotropic medications are prescribed, the nurse checks the database to make sure that the assessment includes all the necessary baseline data. Certain laboratory tests not needed for all clients may be needed for clients receiving specific medications, for example,

pregnancy tests. Some phenothiazines (for example, Thorazine) can enter the fetal circulation and are a vital consideration for assessment. The nurse also obtains information on previous use of the prescribed agent and the client's response to it; known allergies; and other medications used by the client, especially over-the-counter prescriptions, birth control pills, and illegal drugs. The client's reliability may be an important factor when considering self-medication.

In most cases the goals of therapy are to enable the client to be responsible for self-medication and to return to the community. To achieve these, the nurse determines the following:

1. Has the client received information about the medication: name, results to expect, dosage, side-effects?

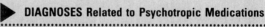

▶ DIAGNOSES Related to Psychotropic Medications

MEDICAL DIAGNOSIS	NURSING DIAGNOSES
Noncompliance with medical treatment	**NANDA**
	Noncompliance
	PMH
	Altered decision making
	Altered judgment
	Noncompliance

DATES	EVENTS
Before 1800	Before the development of psychotropic medications, psychiatric care was limited to custodial care. Clients were committed to asylums where restraint and seclusion were the only methods available to control behavior.
	In India natural products such as powdered root of *Rauwolfia serpentina*, a component of reserpine, were found effective in changing behavior.
1800s	The bromide salt of lithium was used to treat gout and used as a sedative and anticonvulsant. Its toxic effects prevented its use as a treatment for mania in the United States until early 1970.
1950s	Chlorpromazine was synthesized as an antihistamine in France by Charpentier and later was used to treat psychomotor excitement and mania.
	Clinical studies of antitubercular agents led to the discovery that isoniazid and iproniazid were effective in diminishing depression and associated symptoms in psychotic clients.
1959	Librium was introduced in the United States.
1980s	There was a changing awareness among physicians of the role of medications in psychiatric care, with emphasis on research rather than anecdotal notes. It was no longer assumed that clients must tolerate uncomfortable side effects; within limits, medications, dosages, and schedules can be altered based on the client's response. Clients were encouraged to be knowledgeable about their medications.
1990s	More objective assessment tools began to be developed and tested to help quantify and identify client behaviors and drug side effects. Nurses took an active role in the health care team by interacting with clients, assessing clients, and suggesting changes in the treatment plan.
Future	Because *noncompliance* with medication is commonly associated with psychiatric clients, nurses are challenged to identify factors that contribute to noncompliance, to predict those at risk for noncompliance, and to initiate interventions that foster compliance.

2. Are the medications having the desired effects? What data support this?

3. Are side effects occurring? If so, are they tolerable?

4. Is the plan complete and appropriate for the client?

5. How does the client feel about the effects of the medications? Are the client's expectations about the results being met?

6. If side effects cannot be eliminated, can they be controlled or treated, or can the client learn to live with them? Which ones can (or cannot) the client live with?

7. How do family members feel about the medications? Are their expectations being met?

8. How does the client feel if the medications are not effective or produce side effects requiring discontinuance of the agent(s)?

9. Is the client reliable and informed enough to be discharged for self-medication? If not, what alternative plans can be made?

10. Does the client have the finances to purchase the medications when going from inpatient to outpatient care?

11. Does the client have transportation to see the health care provider for medication checks?

General guidelines for teaching clients about psychotropic medications are found in the box on p. 482.

SPECIAL NURSING CONSIDERATIONS

Effects of Psychotropic Medications

The client's age can affect the response to psychotropic medications. In the elderly, medications that cause dry mouth (antidepressants and antipsychotics) can be particularly troublesome because saliva production decreases with age. If the client wears dentures, the potential exists for serious gum irritation. Constipation may alter medication excretion and contribute to use and sometimes abuse of laxatives and enemas, which leads to dehydration and electrolyte imbalances. As body fat increases, the action of medication stored there is lessened in intensity but is prolonged. Reduced renal function can contribute to medication toxicity at lower doses. Reduced vision and hearing may cause misunderstandings about medications and doses. Some drugs also cause blurred vision, creating a serious potential for injury.

The physiological differences and smaller body size of children affect their reactions to psychotropic medications. Cardiac output and blood flow, related to body surface area, result in faster distribution of medications. For these reasons doses for pediatric clients are often determined by ratios of milligram per kilogram of body weight or by the body surface area method.[19] Fortunately, young children seldom need psychotropic medications.

Guidelines for Teaching the Client

1. Caution the client not to "share" medications.
2. Teach the client to inform all health care providers—physicians, nurses, dentists, therapists, pharmacists, chiropractors, and midwives—of all medications being taken.
3. Caution the client that the dosage of any medication should not be decreased, increased, or discontinued without the advice of the health care provider.
4. Remind the client not to double up or catch up with missed doses unless specifically instructed to do so. If in doubt, the client should contact the health care team.
5. Remind the client to keep all medications out of the reach of children. Childproof caps should be used.
6. Instruct the client to avoid drinking alcohol. Most medications discussed in this chapter are central nervous system (CNS) depressants and *cannot* be combined with another CNS depressant.
7. Instruct the client to avoid over-the-counter drugs unless permitted by the physician. This includes cold and cough remedies, allergy medications, aspirin, acetaminophen or other pain relievers, antacids, laxatives, and vitamins.
8. Counsel female clients to use birth control while taking any of these medications because psychotropic medications are usually contraindicated during pregnancy and lactation. If a client suspects she is pregnant, instruct her to consult her physician immediately. If a client wants to become pregnant while using psychotropic medications, advise her to see her physician first.

9. Discuss common side effects with the client. Because everyone may respond differently to a medication, encourage the client to report any unusual sign, symptom, or subjective feeling.
10. Caution outpatients not to keep medicine bottles on the nightstand or in other places where there is a greater likelihood of accidental overdose or repeating a dose in the night. Instruct clients to keep medications in the labeled containers and never to mix different medications in a single container.

Reminders for the Nurse Administering Medications

1. Question the client carefully about any history of medication allergy before therapy begins.
2. Many psychotropic medications are toxic, have high abuse potential, or are frequently used in suicide attempts. Medications are often prescribed in small quantities so the client must return often to have the prescription refilled.
3. Any client may refuse or pretend to take a medication, but this can be a serious problem with psychiatric clients. Missed doses may cause the health care team to increase a dosage or switch to another medication unnecessarily. A client may be storing doses for a later suicide attempt. Carefully supervise all clients to ascertain that doses have actually been taken.
4. In an outpatient setting, be alert for clients who are returning with increased frequency for prescription refills. This may indicate that the medication is being abused or used inappropriately. Carefully assess the depressed or anxious client for suicidal tendencies.

Tolerance, Dependence, and Withdrawal

Tolerance is a state of decreased responsiveness to a medication resulting from prior exposure. It usually requires an increased dosage of the medication. When the continuously increased dosage causes the client to need the medication to maintain normal functioning, and when abrupt cessation results in the characteristic withdrawal syndrome, the condition is called *physical dependence.* Tolerance can occur without physical dependence, but physical dependence without initial tolerance is uncommon. Terms such as *need* and *craving* describe psychological dependence. Information on tolerance, dependence, and withdrawal is included in the discussion of each category of medications when appropriate (see Chapter 16).

ANTIPSYCHOTIC MEDICATIONS

Uses

The antipsychotic medications, often called *neuroleptics,* are used to treat psychoses such as schizophrenia, paranoia, major depressions, and mania. Antipsychotic medications also have antianxiety properties and frequently are prescribed for treatment of severe anxiety. Other conditions treated with antipsychotic medications are intractable hiccups, Huntington's chorea, dementia, and Tourette's syndrome (Table 24-1).

Action and Side Effects

Neuroscientists hypothesize that excessive activity of the neurotransmitter dopamine in certain areas of the CNS leads to psychosis. The antipsychotic agents are thought to block dopamine receptors. The action of antipsychotics is believed to occur in the brainstem reticular formation, which may be a site of dopamine receptor blockade. The brainstem reticular formation controls the inflow, integration, and outflow of information through the brain. For example, schizophrenic clients are extremely aware of peripheral stimuli but have difficulty sorting out their meanings. Many researchers believe that antipsychotic drugs impair the schizophrenic client's ability to respond to peripheral stimuli, while allowing him to respond to direct stimuli.

Alteration of neurotransmission in other areas of the CNS may account for other effects of antipsychotic agents. Dopamine receptor blockade probably leads to endocrine and extrapyramidal side effects. Components of the extrapyramidal system degenerate in Parkinson's disease, and a clinical picture resembling this disease often occurs in clients treated with antipsychotic agents, presumably as a result of dopamine receptor blockade in this area of the CNS. There appears to be a balance of inhibition and excitation in the extrapyramidal system. Dopamine is the transmitter for inhibition, acetylcholine for excitation. The blockade of dopamine receptors leads to an excitation that may be therapeutically diminished with agents that block acetylcholine receptors. Alteration of this balance may lead to motor dysfunction. Chronic use of antipsychotics may produce such an alteration, perhaps leading to tardive dyskinesia or other extrapyramidal side effects (Table 24-2).

The antipsychotic agents differ primarily in potency and side effects (see Table 24-1). The effectiveness of antipsychotic agents is similar; for ease of comparison, doses of

▼ TABLE 24-1 Antipsychotic Medications, Equipotent Dosages, and Side Effects

Generic and Trade Name	Equipotent Dose (mg)	Usual Adult Dose (mg)	Side Effects*			
			Sedation	Orthostatic Hypotension	Anticholinergic	Extrapyramidal†
PHENOTHIAZINES						
Aliphatic						
Chlorpromazine (Thorazine)	100	30-300 bid-qid	+ + +	+ +	+ +/+ + +	+ +
Promazine (Sparine)	200	10-200 q 4-6 hours	+ +	+ +	+ + +	+ +
Triflupromazine (Vesprin)	25	up to 40/day	+ + +	+ +	+ +/+ + +	+ +/+ + +
Piperidine						
Mesoridazine (Serentil)	50	10-50 bid-tid	+ + +	+ +	+ +	+
Thioridazine (Mellaril)	100	25-100 tid	+ + +	+ +	+ +/+ + +	+
Piperazine						
Acetophenazine (Tindal)	20	20 tid	+ +	+	+	+ + +
Fluphenazine (Prolixin)	2	1-5 qd	+/+ +	+	+	+ + +
Perphenazine (Trilafon)	8	2-16 bid-qid	+/+ +	+	+	+ + +
Prochlorperazine (Compazine)	10	5-10 tid-qid	+ +	+	+	+ + +
Trifluoperazine (Stelazine)	4	1-5 bid	+ +	+	+	+ + +
OTHERS						
Butyrophenone						
Haloperidol (Haldol)	2	0.5-5 bid-tid	+	+	+	+ + +
Thioxanthenes						
Chlorprothixine (Taractan)	100	25-50 tid-qid	+ + +	+ +/+ + +	+ +/+ + +	+/+ +
Thiothixene (Navane)	4	2-5 bid-tid	+	+/+ +	+	+ +/+ + +
Dibenzoxepine						
Loxapine (Loxitane)	10	10 bid	+ +	+/+ +	+/+ +	+ +/+ + +
Dihydroindolone						
Molindone (Moban)	10	50-75 qd	+ +	+/+ +	+ +	+ +
Carbamazepine (Tegretol)	—	50-200 qid	+	+	+	—
Clozapine (Clozaril)	—	25-450 qd-bid	+	+ +	+	+

*Relative potency in producing side effects: +, low; + + +, high.
†Excludes tardive dyskinesia, which can be produced to the same degree by all antipsychotic agents.

the medications are based on the chlorpromazine (Thorazine) equivalent—an approximation of the quantity needed to equal the therapeutic effect of 100 mg of chlorpromazine. It does not imply equivalence of adverse effects, which include the following (see also Table 24-10):

Anticholinergic effects (blurred vision, constipation, dry mouth, tachycardia)

Increased lactation in women; gynecomastia in men
Sedation
Cholestatic jaundice
Photosensitivity
Orthostatic hypotension
Allergic reactions (rashes, dermatitis)
Extrapyramidal side effects (Table 24-2)

▼ **TABLE 24-2** Extrapyramidal Side Effects of Antipsychotic Medications

Side Effect	Signs and Symptoms	Difficulties in Assessment	Comments and Treatment
Acute dystonia	Buccolingual reactions (tongue protrusion, grimacing, trismus), opisthotonos, neck twisting, spastic torticollis, abdominal wall spasm, gait abnormalities, scoliosis, lordosis, kyphosis, abnormal eye movements, *oculogyric crisis* (paroxysm of the eyes, eyes held in a fixed position for minutes to hours); may be accompanied by anxiety, tachycardia, respiratory distress, cyanosis, fever; mentation unchanged	Reactions often acute in onset; have been mistaken for tetanus, hysteria, convulsions, meningitis, stroke, strychnine poisoning	Symptoms are most common after parenteral administration in clients under 25 years of age. Symptoms rarely persist but are distressing to client and onlookers. Treatment consists of discontinuing the antipsychotic medication and administering a centrally acting anticholinergic, such as benztropine (Cogentin) or an antihistamine, such as diphenhydramine (Benadryl)
Akathisia	Restlessness, difficulty sitting still, agitation, uncontrolled pacing	May mimic dyskinesia; may be mistaken for psychotic agitation, resulting in inappropriate increases in dose of antipsychotic medication	Treatment consists of reducing the dose of antipsychotic medication and/or administering anticholinergics and/or a sedative such as diazepam (Valium) until symptoms are controlled. If adaptation occurs, antipsychotics can be administered or the dose increased to previous levels
Tardive dyskinesia	Protrusion of the tongue, puffing of the cheeks, chewing movements, involuntary movements of the extremities and trunk, choreiform movements manifested as a single muscle jerk or tic; worsens under stress	Client may try to mask movements by developing semipurposeful movements in response to jerks; poorly fitting dentures in the elderly may result in facial movements resembling tardive dyskinesia; dyskinesia disappears during sleep; tremors have a to-and-fro component, while dyskinesia does not; postures are sustained in dystonia but not in dyskinesia; in severe cases may resemble Huntington's disease	Symptoms are more common with long-term use (more than 1 year), in women, and the elderly. They may be unmasked by suddenly discontinuing medication. No treatment regimen is completely satisfactory, although symptoms *may* gradually lessen if antipsychotics are discontinued. Health care team, with client and family, weigh the potential risks of tardive dyskinesia with psychosis
Parkinsonism	Tremors, rigidity, motor retardation, excessive salivation, shuffling gait, loss of postural reflexes, masklike expression	May be difficult to differentiate between motor retardation, masklike expression, and apathy of parkinsonism and the affect of a major depression	Treatment consists of anticholinergics or amantadine (Symmetrel). Routine prophylactic use of these medications is not recommended

Absorption and Distribution

Chlorpromazine (Thorazine), the prototype of the aliphatics, is only partially absorbed from the gastrointestinal tract after oral administration. Peak plasma levels are usually reached in 2 to 4 hours. (Plasma levels are 4 to 10 times higher after intramuscular injection and are usually reached in 2 to 3 hours.) A significant proportion of the drug is degraded in the intestine, which may account for the diminished absorption when taken orally. Differences in strength, the presence of food in the gastrointestinal tract, and concomitant therapy with drugs such as antacids and antiparkinsonian agents may significantly alter its absorption.

The piperidine group of phenothiazines includes mesoridazine (Serentil) and thioridazine (Mellaril). Side effects within the group are similar (see Table 24-1). Mesoridazine is the only piperidine available in a parenteral (intramuscular) form. Five medications form the piperazine class. In addition to their antipsychotic activity, the piperazines have potent antiemetic properties. Blood dyscrasias and jaundice are less likely to occur with this group of drugs.

Fluphenazine (Prolixin) is available in two depot forms, fluphenazine decanoate and fluphenazine enanthate. The duration of action is approximately 2 weeks, although in some clients 4 weeks between doses may suffice for maintenance therapy. Depot forms are especially useful with noncompliant clients. Depot forms are administered by deep intramuscular (IM) injection in a large muscle mass; the deltoid muscle is avoided.

Haloperidol (Haldol), a butyrophenone, is readily ab-

RESEARCH HIGHLIGHT

Effects of 6 Months of Clozapine Treatment on the Quality of Life of Chronic Schizophrenic Patients

• H Meltzer, S Burnett, B Bastani, and L Ramiriz

PURPOSE

The purpose of this study was to determine the effect of Clozapine treatment on the quality of life of treatment-resistant schizophrenic patients.

SAMPLE

The sample consisted of 38 hospitalized patients who met the DSM-III-R criteria for schizophrenia. Twenty-three of the patients were male, 33 were white, 4 were black, and 1 was Asian American.

METHODOLOGY

The 38 patients began Clozapine treatment between October 1987 and September 1989. Each patient's psychopathology was assessed by the Brief Psychiatric Rating Scale (BPRS). The Quality of Life Scale (QLS) was also administered.

From *Hospital and Community Psychiatry* 41(8):892, 1990.

FINDINGS

By 6 weeks, 14 of the 38 patients (37%) showed an improvement of 20% or more on the BPRS, and by 6 months, 23 patients showed an improvement of 20% or more. An improvement in the total QLS score of 50% or more was noted for 22 of the 38 patients (57.8%). In addition, rehospitalization was dramatically decreased by Clozapine treatment, and 55% of the patients were able to work or go to school.

IMPLICATIONS

The major findings in this study are that Clozapine treatment is associated with significant improvement in the quality of life within a 6-month period. The personal benefits to patients that are apparent in the results of the study should be considered in weighing the risk- and cost-benefit aspects of Clozapine treatment.

---

sorbed when taken orally, reaching peak plasma levels in 3 hours. Peak plasma levels are reached in 1 hour after intramuscular injection. The half-life varies with the route of administration. Haloperidol decanoate is given IM once a month in a dose approximately 20 times the daily oral maintenance dose.

Chlorprothixene (Taractan) is structurally related to chlorpromazine (Thorazine), and thiothixene (Navane) is structurally related to the piperazine group of phenothiazines (see Table 24-1). Loxapine (Loxitane) and molindone (Moban) are each structurally different but produce the same pharmacological responses as the phenothiazines.

Carbamazepine (Tegretol) is an anticonvulsant that has been used to treat bipolar disorder or psychosis in selected clients (see also Table 24-6). Tegretol acts to stabilize cell membranes. The drug does not block dopamine receptors and is not known to produce extrapyramidal side effects. It may produce drowsiness, dizziness, weakness, dry mouth, photosensitivity, hypertension or hypotension, and aggravate preexisting heart disease.[47]

Clozapine (Clozaril) was released for use in the United States in 1990 and is available only through special client management programs. It is an atypical antipsychotic agent; its mechanism of action is that it binds to dopamine receptors. This drug has three serious side effects that limit its use—agranulocytosis, seizures, and respiratory depression. Clients who receive this drug must have frequent hematological monitoring. Because of the side effects, clozapine is not recommended for use until at least two other antipsychotic agents have been tried without success. In addition to seizures and agranulocytosis, side effects include tachycardia, orthostatic hypotension, fever, extrapyramidal side effects, blurred vision, insomnia, depression, and anticholinergic side effects. The usual beginning adult dose is 25-50 mg/day, in divided doses, increased gradually to a dose of 300-450 mg/day. As experience with this drug grows, new information may be available about side effects, dose, and effectiveness; consult the manufacturer's current literature before administration (see the accompanying research highlight).[7,31,43]

Acute Toxicity

Symptoms of acute toxicity may include severe extrapyramidal reactions, as well as blurred vision, hypotension, seizures, and coma. Treatment is supportive and symptomatic. It may be necessary to induce vomiting or perform gastric lavage. Saline cathartics may be prescribed. Respiratory function and cardiovascular functions are monitored. It is essential to maintain blood pressure, but avoid using epinephrine. Overdoses of antipsychotics are seldom fatal in adults. Children may have more serious reactions and are treated with immediate gastric lavage.

Medication Interactions

The antipsychotics are used cautiously with other medications that also depress the CNS, such as antianxiety agents and hypnotics, alcohol, narcotics, analgesics, preanesthetic sedatives, and general anesthetics. If possible, antipsychotics are discontinued temporarily if the client has been given a spinal or epidural anesthetic. Heavy smokers may require a larger dose of an antipsychotic. If antipsychotics are used with a tricyclic or second-generation antidepressant or an anticholinergic, there may be additional anticholinergic activity and CNS depression. Antipsychotics may interfere with the action of guanethidine (Ismelin) by inhibiting antihypertensive effects.

Dosage

Table 24-1 gives the dosage equivalent to 100 mg of chlorpromazine (Thorazine) for the antipsychotics. Dosage must be individualized based on the client's response.

Contraindications

Antipsychotics are contraindicated in children under 3 years of age, comatose clients, and clients with severe CNS depression, severe hypertensive or hypotensive heart disease, or preexisting bone marrow depression. Clients reporting hypersensitivity to a particular agent do not receive it again. Antipsychotics may alter the seizure threshold; use them cautiously in clients with a history of seizures.

Tolerance, Dependence, and Withdrawal

Some tolerance develops to the sedative, anticholinergic, and hypotensive effects of antipsychotic medications, usually after several weeks. Little or no tolerance to the antipsychotic action develops. Medication dependence does not occur, but some physiological adaptation does. Abrupt withdrawal after prolonged therapy often results in nausea, vomiting, diaphoresis, headache, restlessness, and insomnia. Withdrawal symptoms begin in 2 to 3 days and may persist for up to 2 weeks. Slowly withdrawing the antipsychotic may help.

Nursing Implications

When the psychotic client is hospitalized, treatment is generally focused on attaining an effective dosage level. The expected results are a decrease in aggressive, hyperactive behavior and disorganized thought. Observe clients carefully for potential side effects, especially when medication therapy is begun or during periods of dosage adjustment. See Table 24-9 for an outline of drug side effects and nursing interventions.

Weeks or months of treatment may be needed before optimal behavioral changes are seen. Reassure the client and family that early side effects or lack of desired effect is normal. Drowsiness is usually temporary and often diminishes in days to weeks. Teach the client to take regular naps if possible and to avoid driving and using hazardous equipment. Use side rails and a night-light with hospitalized clients.

For dry mouth suggest that clients rinse frequently with water, brush and floss regularly, suck on hard candy (sugar free), and chew sugar free gum. Some clients may wish to try commercially available saliva substitutes. Avoid lemon and glycerin swabs, which are drying and irritating. Dry mouth may contribute to denture irritation of the gums. Assess the client for dry mouth and inspect the mouth regularly. Dry mouth may diminish with time.

Blurred vision is annoying and potentially dangerous. Caution the client to report this side effect if it occurs and to avoid driving and engaging in other hazardous activities until it clears.

Instruct the client to report any difficulty with urination. This problem is more common in the immobilized, those confined to bed, and men with an enlarged prostate gland. Monitor intake and output and encourage an adequate fluid intake (at least 2500 ml/day).

Orthostatic hypotension can be serious. Clients may

RESEARCH HIGHLIGHT

Identifying Akinesia and Akathisia: The Relationship Between Patient's Self-Report and Nurse's Assessment
• RA Michaels and K Mumford

PURPOSE

This study examined the relationship between patient's self-report of drug-induced symptoms of akathisia and akinesia and the assessments of these side effects by nurses.

SAMPLE

The subjects were 52 men and 44 women between the ages of 18 and 55 with a diagnosis of chronic schizophrenia. All were patients in a community mental health center.

METHODOLOGY

Four parts of data were collected. Demographic information, including aspects of the history of the illness, was obtained. Subjects then completed the Medication Response Questionnaire (MRQ), which listed 40 adjectives describing feelings associated with taking antipsychotic medications; subjects rated the degree to which they experienced these feelings on a four-point scale. Finally, a nursing assessment was performed on the subjects, following the format of the Disability Evaluations in Chronic Schizophrenia (DECS).

Based on data from *Archives of Psychiatric Nursing* III(2):97, 1989.

FINDINGS

There was a positive correlation between subjects' self-report of akinesia and akathisia and nurses' assessment of the presence of these symptoms. The correlation was much higher for akathisia, r = 0.670, P = <0.001, than for akinesia, r = 0.287, P = <0.05. This is probably because akathisia is a much more visible side effect, manifested by such behaviors as toe-tapping and changing position.

IMPLICATIONS

Review of all the data supports the belief that the nurse should believe subjective patient reports of distress associated with neuroleptic therapy. Also, patients do not always report subjective complaints. The nurse must carefully weigh subjective and objective data in deciding nursing care approaches. Finally, fostering an ongoing therapeutic relationship with the patient, as well as providing support and education, may help in assessing side effects of neuroleptic drugs.

merely be slightly dizzy when sitting or standing up, or they may actually faint. Monitor blood pressure regularly when therapy is begun and when the dose is increased. Instruct clients to sit at the edge of the bed with their feet on the floor for a minute before trying to stand, ensure that side rails are used at night and supervise walking. Caution clients to avoid hot showers and to wear elastic support stockings. Orthostatic hypotension usually diminishes in time, but until it does, the potential for injury from falls is serious.

Weight gain can become a problem. Weigh the client before medication therapy begins and regularly during the treatment course. Supervise dietary intake, and counsel about calorie restriction if appropriate. Encourage clients to be active and get regular exercise.

Extrapyramidal reactions (Table 24-2) can often be lessened by dosage adjustments or changing drugs, but treating the side effects with additional medications may be necessary (see research highlight). *Tardive dyskinesia* is especially troublesome. It is characterized by irregular movements of the lower facial muscles, jaw, tongue, and extremities. The movements may disappear during sleep, and vary in severity. As many as 10% to 20% of clients receiving antipsychotics for more than 1 year have appreciable tardive dyskinesia. It may appear or become worse when antipsychotics are suddenly discontinued and persist after the medication is stopped. Assess clients carefully for this side

effect, and consult with the physician if clients begin to show signs of tardive dyskinesia. Because there is no effective treatment for this side effect, the health care team must determine, in consultation with the client and family, whether the current medication regimen should be changed if symptoms of tardive dyskinesia begin to appear.[58,50,51] The Abnormal Involuntary Movement Scale (AIMS) is a simple method used to determine tardive dyskinesia symptoms (see the accompanying box).

Tachycardia and electrocardiographic changes can occur. Monitor vital signs regularly and obtain a baseline electrocardiogram. Clients with preexisting heart disease are at greater risk for cardiovascular effects.

Photosensitivity has been reported with many antipsychotic agents. Caution clients to limit direct exposure to the sun and to wear a broad-brimmed hat and sunglasses and to use non-PABA sunscreen when in the sun. Occasionally, in long-term therapy the skin becomes yellowish-brown, changing later to a grayish-purple. Encourage clients and families to report skin changes or allergic reactions.

Additional side effects of antipsychotic agents include signs and symptoms of cholestatic jaundice, such as fever, right upper quadrant abdominal pain, nausea, jaundice, and diarrhea. Teach clients to report these symptoms. If jaundice is suspected, withhold the dose and notify the physician. Agranulocytosis is a rare side effect, with symptoms

▼
ABNORMAL INVOLUNTARY MOVEMENT SCALE (AIMS)

Client Identification   **Date**

Rated by

Either before or after completing the examination procedure, unobtrusively observe the client at rest (for example, in waiting room).
The chair to be used in this examination should be a hard, firm one without arms.
After observing the client, he may be rated on a scale of 0 (none), 1 (minimal), 2 (mild), 3 (moderate) and 4 (severe), according to the severity of symptoms.
Ask the client whether there is anything in his mouth (gum, candy) and if there is to remove it.
Ask client about the *current* condition of his teeth. Ask client if he wears dentures. Do teeth or dentures bother him *now?*
Ask client whether he notices any movement in mouth, face, hands or feet. If yes, ask to describe and to what extent they *currently* bother him or interfere with his activities.

[0 1 2 3 4] Have client sit in chair with hands on knees, legs slightly apart and feet flat on floor. (Look at entire body for movements while in this position.)

[0 1 2 3 4] Ask client to sit with hands hanging unsupported. If male, between legs, if female and wearing a dress, hanging over knees. (Observe hands and other body areas.)

[0 1 2 3 4] Ask client to open mouth. (Observe tongue at rest within mouth.) Do this twice.

[0 1 2 3 4] Ask client to protrude tongue. (Observe abnormalities of tongue movement.) Do this twice.

[0 1 2 3 4] Ask client to tap thumb, with each finger, as rapidly as possible for 10 to 15 seconds; separately with right hand, then with left hand. (Observe facial and leg movements.)

[0 1 2 3 4] Flex and extend client's left and right arms. (One at a time.)

[0 1 2 3 4] Ask client to stand up. (Observe in profile. Observe all body areas again, hips included.)

[0 1 2 3 4] Ask client to extend both arms outstretched in front with palms down. (Observe trunk, legs, and mouth.)

[0 1 2 3 4] Have client walk a few paces, turn, and walk back to chair. (Observe hands and gait.) Do this twice.

From Sandoz Pharmaceuticals, East Hanover, NJ 07936.

TABLE 24-3   Diluents for Antipsychotic Concentrate Forms

Medication	Coffee	Tea	Milk	Water	Acidified Tap Water	Distilled Water	Simple Syrup	Soup	Pudding	Colas	Carbonated Beverages	7-Up	Carbonated Orange Drink	Fruit Juice*	Apple Juice	Apricot Juice	Grape Juice	Grapefruit Juice	Orange Juice	Pineapple Juice	Prune Juice	Tomato Juice	Saline
Chlorpromazine	C	C	C	C			C	C	C		C			C								C	
Fluphenazine	X	X	C	C			C			X	C	C	C	C	X	C		C	C	C	C	C	C
Mesoridazine					C	C											C	C	C				
Perphenazine	X	X	C	C			C			X	C	C	C	C	X	C		C	C	C	C	C	C
Thioridazine				C	C	C								C					C	C			
Trifluoperazine	C	C	C	C			C	C	C		C			C								C	
Thiothixene			C	C							C			C								C	
Haloperidol	X	X		C				C	C	X	C			C									
Loxapine																			C	C			

*Manufacturer states compatibility with fruit juice but does not list specific juices.
C, Compatible; X, not compatible.

of sore throat, fever, and generalized weakness. Instruct clients to report these signs also. Assess clients for blurred vision, increased intraocular pressure, opacities, and photophobia. The physician may obtain baseline ophthalmic examinations before therapy and regularly during therapy. Assess tactfully and sensitively for menstrual irregularities, breast engorgement, changes in libido, and impotence.

Many of the oral concentrates will precipitate when mixed with coffee or tea. Mix these forms with juices, soups, puddings, or other diluents suggested by the manufacturer to improve the taste (Table 24-3). Many of the antipsychotics can cause a contact dermatitis if spilled on the skin. If drugs are spilled during preparation, wash the skin with copious amounts of water.

MEDICATIONS FOR EXTRAPYRAMIDAL SIDE EFFECTS

Uses

Many antipsychotic agents have extrapyramidal side effects (Table 24-2), which resemble symptoms of Parkinson's disease. Assess clients carefully and systematically for these side effects. Enlist the aid of the client in reporting side effects also; see the research highlight, earlier in this chapter, regarding client self-report of side effects. Drug-induced parkinsonism, or pseudoparkinsonism, is characterized by rigidity, akathisia, tremor, akinesia, changes in voice tone, drooling, masklike facial expression, and loss of posture control.

Anticholinergics, antihistamines, and amantadine (Symmetrel) are used to treat the side effects (Table 24-4). When medication side effects are treated with another medication, client response is hard to evaluate. Assess clients carefully for benefit and potential side effects of all medications the client is receiving.

Anticholinergics

Anticholinergics are the medications of choice to treat akathisia, acute dystonia, and parkinsonism. They are not effective against tardive dyskinesia.

The anticholinergics block secretions, depress the tone of the gastrointestinal tract, dilate pupils, paralyze the eye's ability to accommodate, increase heart rate, and counteract the toxicity of cholinergic agents. These actions result in dry mouth; blurred vision; photophobia; flushed, dry skin; increased heart rate; constipation, urinary retention; and mental confusion and excitement. The mental confusion and excitement can manifest as agitation, disorientation, delirium, paranoid reactions, or hallucinations. Anticholinergics are not given to clients with a history of closed-angle glaucoma, urinary or intestinal obstruction, or tachycardia. Anticholinergics are not used prophylactically but are given only when treatment of extrapyramidal side effects is in-

TABLE 24-4   Medications for the Treatment of Extrapyramidal Side Effects

Generic and Trade Name	Usual Daily Oral Dosage Range for Adults (mg)
ANTICHOLINERGICS	
Benztropine (Cogentin)	1-8
Biperiden (Akineton)	2-6
Procyclidine (Kemadrin)	7.5-20
Trihexyphenidyl (Artane)	1-15
ANTIHISTAMINE	
Diphenhydramine (Benadryl)	75-200
DOPAMINE-RELEASING AGENT	
Amantadine (Symmetrel)	100-200

dicated. When given IM or IV, benztropine (Cogentin) is very effective in reversing an acute dystonic reaction.

Antihistamines

Antihistamines may be used to treat extrapyramidal side effects because of their anticholinergic-type actions. Side effects of antihistamines are milder than but similar to those of the anticholinergics, but antihistamines are more likely to produce sedation. Side effects are drowsiness, dizziness, anorexia, nausea, vomiting, euphoria, hypotension, headache, weakness, and tingling of the hands. Like anticholinergics, antihistamines have no effect on tardive dyskinesia.

Antihistamines are well absorbed orally. Their action lasts 4 to 6 hours. They are metabolized to inactive compounds by the liver and kidneys. Diphenhydramine (Benadryl), given orally, IM, or IV, can be used to treat acute dystonic reactions. Antihistamines are used only when treatment of extrapyramidal side effects is needed.

Dopamine-Releasing Agent

Amantadine (Symmetrel), an antiviral drug that promotes the release of dopamine from central neurons, is used infrequently to treat extrapyramidal side effects. Studies show that it may be effective in some clients with tardive dyskinesia.

Amantadine is absorbed well orally. Because the half-life is about 12 hours, it can be given in a single daily dose. Most of the medication is excreted unchanged in the kidneys, so give it with caution to clients with renal impairment.

Side effects are mood changes, dizziness, nervousness, inability to concentrate, depression ataxia, slurred speech, insomnia, lethargy, blurred vision, dry mouth, gastrointestinal upset, and rash. Livedo reticularis (a red-blue, netlike discoloration of the skin, usually of the legs, which worsens in cold weather) is fairly common, especially in women. It may subside or continue through therapy and disappears gradually in 2 to 12 weeks after the medication is stopped. Instruct the client to elevate the legs to reduce severity. Edema of the ankles has also been noted.

Nursing Implications

Monitoring the client receiving an antipsychotic and additional medication to treat the side effects can be challenging. It is often difficult to determine if a particular behavior is related to the initial diagnosis or is a drug side effect. Furthermore, some side effects can be caused by two or more medications simultaneously. The nurse assesses clients systematically and regularly for possible side effects.

NEUROLEPTIC MALIGNANT SYNDROME

Neuroleptic malignant syndrome is a rare, sometimes fatal side effect associated with neuroleptic drug use. Estimates of the frequency of this side effect vary from 0.02% to 2.4%.[39] Symptoms are listed in the accompanying box. Other medical problems that must be ruled out include encephalitis, meningitis, severe parkinsonism, Huntington's chorea, heat stroke, lethal catatonia, malignant hyperther-

---

▼ ······
SYMPTOMS OF NEUROLEPTIC MALIGNANT SYNDROME

Some, but not all, of these symptoms are usually present.
- Elevated body temperature, otherwise unexplained
- Severe extrapyramidal effects such as:
   Muscle rigidity described as being lead-pipe-like
   Severe cogwheel rigidity
   Excessive salivation, drooling
   Flexor-extensor posturing
   Choreiform movements
   Opisthotonus
   Oculogyric crisis
   Difficulty swallowing
   Dyskinesia
- Autonomic system dysfunction manifested by signs such as:
   Hypertension (20 mm rise in diastolic pressure)
   Tachycardia (heart rate 30 beats faster than usual)
   Tachypnea (respiratory rate of 25)
   Excessive diaphoresis
   Incontinence
- Elevated serum creatinine phosphokinase levels

---

mia, and drug allergy. The syndrome may be more common in clients who are dehydrated or receiving depot drug forms.[26,30,42] If this syndrome is suspected, the nurse notifies the physician immediately. The client will require intensive care management. In addition, the nurse discontinues neuroleptics, monitors vital signs and electrocardiogram, and reduces the client's temperature. Drug therapy to treat neuroleptic malignant syndrome includes bromocriptine (Parlodel) and/or dantrolene sodium (Dantrium).

ANTIDEPRESSANT MEDICATIONS

Three major groups of medications are used to treat depression: the tricyclic antidepressants (TCAs), second-generation antidepressants, and monoamine oxidase (MAO) inhibitors.

Tricyclic and Second-Generation Antidepressants
Uses

Although depression is the main indication for the antidepressants, other uses exist such as childhood enuresis, attention deficit disorder with hyperactivity in children, and chronic pain management. Other documented uses are for the treatment of obsessive-compulsive disorder, bulimia nervosa, panic disorder with or without phobias, cocaine withdrawal, and attacks of catalepsy in narcolepsy.[6,24] Some of the newer antidepressants have been found useful in the treatment of some anxiety disorders. Fluoxetine (Prozac) is used to treat obsessive-compulsive disorder. It acts by blocking serotonin uptake, and its side effects include headache, insomnia, anxiety, and nausea. Weight loss may occur. Clomipramine (Anafranil) is also useful in the treatment of obsessive-compulsive disorder and panic attacks.

A recently released antidepressant, sertraline hydrochloride (Zoloft), is chemically different from other antidepressants. Some of its most common side effects are nausea, diarrhea, and headache. Further study is needed to determine results of long-term use.

Action and side effects

Most side effects of TCAs can be attributed to one of three classic pharmacological actions. The agents inhibit the reuptake of norepinephrine, serotonin, or both from the synapse from which they are released after stimulus, thus increasing available monoamine neurotransmitters. TCAs are potent antagonists of certain acetylcholine effects, both in the CNS and in the periphery. Furthermore, the tricyclic drugs antagonize certain central effects of histamine. The side effects of TCAs are shown in the following box.

The elderly may especially have difficulty tolerating side effects of TCAs because of preexisting bowel and bladder dysfunction and sensory deficits. Additionally, the sedating effects of the TCAs increase their risk of falls and hip fractures.[52]

The second-generation antidepressants tend to have fewer anticholinergic side effects and a faster onset of action, compared with the TCAs. Refer to Table 24-5 for a comparison of the sedating and anticholinergic effects produced by the antidepressants.

Absorption and distribution

As a class the TCAs are well absorbed after oral administration. High doses of the compounds, however, may delay their own absorption as a result of a potent anticholinergic effect, which slows gastric motility and therefore absorption from the gastrointestinal tract. TCAs are metabolized by the intestine and liver and slowly eliminated. The plasma half-lives vary from 8 hours for amoxapine (Asendin) to 30 to 60 hours for maprotiline (Ludiomil). Because of their long half-lives, any of the currently used TCAs can be administered once a day.

▼ **SIDE EFFECTS OF TCAs**

- Anticholinergic effects
   Flushing
   Dry mouth
   Blurred vision
   Constipation
- Hemodynamic effects
   Tachycardia
   Electrocardiographical changes
   Orthostatic hypotension, the most common cardiovascular problem experienced by clients[6]
- Increased potential for seizures
- Aggravation of angle-closure glaucoma
- Urinary retention
- Allergic skin reactions
- Hematological disorders
- Tremors
- Weight gain
- Photosensitivity
- Adynamic ileus
- Sedation
- Ejaculation problems
- Anxiety
- Insomnia
- Increased appetite
- Parkinsonian syndrome (with amoxapine only)
- Tardive dyskinesia (with amoxapine only)

Acute toxicity

Acute toxic reactions can occur, especially when these compounds are used by depressed clients in suicide attempts. Doses only 5 to 10 times greater than the therapeutic dose, or 1 to 2 g of the TCAs, may be toxic or fatal.[19] The potentially fatal toxic effect is essentially an anticholinergic (atropine-like) poisoning and is alleviated by physostigmine. The symptoms of toxic reactions follow:
- Confusion, delirium
- Inability to concentrate
- Hallucinations
- Fever
- Dilated pupils
- Hyperactive reflexes
- Seizures
- Coma
- Cardiac effects (tachycardia, bradycardia, dysrhythmias)

Medication interactions

TCAs interact with many medications. When TCAs are administered with barbiturates, benzodiazepines, or alcohol, CNS depression is potentiated. They also block the antihypertensive effect of guanethidine (Ismelin) and clonidine (Catapres). TCA effectiveness may be diminished if the client is a heavy smoker, or if barbiturates or carbamazepine (Tegretol) are given concurrently. When combined with MAO inhibitors, TCAs can contribute to hypertensive crisis and high fever. TCAs with anticholinergics can potentiate anticholinergic effects. With sympathomimetics, TCAs can potentiate sympathomimetic effects. The concomitant use of cimetidine (Tagamet) or ranitidine (Zantac) with TCAs may increase the plasma concentration of the TCA, resulting in toxicity. Concurrent use of fluoxetine (Prozac) with TCAs may increase side effects of the TCAs such as cardiac changes and anticholinergic responses.[54]

Dosage

Therapy generally starts with a low dosage (50 to 75 mg of amitriptyline [Elavil] per day), which is increased every 2 to 3 days by 25 mg until the usual adult dosage of 150 mg (amitriptyline equivalent) is reached. Unresponsive clients may require up to 300 mg/day or more. However, side effects, such as sedation and orthostatic hypotension, may halt dosage increase at relatively low levels (75 mg/day).

Response to TCAs usually occurs in 7 to 10 days, beginning with improved sleep, appetite, and occasionally elevated mood. However, full therapeutic response may require 3 to 4 weeks or longer. The initial treatment period is defined as the 4 to 8 weeks of therapy needed until the client becomes symptom free. Maintenance therapy may be required for 6 months to 1 year. A single dose at bedtime is usually given, especially when drowsiness or dizziness occurs during waking hours. Protriptyline (Vivactil) is an exception because it may produce nightmares or insomnia if administered late in the day. Gradual tapering of the dosage is recommended at the end of therapy. This allows the physician as much as a month to slowly reduce the dosage to 25 to 50 mg/day before discontinuing the drug entirely.

Serum plasma levels may be determined for many of the antidepressants and are drawn a minimum of 8 hours after the last dose. Therapeutic plasma ranges for some of the antidepressants are as follows: amitriptyline (Elavil) 110 to 250 mg/ml, desipramine (Norpramin) 125 to 300 mg/ml, imipramine (Tofranil) 200 to 350 mg/ml, and nortriptyline (Pamelor) 50 to 150 mg/ml.[24] Consult laboratory results for plasma levels before administering doses.

Contraindications

TCAs should be avoided during the acute recovery period after a myocardial infarction. Clients with a history of cardiovascular disorders require careful monitoring because of increased risk of dysrhythmias or heart block. Careful consideration is given to clients with a seizure disorder, since the seizure threshold may be lowered with the use of some TCAs. The use of antidepressants in some clients with bipolar disorder may produce rapid cycling between mania and depression. TCAs may have to be discontinued for these persons. Psychosis may be activated in the client with schizophrenia when TCAs are administered.

GUIDELINES FOR A TYRAMINE-RESTRICTED DIET

A high tyramine content is most commonly found in foods that are aged or fermented. An estimated 2% to 5% of clients receiving MAO inhibitors experience hypertensive reactions.[34] Ideally, the client should maintain a tyramine-restricted diet during treatment with MAO inhibitors and for at least 2 weeks after MAO inhibitors have been stopped.

Foods to Avoid

Avocados
Yogurt
Most cheeses, particularly aged or matured types
Smoked or pickled fish, poultry, or meat
Fermented sausage (bologna, pepperoni, salami, summer sausage)
Chicken or beef liver pate
Broad bean pods (fava beans)
Overripe fruit
Yeast or protein extracts (brewer's yeast, marmite)

Beverages to Avoid

Sherry   Liqueurs   Beer
Red wine   White wine
Reduced-alcohol and alcohol-free wine and beer
Large quantities of beverages containing caffeine (such as coffee, tea, cola soft drinks)

Foods to Take in Moderation

If eaten when fresh and in moderation, these are unlikely to cause serious problems:
Sour cream   Soy sauce
Cream cheese   Chocolate
Cottage cheese

Medications to Avoid

Cough medicine   Allergy remedies
Cold medications   Hay fever medications
Appetite suppressants   "Pep pills"
Sedatives   Anesthetics
Muscle relaxants   Narcotics
Contact the physician first before taking any over-the-counter or prescribed medications.

Tolerance, dependence, and withdrawal

TCAs are not addictive and seem to have low abuse potential. Abrupt cessation of treatment may produce withdrawal symptoms such as headache, GI disturbances, excitation or malaise, and vivid dreams.

Monoamine Oxidase Inhibitors
Uses

Although MAO inhibitors have been used to treat depression longer than TCAs, they are given to only a small percentage of clients. Side effects and interactions with food have limited their usefulness more than lack of effectiveness.

Action and side effects

The exact mechanism of the MAO inhibitor antidepressant effect is unknown. MAO is an enzyme involved in the metabolism of serotonin and catecholamine neurotransmitters such as epinephrine, norepinephrine, and dopamine. Reduced MAO activity increases concentration of these neurotransmitters in the CNS, which is thought to be the antidepressant mechanism. Onset of action may occur as early as 7 to 10 days, but a complete therapeutic effect may take 4 to 8 weeks.

The major side effect of the MAO inhibitors is the hypertensive crisis caused by eating foods that contain a high concentration of tyramine. Symptoms generally are high blood pressure, headache, nausea, vomiting, stiff neck, muscle twitching, chills, and diaphoresis with pallor. Cerebral hemorrhage and death may result. The nurse instructs the client and family not to eat foods that contain tyramine (see the accompanying box and Figure 24-1).

MAO inhibitors lower blood pressure and have been used as antihypertensives. Like TCAs, MAO inhibitors can cause dry mouth, constipation, urinary retention, skin rashes, hypotension and tachycardia, and increased intra-

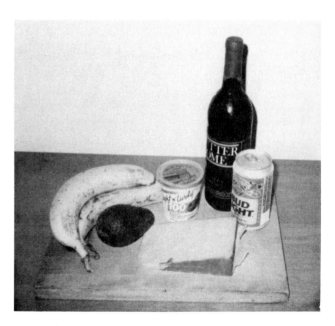

FIGURE 24-1 Foods to avoid when taking MAO inhibitors.

ocular pressure. Clients with dementias are generally not prescribed MAO inhibitors because of the difficulty memory loss poses in adhering to specific dietary and pharmacological restrictions.[52]

Absorption and distribution

MAO inhibitors are well absorbed from the gastrointestinal tract. They are metabolized in the liver and eliminated in the urine.

Acute toxicity

Symptoms of overdose may not be apparent for 12 hours after ingestion. It may take 24 to 48 hours for maximum effects to occur. Death may result from overdose. Symptoms of overdose include, but are not limited to, the following:

- Severe anxiety
- Convulsions
- Muscle stiffness
- Confusion
- Cool, clammy skin
- Slowed reflexes
- Respiratory depression or failure

Immediate hospitalization and close client monitoring following overdose is essential. Mechanical ventilation, IV diazepam (Valium), IV fluids, and a dilute pressor agent, antipyretic, and dantrolene sodium for hypermetabolic symptoms may be included in treatment of overdose.

Medication Interactions

MAO inhibitors are not combined with TCAs; sympathomimetics, including over-the-counter cough and cold preparations; alcohol; amphetamines; narcotic analgesics; barbiturates; or anesthetics. During a medication change or before surgery, MAO inhibitors are generally withheld for 10 to 14 days.

Dosage

MAO inhibitors are usually prescribed for those clients who have not responded to other antidepressants. See Table 24-5 for the usual dosage range.

Contraindications

The use of MAO inhibitors is contraindicated in active alcoholism, since CNS depression may be increased, and tyramine content in some alcoholic beverages may produce a hypertensive reaction. MAO inhibitors are not recommended for clients receiving antihypertensive medications because hypotensive effects may be more pronounced. A more severe hypertensive crisis may also occur in these clients if they fail to adhere to dietary restrictions.

Tolerance, Dependence, and Withdrawal

Withdrawal symptoms may occur and include agitation, tachycardia, headache, nausea, and possibly confusion.

▼ **TABLE 24-5** **Medications for Mood Disorders: Antidepressants and Antimanics**

Generic and Trade Names	Daily Dose (mg) Range During Initial Treatment	Sedation*	Anticholinergic Symptoms*
TRICYCLICS			
Amitriptyline (Elavil)	75-300	+ + +	+ + +
Amoxapine (Asendin)	75-300	+	+
Clomipramine (Anafranil)	25-250	+	+ +
Desipramine (Pertofrane, Norpramin)	75-200	+	+
Doxepin (Sinequan)	75-300	+ + +	+ + +
Imipramine (Tofranil)	75-300	+ +	+ +
Nortriptyline (Aventyl, Pamelor)	20-100	+ +	+
Protriptyline (Vivactil)	15-60	+	+ +
Trimipramine (Surmontil)	75-300	+ + +	+ +
SECOND GENERATION			
Bupropion (Wellbutrin)	200-450	+	+
Fluoxetine (Prozac)	20-80	+	+
Maprotiline (Ludiomil)	75-300	+ +	+ +
Trazodone (Desyrel)	75-600	+ +	+
MAO INHIBITORS			
Isocarboxazid (Marplan)	20-30		
Phenelzine (Nardil)	45-90		
Tranylcypromine (Parnate)	20-30		
ANTIMANICS			
Carbamazepine (Tegretol)	600-1600		
Lithium (Eskalith)	600-2100		

*Relative potency in producing side effects: +, low; + + +, high.

Gradual withdrawal from tranylcypromine (Parnate) is necessary to prevent reappearance of original symptoms.

Nursing Implications

Work closely with the client and family when antidepressants are prescribed. Many side effects encountered early in treatment diminish in days to weeks. As the client begins to improve, assess him for suicidal tendencies. The client who feels better may develop the emotional energy to plan suicide.

Drowsiness is usually temporary and often diminishes as the client develops tolerance to the medication. Caution against driving or operating hazardous equipment. Daily naps may be appropriate. Changing the time of medication administration to bedtime may also be possible. Keep side rails up at night, and provide a night-light. Caution the client to avoid other medications that also produce drowsiness, such as cold remedies, alcohol, sleep medications, and other prescription drugs. If blurred vision occurs, the client should report it.

Anticholinergic side effects are treated symptomatically. To relieve constipation increase daily fluid intake to at least 2500 ml, increase dietary intake of high-fiber and other foods known to stimulate defecation, and exercise regularly. Suggest that clients avoid excessive caffeine. Occasionally, especially in the elderly, adynamic ileus has been reported. Assess the client who complains of constipation or abdominal pain for bowel sounds.

Weight gain may result from an actual medication effect or an improved sense of well-being and increased appetite. A calorie-restricted diet may be needed. Teach clients about well-balanced diets, with a focus on decreasing unnecessary high-calorie food items. Encourage daily exercise.

Orthostatic hypotension can be serious because of the potential for injury. Take the client's blood pressure sitting and standing one-half hour after administering medication. Monitor blood pressure regularly during medication therapy. Tachycardia and other cardiovascular effects can occur, especially in the elderly and those with a history of cardiovascular disease. Monitor clients for changes in heart rate or rhythm.

Confusion, urinary retention, and aggravation of angle-closure glaucoma can also occur, especially in the elderly. Before therapy begins, obtain a careful history of glaucoma. Monitor fluid intake and urinary output, and instruct the client to report any difficulty urinating. If urinary retention occurs, it may be necessary to catheterize the client.

The nurse carefully assesses confusion, especially in the elderly, and does not automatically attribute it to the natural aging process. Nursing measures for the confused client include reorientation to the environment, keeping staff assignments consistent and the environment well lit, and accompanying the client when walking.

Sexual dysfunction commonly occurs with antidepressant use, resulting in delayed, inhibited, or retrograde ejaculation and impotence. The nurse is especially sensitive in assessing sexual problems, since clients are often reluctant to discuss them. Clients may stop taking their medications because of these adverse effects. In some cases, sexual problems are caused by the specific medication or dose prescribed, and a change in either or both may alleviate the problem. However, it may be necessary to help others accept this side effect. Nurses may be able to suggest other ways for the client to achieve sexual gratification. Selected clients may be referred to qualified sex therapists.

Teach clients receiving MAO inhibitors about the hazards of foods with a high tyramine content. Symptoms of tyramine-induced hypertensive crisis are severe headache, hypertension, tachycardia, palpitations, nausea and vomiting, and a stiff or sore neck. Since hypertensive crisis can be life threatening, clients need to seek medical help immediately. Phentolamine, propranolol, or parenteral chlorpromazine (Thorazine) is given to counteract the hypertension.

Changes in blood glucose level have been reported. Caution diabetic clients to monitor blood sugar carefully. A change in diet or dose of insulin may be necessary.

A variety of other side effects are rare. Unexplained bleeding or excessive bruising may be symptoms of thrombocytopenia. Jaundice, abdominal pain, or change in stool color may indicate liver dysfunction. Photosensitivity may occur. Fever, chills, malaise, and a sore throat may be symptoms of agranulocytosis and need to be reported.

Antidepressants can lower the seizure threshold; caution clients with a history of seizures about this. Fine tremor and ataxia, if they persist, may necessitate a change in medication or dosage. A variety of other side effects may also occur, including anxiety, restlessness, hypomania, and psychotic behavior. If any unexpected behavior appears, notify the physician, who may change the medication or dosage. See Table 24-9 for a summary of side effects and related nursing interventions.

ANTIMANIC MEDICATIONS

Uses

Lithium is the medication of choice to treat mania and bipolar disorders. Approximately 80% of clients treated with lithium respond. When lithium is ineffective, carbamazepine (Tegretol) may be used (Table 24-5).

Lithium
Action and side effects

Lithium abolishes the excitement, euphoria, and insomnia of mania without causing sedation. It produces many neurochemical changes in the CNS, which may be related to its interaction with the distribution of sodium and potassium across the cell membrane. Unlike other psychotropic medications, side effects are closely associated with serum levels. The nurse should monitor serum levels frequently at first, monthly once the maintenance dose is reached, and finally quarterly. Table 24-6 lists the side effects common at various serum levels of lithium. In prolonged treatment the side effects listed in the box on p. 494 may occur.

Lithium is excreted in the kidney and may produce irreversible renal changes. Therefore it is used cautiously in clients with compromised kidney function, in those requiring fluid restrictions, and in the elderly. Clients who have sodium deficiency or who are receiving diuretics may be predisposed to lithium toxicity. Use lithium cautiously

▼ **TABLE 24-6**   Serum Lithium Levels and Side Effects

Blood Level (mEq/L)	Symptoms
Below 1.5	Nausea
	Dry mouth
	Malaise
	Fine hand tremor
	Increased thirst
	Polyuria (increased urination)
1.5-2.0	Drowsiness, lethargy
	Vomiting, diarrhea
	Abdominal pain
	Lethargy
	Dizziness
	Slurred speech
	Confusion
	Ataxia
2-2.5	Anorexia
	Persistent nausea and vomiting
	Blurred vision
	Fasciculations (muscle twitching)
2.5-3.0	Choreiform and athetoid movements
	Urinary and fecal incontinence
	Myoclonic twitches or movements of an entire limb
Above 3.0	Generalized convulsions (seizures)
	Cardiac arrhythmias
	Hypotension
	Peripheral vascular collapse
	Death

▼ **SIDE EFFECTS OF LITHIUM**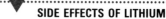

Thyroid enlargement or hypothyroidism
Polyuria
Polydipsia
Transient hyperglycemia
Headache
Peripheral edema
Weight gain
Hair loss
Metallic taste
Rashes, skin reactions
Increases in white blood cell count
Electrocardiographic changes

in clients with cardiovascular or renal disease, the dehydrated, or those receiving diuretics.

Absorption and distribution

Lithium is readily absorbed from the entire gastrointestinal tract, with plasma levels reaching a maximum in 1 to 3 hours. The compound is excreted by the kidneys and has a half-life of 17 to 36 hours in normal sodium concentrations. When plasma sodium levels are low, lithium is less effectively cleared from the body, and toxic reactions can result. Therapeutically effective plasma levels of lithium lie between 0.6 and 1.2 mEq/L of plasma but can be as low as 0.2 mEq/L in the elderly. Serious toxicity can result from plasma levels above 2 mEq/L.

Tremor and nausea have been associated with the rapid absorption of lithium. Absorption can be slowed by using a sustained-release formula, which produces peak plasma levels in 4 to 6 hours, compared with 1 to 2 hours for the regular formula.

Medication interactions

Avoid concurrent use of lithium and iodine. Caution clients to avoid preparations containing iodides (such as cough medicines and multivitamins). Indomethacin (Indocin) and phenylbutazone elevate serum lithium levels. It is important to observe for changes in serum lithium levels when these or other nonsteroidal antiinflammatory medications are given with lithium.

Acute toxicity

Lithium poisoning has no specific antidote. When frank toxic reactions occur or plasma levels exceed 2 mEq/L, the medication is discontinued and fluid and electrolyte replacement initiated.

Dosage

Lithium dosage is guided by plasma levels. During initiation of lithium therapy in an acute manic episode, dosage is usually aimed at a plasma level near 1.2 mEq/L, which generally requires 600 to 1800 mg of lithium carbonate per day. Maintenance dosage is usually lowered to 900 to 1200 mg per day to obtain plasma levels of 0.5 to 1.3 mEq/L 8 to 12 hours after the last dose. Clients occasionally cannot tolerate this amount and are maintained on lower dosages. Because of coexisting illnesses, not all clients are candidates for lithium therapy. A "prelithium workup" establishes normal parameters to monitor during therapy (Table 24-7).

Contraindications

Lithium is used with caution in pregnant or lactating women. Since congenital abnormalities can result from the use of lithium, it is generally avoided at least during the first trimester. Lithium is excreted in breast milk, so women are not encouraged to breast-feed. Some clients develop hypothyroidism while on lithium; thyroid studies are monitored before the start of therapy and periodically while therapy is continued. Renal damage and/or diabetes insipidus may also develop. See Table 24-7 for the prelithium workup.

Nursing implications

Ten days to several weeks may be needed to obtain a serum level between 0.6 and 1.2 mEq/L. Gastrointestinal irritation, tremors, muscle weakness, tinnitus, vertigo, weight gain, thirst, and polyuria may occur. Many clients develop tolerance and may be symptom free within a week. Stress to the client and family the importance of returning to have serum levels measured, and explain the signs of lithium toxicity (see Table 24-6). Teach clients that it is the persistent blood level of the lithium that produces the desired result and that they must continue to take the lithium as prescribed even when they feel better. Also, emphasize the importance of not doubling up for missed doses, which may cause the client to experience a toxic drug level.

Weigh clients before therapy. Excessive weight gain or edematous swelling of wrists and ankles can occur. Teach the client to keep a weekly weight record. Assess for edema, and, if necessary, measure the client's wrists and ankles regularly. Monitor blood pressure regularly. If weight gain is excessive or troublesome to the client, and it is not due to fluid retention, teach the client about a calorie-restricted diet, and encourage daily exercise. Counsel as needed about the health risks of weight gain.

Lithium is not contraindicated in diabetic clients, but it may increase the serum insulin level. The drug may also cause polydipsia and polyuria. Monitor the blood glucose levels and serum electrolyte levels to help avoid additional problems. Monitor intake and output as needed.

Lithium may reach toxic levels in the kidney in the presence of dehydration or electrolyte depletion. Instruct the client to seek medical attention for prolonged diarrhea or vomiting and to avoid activities that cause excessive sweating. Stress the importance of an adequate fluid intake (approximately 2500 ml/day). Assess for signs of altered kidney function: fluid retention, unexplained weight gain, new signs of lithium toxicity, polyuria, or nocturia. Monitor weight, intake and output, serum electrolytes, urinalysis, blood urea nitrogen, creatinine clearance, and blood pressure.

Some clients find persistent hand tremors embarrassing. Suggest that the client decrease caffeine consumption or, on physician's approval, take most of the daily lithium dose at bedtime or reduce the dose slightly.

Metallic taste may be a nuisance but is not serious. Taking lithium with meals may lessen nausea (ideally, clients take their dose(s) at approximately the same time each day).

Lithium is available from several manufacturers and has several similar-sounding brand names. Sustained-release and liquid forms cannot be substituted for regular oral forms without the physician's approval and dosage adjustment. Teach clients to take only the lithium preparation prescribed.

▼ **TABLE 24-7** **Prelithium Workup**

Sample	Specific Test
Blood	Hemoglobin
	White blood cell differential
	Serum electrolytes
	Serum calcium and phosphate
	Blood urea nitrogen (BUN)
	Creatinine
	Thyroid function (serum thyroxine, thyroid stimulating hormone)
Urine	Complete urinalysis
Other	Electrocardiogram
	Weight
	Blood pressure
	Pregnancy (when in doubt)

Carbamazepine

As noted in Table 24-5, carbamazepine (Tegretol) is an anticonvulsant that may be effective in clients unable to take lithium. Lithium remains the drug of choice for bipolar disorder.

ANTIANXIETY MEDICATIONS

Antianxiety medications are widely used to reduce anxiety. The major category of antianxiety agents is the benzodiazepines. Three nonbenzodiazepines, buspirone (BuSpar), hydroxyzine (Atarax), and meprobamate (Equanil), are also used.

Uses

Antianxiety, or anxiolytic, medications are used primarily to diminish anxiety. Benzodiazepines are also used in acute alcohol withdrawal and impending delirium tremens. In larger doses benzodiazepines produce sedation and are potent anticonvulsant agents. Flurazepam (Dalmane) is one benzodiazepine used solely to induce sleep and not to treat anxiety. Other benzodiazepines, temazepam (Restoril), triazolam (Halcion), and quazepam (Doral) are also preferred hypnotics in the management of insomnia. First marketed in the United States in 1990 as a long-acting benzodiazepine sedative-hypnotic, quazepam is used for the treatment of insomnia associated with difficulty falling asleep, frequent nighttime awakening, or early morning awakening. Intravenous diazepam (Valium) is the drug of choice to treat status epilepticus. The benzodiazepine anticonvulsant clonazepam (Klonopin) is used in the management of panic disorder. Benzodiazepines are also used as muscle relaxants and as a light preoperative anesthetic. The effectiveness of benzodiazepines to manage anxiety long-term (greater than 4 months) has not been evaluated.[2]

Benzodiazepines
Action and side effects

In general benzodiazepines act as CNS depressants. They are believed to enhance or facilitate the inhibitory neurotransmitter action of gamma-aminobutyric acid (GABA), which mediates both presynaptic and postsynaptic inhibition in all areas of the CNS. Since GABA is inhibitory, receptor stimulation increases inhibition and blocks both cortical and limbic arousal. The most comon side effects are listed in the accompanying box.

▼ **SIDE EFFECTS OF BENZODIAZEPINES**

Sedation	Tremor
Hangover	Urinary incontinence
Ataxia	Constipation
Dizziness	Fatigue
Blurred vision	Dysarthria
Diplopia	Muscle weakness
Hypotension	Dry mouth
Amnesia	Nausea
Slurred speech	Vomiting

The benzodiazepines are capable of producing a range of CNS depression from mild sedation to coma. They have minimal effect on the autonomic nervous system, the cardiovascular system, or respirations in normal doses. Respiratory distress, apnea, and cardiac arrest have been reported but usually only after intravenous administration. Only three benzodiazepines have parenteral forms: chlordiazepoxide (Librium), diazepam (Valium), and lorazepam (Ativan).

The elderly are likely to experience side effects more profoundly because they metabolize the benzodiazepines less readily, causing the drug to remain in the body two to three times longer. The drug dose is usually reduced for the elderly and those with liver disease.[19,38]

The benzodiazepines are preferred as antianxiety agents over the barbiturates or meprobamate because they have lower abuse potential, are less sedating, and are less toxic in acute overdose. No one benzodiazepine is more effective than another in adequate dosage. Pharmacokinetic differences may be more important in deciding the drug of choice. All benzodiazepines are controlled substances and are schedule IV drugs.

Absorption and distribution

All benzodiazepines except prazepam (Centrax) and oxazepam (Serax) are absorbed rapidly when given orally, reaching peak plasma concentration in 1 to 3 hours. Prazepam and oxazepam are slower in reaching peak plasma concentration; prazepam, the slowest, requires up to 6 hours. Lorazepam (Ativan) is the only benzodiazepine absorbed rapidly and completely after intramuscular injection.[19] Elimination half-lives of benzodiazepines and their metabolites vary widely from client to client. Most benzodiazepines have prolonged duration of effects and are slowly eliminated.

Benzodiazepines are absorbed well from the gastrointestinal tract and are widely distributed into body tissue. They cross the blood-brain barrier and are highly bound to plasma protein. Since protein binding is reduced in clients with cirrhosis and renal insufficiency, these clients require a reduced dosage.[19]

Benzodiazepines are transformed in the liver. Rates and patterns vary considerably among healthy and sick clients. Some benzodiazepines are broken down to two or more active metabolites. When metabolites are active, biotransformation extends the half-life (Table 24-8). Benzodiazepines accumulate until a steady state is reached in days to weeks. Clients receiving long-term therapy are evaluated carefully for weeks after therapy is begun because medications with long half-lives may accumulate excessively.

Lorazepam (Ativan) or oxazepam (Serax) ar preferred to treat symptoms of anxiety or insomnia in the geriatric client and the client with liver disease. These drugs have relatively short elimination half-lives and active metabolites are nonexistent.

Acute toxicity

Pure benzodiazepine overdosage is nonlethal in most clients. However, the combination of benzodiazepines with other CNS depressants, particularly alcohol, often produces a hazardous CNS depression.

Medication interactions

Additive sedation may occur when benzodiazepines are given with other CNS depressants, including other antianxiety or hypnotic medications, alcohol, tricyclic antidepressants (TCAs), narcotic analgesics, antipsychotics, antihistamines, and over-the-counter sleep and cold medications. Benzodiazepines are given carefully with cimetidine (Tagamet) or disulfiram (Antabuse) because these drugs may

▼ **TABLE 24-8**   Antianxiety Medication, Dosages, and Half-lives

Generic and Trade Name	Usual Daily Oral Dosage Range (mg) for Adults		Average or Range (hr) of Parent Compound Half-life
	Antianxiety	Hypnotic	
BENZODIAZEPINES			
Alprazolam (Xanax)	0.5-4	—	12-15
Chlordiazepoxide (Librium)	10-100	—	10
Clonazepam (Klonopine)	1.5-20	—	18-50
Clorazepate (Tranxene)	7.5-60	—	—
Diazepam (Valium)	2-30	—	20-70
Flurazepam (Dalmane)	—	15-30	—
Halazepam (Paxipam)	20-120	—	14
Lorazepam (Ativan)	0.5-9	1-4	10-20
Oxazepam (Serax)	30-120	—	5-15
Prazepam (Centrax)	10-60	—	—
Quazepam (Doral)	—	7.5-15	39
Temazepam (Restoril)	—	15-30	10-12
Triazolam (Halcion)	—	0.25-0.5	2-6
NONBENZODIAZEPINES			
Buspirone (BuSpar)	15-60	—	2-3
Hydroxyzine (Atarax)	75-400	—	3
Meprobamate (Equanil)	1200-1600	—	10-24

reduce benzodiazepine clearance and therefore prolong half-lives, resulting in drug accumulation. Cigarette smoking may decrease the sedative effects of benzodiazepines.

Use caution in administering benzodiazepines to clients with Parkinson's disease receiving levodopa because some clients, when given chlordiazepoxide (Librium) or diazepam (Valium), have experienced a reduction in the control of parkinsonism symptoms. Diazepam (Valium) half-life may change when it is administered with isoniazid (Laniazid), rifampin (Rifadin), low-dose estrogen-containing oral contraceptives, or valproic acid (Depakene).

Dosage

Because anxiety symptoms are episodic and fluctuating, dosage is often titrated to the severity of symptoms. Benzodiazepine dosage, tailored to the individual, rarely exceeds 30 mg per day of diazepam (Valium) or its equivalent. Treatment is usually begun at a low level and carefully titrated upward until the desired effect (client's ability to cope and reduction of avoidance behavior) is obtained.

Contraindications

The use of benzodiazepines is contraindicated in clients with angle-closure glaucoma because of the anticholinergic effects. Clients with myasthenia gravis may experience an exacerbation of symptoms with benzodiazepine use. Paradoxical reactions may occur in psychotic clients. Benzodiazepines are contraindicated in clients with severe chronic obstructive pulmonary disease and organic brain disease. Clients with impaired renal or hepatic function require careful monitoring because drug elimination may be prolonged.

Tolerance, dependence, and withdrawal

Tolerance may develop during long-term therapy, manifested as decreased side effects or a need to increase the dose to induce sleep or maintain clinical benefits. Benzodiazepines are now recognized as being capable of producing drug dependence. Alcohol combined with sedative-hypnotic drugs or antianxiety drugs is the most common pattern of drug abuse.[19]

To avoid a withdrawal syndrome, treatment with benzodiazepines should not be abruptly discontinued. Minor withdrawal symptoms are anxiety, apprehension, insomnia, dizziness, and anorexia. Because these are also the common symptoms of anxiety, it is difficult to decide clinically whether they are signs of withdrawal or a recurrence of the previous disorder as a result of premature termination of therapy. If therapy has lasted less than 1 month at the traditional therapeutic dosage, physical dependence is unlikely. If higher doses have been given for longer periods, the benzodiazepine is gradually withdrawn over 1 to 2 weeks to eliminate the possibility of a withdrawal syndrome.

Signs of a more severe physical dependence are those already described plus (in order of severity) nausea, vomiting, muscle weakness, tremor, postural hypotension, hyperthermia, muscle twitches, convulsions, and confusion or psychoses.

The antianxiety medications in general serve as strong reinforcing agents, and many anxious clients become psychologically dependent on them. This dependence may range from enjoying the effects to centering one's life-style on the use of the medication. It becomes difficult for the physician to distinguish between psychological dependence and the need for extended therapy. As psychological dependence intensifies, the drive to obtain the medication increases, and tolerance is therefore likely.

As noted earlier, quazepam (Doral) is a recently developed drug, and its safety and effectiveness in clients under 18 has not been established. Its use in pregnancy and for nursing mothers is contraindicated because it may cause fetal damage, and it is excreted in breast milk. Cimetidine (Tagamet) may slow the metabolism of quazepam, causing its effects to be extended. More common side effects include daytime sedation and headache. Other side effects are dizziness, fatigue, and dry mouth.

Nursing implications

Antianxiety medications are useful for temporary relief of symptoms associated with anxiety. They are not considered to be a cure for anxiety. Hence it is important for the nurse to teach the client other ways of coping with anxiety (see Chapter 10).

Caution clients against the use of alcohol and other drugs that may produce CNS depression while taking these medications. Warn clients to consult their physician before making any changes in their medication dose or frequency. Advise client to avoid driving and operating dangerous equipment if drowsiness occurs. Make clients aware of the importance of keeping drugs out of the reach of children and not sharing medication with others.

Provide side rails and assist with ambulation, especially with the elderly. Monitor vital signs and liver and renal function tests.

Meprobamate

Meprobamate (Equanil) was the first widely prescribed antianxiety drug. It is less potent than the benzodiazepines, and long-term use of large doses produces dependence, limiting its usefulness. Withdrawal symptoms range from insomnia and anxiety to hallucinations and seizures. It does not break down in the liver to significant major metabolites.

Hydroxyzine

Hydroxyzine (Atarax, Vistaril), an antihistamine with sedative and antiemetic properties, is less effective than benzodiazepines in treating anxiety, but since it is not a controlled substance, it is suitable for selected clients. Side effects are uncommon; drowsiness is transient; and fatal overdose is rare. Withdrawal reactions have not been reported.

Buspirone (BuSpar)

Buspirone is not a benzodiazepine and produces fewer and less severe adverse CNS effects than the benzodiazepines and barbiturates.[19] It possesses little abuse or dependence potential. When compared with other anxiolytics, onset of action is slower with buspirone, and a decrease in symptoms takes 1 to 2 weeks. This needs to be included in client teaching to minimize clients' discouragement. Bus-

▼ **TABLE 24-9** **Common Side Effects and Suggested Nursing Interventions for Psychotropic Medications**

Side Effect	Group of Drugs	Nursing Interventions
ANTICHOLINERGIC		
Dry mouth	AP TCA MAOI APARK	Offer to give the client frequent sips of water or other beverages; because weight gain is often a problem, low-calorie beverages are preferred. Suggest that the client suck on hard candy or mints or chew gum; again, low-calorie or sugarless forms are preferred. Frequent toothbrushing or rinsing the mouth with a pleasant mouthwash or other solution may help eliminate a bad taste in the mouth. Commercially prepared saliva substitutes are available; consult a pharmacist.
Constipation	AP TCA MAOI APARK	Monitor and record the frequency of bowel movements. Encourage the client to increase the dietary intake of bran, fresh fruits, prunes, or other foods known by the client to stimulate defecation. Have the client increase fluid intake to 2500 to 3000 ml per day if not contraindicated by other medication conditions. Encourage the client to increase his level or activity by walking or engaging in other forms of exercise. Consult with the physician about prescribing stool softeners or bulk-forming agents if above measures are not appropriate in individual clients.
Blurred vision	AP TCA MAOI APARK	Caution the client to avoid driving or operating hazardous equipment until the blurring clears. If blurred vision persists, notify physician, since it may indicate a need to change drugs or reduce dosages. Persistent or suddenly occurring blurred vision may also indicate a need for the client to see an ophthalmologist.
Urinary retention	AP TCA	Although this side effect is possible at any age, it is usually more of a problem in the elderly, the immobilized, and in men with enlarged prostate glands. Monitor intake and output. Assess client for difficulty voiding, subjective complaints of incomplete bladder emptying. Notify physician if retention is suspected; catheterization may be necessary. Suggest that the client void before taking ordered doses of medication. Teach the client to notify the health care provider if retention is suspected.
Diaphoresis	TCA	Maintain adequate fluid intake (usually over 2500 to 3000 ml/day). Assess for electrolyte imbalance and monitor serum electrolytes.
ENDOCRINE AND METABOLIC		
Weight gain	AP TCA MAOI	Weigh the client weekly; instruct the client to monitor and record weight at home on a weekly basis. Provide dietary instruction about nutritious but low-calorie meal planning. Assist in the development of a regular exercise program.
Hyperglycemia and hypoglycemia	TCA AP	Monitor blood sugar carefully and frequently in diabetic clients. Consult physician about modifications in prescribed diet, insulin dose, or dose of oral hypoglycemic agent as necessary.
Increased or decreased libido; changes in ability to ejaculate or maintain erection	AP TCA LI	It may not be possible to eliminate these side effects. If they occur, provide emotional support to client and spouse as appropriate. These side effects may contribute to poor medication compliance if the client views them as severe problems. Altering the drug dose or switching medications may be helpful; consult the physician.
Menstrual irregularities	AP	Refer women for gynecological exam if appropriate. Advise the use of birth control measures to avoid unwanted pregnancy.
Gastric irritation	TCA LI	Alter the prescribed times for taking doses to coincide with meals. Decrease the size of the dose and administer more frequently. Change the medication form (for example, switch to liquid from tablets).
NEUROLOGICAL		
Drowsiness and sedation	AP TCA MAOI APARK	Caution the client to avoid driving or other dangerous activities requiring mental alertness until the degree of drowsiness can be evaluated. With some medications or with some clients drowsiness may be a desirable effect. Daytime drowsiness, especially with antidepressants, may indicate the need to increase the nighttime dose or give the entire day's dosage at bedtime. Persistent drowsiness may indicate the need to change the medication or dose; this requires careful clinical judgment. Drowsiness may lessen with time. Encourage the client to continue the medication for several weeks at least.

AP, Antipsychotic agents; *TCA,* tricyclic and second generation agents; *MAOI,* monoamine oxidase inhibitors; *APARK,* antiparkinsonian agents; *LI,* lithium.

▼ **TABLE 24-9** Common Side Effects and Suggested Nursing Interventions for Psychotropic Medications—cont'd

Side Effects	Group of Drugs	Nursing Interventions
CARDIOVASCULAR		
Orthostatic hypotension	AP	Instruct the client to rise slowly from a lying to a sitting or standing position.
	TCA	Keep side rails up for hospitalized clients. Suggest they call for assistance when getting up
	MAOI	until they have learned to manage the problem.
	APARK	Elastic stockings may be helpful.
		Instruct the client to avoid hot showers or baths, since they may cause vasodilation and aggravate the problem.
		Monitor the blood pressure when drug therapy is started and during periods of dosage adjustment.
Tachycardia	TCA	Monitor the pulse two to four times daily until stable.
	APARK	Withhold the dose if the resting pulse before a dose is 120 or greater (or follow institutional policy regarding this).
	LI	If appropriate, teach the client to record the pulse regularly at home.
		Instruct the client to avoid excessive caffeine intake.

pirone is metabolized in the liver and excreted in the urine. Therefore it is used with caution in clients who have impaired hepatic function. Because of a possible increase in blood pressure, the concomitant use of buspirone with an MAO inhibitor is currently not recommended. Additionally, it is suggested that at least 10 days elapse between therapy with an MAO inhibitor and buspirone. Increased serum levels of haloperidol (Haldol) may result when given with buspirone. The simultaneous use of these drugs is currently not recommended. See Table 24-9 for a review of common side effects and nursing interventions for psychotropic medications.

NONCOMPLIANCE

Noncompliance is a client's failure to carry out a prescribed health care plan. NANDA's defining characteristics are listed in the accompanying box. A corresponding diagnosis in the DSM-III-R is noncompliance with medical treatment. The diagnosis is made, according to the DSM-III-R, when a client fails to follow a prescribed diet because of religious beliefs or makes decisions about the advantages and disadvantages of the proposed treatment based on personal value judgments or denial of illness.[4]

Readmission commonly results from medication noncompliance, particularly for schizophrenic clients who do not understand that they are sick and who cease taking medication when it is needed most. According to figures cited by Collins-Colon (1990),[20] 80% to 90% of discharged psychiatric clients are placed on medication. Additionally, it is estimated that over 50% of clients diagnosed with schizophrenia relapse in the first year, and that two years after hospitalization close to 70% relapse.[52] Although relapse may occur in clients who are compliant with their medication regimen, maintenance of neuroleptic treatment is the most significant variable in decreasing relapse rates for schizophrenia clients.[51] Also, many chronically mentally ill (CMI) clients now live in the community, making medication self-management important in reducing repeated episodes of acute psychiatric illness and rehospitalization.

▼ **NONCOMPLIANCE**

DEFINITION

The state in which an individual who has expressed the desire and intent to adhere to a therapeutic recommendation does not adhere to the recommendation.

DEFINING CHARACTERISTICS

- **Physical dimension**

  Display of noncompliant behavior

  Evidence of development of complications

  Evidence of exacerbation of symptoms

  Failure to keep appointments or follow through on referrals

  Failure to progress or achieve therapeutic goals

  Experiencing side effects from therapy

  Distance or lack of transportation

- **Intellectual dimension**

  Statements by client or significant others describing noncompliant behavior

  Objective tests indicating noncompliant behavior (physiological measures or detection of markers)

  Perception that the costs outweigh the benefits of the therapeutic recommendation

  Knowledge deficit

- **Social dimension**

  Nonsupportive family

  Unsatisfactory relationship with caregiver

  Lack of confidence in professional and technical capabilities of health care providers

- **Spiritual dimension**

  Incongruence between the therapeutic recommendation and the client's personal value system

  Conflicts with general health motivations, cultural influences, or spiritual beliefs

Modified from McFarland G, McFarlane E: *Nursing diagnosis and intervention: planning for patient care,* ed 2, St. Louis, 1993, Mosby–Year Book.

Consequently, medication compliance is an important issue for the nurse.

Davidhizar and McBride[22] cite the following errors in medication adherence for outpatients:

1. Errors in administration
2. Omitting medication
3. Stopping medication
4. Self-adjustment of dosage

The following case example illustrates the characteristics of the nursing diagnosis of noncompliance.

▼ Case Example

Donald, a physician, was found at age 46 to have bipolar disorder. Over the years his increasingly prolonged and pronounced periods of mania caused his family to urge him to seek psychiatric care. He was hospitalized, and therapy included lithium titrated to the desired serum level. The lithium produced a pronounced change in behavior, which Donald stated was subjectively more pleasant. He was discharged. When he returned for an appointment in 3 weeks, serum lithium levels were significantly lower than expected. He said that the fine hand tremor caused by the lithium made him appear old; he felt people would not have confidence in a physician "whose hands tremble all the time." He also felt that as a physician he should be "strong enough to handle this illness without medications," and that "people shouldn't come to rely on drugs for well-being."

The following factors may be used to predict with minimal reliability whether a client will adhere to a medication regimen:

1. Chronic illness
2. Symptom suppression (as opposed to curative action) by the medication
3. Delayed relapse with cessation of the medication
4. Ambivalent feelings toward dependence issues
5. Need for multiple medications
6. Social isolation

NURSING IMPLICATIONS

Many clients treated with psychotropic medications are ambivalent about medication. They may associate these medications with illegal drug use or be suspicious about taking any prescribed medication. Following are other variables that influence client compliance:

1. Lack of understanding of diagnosis and treatment
2. Denial of illness
3. Fear of experiencing or actually experiencing side effects of medication
4. Fear of dependence on medication
5. Desire to remain ill to receive secondary gains
6. Feeling a loss of control over body
7. Negative relationship with health care team
8. Lack of family support
9. Cost
10. Complicated medication regimen

The nurse asks the following questions to prepare the client for discharge and self-management[14]:

1. What physiological dysfunction does the client appear to have that may interfere with carrying out the treatment regimen?
2. What beliefs does the client have about the illness or effectiveness of treatment?
3. Does the client have medication-induced side effects that make compliance difficult?
4. Does the regimen make compliance difficult?
5. Does the client have the necessary knowledge to carry out the regimen?
6. Does the client have the necessary skills to carry out the regimen?
7. Does the client's social support system or daily routine interfere with compliance?

One criterion for discharge is the client's ability to deal with activities of daily living. The client needs to be able and willing to adhere to the medication regimen. It is acknowledged that no single intervention is adequate to improve medication compliance but that a combination of interventions is necessary to improve long-term compliance.[35] Medication education is one way to increase clients' knowledge and skill regarding medication management and to encourage client participation in treatment.[20] Necessary information needed by clients includes the name, color, and kind of medication, symptoms it will help control, dosage, and time for administration, major side effects, and possible effects of discontinuing the medication.[22] In addition, the nurse helps the client to develop a plan for obtaining and maintaining a supply of the medication, how to remember to take it, and what to do if symptoms develop that may be medication related.[22] There is evidence that providing both written and verbal instructions may be most beneficial. Medication cards (see the accompanying box) are helpful, and group teaching sessions may also be appropriate.

Strategies that may enhance teaching effectiveness include providing small amounts of information throughout the course of hospitalization, frequently reviewing and reinforcing prior information, teaching by someone who is trusted by the client, and tailoring strategies based on the client's symptoms and cognitive functioning.[22] The use of

▼ SAMPLE MEDICATION CARD

Your medication is *Elavil*. Your dosage is *75 mg three times each day with meals.*

Action

This medication will increase your energy level and decrease your depressed feeling.

Effects and Precautions

1. You may experience drowsiness, blurred vision, dry mouth, and constipation while taking this medication.
2. It may take 2 to 3 weeks before you begin to feel less depressed. It is essential that you continue taking the medicine even though you do not feel any benefits.
3. Do not use alcohol while taking this medicine because of possible serious interaction of your medication with the alcohol.
4. Do not use any over-the-counter medications without informing your physician.
5. Do not drive a car until you are sure the medicine does not make you drowsy.
6. Notify your physician if you are constipated or have difficulty passing urine. Use a stool softener (Colace) and eat a diet high in fiber.
7. Do not change the dosage of your medicine without informing your physician, and do not give the medicine to anyone else.

RESEARCH HIGHLIGHT

Invitation to Compliance: The Prolixin Brunch

• T Cassino, L Apellman, J Heiman, J Shupe, and H Sklebar

PURPOSE

This study was designed to investigate the effect of a reward system on medication compliance.

SAMPLE

Subjects were 35 clients (27 males and 8 females) in an Intensive Community Support Program. All were described as chronically mentally ill, with 33 having a diagnosis of schizophrenia and 2 with a major affective disorder. All were receiving Prolixin Decanoate IM, usually on a schedule of once every other week.

METHODOLOGY

Subjects were previously assigned to a Tuesday time of drug administration, or a Thursday time, and they remained in these groups. For 9 weeks, compliance was noted. Compliance was defined as appearing for the injection within the 1-hour time slot scheduled for the patient; noncompliance was defined as failure to show up, wrong day, or incorrect time. After the first 9 weeks, a snack was provided during the hour scheduled for the patients. The Tuesday morning group received a breakfast-type snack (for example eggs, donuts, and juice) and the Thursday afternoon

Based on data from *Journal of Psychosocial Nursing and Mental Health Services* 25(10):15, 1987.

group received snacks such as hamburgers, pizza, and grilled cheese sandwiches. Compliance was noted during the 17-week snack period, and again during a 9-week period of no snack immediately after the 17-week period.

FINDINGS

The compliance rates for the Tuesday group for the 3 successive time periods were 58%/76%/61%. For the Thursday afternoon group, the compliance rates were 56%/59%/61%.

IMPLICATIONS

Compliance rates increased significantly for the Tuesday morning group when a morning-type snack was provided, but less so for the afternoon group. Providing rewards may improve patient compliance. The scheduled times for outpatient drug administration may have an influence on compliance or on the effect of the reward used. The effectiveness of the snack may also relate to the support and socialization that occurred during the 17 weeks that snacks were provided. Further research is needed to evaluate the effectiveness of rewards on patient compliance with drug regimes.

▼ **TABLE 24-10   NURSING CARE PLAN**

GOALS	OUTCOME CRITIERIA	NURSE INTERVENTIONS	RATIONALES
NURSING DIAGNOSIS: Noncompliance related to side effects of medication			
LONG TERM			
To adhere to medication regimen in an informed and responsible manner	Verbalizes accurate information about risks and benefits of medications		
SHORT TERM			
Establish trusting relationship with caregiver	Demonstrates trusting relationship with caregiver by stating fears and discomforts associated with medications	Be honest Inform client about effects of medications Use therapeutic communication, e.g. reflecting, clarifying	Showing warmth; accurate information increases trust and facilitates change
Verbalize feelings about taking medications	States feelings about taking medications	Facilitate expression of feelings, both positive and negative	Expressing feelings in an atmosphere of trust allows the nurse to assess factors that block compliance
State information about condition and need for medications	Verbalizes information about condition and need for medications	Assess perception of illness and promote realistic perception by giving accurate information	Inaccurate perception or denial of illness may result in noncompliance

role playing and return demonstration, brief lectures with audiovisual aids, and games in a group setting may also help clients become more self-reliant.[20] The support and opportunities for peer discussion and reinforcement as part of the group process may also influence compliance (see the research highlight on p. 501). Involvement of the client's family or other support system may improve compliance.

Compliance is under the client's control but is influenced by factors such as professionals' attitudes.[52] An approach that conveys an attitude of partnership and not authority is necessary.[22] Medication compliance is not inherently "good" or "bad" and by itself does not guarantee freedom from illness.[22] "Medicated relapses" are estimated to be between 18% and 48%.[51] Recognizing that medication compliance may be impossible, especially for the schizophrenic client, and maintaining respect for the client's autonomy and freedom to make personal choices will prevent the nurse from blaming the client or others for noncompliance.[22,51] A nursing care plan for noncompliance is presented in Table 24-10.

BRIEF REVIEW

The four major categories of psychotropic medications are the *antipsychotic agents,* the *antianxiety agents,* the *antidepressant agents,* and the *antimanic agents.* The *antiparkinsonian agents* are also discussed because of their effectiveness in lessening the side effects of psychotropic medications.

The antipsychotic agents are most effective for clients with schizophrenic and paranoid disorders, major depressions, and mania. The antiparkinsonian agents are given to clients with extrapyramidal symptoms resulting from their antipsychotic medications. The tricyclic and second generation antidepressants and the monoamine oxidase (MAO) inhibitors are the most commonly used antidepressants. MAO inhibitors are prescribed less often than TCAs because hypertensive crisis may occur when a client receiving MAO inhibitors eats food containing tyramine. For clients with bipolar disorder, lithium is effective in treating manic episodes. Serum levels of lithium are frequently monitored to avoid toxicity. Antianxiety medications are widely used for reducing anxiety. They are also commonly misused and abused. Because of their long half-life, these medications may accumulate excessively in the body and remain for weeks after therapy is begun. The combination of antianxiety medications and other CNS depressants, such as alcohol, can be fatal. Tolerance and dependence may develop with long-term use.

Noncompliance with a medication regime is a problem with psychiatric clients, particularly schizophrenic clients. Noncompliance results in frequent readmissions to the hospital. Medication cards and group teaching sessions may help clients comply.

REFERENCES AND SUGGESTED READINGS

1. Advice for the patient: USPDI, Rockville, Md, 1990, United States Pharmacopeial Convention, Inc.
2. AHFS Drug Information 90, Bethesda, Md, 1990, American Society of Hospital Pharmacists.
3. Aman MG, Singh NN, Fitzpatrick J: The relationship between nurse characteristics and perceptions of psychotropic medications in residential facilities for the retarded, *Journal of Autism and Developmental Disorders* 17(4):511, 1987.
4. American Psychiatric Association: *Diagnostic and statistical manual of mental disorders,* ed 3, revised, Washington, DC, 1987, The Association.
5. Antai-Otong D: Concerns of the hospitalized and community psychiatric client, *Nursing Clinics of North America* 24:665, 1989.
6. Baldessarini RJ: Current status of antidepressants: clinical pharmacology and therapy, *Journal of Clinical Psychiatry* 50(4):117, 1989.
7. Barrett N, Ormiston S, Molyneux V: Clozapine: a new drug for schizophrenia, *Journal of Psychosocial Nursing and Mental Health Services* 28(2):24, 1990.
8. Beare PG: Psychotherapeutic drugs: implications in occupational health nursing, *AAOHN Journal* 35(9):394, 1987.
9. Beebe LH: Reframe your outlook on recidivism, *Journal of Psychosocial Nursing and Mental Health Services* 28(9):31, 1990.
10. Beeber LS: It's on the tip of the tongue: tardive dyskinesia, *Journal of Psychosocial Nursing* 26(8):32, 1988.
11. Beeber LS: Undesirable weight gain and psychotropic medications, *Journal of Psychosocial Nursing and Mental Health Services* 26(10):39, 1988.
12. Beeber LS: Update on medications for the treatment of anxiety, *Journal of Psychosocial Nursing* 27(10):42, 1989.
13. Bostrom AC: Assessment scales for tardive dyskinesia, *Journal of Psychosocial Nursing and Mental Health Services* 26(6):9, 1988.
14. Brief DJ, Dorman JE: Noncompliance: understanding and intervening when clients fail to follow the treatment plan. In Backer BA, Dubbert PM, Eisenman EJP, editors: *Psychiatric mental health nursing,* ed 2, Monterey, Calif, 1985, Wadsworth Health Sciences Division.
15. Carey N, Jones SL, O'Toole AW: Do you feel powerless when a patient refuses medication? *Journal of Psychosocial Nursing and Mental Health Services* 28(10):19, 1990.
16. Carpenito LJ: *Nursing diagnosis: application to clinical practice,* ed 4, Philadelphia, 1992, JB Lippincott.
17. Cassino T and others: Invitation to compliance: the Prolixin brunch, *Journal of Psychosocial Nursing* 25(10):15, 1987.
18. Chafetz L: Recidivist clients: a review of pilot data, *Archives of Psychiatric Nursing* 2(1):14, 1988.
19. Clark JB, Queener SF, Karb VB: *Pharmacological basis of nursing practice,* ed 3, St. Louis, 1990, Mosby–Year Book.
20. Collins-Colon T: Do it yourself medication management for community based clients, *Journal of Psychosocial Nursing and Mental Health Services* 28(6):25, 1990.
21. Dauner A, Blair DT: Akathisia: when treatment creates a problem, *Journal of Psychosocial Nursing* 28(10):13, 1990.
22. Davidhizar R, McBride A: Teaching the client with schizophrenia about medication, *Patient Education and Counseling* 7:137, 1985.
23. DeLuca A and others: Neuroleptic reduction helps prevent relapse, *Journal of Psychosocial Nursing* 26(8):13, 1988.
24. Drug information for the health care professional: USPDI, Rockville, Md, 1990, United States Pharmacopeial Convention, Inc.
25. Durel SH, Munjas BA: Client perception of role in psychotropic drug management, *Mental Health Nursing* 4:65, 1982.
26. Epperly TD, McGlaughlin VG, Leo KU: A hazardous side effect of neuroleptics: diagnosis and treatment, *Geriatrics* 45(8):58, 1990.
27. Glassman R, Salzman C: Interactions between psychotropic and other drugs: an update, *Hospital and Community Psychiatry* 38:236, 1987.

28. Glod C, Beeber L: Prozac: pros and cons, *Journal of Psychosocial Nursing and Mental Health Services* 28(12):33, 1990.

29. Gomez GE, Gomez EA: The special concerns of neuroleptic use in the elderly, *Journal of Psychosocial Nursing* 28(1):7, 1990.

30. Guze BH, Baxter LR: Current concepts: Neuroleptic malignant syndrome, *The New England Journal of Medicine* 313(3):163, 1985.

31. Hamilton D: Clozapine: a new antipsychotic drug, *Archives of Psychiatric Nursing* IV(4):278, 1990.

32. Harris E: The antidepressants, *American Journal of Nursing* 88:1512, 1988.

33. Harris E: The antipsychotics, *American Journal of Nursing* 88:1508, 1988.

34. Harrison WM and others: MAOIs and hypertensive crisis: the role of OTC drugs, *Journal of Clinical Psychiatry* 50(2):64, 1989.

35. Haynes RB, Wang E, Gomes M: A critical review of interventions to improve compliance with prescribed medications, *Patient Education and Counseling* 10:155, 1987.

36. Health Letter, drug alert: Antipsychotic clozapine (Clozaril) may arrest breathing on first doses, Public Citizen Health Research Group, 1991.

37. Jackson RT, Haynes-Johnson V: Nutritional management of patients undergoing long-term antipsychotic and antidepressant therapies, *Archives of Psychiatric Nursing* II)(3):146, 1988.

38. Jeste DV, Krull AJ, Kilbourn K: Tardive dyskinesia: managing a common neuroleptic side effect, *Geriatrics* 45(12):49, 1990.

39. Karb VB, Queener SF, Freeman JB: *Handbook of drugs for nursing practice,* St Louis, 1989, Mosby—Year Book.

40. Keck PE and others: Risk factors for neuroleptic malignant syndrome, *Archives of General Psychiatry* 46:914, 1989.

41. Kerr LE: Oral liquid neuroleptics, *Journal of Psychosocial Nursing and Mental Health Services* 24(3):33, 1986.

42. Levenson JL: Neuroleptic malignant syndrome, *American Journal of Psychiatry* 142(10):1137, 1985.

43. Marder SR, Van Putten T: Who should receive clozapine? *Archives of General Psychiatry* 45:865, 1988.

44. Masters JC, Spitler R: Neuroleptic malignant syndrome, *Journal of Psychosocial Nursing and Mental Health Services* 24(9):11, 1986.

45. Meador-Woodruff JH: Psychiatric side effects of tricyclic antidepressants, *Hospital and Community Psychiatry* 41(1):84, 1990.

46. Michaels RA, Mumford K: Identifying akinesia and akathisia: the relationship between patient's self-report and nurse's assessment, *Archives of Psychiatric Nursing* III(2):97, 1989.

47. Norris AE, Disalver SC, Del Medico VJ: Carbamazepine treatment of psychosis, *Journal of Psychiatric Nursing* 28(12):13, 1990.

48. Puskar KR and others: Psychiatric nursing management of medication-free psychotic patients, *Archives of Psychiatric Nursing* IV(2):78, 1990.

49. Roth HP: Current perspectives: Ten year update on patient compliance research, *Patient Education and Counseling* 10:107, 1987.

50. Scrak BM, Greenstein RA: Tardive dyskinesia: evaluation in a nurse managed Prolixin program, *Journal of Psychosocial Nursing and Mental Health Services* 24(5):10, 1986.

51. Scrak BM, Greenstein RA: Tardive dyskinesia, *Journal of Psychosocial Nursing and Mental Health Services* 25(9):25, 1987.

52. Sulliger N: Relapse, *Journal of Psychosocial Nursing and Mental Health Services* 26(6):20, 1988.

53. Taft LB, Barkin RL: Drug abuse? Use and misuse of psychotropic drugs in Alzheimer's care, *Journal of Gerontological Nursing* 16(8):4, 1990.

54. Townsend MC: *Drug guide for psychiatric nursing,* Philadelphia, 1990, FA Davis.

55. Vaughan DA: Interactions of fluoxetine with tricyclic antidepressants, *American Journal of Psychiatry* 145:1478, 1988.

56. Youssef FA: Compliance with therapeutic regimens: a follow-up study for patients with affective disorders, *Journal of Advanced Nursing* 8:513, 1983.

ANNOTATED BIBLIOGRAPHY

Barrett N, Ormiston S, Molyneux V: Clozapine: a new drug for schizophrenia, *Journal of Psychosocial Nursing and Mental Health Services* 29(2):24, 1990.

The authors review a new antipsychotic medication recently released by the Food and Drug Administration for the treatment of schizophrenia. The psychopharmacodynamics, side effects, and implications for nursing are described and case studies are presented.

Hooper J, Herren C, Goldwasser H: Neuroleptic malignant syndrome: recognizing an unrecognizable killer, *Journal of Psychosocial Nursing and Mental Health Services* 27(7):13, 1989.

The authors discuss a serious complication associated with taking psychotropic medications, neuroleptic malignant syndrome. Death may result when untreated. Early symptoms are described

Jackson R, Haynes-Johnson V: Nutritional management of patients undergoing long-term antipsychotic and antidepressant therapies, *Archives of Psychiatric Nursing* 2(3):146, 1988.

The authors discuss the relationship between antipsychotic and antidepressant medications, their side effects, and nutritional management.

Scrak B, Greenstein R: Tardive dyskinesia, *Journal of Psychosocial Nursing and Mental Health Services* 25(9):24, 1987.

The authors report on the occurrence of tardive dyskinesia in a nurse-managed prolixin clinic. Estimates range from 10% to 20% (from the Task Force Report of the American Psychiatric Association) to as high as 50%.

Skidmore-Roth L: *Mosby's 1991 nursing drug reference,* St Louis, 1991, Mosby—Year Book.

An up-to-date nursing drug reference book that allows easy access to drug information and nursing considerations that specifically tell the nurse what to do.

Judith A Saifnia

After studying this chapter, the student will be able to:

- Define milieu therapy
- Describe the historical background of milieu therapy
- Discuss characteristics of nurses working in a therapeutic milieu

- Utilize the nursing process to provide a therapeutic milieu for care
- Identify methods for evaluating therapeutic milieu

Two major approaches to establishing a therapeutic treatment environment have been developed: the therapeutic community and milieu therapy. Although many treatment strategies used in these two approaches are the same, some distinctions can be made based on specificity and philosophy.

The *therapeutic community* is a structured environment with a specific philosophy of care and a focus on health rather than illness. The client is regarded as a responsible member of a social group. The treatment setting is viewed as a community of both staff and clients. All members interact democratically to achieve therapeutic outcomes. The goal of this approach is to develop insight into behavior through feedback received from the whole population of clients and staff.[14]

Milieu therapy is the scientific planning of an environment for therapeutic purposes. *Milieu* is a French word meaning environment or setting. Specific milieu factors and social interactions are structured to form a total treatment approach. The goal of this approach is to develop social and emotional skills beneficial in everyday life.[14]

The difference between these two approaches is one of emphasis. Although the goal of the therapeutic community is insight, the desired end result is improvement in behavior. Likewise, evaluation of thoughts and feelings is often incorporated in the milieu therapy setting to achieve the desired behavioral changes. Because of this overlap and the resulting confusion, Herz[19] suggested using the broader term of *therapeutic milieu* to describe all milieu treatment approaches. *Therapeutic milieu* refers to the general setting where treatment occurs, not the philosophy of treatment. For each environment the specific goals and treatment strategies serve as criteria for the evaluation of effectiveness.

In this chapter the terms *milieu therapy* and *therapeutic milieu* are used interchangeably. Therapeutic community is used to refer to the classic approach developed by Jones.[23] The distinguishing feature of Jones' therapeutic community is its emphasis on the way in which the total resources, including staff, clients, their relatives, and the institution are involved in treatment. Jones' approach focuses on open communication among staff and clients.

THEORETICAL APPROACHES

To examine the multifaceted dimensions of a psychiatric treatment environment, a holistic approach that incorporates information from various fields is necessary. This approach is based on the view that both personal and environmental factors determine behavior. Individual behavior cannot be predicted by personal factors alone; environmental factors are also considered.

Historically, the domestic service pattern of custodial care and the medical intervention pattern have been the theoretical models used to provide a therapeutic milieu. Currently, the social interaction pattern is gaining acceptance.

In the social interaction pattern, the physician, client, and staff are viewed as team members who all have information that is valuable to the client's care. All nursing personnel, including technicians, have an active role in maintaining a therapeutic social milieu. Every interaction with the client is seen as having potentially beneficial outcomes.

The principles of the interaction pattern have been identified as follows[53]:

1. The health of each individual is to be realized and encouraged to continue.

HISTORICAL OVERVIEW

DATES	EVENTS
Late 1700s	Pinel coined the term "moral treatment" to describe his new approach to psychiatric care, which included removing chains, using accepting attitudes, and setting examples of appropriate behavior and humanitarianism.
Early 1800s	Tuke established the York Retreat based on an atmosphere of kindness, meaningful employment of time, regular exercise, a family environment, and treatment of clients as guests.
Late 1800s	The predominant service pattern in psychiatric institutions was the domestic service pattern in which care was custodial and the staff performed essentially housekeeping tasks.
Early 1900s	Attention to hospital atmosphere declined, resulting in the development of environments that were benignly custodial or more destructively controlling, much like a prison.
1930	Sullivan[55] began to experiment again with varying the treatment milieu by selecting staff members who were sympathetic and interacted well with psychotic clients.
1939	Menninger and others[37] developed "prescribed" attitudes based on psychoanalytical principles that determined staff interaction patterns.
1940s	The predominant service pattern was the medical intervention pattern in which staff, including nurses, served as the physician's agents in providing care.
1946	Main[33] coined the term "therapeutic community" to describe the approach of resocialization of neurotic individuals through social interactions.
1948	Bettleheim[4] coined the term "milieu therapy" to describe his use of the total environment for treatment of disturbed children.
1953	Jones[23] used the therapeutic community approach in two experimental units for the treatment of antisocial personality disorders in which the social environment was seen as the primary treatment modality.
1960s	All nursing personnel had an active role in maintaining a therapeutic social milieu.
1970s	Treatment environments were tailored to meet the needs of the particular population they served.
1990	The development of milieu therapy based on research to identify the milieu structure most effective for specific treatment groups.
Future	Better integration of hospital and community psychiatry will provide for more efficient and more effective care for the mentally ill in the community.

2. Every interaction is an opportunity for therapeutic intervention.
3. The client's environment is a significant component of his treatment.
4. Each client owns his behavior.
5. Peer pressure is a useful and powerful tool.
6. Inappropriate behaviors are dealt with as they occur.
7. Restriction and punishment are avoided.

This pattern emphasizes the healthy personality, individual responsibility, positive reinforcement, and the use of the whole group for behavior control. The group must interact in a democratic style to be beneficial.

The *democratic style* of leadership emphasizes use of resources within the group. The intent is to create a climate in which members can openly express themselves, share their diversity without fear of rejection or excessive conflict, and employ their individual skills and talents to accomplish mutual tasks.[50] The democratic leader facilitates member participation. The importance of this role in promoting positive client outcomes has been demonstrated in many studies.

Devine[15] asserted that as milieu therapy becomes more popular, nurses have even more opportunity to "take initiative in organizing effective therapies." Holmes and Werner[22] described this role as follows:

. . . an exciting adventure, marked by loss of traditional nursing roles, blurring of roles of all disciplines, increased responsibility for therapy on the part of both patients and staff, more intense staff-patient relationships, and a whole complex of problems for nursing that we are just beginning to explore.

This new adventure is not without anxiety and uncertainty. However, the nurse is now able to contribute to efficient social milieu functioning and therapeutic effectiveness.

CHARACTERISTICS OF MILIEU THERAPY

The concept of milieu therapy developed from a desire to counteract the negative, regressive effects of institutionalization: reduced ability to think and act independently, an adoption of institutional values and attitudes, and loss of commitments in the outside world.[54]

Several strategies have been developed to counter these negative effects. They include (1) distribution of power, (2) open communication, (3) structured interactions, (4) work-related activities, (5) community and family involvement in the treatment process, and (6) adaptation of the environment to meet developmental needs.

Distribution of Power

The milieu therapy approach involves "flattening" the control hierarchy so all participants have a voice in decision making. Decisions are made according to the democratic process in client government meetings. This process may include the whole population of the treatment unit, or a governing council may make the final decisions based on input from various smaller groups of clients and staff members.

There is much discussion in the literature about how "flat" the hierarchy of decision making needs to be. On one hand it can be argued that a unilateral decision is contrary to the therapeutic community philosophy. On the other hand, some clients have regressed too much to participate in decision making. Staff in many treatment settings subscribe to the belief that clients are capable of decision making but act as if clients are not. This creates an antitherapeutic double-bind situation.[49] In a study conducted on three different psychiatric settings in a Veterans Administration Medical Center, Bell and Ryan[2] found that staff values may conflict with therapeutic community ideals. For example, staff felt responsible for controlling client behavior and intervening in decision-making processes while the values of the milieu were directed more at staff supporting independent decision making by clients. It appears the best way to resolve this dilemma is to identify a program's treatment goals and relate autonomous decision making to these goals. In any social structure, decisions need to be made when they can most effectively achieve the goals of that structure. For example, if the goal of a unit is short-term intensive treatment of severely disturbed individuals, many decisions will involve medical intervention. The physician logically makes these decisions. Alternately, if the goal of the unit is to provide service to clients remaining in the community in productive social roles, the clients may make most of the treatment decisions.

The ultimate goal of any treatment program is client autonomy. This may be achieved through a stepwise progression through a number of treatment programs or by gradually increasing independence within a given program. Consciously incorporating a plan for increasing independence is a means to achieve client autonomy.

Open Communication

Although the importance of open communication has been widely recognized in literature, it is still not a reality in many settings. One reason for this may be the insecurity of persons in authority. Open communication requires risk taking. Questioning and criticism may be threatening, whereas there is little to risk if no feedback is allowed.

For example, when the client questions the decision to extend his hospitalization an additional week, the nurse replies, "Your physician thinks it's best for you to stay in treatment a little longer." The nurse's insecurity and authoritarianism prevent her from responding to the client's concerns about the extended hospitalization.

In the traditional medical model of intervention, all information is directed to the physician, who makes the decisions. These decisions are then passed down in the form of edicts. Information about a client's background and problems are considered "confidential," meaning that only the physician has the right to that knowledge.

In the therapeutic milieu, treatment decisions are often made by the clients themselves, who therefore need information to make effective decisions. It is not necessary to communicate personal information but clients and staff need to be aware of individual treatment goals to ensure that everyone is working toward the same goals. In this atmosphere, exclusive confidentiality is replaced by mutual trust, honesty, and open communication.[34]

The development of open communication is difficult at times. Cultural norms, personal defenses, and established communication patterns may block communications. Opening communication channels requires taking risks and learning new patterns of expression. All members of the health care team need to work together to provide a safe atmosphere for this to occur.

Structured Interactions

K.A. Menninger[37] pioneered the concept of structured interaction patterns in the form of attitude therapy. The attitudes he prescribed are described in Table 25-1.

An advantage of the structured interaction approach is that all staff members approach the client in a consistent manner, acknowledging specific diagnostic areas, thereby shortening treatment time. The difficulty with this approach is that once a diagnosis is made and an attitude prescribed there is little flexibility in the interaction pattern. Day-to-day fluctuations in the client's condition may not be accounted for, and staff members sometimes seem stilted in their responses to clients.

Currently, a behavioral intervention technique is used in many settings. Problem behaviors are identified, and individual approaches are specified. For example, a client with a bipolar disorder may display several problem behaviors. In the manic phase of illness he may talk excessively, interrupt the activity of others, and constantly move about. These behaviors are best managed with a kind, firm approach that sets limits and directs the client's energy into productive activity. On the other hand, during the depressive phase, he may be withdrawn and passive. By using an active, friendly approach, staff members make contact with him and encourage interaction and activity.

▼ **TABLE 25-1**   **Approaches Used in Attitude Therapy**

Attitude	Description	Example
Indulgence	Extremely flexible; all reasonable requests are granted and divergence from expected behavior is accepted	Favorite foods are obtained, wine provided, hugs are given frequently, and extra time is spent with client
Active friendliness	Staff take the initiative in interactions and show special interest in the client	The nurse approaches a client who is working on a ceramic project. She calls him by name, comments on the colors, the usefulness of the article, and the feelings that accompany having accomplished a task successfully
Passive friendliness	Staff allow the client to take the initiative in interactions; staff convey the message that they are available, but they wait for the client to approach before responding	The client seeks out his primary nurse and shares information about his plans for a weekend pass.
Matter-of-factness	Suggests an element of casualness in interactions, especially regarding requests, pleas, or manipulative maneuvers; emotional responses and reassurance are avoided	Client: "I'll go to occupational therapy when I finish this letter." Nurse states, "It is time to go to occupational therapy now."
Watchfulness	Observation is continuous either openly or unobtrusively, as the situation indicates	Clients suspected of feigning symptoms, such as seizures, or suicidal clients are watched closely
Kind firmness	Approach is direct, clear, confident; rules and regulations are calmly cited in response to infractions and requests; directions are specific and concise with the expectation that they will be followed	"You will not be allowed to watch TV after 10 PM. These are the rules we agreed on for this unit."

The behavioral intervention technique has several advantages over traditional attitude therapy. Specific behaviors can be targeted for change, and plans can accommodate fluctuations in the client's condition, indicating specific approaches for each behavior. Also, staff interactions can be more spontaneous, based on current conditions. It is useful to write a contract that defines client and staff responsibility in reaching goals.

Work-Related Activities

Milieu treatment programs include work-related activities as a part of the treatment process. The focus of these activities is on benefits to the client rather than to the agency. Work under realistic circumstances and for appropriate rewards is probably the best central activity for all clients.

Several factors contribute to effective work therapy programs. First, clients need to choose the type of work they wish to perform. Second, work activities should be geared toward developing skills that will be useful in actual job situations. The current trend is to place clients on the job and provide funds for staff support in the work environment.[30] Third, a variety of activities provides the opportunity to test different areas for future job interests.[16]

Community and Family Involvement

As a result of more effective medications and humane treatment philosophies, community mental health centers emerged. Hospitalization is considered desirable only for acute illnesses. For easy accessibility, mental health centers are placed conveniently within a neighborhood.[9]

According to the milieu treatment approach, clients are kept in their usual environment, for example, a day treatment center or halfway house, and continue most of their routine activities while receiving treatment. Recent research has shown that this approach reduces costs as well as enhances benefits.[52] An attempt is made to involve all family members in the treatment process. If one family member is hospitalized, an attempt is made to continue family involvement. Visits to the hospital, home passes for the client, and family therapy sessions offer increased opportunity to practice newly acquired interaction skills, while staff members are available for support. Discharge is also coordinated with the family. Some treatment units have extended the concept of family to admitting the entire family to the hospital for treatment (for example, families in which there is child abuse). This may be considered radical; however, it is an effective way to improve family interaction and minimize the isolation resulting from hospitalizing one family member.

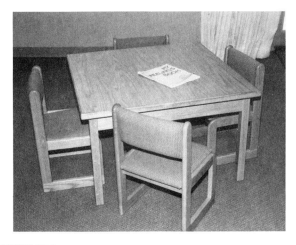

FIGURE 25-1 Scaled down furniture helps children adapt to their environment.

Adaptation of the Environment to Meet Developmental Needs

To develop his full potential, an individual must have an environment adapted to his current needs. Adapting the environment to meet these multiple needs is challenging due to the extension of milieu therapy to all age groups and the inclusion of families with individuals of varying ages within the treatment milieu.

Children

The most apparent environmental change necessary to accommodate children is a change in size of furnishings. Beds, chairs, tables, dressers, and play equipment that are designed for changing sizes facilitate a positive relationship with the environment and encourage activity and exploration (Figure 25-1).

Initially infants appear to respond better to black-and-white designs and patterns than to colors.[1] As they mature, they recognize brighter colors first, with examples of contrasting colors being more easily comprehended.

Meaningful sound is important, even to a newborn. The most valuable sound is that of human voices directed to the child.[2] Excessive sound is harmful to concentration, whereas silence results in sensory deprivation.

Play equipment is important for children because toys can counteract sensory deprivation, relieve tension and feelings of hostility and aggression, and provide an avenue to "work through" problems and conflicts.[7] Blocks, puzzles, and games, as well as crayons, paint, chalk, clay, scissors, and paper encourage skill development and creative self-expression. Chapters 34 and 35 give useful suggestions for enhancing the milieu of infants and children.

Adolescents

One of the major needs of the adolescent population is a communal area for interaction with peers. Decreasing the level of noise in this area is important but should not be so great as to diminish sensory input. Soft surfaces and malleable furnishings, such as beanbag chairs, accommodate adolescents who often sit on the floor or in odd positions on furniture. Other accommodations include stereo systems, advanced creative materials such as oil paint and canvas, games and cards appropriate to their level, and sports equipment to encourage expenditure of excess energy. Individual bulletin boards encourage the display of personal items; soft drinks and simple foods promote social interaction; and participation in food preparation encourages responsibility.

Adults

Differences in the amount of responsibility granted to various types of psychiatric clients have been identified. Clients (adults or children) who are regressed or who are overwhelmed need more structure and support; other clients benefit from a program that promotes autonomy and responsibility. A program that provides a stepwise increase in responsibility would be an effective solution (Table 25-2).

▼ **TABLE 25-2** Progressive Levels of Responsibility According to Client's Self-Care Capacity

Classification Level	Characteristics of Clients Assigned to this Level
Level I	Displays a destructive behavior to self, others, or the environment
	Disoriented as to time, place, and person
	Unable to function in group therapy
	Exhibits poor personal hygiene
Level II	Does not display destructive behavior
	Knows the current date, time, and place
	Attends at least one therapeutic group daily
	Attempts to maintain good personal hygiene and grooming
Level III	Attends all therapeutic activities
	Participates actively in community meetings and serves on at least one client committee
	Develops a self-directed behavior plan to change or resolve a personal problem
	Knows the names of all medications and the times they are to be taken
	Participates in a family session
Level IV	Takes an active role in assisting other clients to gain level changes
	Demonstrates willingness to serve as an officer on the client committee
	Assumes a leadership role in the community, acts as a positive role model, and ensures that other clients are prompt in their attendance of regularly scheduled activities and group meetings
	Initiates discussions with the mental health team concerning discharge planning

One approach to differing levels of responsibilities is to divide clients into small groups according to their developmental needs. More regressed clients focus on physical and safety needs, and more advanced individuals concentrate on social, esteem, and self-actualizing needs. Individuals progress to more advanced levels as their needs indicate. While more research is needed in this area, these approaches suggest several possibilities for varying the treatment program to meet changing needs.

Aged persons

It has been found that the elderly are more vulnerable to their environmental content because of age-related physical and emotional changes.[39] Environmental alterations that promote safety and orientation are of primary importance for the aged. Adequate lighting, nonskid surfaces, color coding of doorways, and curved mirrors at junctions can greatly assist the elderly to safely maintain orientation and mobility. Yellow-green color vision is retained the longest; therefore steps and protrusions such as doorknobs can be identified by these colors to promote safety.[2]

Diminished visual ability requires the use of brighter colors and 25% more illumination.[1] This can be provided by natural light, additional reading lights, and indirect nonglare artificial lighting. The aged have less ability to accommodate sudden increases in light; therefore windows need to be well shaded and artificial lighting placed on a dimmer switch so that a gradual change in lighting is possible.

Older individuals have a decreased ability to distinguish meaningful sound. The hum of heating, ventilating, air-conditioning systems, refrigerator units, toilets, and other appliances can be modified to decrease this background sound. Rather than increasing the volume on televisions, radios, and sound systems, earphones may be used to improve hearing without increasing environmental noise.

Often contact with the outside world is limited; therefore special attempts are made to improve input. Windows are valuable in maintaining visual contact with the outside world, and the weather provides a common topic of conversation. For those who are bedridden, the ceiling can be treated as a fifth wall and designed to enhance sensory input. Entrance hallways and other hubs of activity such as nurses stations provide needed social contact. Furniture arrangements that provide face-to-face contact or round table discussions promote social interaction.

The facility location used by the elderly is especially important. It is most desirable for the elderly to remain in a familiar neightborhood so they feel safer and have an established support system. However, a once-supportive neighborhood may deteriorate. Friends and family relocate or die, crime may increase, and neighborhood shops may change hands. These factors can force relocation. New surroundings need to replace the social network that was left behind, and transportation needs to be provided to maintain old ties.[51]

Settin[51] contended that perceived control over the environment is the most important factor in maintaining the physical and emotional status of the elderly. Freedom of choice, appropriate sensory stimulation, physical activity, social interaction, and social status contribute to a sense of control and environmental mastery.

CHARACTERISTICS OF THE MILIEU THERAPIST

In the interaction pattern of milieu therapy a great deal of role blurring occurs. Any individual, including the client, can assume a leadership position. Some people work well in this environment while others are threatened by the lack of structure (Table 25-3).

NURSING PROCESS

The physical, intellectual, and social aspects of the environment all contribute to the emotional atmosphere. Therefore the order of the dimensions has been changed in this chapter to provide a more logical flow of information.

Assessment

Physical dimension The physical aspects of the treatment environment include all concrete features of the external world. These features include the organization, structure, and interaction of many spatial components. The study of this interrelationship, called *proxemics,* is subdivided into three aspects: fixed feature space, semifixed feature space, and informal space.[16]

Fixed Feature Space The internal and external design of a building and its relationship to other buildings and environmental factors constitute the "fixed" or permanent elements in space. The arrangement of these elements strongly affects interactions that influence therapeutic outcomes. The importance of locating the treatment facility close to the community it serves has already been mentioned. Also important is the internal structure and dimensions of a treatment facility. To provide a humanizing environment, newer hospitals provide greater privacy with smaller wards, each with bathrooms, showers, and personalized space to store individual belongings (Figure 25-2).

Semifixed Feature Space Objects that have some degree of mobility are regarded as semifixed. These are the "props" that promote a certain degree of freedom within the environment such as furniture, partitions, folding doors, and planters.

Certain furniture arrangements (such as long benches found in railway stations) tend to decrease social interaction, while others (such as tables at a sidewalk cafe) tend to pull people together. Those who sit at the corners of a table at right angles to each other tend to speak more than those sitting next to each other and more than those sitting across the table from each other. The importance of the environment as a therapeutic agent is discussed in the research highlight on p. 511.

Informal Space Informal space, or personal distances maintained in interpersonal encounters, is probably the most significant use of space for the individual (see Chapter 6). Humans, like animals, have territorial needs. They claim a certain space and defend it against intrusion. However, unlike animals, people vary and are flexible. The proper distance between persons varies by culture. For example, a German may consider an entire room his private space and be offended if someone enters it.

▼ **TABLE 25-3** **Characteristics of the Milieu Therapist**

Productive	Nonproductive
Shares problems within a context that will benefit others	Talks about personal problems without regard to the impact on others
Recognizes the risks involved in honest communication and works to minimize these risks	Interprets openness and honesty as a license to be hurtful or vindictive
Communicates an empathic understanding of others' problems	Sees others' problems only in terms of own difficulties
Is warm and supportive without excessive attachment	Is rejecting or becomes overly involved with others
Accepts responsibility for own actions and admits mistakes	Blames others for mistakes and failures
Works to solve problems independently; asks for assistance when problems exceed own scope or resources	Demands attention and assistance from others for any difficulty
Is self-directed in selecting activities that contribute to organizational goals	Avoids work and responsibility and relies on others for direction
Believes that others enjoy work and responsibility when given the opportunity to participate in goal setting	Believes that others need to be coerced and controlled to complete tasks
Sees their contribution in terms of the "whole"	Focuses only on own task
Works with others to achieve consensus in decision making	Makes unilateral decisions
Shares information at the appropriate time and with the appropriate people	Selectively communicates information for manipulative purposes
Acknowledges anxiety and uses resources to cope effectively	Becomes defensive in the face of anxiety
Seeks feedback about abilities and performance	Interprets feedback as criticism to be avoided
Has a sense of self-worth and self-respect	Is either egotistical or self-deprecating
Readily adapts to change	Resists change and works to maintain the status quo
Functions comfortably in various roles; acts as either a leader or a follower as the situation dictates	Strongly prefers one role assignment; adheres to a position of leader or follower regardless of the situation
Accepts conflicts and confrontation as normal aspects of life and handles them effectively	Avoids conflict and confrontation or becomes agitated when they occur
Believes that all people can change, grow, and function more effectively	Believes that the individual has little control over mental illness and that it is a permanent, recurring condition

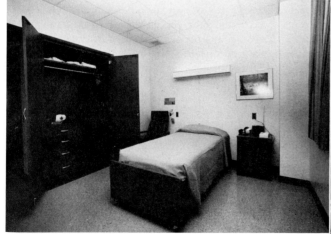
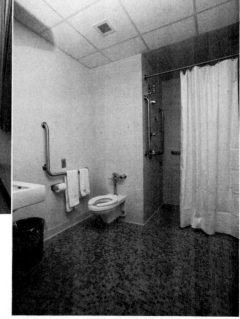

FIGURE 25-2 Personal privacy at the new John L McClellan Memorial Hospital, North Little Rock. **A,** Private room with individual storage space. **B,** Private bathroom. (*Courtesy Brian House.*)

RESEARCH HIGHLIGHT

The Ward Milieu and its Effect on the Behavior of Psychogeriatric Patients

• R Minde, E Haynes, and M Rodenberg

PURPOSE

This study was based on previous research that showed that relatively minor changes in the environment can result in significantly improved psychosocial functioning in psychogeriatric patients. In this study the following questions were examined: (1) What was the role of planned activities versus purely environmental changes? (2) Are there subgroups of patients who responded differently to such interventions? (3) What role does the attitude of nursing staff play in the process?

SAMPLE

The sample consisted of 36 psychogeriatric patients in a 400 bed mental hospital. Sixty-nine percent of the patients were demented, and 31% were chronic schizophrenics. The average age was 75.8 years. The setting was a geriatric unit that consisted of a long tiled hall flanked by rooms on both sides with a locked door at one end and a sunroom at the other.

METHODOLOGY

The stark institutional environment with its bare walls and basic chrome furniture was replaced by a "country kitchen" look, using a wooden table with a tiffany lamp overhead, rockers, and planters. This process of normalizing the institution ensured that in addition to good medical and nursing care, patients lived as normally as possible.

From *Canadian Journal of Psychiatry* 35(2):133, 1990.

Observations were made of patients' use and behavior while in the "country kitchen." This quasinatural approach does not lend itself to systematic scrutiny, but by comparing results with findings from previous research, researchers found a number of issues for further investigation.

FINDINGS

There were no major diagnostic differences in patient populations; however, behavioral differences were substantial. In general, patients looked relaxed and happy, behaved more appropriately, and some preferred to sit with visitors in this room. Changes concerned staff as much as patients and resistance by staff to changes was noted. Secondary gains associated with a pleasant place to work was reflected in workers interactions with patients and in satisfaction with their work.

IMPLICATIONS

This project suggests that even very impaired and behaviorally difficult patients can enjoy a better quality of life in an environment that is responsive to their needs. It also highlights the importance of the environment as a therapeutic agent.

Intellectual dimension

Sensory Features   The intellectual aspects of the environment are an extension of the physical properties. They include color, light, sound, texture, temperature, odor, and taste. The quality of the intellectual environment is determined by the amount and clarity of sensory stimulation. The number of stimuli becomes a problem at either end of the continuum—excessive stimuli (sensory overload) or lack of stimulation (sensory deprivation).

The intellectual quality of a psychiatric treatment setting is important because perceptual distortion may be part of mental illness. Shapes, color, lighting, and textures need to be distinct and corridors and spaces clearly defined.

The major impact of color appears to be on arousal. For the normal individual, warm colors (red, pink, orange, yellow) tend to produce arousal, whereas cooler colors (green, aqua, blue) tend to induce relaxation and self-reflection. Based on this information, it is logical to assume that blue will tranquilize an agitated client, and red will stimulate a withdrawn one. However, the reverse has been shown. A manic client is often calmed by a hot color, not a cool color.[58] One explanation is that an individual prefers to be in an atmosphere that suits his mood. A color scheme that parallels a mood may be comforting. Therefore an agitated client may feel more at ease in a bright atmosphere,

provided that there is not also overstimulating noise and activity to distract him.

In addition, variation in color is important. Rooms with different colored walls are more interesting than a room painted all one color.[6] Variation in the intensity of color can also add interest, for example, one wall dark yellow and the other three pale yellow.

Closely related to color is lighting. Natural lighting is most beneficial. When natural light is not possible, artificial lighting needs to stimulate the effects of natural light, such as soft, indirect light that avoids spotlight effects. Artificial light should contain the full spectrum of daylight color to avoid harmful effects.

The duration of exposure to light is also important. Constant light throughout the day and night can alter circadian rhythms, affecting various biological functions and emotional adjustment. Difficulty with sensory integration and orientation has been demonstrated in intensive care units with uncycled lighting.

Noise in the treatment setting is defined as unpleasant, unwanted, or intolerable sound. The sensory impact of noise is hearing loss. High-intensity sound also has social and emotional consequences. Workers continually exposed to very high-intensity noise have an increased incidence of nervous complaints, argumentativeness, sexual impotence, mood changes, and anxiety. They may also show decreased ability to perform complex tasks, reduced willingness to be neighborly, and failure to inhibit aggression. Annoyance has been found to increase as noise levels increase. Background sounds of up to 50 decibels (the level of an air conditioner) annoy only a few people. A level of 70 decibels (a vacuum cleaner) irritates a high percentage of hearers, and noise of 110 decibels (a riveting machine) is likely to bother almost everyone. While negative effects of noise were found in apparently normal individuals, respondents with psychiatric problems at the time they were surveyed were even more likely to report noise annoyance than individuals without psychiatric difficulties.[10]

Hard surfaces frequently used in hospitals reflect sound, adding to the client's difficulty in face-to-face social relationships. Such surfaces may distort human voices or heighten the irritating qualities of sounds, making it difficult for clients to determine from where a voice is coming. A client who is facing away from a person to whom he is speaking may be merely speaking toward what he perceives as the source of the other person's voice. On the other hand, institutional spaces should not be acoustically softened so much that they eliminate all echoes.

A noisy environment has been found to increase the motor and verbal performance of withdrawn clients. Perceptual organization and sleep patterns are also improved, allowing for medication reduction.[46] The reverse is true for active clients. Therapeutically, one is again faced with the challenge of providing a balance of enough noise to stimulate withdrawn, depressed clients without overstimulating agitated, active clients.

Temperature control is basic to well-being. The comfort zone for greatest productivity varies from 64° to 74° F. There are individual differences in this preference, and the aged adult seems not to tolerate cold and heat less as a younger individual.

Extremes in external termperature continue to affect hospital admissions. Besides increases in physical illness, mental illness also is affected by extremes in heat and cold. Psychiatric admissions peak in summer and winter.

Increases in schizophrenia, hypotension, depression, fatigue, confusion, headaches, hypoglycemic spells, and ataxia are related to combinations of heat and high humidity or heat and wind.[29] As knowledge of the impact of weather on body functions and mental health increases, it can be used to promote well-being.

Texture, the quality of roughness or smoothness of a material, has visual, acoustic, and tactile impacts. Visually, variations in roughness and smoothness contribute to orientation, making existing objects and surfaces distinct. Acoustically, more highly textured surfaces such as carpeting and textiles dampen noise, while smooth, hard surfaces reflect noise, causing it to reverberate. Tactilely, soft, nubby surfaces are comforting and warm, whereas hard, smooth surfaces are not.

Although soft textures have more therapeutic benefit, psychiatric treatment settings have most frequently used vinyl upholstery, metal, tile, plastic, and similar smooth materials because of their easy maintenance and durability.

Odor affects individuals both consciously and unconsciously. A strong odor may actually cause pain, whereas a pleasant odor is comforting. Long-term memory is closely connected with smell. For example, the smell of a rose can trigger memories of romantic occasions. Sexual arousal has also been linked with the partner's smell.

In the treatment setting, as elsewhere, both people and materials emit odors. The smell can be pleasant or distasteful, depending on cleanliness, disease, and other factors such as cigarette smoke. Room deodorizers used to mask these smells often have a biting, synthetic odor that can contribute to the problem rather than alleviate it.

There is no substitute for cleanliness and fresh air in eliminating unpleasant odors. Heightened awareness and perceptual distortions such as olfactory hallucinations in the mentally ill make it especially important to be aware of the impact of odor in treatment settings.

The current movement for smoke-free environments in psychiatric hospitals has received considerable attention lately. Studies have revealed a striking prevalence of smoking among psychiatric clients, and clients appear to be ambivalent about curtailing their use of tobacco. Concerns about smoking include fire setting, self-inflicted injuries, health risks, aggression toward other clients and staff during attempts to procure smoking materials, institutional maintainence costs, and the ethical dilemma of using tobacco as a reinforcer for behavioral change. Attempts to curtail smoking have lagged behind those in other medical settings. However, the antismoking movement is gaining momentum, and more psychiatric hospitals are now providing a smoke-free environment for their clients.

Although the discussion of taste is more related to the subject of nutrition, a few points can be made in relation to the treatment setting. The mentally confused may experience perceptual distortions such as the tasting of color *synesthesia*. Although these behaviors cannot be totally controlled, an awareness of them is necessary.

Design Features Several design features can be used to promote orientation. Patterns in floor coverings and furnishings may be used to identify personal space. These can serve as orientation supports to assist confused individuals in identifying their spatial relationship to others. Furniture size and arrangement can also contribute to defining personal space.

Differences in distances between visual planes need to be emphasized. For example, the distance between a balcony and the wall behind it can be made obvious by using contrasting colors, varying textures, or different lighting levels. Perceptual clarity is especially important for stairways to prevent accidents resulting from confusion.

Social dimension One of the most significant environmental aspects to consider in relation to therapeutic milieu is the social aspect. The social system of a treatment milieu includes the roles of individual members, the organization of these roles into a social system based on leadership style, communication patterns that develop, and staff/client ratio.

The function of the caregiver is to respond to the needs of the client who is seeking assistance. Within psychiatric treatment settings, the following professional caregiving roles have evolved.

A *psychiatrist* is a physician who specializes in the treatment of mental disorders. Training and certification prepare the psychiatrist for diagnosis of mental disorders and prescription of treatment, especially medications. Depending on their background and interest, some psychiatrists participate in various modes of psychotherapy such as individual, family, and group therapy. In most settings the psychiatrist is considered the leader of the treatment team.

The *psychoanalyst* has the unique ability to perform analysis. The goal of analysis is a complete understanding of the client's background and motivation for behavior, leading to changes in current behavior. Because both the training and the treatment by this method are very time consuming, less psychoanalysis is practiced today than in the past.

The *clinical psychologist* contributes to the team through selection, administration, and interpretation of psychological tests. Clinical psychologists are prepared to conduct and guide research in the field of mental health, to design behavior management programs, and to conduct psychotherapy.

Psychiatric social workers deal with the social problems of the clients including family relationships, housing, financial support, and placement with community agencies. The needs of the client are determined after a detailed social history has been obtained. Interventions include participation in individual, family, and group psychotherapy.

The *psychiatric nurse* performs many traditional functions such as assessment and intervention in medical problems, distribution of medications, and supervision of treatments. However, the role has been expanded to include many other functions. The psychiatric nurse is in charge of milieu management 24 hours a day. Every aspect of daily living is an opportunity for therapeutic intervention. Personal hygiene, meals, bedtime, social interactions, and therapy activities all provide opportunities for remedial approaches. The psychiatric nurse plans for these activities and supervises psychiatric technicians and practical nurses in delivering this care.

As an active member of the psychiatric team, the nurse contributes observations on and suggestions for the planning of individual treatment. The nurse also participates in program planning. Much of the responsibility for coordination of team activity rests on the nurse.

The background and preparation of psychiatric nurses vary. The master's degree prepares the nurse for the most autonomous role, the *clinical specialist.* The clinical specialist is trained to direct individual, group, and family therapy, as well as to provide consultation and educational support to other nurses.

Registered nurses, regardless of educational background, serve multiple roles. They manage the ward milieu, work with clients individually, lead groups, participate in community meetings, coordinate medical care (with physicians), dispense routine medications, and make decisions as to the administration of PRN medications, make discharge arrangements, and work with families. In addition, they provide leadership in interdisciplinary team meetings, and are the professionals who most often implement team decisions.

The role of the *practical nurse* in the psychiatric setting has not been clearly defined. In some settings it may be closely related to that of the registered nurse. In others it has more similarity to the psychiatric technician. In all cases the psychiatric nurse helps determine the practical nurse's role.

The *psychiatric technician,* also known as psychiatric assistant or aide, performs much of the direct care but has the least preparation. Psychiatric technicians function under the supervision of the nurse and assist in providing for the basic needs of clients. In addition, they often supervise leisure activities, have responsibility for maintaining a therapeutic environment, and may participate in individual and group therapy activities.

The *dietician* is concerned with the nutritional needs of the client. Besides providing attractive, nutritious meals, dieticians participate in education programs to improve eating habits and meal preparation. They also contribute to planning therapeutic intervention in food-related illnesses such as anorexia nervosa, bulimia, pica, rumination, and obesity.

The *occupational therapist* contributes significantly to remedial learning activities such as the activities of daily living, the development of work tolerance, the development of muscle strength and skills, resocialization, and prevocational assessment. The occupational therapist contributes much to the overall sense of well-being by increasing clients' productivity and creativity.

There are many other specifically trained activity therapists in areas such as art, dance, poetry, and music who provide recreational and expressive outlets for clients.

Housekeepers, secretaries, clerks, dietary aides, and canteen personnel contribute to the functioning of any setting and influence interactions that set the tone of the treatment milieu. The varied backgrounds and personalities of this group can add much to the richness of the environment.

Although each of the caregiver roles described has separate functions, many of them overlap. One area in which there is much overlap is in individual, family, and group therapy where many members of the team participate. The delegation of specific functions is largely determined by the social structure and leadership style of the treatment setting.

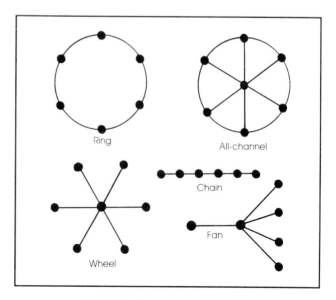

FIGURE 25-3 Communication patterns.

Communication Patterns Communication patterns are closely related to the social structure of the treatment setting. Several patterns have been identified: fan, chain, ring, wheel, and all-channel (Figure 25-3). In the *fan pattern,* messages originate at one source and are directed downward to several receivers who do not interact with each other. They may only respond to the central message sender. In the *chain pattern,* messages are initiated at one point and are passed from one receiver to the next until the message reaches the end of the chain. Feedback must return through the reverse sequence of receiving. The *ring pattern* is similar to the chain pattern except that the last receiver reports to the sender. Messages and feedback follow a cyclical pattern. In the *wheel pattern,* messages originate at a central position. Interaction may occur between the message sender and any one of the receivers as well as between the receivers positioned next to each other. In the *all-channel patterns,* messages may originate at any point and all members may interact. The fan network is most likely to develop in groups with autocratic leadership; chain and ring networks are common with laissez-faire leadership, and wheel and all-channel communications are most common in democratic groups.

The type of communication network determines the number and nature of messages sent by members in various positions, the speed of organization, and problem-solving skill. Groups make fewer errors and organize more rapidly in the all-channel and wheel patterns and make progressively more errors and organize less rapidly in the fan, chain, and ring networks.

The network of communication also affects the roles within a group. The person who occupies the position nearest the center of the network is the one most likely to be recognized as leader. This implies that centrality is more important than position within the formal hierarchy of leadership.[36] While observing communication patterns on a psychiatric ward, McKeighen[36] found that the actual leader was the ward clerk, rather than the psychiatrist or head nurse, who were the official leaders. The recognition of informal leaders helps identify sources of information and clarify confusion when problems in communication arise.

Group morale is affected by communication networks. The individual in the central position will have the greatest understanding of the overall plan of action and will be most satisfied with his job. The person farthest from the center will have the least knowledge and the lowest morale.[36] Therefore the more equality in communication of information, the greater the morale of the whole group.

As part of the communication process, it is important to distinguish between constructive and destructive conflicts and to intervene to promote constructive conflict resolution. Destructive conflict occurs when it directs energy from more important activities, destroys the morale of the group, disrupts group cohesion by polarizing members, deepens differences in values, and produces negative behavior such as name calling and fighting.[17] Constructive conflict opens up and clarifies issues, results in solution of problems, increases individual involvement, enhances authentic communication, releases pent-up emotions, builds cohesiveness, and promotes individual growth.

Staff/Client Ratio A concrete factor that affects social interaction in a treatment setting is the staff/client ratio.

Moos[41] found that the more clients per staff member on a psychiatric ward, the more emphasis that was placed on staff control and the less on support and spontaneous communication. Moos also related negative factors to large numbers of clients regardless of ratio. He concludes that a decreased number of staff members and an increased number of clients have several negative effects:

1. There is greater pressure to develop a more rigid structure.
2. Staff members' need to control and manage is increased.
3. The degree of client independence and responsibility, the amount of support given, and the involvement of staff members with clients are decreased.
4. There are fewer spontaneous interactions between clients and staff.
5. There is decreased understanding of clients' personal problems and less open handling of angry feelings.

Thus the staff/client ratio is extremely significant in developing positive social interactions.

Emotional dimension The emotional atmosphere can be sensed almost immediately when one enters a treatment setting. Descriptive phrases are often used for this emotional sense: "I feel comfortable here," "Everyone is so relaxed," "Everyone works well together," and "Everything is taken care of." Bradford[7] developed a more systematic list of adjectives to describe the emotional atmosphere of a group. These have been adapted to apply to a treatment setting (Table 25-4).

Moos[41] identifies spontaneity, support, and involvement as the most beneficial qualities for treatment. Spontaneity describes the extent to which the environment encourages clients to act openly and to freely express their feelings. Support indicates the amount of helpfulness and understanding of client needs that the staff and other clients show. Involvement describes how active and energetic clients are in the social functions of the treatment setting.

Moos states that in treatment settings with an involved, supportive, spontaneous atmosphere, clients are more satisfied, like one another and staff members more, believe that their experiences are relevant to personal development, are more self-revealing, more openly express anger, and are less submissive.

Spiritual dimension Although providing a specific place for worship is important, the entire treatment environment can provide the background for meeting spiritual needs. Important in this assessment is the provision of quiet spaces and opportunities for relating to nature and to other people.

The factors identified in this section form the basis for assessment of the characteristics that promote positive outcomes in milieu therapy. They also serve as a guideline for evaluation of actions. A summary of these factors for assessment is presented in the box on p. 516.

Analysis
Nursing diagnosis

Many factors interact to create an impression of the treatment milieu impact. Although standardized nursing diagnoses have not been developed for environmental factors, examples of patterns that could be seen as nursing

▼ **TABLE 25-4**   **Types and Characteristics of Emotional Atmospheres**

Type	Characteristic
Rewarding	When members have worked together well on the task they set for themselves, they feel that they have gained from the experience. The members may feel rewarded if they have accomplished something, even though the task is still incomplete.
Sluggish	Often members try hard to deal with the tasks at hand but "just can't get going."
Cooperative	Members work together harmoniously. Members seem to share goals and support one another in attaining goals.
Competitive	Several members seem out to win their own points, with the result that action can only proceed out of a "win-lose" approach.
Play	Play is the opposite of being task oriented. It exists when the members avoid tasks and cannot seem to shake off a light-hearted, nonserious attitude long enough to get anything done.
Work	When the members devote themselves to tasks in a purposeful manner, the atmosphere is one of work. This may be true regardless of what other impressions result as well; for example, it is possible to fight or not accomplish the task and still "work" hard.
Fight	Often members find themselves in complete disagreement regarding the topic to be discussed, decisions to be made, or action to be taken.
Flight	Members pursue inappropriate or outside topics, horseplay, or a bull session as a means of avoiding the real task at hand (which may be threatening or unpleasant).
Tense	Members feel pressures from limited time, conflict between members, or personally threatening topics.
Relaxed	Members work together in a harmonious manner with little tension or conflict.
Cold	Insensitivity to emotional needs is apparent. Defense mechanisms are used to avoid contact. Clichés substitute for support.
Warm	An emotionally supportive climate that promotes appropriate expression of feelings and the development of mutual trust.

Modified from Bradford L: *Class syllabus,* Searcy, Ark, 1978, Harding University School of Nursing.

diagnoses for milieu treatment are presented here:

1. Overcrowded and overconcentrated hospital ward
2. Failure to provide individual privacy in bathrooms
3. Assignment of clients to bedrooms (clients not allowed to choose roommates)
4. Stark white walls, resulting in glare
5. Smooth and hard textures
6. Lack of orientation supports
7. Authoritarian power structure that prevents client involvement in decision making
8. Blocking of interaction by formal communication channels
9. Low group morale
10. Cold and competitive emotional climate
11. Blocking of emotional expression by staff members' use of clichés
12. Punishment of aggressive acting out rather than management to promote emotional growth
13. Locking of bedroom doors in the daytime to prevent withdrawal, resulting in lack of a quiet place for meditation
14. Lack of recognition, display, or development of creative abilities of clients
15. Lack of provision for contact with nature
16. Lack of participation in goal setting and limited knowledge of overall treatment objectives

Planning

The care plan (Table 25-5) provides examples of long- and short-term goals, outcome criteria, interventions, and rationales related to the therapeutic milieu. These serve as examples of the planning stage in the nursing process. The therapeutic milieu is the identified client in the care plan.

Implementation

Physical dimension A nurse participating in the design or renovation of the setting can greatly affect the therapeutic physical environment. The nurse translates human needs into dimensional terms. For example, the size of the dayroom is especially important in both outpatient and inpatient facilities since this is the hub of activity. This space needs to accommodate a variety of activities. A nurse's input concerning the number of activities and interactions that occur can determine if the design is functional.

Not all nurses will have the opportunity to participate in designing or renovating a treatment area. However, much can be accomplished by arranging semifixed features to promote interaction and provide privacy. Shower curtains, lockers for personal items, bulletin boards to display personal artwork and pictures, and bedside lamps can be added at little cost.

Intellectual dimension The nurse may interpret the needs of the client population for design experts with knowledge of color, texture, and lighting. Some important client needs include the level of mental confusion, common behavioral problems such as withdrawal or acting out, the developmental level of clients, the type of activity that will occur in the setting, and the type of graphics, maps, and color coding necessary to provide orientation.

Maps of the area, color coding of specific areas, name plates on doors, and wall graphics can be designed to con-

NURSING ASSESSMENT TOOL

Milieu Therapy

Physical Dimension

Where is the treatment facility located in relation to the community it serves?

Are there planned interactions, such as outings, sports events, entertainment, and discussion groups, that involve both members of the treatment unit and community members?

Is transportation provided to facilitate interaction?

What is the floor plan of the building?

Does the physical layout provide areas of privacy?

Are there areas that promote interaction?

Is the furniture arranged to promote interaction?

Is there enough space to provide for individualized contact needs?

Intellectual Dimension

What colors are used in the environment?

Are the colors varied according to the activity of the area?

Are contrasting colors used to distinguish different visual planes?

Is the color balanced to reproduce the spectrum of daylight?

Does the lighting glare or have spotlight effects?

Is there natural lighting from windows, doors, or skylights?

What time are the lights turned on and off? Does this follow the natural circadian rhythms of the body?

What is the noise level of the environment?

Are areas provided for quiet and noisy activities?

Is the temperature of the area within the comfort zone?

Are provisions made for individual temperature control such as thermostats in bedrooms, offices, and treatment rooms?

How is the indoor temperature modified in relationship to external weather changes?

Is the humidity controlled?

Do the textures used reflect or absorb light and noise?

Are the surfaces cold or warm in appearance and touch?

Are the surfaces durable?

What odors are noticeable?

Is there a provision for circulation of fresh air?

Is the environment kept clean and waste disposed in closed areas?

Are there plants that absorb odor and give off oxygen?

Are synthetic materials used extensively?

Does the design of the building promote orientation, or is it easy to get lost?

Are there aids such as direction signs, clocks, calendars, and posted schedules to promote orientation?

What are the ward rules? Are they rigid or flexible?

What information is given to a new client arriving in the area?

Do clients have the opportunity to choose areas that are most comfortable to them?

Are clients and staff members of all levels involved in decision making?

Social Dimension

What are the formal roles of the members?

What are the functions (job descriptions) of the various members of the team?

Are the roles clearly distinct, or are there overlapping functions?

What is the formal administrative hierarchy?

What style of leadership is used?

What is the primary pattern of communication (who talks to whom and how frequently)?

Is the informal communication pattern the same as the formal hierarchy of communication?

Is the established pattern of communication efficient in speed, accuracy, and problem-solving capability?

What is the effect of the communication pattern on group morale?

Is there an attempt to assist clients to maintain community and family commitments?

Are family members involved in the treatment process?

What is the staff/client ratio?

What type of interaction pattern does the staff/client ratio promote?

Emotional Dimension

What is the emotional climate of the treatment environment? (How do you feel in the setting?)

What factors influence the emotional climate?

What blocks and facilitates the group interaction?

Does the climate allow for spontaneous expression of feelings?

What are the limits set on expression?

How is behavior that goes beyond the set limits handled?

Is support given for working through personal problems?

Is a sense of pride, camaraderie, and enthusiasm apparent?

Spiritual Dimension

Is a place provided for meditation and religious activities?

Is a time allotted for quiet meditation and participation in religious activities if desired?

Is the staff willing to listen to explorations of the meaning of life and illness?

Do the architectural lines of the setting inspire transcendence?

Do the space and the arrangement of the furnishings promote meaningful relationships?

Is the staff available for interactions?

What is the relationship of the facility to the natural setting?

Have natural items been included in the decor?

Are opportunities provided for creative expression?

Is there a sense of peace, harmony, and balance in the setting?

Do interactions promote self-fulfillment?

---

tribute to perceptual clarity. Clocks and calendars need to be clearly visible in each area, and bulletin boards for posting treatment schedules, mealtimes, visiting hours, recreational events, and other routines need to be readily available. All of these factors combine to promote perceptual clarity and orientation.

Such decisions as when the television and lights are turned off, what activities are planned, and who can come and go in the treatment setting also have great impact on the milieu.

Several special forms of therapy have been developed to take advantage of sensory stimuli. High light levels that extend daylight time have been beneficial in treating winter depressions.[18] Sound has been used to stimulate withdrawn individuals. Exposure to a noisy environment has improved both perceptual organization and sleep patterns.[46]

Music therapy provides sensory and expressive benefits. Occupational art, recreational, and sensory integration therapy have tactile inputs. The nurse is often responsible for making referrals, encouraging client participation, and coordinating the team members involved.

Social dimension Social interventions are primarily directed toward increasing interaction, improving communication, and promoting involvement in decision making

▼ TABLE 25-5 NURSING CARE PLAN

GOALS	OUTCOME CRITERIA	INTERVENTIONS	RATIONALES
NURSING DIAGNOSIS: Altered thought processes: confusion related to failure to provide orientation guides			
LONG TERM			
To provide orientation guides	Orientation guides are provided to all clients		
SHORT TERM			
To have clients and staff develop orientation guides	Orientation guides are planned and developed by clients and staff	Identify areas for placement of bulletin boards, clocks, and calendars	To facilitate orientation to time, date, and scheduled activities
		Color code functional areas	For ease in identifying areas
		Use graphics and maps	To aid in orientation and prevent dependence
		Include rules and regulations in guides, available services, a general map, and routine schedules	To prevent confusion
To have experts participate in the planning (consultants, interior designers)	Experts are consulted in the planning	Consult with experts for planning placement of bulletin boards, clocks, calendars, schedules, and most effective colors	To facilitate orientation
To orient clients to unit using orientation guides	Clients are oriented to unit and given guides	Staff and clients participate in orienting new admissions to units and provide guides to each resident	To prevent confusion, to increase autonomy, to decrease anxiety, and to provide supportive persons

---

RESEARCH HIGHLIGHT

Social Skills Training for Acute Inpatients

• K Mueser, S Levine, A Bellack, M Douglas, and E Brady

PURPOSE

The purpose of this study was to explore the feasibility of conducting social skills training with a mixed population of psychiatric inpatients hospitalized for treatment of an acute symptom exacerbation.

SAMPLE

The sample consisted of 115 patients—52% female, 65% white, and 57% single. Most had diagnoses of schizophrenia (25%), schizoaffective disorder (32%), or bipolar disorder (15%).

METHODOLOGY

Social skills groups were led by two therapists who conducted 1-hour sessions three times a week. The group focused on two skills useful for resolving interpersonal conflicts: compromise and negotiation and negative feelings. Patients usually remained in the group for 2 weeks. Following each session, each therapist completed ratings of each patient's social skills, performance, attention, and cooperation using a 5-point Likert scale. Periodic reliability checks were conducted and ranged from 0.64 to 0.89.

From *Hospital and Community Psychiatry* 41(11):1249, 1990.

FINDINGS

To determine whether the group resulted in improvements in performance, cooperation, and attention, MANOVA was performed with ratings from the first and last session as the repeated measures. There was no change in attention or cooperation over sessions. Patients who engaged in more than five role plays demonstrated greater improvements in social skill performance than those who engaged in fewer role plays. Males improved their performance more than females.

IMPLICATIONS

The findings suggested that social skills training may be a feasible psychosocial intervention when conducted with acutely ill psychiatric inpatients. Improvements in social skills were related to participation in greater numbers of role plays not in the number of sessions attended, suggesting the importance of behavioral rehearsal. The study supports the role of social skills training for acutely ill psychiatric patients.

(see the research highlight on p. 517). Conflict resolution and confrontation are sometimes necessary to overcome barriers that prevent these interventions.

Intervening in communication patterns is most effective if it begins at the top of the chain of command. The style of communication one chooses depends most on the style chosen by the person next highest in the organizational chain.[26] If the top person does not allow feedback, this blocks feedback along all other channels and may result in frustration and a deterioration in morale.

When it is not possible to alter communication patterns at the top levels, informal patterns of communication develop in the form of rebellion and lack of productivity. However, an effective informal leader may be able to relieve some of the tension by allowing venting of frustration and promoting group interaction outside the sanctions of formal control. Unfortunately, if an authoritarian interaction pattern is firmly entrenched, it may be the only option.

In any communication system, conflicts emerge. Constructive conflict resolution requires use of confrontation to bring the issues into the open where mutual goal setting can be achieved. Several principles enhance the effectiveness of confrontation[24]:

1. Face-to-face interaction involving all the major participants is necessary to clarify communications.
2. Confrontation needs to occur as soon as possible after the conflict has developed. Delays in confrontation allow for polarization and the development of defenses.
3. A skilled neutral leader is necessary to analyze the factors contributing to the conflict and to plan the circumstances and timing for the confrontation to occur.
4. A setting that allows the expression of feeling without fear of reprisal is important.
5. The confrontation needs to be timed so that feelings are not too strong and overwhelming but sufficient to motivate change if growth is to occur.

The major participants need to be willing to look at themselves, examine their roles, express themselves openly, listen to other points of view, and change for conflict resolutions to result in growth. These principles provide the ideal conditions for conflict resolution. Sometimes it is necessary to diffuse strong emotions and wait for a more favorable climate. The circumstances may not always be the most desirable, and individuals may not always be willing to change. The most important factors in conflict resolution are an acceptance of conflict as a natural occurrence and a willingness to face the emotional turmoil that results.

Emotional dimension To achieve the climate of support, involvement, and spontaneity necessary for therapeutic outcomes, it is important to develop a sense of harmony, cooperation, and group cohesiveness. Group cohe-

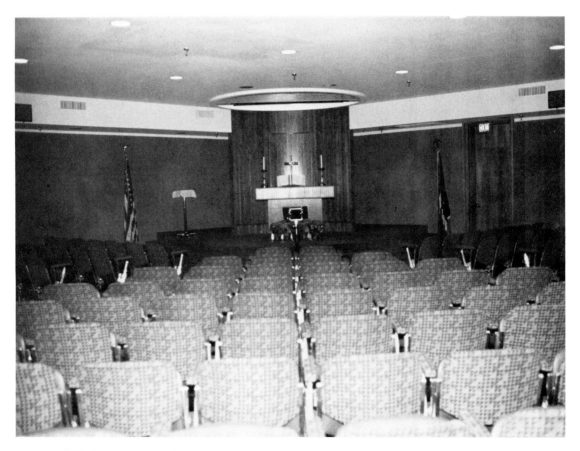

FIGURE 25-4 Focal point enhances meditation at the new John L McClellan Memorial Hospital, North Little Rock. (*Courtesy Brian House.*)

siveness holds a group together, helps it over the rough spots, allows it to fend off outside threats, and helps group members change and grow.[32] The two factors consistently identified in the literature as promoting group cohesiveness are acceptance and liking among group members and the pursuit of common goals.

People tend to like people who are similar to themselves. Similarity of group members may be enhanced by selection of a homogeneous group or by providing an opportunity to explore common interests and backgrounds through group interaction. Homogeneity may be promoted through screening criteria that select members with common goals or problems. When this is not possible, or when there is a large group in which diversity is inevitable, smaller subgroups with similar membership, which respect individual differences, may be created. Heterogeneity among group members can also contribute to therapeutic outcomes as members learn to listen and empathize with others.

For people to like each other they must know each other. This means that there must be an opportunity to spend time together. One way to achieve this is through working on a mutual project.

Another major factor affecting group cohesiveness is the development of common goals. In the treatment setting it seems logical that all group members work toward the common goal of improved mental health. However, individual clients may be pursuing their own development at the expense of others. A common error in the mental health field is to promote emotional expression at all costs. Many techniques have been developed to encourage emotional expression. Yet indiscriminate emotional expression can lead to ostracism from the group or to dissolution of the social network. For emotional expression to be productive, it needs to enhance not only individual well-being but also that of the social group.

Community meetings and group therapy sessions can be used to identify group goals and promote adherence to the group task. For an individual to adhere to group goals, the goals need to be explicitly formulated, the path for attainment needs to be clear, and there needs to be a likelihood that they can be successfully attained.[32] The process of mutual goal setting, as well as the interaction necessary for goal achievement, can do much to enhance group cohesiveness and promote a positive emotional climate.

Spiritual dimension Interventions that enhance the spiritual qualities of the environment are directed toward maximizing the meaningfulness of the treatment experience, developing a sense of transcendence, increasing relatedness to other people and nature, and promoting freedom and creativity of expression.

Meaningfulness is determined by the relevance of the program to the individual. When a client's goals cannot be met in a program, he needs to be transferred to a more appropriate treatment group. This has the twofold effect of enhancing individual meaningfulness and preserving group cohesiveness. A person who is unhappy in a group can create disharmony.

The need for both transcendence and relatedness involves creating a balance between aloneless and interaction. The physical environment can be structured to provide both private places for contemplation and reflection and larger areas for group interaction.

It is important to provide a quiet space and time to contemplate the meaning of life and to renew hope for the future. An enclosed space that blocks an external view creates a womblike effect, which promotes an inward focusing of attention. Lighting may be dimmed by the use of colored glass, and low levels of interior lighting may be used in this area. A single focal point such as a brighter source of light may be used to capture attention. In a chapel the altar makes a natural focal point[35] (Figure 25-4).

The need for transcendence can be supported through vertical lines in the architectural design. McClinton[35] stated that the vertical line is inspiring, uplifting, emotional, and mystical. Strong design elements such as beams or windows focus attention upward and create a sense of transcendence and relatedness to the universe beyond (Figure 25-5).

Relatedness to God may be enhanced through worship and communion in a chapel setting. Providing an individualized religious experience is most frequently seen as a duty of the chaplain service; however, nurses can work with this service to assist clients in meeting spiritual needs.

Factors that promote relatedness to others range from furniture groupings that promote interaction to developing open channels of communication. Planned activities can encourage interaction of withdrawn and isolated members,

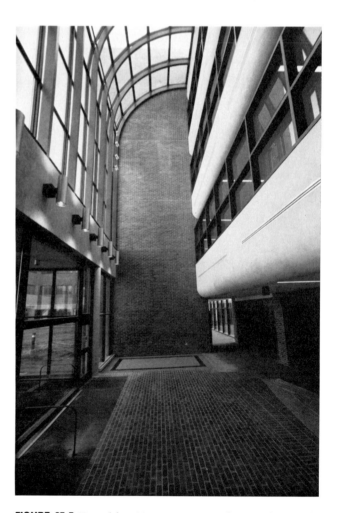

FIGURE 25-5 Upward focusing creates a sense of transcendence at the new John L McClellan Memorial Hospital, North Little Rock. *(Courtesy Brian House.)*

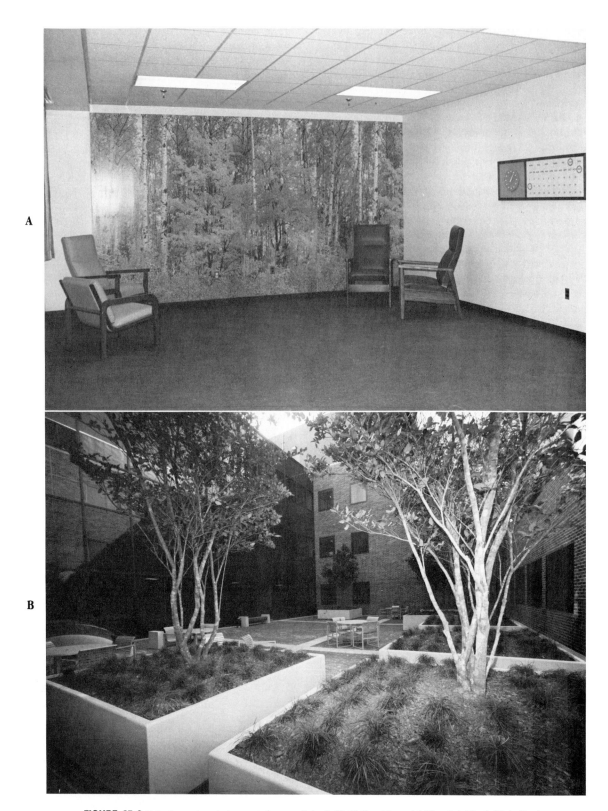

FIGURE 25-6 Bringing nature indoors at the new John L McClellan Memorial Hospital, North Little Rock. **A,** Mural of natural scene in dayroom. **B,** Enclosed patio with plants and trees. *(Courtesy Brian House.)*

▼ TABLE 25-6   Scales for Objective Evaluation of Environmental Interventions

Scale	Author	Environmental Factors Measured
Behavioral Mapping	Ittelson, Rivlin, and Proshansky	Eighteen categories of observable behavior
Ward Atmosphere Scale	Moos	Order and organization, clarity of expectations, staff control; autonomy, practical orientation, personal problem orientation; involvement, support, spontaneity, anger, aggression
Opinion about Mental Illness	Cohen and Struening	Authoritarianism, benevolence, mental hygiene ideology, social restrictiveness, interpersonal causes of mental illness
Ward Information Form	Kellam, Schmelza, and Berman	Disturbed behavior, adult status, patient/staff ratio, social contact, ward census
Group Climate Questionnaire	Johnson	Genuineness, understanding, valuing, accepting
Ward Value Scale	Almond, Keniston, and Boltax	Openness, involvement, responsibility, faith in ward

while enforced quiet time can encourage contemplation for those who are always with a group.

Contact with nature can be provided by choosing a naturally beautiful setting, using landscaping to enhance the setting, using large windows that provide a view of the natural environment, and "bringing nature indoors" by using plants, flowers, and pictures of natural scenes (Figure 25-6).

The development of relatedness to humanity is a self-actualizing process that includes the desire for order, harmony, truth, and beauty. The creativity needed for this process is best nurtured in an environment that provides daily freedom of expression and choice. Whitehead and others[58] saw exercise of choice as a major factor in prevention of the negative effects of institutionalization. Opportunities to choose are important in sustaining autonomy and self-worth and can be facilitated in the environment.

Creativity results when all of the environmental aspects combine to promote individual growth and expression. The creativity of a treatment group reflects the capacity of the group to balance the opposing needs of the members, develop cohesive interactions, resolve conflicts productively, and effectively use the members' intellectual and physical resources to accomplish goals.

RESEARCH HIGHLIGHT

An Analysis of Methodology in Follow-Up Studies of Adult Inpatient Psychiatric Treatment
• S Pfeiffer

PURPOSE

The purpose of this study was to examine methods used in clinical follow-up studies of inpatient psychiatric treatment with the aim of providing a basis for objective evaluation of accumulated empirical evidence supporting the efficacy of such treatment. A second goal was to provide recommendations for future outcome investigations.

SAMPLE

The 70 studies selected for review were located by a computerized bibliographical search of the Medical Literature Analysis and Retrieval System and the Psychological Information Data Base.

METHODOLOGY

The 70 studies were coded by a trained research assistant. A second research assistant coded 8 studies to evaluate rater accuracy. Reviews were grouped into 3 categories: (1) patient characteristics, (2) descriptions of treatment, and (3) methodological considerations.

From *Hospital and Community Psychiatry* 41(12):1315, 1990.

FINDINGS

Only 1% of the studies included all 5 types of data required for an adequate description of the patient population. Fifty-six percent of the studies did not describe the treatment regimen. An overwhelming majority of the 70 studies (95%) had only 3 or fewer of the important methodological features.

IMPLICATIONS

This study provides empirical justification for offering suggestions for future outcome investigations. These suggestions include the following: more detailed description of the sample patients, more careful delineation of patient treatment regimens, use of state-of-the-art published instruments rather than in-house developed scales, and the use of power analysis to compute the number of subjects needed. In short, if it is hoped to develop more effective programs for patients in need of psychiatric inpatient treatment, more carefully designed investigations are essential.

Evaluation

Evaluation of a therapeutic milieu is based on observation of desired outcomes. Several scales have been developed to objectify observations (Table 25-6). These can be effective tools in both assessment and evaluation. Recommendations for evaluating outcomes of inpatient treatment in psychiatric hospitals are described in the research highlight on p. 521.

Evaluation of environmental interventions is most effective when all members of the group participate in the process. By looking at behavior and its consequences, the group can develop new awareness of effective action and interaction. This awareness can form the basis for personal growth.

BRIEF REVIEW

Milieu therapy originated in the eighteenth century with the concept of "moral treatment" developed by Dr. Philippe Pinel. This approach replaced the custodial, often punitive method of treatment employed at that time. Menninger, Main, Jones, and Bettelheim extended milieu therapy to every age group, diagnostic category, and treatment setting.

Nursing intervention in the therapeutic milieu requires knowledge of the factors that affect therapeutic outcomes. The significant physical aspects include the external and internal design of the treatment setting as well as furniture and other movable objects that are most effective when they promote constructive relationships between the members of the treatment community and the surrounding neighborhood.

The intellectual aspects of color, lighting, sound, temperature, texture, odor, and taste can be integrated to form a coherent environment that promotes stability and comfort and avoids ambiguity, complication, and sensory overload.

The social aspects of the therapeutic milieu include the organization of roles of individual members into a social system based on leadership style, the communication patterns within the system, and the staff/client ratio.

The emotional aspects include development of a positive emotional climate with elements of spontaneous expression and support of others.

The spiritual aspects provide relatedness to God, others, and nature by arranging the environment to encourage interaction and using a natural setting with natural scenes and materials.

Assessment of the factors mentioned is followed by the development of nursing diagnoses and establishment of goals and outcome criteria. Interventions focus on identified problems in each aspect of the treatment milieu and on stated goals. Examples of interventions include the following: designing a treatment setting, interpreting sensory stimuli for clients, promoting healthy conflict resolution, sharing common activities and development of goals, and promoting relatedness.

Evaluation of interventions rests on objective evaluation of multiple interacting environmental factors. This includes recognition of the role of the intervener within the total process of change.

REFERENCES AND SUGGESTED READINGS

1. Beck WC, Meyer RH: *The health care environment: the user's viewpoint,* Boca Raton, Fla, 1982, CRC Press.
2. Bell MD, Ryan ER: Where can therapeutic community ideals be realized? An examination of three treatment environments, *Hospital and Community Psychiatry* 12:1290, 1985.
3. Benfer BA, Schroder PJ: Nursing in the therapeutic milieu, *Bulletin of the Menninger Clinic* 49(5):451, 1985.
4. Bettelheim B, Sylvester E: The therapeutic milieu, *American Journal of Orthopsychiatry* 18:191, 1948.
5. Blake FE, Wright FH, Waechter EH: *Nursing care of children,* Philadelphia, 1970, JB Lippincott.
6. Bonier RJ: Staff countertransference in an adolescent milieu treatment setting, *Adolescent Psychiatry* 10:382, 1982.
7. Bradford L: Class syllabus, Searcy, Ark, 1978, Harding University School of Nursing.
8. Brown LJ: The therapeutic milieu in the treatment of patients with borderline personality disorders, *Bulletin of the Menninger Clinic* 45(5):377, 1981.
9. Church OM: From custody to community in psychiatric nursing, *Nursing Research* 36(1):48, 1987.
10. Cohen S: Sound effects on behavior, *Psychology Today* 15(10):38, 1981.
11. Collins JF and others: Treatment characteristics of effective psychiatric programs, *Hospital and Community Psychiatry* 35(6):601, 1984.
12. Cotton NS, Geraty RG: Therapeutic space design: planning an inpatient children's unit, *American Journal of Orthopsychiatry* 54(4):624, 1984.
13. Cox KG: Alzheimer's disease: milieu therapy, *Geriatric Nursing* G(3):152, 1985.
14. Cumming E: Therapeutic community and milieu therapy strategies can be distinguished, *International Journal of Psychiatry* 7:204, 1969.
15. Devine BA: Therapeutic milieu/milieu therapy: an overview, *Journal of Psychiatric Nursing* 3:24, 1981.
16. Hall ET: The anthropology of space: an organizing model. In Proshansky HM, Ittelson WH, Rivlin LG, editors: *Environmental psychology: man and his physical setting,* New York, 1970, Holt, Rinehart and Winston.
17. Hart LB: *Learning from conflict: a handbook for trainers and group leaders,* Reading, Mass, 1981, Addison-Wesley.
18. Hellman H: Guiding light, *Psychology Today* 16(4):22, 1982.
19. Herz MI: The therapeutic milieu: a necessity, *International Journal of Psychiatry* 7:209, 1969.
20. Herz MI: The therapeutic community re-examined, *Hospital and Community Psychiatry* 32(2):81, 1981.
21. Hiatt LG: The color and use of color in environments for older people, *Nursing Homes,* p 18, May-June 1981.
22. Holmes M, Werner J: *Psychiatric nursing in a therapeutic community,* New York, 1966, Macmillan.
23. Jones M: *The therapeutic community,* New York, 1953, Basic Books.
24. Jones M: *Beyond the therapeutic community,* New Haven, Conn, 1968, Yale University Press.
25. Keltner NL: Psychiatric management: a model for nursing practice, *Perspectives in Psychiatric Care* 23(4):125, 1985.
26. Kepler TL: Mastering the people skills, *Journal of Nursing Administration* 10(11):15, 1980.
27. Kernberg O, Haran C: Interview: milieu treatment with borderline patients: the nurse's role, *Journal of Psychosocial Nursing and Mental Health Services* 22(4):29, 1984.
28. Kirshner LA, Johnston L: Current status of milieu psychiatry, *General Hospital Psychiatry* 4(1):75, 1982.
29. Klosterman VJ: The psychological effects of weather, *Journal of Psychiatric Nursing and Mental Health Services* 17(1):25, 1979.

30. Land SK, Cara E: Vocational integration for the psychiatrically disabled, *Hospital and Community Psychiatry* 40(9), September 1989.

31. Lehman AF: Strategies for improving services for the chronically ill, *Hospital and Community Psychiatry* 40(9):916, September 1989.

32. Loomis ME: *Group process for nurses,* St Louis, 1979, Mosby–Year Book.

33. Main TF: The hospital as a therapeutic institution, *Bulletin of the Menninger Clinic* 10:66, 1946.

34. Margo GM, Manring JM: The current literature on inpatient psychotherapy, *Hospital and Community Psychiatry* 40(9):909, September 1989.

35. McClinton KM: The changing church: its architecture, art, and decoration, New York, 1957, Morehouse-Gorham.

36. McKeighen RJ: Communication patterns and leadership roles in a psychiatric setting, *Perspectives in Psychiatric Care* 6(2):80, 1968.

37. Menninger KA and others: *A manual for psychiatric case study,* ed 2, New York, 1962, Grune & Stratton.

38. Menninger WC: Psychoanalytic principles in psychiatric hospital therapy, *Southern Medical Journal* 32:348, 1939.

39. Minde R, Haynes E, Rodenburg M: The ward milieu and its effect on the behaviour of psychogeriatric patients, *Canada Journal of Psychiatry* 35:133, March 1990.

40. Molina JA: Psychobiosocial "maps": a useful tool in milieu therapy and psychiatric education, *Journal of Clinical Psychiatry* 43(5):182, 1982.

41. Moos RH: *Evaluating treatment environments: a social ecological approach,* New York, 1974, John Wiley & Sons.

42. Mosher LR and others: Milieu therapy in the 1980's: a comparison of two residential alternatives to hospitalization, *Bulletin of the Menninger Clinic* 50(3):257, 1986.

43. Mulvihill DL: Milieu therapy in a children's unit, *Canadian Journal of Psychiatric Nursing* 24(4):17, 1983.

44. Olds J: The inpatient treatment of adolescents in a milieu including younger children, *Adolescent Psychiatry* 10:373, 1982.

45. Osmond H: Function as the basis of psychiatric ward design, *Mental Hospitals* (architectural suppl) 8:23, 1957.

46. Ozerengin MF, Cowen MA: Environmental noise level as a factor in the treatment of hospitalized schizophrenics, *Diseases of the Nervous System* 35:241, 1974.

47. Pfeiffer SI: An analysis of methodology in follow-up studies of adult inpatient psychiatric treatment, *Hospital and Community Psychiatry* 41(12):1315, December 1990.

48. Rosenbaum M: Violence and the unstructured psychiatric milieu, *Hospital and Community Psychiatry* 41(7):721, July 1990.

49. Sacks RH, Carpenter WT: The pseudotherapeutic community: an examination of antitherapeutic forces on psychiatric units, *Hospital and Community Psychiatry* 25:315, 1974.

50. Sampson EE, Marthas M: *Group process for the health professionals,* ed 2, New York, 1981, John Wiley & Sons.

51. Settin JM: *Gerontologic human resources: the role of the paraprofessional,* New York, 1982, Human Sciences Press.

52. Shanks J: Mental illness services in Britain: counting the costs, weighing the benefits, *Hospital and Community Psychiatry* 40(9):878, September 1989.

53. Skinner K: The therapeutic milieu: making it work, *Journal of Psychiatric Nursing and Mental Health Services* 17(8):38, 1979.

54. Sommer R, Osmond H: Symptoms of institutional care, *Social Problems* 8:345, 1960.

55. Sullivan HS: Sociopsychiatric research: its implications for the schizophrenic problem and for mental hygiene, *American Journal of Psychiatry* 10:977, 1931.

56. Szekais B: Using the milieu: treatment-environment consistency, *Gerontologist* 60(4):7, 1985.

57. van Bilsen HP, van Emst AJ: Heroin addiction and motivational milieu therapy, *International Journal of the Addictions* 21(G):707, 1986.

58. Whitehead C and others: The aging psychiatric hospital: an approach to humanistic redesign, *Hospital and Community Psychiatry* 27:781, 1976.

ANNOTATED BIBLIOGRAPHY

Devine BA: Therapeutic milieu/milieu therapy: an overview, *Journal of Psychosocial Nursing and Mental Health Services* 3:24, 1981.

Following a historical overview of milieu therapy, the author defines the concepts of milieu therapy and therapeutic community. Principles of milieu therapy are discussed, and the nurse's role in designing and implementing a therapeutic milieu is presented. The author also reviews research findings related to milieu therapy.

Geller J, Kaye N: Smoking in psychiatric hospitals: a historical view of a hot topic, *Hospital and Community Psychiatry* 41(12):1349, 1990.

This report traces the history of the antismoking movement beginning in the 1800s. Early manuscripts demonstrated questions about tobacco usage indicating that the movement toward smoke-free environments is neither newly conceived nor newly controversial.

Greenman M, McClellan T: Negative effects of a smoking ban on an inpatient psychiatric service, *Hospital and Community Services* 42(4):408, 1991.

The authors suggest that problems associated with implementation of a no-smoking policy have been underreported. Four cases illustrating problems in treating highly disturbed, nicotine-dependent clients are presented and recommendations for clients who cannot tolerate the abrupt cessation of smoking are made.

Kirshner LA, Johnston L: Current status of milieu psychiatry, *General Hospital Psychiatry* 4(1):75, 1982.

Historical trends in the use of environment in treatment of mental illness are integrated with social science and empirical research studies of milieu. Research is reviewed that documents the significant effects of milieu on treatment outcomes. Also discussed is the importance of the direction of future research efforts toward more specific parameters of milieu in interaction with different diagnoses or client populations.

Margo G, Manning J: The current literature on inpatient psychotherapy, *Hospital and Community Psychiatry* 40(9):909, 1989.

In a review of the literature on inpatient psychotherapy, the authors discuss the shortened length of stay and the interdisciplinary team approach as factors affecting psychotherapy in the inpatient setting. The importance of the therapeutic community is emphasized.

Shanks J: Mental illness services in Britain: counting the costs, weighing the benefits, *Hospital and Community Services* 40(9):878, 1989.

The author presents studies conducted in Britain that provide information on costs and benefits of care in the community for people with severe mental illness. Evidence suggests that community care is likely less expensive and more beneficial than institution-based care.

Doris E Bell

Sophronia R Williams

After studying this chapter, the student will be able to:

- Identify significant events in the evolution of community mental health nursing
- Discuss theoretical approaches to community mental health nursing
- Identify significant legislative events in the Community Mental Health Movement
- Discuss characteristics of the community mental health–psychiatric nurse

- Use the nursing process to provide nursing care to clients in community-based settings
- Describe the indirect and direct roles of the community mental health nurse
- Describe the role of the community mental health nurse in specialized populations
- Identify current research findings relevant to community mental health nursing

It has been 35 years since the landmark legislation that brought the concept of community mental health to the forefront of mental health. There was great excitement with federal commitment to mental health in the early 1960s. Changes were going to be made in mental health service delivery, settings for delivery of service, and personnel involved in the delivery of service. There was going to be a commitment to deinstitutionalization, a commitment to comprehensive service delivery, and a multidisciplinary approach to providing care to the chronically mentally ill.[32]

The enthusiasm and dedication of the 1960s was soon replaced by the problems of the 1970s and 1980s—the lack of treatment facilities for the chronically mentally ill, the inability to deal with the effects of substance abuse in mentally ill people, the continuing power struggles between the core mental health professions over turf, inability to provide both long-term and short-term physical care in the community for chronically mentally ill clients, and lack of funding for basic needs such as housing, food, education, recreation, and vocational rehabilitation services. The community mental health movement entered the 1990s being described as a nonsystem of care with little incentive to coordinate services or funding most of the time.

The 1990s have ushered in changes. The community mental health movement has started to refocus on the needs of the seriously mentally ill again and to promote community-based housing, job programs, and education for the mentally ill in the community.[32] Attention is being given to the caregivers and families of the chronically mentally ill and the importance of collaboration between service providing agencies is being stressed. Private foundations such

as the Robert Woods Johnson Foundation are becoming involved in the care of the chronically mentally ill. The Robert Woods Johnson Foundation is providing grants, loans, and rent subsidies to nine cities to develop central mental health authority to deliver a variety of services to the chronically mentally ill population.[32]

Community mental health nurses have a central role in this new focus in community mental health. They are the mental health professionals that emphasize the concept of continuous, comprehensive care and provide this care for the chronically mentally ill by using direct and indirect interventions, such as case management, psychotherapy, and psychosocial education, and programming for individuals and community.

HISTORICAL ASPECTS OF THE COMMUNITY MENTAL HEALTH MOVEMENT

The community mental health movement changed the way psychiatric treatment was offered in the United States. There were several developments that provide the emphasis for this movement: the development and use of psychotropic drugs, the resulting idea that the chronic mentally ill population could be in a less restrictive environment, and a less restrictive environment meant living in the community close to their homes. Another force was the growing concern about the civil rights of the clients and the changes in several states' commitment policies. Financial concern was still another force. The states and local governments wanted to shift the fiscal burden for the mentally ill to the federal government.[49]

HISTORICAL OVERVIEW

DATES	EVENTS
1200	Community care for the mentally ill was evident in Gheel, Belgium, when people were placed with families for mental health care.
Late 1940s	Community-based mental health care projects were developed at the Menninger and Yale clinics.
1957	Community mental health–psychiatric nursing was provided in the hospital and community.
1963	The Community Mental Health Centers Act was passed. A community-based system of mental health care was established with community mental health centers as the locus of services.
1969	The number of community psychiatric nursing services increased.
1975	Nurses working in community mental health centers were largely generalists.
1980	The number of psychiatric clinical specialists working in community mental health centers increased.
1982	Several subspecialties of community mental health nursing were developed, such as geropsychiatric and liaison nursing. These were developed as the result of funding emphasis and needs of the different agencies providing care in the community.
1985	The chronically mentally ill and substance abuse clients became a priority for care in the community. Nursing developed subspecialties to educate nurses to meet the care challenge.
1988-1990	Home health nursing emerges as a subspecialty of community mental health nursing.
Future	The chronically mentally ill homeless and psychosocial needs of victims of AIDS will become a priority for community mental health nursing.

In 1963, for the first time, the chronically mentally ill individuals were eligible for federal financial support in the community. Supplemental Security Income administered by the Social Security Administration provided money for the mentally ill to live in the community. Medicaid paid for the cost of inpatient care in the community. The community mental health center legislation was passed and provided for construction of community mental health centers. The centers were mandated to offer five essential community services in order to receive the funds:

1. Inpatient care
2. Partial hospitalization, which includes day hospitalization and night hospitalization
3. Outpatient treatment
4. Emergency care (24-hour treatment)
5. Consultation and educational services to the community

In 1975, the Community Mental Health Center Amendment of 1975 was enacted. This Act gave more money to the community mental health centers for construction and operation. Guidelines were added to clarify services offered by the centers, and five other services were added:

1. Follow-up care for client's discharged from mental institutions
2. Mental health diagnostic treatment, liaison and follow-up services for children, adolescents, and the elderly
3. Screening services for people needing mental health services

4. Prevention, treatment, and follow-up of alcohol and drug abuse
5. Transitional living arrangements for the newly discharged mentally ill clients who need help to adjust to living on their own and the clients unable to live on their own

In 1981 The Omnibus Budget Reconciliation Act was passed, and it repealed the 1975 and 1980 Acts. Federal funding was reduced for health care and the states were encouraged to use block grants to fund community mental health centers. This resulted in reduction of services offered by the centers. The following services were left:

1. Outpatient care
2. Partial hospitalization
3. 24-hour inpatient care
4. Emergency care
5. Consultation and education to community
6. Screening services[34]

After the 1981 Omnibus Budget Reconciliation Act was passed, federal funding for mental health care became program focused. Legislation is summarized in Table 26-1.

Since 1988, federal funding for community mental health care has focused on the chronically mentally ill, the elderly, the homeless, persons who abuses substances, and the victims of AIDS. Efforts are being made to identify the mental health needs of these populations and to provide care in an acceptable manner. Funding is being provided for housing, food, transportation, and basic medical and rehabilitation services.

▼ **TABLE 26-1**   Legislative Developments in the Community Mental Health Movement

Year	Legislative Act	Year	Legislative Act
1963	*The Community Mental Health Centers Act* was passed during President Kennedy's administration to provide matching funds with the states for 3 years to build community mental health centers (CMHCs).	1987	*The Steward B McKinney Homeless Assistance Act* provided block grants for outpatient services to the homeless, with special emphasis on elderly, handicapped, chronically mentally ill, and families with children.
1975	*The Community Mental Health Center Amendments of 1975* extended the funding of the community mental health centers and provided guidelines for services for the mentally ill.	1988	*The Anti-Drug Abuse Act* provides funds for block grants to states for alcohol, drug abuse, and mental illness prevention and treatment.
1977	President Carter organized the *President's Commission on Mental Health.* The purpose of the Commission was to make recommendations on the mental health needs of the nation. For the first time in history, nursing was included as one of the five professions serving on this Commission.	1988	*The Stewart B McKinney Homeless Assistance Amendments Act of 1988* provides funds for state and local governments for health care assistance to the homeless, including mental health block grant programs, community demonstration projects for mental health services, and alcohol and drug abuse treatment. It also provides funds for VA domiciliary care for homeless veterans and rehabilitative services for chronically mentally ill homeless veterans.
1980	*The Community Mental Health Center Act of 1980* was enacted to coordinate the state hospital system and the community mental health centers.	1989	*The Omnibus Budget Reconciliation Act of 1989* provided Medicare coverage to community mental health centers, clinical psychologists, and nurse practitioners.
1981	*The Omnibus Budget Reconciliation Act* was passed for the purpose of reducing federal spending on health care and to give states more flexibility in providing health care. States were encouraged to use block grants (specific programming grants) to finance mental health care.	1990	*The Mental Health Amendments of 1990* provide funds for NIMH grants to states for development and implementation of plans to improve community-based mental health services for the mentally ill.
1986	*The State Comprehensive Mental Health Service Plan Act of 1986* provided funds for Human Health Services grants (block grants) to states for planning and implementation of comprehensive mental health and social services for clients who were chronically mentally ill, including deinstitutionalized and homeless individuals.	1991	*The Ryan White Comprehensive AIDS Resources Emergency Act of 1990* provides funds to health care providers for AIDS early intervention services.

One of the major problems in community mental health care is the cost, but it can be operationalized in a cost-effective manner. There are two factors to consider in keeping costs within limits. The first factor is the lack of coordination between levels of state and local government. This lack of coordination is also seen at the federal level with funding sources between the levels of federal and state government having different goals. The federal government is paying for in-hospital services, not community services, yet the states are encouraged to focus on community care. The second factor is the attempts at cost shifting. States are trying to shift the cost of caring for the mentally ill to the federal Medicaid program. Since that program does not pay for care in the state mental hospitals, these state hospitals are being emptied and closed, forcing inpatient care on nursing homes and general hospitals.[49] One of the approaches to solving these problems has been case management.

COMMUNITY MENTAL HEALTH–PSYCHIATRIC NURSING

Community mental health–psychiatric nursing is the application of specialized knowledge to populations and communities to promote and maintain mental health and to rehabilitate populations at risk that continue to have residual effects of mental illness. These at risk populations include the chronically mentally ill who are discharged from the mental hospitals and the young adult chronic client who has not been hospitalized. Other possible populations at risk are the elderly, the abused, the homeless, the person who abuses substances, and the victims of AIDS.

Community mental health nursing focuses on the community rather than individual clients. Thus community mental health nursing emphasizes preventive interventions—interventions that decrease the number of stressors in the environment, reduce the effects of stress on populations of persons at risk, and incidents of mental disorder using a primary prevention approach.

There are three levels of prevention—primary, secondary, and tertiary. *Primary prevention* is divided into two categories, disease prevention and health promotion. The goal of this level is to decrease or remove sources of stress and to increase the strength of the at risk population to cope with the stress and, in this way, prevent mental illness. Nursing activities are directed toward identification of people at risk for mental illness; identification of stressors, both actual and potential; and development of programs that decrease, remove, or modify risk factors through education, positive reinforcement, assertiveness training, and self-help groups. Examples of primary prevention include:

1. Providing classes for adults with elderly parents or people who provide caregiving services to older adults to help them learn about the normal aging process and community services available to cope with the stress of being responsible for an elderly person
2. Providing consultation services to self-help groups
3. Teaching individuals to talk about feelings rather than acting out feelings

Secondary prevention involves early recognition of illness and prompt treatment, with the goal of decreasing the impact and duration of the illness. Nursing activities involve early case finding through screening and periodic examinations of populations at risk, monitoring of clients, and direct service. Examples of secondary prevention include:

1. Providing counseling services to caregivers of abused children and the children
2. Providing intake screening and assessment of clients in emergency rooms
3. Teaching techniques of stress reduction to community groups, such as fire fighters, airline pilots, health workers
4. Providing screening services in shelters for the homeless mentally ill

Tertiary prevention involves decreasing or prevention of long-term impairment from disease. The goal is to reduce the effect of the disease on the client. Nursing activities include reeducation and resocialization of clients. Rehabilitation services are used to help the client to become productive members of the community. Examples of tertiary prevention include:

1. Providing discharge planning for groups of young chronically mentally ill clients
2. Monitoring follow-up care for the chronically mentally ill in shelters, halfway houses, and nursing homes
3. Teaching work-readiness skills or psychosocial education to the mentally ill
4. Serving as an advocate for psychiatric educational programs for caregivers

Clients were moved out of the large mental hospitals into the community *(deinstitutionalization)*. The focus of care changed from custodial care and management to prevention and rehabilitation. The client population shifted to include not only the chronically mentally ill but clients with Alzheimer's type of dementia, the homeless, the unemployed, the elderly, the abused, and persons who abuse substances. This change in client population and treatment setting has increased the need for the services of the community mental health nurse. Since 1980 three new subspe-

cialties in community mental health have emerged: geropsychiatry, liaison nursing or mental health consultant, and psychiatric home health nursing. This trend toward development of subspecialties will continue primarily because of the development of new knowledge in mental health, public concern, and funding priorities.

CASE MANAGEMENT

Providing services to the mentally ill so that they can function in the community has been described as fragmented and uncoordinated. Before deinstitutionalization, the provision of food, shelter, clothes, health care, supervision, and protection were all offered in a single location by the mental hospital. Now, after deinstitutionalization, these services have become the responsibility of numerous formal and informal government and community agencies. The need to coordinate these services had led to the development of case management.[3]

Case management is an approach to providing treatment for the chronically mentally ill in the community and an effort to provide cost containment and accountability. The goal of case management is to enhance the quality of life of the chronically mentally ill, facilitate their survival in the community by making sure their basic needs are met, encourage personal growth, promote community participation, and foster recovery from or adaptation to mental illness.[30] Case management has been defined as a system of health assessment, planning, service procurement, delivery, coordination, and monitoring through which multiple service needs of clients can be met.

There are two models of case management used in nursing. The rehabilitation model focuses on services being provided as part of a time-limited, private benefit plan with the goal of returning the client to a productive role in society. The case manager's main function is to act as a broker of services to link clients with needed services. The second model's main focus is supportive; it is not time-limited, and an advocacy model is used to link needed services to clients. Case managers not only coordinate and link needed services to clients, they also provide intermittent psychotherapeutic interventions, such as ways to handle roommate conflicts. This is important, since most clients do not continue in traditional long-term psychotherapy, and helping clients to handle everyday stressors can avert possible relapses. One of the advantages of case management that lasts over an extended time is a therapeutic alliance or trust that is gradually established between the client and the case manager. This alliance is used to facilitate the client's survival in the community. The case manager knows and understands her clients' strengths and weaknesses, and has an understanding of the informal support system, such as parents, siblings, and spouses. The therapeutic alliance between the case manager and the client helps the manager to provide continuous care that is flexible and meets the identified needs of the client, not the needs of systems providing the services.

THEORETICAL APPROACHES

There are several theoretical approaches that have relevance for community mental health nursing. A discussion of the systems and ecological approaches follows.

Systems

Systems theory, introduced by Ludwig Von Bertalanffy in 1933, is a universal approach that is applicable to many disciplines and allows human beings to be seen as complex wholes, therefore resolving the mind-body dispute. It can also be used to explain the relationship between human beings and their environment. Systems can be natural or artificial. Webster's Dictionary defines *system* as "a set or arrangement of things so related or connected as to form a unity or organic whole." Systems have certain characteristics of interest to nursing.

1. Hierarchic order indicates that each system is part of a greater system and also has components or subsystems, for example, city-state-country, individuals-families-community.

2. Systems are open and closed. They have boundaries that enclose them from the environment. In closed systems, there is no constant flow of energy and information between the system and the environment. The human being is an open system, and in an open system information flows freely between the system and the environment. This exchange of information and energy across the boundaries of the system is achieved with the system retaining its basic pattern or form. The system's ability to compensate and accommodate the information helps the system to maintain itself or keep a steady state and make needed changes for continued functioning. When the system cannot maintain its dual function of keeping a steady state and making the necessary changes, the system or part of the system will malfunction.

3. The subsystems or components of a system are interrelated and interdependent, and a change in one part causes a change in the other subsystems. For example, during employee layoffs there can be an increase in domestic violence; depression; suicide; robberies caused by financial need; feelings of helplessness, powerlessness, and hopelessness; and expressions of anger and hostility toward oneself and others.

▼ Case Example

Mr. Jones, a 50-year-old man, had been working at Plant A for 30 years. During this time, he had progressed to a salary of approximately $40,000 per year. He is married with two teenagers, both enrolled in the local high school. One son is graduating and preparing to go away to college. Mr. Jones was laid off from the plant in May 1990 and has not been able to get another job. Mr. Jones becomes despondent and stays in his bedroom, not dressing, refusing to eat, sleeping very little, and blames himself for the laying off of 200 people at the plant.

Mrs. Jones, a homemaker up to this point, decides to improve the family's financial situation and get help for her husband. A local community mental health center was contacted, and Mr. Jones is referred to an inpatient unit at the hospital, with outpatient treatment at the clinic upon discharge from the hospital. Mrs. Jones is helped by the nurse counselor at the mental health center to start college part-time, work in a department store part-time, and feel comfortable with her new role in the family.

The eldest son, who had planned on going away to school, was told that the family could not afford a university, and he must now go to the local community college and will be expected to help finance his education. The youngest son has reacted to the changes in the family by being sullen and hostile at school, picking fights, and refusing to do homework. He is picked up by the police for stealing in the local mall and referred through the Juvenile Court System to the same mental health center his father and mother attend.

This situation illustrates how changes in one system can affect other systems and subsystems. Mr. Jones, or the individual, is affected by the changes in industry, and this affects his family system. The role and function of each member of the family is changed. The changes in the family system affect the other systems in the community. The mental health system has to offer new services, ones for women and children. The educational and industrial systems have to change to allow for part-time instead of full-time progression and employment.

4. A system is more than the sum of its parts or components. In analysis of a system, the nurse assesses the system looking at all the subsystems and their interrelationships plus how the system relates to other systems, which includes looking at its functions and goals.

5. Feedback is a process that includes both input and output. Output discharged by a system is returned by external sources in the form of input to the system. There are two types of feedback (1) negative, which produces change in order to correct errors and leads to increasing order and complexity in the system and (2) positive, which maintains the status quo by validating or reinforcing current operations of a system. For example, Mr. and Mrs. Jackson have been married for 4 years. For the last 3 years, Mr. Jackson has been drinking heavily and physically abusing Mrs. Jackson. Mrs. Jackson has talked to family and friends, and they have all told her to stop complaining, that Mr. Jackson's behavior was not unusual; she should try harder to understand. After several months of questioning Mr. Jackson's behavior, Mrs. Jackson accepted the abuse and no longer questioned it. Mrs. Jackson, by chance, watched a television program on abuse and afterwards started again to wonder about her husband's behavior toward her.

Mrs. Jackson had been receiving positive feedback from her family and friends regarding the functioning of Mr. Jackson. This input, or feedback, maintained or validated the system (marriage) operation. The information (input) from the television program was negative and led Mrs. Jackson to question her decision about the correctness of her husband's behavior.

Ecological

The ecological approach builds on the systems theory approach to the study of human behavior. The term "ecology" was first proposed in 1869 by a German biologist, Ernst Haeckel, to mean the study of the relationship between an organism and its environment. Through the years the ecological concept has gained wide acceptance in both the biological and the behavioral sciences as a way to study the total environmental effect on organisms. The ecological model emphasizes a holistic view of people and their total environment, noting the interactive nature of community functioning.

Human ecology, which refers to the study of people and their interdependence with the environment, is composed of essentially three parts: a philosophy, a set of principles, and an attitude. The human ecological philosophy values the study of people as holistic organisms continually affecting and being affected by their environment. The environment includes the external and the internal environment of a person. Thus a change in either environment influences a person's equilibrium. Within this framework, mental health and mental illness can be judged only in relation to the context in which they occur. Essentially all problems of people are specific to the individual and his or her particular situation.

Principles of ecology, derived from systems theory, explain how people live together within the confines of their environment. Three principles of ecology—adaptation, cycling of resources, and succession—elaborate on the philosophy and further explain the interaction between people and their environment. People strive to adapt to environmental stimuli to maintain system stability. People's behavior depends on the relationship between their system stressors and their adaptive abilities. Favorable ecological conditions (adaptors) motivate a person toward a state of health or positive adaptation, whereas unfavorable influences direct the person toward illness or maladaptation. However, each person has a finite supply of adaptive responses; the rate and variability of stressors include the quality of adaptive response. Too much change too fast can disrupt system stability. The ecological attitude refers to a respect or an appreciation for the total universe.

All systems have a finite system of physical and psychosocial resources. These resources may be tangible, such as shelter, or intangible, such as a positive, nurturing emotional climate. Because people do not have unlimited reserves of coping capacity or resources, communities need to provide mechanisms to cycle their resources before they are depleted.

The principle of succession holds that living systems are never stable or static but rather are in a constant state of change. Succession means that a state of openness and receptivity exists in the environment; this diminishes predictability and also increases the need for reserves of adaptive energy.

The focus of an ecological approach is on the essential holism of human problems. Both an ecological view and a holistic view imply that the health of a person is more than

the sum of a person's body parts. Likewise the health of the community is more than the total of all residents. The community serves as a potential source of strength when an individual faces assaults against maintaining equilibrium. The community is the support system for human existence and ultimately the basis for all survival. The theoretical approaches are summarized in Table 26-2.

THE ROLE OF THE COMMUNITY MENTAL HEALTH NURSE

The role of the nurse in the community mental health movement has been difficult to define. Community mental health nursing practice is no longer confined to the community mental health centers. Many times, the nurse's role in the movement has blurred with the traditional functions and roles of the other mental health professionals. The task and functions of psychiatric nurses in community mental health are often indistinguishable from those performed by the psychologist, social worker, and the psychiatrist. Nursing's practice has run the gamut from clients with AIDS, crack cocaine babies, and rural mentally ill, to the chronic, homeless, and mentally ill roaming the urban streets. Nurses provide crisis intervention, psychotherapy, case management, and psychosocial rehabilitation services to their clients. Because of the nurses' wide range of activities in the community mental health movement, nurses need a variety of skills.

In the 1982 American Nurses' Association's Guidelines for Psychiatric Nursing and Mental Health Nursing, Standard 10 outlines the role of nurses in the community health system:

The nurse participates with other members of the community in assessing, planning, implementing, and evaluating mental health services and community services that include the promotion of the broad continuum of primary, secondary, and tertiary prevention of mental illness.

The Guidelines also specify that the role of the nurse in the community mental health system is within the scope of practice of the clinical specialist, a nurse with a master's degree in psychiatric–mental health nursing. Therefore the preferred qualifications for nurses working in community mental health settings are that they be registered nurses who are either graduates from a master's or doctoral program in psychiatric–mental health nursing with a clinical specialization. Other nurses also work in community mental health, and these nurses are called *generalists.* They are either diploma, associate degree, or baccalaureate degree graduates and have acquired increased specialized knowledge and skills in psychiatric–mental health nursing through continuing education programs, workshops, and experience.

The work setting and functions of the nurse in community mental health depend on the nurse's educational preparation, skills, and experience. The nurse using the title "Community Mental Health Nurse" may be employed in many different settings, including but not limited to community mental health centers, adult day care centers, home health agencies, shelters for the homeless, and school systems. In these diverse settings, nurses function in various direct and indirect roles. *Direct practice roles* involve the

▼ **TABLE 26-2** **Summary of Theoretical Approaches**

Theory	Dynamics
Systems	The community is composed of numerous subsystems that are in constant interaction, with compensatory changes occurring as the various components interact with each other.
Ecological	The people in the community and their environment are interdependent. A change in the internal or external environment influences the person's equilibrium.

▼ **TABLE 26-3** **Direct and Indirect Roles with Related Functions**

Roles	Functions
DIRECT	
Clinician	Provide direct technical nursing care; dispensing and monitoring of medication; screening and evaluating clients; testifying in court; providing aftercare for clients; teaching the chronically mentally ill simple skills such as budgeting, use of public transportation, and housekeeping.
Therapist	Establish and lead support groups. Provide various types of psychotherapy. Provide therapy to caregivers of chronically mentally ill clients with AIDS and the elderly.
Educator	Teach residents of the community about stress reduction. Provide skill-training classes. Serve as a resource for the community in mental health.
Case Manager	Assessment of client needs, strengths, and deficits and development of a treatment plan. Linkage of client with needed services and monitoring of service delivery and act as client advocate. The goal is to support the client in the community.
INDIRECT	
Consultant	Provide knowledge to other professionals and paraprofessionals who are working directly with clients, e.g., nursing home staff who need to learn how to handle aggressive behavior of the chronically mentally ill or the wandering behavior of Alzheimer's clients.
Case Manager	Act as a broker for groups of clients and help them to obtain the services (health, housing, transportation, financial, and educational) they need and monitor the delivery of the services. The goal is to help the clients become productive members of society.
Researcher	Identify clinical problems suitable for research and utilize current research in clinical practice.
Educator	Act as a resource person for other professionals. Keeping other professionals aware of nursing research that has relevance for community mental health. Provide continuing education programs for other professionals.
Change Agent	Provide the leadership in the community by forming coalitions of concerned citizens to affect health care legislation. Participate in community organizations that plan programs of care.

nurse working directly with populations at risk. *Indirect roles* involve the nurse providing clinical expertise and knowledge to other health care providers who use that knowledge to meet the mental health care needs of the community. For example, the nurse may provide an indirect service to health care providers in nursing homes, adult day care settings, in the school systems, or to policy and program planners. The focus of indirect service is prevention of mental illness. The direct and indirect roles in which the nurse functions are presented in Table 26-3.

One of the indirect roles of the community mental health nurse is that of educator. The following example illustrates the educator role. A 5-day, 30-hour mental health training program was presented by mental health nurses to seven groups of primary care nurses. The purpose of the program was to increase the primary care nurses' knowledge and skills about depression. The program emphasized criteria for assessing depression, psychopharmacological and psychotherapeutic content, and care coordination and referral resources. As a result of the program, participants became more skilled in recognizing depression symptoms and potential suicide. This had a positive effect on client care by providing more timely access to mental health treatment.[6]

GOALS

The goals of community mental health nursing are derived from the needs of clients and from knowledge and research about the prevention and treatment of mental disorders. The goals are diverse and include, but are not limited to, the following:

1. To provide prevention activities to populations and communities for the purposes of promoting mental health and securing participation in self-help activities (primary prevention)
2. To provide opportunities for interventions as early as possible when families, special interest groups, and communities experience a level of stress, tension, and lack of organization that affects their abilities to handle affairs of daily living and to work in satisfying and effective ways (secondary intervention)
3. To provide corrective learning experiences for client groups who have deficits and disabilities in the basic competencies needed to cope in society and to help individuals develop a sense of self-worth and independence (tertiary intervention)
4. To anticipate when populations become at risk for particular emotional problems and to identify and change social and psychological factors that diversely affect people's interaction with their environments (primary prevention)
5. To develop innovative approaches to primary prevention activities
6. To assist in providing mental health education to populations at large to demystify stereotypes about mental health and illness and to teach people how to assess their mental health
7. To provide leadership in the field of community mental health nursing as the care of the mentally ill becomes entirely a community-based endeavor

▼ **TABLE 26-4** **Categories of Homeless**

Chronic Disability	Personal Crisis	Economic Conditions
Alcoholics	Victims of domestic violence (elderly, women, and children)	Newly laid off workers
Persons who abuse chemical substances	Runaway teenagers	Part-time workers
Chronically mentally ill	Victims of divorce	Elderly
	Individuals with chronic health problems	Single parents
	People recently discharged from hospitals and jails, with no permanent housing	

SPECIAL POPULATIONS

Community mental health nurses provide care to many special populations, including the homeless, individuals at high risk for AIDS, rural populations, the elderly, and the abused.

The Homeless

There are approximately 4 million homeless people in the United States, and this number is thought to be increasing yearly. The reasons for this increase are complex. They include social, economic, and political factors. The homeless have been divided into three categories—people with chronic disability, personal crises, and economic problems[41] (Table 26-4).

Homelessness has been described as a process that exists on a continuum (Figure 26-1); one that leads to residence in the street, a public shelter or mental institution; a lifestyle characterized by absence of adequate housing and affiliation bonds to family, friends and community.[18,27,36] Basic needs of the homeless include food, adequate low-cost housing, appropriate clothing, access to both physical and mental health services, educational opportunities, job training, and social services. Major problems include substance abuse, which includes both alcohol and crack cocaine, as well as high risk for contracting human immunodeficiency virus (HIV), the etiological agent of acquired immunodeficiency syndrome (AIDS).[36]

Who are the homeless? They are the bagladies, people sleeping on steam grates or bathing in public facilities and eating out of garbage cans. They are the invisible subpopulation in the urban and rural areas, the "nobodies" seen yet not "acknowledged" as part of the community.

Before the late 1970s, the homeless were characterized as older men who were either alcoholics or had a history of alcohol abuse. They were the "hobos" and "skid row" characters romanticized in the 1940 and 1950 movies, the people who "panhandled" on the urban street corners and the train and bus terminals. They moved from place to place, living a marginal existence. Over the past 15 years, the homeless population has changed. They are of all ages and races, with varied backgrounds and educational levels. The homeless include men, women, teenagers, and families with children. There is also an increased number of chronically mentally ill individuals, many of whom are schizophrenic and homeless as a result of deinstitutionalization.

Some young adult severely mentally ill individuals who have either never been hospitalized or were hospitalized only briefly are among the homeless.[36,57]

The Homeless Mentally Ill

The failure of deinstitutionalization has been given as the reason for the increased number of mentally ill persons being counted as part of the homeless population. Many professionals question the reason for the chronically mentally ill being such a large percentage of the homeless population. Are the mentally ill homeless because of their illness, or are they mentally ill because of the effects of homelessness? Many times the bizarre behaviors of the homeless mentally ill may not be an indication of illness; instead they may be an attempt to master the environment. For example, burning paper money at night may be an effort to prevent being robbed.[27,41]

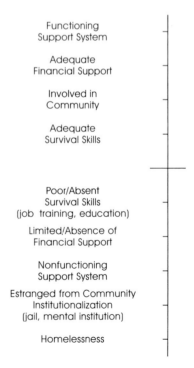

Functioning
Support System

Adequate
Financial Support

Involved in
Community

Adequate
Survival Skills

Poor/Absent
Survival Skills
(job training, education)

Limited/Absence of
Financial Support

Nonfunctioning
Support System

Estranged from Community
Institutionalization
(jail, mental institution)

Homelessness

FIGURE 26-1 Homeless continuum (movement toward homelessness).

The chronically mentally ill homeless have been described as having the following characteristics[5,25,28,40]:

1. Mobile—frequent movement from one residence to another, one geographic area to another, and having episodic homelessness
2. Social isolates and disaffiliated
3. Vulnerable to stress and abuse
4. High level of alcohol and drug abuse
5. Ineffective coping skills—difficulty in performing activities of daily living, financial management, and personal hygiene
6. Difficulty in articulating needs for services, which includes vocational and educational opportunities
7. Noncompliance in taking medication

The American Psychiatric Association Task Force on the Homeless Mentally Ill recommendations for care of the chronically mentally ill in the community includes the following[34]:

1. Basic needs of food, shelter, and clothing
2. Appropriate supervised housing in the community
3. Comprehensive and accessible psychiatric and rehabilitative services
4. Accessible medical care and crisis intervention services
5. A support system in community for clients
6. The development of laws and procedures that guarantee clients' rights to treatment in the community
7. Improve coordination between funding sources and implementation agencies
8. Education of professionals and paraprofessionals to provide community care
9. Provide for general social services
10. Hospitalization for clients that need these services
11. Research etiology and treatment of homeless chronically ill
12. Accurate epidemiological data
13. Increase funding for long-term community care

Community mental health nurses have been identified as some of the best prepared mental health professionals to monitor and provide services to the chronically mentally ill, including the homeless subgroup. Nurses should participate not only in direct care but also in indirect care by being involved at the state and national levels in the planning of services for this population.[31,43]

High-Risk Population for Acquired Immunodeficiency Syndrome (AIDS)

Acquired immunodeficiency syndrome (AIDS) is at epidemic proportion in the United States and is one of the nation's most serious health problems. It is estimated that approximately 1.5 million Americans are infected with human immunodeficiency virus (HIV); the percentage of these persons who will develop AIDS is unknown, but high.[13] The prevalence of HIV in the homeless is thought to be double that found in the general population and higher in the chronic mentally ill subgroup of the homeless.[12] Homeless women are especially high risk for AIDS because of the high frequency of unsafe sexual contact. This contact is either through mutually agreed sex, rape, or use of sexual activity as a way to get money and shelter.

The mode of transmission of HIV includes the following:

unsafe sexual practices (nonuse of condoms); sharing of intravenous needles, which is the most common form of blood exposure; body fluid contact on unprotected skin and mucous membranes; and mother-to-child transmission from an infected mother to her fetus.

To prevent sexual transmission, the only absolute method is not to be sexually active. Other sexual practices that are unlikely to transmit HIV include mutual masturbation; dry kissing; body-to-body rubbing; and use of condoms when engaged in oral, vaginal, or anal sex. For IV drug users, no sharing of needles, and washing needles and syringes with bleach before use helps to prevent transmission. Ways to prevent other modes of transmission of HIV include use of gloves to prevent body fluid contact on skin.

Strategies for preventing and treating HIV infection are inadequate (see the research highlight on p. 533). Community mental health nurses acting as this population's case managers can be advocates for this population to make sure educational programs are offered, utilize the system to coordinate needed services, monitor outcomes, and teach prevention strategies such as the use of condoms and nonsharing of needles; teach the social skills needed to negotiate for services; and the verbal skills needed to protect themselves in interpersonal situations.

Rural Populations

People living in the rural areas of the United States have a great need for mental health services. The Commission on Mental Health[41] stated:

Rural communities tend to be characterized by higher than average rates of psychiatric disorders, particularly depression, by severe intergenerational conflict, by restricted opportunities for developing adequate coping mechanisms for facing stress and problem solving, by an exodus of individuals who might serve as effective role models for coping, by an acceptance of conditions as being beyond individual controls, and by acceptance of fatalistic attitudes and minimal subscription to the idea that change is possible. (p. 904)

Yet, many times, the mental health needs of rural people are not met, or they have been limited to crisis intervention, outreach programs, and long-term hospitalization.

There are several factors that account for this situation. The great distance rural clients have to travel to reach mental health facilities; the reluctance of the rural population to accept the need for mental health care because of the stigma attached to mental illness; the shortage of mental health personnel; and the fragmented, inaccessible mental health and social services found in many rural communities. To provide effective mental health services to the rural communities in the United States, the community mental health nurse needs to be aware of the value systems of the people. These values include strong individualism, emphasis on primary relationships and family ties, traditionalism, fatalism, the strong work ethic, conservative beliefs, and strong religious values.[47] These values influence the identification of certain behaviors as pathological and effect the type of treatment sought and accepted. The ecological systems approach can be used in assessment and planning for treatment of the problems and identification of high-risk populations in the rural communities.

RESEARCH HIGHLIGHT

Preventing and Treating Human Immunodeficiency Virus Infection in the Homeless

• M Fetter and E Larson

PURPOSE

The purpose of the study was to gather data from health care providers to the homeless regarding factors associated with the prevention and treatment of HIV infection in homeless persons.

SAMPLE

The sample consisted of health care providers at 19 agencies funded by a national foundation to deliver health care and related services to homeless people. The agencies were located in major metropolitan areas. The estimated populations of homeless at the agencies ranged from 700 to 70,000 people per night, with a median of 5000 per night.

METHODOLOGY

A questionnaire, developed and administered by the principal investigator, was used as a guide for telephone interviews. The questionnaire contained 21 questions related to the target city and its homeless population, and factors and activities related to the prevention of HIV in-

fection. The response rate was 100%; responses were coded, sorted, and compared.

FINDINGS

Prevention and treatment activities included testing, counseling clients and sexual partners of high-risk persons, educational programs, primary care to the clients, and referral services. There were problems with obtaining reliable data regarding the prevalence of IV drug use and HIV seropositive in the homeless. Formal evaluation of services was needed. There was also a gap in AIDS education for the homeless according to the types (financed) of shelter, for example, religiously affiliated shelters usually prohibited condom distribution but city financed shelters did not. Lack of day care, respite, hospice, and case management for homeless individuals with HIV infection was also noted.

IMPLICATIONS

The services that are available for the prevention and treatment of HIV infection in the homeless need to be improved. Mental health nursing, clinical research, and public policy have a role in the prevention and treatment of HIV infection in the homeless.

Based on data from *Archives of Psychiatric Nursing,* 4(6):379, 1990.

Elderly

The current estimate is that there are more than 31.0 million persons over the age of 65 living in the United States. By the year 2030, the elderly will represent more than 20% of the United States population.[2] Most of these elderly Americans live in the community, with 2% in nursing homes or long-term care facilities. Approximately 15% to 25% of the elderly living outside of long-term care facilities have need for mental health services and 60% to 80% of the elderly living in long-term care facilities have mental behavior problems.[19]

Providing mental health services to the elderly in the community is challenging for several reasons. Decreased mobility in the elderly make many services inaccessible, the stigma associated with mental illness in the minds of many older people, the lack of trust in the effectiveness of the service by the elderly, and the ageism biases on the part of many mental health professionals leads to nonuse of mental services when they are provided. Other reasons for difficulty include the belief of the elderly and many mental health professionals that mental illness and cognitive problems such as changes in memory are a normal factor in aging; therefore treatment is not needed. Many times physical and psychiatric diseases have the same symptoms, plus physical disease may have psychiatric symptoms before physical symptoms appear. The tendency of elderly people to describe all illness in terms of physical complaints reinforces the emphasis on physical care. In addition, many

medications such as reserpine, guanethidine, steroids, digitalis, and diuretics can cause psychiatric symptoms that result in the elderly being labeled as mentally ill when a change in their medication will erase the problem.[1]

The two most common psychiatric disorders of the elderly are dementia of the Alzheimer-type and depression. Depression is one of the most treatable psychiatric disorders, but many times in the elderly it is overlooked and undertreated. Reasons for the misdiagnosis and/or lack of diagnosis of depression in the elderly include the difficulty in differentiating symptoms of depression from symptoms of early dementia, the acceptance of the symptoms of depression as a consequence of the normal aging process by many elderly and health professions, the fact that many times the depressed elderly clients' symptoms include cognitive complaints such as disorientation, agitation, memory loss, and preoccupation with vague physical symptoms such as constipation, headaches, muscle pain, and gastrointestinal upset rather than complaints of depression, such as sadness, guilt, and loss of interest in family and friends. There is no specific diagnostic test for depression, but screening tests such as the Beck Depression Inventory (BDI) and the Geriatric Depression Scale (GDS) are useful in the elderly population. Treatment includes psychotherapy, psychopharmacology, as well as electroconvulsive therapy on an inpatient or outpatient basis.[6,8,40]

Dementia of the Alzheimer-type is the most common dementia found in elderly people living in the community.

Approximately 2 million people in the United States suffer from this dementia, which leads to progressive loss of mental faculties. It is estimated that 1 million of the 1.5 million persons in nursing homes suffer from this disease and, by the year 2000, over 7 million people will have dementia.[16,40] The etiology of Alzheimer's is unknown, but there are several theories (see Chapter 33).

For the community mental health nurse, the goal of care is to help people with Alzheimer's function in the home and community as long as possible and to educate the community about the disease and needs of the client. The focus is on the families and professional and nonprofessional caregivers of the Alzheimer's clients.

Mental health care of the elderly in the community has a two-prong focus. The first is to help the elderly cope and adapt to their environment. To meet this goal, community mental health nursing focus is on (1) providing community education, which includes coping skills for at-risk populations and the community; (2) providing guidance for predictive life crises; (3) acting as an advocate for the elderly by working for changes in social policy that effect elderly negatively.

The second part of the two-prong focus is providing support to the professional and nonprofessional caregivers, which includes the family of the elderly by emphasizing the importance of the caregiver's role and need for community services to support this role. Community services needed include home-delivered meals, housekeeping services, home health care, respite care, adult day care, transportation, mental health counseling, psychological education, and support groups.[16]

The Abused

Violence is a community health problem. Human abuse is one form of violence seen in the community. Human abuse is an expression of hostility against oneself and others. Abuse occurs regardless of age, sex, education, and social economic levels. Types of abuse include spouse abuse, child abuse, sibling abuse, and elderly abuse.

There are several forms of abuse: physical; psychological; and neglect, or omission. Physical abuse involves actual physical contact between the abuser and the victim or the vulnerable person. Sexual abuse is a form of physical abuse and can range from fondling to rape. Psychological abuse involves threats, demands, and gestures that indicate the victim can be harmed. The third form of abuse is neglect, or omission, which takes the form of withholding needed necessities from the victim. These necessities can be food, shelter, medicine, or anything that the omission of will cause the victim discomfort or threaten his or her well-being, either psychologically or physically.

It is common for the abuser to be a close friend or family member of the victim. Because of this, many times the victim has fear of retaliation or guilt about somehow provoking the attack. This fear of the abuse being repeated and the stigma of having someone close do these things many times prevents the victim from reporting the crime (see Chapter 34).

The role of the community mental health nurse is to prevent abuse by helping the community become aware of factors that influence or support violence, and to help the community to provide resources that support effective coping with life stressors and reduce the destructive elements in the community. Mutual help groups, parenting groups, and public education about abuse all help at-risk populations to cope. Work with communities to get public policy and laws changed to ensure availability of needed services and resources for both the abusers and the abused. Temporary shelters, sources of emergency funds, emergency transportation, counseling, and legal aid are all examples of resources and services needed in communities to deal with abuse. The overall goal of community mental health nurses is to increase community awareness of the abuse, regardless of the form or at-risk population, and to mobilize the community resources to prevent, solve, and manage the abuse.

NURSING PROCESS

The system and ecological theory emphasizes that the community is a system. As a system, the community is approached as a whole, interacting and reacting within a constantly changing environment. Therefore the community mental health nurse assessment involves an analysis of the total system and all its subsystems, plus an analysis of relationships with other systems and their effect on each other.

Assessment

Physical dimension The physical features of the community's environment directly and indirectly influence the resident's mental health. The residents have a need to grow and develop in a clean, safe, and uncrowded environment, free of excessive noise. The nurse understands that noise is essential to stimulate and maintain community functioning; however, excessive amounts can be detrimental to mental health. For example, excessive noise disrupts the performance of tasks that require concentration, increases errors in completing tasks, and causes decreased reading levels in children. Unpredictable noise can lead to increased aggression.[42] Sudden noises excite an individual's autonomic nervous system and temporarily disrupt his equilibrium.

Workers continuously exposed to high-intensity noise show an increased incidence of nervous complaints, nausea, headaches, instability, argumentativeness, sexual impotence, mood changes, and anxiety.[15] Industrial facilities in the community that have a high noise level may disrupt the residents' sleep patterns.

The nurse also determines the availability and accessibility of mental health services in the community. For example, how accessible, by public transportation, are the community health centers and other aftercare facilities? The deterioration of public transportation in the central city reduces the means residents use to get around, especially the elderly, poor, and youth. Residents of the community are less likely to use mental health services if they cannot be reached by public transportation.

When doing an assessment of the community the nurse attends to the number of persons with physical and psychological illness and disabilities. Physical and psychological illnesses cause emotional distress for the ill person and the person caring for him. The nurse also determines the residents at risk for developing physical and psychological disorders and disabilities that may affect their mental functioning.

Emotional dimension When assessing the emotional climate of the community, the nurse may observe fear when residents do not feel safe. The nurse collects data about the law enforcement services and patterns of patrolling the community. Such services need to be sufficient and allocated in ways that protect the safety and lives of the residents as well as their property. Break-ins, robberies, and rapes increase the fear and anxiety of community residents. High crime rates and a general feeling that their community is unsafe may also lead residents to feel despair and anger.

The nurse can gain a sense of the emotional climate by observing the freedom with which the residents use the streets and how they secure their homes. For example, if many of the homes have bars on the windows and doors, the residents feel unsafe. When walking in a community, is there a feeling that streets are safe or a feeling of impending assault?

The nurse assesses outlets the community provides for the expression of anger. For example, is there a gymnasium, recreation center, or basketball court that allows for indirect expression of anger? The nurse notes if there are discussion groups at facilities in the community that allow for verbal expression of anger and if residents are permitted to disagree during discussion of community issues. Generally, residents in a community are encouraged to control their anger or release anger in a productive manner through clubs, church groups, and professional groups formed to promote harmony and provide opportunity to talk about stress and not act out anger. The community may even deny that anger exists among its residents. The media may not report examples of anger but instead promote and report only examples of harmony. Evidence of anger in the community includes violence against a person (abuse) and property. When observing behavior in a school setting, the nurse may note anger expressed as acting out behavior and angry interactions with teachers. Yet, children in schools are punished for expressing anger many times by being spoken to in an angry manner, thus reinforcing the behavior. Unemployed men and women who feel powerless may respond with anger and strike out verbally or physically toward others.

Improvements in the community's response to clients' needs may give rise to feelings of hope. However, new community programs or urban development programs involving relocation of residents may leave them with feelings of anger and hopelessness.

The total community may express grief in response to losses that result from natural disasters such as floods, earthquakes, and tornadoes. During such experiences, the residents may be unable to support one another and need assistance from the nurse. The nurse assesses the strength and resources available to the community and encourages community use of the resources. While this is happening, the nurse may observe that the residents of the community express a kindred or fellow survivor feeling as they work together to rebuild the community.

Intellectual dimension The nurse assesses the residents' responses to changes such as an increased level of unemployment, the role of women, and the ethnic mix of community residents. Some communities may be so resistant to change that their mental health is adversely affected. In general, change improving the image of the community is viewed as positive, whereas change to a lesser status tends to have a negative influence. Some communities welcome innovations, whereas others are committed to the way they have always done things. When people and organizations introduce new ideas not involving the thinking of the residents, they are likely to encounter resistance and may be ostracized by the mainstream of the community.

Assessment of the educational services in the community is important. Educational services are needed for all residents: preschool children, school-age children, college-age young adults, and adults returning to school and continuing education courses, including those that meet the needs of retirees. The nurse learns about the availability of technical and vocational opportunities and determines if job retraining programs are available for the unemployed.

The nurse finds out how education is valued and what efforts are made by parents and community members to help young residents complete high school, attend college, or acquire skills that prepare them for employment. If education is devalued, some young adults may leave the community for education and employment. This action greatly affects the stability of the community.

The nurse assesses the community's coping behavior in relation to information seeking, direct action, inhibition of action, intrapsychic processes, and turning to others.[15] In appropriate information seeking, the residents are assertive in trying to find out what problems exist and what can be done to solve the problems. The residents engage in direct action when they do something about the problem, whether or not the action is effective. Rather than engage in action impulsively or ill advisedly, the residents, using skillful coping resources, postpone action until they have sufficient information. Denial, avoidance, and intellectualization are intrapsychic processes the residents use when they are limited in what they can do about problems. Realizing they cannot solve the problems in isolation, residents turn to one another for supportive relationships as a form of coping.

Social dimension The structure of buildings in the physical environment affects health. Architectural variables, including the distance between houses, affect social formation and friendship patterns. Neighbors meet and form friendships more readily if their dwellings face a common courtyard or if they use the same communal areas, such as a swimming pool or laundry room.[21] The nurse attends to the size of buildings in the community. In taller buildings there seems to be a higher crime rate and lower levels of overall tenant satisfaction. This may be caused by a reduced potential to see or identify intruders, the impersonal image of the tall structures, and a lack of a feeling of territory in such buildings. The size of the community also needs to be assessed. Residents of a small community may have a stronger support system because they are likely to know other people in the community. In a large community the residents are less familiar with neighbors and may feel isolated.

▼ **TABLE 26-5   NURSING CARE PLAN**

GOALS	OUTCOME CRITERIA	INTERVENTIONS	RATIONALES
NURSING DIAGNOSIS: Fear related to lack of safety for residents			
LONG TERM			
To provide a safe community	Accepts and adapts to changes in the community	Encourage residents to express feelings (negative and positive) about changes in the community	Encouraging residents to express their feelings will allow for correcting any cognitive distortions and decreasing any anxiety about the changes
		Invite residents to work on committees implementing the changes	Gives a sense of responsibility and commitment to changes
		Encourage expression of mistrust and threats to security	Reduces anxiety
	Initiates safety measures	Invite a member of the police force to come to a group meeting and discuss safety measures	Provides information and strategies for control Increases feelings of power over environment
	Demonstrates awareness of changes in safety	Encourage residents to participate in planning the changes in their community	Encourages feelings of control over the environment and commitment to plans
		Get news media to interview residents talking about changes in their community	Provides widespread dissemination of information about changes
	Demonstrates comfort in the community	Involve residents in organizing an evening walk through the community	Provides opportunity for socialization and reinforces the attitude that the community is safe
SHORT TERM			
To monitor the safety of the community	Recognizes need for safety measures	Encourage residents to discuss the type and number of crimes being committed in their community and strategies for prevention of crimes	Provides information and increases feelings of control and power over the environment
		Have television and news media write articles about community safety problems	Allows for communication to larger number of community residents
	Verbalizes understanding of problem	Provide each resident with a list of possible hazards in their community to review and discuss	Provides for involvement and feelings of control
		Encourage discussion of threats to security based on experience	Decreases anxiety and increases security
	Reports strange activity in community	Provide each resident with the emergency police number, names and telephone numbers of neighbors	Increases feelings of control over the environment and involvement with others
		Discuss importance of neighbors knowing each other and activities that happen daily in the community	Provides feeling of security and support
	Acquires watchdog	Review safety measures used by other community groups. Get the animal shelter to donate dogs to residents to use as watchdogs	Provides information to be used for decision making Provides a feeling of safety and companionship

TABLE 26-5 NURSING CARE PLAN —cont'd

GOALS	OUTCOME CRITERIA	INTERVENTIONS	RATIONALES
	Participates in crime watch program	Explain the purpose of a crime watch program and the importance of citizen participation	Provides information and an opportunity for involvement and feelings of control
		Distribute crime watch signs for members to display in community	Deters criminal activity in the community
	Enlists support of community members	Encourage residents to discuss issues of community safety with other groups, e.g., churches, clubs, school, and to bring one other person to safety meetings	Provides involvement and feelings of control over environment

The formal and informal communication system within the community is assessed. First, it is necessary to determine what media are available and their general rate of use. Next, it is useful to determine the quality and tone of the communication system. Questions may be raised about whether newspapers, radio, and television promote community harmony and competence or address the needs of predominantly one or selected groups in the community. In some communities, news reports receiving priority deal with crime, danger, and scandal. When residents are primarily exposed to negative messages, they are more likely to experience stress than if the media blend negative and positive factors. Informal channels of communication provide vital information about the community. Often people learn more about the community at the beauty shop, barber shop, or a bridge party than through multiple formal sources.

Population density leading to overcrowding or isolation can affect mental health. In general, the more people living in a community, the greater the stimulation, demands on one another, and general level of frustration. Areas of high density have been related to increases in mortality, level of juvenile delinquency, and admissions to psychiatric hospitals.[44] Culture influences whether crowding is perceived negatively or positively; some groups are able to tolerate closer physical proximity to family and friends. The opposite of overcrowding, isolation, may cause people to feel bored and alienated. These feelings can lead to withdrawal and lack of concern for the comunity, which can foster crime and violence in the community because no one feels responsible.

Spiritual dimension The community is assessed as to the number, availability, accessibility, and variety of religious institutions. The spiritual needs of all residents of the community may not be met when only a limited number of religious institutions are present in the community. Religious preferences and religious practices, regardless of denomination, have been associated with lower rates of mental disorders.[39] Nonreligious groups may be considered populations at risk because of a lack of social support, par-

ticipation, and control that being a member of a religious group might contribute. Communities vary in provision of peace and solitude for residents. Some have beautiful parks, lakes, or walkways where residents can rest, meditate, or commune with God or a higher power; others do not.

The nurse attends to subtle cues that provide information about a community's spirituality. For example, are there signs advertising open forums, speakers, and musical presentations of a spiritual nature? Are gatherings with a spiritual orientation appreciated and well attended?

Analysis
Nursing diagnosis

The following list provides examples of NANDA-accepted nursing diagnoses with causative statements.
1. Potential for violence to others related to inadequate police patrol
2. Diversional activity deficit related to lack of recreational facilities
3. Social isolation related to a climate of mistrust
4. Knowledge deficit related to inadequate educational institutions
5. Spiritual distress related to lack of religious affiliation

Planning

Table 26-5 gives an example of a nursing care plan with long-term and short-term goals, outcome criteria, interventions, and rationales related to community mental health nursing. These serve as examples of the planning stage of the nursing process.

Implementation

Physical dimension The nurse participates in encouraging the improvement and availability of mental health facilities and services by presenting statistics on mental health needs and the lack of current resources. She works with community organizations, such as local agencies on aging, to arrange for transportation to the community mental health centers and other aftercare services.

The nurse may intervene in problems with reading skills among children through treatment or referral of individuals. Determining ways to restrict uncontrollable noises near schools and residential areas may prevent the problem. Nurses can join forces with other mental and environmental health workers to build a strong case for adequately insulating schools and residences, and for establishing and enforcing appropriate building and zoning codes.[42]

Special implementations within the physical dimension include heightening community awareness of the need for safe playgrounds, parks, museums, and zoos where children can explore their world as well as learn and practice age-appropriate physical activities in a safe and carefully monitored setting. Since accidents are a major cause of injury and death, mental health–psychiatric nurses need to work with communities to provide safety in streets, prevent crime, regulate the use of guns, and decrease personal violence.

The nurse can write a column or an article in the neighborhood newspaper that focuses on safety needs. The nurse also solicits participation from the police to provide or refer residents to seminars on home security, personal defense, and gun control. Police and the nurse can assist residents in developing a neighborhood watch program to increase safety in the community.

Initially, the nurse intervenes in family violence by arranging for the abused spouse and children to go to a protected environment such as a domestic violence shelter. Then intervention focuses on providing emotional support while the spouse considers options such as family therapy or leaving the abusive situation. (See Chapter 34 for discussion of family violence or abuse.)

Attention to the workplace, where major hazards include chemicals, dusts, fumes, noise, heat, radiation, and vibration, is particularly important. In some factories workers are expected to complete their assigned activities in crowded, overheated, and poorly ventilated areas. A nurse can document the detrimental effects of such working conditions, lead or participate in planning a healthier work environment, and develop educational programs to increase workers' awareness of hazards in the work environment.

Emotional dimension Intervention in the emotional dimension is directed at making the community a place in which residents can experience feelings of joy, hope, compassion, and responsibility for self and others, and in which they can deal effectively with such feelings as fear, anger, guilt, anxiety, hopelessness, and despair. Institutions greatly influence the emotional tone of the community. Community mental health–psychiatric nurses play a vital role in helping agencies and institutions such as day care centers, schools, hospitals, and social agencies in recognizing a need for emotional expression among residents and an environment free of undue stress, ambiguity, and feelings of alienation or rejection.

A particularly useful way to meet emotional needs is through self-help or mutual-help groups. Essentially, *self-help* means supporting and encouraging people to take control of and responsibility for their own lives and health. The recipients of self-help also give assistance; participants help others as well as themselves.

Self-help groups are voluntary and involve face-to-face interactions in which participants have equal amounts of power and serve as a point of reference and support for one another. They provide social support to members through the establishment of a warm and caring group and increase members' coping skills by providing information and by sharing of similar experiences.

Support groups that can prove beneficial in most American communities are those for isolated or disrupted families, new mothers, widows, teenagers (especially teenage mothers), people who want to learn more effective ways of handling stress, and discharged mentally ill clients.

Active participation in self-help groups provides members an opportunity to use their personal strengths to exert greater control over their health. Members feel valued, in control, capable and successful, frequently for the first time in a long time. The use of self-help groups by professionals often necessitates learning a new role. Traditionally, mental health professionals have led groups. However, the key to effective self-help is for the professional members to aid in establishing the group and then decrease involvement so participants can assume responsibility. The value of such groups will increase, since they are inexpensive, available, and responsive to members' unique needs. Professionals facilitate recognition of the need for such groups, aiding in their implementation and evaluating their effectiveness.

Intellectual dimension In many instances the goal of community-oriented health education is to increase the degree of self-responsibility among the residents. Many opportunities for intellectual enrichment can be identified. For example, aging parent classes can enrich the health of older adults. These classes teach coping skills and provide adult children an opportunity to discuss their feelings and fears about their new role as caregiver.

When working with adult children as caregivers, the nurse can lead group discussions that focus on normal aging and its importance for mental health. Pamphlets can be distributed that cover principles of aging; this information can serve as a focus for group discussions. The nurse can also show films or use television programs on effective caregiving and lead a discussion of the topic afterward.

Social dimension The development of organizations providing opportunities for people to learn and practice interacting with one another is a useful approach to implementing plans in the social dimension. For example, in one town of about 50,000 residents, all youth in the junior high grades were involved in "rap groups" led by mental health volunteers. Over several years the nurse consultant with the city's mental health center had been able to develop a network in which all seventh, eighth, and ninth graders, in groups of 10 to 12 each, had a chance to informally discuss with an interested adult any topic of interest for 1 hour a week. Volunteers also met regularly with a mental health center counselor for supervision and encouragement. This program was the result of one nurse's dream and goals for enriching the mental health of young people in her community. This same type of rap group approach was also used in elementary schools.

Community mental health—psychiatric nurses can participate in the implementation of a variety of community groups based on a thorough assessment of community characteristics, needs, and resources. Groups not only serve to enrich coping abilities but can also work toward improving the overall health and competence of the community. Nurses can participate with other mental health professionals and community groups in planning any of the following types of projects.[18]

1. Building projects including schools, homes, airports, shopping centers, and recreational and health care facilities
2. Programs for special populations such as children, adolescents, the elderly, the handicapped, minorities, migrant workers, immigrants, chronically mentally disturbed people, and the homeless who are emotionally ill
3. Legislation affecting social practices including substance abuse, retirement, deinstitutionalization, unemployment, and job training
4. Regulatory bodies responsible for building codes, safety procedures, professional practices and policies, and investigation of accidents and disasters
5. Contingency groups formed to plan for epidemics, influx of migrants, and terrorism

Other community efforts to meet social needs include the development of neighborhood or lay networks in which residents turn to members of their own community for support and encouragement. Community mental health–psychiatric nurses can serve as catalysts in helping organize and encourage residents to form such networks.

In addition, nurses can work with or serve as consultants to a variety of social groups and institutions to help them recognize their full potential for meeting the social needs of participants. Groups such as Boy Scouts and Girl Scouts can be encouraged to recruit members not only from those eager to join but also from children who are isolated and feel alienated from their peers because of their social status, disabilities, homelessness, or other factors that may differentiate them from the general population of their peers.

Spiritual dimension Churches and synagogues, social groups, and other institutions influence the philosophy and orientation toward life of residents of the community. Community mental health–psychiatric nurses can serve as catalysts or consultants to assist religious and other groups to recognize their role and value in helping people cope creatively and effectively with life stressors. Religious leaders provide face-to-face counseling to people dealing with stressors. These leaders are often skilled in dealing with the whole range of needs of members of their congregations. However, some clearly may profit from the consultation provided by a nurse.

Religious institutions possess rich opportunities to strengthen the spirituality of members. Lay members of these institutions can also provide care and support to community groups. For example, churches and synagogues can develop helping groups for newcomers, widows, members of divorcing families, parents of handicapped children, released prisoners, or discharged psychiatric clients.

Evaluation

Community program evaluation is often completed over an extended time and at intervals. For example, if a community goal was to decrease the effects of noise on children living near the airport, evaluation may occur at intervals of 6 months or 1 year. Changing building codes and increasing insulation in homes and schools are lengthy processes;

therefore accurate evaluation of the goal takes time and repeated measures. Such measures provide information about how long people and communities "feel better" and how resistant they remain to stressors.

Evaluation of community programs answers questions such as: How well did the project work? How many people (communities) benefitted? Specifically, what gains were noted? Evaluations are often most effective when they represent the thinking of the whole planning group.

Evaluation of community-oriented efforts seeks to measure either the organizational structure and its impact on the program's quality, effectiveness of the process, or the outcome derived from the program or project. Evaluation of the structure involves asking questions such as Were there enough resources supplied? Were the resources supplied in a timely manner? This approach is used to determine the impact of the organizational patterns on the delivery of services. Process evaluation examines the roles and activities of the participants and determines to what extent their efforts have been positive or negative. The process approach is used to determine problem areas. In contrast, outcome appraisal methods look at the results of the project and raise questions, for example, about the degree to which noise levels were decreased and how many parks were developed.

BRIEF REVIEW

Community mental health nursing is directed toward the mental health needs of the total community. Special attention is given to high-risk populations, which include the elderly, the abused, the homeless, and individuals at high risk for AIDS. Systems theory and ecological theory can be effectively applied to mental health nursing in the community. The community is viewed as a system in interaction with other systems. Change and adaptation are ongoing processes in the community.

The nurse assumes direct and indirect practice roles in the community. Nurses bring about changes in the community through use of various treatment modalities, such as self-help groups. Nurses also make a contribution to the mental health of the community by sharing their knowledge and clinical expertise with other health care providers. The goals of the community mental health–psychiatric nurse are based on the needs of the community and are directed toward promotion of health and prevention of long-term disabilities.

REFERENCES AND SUGGESTED READINGS

1. Abraham IL and others: Outpatient psychogeriatric nursing services: an integrative model, *Archives of Psychiatric Nursing* V(3):151, 1991.
2. American Association of Retired Persons: *A profile of older Americans,* Washington, DC, 1990.
3. Anthony W and others: Clinical care update: the chronically mentally ill, case management—more than a response to a dysfunctional system, *Community Mental Health Journal* 28(3):20, 1989.
4. Bachrach LL: The challenge of service planning for chronic mental patients, *Community Mental Health Journal* 22(32):170, 1986.
5. Bachrach L: The chronic patient: planning high-quality service, *Hospital and Community Psychiatry* 42(3):268, 1991.
6. Badger T and others: Assessment and management of depres-

sion: an imperative for community-based practice, *Archives of Psychiatric Nursing* 4(4):235, 1990.

7. Baker F, Douglas C: Housing environments and community adjustment of severely mentally ill persons, *Community Mental Health Journal* 26(6):497, 1990.

8. Belcher J, DiBlasio F: The needs of depressed homeless persons: designing appropriate service, *Community Mental Health Journal* 26(3):15, 1990.

9. Bellack AS and others: A comprehensive treatment program for schizophrenia and chronic mental illness, *Community Mental Health Journal* 22(3):175, 1986.

10. Bloom BL: *Community mental health: a general introduction,* ed 2, Monterey, Calif, 1984, Brooks/Cole Publishing.

11. Carling PJ and others: Psychosocial rehabilitation program as a challenge and an opportunity for community mental health centers, *Journal of Psychosocial Rehabilitation* 10(1):39, 1986.

12. Carmen E, Brady S: AIDS risk and prevention on the chronic mentally ill, *Hospital and Community Psychiatry* 41(6):652, 1990.

13. Centers for Disease Control: First 100,000 cases of acquired immunodeficiency syndrome, *Mortality and Morbidity Weekly Report* 38:561, 1989.

14. Chamberlain R, Rapp C: A decade of case management: a methodological review of outcome research, *Community Mental Health Journal* 27(3):171, 1991.

15. Cohen F, Lazarus RS: Coping with the stresses of illness. In Stone GC, Adler NE, editors: *Health psychology: a handbook,* San Francisco, 1979, Jossey-Bass.

16. Collins C and others: Knowledge and use of community services among family caregivers of Alzheimer's disease patients, *Archives of Psychiatric Nursing* 5(2):84, 1990.

17. Crosby RL: Community care of the chronically mentally ill: a theory for practice, *Journal of Psychosocial Nursing and Mental Health Services* 25(1):33, 1987.

18. Drake RE, Wallach MA, Hoffman JS: Housing: instability and homelessness among aftercare patients of an urban state hospital, *Hospital and Community Psychiatry* 40:46, 1989.

19. Dellasega C: Meeting the mental health needs of elderly clients, *Journal of Psychosocial Nursing and Mental Health Services* 29(2):10, 1991.

20. Ebben P, Bliss D, Perlman B: Problems and issues in community mental health services delivery in the 1990s, *Community Mental Health Journal* 27(3):225, 1991.

21. Festinger L, Schacter S, Back K: *Social pressures in informal groups,* Stanford, Calif, 1950, Stanford University Press.

22. Fetter M, Larson E: Preventing and treating human immunodeficiency virus infection in the homeless, *Archives of Psychiatric Nursing* 4(6):379, 1990.

23. Fraser MW and others: The community treatment of chronically mentally ill: an exploratory social network analysis, *Journal of Psychosocial Rehabilitation* 9(2):35, 1985.

24. Gold Award: A network of services for the homeless chronic mentally ill, *Hospital and Community Psychiatry* 37(11):1148, 1986.

25. Goldfinger S: Introduction: Perspectives on the homeless mentally ill, *Community Mental Health Journal* 20(5):387, 1990.

26. Gomez G, Gomez E: Chronic schizophrenia: The major mental health problem of the century, *Perspectives in Psychiatric Care* 27(1):7, 1991.

27. Grunberg J, Eagle P: Shelterization: how the homeless adapt to shelter living, *Hospital and Community Psychiatry* 41(5):521, 1991.

28. Harris M, Bachrach L: Perspectives on homeless mentally ill women, *Hospital and Community Psychiatry* 41(23):253, 1990.

29. Hutton FM: Self-referrals to a community health centre: a three year study, *British Journal of Psychiatry* 147:540, 1985.

30. Kanter J: Clinical case management: definition, principles, components, *Hospital and Community Psychiatry* 40(4):361, 1989.

31. Krauss J: New concepts of care, community, and chronic mental illness, *Archives of Psychiatric Nursing* 111(5):281, 1989.

32. Krauss J: Put the community back in mental health, *Archives of Psychiatric Nursing* 15(1):1, 1991.

33. Kuper J: Big ideas and little ones, *Community Mental Health Journal* 26(2):217, 1990.

34. Lamb HR, editor: *The homeless mentally ill: a task force report of the American Psychiatric Association,* Washington, DC, 1984, American Psychiatric Association.

35. Lamb HR: Community treatment for the chronically mentally ill, *Hospital and Community Psychiatry* 42(2):117, 1991.

36. Lamb HR, Lamb D: Factors contributing to homelessness among the chronically and severely mentally ill, *Hospital and Community Psychiatry* 41(3):301, 1990.

37. Lancaster J: *Community mental health nursing: an ecological perspective,* St Louis, 1980, Mosby–Year Book.

38. Lewis R: Undesirable neighbors, *American Journal of Nursing* 86(5):535, 1986.

39. Levy L, Rowitz L: *Ecology of mental disorders,* New York, 1972, Behavioral Publications.

40. Martin R: Update on dementia of the Alzheimer-type, *Hospital and Community Psychiatry* 40(6):593, 1989.

41. McFarland G, Thomas M: *Psychiatric mental health nursing: applications of the nursing process,* Philadelphia, 1990, JB Lippincott.

42. Monahan J, Vaux A: Task force report: the macroenvironment and community mental health, *Community Mental Health Journal* 16:14, 1980.

43. Pothier P and others: Dilemmas and directions for psychiatric nursing in the 1990s, *Archives of Psychiatric Nursing* 4(5):284, 1990.

44. Price RH and others, editors: *Prevention in mental health: research, policy, and practice,* vol 1, Beverly Hills, Calif, 1980, Sage Publications.

45. Steiner D, Marcopulos B: Depression in the elderly: characteristics and clinical management, *Nursing Clinics of North America* 25(3):585, 1991.

46. Susser E, Goldfinger S, White A: Some clinical approaches to the homeless mentally ill, *Community Mental Health Journal* 20(5):463, 1990.

47. Swan J, Fox P, Estes C: Geriatric services: community mental health center boom or ban, *Community Mental Health Journal* 25(4):327, 1989.

48. Swift C: Task force report: National Council of Community Mental Centers task force on environmental assessment, *Community Mental Health Journal* 18:7, 1980.

49. Torrey EF: Economic barriers to widespread implementation of model programs for the seriously mentally ill, *Hospital and Community Psychiatry* 41(5):526, 1990.

50. Wagner J, Hackenberg A: Highlights of the 41st Institute on Hospital and Community Psychiatry, *Hospital and Community Psychiatry* 41(1):19, 1990.

ANNOTATED BIBLIOGRAPHY

Badger T and others: Assessment and management of depression: an imperative for community-based practice, *Archives of Psychiatric Nursing* 4(4):235, 1990.

This article describes a mental health training program for primary care nurses that addresses primary and secondary prevention issues of depression. The authors propose a community-based educational program that can be offered by psychiatric liaison nurses. They emphasize the use of educational material that is culturally and developmentally sensitive.

Calsyn RJ, Morse G: Homeless men and women: commonalities and a service gender gap, *American Journal of Community Psychology* 18(4):597, 1990.

This article is a report of a research study that examined gender differences among homeless persons on a host of variables. Findings that are useful in planning to meet the needs of the homeless population based on gender, especially in the area of service utilization, are presented.

Carmen E, Brady S: AIDS risk and prevention for the chronic mentally ill, *Hospital and Community Psychiatry* 41(6):652, 1990.

This article describes the high-risk population for AIDS and the barriers to health education. Measures for AIDS prevention for the chronically mentally ill in the community are presented.

Chafetz L, Barnes L: Issues in psychiatric caregiving, *Archives of Psychiatric Nursing* 3(2):61, 1989.

This research article reports the results of a descriptive study of 20 family caregivers of psychiatrically disabled individuals. The families were from community agencies and hospitals. Major concerns and needs for support were identified.

Rife JC and others: Case management with homeless mentally ill people, *Health and Social Work* 16(1):58, 1991.

The article reports the findings of a National Institute of Mental Health (NIMH) services demonstration project that used a mobile case management team to serve the homeless mentally ill. Implications for providing case management services to homeless mentally ill people are presented.

Sophronia R Williams

After studying this chapter, the student will be able to:

- Define crisis
- Define crisis intervention
- Describe the historical development of crisis intervention
- Describe selected theoretical models of crisis intervention

- Discuss the characteristics of the crisis therapist
- Discuss the characteristics of crisis intervention
- Apply the nursing process in crisis situations
- Identify current research findings related to crisis situations

Crisis is an inevitable aspect of human existence. Individuals are constantly confronted with potentially crisis-producing events that threaten their level of functioning. The ongoing changes and pressures in today's society test the person's ability to effectively use problem-solving behaviors and may cause the individual to experience a crisis situation that cannot be resolved without professional assistance.

A *crisis* occurs "when a person faces an obstacle to important life goals that is, for a time, insurmountable through the utilization of customary methods of problem solving."[16] Situational supports may help prevent the crisis or decrease the intensity of the reaction to the crisis, but in today's mobile society family and close friends often are not accessible to provide support. Individuals then turn to mental health professionals for crisis intervention. *Crisis intervention* is an active entering into the life situation of a person, family, or group who is experiencing a crisis to decrease the impact of the crisis event and to assist the individual to mobilize his resources and regain equilibrium.[39]

Nurses are constantly confronted with clients who are in a potential state of crisis. Regardless of the area in which they work, nurses are available to implement the concepts and techniques of crisis intervention with a mother who has given birth to a physically or mentally handicapped child, in the emergency room, with an automobile accident victim, and with families of clients who have had surgery or a heart attack and are told "nothing more can be done."

THEORETICAL APPROACHES

Psychoanalytical

Eric Lindemann's initial contributions[49] to the theory of crisis intervention are based on his scientific investigation of the behavior of people experiencing an acute grief reaction. The sample of 101 people studied consisted of disaster victims of the 1942 Coconut Grove fire in Boston and their close relatives, clients with psychoneuroses who had lost a relative during the client's treatment, relatives of members of the armed forces, and relatives of clients. Lindemann concluded that grief and bereavement as a response to loss by death lead to a crisis in almost all individuals, and most will experience a *normal grief reaction*.

A bereaved person who experiences a normal grief reaction manifests a characteristic syndrome that consists of (1) somatic distress, (2) preoccupation with the image of the deceased, (3) expression of guilt and hostility, (4) disorganization in daily patterns of activity, generally with a decrease in level of activity, and (5) sometimes identification with the deceased. The duration and intensity of the grief reaction vary among individuals, depending on the extent to which the person successfully completes the grief work.

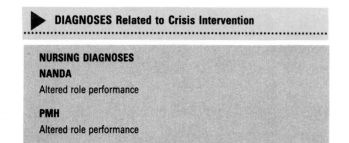

▶ **DIAGNOSES Related to Crisis Intervention**

NURSING DIAGNOSES

NANDA
Altered role performance

PMH
Altered role performance

DATES	EVENTS
1906	First recorded instance of "crisis intervention" concerned Freud's treatment in six visits of client with partial paralysis in an arm.
1940s	Principles and techniques of crisis intervention were derived from the use of supportive techniques to treat soldiers suffering from crises related to combat during World War II. Psychiatrists, on their return home after the war, used the techniques that were effective with soldiers to deal with survivors of civil and military disasters.
1944	Lindemann's classic study of bereaved victims of the Coconut Grove nightclub fire established a format for the study and development of crisis theory and practice.
1948	Lindemann refined his crisis concepts and organized an innovative community mental health program in Boston. Caplan elaborated on Lindemann's model and became known as the father of modern crisis intervention.[33]
1950s	The development of crisis intervention paralleled brief or short-term psychotherapy.
1950s-1960s	Caplan developed his interest in crisis situations out of his early work with immigrant mothers and children in Israel after World War II. Caplan's approach to crisis intervention was set in the format of primary, secondary, and tertiary levels of intervention at the Harvard School of Public Health.
	Parad, Rapoport, Jacobson, and Aguilera, building on the work of Lindemann and Caplan, refined crisis theory and developed treatment models for crisis in marital and family conflicts and in suicide prevention.
	The Community Mental Health Act of 1963 influenced the development of crisis intervention. One requirement of the Act was that community facilities provide emergency services.
Mid-1960s	Crisis intervention became a treatment modality in its own right.
1970s	Caplan focused his attention on natural and mutual support systems in the community that could be used to prevent or ameliorate the destructive aspects of crisis situations.
1980s	Nurses have increased their involvement with crises in a variety of inpatient and outpatient settings.
1990s	Rapid, increasingly complex social changes threaten people's stability and coping behavior, increasing the need for nurses to give priority to crisis intervention as a means of preventing psychiatric problems.
Future	There will be increased use of crisis intervention techniques to prevent rehospitalization of individuals with chronic mental illness.
	Mobile crisis intervention services will be used as an outreach approach to provide treatment for individuals who cannot or will not use other types of crisis services.

Normal grief work begins when the individual frees himself from ties to the deceased, readjusts to his social environment, and establishes new and satisfying relationships. Although this process may be accomplished without professional assistance, some individuals with a normal grief reaction need professional help. Lindemann found that with the guidance of a mental health professional in 8 to 10 interviews and within 4 to 6 weeks, these individuals successfully completed grief work.

Lindemann found that survivors of the Coconut Grove disaster who developed serious psychopathological conditions had failed to go through the normal process of grieving. This led him to describe *morbid grief reactions*, in which individuals experience either a *delayed* or a *distorted* reaction. People may delay or postpone their reaction to the loss for a few weeks or longer. A distorted

reaction may be an immediate response to bereavement and includes overactivity without a sense of loss, taking on symptoms belonging to the last illness of the deceased, the development of a medical problem, and agitated depression.

Lindemann believed that his work with the bereaved was basic to the development of a conceptual framework related to emotional crises. He viewed the birth of a child and marriage as examples of events that could generate sufficient emotional strain to lead to crises. The preventive intervention that is effective with bereavement can also be applied to these events. He believed that when crises are properly managed, prolonged and serious alteration in social functioning can be avoided.

One aspect of crisis theory that Lindemann introduced and that Caplan described in depth is the different types of crises. He acknowledged the influence of Erikson's model[25] of developmental (maturational) and situational (accidental) crises on his theories about life crises.

Caplan defined *developmental crises* as transitional periods in personality development characterized by disturbances in cognitive and affective functioning. These crises are experienced by everyone as they learn to adjust to the new expectations related to the various maturational periods in life. The discussion of Erikson's developmental stages in Chapter 4 includes examples of this type of crisis.

A sudden, unexpected threat to or loss of basic resources or life goals is a *situational crisis*. These crises are not as common as the developmental ones and are characterized by periods of psychological and behavioral disorganization that occurs when the individual is unable to cope by his usual behavior. Such crises may be precipitated by fires, floods, earthquakes, and other natural disasters that affect large numbers of people. The Coconut Grove fire is an example of a disaster that led to a crisis. Loss through divorce, the death of a loved one, and a job promotion or demotion are also examples of events that may trigger a situational crisis.

Caplan[17] observed the reactions of clients with psychiatric disorders to situational crises such as the death of a significant other, the loss of a job, or becoming a parent. These problems were new to the clients, and their usual coping behavior did not work. Clients who dealt with the problem in adaptive ways seemed healthier after than before the crisis. Based on his observations, Caplan concluded that there are universal responses to crises. An individual with a relatively stable personality may change in ways that are unexpected during a crisis. The outcome of the crises may be a positive change in personality, in which case the crisis was a period of opportunity, or the crisis may result in decreased efficiency in the individual's ability to cope. These notions lead to the view of crisis as a transitional period that affords the individual both an opportunity for personality growth and the danger of greater vulnerability. Either response to the crisis is determined by the individual's handling of the situation.

Caplan believed that mental disorders may decrease if individuals are assisted in improving their problem-solving skills, which in turn increases their ability to deal effectively with stress. He considered a crisis a turning point toward or away from mental disorders and believed that intervention at the point of crisis can prevent later serious mental illness. Caplan viewed crisis intervention as a major technique of *preventive psychiatry*. Preventive psychiatry focuses on using theoretical knowledge and skills to plan and implement programs designed to achieve three categories of prevention: *primary*, *secondary*, and *tertiary*.[17]

Primary prevention involves decreasing the incidence of psychiatric illness in the community. It is designed to intervene in hazardous situations with the goal of preventing the development of psychiatric disorders. Thus an aspect of primary prevention is the promotion of general mental health. The goals of primary prevention are achieved by activities such as providing educational programs to groups in the community, consultation to school teachers, identifying groups at risk, and designing and implementing programs to prevent psychiatric disorders. For example, sex education for teenagers who are at risk for pregnancy is a type of primary prevention.

The focus of secondary prevention is early diagnosis and prompt and effective treatment to reduce the duration of a significant number of psychiatric disorders. When people in crisis receive early effective intervention and regain equilibrium, their chances for developing a long-term disability decrease. When the first psychiatric illness of a young adult is treated early and effectively, he may not develop a chronic psychiatric problem. Individuals who need treatment for psychiatric problems may be identified through screening large populations referred for treatment. One setting in which screening procedures are conducted is the school. Educating the public to recognize early signs of psychiatric disorders may be effective for secondary prevention. Individuals who require secondary prevention may be hospitalized or may engage in some form of psychotherapy.

Tertiary prevention refers to the reduction of long-term disability that may result from psychiatric disorders. Individuals with chronic psychiatric illnesses benefit from tertiary prevention. Rehabilitation programs are designed for tertiary prevention.

Jacobson, Strickler, and Morley classified two types of treatment approaches to crisis: the generic approach and the individual approach.[41] The *generic approach* is based on the premise that certain identifiable patterns of behavior are characteristic of each type of crisis and that psychological tasks specific to the type of crisis are required if the crisis is to be successfully resolved. Treatment of the crisis is focused on the characteristic course rather than the psychodynamics of the particular crisis type. Treatment also is designed for the target group rather than a specific individual. For example, in the crisis of a child with terminal cancer the mother must accomplish the psychological task of accepting that the child will likely die and must prepare for the impending loss.

The client and therapist participate together in the problem-solving process. The generic approach to problem solving encourages the use of adaptive behavior, includes general support, and allows for manipulation of the environment and anticipatory guidance. Jacobson and others[41] believed that because of the specificity of the approach, it can be used by nonprofessionals and others not trained in crisis intervention.

The *individual approach* emphasizes assessment of the intrapsychic and interpersonal process of the person in crisis by a mental health professional. The crisis therapist focuses on identification of the precipitating factors and examines reasons the individual's usual coping mechanisms are no longer effective. Once the therapist achieves these goals she determines the intervention that is necessary to improve the client's coping abilities. The therapist knows the psychodynamics of crisis. Various situational crises that a person experiences may be treated effectively with the individual approach, as this approach is directed toward the individual's unique situation.

Baldwin[3] developed a classification system that describes six general types of crises in relation to the degree of psychopathology, the cause of the crisis, and implications for effective interventions. As each type moves from a lesser to a greater degree of psychopathology, the cause becomes more internal than external. The model is based on the assumption that crisis intervention requires assessing the emotional crisis rather than making a diagnosis in a tradi-

▼ **TABLE 27-1** Classification of Emotional Crises

Class	Type	Characteristics	Source	Example
1	Dispositional crises	Caused by distress that arises from a problematic situation in which intervention is not directed at the emotional level	External	Providing information to a mother about parenting classes
2	Anticipated life transition crises	Relates to normal life transitions over which the person may or may not have control	External	Getting married; midlife career changes; retirement
3	Crises resulting from traumatic stress	Precipitated by externally imposed stressors that are unexpected and uncontrolled	External	Rape; sudden death of a family member; sudden loss of job
4	Maturational or developmental crises	Relates to an attempt to achieve emotional maturity by completing developmental task; involves a struggle with a deep-seated, unresolved issue	Internal	Emancipation from an overprotective parent
5	Psychopathological crises	Preexisting psychopathological condition precipitates the crisis or complicates resolution of crisis	Internal	Client with severe anxiety disorder or pathological dependence
6	Psychiatric emergency crises	Severe psychiatric disorder with severe impairment; incompetent; danger to self or others	Internal	Psychosis; drug overdose; acutely suicidal

tional psychiatric sense. The classification of the crisis, the characteristics, and an example of each type are presented in Table 27-1.

Systems

An aspect of Caplan's work is based on systems theory. The first to relate homeostasis to crisis reactions, Caplan recognized that a goal of human functioning is to maintain a homeostatic balance with the environment. The individual is constantly faced with situations that threaten his balance. Usually the individual readily activates habitual problem-solving activities that effectively restore a steady state. When one is faced with a crisis, however, the usual habitual mechanisms cannot reestablish equilibrium within the usual time span. When unsuccessful in solving the problem the individual enters the phases of a crisis. Caplan[17] elaborated on crisis therapy by describing four characteristic phases of a crisis. The stages and responses are depicted in Figure 27-1.

Parad[60] introduced the idea that the person must perceive the precipitating event as stressful before it becomes a crisis. This premise is discussed later in the chapter. Parad and Resnik,[62] using a different approach than Caplan's characteristics of a crisis, described the crisis sequence in terms of time periods: the precrisis, the crisis or upset, and the postcrisis (Figure 27-2). During the *precrisis period* the individual maintains his equilibrium through his usual coping methods. He may have minor stresses, but they are not perceived as threatening to his life goals. A threat to life goals is a hazard to the individual's basic security needs such as body integrity, love, or a sense of security. If the person perceives an event as a threat to life goals and one with which he is unable to cope, he enters the *crisis period*.

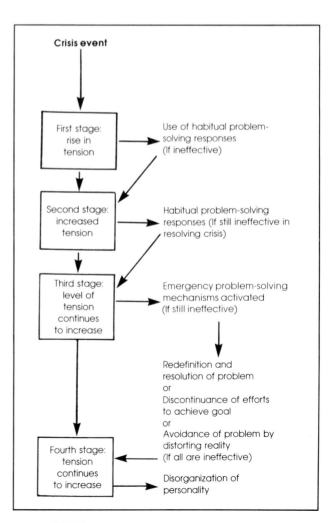

FIGURE 27-1 Caplan's developmental stages of a crisis.

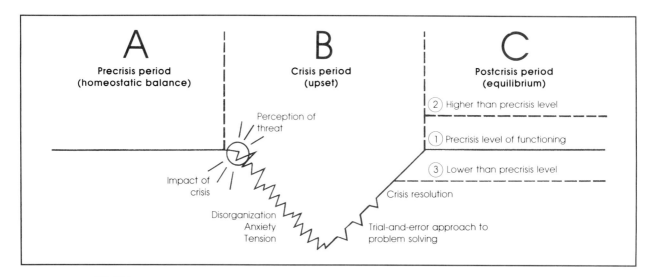

FIGURE 27-2 Crisis sequence diagram. *(Modified from Parad HJ and others. In Resnik HLP, Ruben HL, Ruben DD, editors: Emergency psychiatric care; the management of mental health crises, Bowie, Md, 1975. Reprinted with permission of Charles Press, Division of Robert J Brady Co, from the copyrighted work Emergency Psychiatric Care.)*

The crisis period begins at the time of the impact of the crisis.

During a crisis the individual experiences disorganization, tension, and anxiety and uses various trial-and-error responses to resolve the crisis. *Crisis resolution* is the development of effective adaptive and coping devices based on the client's use of his own resources through the intervention of health care professionals and with assistance from family and significant others.[62]

With resolution of the problem the individual experiences a *postcrisis period*. This period is characterized by a return to the steady state, and the individual may resume his precrisis level of functioning or perhaps a higher or lower state of functioning, depending on the effectiveness of the crisis resolution. The theoretical approaches are summarized in Table 27-2.

CHARACTERISTICS OF CRISIS INTERVENTION

Client Selection

The initial consideration in client selection is the determination that the client is experiencing a crisis. A traditional and still widely accepted criterion for selection is that the client is dealing with a recent, sudden life situation that requires immediate attention and that the client cannot solve himself. The client must have a clearly defined environmental stress such as the loss of a job, acute bereavement, marital discord, or suicidal gestures that can be resolved rapidly.

Some therapists believe that only clients who are fairly well integrated and who have never had a psychiatric illness can receive the maximal benefits from crisis intervention. Other therapists select clients with previous psychiatric problems who are now experiencing a crisis. Still others include clients who are experiencing their first psychotic breakdown and those with chronic psychiatric symptoms

who are in remission.[48] Janosik[42] believed that chronically depressed clients, alcoholics, individuals with psychoses, and withdrawn persons without reliable social networks are not appropriate candidates for crisis intervention.

It is generally accepted that crisis intervention techniques are effective with individuals in crisis regardless of their socioeconomic background. However, the client must have the ability and motivation to participate in the problem-solving process. The client's level of motivation is determined in part by the extent to which he shares information and the specific information that he shares. Some therapists expect the client to acknowledge a target problem in two or three sessions or the therapy is terminated.[22]

In addition to individuals, families are suitable candidates for crisis intervention. To be selected for crisis intervention the family must accept the crisis situation as a family problem, regardless of the precipitating event or the family member who is perceived as responsible for the crisis.[22]

The therapist uses her knowledge of *crisis-prone persons* as an aid in the selection of clients. The crisis-prone person has been described as an individual who has no available support system or is unable to use one, if it does exist, in his efforts to cope with everyday stress.[62] The person lives a marginal existence and may manifest the following interrelated problems:

1. Difficulty in learning from experience
2. History of frequent crises and unsuccessful resolution of the crisis because of the person's poor coping skills
3. History of previous psychiatric disorders or serious emotional instability
4. Low self-esteem, which the individual may attempt to disguise by provocative behavior
5. Impulsiveness, manifested by taking action before the person thinks through the consequences
6. Poor work history in an unfulfilling job that results in a marginal income
7. Faulty marital and family relationships

8. Alcohol and drug abuse
9. Tendency to have numerous accidents
10. Frequent contacts with law enforcement agencies
11. A tendency to change residence frequently

Therapeutic Settings

Crisis intervention is provided in a variety of settings. The nurse has many opportunities to perform crisis intervention in formal settings such as emergency rooms. In these settings, the nurse may encounter relatives of accident victims and of clients who may be faced with a serious life-threatening illness, such as a heart attack, who are in need of crisis intervention. Rape victims, clients who have made suicide attempts or threats, individuals with homicidal behavior, and those who have experienced drug overdoses are possible clients for crisis intervention in the emergency room setting. In some instances, the nurse refers the client to a crisis team in the emergency room after she does a cursory assessment and establishes that the client may be in crisis.

Crisis intervention centers and crisis units in community mental health centers are other formal settings in which the nurse conducts crisis intervention. In these settings, ambulatory clients who are making suicidal threats or are experiencing a situational crisis, such as a grief reaction in response to a loss, an unwanted pregnancy, or reactions to environmental disasters, such as tornadoes and floods, are candidates for crisis intervention. Other candidates include individuals who need assistance with their adjustment to a development crisis, for example, adolescent turmoil. The nurse may function in formal agencies for special populations such as adolescents, children, and families when these agencies use crisis intervention as a treatment modality.

Another formal setting in which the nurse frequently intervenes in crisis is on units in the general medical hospital. Clients may react to impending surgery with a crisis reaction, especially when the surgery will result in the loss of a body part and other changes in body image. The stresses associated with any physical illness may precipitate a crisis that requires the nurse to use her knowledge and skills in crisis intervention. Families may need crisis intervention directly after the death of a family member.

Telephone hot lines are semiformal approaches to providing crisis intervention. They may provide crisis intervention services on a 24-hour, 7-day-a-week basis. Generally, trained nonprofessional volunteers operate the telephone services, with consultation from members of a professional mental health staff. Among the consultation services provided by way of telephone hot lines are suicide prevention and crisis intervention for rape victims.

Special Characteristics and Process

Most major crisis theorists accept Caplan's premise that a crisis situation is self-limiting, lasting from 1 to 6 weeks.[17] The average crisis lasts 4 weeks; however, the 1- to 6-week time frame for the therapeutic process is flexible, varying according to the needs of the client.

The focus of treatment is the individual's current life experiences that relate to the crisis. The client's previous

▼ **TABLE 27-2   Summary of Theoretical Approaches**

Theory	Theorist	Dynamics
Psychoana-lytical	Lindemann	Grief and bereavement in response to death leads to a crisis.
		The response to death as a crisis may be a normal grief reaction or a morbid grief reaction: a delayed or distorted response.
	Caplan	There are developmental and situational crises.
		A crisis may lead to decreased efficiency in one's ability to function, or may be experienced as an opportunity for growth.
		Crisis intervention is a major type of preventive psychiatry: primary, secondary, and tertiary prevention.
	Jacobson and others	Generic approach: Each type of crisis has identifiable patterns of behavior and characteristics and specific psychological tasks for successful intervention.
		Individual approach: Emphasizes an assessment of the intrapsychic and interpersonal process of the person in crisis.
	Baldwin	Classification system that describes six types of crises in relation to degree of psychopathology, the cause of crisis, and implications for effective interventions.
Systems	Caplan	A crisis is a threat to homeostasis.
		The individual's usual problem-solving activities cannot restore equilibrium.
	Parad and Resnik	The event that precipitates a crisis must be perceived as stressful by the individual.
		There are three time periods in a crisis sequence: precrisis, crisis, and postcrisis.

experiences related to unresolved conflicts are a part of the therapeutic work only to the extent that they influence the current crisis situation.

Balancing factors

Three interrelated *balancing factors* contribute to the production of a crisis and influence the outcome of the crisis.[1] These balancing factors, which occur between the perceived effects of a stressful situation and the resolution of the problem, are (1) perception of the event, (2) available situational supports, and (3) coping mechanisms. The upper portion of the paradigm in Figure 27-3 illustrates the "normal" initial reaction of an individual to a stressful event. The presence or absence of these factors affects the return of equilibrium. In column A of Figure 27-3, the balancing factors are operating and crisis is avoided. In column B, one or more of these balancing factors are absent. Resolution of the problem may be blocked, thus increasing disequilibrium and precipitating a crisis.

In Figure 27-4 the paradigm is applied to Tom and Mark who were affected differently by the same stressful event. Both men recently became unemployed due to a production slow down. The supervisor told each man the reason for the layoff. The men have worked at the company for 7 years and had less seniority than other employees in the department. Each man's wife was employed outside the home. Tom is concerned about the layoff but does not experience a crisis. Mark reacts to the layoff with a crisis. What accounts for the differences in their responses to the same stressful event?

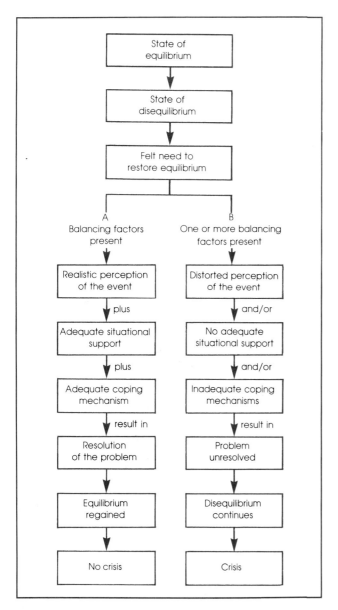

FIGURE 27-3 Paradigm: the effect of balancing factors in a stressful event. (*Modified from Aguilera DC: Crisis intervention: theory and methodology, ed 6, St Louis, 1990, Mosby–Year Book.*)

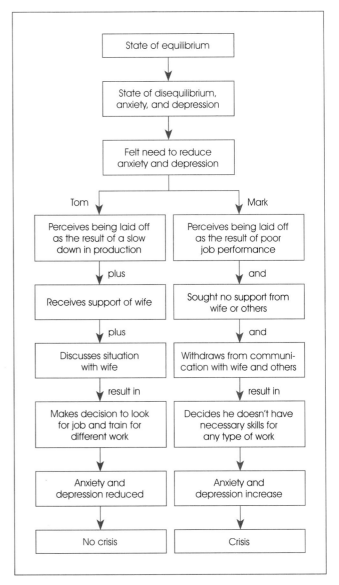

FIGURE 27-4 Paradigm applied to case study. (*Modified from Aguilera DC: Crisis intervention: theory and methodology, ed 6, St Louis, 1990, Mosby–Year Book.*)

Perception of the event

An individual's perception of a stressful event plays a major role in determining the nature and degree of his response to the event. The perception of the crisis event is determined in part by the extent to which the event is a threat to the individual's values and life goals. The crisis event may be perceived as a threat to basic needs that are related symbolically to needs that led to a conflict earlier in life. In this instance the predominant emotional response to the threat is anxiety. The crisis situation may be perceived as a loss. The loss may be real or it may be experienced as a deprivation. The response to the perceived loss or deprivation is a feeling of depression. If, on the other hand, the crisis is perceived as a challenge,[65] the individual mobilizes his energy and engages in purposeful problem-solving activities. Examples of challenges may be getting married, job promotions, and parenthood.

The individual's perception of the event may be realistic or distorted. If the person perceives the crisis event realistically, he will recognize the relationship between the event and his feelings of stress. He can then participate in problem-solving activities directed toward successful resolution. A distorted perception of the crisis situation leads to continued feelings of tension, and his attempts to resolve the problem are futile. These individuals do not recognize the relationship between the crisis event and their stress.

Differences in Tom's and Mark's perceptions in terms of the threat of the event to their means of livelihood account for the differences in their response behavior. Tom perceived the supervisor's actions as justifiable because there had not been sufficient work to keep them busy. He soon began looking for work and was willing to train for another type of job, if necessary. On the other hand, Mark believed the supervisor fired him because his work was not up to par. He thinks he does not have the skills necessary for another job. Tom's appraisal of the situation led him to anticipate success in his efforts to get a job. He experienced the event as a challenge and engaged in problem solving. Mark appraised the situation as overwhelming; he felt helpless and resorted to the use of intrapsychic defense mechanisms to distort the reality of the situation.

Situational supports

Situational supports, a second balancing factor, refer to available persons in the environment who can be depended on to help the individual solve problems. The situational supports become the individual's signficant others, and from them the individual learns to seek advice and support in solving daily problems. Individuals may readily develop dependent relationships with support persons who protect them from feelings of insecurity and thus reinforce their feelings of ego integrity.

Any perceived failure to obtain adequate support to meet one's needs may provoke or compound a stressful situation. Negative support can be equally detrimental to the person's self-esteem. When self-esteem is lowered by a threatening situation, the individual seeks out situational supports. When there is a loss or a threatened loss of a supportive relationship, the individual feels vulnerable. If faced with a stressful situation when there is lack of situational support, the person may experience a state of disequilibrium and possible crisis.

Tom had someone for support during the stressful event. He discussed the situation with his wife and together they decided how they could manage until he found a job. Mark anticipated a negative response from his wife, so he did not tell her about the layoff. He discussed the situation with no one; he felt alone, hopeless, and helpless.

Coping mechanisms

Coping mechanisms are the third balancing factor that affects an individual's ability to restore equilibrium after a stressful event. The individual's use of intrapsychic ego defense mechanisms to deal with stress and anxiety are discussed in Chapter 10. Coping mechanisms differ from intrapsychic ego defense mechanisms in that coping mechanisms may be consciously or unconsciously motivated, and they are used to deal with the minor stresses of everyday life. They also are attempts to solve the problem rather than to avoid it.

Through the process of daily living, individuals are confronted with what Menninger and others[53] referred to as *minor emergencies,* or problems that create disequilibrium. Through experience and by learning about their potentialities, individuals develop techniques for dealing with minor external and internal stresses. One way to deal with these stresses is by using the coping mechanisms of everyday living as stabilizers.

Various adaptive and maladaptive coping mechanisms are available when people experience minor emergencies or problems. They may try to think out their problems or talk about them with a friend. Some cry or try to get rid of their feelings of anger and hostility by swearing, kicking a chair, or slamming doors. Others may get into verbal battles with friends. Some may react by temporarily withdrawing from the situation to reassess the problem. The individual has used each of these mechanisms at some time in the developmental past and found them effective to maintain emotional stability. Thus the mechanism became part of the person's life-style in dealing with the stresses of daily living.

Maladaptive coping mechanisms may sometimes resemble ego defense mechanisms. Examples of such mechanisms are excessive fantasy, magical thinking, and withdrawal from reality.

Tom coped by talking to his wife; this approach reduced his tension and anxiety. He was able to engage in problem solving and make plans for getting another job. His tension and anxiety were reduced, equilibrium was restored, and he did not have a crisis.

Mark was uncommunicative. He used maladaptive coping skills by withdrawing. His anxiety and depression increased. He was unable to solve the problem and he went into a crisis.

A person who is in crisis usually seeks crisis intervention within 1 or 2 weeks of the precipitating event. Often, the event that led to the crisis happened within the 24 hours before the individual's arrival for therapy. By the time the client seeks crisis intervention, he is more vulnerable and capable of being influenced by others than when his equilibrium is in balance. Intervention at this point in the crisis can prevent later serious mental illness or the development of maladaptive patterns of behavior. Minimal interaction by the nurse can have maximal effect on the client's coping mechanisms and problem-solving activities. This influence promotes or impedes further development of the client's mental health. The client needs immediate attention. The longer the delay between the time the client requests help and the time he receives assistance, the greater the opportunity for the person to distort the crisis event.

The initial phase of crisis intervention is crucial to resolve the crisis. Sometimes this phase lasts only one session because with the nurse's assistance the client identifies and resolves the problem. Problem identification and resolution are the crux of crisis intervention. The focus of the therapeutic process is the client's perception of the problem. Anxiety affects the individual's perception of situations and his ability to solve problems. Clients in crisis are often experiencing a severe to panic level of anxiety. Thus their perceptual field is limited and problem-solving abilities become increasingly ineffective.

During the initial phase of therapy and preferably during the first session, the nurse actively guides the client in identifying the precipitating event that led to the crisis and the basis for his perception of the event as a crisis. The nurse needs to be persistent in learning the reason the client is seeking crisis intervention at this time. The nurse may ask directly, "What is your reason for seeking help *now* or *today*?" Another question that may be asked is, "What has happened in the last hour, day, or week to upset you?"

During the initial contact with the client, the nurse conveys to the client hope that the crisis can be resolved successfully. The nurse participates with the client in exploring his problem and clearly defines the goals for treatment and the activities necessary to achieve the goals.[66] The nurse communicates verbally and nonverbally that she will work *with* the client in resolving the crisis and regaining hope. With this support the client can leave the first session with the feeling that he can participate in solving the crisis. In subsequent sessions the nurse plans and implements specific treatment for the client that takes into consideration the client's motivation, strengths, and capabilities. The specific treatment is determined by the precipitating problem. For example, if the crisis is in response to a loss, the nurse guides the client in grief work.

Crisis intervention is terminated when the client has resolved the crisis. Some nurses use the maximum of six sessions as a criterion for termination. If in these instances additional therapy is needed, the client is referred for another type of therapy, such as short-term psychotherapy.[61] Preplanned follow-up interviews are recommended as an aspect of the termination phase. These interviews provide information about the extent to which the crisis is successfully resolved and serve as a safeguard if the client needs additional therapy. The client needs to terminate therapy with the feeling that the therapist is available if necessary.

CHARACTERISTICS OF THE CRISIS INTERVENTION THERAPIST

Qualifications

Many nurses have attended workshops or lectures on crisis intervention and therefore possess the basics of crisis intervention techniques. Nurses who work in community mental health centers and conduct therapy with clients who seek crisis intervention are required to have extensive education and training. In general, to qualify academically to perform therapy with clients in crisis, nurses need to have (1) 2 years of experience in an inpatient psychiatric hospital, (2) a master's degree in psychiatric nursing, and (3) a year of intensive training in crisis intervention at a community mental health center.

An increasing number of paraprofessionals with various levels of basic training and educational preparation are working in crisis centers. They are provided additional education and training that qualify them to perform crisis intervention in the role of mental health worker.

Irrespective of the academic preparation, all individuals who perform crisis intervention need to have knowledge and understanding of human behavior. More important, the precarious nature of crisis situations requires all persons working with clients in crisis to possess certain personal characteristics. The nurse needs to be a warm and caring person who is able to use herself as a therapeutic tool. Because crisis situations are intense and can be anxiety provoking for the therapist, an ability to tolerate intense painful emotions and keep the focus on the client are important attributes. She needs personal resources for coping with anxiety and other emotions so that she can assist the client.

The nurse needs to be confident in her ability to help the client in crisis. The feeling of confidence helps the client feel secure. A willingness to assume responsiblity for the client who may be unable to assume full responsibility for himself is an essential characteristic of the crisis nurse. She needs to be flexible and ready to respond at any time to a crisis situation. This means the nurse must be able to think quickly and achieve goals with little preparation time. Flexibility in the use of various commmunication techniques is also important. The nurse needs to be sensitive to the client's needs and relate to him positively.

Goals

A maximal goal is to help the client function at greater than the precrisis level. However, the nurse hopes to achieve a minimum of three basic goals. An immediate goal is to reduce the impact of the crisis. The nurse gives immediate attention to the anxiety, the tension, and the feeling of being out of control that the client is experiencing *now*.[62] She intervenes to protect the client from injuring himself and others, to reduce anxiety and guilt, and to prevent further disorganization. The second therapeutic goal is to provide an opportunity for the client to deal with the *nuclear problem*, using his previous problem-solving skills. A third goal is to assist the client in returning to his precrisis level of functioning. The nuclear problem is the underlying cause of the client's reaction to the precipitating event.

Role

The role of the crisis nurse differs from that of the nurse in traditional therapy roles because of the need to achieve the goals of therapy in a short time. An important role of the nurse is to rapidly establish a therapeutic relationship in which she and the client work to resolve the problem. The active involvement of the client conveys that the client's thoughts and ideas are important and that he has the potential for solving his problems.

The nurse's role includes quickly and accurately assessing the situation and quickly establishing a tentative formulation of the client's problem. She uses the information the client shares and her understanding of human behavior to identify the problem. At times the nurse needs to make life-and-death decisions quickly. Thus quickness and accuracy are crucial for effective and safe functioning.

In crisis intervention, the nurse assumes an active, direct, and involved role. She actively guides the client in exploring the problem. Instead of the passive use of reflection that characterizes some traditional forms of therapy, the nurse uses active and direct techniques such as confrontation and interpretation. She shows therapeutic involvement through empathic understanding of what the client is experiencing. The judicious use of touch is an example of the involvement of the crisis nurse with the client.

Even though the client participates in the process of crisis intervention, the role of the nurse is to demonstrate that she has the situation under control and is able to offer the client direction out of the problem. The nurse uses her role as resource person and teacher to assist in guiding the client toward resolution of the problem. The role of the nurse also includes providing whatever nurturing the client needs to reestablish equilibrium. While enacting this role the nurse avoids fostering unwarranted dependence.

NURSING PROCESS

Assessment

Physical dimension Clients generally manifest physical problems characteristic of depression and anxiety. Many of these physical symptoms are seen in the somatic reactions to grief described by Lindemann. The nurse collects data about any alteration of the client's sleep pattern, appetite, and weight. The individual in crisis may be unable to sleep for a few nights or for a few weeks, depending on the length of time he has been experiencing the crisis. Difficulty falling asleep, restless sleep with frequent awakening during the night, or early morning awakening are sleep patterns that may be typical for an individual in crisis. The client may have a poor appetite or complete loss of desire for food. The lack of sufficient food intake may lead to weight loss. A direct result of the sleep disturbances, poor appetite, and weight loss may be changes in body image. The individual may have dark circles and bags under the eyes. He may also be debilitated, with a low energy level and general physical deterioration.

Because of overwhelming anxiety, the client may think there is something physically wrong. During the assessment the individual may complain of stomach discomfort or a nervous stomach. The nurse may note more than the usual amount of gesturing and frequent shifting of seat position in response to the anxiety. The client may express his anxiety by foot and finger tapping. The physical symptoms related to anxiety may result in hyperventilation. Other physical manifestations of anxiety are discussed in Chapter 10.

Emotional dimension The individual's emotional reactions to the crisis experience are varied and require careful assessment. He may be in a state of severe emotional upheaval and feel out of control. Based on systems theory, the nurse attends to the client's state of equilibrium. The crisis creates disequilibrium and anxiety. Because individuals often perceive the event that precipitated the crisis as a threat to their survival, anxiety is one of the cardinal signs of a crisis. The nurse assesses the level of anxiety to determine the person's ability to participate in the problem-solving process. Anxiety may range from a moderate to panic level. With a moderate level of anxiety, the individual can participate in problem solving when directed to do so. As the anxiety increases to a severe level, the individual needs much assistance to problem solve. When anxiety reaches a panic level, the person is unable to problem solve, even with direction. The nurse needs to obtain information about the duration of the crisis. According to Caplan, the longer the individual has been unsuccessful in solving the problem, the higher the level of anxiety when the individual presents in crisis. The manifestations of anxiety described in Chapter 10 provide additional characteristics of the client in crisis.

Depression is another emotional state typically experienced by the individual in crisis because of the frequency with which the crisis is precipitated by a loss. During the first few minutes of the assessment, the nurse determines whether the client has engaged in any self-destructive acts such as threatened or attempted suicide. Suicide attempts and threats in conjunction with crisis are common. Even when the likelihood of suicide seems remote, the nurse assesses the person's current thoughts about self-destruction as well as past behavior when he was seriously depressed. The means of suicide are usually more available to this person than to a hospitalized client. If the client has made a suicide attempt (e.g., has taken pills), the nurse's first concern is the physical rather than the emotional state. Rapid assessment of the suicide plan according to the guidelines discussed in Chapter 14 is crucial. The potential for committing suicide is greater when the client has a plan. Thus the nurse asks the client what plan he has for committing suicide. How he plans to carry out the act helps determine the seriousness of the intent. For example, a plan to use a gun or jump from a building is more serious than taking an overdose of psychotropic medications. The nurse also needs to learn when the client plans to commit suicide. Plans for doing so in the middle of the day while members of the family are up and about may not be as serious as plans to do so after they retire.

In crisis intervention the nurse may need to assess the behavior of a suicidal client on the telephone. The box on the next page gives an approach for responding to telephone calls from a suicidal client.

Once the suicidal behavior or potential for it has been assessed, the nurse assesses the depressive behavior. The degree and duration of depression experienced by a person in crisis varies. The nurse attends to the severity of the depression to determine whether the client needs to be hospitalized. It is not uncommon for the individual to have profound feelings of despair and dejection. The person in crisis often feels hopeless because of his inability to resolve the crisis and the belief that no one can help him. Based on Caplan's theory, the nurse assesses for disorganization of the client's personality as his feelings of helplessness and

▼ ....
RESPONSE TO CALLS FROM SUICIDAL CLIENT

1. *Establish a relationship during which you maintain contact with the client and obtain information.* Assure the caller of your availability by listening nonjudgmentally. Convey interest and concern.
2. *Identify and clarify the problem.* The caller may be disorganized and confused and may need structure to help him determine what is important.
3. *Evaluate the suicidal potential to determine how close the caller is to harming himself.* Evaluate the information obtained in terms of factors such as age, sex, and suicide plan.
4. *Assess the caller's strengths and resources.* Use the information obtained to develop a therapeutic plan.
5. *Formulate a constructive plan and mobilize the caller's resources and those of others.* The resources available to the client may include family and close friends. Referral to a crisis clinic or recommendation of immediate hospitalization may be indicated. Arrange for these services.

hopelessness increase. The individual may cry uncontrollably and for prolonged periods, making it difficult for him to provide information.

Along with depression the individual may experience guilt and shame. Sometimes the guilt and shame are the client's responses to his need to seek professional assistance.

The client may express crisis by inappropriate anger directed toward other people, especially those who are trying to help. The anger may be brief but destructive enough to be considered homicidal. Most homicides occur in the home and may be the culmination of long-standing spouse abuse or parent-adolescent conflicts. The situation that initiated the homicidal ideas may become stressful enough to motivate the individual to seek crisis intervention. A person who has an aggressive, impulsive personality is a likely candidate for carrying out the homicide. When assessing the client's behavior, it is important to remember that an act of homicide may not be premeditated. Following are clues to homicidal intent or attempt[64]:

1. Threats made by the aggressor, such as "I will kill you next time."
2. A report that fights are generally limited to the kitchen or bedroom.
3. The presence of weapons in the home, especially guns.
4. An aggressor with impulsive behavior and a bad temper. After striking out, the person may insist that he did not intend to harm the victim.
5. A victim who tends to encourage the fights with belittling remarks.
6. A history of previous fights between the victim and the aggressor.
7. Injuries so serious that they might have resulted in death.

Chapter 11 discusses anger more fully.

Intellectual dimension The initial focus when assessing the intellectual dimension is eliciting the individual's perception of the crisis event. Using Parad's ideas, the nurse considers the situation a crisis if the client perceived the precipitating event as stressful. The client's perception may be realistic. Because of the intensity of the stress related to the crisis, however, individuals frequently distort the precipitating event. According to Caplan, this distortion of reality may lead to avoidance of the problem. The opportunity for distortion increases as the client waits for his request for assistance to be met. The less distorted the client's description of the crisis event, the more likely the problem can be solved.

When using the individual approach of Jacobson and associates, the nurse assesses the intrapsychic processes of the individual in crisis. The nurse may observe a narrowing of the person's perception in response to anxiety. When the situation is perceived unrealistically, the individual may resort to the use of intrapsychic defense mechanisms, such as repression and denial, in his efforts to cope. Attack, flight, or compromise are direct modes that may be used to cope when the situation is perceived realistically.

The nurse examines the mental status of the client. The client's ability to recall and to give an account of events leading to the crisis provides information about his intellectual activity. His level of anxiety may be severe and may greatly interfere with his recall of the events. In other instances the client may readily give an account of the situation. When the intellectual functions are intact and the client is alert, he is better able to participate in the problem-solving process.

The clarity with which information is communicated is assessed. In addition to crying, which was mentioned earlier as a possible barrier to verbal communication, the client may be unable to express his thoughts because of muteness. The muteness may result from feeling overwhelmed by the crisis situation. Anger may also interfere with the client's ability to give a logical account of the events that led to the crisis. The client may explode with a barrage of angry questions related to the misinterpretation of the crisis situation. The anger may motivate the client to work on resolving the crisis situation.

The individual's level of motivation to participate in crisis intervention is assessed in terms of his willingness to help himself. The individual can be asked directly whether he feels able to help work on his problems by performing certain tasks. For example, to assess the level of motivation the nurse asks the client directly to think about what led to the crisis. She can also elicit the client's willingness to participate in sharing the thoughts and feelings he is experiencing now. When assessing the level of motivation the nurse takes into consideration the emotional state and the intellectual functions that may be affected by the crisis and allows time for the client to respond.

Social dimension An individual in crisis usually experiences noticeable impairments in the social aspects of his life. Jacobson's individual approach that focuses on the person's interpersonal process provides a useful framework for the nurse's assessment of the client's relationship with family, friends, and co-workers. The nurse determines the quality of these relationships and if they are sufficient to meet the individual's need for social support. Because the availability of social supports is important when making plans to prevent or minimize the recurrence of problems, an assessment of who comprises the client's social network and the accessibility and reliability of social supports is essential. The composition of the social support is not as crucial as the accessibility of support.

The dependence needs of a client may be intensified when the client has to turn to another person for assistance. As the client seeks a crisis nurse to help him solve his problems, he may talk about feelings of helplessness and convey a need to be taken care of. In a crisis situation the client is more helpless and more amenable to being helped than at any other time in his life.

The nurse determines whether certain events have led to a situational crisis as described by Caplan, for example, the discovery of an extramarital relationship or the threat of or actual occurrence of a divorce. These events may be perceived as a loss or threatened loss and may lead to depression. A crisis may result from the loss of a job, a promotion, or retirement. A job change accompanied by a lower salary may also lead to a crisis.

A change in living arrangements may lead to a crisis. The person may have moved to another city or state or to another place of residence within the same city. In each instance the relocating requires changes such as meeting new neighbors and making new friends. This change can be handled effectively, or the person may experience a crisis when the change is viewed as a loss.

When performing an assessment, the nurse also considers the possibility of a developmental crisis as described in Caplan's theory. She collects data about how the client adjusted to maturational changes. For example, the client may be in crisis in response to retirement and the accompanying changes in role. The parents' role change from rearing a latency child to an adolescent can trigger a crisis.

Based on Parad's theory, it is important for the nurse to assess the client's self-concept, as a threat or attack on his sense of security can cause a crisis. The individual who is in crisis may have a negative self-concept and the stress of a crisis further alters his self-concept. All of the previously discussed changes in the individual's social life can lower his opinion of himself. The fact that the client has to seek professional help may contribute to his negative self-concept.

Spiritual dimension The role of religion in the client's life needs to be assessed. If the client has thoughts of suicide these feelings may be in conflict with his spiritual orientation and can lead to feelings of guilt and shame. At the same time the client in crisis may think that his life is meaningless because he is unable to resolve the crisis. When the precipitating event is related to a loss, the client may feel isolated and alone. Because of his feelings of helplessness and hopelessness, he may think his God or spiritual leader has forsaken him. The disorganization and loss of control in response to the impact of the crisis may further increase his doubt about his self-worth.

The questions in the accompanying box provide a useful guideline for assessing the five dimensions of a client in crisis.

Analysis
Nursing diagnosis

Altered role performance is a nursing diagnosis approved by NANDA that applies to crisis intervention. The defining characteristics are listed in the box on p. 554.

The following case example demonstrates the nursing diagnosis described in the box on p. 554.

▼ **QUESTIONS RELATED TO AN ASSESSMENT OF THE FIVE DIMENSIONS OF A CLIENT IN CRISIS**

Physical Dimension

How is your appetite?
When did you first notice a change in your appetite?
What is your sleeping pattern?
How long have you had restless nights?
How much weight have you lost?

Emotional Dimension

What changes have recently taken place in your life?
　Loss of a significant other?
　Loss of a job?
　Job promotion?
　Illness?
　Accident?
How do you feel about having to seek help?
How do you feel about your life situation?
　Scared?
　Anxious?
　Depressed?
　Overwhelmed?
　Fearful you might hurt yourself or someone else?

Intellectual Dimension

What does the crisis event mean to you?
In what way is the crisis event going to affect your future?
What do you usually do when you are upset?
　Anxious?
　Depressed?
How did you try to cope with this crisis situation?
If you used your usual method, what are your thoughts about why it didn't
　work?
What do you think would help you to feel better now?

Social Dimension

With whom do you live?
Where does your closest friend live?
How often do you see your best friend?
Whom do you trust?
Who is your closest friend in your family?
How long have you lived in your present neighborhood?
How do you feel about yourself?

Spiritual Dimension

What is your religious preference?
What kind of religious activities do you participate in when you are upset?
How often do you talk with your clergyman?
How has life treated you?
What are your purposes in life?

▼ ALTERED ROLE PERFORMANCE

DEFINITION
Disruption in the way one perceives one's role performance.

DEFINING CHARACTERISTICS
- **Physical dimension**
  Change in physical capacity to resume role

- **Intellectual dimension**
  Change in self-perception of role
  Denial of role
  Change in others' perception of role
  Conflict in roles
  Lack of knowledge of role

- **Social dimension**
  Change in usual pattern or responsibility

Modified from Kim MJ, McFarland GK, McLane AM: *Pocket guide to nursing diagnoses*, ed 5, St Louis, 1993, Mosby—Year Book.

▼ Case Example

Martha, a married mother of two children, works as a legal secretary for a law firm. She presents at the crisis center complaining of anxiety, inability to sleep, and increasing difficulty managing her job and her household and parenting responsibilities. As the nurse explores Martha's perception of the problem, the nurse learns that until 3 weeks ago, when Martha's husband received a promotion at his job, he had helped out with the household chores. Now because of the demands of his job and the need to sometimes work late hours, her husband says he doesn't have time to help with the housework. Martha says they cannot afford to hire help. She expresses doubt that she can handle the extra responsibility for the housework and care for the children. She says she is overwhelmed and came to the crisis center for help with the problem. The change in Martha's responsibility for the housework is perceived as altered role performance and has led to a crisis.

The following list provides examples of NANDA-accepted nursing diagnoses with causative statements related to crises:
1. Potential for violence to self related feelings of hopelessness
2. Impaired social interaction related to lack of social support secondary to relocation to another city
3. Sleep pattern disturbance related to anxiety
4. Severe anxiety related to failure in examination secondary to insufficient time for study
5. Alteration in thought processes related to feelings of despair

Planning

Table 27-3 provides a nursing care plan with long-term goals, short-term goals, outcome criteria, interventions, and rationales related to crisis intervention and are examples of the planning stage of the nursing process.

Implementation

Physical dimension The nurse informs the client that his sleep disturbances will most likely improve after the crisis resolves. However, until such time measures such as taking a warm bath and drinking warm milk before going to bed are helpful. Relaxation exercises may also induce sleep. If sedatives are prescribed to help the client sleep, the amount of medication prescribed is small in the event the client is suicidal. When there is loss of appetite, the nurse suggests that the client prepare his favorite foods and eat as much as he can tolerate at each meal. He may also eat high-calorie snacks between meals to increase his food intake. Once the client is able to sleep restfully and eat sufficient amounts of food, he will regain his weight and the problems with his body image may be resolved.

When the physical symptoms are related to anxiety, the nurse assures the client that the problems will subside after his anxiety is relieved. When the client experiences hyperventilation, the nurse increases the effectiveness of his breathing by providing the client with a paper bag, instructing him to place the bag over his nose and mouth and to breathe with the bag in place. The nurse remains with the client until his regular breathing returns.

Emotional dimension The nurse needs to proceed with caution in establishing rapport with the client who is depressed and is expressing feelings of hopelessness. She allows the client to talk at his own pace and listens for themes related to the precipitating event.

The nurse communicates with the client in a hopeful, empathic manner. The client often feels some relief when the nurse communicates that she understands his problem. She encourages the client to talk about the loss that contributed to the depression. She reinforces appropriate coping behavior, such as crying. The client needs privacy when crying and the nurse offers or has available facial tissue for the crying client. Skillful use of verbal and nonverbal communication is supportive for the client coping with a loss. Listening, touch, and the nurse's physical presence are important nonverbal interventions. Empathic verbal responses are reassuring and comforting for the client in crisis who is dealing with a loss.

The client may need help to initiate or complete the grieving process after the loss of a significant other. Discussing the steps in the grieving process and related thoughts and feelings enables the client to begin to work through the stages during crisis intervention with the understanding that he can complete grief work. The nurse conveys to the client that depression in response to a loss is seldom resolved in one session. She schedules the client to return for additional sessions. The research highlight on p. 556 provides an example of the intervention in grief work.

Because suicide or suicide attempts are most frequent in clients in crisis who are depressed, the nurse is constantly alert for signs of suicide. Hospitalization may be indicated if the suicidal client is (1) a high risk for suicide, (2) lacks reliable social supports, or (3) has symptoms so severe that he requires constant observation. When the suicidal risk is low, the client is encouraged to talk about reasons for his feelings and explore alternate coping behaviors. The nurse inquires about the family's ability to support the client if he returns home. If people are available and supportive,

▼ **TABLE 27-3   NURSING CARE PLAN**

GOALS	OUTCOME CRITERIA	INTERVENTIONS	RATIONALES
NURSING DIAGNOSIS: Alteration in role performance related to ineffective social adjustment after divorce			
LONG TERM			
To develop plans for a satisfying life as a divorcee	Establishes other forms of life satisfaction	Encourage to participate in activities of interest such as sports, social organizations	Involvement in such activities contribute to resolving feelings related to loss
	Uses existing support system	Encourage to maintain contact with relatives and friends	Social support (relatives and friends) can help client feel he is not alone
	Develops new relationships	Assist to identify approaches to meeting people	Knowledge of ways to meet people may hasten meeting and integrating new people into his life
SHORT TERM			
To deal with feelings that accompany the divorce: anger, grief, guilt	Verbalizes feelings about the divorce	Provide a safe environment in which to express feelings	Client needs to feel he will not be rejected or lose control if he expresses feelings
	Accepts realistic responsibility for the divorce without feelings of self-blame	Provide opportunity for realistic evaluation of feelings of self-blame	Realistic appraisal of blame may enhance self-esteem and resolution of feelings related to the divorce
NURSING DIAGNOSIS: Impaired social interaction related to lack of support resulting from relocation to another city			
LONG TERM			
To become friends with at least two people in 6 weeks	Invites neighbors to home for a social event such as coffee	Encourage to initiate interaction with neighbors	The ability to make friends increases when one reaches out
	Joins social organizations of interest	Identify source for obtaining information about social organizations	Knowledge about what is available is basic to selecting an organization to join
	Participates in social activities involving people at work and at church	Encourage client to inquire about social activities associated with work and church	An invitation to participate is likely to be extended when interest is shown
SHORT TERM			
To use existing situational supports while developing new ones	Telephones relatives or close friends at least once every 2 weeks for 6 weeks	Determine if she can financially afford to make the calls	Without sufficient funds the individual cannot achieve the goal and may feel like a failure
	Shares reactions to new experiences in letters to family and friends	Discuss benefits from communicating with social supports (friends/family)	Knowledge of benefits can be a motivator to follow through with communicating with social supports

RESEARCH HIGHLIGHT

Comparison of Two Group Interventions for the Bereaved
• RE Constantino

PURPOSE

This study was conducted to compare differences in the levels of depression and levels of socialization among three groups of bereaved widows using two group interventions: bereavement crisis intervention and group social activities.

SAMPLE

The sample consisted of 117 widows ranging in age from 50 to 79 years, with a mean age of 57.98. Ninety-eight percent of the sample was white. There were 11 blacks, 3 Hispanics, 3 Asians or Pacific Islanders, and 2 American Indians or Alaskan natives. Each subject had to be able to read and understand English, come to the School of Nursing setting, and fill out the questionnaire. Length of widowhood was not controlled. The sample was obtained by radio and newspaper advertisements or were referred to the study by health, social, church, and community agencies.

METHODOLOGY

Using a list of random numbers, the subjects were assigned randomly to the three study groups: the social adjustment group (36), the bereavement crisis intervention group (44), and the control group (37). The two group interventions were conducted by doctoral students in a university school of nursing. The group leaders were given a 2-week, training program (total of 16 hours). The bereavement crisis intervention group followed a planned and sequential 6-week series of 1.5 hour group sessions per week. The social adjustment group was task oriented and engaged in planned social activities for 6 weeks: trips to flower show, play, planetarium, art museum, aviary, and restaurants.

Based on data from *Image: Journal of Nursing Scholarship* 20:2, 1988.

A three-group, five-testing interval design was used to determine changes in levels of depression and socialization before and after interventions. Participants were tested at intake; at 6 weeks after interventions; and at 3-, 9-, and 12-month intervals. Depression levels were measured by two scales; the Beck Depression Inventory (BDI) and the Depression Adjective Check List (DACL). Socialization levels were measured by the Revised Social Adjustment Scale (RSAS).

FINDINGS

There was a statistically significant difference in the changes in depression scores among widows receiving crisis intervention, widows in the social adjustment group, and those in the control group. As measured by the BDI, depression decreased more in the bereavement crisis intervention group than in the other two groups. The BDI and RSAS mean scores for the bereavement crisis intervention group decreased from intake across the time interval, indicating that this group became less depressed and more socially adjusted after 6 weeks of bereavement crisis intervention. However, this intervention was effective only while it lasted; it did not have a long-term therapeutic effect on widows who received it.

IMPLICATIONS

Six weeks of bereavement crisis intervention, an organized type of group treatment that provides an opportunity for widows to share experiences, is more beneficial than a socialization group in decreasing depression and increasing socialization when conducted by nurses trained in this type of treatment approach. Because of the time-limited benefits, additional treatment is needed.

---

she gives the client the telephone number for the crisis hotline before he leaves and asks him to return to the crisis center for additional sessions.

If a client who is suicidal seeks crisis intervention without his family, the nurse accepts responsiblity for alerting relatives or close friends. These support persons can assume some of the responsiblity for preventing suicide. A suicidal client needs always to be accompanied by relatives or friends when he leaves the hospital. If hospitalization is indicated the client and family are also encouraged to express their thoughts and feelings about this decision.

The nurse assists the client in expressing his feelings of anxiety, anger, and guilt. Once she assesses the level of anxiety, she implements plans accordingly. The nurse intervenes with the client with a severe to panic level of anxiety by providing a calm environment with limited stimuli. The room should be well lighted to decrease shadows. The nurse explains the approach to treatment used in the crisis setting and orients him to his surroundings to de-

crease the strangeness of the situation. It is important for the nurse to remain calm and to approach the client in a warm, unhurried manner. The nurse speaks clearly and uses simple language. She communicates to the client that the feelings he is experiencing are normal. The client's painful emotions need to be vented thoroughly before the nurse attempts to obtain the facts of the precipitating event. Expressing these feelings lets the client in crisis gain mastery over his emotions. The nurse skillfully encourages and guides the client toward venting his feelings by using questions and techniques that elicit emotions. For example, when the client says he feels as if he is losing his mind, the nurse may respond, "Describe for me what this feels like." The exploration of statements related to the client's painful feelings helps the nurse determine if the client's statement relates to what he is actually experiencing or if the statement is only a figure of speech.

The client who is experiencing guilt is allowed to express these feelings in an accepting atmosphere. The nurse avoids reassuring the client too rapidly, as such a response may stop the client from expressing his feelings. Listening attentively and making empathic responses assist in alleviating the guilt. The nurse lets the client know that coming for help with his crisis is a sign of strength, not weakness. Thus she readily and actively implements the techniques for anxiety reduction. If none of the techniques reduces the anxiety, the nurse requests an order for antianxiety medication.

The basic principles to apply when intervening in the behavior of the angry client are the same as those discussed in Chapter 11. The nurse gives the client permission to express anger that has been suppressed possibly because of feelings of guilt. The client may have a greater fear of losing control in a crisis setting that provides fewer external controls than does an inpatient setting. Thus the nurse conveys confidence in her ability to help the client express his anger within reasonable limits. For example, the nurse verbally communicates to the client that he may express anger appropriately and that she will set limits on the behavior before he hurts himself or another person. Venting, discussed in the intellectual dimension, is effective in helping the client achieve the emotional catharsis that reduces tension.

Intervention in the behavior of a homicidal client is direct. Once the nurse has made an assessment she decides whether the client needs to be hospitalized. As with the suicidal client, if the client requires hospitalization, the client and the relatives are told. Relatives sometimes assume responsibility for getting the client to the hospital. If the client's homicidal behavior can be treated through crisis intervention, the nurse provides an opportunity for the client to talk about his anger in a controlled, safe environment. She provides general support by active listening and functioning essentially as a sounding board.

Intellectual dimension With a decrease in the client's emotionality, the nurse focuses on restoring the client's cognitive functioning. This intervention enhances the client's ability to discuss his perception of the precipitating event. The nurse directs intervention toward helping the client gain an intellectual understanding of his crisis; the client is guided to examine and understand the here-and-now factors that contribute to the crisis.

Cognitive restoration is a process by which the nurse communicates to the client in crisis an explanation of the cause of the crisis.[22] The nurse also shares with the client reasons that his usual coping behaviors are ineffective.

There are two therapeutic techniques for achieving cognitive restoration: causal connecting statements and interpretation.[22] A *causal connecting statement* is the process by which the nurse helps the client relate the cause and effect between two events that are an outcome of the client's specific feelings, behavior, or responses. In essence, the causal connecting statement ties together the cause and effect of the client's related events and responses. Following is an example of a causal connecting statement:

Nurse: *What's important for you to talk about today?*
Client: *Why I feel so hopeless. I can't see how I can get out of it. I just sit and think and think but can't come up with any answer on how to get myself straightened out. But I have to do something. It's very bad.*
Nurse: *What's bad?*

Client: *That before I tried to get out of it by cutting my wrist.*
Nurse: *(Causal connecting statement.) It sounds like you feel helpless to do anything about your feeling of hopelessness and when the pain becomes unbearable you attempt to take your own life.*

Causal connecting statements differ from interpretation in that explanations are based on the client's overt communication rather than on unconscious inferences.

The second basic technique of cognitive restoration is *interpretation.* "Interpretation is the crisis therapist's explanation of the unconscious cause and meaning of the client's feelings and behavior for the purpose of the client's self-understanding and reestablishment of cognitive control."[22] The explanations are based on the information the client provides in response to the nurse's questions regarding when and why the crisis occurred. Interpretation restores order and structure to the client's emotional behavior and thus improves his cognitive functioning.

Interpretation enables the client to become conscious of feelings and behaviors that are unconscious. He is offered reasons and causes for his behavior. Deep unconscious interpretation is not necessary in crisis intervention. Instead, when cognitive restoration is used in crisis intervention, there are two forms of interpretation: (1) informing the client of behavior of which he is unaware that involves his current life situation, such as interpersonal relationships with significant others or conflicts in goals; and (2) examining with the client the relationship between his past and present behavior. An example of interpretation is as follows:

Client: *I need to talk about how to defend myself and not do everything I'm asked to do. At work, I can't say no. I'm always the good guy.*
Nurse: *I wonder where these feelings about being good come from.*
Client: *For me, I guess it's in my nature. I grew out of it once, but it came back.*
Nurse: *Is it possible that when you were a kid, you were expected to be good?*
Client: *No, I don't think so . . . but yes, I guess so. I was always being good—at home and at school—and people liked me.*

Confrontation is a technique that may be used for intervention in rigid thinking. This method is used when the client resists facing the reality of the situation, which may include feelings and behavior. The goal of confrontation is to help the client accept some aspects of reality that he prefers not to face. In crisis intervention, supportive measures rather than attack are used with confrontation. The intervention begins slowly with the use of mild confrontation. If the client does not respond, a more direct approach is used. For mild confrontation, the nurse may begin by saying to the client, "For some reason you seem not to want to act on your verbalized desire to change your behavior." If this response is ineffective, the nurse will be more direct and say, "Knowing that your behavior is interfering with your functioning and you are asking for professional assistance, perhaps you need to look at what is preventing you from working on the problem." If the rigid thinking continues, the nurse sets limits or takes direct action. An example of a response is, "You will begin working on the problem, or the crisis intervention will be terminated."

Venting is one of the most useful techniques for crisis intervention. Venting allows the client to speak freely about his thoughts and feelings related to the crisis situation. This technique is one of the most effective ways of reducing tension and anxiety. By reliving the crisis experience through active verbalization, the client often perceives the problem in a different perspective and returns to his precrisis level of functioning. Venting involves exploration of the content of the client's communication without controlling the conversation. To explore the communication the nurse may say, "I can see that your marriage was important to you. Describe for me exactly how you feel now that the divorce is final." When the client is extremely depressed or is minimally responsive because of a drug overdose or other reasons, the nurse assumes an active role in which she guides the client to verbally express his thoughts and feelings.

Focused activity actively focuses the client toward his adaptive coping abilities and away from maladaptive ones. This method may be used with venting. The client is allowed to share his thoughts and feelings with emphasis on his strengths. This technique is useful in crisis intervention, as the nurse needs to learn about the client's adaptive coping abilities within a short time to guide him to capitalize on his strengths as he participates in the problem-solving process.

Another intervention that can be used is *clarification*. Clarification is designed to guide the client to focus on his problem or to recognize the inconsistencies or gaps in what he is saying, which the nurse points out. Clarification helps the client expand his perception of the crisis event. Discussing new problems as well as exploring feelings the client did not want to recognize may be outcomes of this intervention.

All of the intervention techniques allow the nurse and client to work on crisis resolution. However, the nurse guides the client in active, deliberate problem-solving activities. The nurse provides the client with knowledge about the steps in the problem-solving process and assists him in examining the effectiveness of his problem-solving behavior.

Social dimension The nurse implements plans designed to restore the client's social functioning to at least the precrisis level. If the crisis was precipitated by the loss of a significant person, the client may need to reopen his social world and meet new people to fill the void. When the client derives support and gratification from the new relationships similar to that which he obtained from the lost one, the new relationships can be especially effective in helping the client resolve the crisis. To avoid possible unrealistic expectations of the new relationship by the client, the nurse clearly conveys that the new relationship will not be the same as the lost one.

The client may need assistance learning how to strengthen existing relationships and thus his situational supports. Sometimes the client only needs to develop an awareness of how he can better use the existing support systems. The nurse may use the social worker as a resource when implementing plans for social supports.

The nurse helps the client become aware of and plan to use social activities of interest as a possible resource for meeting people as well as an outlet for reducing tension.

If the client once belonged to social organizations in the community, he can resume his involvement in these organizations.

The nurse assists the client in crisis to improve his self-concept by conveying respect for him as a person. Addressing the client by his surname unless he gives you permission to do otherwise is one way to convey respect. Accepting the client as a person who deserves the nurse's time contribute to improving the client's self-concept. The nurse communicates her acceptance to the client, for example, when she reinforces his strengths and conveys her confidence in his ability to participate in the problem-solving process. Allowing the client to do what he can for himself also contributes to improving his self-concept and decreases the client's dependence on the nurse. Whatever the outcome of the work on the crisis, the nurse recognizes the client's constructive contributions to these outcomes. Acceptance of the client as a person of worth entails acceptance of his painful feelings regardless of the content.

Environmental modification focuses on making changes in the client's environment that decrease stress and the potential for another crisis.[22] Because changing the client's environment involves other people in his life, the nurse may need to work with the client's spouse, employer, or parents. The client's environment may be modified when he lives alone and is no longer able to carry out his activities of daily living without supervision. Living arrangements may be sought for an adult child who still lives with his parents if the parent-child conflict is perceived as the precipitant of the client's crisis. Sometimes environmental modification means recommending that the client be placed temporarily in a hospital because the client's problem was not resolved sufficiently for him to function effectively at home. Modification of the environment may involve arranging for the client to have accessible situational supports. Knowledge of community resources, social agencies, businesses, and organizations contributes to the nurse's effective use of this technique.

Anticipatory guidance is a technique that is useful in helping the client prepare for and adjust satisfactorily to changes in his life. This technique involves assisting the client to anticipate certain events and prepare to cope with them in a constructive and adaptive way. This technique is especially useful for intervention in normal maturational crises. Examples of anticipatory guidance are premarital counseling for the engaged couples and parenting classes for first-time parents.

Spiritual dimension A major intervention related to the spiritual dimension is to work with the client in generating a feeling of hope. Nursing measures for achieving this goal are discussed in Chapter 14. The nurse functions as a stabilizing force and provides external control that may strengthen the client's sense of personal worth as he works toward reestablishing equilibrium and control over his cognitive functioning. Religious organizations and the individual's religious leader may serve as resources in helping him deal with a crisis of bereavement and other losses. The client may arrive for crisis intervention with members of his church or synagogue. He may need a quiet, private place to participate in prayer with these individuals. The therapist takes her cues from the client in terms of how much time and privacy is essential to fulfill his spiritual needs.

Evaluation

The nurse and the client evaluate the resolution of the crisis. They discuss whether the client achieved the goal of returning to his precrisis level of functioning or learned new, more effective coping skills. The nurse discusses with the client realistic plans for the future in terms of his perception of his progress, his support system, and the coping mechanisms he is now using. The nurse reinforces the strengths the client exhibited during his work toward resolution of the crisis. At the same time, she and the client explore ways in which he can continue to grow.

If the client did not resolve the crisis during crisis intervention, the nurse determines the assistance the client still needs and makes a referral for another type of professional help. Depending on the client's needs, the nurse may make a referral for service such as short-term psychotherapy, long-term psychotherapy, or hospitalization.

BRIEF REVIEW

Lindemann and Caplan were pioneers in the development of crisis intervention as a form of intensive brief therapy, usually consisting of one to six sessions. The therapy was designed for individuals facing a sudden loss of the ability to cope with a life situation. Any change or loss can precipitate a crisis. A crisis may be developmental or situational. Examples of developmental crisis are a child's first day of school, movement into adolescence, and retirement. Situational crisis may be precipitated by changes such as a divorce, a change of job, a promotion, and the loss of a significant other through separation or death.

The focus of crisis intervention is the crisis situation. The goals of therapy are resolution of the immediate crisis and restoration of the individual to his precrisis level of functioning and, it is hoped, to a higher level of functioning. The nurse is an active and direct participant in this process. The client and the nurse work together on solving the immediate problem. They focus on the here and now rather than reflecting on the individual's past.

Nurses are ideally suited to use crisis intervention techniques. They are with clients in hospitals and in the community. They are also adept at problem solving, which is the basis of crisis intervention.

REFERENCES AND SUGGESTED READINGS

1. Aguilera DC: *Crisis intervention: theory and methodology*, ed 6, St Louis, 1990, Mosby—Year Book.
2. Baird SF: Helping the family through a crisis, *Nursing* 17(6):66, 1987.
3. Baldwin BA: A paradigm for the classification of emotional crises: implication for crisis intervention, *American Journal of Orthopsychiatry* 48(3):538, 1978.
4. Barasch DA: Defusing the violent patient—before he explodes, *RN* 47(3):34, 1984.
5. Beckingham AC, Baumann A: The ageing family in crisis: assessment and decision-making models, *Journal of Advances in Nursing* 15(7):782, 1990.
6. Belbe LH: Reframe your outlook on recidivism . . . crisis stabilization unit is a community alternative to psychiatric hospitalization, *Journal of Psychosocial Nursing and Mental Health Services* 28(9):31, 1990.
7. Bengelsdorf H and others: A crisis triage rating scale: brief dispositional assessment of patients at risk for hospitalization, *Journal of Nervous and Mental Diseases* 172:424, 1984.
8. Bengelsdorf H, Alden DC: A mobile crisis unit in the psychiatry emergency room, *Hospital and Community Psychiatry* 38:662, 1987.
9. Bluhm J: Helping families in crisis hold on, *Nursing* 17(10):44, 1987.
10. Bond GR and others: A comparison of two crisis housing alternatives to psychiatric hospitalization, *Hospital and Community Psychiatry* 40(2):177, 1989.
11. Bonneson ME, Hartsough DM: Development of the crisis call outcome rating scale, *Journal of Consulting and Clinical Psychology* 55:612, 1987.
12. Bowie SI, and others: Blitz rape and confidence rape; implications for clinical intervention, *American Journal of Psychotherapy* 44(2):180, 1990.
13. Brent DA and others: Risk factors for adolescent suicide: a comparison of adolescent suicide victims with suicidal inpatients, *Archives of General Psychiatry* 45:581, 1988.
14. Britton JG, Mattson-Melcher DM: The crisis home: sheltering patients in emotional crisis, *Journal of Psychosocial Nursing and Mental Health Services* 23(12):18, 1985.
15. Brownell MJ: The concept of crisis: its utility for nursing, *Advances in Nursing Science* 6(4):10, 1984.
16. Caplan G: *An approach to community mental health*, New York, 1961, Grune & Stratton.
17. Caplan G: *Principles of preventive psychiatry*, New York, 1964, Basic Books.
18. Cohen LH, Claiborn WL, Specter GA, editors: *Crisis intervention*, ed 2, New York, 1983, Human Sciences Press.
19. Constantino RE: Comparison of two-group interventions for the bereaved, *Images: The Journal of Nursing Scholarship* 20:2, 1988.
20. Cox JF and others: A model for crisis intervention services within local jails, *International Journal of Law and Psychiatry* 11(4):391, 1988.
21. Diekstra RF, Engels GI, Methorst GL: Cognitive therapy of depression: a means of crisis intervention, *Crisis* 9(1):32, 1988.
22. Dixon SL: *Working with people in crisis: theory and practice*, St Louis, 1979, Mosby—Year Book.
23. Dubin WR, Sarnoff JR: Sudden unexpected death: intervention with survivors, *Annals of Emergency Medicine* 15(1):54, 1986.
24. Ebersole P, Flores J: Positive impact of life crises, *Journal of Social Behavior and Personality* 4(5):463, 1989.
25. Erikson EH: *Childhood and society*, New York, 1950, WW Norton.
26. Essa M: Grief as a crisis: psychotherapeutic interventions with elderly bereaved, *American Journal of Psychotherapy* 40(2):243, 1986.
27. Everstine DS, Everstine L: *People in crisis: strategic therapeutic interventions*, New York, 1983, Brunner/Mazel.
28. Fisher HL: Psychiatric crises: making the most of an emergency room visit, *Journal of Psychosocial Nursing and Mental Health Services* 27(11):4, 1989.
29. France K: *Crisis intervention: a handbook of immediate person-to-person help*, ed 2, Springfield, Ill, 1990, Charles C Thomas.
30. Geissler EM: Crisis: what it is and is not, *Advances in Nursing Science* 6(4):1, 1984.
31. Gillig MD, Dumaine M, Hillard JR: Whom do mobile services serve? *Hospital and Community Psychiatry* 41(7):804, 1990.
32. Gilliland BE, James RK: *Crisis intervention strategies*, Pacific Grove, Calif, 1988, Brooks/Cole Publishing.
33. Gingerich WJ, Gurney RJ, Wirtz TS: How helpful are helplines? A survey of callers, *Social Casework* 69:634, 1988.
34. Gutstein SE and others: Systemic crisis intervention as a response to adolescent crises: an outcome study, *Family Process* 27(2):201, 1988.

35. Hayes G, Goodwin T, Miars B: After disaster: a crisis support team at work, *American Journal of Nursing* 2(2):61, 1990.
36. Hayes S and others: Crisis counselling, *Lamp* 47(1):30, 1990.
37. Hoff LA: *People in crisis: understanding and helping*, ed 3, Redwood City, Calif, 1989, Addison-Wesley.
38. Hradek EA: Crisis intervention and suicide, *Journal of Psychosocial Nursing and Mental Health Services* 25(10):20, 1987.
39. Jacobs LS: Crisis screening and diversion services, *Hawaii Medical Journal* 48(3):73, 1989.
40. Jacobs D, Mack JE: Case report on psychiatric intervention by mail: a way of responding to suicidal crisis, *American Journal of Psychiatry* 143(1):92, 1986.
41. Jacobson G, Strickler M, Morley WE: Generic and individual approaches to crisis intervention, *American Journal of Public Health* 143(1):92, 1986.
42. Janosik EH, editor: *Crisis counselling: a contemporary approach*, Belmont, Calif, 1984, Wadsworth.
43. Johnson J: Psychiatric nursing in a crisis center: standards and practice, *Nursing Management* 17(8):81, 1986.
44. Kennedy B: Gold award: stabilizing teens in crisis and fortifying their support network, *Hospital and Community Psychiatry* 38(11):221, 1987.
45. Kirk AK, Stanley GV, Brown DF: Changes in patients' stress and arousal levels associated with therapists' perception of their requests during crisis intervention, *British Journal of Clinical Psychology* 11(4):363, 1988.
46. Kresky-Wolff M and others: Crossing place: a residential model for crisis intervention . . . severe psychiatric crises, *Hospital and Community Psychiatry* 35(1):72, 1984.
47. Kurlowicz LH: Violence in the emergency department, *American Journal of Nursing* 90(9):34, 1990.
48. Lieb J, Lipsitch II, Slaby AE: *The crisis team: a handbook for the mental health professional*, New York, 1973, Harper and Row.
49. Lindemann E: Symptomatology and management of acute grief, *American Journal of Psychiatry* 101:101, 1944.
50. Lindemann E: The meaning of crisis in individual and family living, *Teachers College Record* 57:310, 1956.
51. Losee N and others: *Crisis intervention in the elderly*, Springfield, Ill, 1988, Charles C Thomas.
52. McGee RF: Hope: a factor influencing crisis resolution, *Advances in Nursing Science* 6(4):34, 1984.
53. Menninger K, Mayman M, Pruysen P: *The vital balance: the life process in mental health and illness*, New York, 1967, The Viking Press.
54. Mitchell JT: Assessing and managing the psychologic impact of terrorism, civil disorders, disasters and mass casualties, *Emergency Care Quarterly* 2(1):51, 1986.
55. Moore AC: Crisis intervention: a care plan for families of hospitalized children, *Pediatric Nursing* 15(3):234, 1989.
56. Morley WE: Theory of crisis intervention, *Pastoral Psychology* 21(203):14, 1970.
57. Morley WE, Messick JM, Aguilera DC: Crisis: paradigms of intervention, *Journal of Psychiatric Nursing and Mental Health Services* 5:538, 1967.
58. Olfson M and others: A controlled evaluation of inpatient crisis treatment for acute schizophrenic episodes, *Psychiatric Quarterly* 61(2):143, 1990.
59. Neville D, Barnes S: The suicidal phone call, *Journal of Psychosocial Nursing and Mental Health Services* 23(8):14, 1985.
60. Parad HJ: The use of time-limited crisis intervention in community mental health programming, *Social Services Review* 40:275, 1966.
61. Parad HJ: Crisis intervention. In *Encyclopedia of social work*, vol I, ed 16, New York, 1971, National Association of Social Workers.
62. Parad HJ, Resnik HP: The practice of crisis intervention in emergency care. In Resnik HP, Ruben HL, Ruben DD, editors: *Emergency psychiatric care; the management of mental health crisis*. Bowie, Md, 1975, Charles Press Publishers.
63. Parad HJ and others: Crisis intervention and emergency mental health care: concepts and principles. In Resnik HLP, Ruben HL, Ruben DD, editors: *Emergency psychiatric care: the management of mental health crises*, Bowie, Md, 1975, Charles Press Publishers.
64. Polak PR, Reres M, Fish L: The management of family crisis. In Resnik HLP, Ruben HL, Ruben DD, editors: *Emergency psychiatric care: the management of mental health crises*, Bowie, Md, 1975, Charles Press Publishers.
65. Rapoport L: The state of crises: some theoretical considerations, *Social Support Review* 36:211, 1962.
66. Rapoport L: Crisis intervention as a mode of brief treatment. In Roberts RW, Wee RH, editors: *Theories of social casework*, Chicago, 1970, The University of Chicago Press.
67. Rubin JG: Critical incident stress debriefing: helping the helpers, *Journal of Emergency Nursing* 16(4):255, 1990.
68. Schram PC, Burti L: Crisis intervention techniques designed to prevent hospitalization, *Bulletin of the Menninger Clinic* 50(2):194, 1986.
69. Smith LL: *Crisis intervention theory and practice: a sourcebook*, Washington, DC, 1976, University Press of America.
70. Stelzer J, Elliott CA: A continuous-care model of crisis intervention for children and adolescents, *Hospital Community Psychiatry* 41(5):562, 1990.
71. Stroul BA: Residential crisis services: a review, *Hospital and Community Psychiatry* 39(10):1095, 1988.
72. Taplin JR: Crisis theory: critique and reformulation, *Community Mental Health Journal* 7(1):13, 1971.
73. Wheeler BR: Crisis intervention: recognizing and helping patients overcome anxiety, *Journal of Association of Operating Room Nurses* 47(5):1242, 1988.
74. Zener KA: Some basic assumptions of crisis intervention, E.F.A., *Journal of Crisis Intervention* 2(3):16, 1985.

ANNOTATED BIBLIOGRAPHY

Aguilera DC: *Crisis intervention: theory and methodology*, ed 6, St Louis, 1990, Mosby–Year Book.

The sixth edition of this practical book presents one of the most comprehensive discussions of the basic theory and principles of crisis intervention. Attention is given to a wide range of events that may precipitate a crisis with a discussion of related theoretical concepts and the problem-solving process. Case material is well integrated throughout the book. A chapter is devoted to crisis intervention in AIDS, a current health problem. This book is a valuable reference for nursing students and other health care professionals.

Lindemann E: *Beyond grief: studies in crisis intervention*, New York, 1979, Jason Aronson.

This book contains a collection of Lindemann's papers, including his classical work on the symptoms and management of acute grief. The articles will be of interest to nurses working in various clinical settings, since crisis events such as surgery, ulcerative colitis, and moving are discussed. He also addressed preventive intervention and social changes.

Narayan SM, Joslin DJ: Crisis theory and intervention: a critique of the medical model and proposal of a holistic nursing model, *Advances in Nursing Science* 2:27, 1980.

The authors critique Lindemann's and Caplan's theoretical models of crises, emphasizing the problems of the models related to disease and symptom treatment. The holistic nursing model of crisis proposed by the authors is based on depletion of health potential, which is viewed as an aspect of the health continuum. They provide a useful comparison of the medical and holistic nursing models of crisis.

CHAPTER
28
Group Therapy

Ethel Rosenfeld

After studying this chapter, the student will be able to:

- Define group therapy
- Describe the involvement of nursing in group therapy from a historical perspective
- Describe theoretical frameworks for group therapy
- Use the nursing process in group therapy
- Identify types of group therapy available through the life cycle
- Identify current research findings relevant to group therapy

Any group—family, school, work, or community—is a collection of individuals who are to some degree interdependent. Groups, then, are naturally appropriate for preventing and treating mental health problems involving interactions with others. Three kinds of groups are discussed in this chapter: group therapy, therapeutic groups, and adjunctive groups.

Group therapy focuses on self-awareness, improving interpersonal relationships, and making behavioral changes. Therapeutic groups deal with emotional stress associated with physical illness or developmental crises. An adjunctive group uses special activities to increase socialization, sensory and intellectual stimulation, and orientation to reality. The nurse's knowledge about the different types of groups and group process increases effectiveness in working with groups of clients.

GROUP THERAPY

Group therapy is a treatment method in which clients meet at planned times with a qualified therapist to focus on becoming self-aware and self-understanding, improving interpersonal relationships, making behavioral changes, or all three. The group is based on philosophical concepts and theories, with specific content and outcome goals. Positive, creative change is the major purpose. Clients need to want to change some aspect of themselves and be willing to take the necessary steps to change. This may involve recognizing and accepting aspects of themselves that benefit from change or learning to make decisions to enhance the quality of their relationships.

Group therapy is generally categorized according to the group objectives. The kind of group reflects the therapist's theoretical framework. This framework also reflects the role

the therapist assumes, the terminology used, and the focus of the group.

Groups usually have one or two leaders. The following lists the advantages of both types:

ONE LEADER	CO-LEADERS
No clash in leadership style or theory base	Feedback and validation are mutually shared.
Greater autonomy	Group strategies are planned together.
	One leader can assess group as a whole while the other works with one person.
Greater financial gain	Co-leaders relating to each other openly and honestly can be role models.
	When co-leaders are a man and a woman, clients' old feelings about parents may be more readily worked through.
	Dependence on co-leaders is shared.
	If one leader is absent, the other can maintain the group.

Typically, therapy groups are composed of five to ten members (Figure 28-1). A group of seven or eight members is considered ideal. A therapy group with fewer than five yields less effective interaction; more than ten means less focus on individuals, diluting group potency and effectiveness.

The frequency and length of sessions depend on goals and membership. Groups of clients with a short attention span or who withdraw as a way of coping meet two or three times a week for an hour or less; most groups are held weekly. An hour and a half is needed to get beyond the slow starting phase into the working part of the session and to give clients time to deal with specific needs. Some

HISTORICAL OVERVIEW

DATES	EVENTS
1900s	Joseph Pratt introduced a type of group therapy by his attempts to educate tuberculosis patients, alleviate their feelings of discouragement, and raise their morale. His repressive-inspirational approach used informal discussion, biblical and philosophical readings, and poetry.
	Jacob Morino coined the term *group psychotherapy* and introduced psychodrama as a therapeutic modality.
1940s	SR Slavson founded the American Group Psychotherapy Association (AGPA).
	Group therapy flourished during World War II because of the shortage of psychiatrists and psychologists. Treating battle victims in groups was an expedient way of reaching large numbers of clients.
1950s	The effectiveness and economy of treating groups gradually led to the integration of group psychotherapy into the education and practice of nurses, social workers, psychiatrists, and psychologists.
1967	The American Nurses' Association statement on psychiatric nursing practice stated that clinical nursing specialists can function as group therapists when graduate study included theory, supervision, and clinical practice related to group therapy.
1990s	Group therapy is now practiced by many kinds of practitioners, and there are groups for almost everything—to lose weight, to quit smoking, to be a more effective single parent, to cope with divorce or death, to change behavior, to improve management skills, to share common feelings, and so on. Nurses have unlimited opportunities to practice group therapy.
Future	High levels of stress, faulty interpersonal relationships, and rising health care costs will continue to influence the need for nurses to work with groups of clients, scientifically documenting the group's effectiveness and evaluating the outcome of treatment.
	Increasing numbers and kinds of self-help groups will develop as resources for mutual support.

group leaders believe that members use whatever time is allotted—if the time is shorter, participants start to work more quickly. All therapists agree on the importance of beginning and ending on time. If a portion of group work is left uncompleted, it is continued at the next session, or, if appropriate, the leader works individually with a member before the next meeting (since the leader is responsible for the emotional safety of the client).

The duration of a group depends on its goals and membership. Groups with a specific task or function may have a set number of meetings, such as once a week for 6 weeks or 6 months. Groups that are intensive and insight oriented may meet for 1 to 3 years. *Marathon groups* meet for several days in a row or an entire weekend.

THEORETICAL APPROACHES

Psychoanalytical

Psychoanalytical groups focus on the analysis and interpretation of transferences, defenses, and resistances. Dreams, slips of the tongue, free associations, and defense mechanisms are seen as clues to unconscious motivation. The overall goal is to reconstruct personality through the development of insight. Through time the therapist focuses on the problems of individual members. Others benefit by recognizing some of these problems as theirs and realizing the need to change patterns of feeling, thinking, and behaving. The group gives support as members grapple with new ideas and choose new life directions.

Transactional Analysis

Transactional analysis (TA) is a unique form of group therapy rooted in psychoanalytical thought that focuses on learning and doing and is health oriented rather than illness oriented. Communication among group members is examined, and each member's "script" becomes apparent in all behaviors used during sessions. Each person develops contracts with the therapist to change specific problematic aspects of life. Questions asked by the therapist and other members may include: "How will you make this change? When will you start? How will we know that you have made the change?" When one contract is fulfilled, a new one is made.

Interpersonal

Interpersonal groups emphasize members relating to each other, how each perceives the relating, and the impact of the relating. Anxiety generated by the group experience is a major focus. Sources of anxiety from the client's past and from group dynamics are identified. As the anxiety is openly addressed, it becomes less significant. The acceptance of each member as worthy and valuable allows all to develop increased security and self-esteem and strengthens them for the future.

Client- or Group-Centered

Client- or group-centered groups assume that clients have the ability and responsibility to make needed and

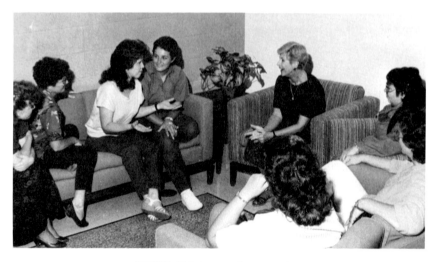

FIGURE 28-1 A group therapy session.

wanted changes. Each person seeks his true self and with group support removes his social facade to expose his inner core. Members and therapist are viewed as equals, the therapist being the most experienced member. The therapist relates to the group with genuineness, empathy, and warmth, encouraging all to participate the same way. Emphasis is on the healthy aspects of the self and on using all of oneself to experience the present reality.

Existential

Clients whose lives lack direction and meaning often find existential groups valuable. They focus on members knowing their inner world, their interpersonal world, and their natural world to bring them together in a meaningful way. Members build emotional strength as they increase awareness by sharing major life events. They are encouraged to be genuine and open (authentic) and to involve themselves in living joyously and passionately. The therapist is considered an equal and shares herself openly. The therapist is a role model of authentic relating and deep investment in living.

Gestalt

Gestalt group therapy focuses on the individual becoming a whole person through autonomy, which stems from self-awareness. Clients learn techniques and exercises to heighten awareness and assist in recognizing feelings hidden from self. They are encouraged to fully experience their feelings in the group, thereby resolving incomplete emotional experiences. Gestalt groups seem particularly effective for clients who are depressed or anxious or who have constrained, restricting patterns of living.

General Systems

According to general systems theory (GST), each group member is a system that interacts with other systems to become part of the larger group system. The group develops over time to become relatively stable. Goals for systems groups help members restore or enhance their own autonomy by more effectively opening and closing their boundaries. The therapist monitors and regulates the group and assists with the opening and closing of individual and group boundaries.

Askelepian

The Askelepian approach is useful for extremely self-centered, impulsive, and manipulative clients who do not usually benefit from group therapy as traditionally conducted. In fact, these clients are likely to be destructive elements in the group process. Askelepian (from the Greek askelapeius, "place of the last resort") groups are held several times weekly. Goals are for members to (1) acknowledge their own behavior, (2) make contracts to change unhealthy behaviors, and (3) emphasize social responsibility over personal wishes and needs. The leader starts by confronting ("indicting") a member about a negative behavior displayed since the last meeting. The other members reinforce the indictment ("rat packing"). The confrontation continues until the member acknowledges the truth of it. The leader then helps the client understand the behavior and to make plans with the client for positive change. If the client is ready, a contract may be drawn up, in which the client agrees to make certain changes, specifying exactly how and when, knowing that the contract will be discussed at the next meeting. This member then proceeds to indict another group member, and the sequence is reenacted. The group continues until all indictments are made and worked through. Leaders are not excluded from indictment. The leader is a role model of open, honest, confronting, responsible behavior and demonstrates that she is not easily manipulated. At the end of each session warm, caring verbal and physical responses are shared by group members and leader.

Because these groups are part of a larger therapeutic community (hospitals, halfway houses, and group homes, for example), behavioral change can be assessed daily over a long time by the other group members and by the leader.

▼ **TABLE 28-1**   **Organization of Groups by Theoretical Frameworks and Theorists**

Theory/Theorist	Dynamics	Role of Leader	Focus of Group
PSYCHOANALYTICAL			
Sigmund Freud	Personality is determined by biological and environmental forces. Behavior is based on unconscious motivation. Neuroses develop from unmet needs in one's past.	Authority figure; neutral sounding board; active listener; calls attention to group process; challenges defenses; focuses on individuals within the group and also needs of the total group	*General:* Primarily cognitive; insight oriented; expecting reconstruction of personality structure *Specific:* Freeing the libido (positive life energies related to love, energy, and sex) Maintaining a balance among the id, ego, and superego Breaking down defenses against anxiety Dealing with early life and past traumatic experiences and their relationship to current thinking and behavior Transferences and resistances Dream content
TRANSACTIONAL ANALYSIS (TA)			
Eric Berne	Personality is determined by all past experiences. One can be fully in charge of the directions taken in life.	Facilitator; teacher; active or inactive depending on group process; focuses on individuals within the group and also needs of the total group; recognizes and points out ego states in use by group members; assists members to choose more effective modes of behavior; gives permissions and protection to clients in the process of change; relates to group openly and without use of games	*General:* Cognitive, affective, conative, insight oriented; expecting reconstruction of personality structure *Specific:* Ego states used (parent, adult, and child) Transactions used (complementary, crossed, or ulterior) Life script Strokes given and received Games played Congruence in feeling, thinking, and behaving Autonomy Awareness, spontaneity, and intimacy Individual contracts for change Assuming responsibility for self
INTERPERSONAL			
H.S. Sullivan Hildegard Peplau	Behavior is the result of interaction of many forces. Interpersonal security is a basic need. Processes that take place in the interpersonal field are central to understanding human behavior. Self-concept is obtained from reflected appraisals from significant people in one's life.	Participant-observer; focuses on group process; catalyst; encourages; strengthens self-esteem of members	*General:* Cognitive, affective; insight oriented; expecting reconstruction of personality structure *Specific:* Interactional patterns of member with family and with group Relationship of past distorted experiences to current problems (transferences) Consensual validation of behavior to correct distortions in growth derived from early anxieties, (parataxic distortion)
CLIENT-CENTERED			
Carl Rogers	Behavior results from self-concept. People are basically good. Wholeness results from becoming fully onself. Clients have the ability and responsibility to change. Clients and leader are equals.	Nondirective; open; congruent; reflective; "being with" clients with genuineness, empathy, and warmth; focuses on group process and individuals in the group	*General:* Affective *Specific:* Awareness; perceptions of oneself and one's world Here and now Unconditional positive acceptance of oneself and others Self-actualization Responsibility for oneself Empathy, genuineness, and warmth in relating

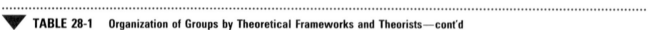

TABLE 28-1   Organization of Groups by Theoretical Frameworks and Theorists—cont'd

Theory/Theorist	Dynamics	Role of Leader	Focus of Group
EXISTENTIAL Rollo May Hugh Mullen Josephine Paterson Loretta Zderad	Life is open to choice. Each person is unique and of value. Each person shares commonalities with others. There is mutual growth of self and others through being together and experiencing each other.	Nondirective; guiding; sharing of self; intimate contract with the group as a whole	*General:* Affective; experiencing and relating to others *Specific:* "Being with"; "being here" Themes of death, despair, nothingness, fate, anxiety, guilt, joy, and commitment (the meaning of life) Becoming all that one is capable of being
GESTALT Frederick Perls	One needs to live fully in the present. Self-awareness is the avenue to personal autonomy. One can recognize and experience wholeness of self and in one's world.	Active; directs structured exercises; works with one member at a time on the "hot seat"; confronts; supports	*General:* Affective, conative *Specific:* Awareness of feelings and behavior of self and others' responses Completion of unfinished business through fantasies, dreams, experiencing past experiences now, and working through impasses Here and now Authenticity; spontaneity Responsibility for self
GENERAL SYSTEMS Ludwig von Bertalanffy	The world is composed of systems, subsystems, and supersystems. Systems function to maintain wholeness, achieve self-regulation, and achieve self-transformation to higher levels of adaptation. Systems achieve the above by opening and closing their boundaries and then exchanging energy and information with their environments. Group members are open systems and the subsystems of the group; in turn, the group is an open, living system. The group is autonomous and capable of changing itself.	Group member; acts in terms of own living structure; a catalyst	*General:* Cognitive and affective *Specific:* Systems of individual personalities composing group Larger system in which group operates; autonomy and determining boundaries Searching for deeper structure Acceptance of uncertainty
ASKELEPIAN	Leader and members confront each other about negative behavior. Confrontation continues until member acknowledges the behavior. Plans are made for positive change.	Confronter: demonstrates open, honest, responsible, nonmanipulative behavior	*General:* Affective *Specific:* Awareness of behavior and effects on others. Accepts responsibility for behavior with contract made to change behavior.

Eclectic

Many group therapists combine aspects of more than one theory for an eclectic approach (see Chapter 4). The therapist using this approach is familiar with various theories and blends them purposely to express her philosophical beliefs and the group purpose. Table 28-1 summarizes groups by theoretical framework.

THERAPEUTIC GROUPS

Therapeutic groups deal with emotional stress from physical illness, normal growth and development crises, or social maladjustment. Examples are groups for expectant mothers, people who have lost their spouse through divorce or death, the terminally ill, and people with similar health problems. The main purposes of groups are (1) to prevent health problems, as in the groups for expectant and new mothers; (2) to educate and develop group members' potentials, as in groups for clients with chronic illnesses or disabilities; and (3) to enhance quality of life, as in groups for the terminally ill. Participants can be inpatients, outpatients, or people in the community. Nurses are commonly leaders of these groups because of their work in all kinds of settings, their understanding of the interaction of physical and emotional parts of the self, and nursing's emphasis on health teaching.

Many therapeutic groups are self-help groups—groups without leadership by a health professional (although some are held jointly by health professionals and lay people (see research highlight). Almost all self-help groups use the repressive-inspirational approach. They attempt to replace unwanted feelings and behaviors with healthier ones, using group teaching, counseling, and peer support. Some examples of self-help groups are represented in Table 28-2.

ADJUNCTIVE GROUPS

Adjunctive groups deal with selected needs of individuals, such as cognitive stimulation, sensory stimulation, orientation to reality, and socialization. These groups are

---

RESEARCH HIGHLIGHT

Therapeutic Processes in Peer Led and Professionally Led Support Groups for Caregivers
- R Toseland, C Rossiter, T Peak, and P Hill

PURPOSE

The purpose of this study was to compare outcomes of support groups for caregivers of frail older persons when led by peer leaders or by professional leaders.

SAMPLE

The sample consisted of four support groups, two peer led and two professionally led. These groups were part of an NIMH funded study that included 130 participants and 14 groups. Sizes of groups and participant ages were unlisted.

METHODOLOGY

All four groups met for eight weekly, 2-hour sessions. All groups used supportive interventions and, to a lesser degree, education-discussion and problem solving. Professional leaders received 6 hours of training, a protocol, background reading material, and weekly telephone consultation with project staff who listened to group audiotape recordings. Peer leaders were chosen for their experience in caregiving and were members and leaders of self-help groups. They received 4 hours of training, a brief protocol, and background reading. Project staff were general consultants, helping formulate their plans for group leading and for problem resolution encountered in group. Peer-led groups were less structured, using a self-help approach that promotes mutual support, sharing of common concerns, and exchange of information and coping mechanisms found useful by caregivers. Measurement of group process was through audiotape analyzing, standardized rating forms, and qualitative content analysis by three project staff listening to every group audiotape at least once and sharing weekly meetings to discuss group processes.

Based on data from *International Journal of Group Psychotherapy* 40:3, 1990.

FINDINGS

Both peer and professionally led groups were similar in (1) group content style, relationships, and use of low confrontation; (2) exploration, encouraging, and leader-shared information; and (3) finding respite from caregiving, reduction of isolation, ventilation, support, validation of experience, and affirmation of coping ability. Peer-led groups offered more specific content in relation to resources and services, general themes and issues, superficial conversation, not inviting exploration or questioning, there-and-then interactions, leader-to-member interaction, social interaction, and modeling. Professionally led groups offered more focus on individuals in the group, member concerns or member relationships with other group participants, here-and-now interactions, invitations to explore and give feedback, problem solving, work focus, sharing, cohesion, and help with specific problems. Qualitative analysis of group outcome data revealed no significant difference between peer and professionally led groups. Follow-up study, including a no-treatment control group, revealed that changes persisted one year after intervention.

IMPLICATIONS

Findings suggest that the therapeutic processes shared by both groups were the effective therapeutic ingredients. Both types of leaders were highly effective in meeting member needs. Unaddressed issues needing attention in future research include (1) amount of active facilitation optimal in short-term support groups for caregivers, (2) amount of attention that should be paid to group-as-a-whole skills, (3) appropriateness of therapy in support groups, and (4) appropriate role of professionals and peers in support groups.

▼ **TABLE 28-2**   **Examples of Self-help Groups**

Type	Purpose or Goal
Alcoholics Anonymous (AA)	To help alcoholics maintain sobriety and to help others abstain from drinking
Al-Anon and Alateen	To assist the spouse and children of alcoholics to understand the drinker and to develop healthy life-styles for themselves despite the problems of the alcoholic
Synanon	To encourage drug-free living by using heavy confrontation in residential centers for drug abusers
Gamblers Anonymous (GA)	To help gamblers stop gambling, using the principles of AA
Neurotics Anonymous (NA)	To assist self-acknowledged neurotics with emotional problems, using the principles of AA
Recovery	To encourage reintegration into community after psychiatric hospitalization, using Low's concepts from "Mental Health through Will-Training"
National Alliance for the Mentally Ill (NAMI)	To help families and friends of the severely or chronically mentally ill understand their illnesses and to give support to each other as caregivers and advocates
Parents Anonymous (PA)	To help abusive parents learn healthy parenting and to give support to each other
Parents Without Partners (PWP)	To help single parents improve parenting and to support each other through teaching and social activities
Weight Watchers International	To promote weight loss through peer support while learning and practicing new patterns of eating and more active life-styles
Manic-Depressive Group	To support persons diagnosed as manic depressive (bipolar disorder) and provide information on the disease
Obsessive-Compulsive Group	To give peer support, to share resources for help, to learn about the disorder and ways to deal with it

often adjuncts to group therapy or therapeutic groups (Table 28-3).

CHARACTERISTICS OF THE GROUP THERAPIST

Qualifications

Three areas prepare a person to lead group therapy safely and effectively: (1) theoretical preparation through formal courses, lectures, reading, and workshops; (2) supervised practice in the role of co-leader and leader; and (3) experience as a group therapy member.

Nurses should be leading group therapy sessions only when prepared by these areas. Their functioning within the group is not different from that of other prepared professionals, except that their background gives them familiarity with all aspects of client care.

The American Nurses' Association (ANA) statement on psychiatric nursing practice states the clinical specialists can function as group therapists. Certification by the ANA as a clinical specialist in psychiatric–mental health nursing assures that the nurse is qualified and competent as a group therapist.

The American Group Psychotherapy Association (AGPA)

▼ **TABLE 28-3**   **Goals, Types, and Activities of Adjunctive Groups**

Goal	Type	Activities
To foster cognitive stimulation	Bibliotherapy	Use articles, books, poems, and newspapers to stimulate thinking and foster relating to others
To foster sensory stimulation	Music, art, and dance groups	Provide outlets for expression of feelings
	Relaxation groups	Focus on learning relaxation techniques using modalities such as deep breathing, muscle relaxation, and guided imagery
To foster reality orientation and socialization	Remotivation groups	Use a 5-step format to orient withdrawn and regressed clients to reality
	Reality/orientation groups, validation groups	Focus on orientation to time, place, and person and right and wrong to help clients meet needs
	Reminiscent groups	Focus on remembering past experiences, to assign positive meanings to them

is the principal accrediting organization for group therapists. Membership is open to qualified therapists or counselors with a master's degree.

Many nurses lead therapeutic and adjunctive groups. Requirements for these types of groups are specific knowledge of the problems and concerns of the clients, an understanding of the methods used in the specific group, and skill in functioning as leader.

Roles

Task role functions

First, the leader identifies the need for a specific group. In an inpatient or outpatient setting the leader meets with the staff members to explain the purposes and plans for the group. Their goodwill is important; they can encourage and support the ongoing group or impede its progress if they feel ignored.

The leader also makes room arrangements. The room needs to be quiet, free from distractions, and large enough to hold a comfortably spread circle of chairs, without a table. (A table restricts the ability to see nonverbal communication.)

The leader selects group members according to group purpose. She interviews the client to assess needs and behaviors. Clients want to know what they can gain from group involvement and what to expect in the sessions. They need ample time to voice their hopes and fears and to become familiar with the goals of the group.

The leader also decides whether the group will be open or closed. Open groups, the most common form, allows clients to terminate when they are ready, although the group itself continues. In closed groups the duration is decided in advance or by the consensus of the leader and the group members.

Maintenance role functions

The therapist's maintenance role functions are to continually observe group process, assess levels of anxiety, and establish direction. The therapist is the one person known by all members and therefore can be the mutual supporter of all participants as they begin a new venture together.

In the early stages of group development, many therapists take an active role. They give positive recognition to clients who initiate interactions; they make verbal observations, question, and summarize what has taken place. At times the therapist may purposely remain silent so that members will deal with each other more directly or experience the silences of group interaction. The therapist guides the group but does not control it. Thus the members take responsibility for group actions and reactions and for personal decisions. When the group becomes cohesive, the leader takes a less active role but continues to be a resource person, supporter of change, and role model of healthy behavior.

New therapists are likely to make some mistakes. Table 28-4 gives examples of common mistakes and helpful leader responses.

....

▼ **TABLE 28-4   Pitfalls and Helpful Responses for the Novice Group Therapy Leader**

Pitfalls	Examples	Helpful Responses
A need to structure the group	**Leader:** *(At beginning of each group)* We'll do our usual start of going around the group, telling others who you are and what you feel right now.	Leader quietly waits for group members to begin the session.
Denying or ignoring nonverbal behavior	**Member:** *(Smiles, with eyes tearing)* This week has been so much better for me! **Leader:** That's great! What did you do differently?	**Leader:** Oh? Then what are your tears all about?
A need to give advice from nursing knowledge or personal experiences	**Member:** My foot is hurting today because I have an ingrown toenail. **Leader:** There are several ways you can deal with that. You can lift a corner of the nail and . . .	Leader listens and waits to see how group members move in to respond.
Role reversal: focus of group on leader's needs	**Member:** *(To leader)* You look sad today **Leader:** Well, yes. I heard yesterday that my child is going to need surgery soon.	Leader looks at group members, neither denying nor reinforcing.
Revealing self	**Member:** *(To leader)* Are you married? **Leader:** Yes, for 25 years. I also have three children and four grandchildren who are my pride and joy!	**Leader:** Yes, I am. I wonder what made you think of that right now?
Intellectualizing	**Leader:** Maslow says that . . .	Leader quietly encourages expression of feelings; identifies, where needed, what is occurring; and monitors group process.
A need to be liked by the group members	Leader is primarily reassuring, warm, and protective; encourages, "happy talk."	Leader encourages expression of all kinds of feelings toward leader and other group members.

....

CHARACTERISTICS OF GROUP THERAPY

Client Selection

People who profit most from group therapy value and desire personal change, want to know more about their own feelings and to understand others better, and have high expectations for the outcome.[40] Following is a case example of someone who benefited from group therapy.

▼ Case Example

Theresa is the only child of a conservative, middle class couple. Her mother taught her from an early age to be personable and outgoing and emphasized the importance of physical attractiveness. Theresa learned her lessons well. She "rarely met a stranger," and she led an active social life in college. Soon after graduation she married a successful businessman. He was very involved in his work and became more and more disinclined to participate in social and recreational activities with Theresa. She was often alone, feeling restless and bored. In time Theresa filed for divorce. Because of her unhappiness with her life, she sought the services of a psychotherapist. After careful assessment of needs, the therapist placed Theresa in group therapy with seven other men and women. In the group Theresa appeared outgoing, but her relating was superficial. She was verbal, liked to be the center of attention, and seemed overly concerned with appearances. After a few sessions she was confronted about her behavior. Theresa's response was to cry, sobbing loudly that no one was trying to understand her. The others listened but maintained that her facade was such that she did not allow them to know her as a real person. They pointed out her superficiality and her entertaining or coy remarks that actually served to cover her feelings.

Slowly, Theresa began sharing her feelings of loneliness. She asked for help in becoming more a real part of the group. She was encouraged to honestly identify her own feelings in relation to events occurring in the group and to voice them, even when they had a negative connotation. In addition, she agreed to really listen to others responding to her and to accept their concern and caring.

In time, as Theresa continued to participate, she became a role model of open, forthright behavior. She remained in this group for 16 months. She continued to make subtle but increasingly apparent changes in self-esteem, and her behavior was more appropriate and deeper when relating to the others.

Theresa's regular mode of relating to others was openly confronted. The group let her know she was a worthwhile individual who did not need to hide behind a facade and encouraged her to try new ways of relating that proved to be more effective. In the process she became a vital group member.

Not everyone is a candidate for group therapy. For example, those who are not "psychologically minded"—who are strongly disinclined or resistant to therapy—do not benefit. Also excluded are psychotic individuals whose autistic thinking, bizarre communications, and short attention span disrupt the group process. Following are reasons used by some people who do not wish to become group members:

1. They are too uncomfortable in groups and may not tolerate the atmosphere.
2. They become irritated with members who have special problems.
3. They are unwilling to share the leader with other group members.
4. They want more time for personal work and do not think they benefit from listening to others.

These people may profit from individual sessions with a therapist or from such sessions concurrent with group therapy. The following is a case example of a person who was not ready for group therapy.

▼ Case Example

Randy was a shy, aloof 20-year-old whose mother brought him to a therapist for help in becoming more comfortable with others. Usually, Randy avoided other people whenever possible. In college he was a loner, typically returning to his room immediately after each class. The therapist decided to place Randy in group therapy with six other people who were accepting and welcomed him as a group member. Randy was extremely uncomfortable. He would tremble and shake and would move his chair outside the group circle. When gently confronted about this behavior, he would become agitated. He would then leave the room to pace in the hall until called back in. Because of Randy's increasing anxiety, the therapist decided to remove him from the group and see him in individual weekly sessions. The therapist was quiet, warm, and supportive. Gradually, Randy responded and talked about his anxieties and feelings of low self-esteem. After 3 months he asked to become a part of the group therapy sessions again.

Randy was not able to respond to the give and take of group process, although the other members were warm and responsive. His anxiety increased until he physically removed himself from the others. He was willing to relate to the therapist alone, however, and in time he acknowledged his anxious feelings and low self-esteem. Moreover, he took the initiative to return to the group, which indicated development of inner strength and readiness for increased risk taking.

The factors of group therapy most commonly identified as beneficial by clients in research studies are (1) encouragement to ventilate feelings (catharsis), (2) close identity with the group, (3) giving feedback to other group members, (4) receiving of feedback from other group members, and (5) self-understanding.[32]

Group membership can be *heterogeneous* (a variety of ages, backgrounds, behaviors, and needs) or *homogeneous* (similar backgrounds, needs, behaviors). An advantage of a heterogeneous group is the stimulation created by variety. Values, beliefs, and ways of doing things differ, causing the client to look at options. The anxiety generated can be a catalyst for constructive action, with resultant emotional and behavioral change. However, extreme differences in basic values and behaviors of group members can cause schisms in a group. In addition a balance of behaviors is needed. For example, one or two very depressed individuals may do well in a typical group; they can benefit from the caring and gentle prodding of the others to get reinvolved in living. But several depressed individuals in one group can slow down the process. Such feelings can be contagious. Other members may refuse to identify with the group. A number of hyperactive clients can totally disrupt a group, stimulating each other to a point at which the group goals cannot be met; but one hyperactive person in a group may do well.

Homogeneous groups can become cohesive more quickly because of shared feelings and needs. However, most clinicians believe these groups tend to remain more superficial and are ineffective in altering character structure when this is the intent of the group.[49]

Stages of Group Development

Regardless of the theoretical framework, all types of group therapy have an orientation phase, a working phase, and a termination phase (Table 28-5). Each phase will be discussed, with emphasis on group behaviors and tasks.

In the *orientation phase*, contracts are established. Contracts are the rules, rights, and responsibilities of members and group leaders. They may be written or verbal and need to be understood and accepted by all. Following are examples of contractual components:

1. Awareness of duration, frequency, and length of sessions
2. Commitment to the group, demonstrated by regular attendance, punctuality, and active participation
3. Regular payment of fees or arrangements made for payment
4. Group rules
   a. Maintaining confidentiality (Anything occurring in the group is to be kept there; members do not gossip about each other or even divulge each other's names.)
   b. Encouraging verbal expression of all kinds of feelings
   c. Prohibiting physical violence or use of drugs during sessions
   d. Only one person speaking at a time
   e. Dealing with anxieties engendered by the group process instead of backing away
   f. Taking responsibility for change in themselves

Contracts may also specifically state expectations of both therapist and members. Clients state what they want to change about themselves, and the therapist states how she can help the client reach these goals. Goals inevitably change as the group progresses, as needs are met, and as new needs emerge.

Information is given and received, and *group norms* (acceptable group behaviors) are established during the orientation phase. Some members may test other members to determine how much trusting can take place. For example, a member may share some negative personal information, such as having had a child out of wedlock or having abused drugs in the past. Some may test group rules by coming irregularly or late and seeing if they are reprimanded or rejected. Also in this phase conversation may lapse into awkward silences, with frequent stops and starts. The message to the group leader is unspoken but strong: "take over and keep the ball rolling."

The task for group members in this stage is to achieve a sense of identification or belonging to the group. The leader is the catalyst or unifier by spelling out the rules, refusing to control the group, pointing out the process taking place, and encouraging verbalization of all kinds of feelings. The leader's clear message to the group is that this is their group; her strengths, needs, or leadership style do not hold it together. Rather, each member is responsible for all that occurs.

Anxiety is the prominent feeling in this first stage. The newness of the situation is threatening, but the group is a safe place to examine anxiety and what fosters it and to learn to deal constructively with it. The leader is wise to let the group take care of its own anxieties, unless they are excessive. When the group falls silent or otherwise feels tension, each member chooses a response to deal with the anxiety. The leader assesses what is occurring and may comment on the group process. She encourages members to be aware of their defenses and to face the threatening situation directly, without their defenses. At these times members are most open to making positive changes in themselves.

Trust cannot develop until group members begin to know each other. Testing takes place until individuals feel safe expressing their feelings and needs. If this sense of

▼ **TABLE 28-5   Group Phases, Leader and Member Tasks, and Group Behaviors**

Phase	Leader Tasks	Member Tasks	Group Behaviors

Orientation	Serve as catalyst:
	  Encourage verbalization of
	    feelings
	  Summarize process of group
	  Refuse to control group
	  Clarify work and goals of
	    group
		Identify with group
		Develop trust with group
		  Deal with anxiety
		  Verbalize thoughts and
		    feelings
			Relate superficially
			Test group rules
			Test each other
			Stay silent
			Intellectualize
			Depend on leader
			Compete for leader's attention

Working	Serve as role model:
	  Listen intently
	  Respond honestly
	  Support members' exposure
	    of feelings
	  Confront negative behaviors
	  Clarify work and goals of
	    group
		Maintain trust:
		  Expose innermost feelings
		Develop interdependence
		  with group members
		Develop responsibility for
		  own behaviors
			Relate intensely
			Attempt to avoid problem areas
			Manipulative behaviors
			Listen actively
			Confront each other
			Express all kinds of feelings
			Try out new behaviors
			Support positive changes in each other

Termination	Serve as resource person Process group efforts Share perceptions about what is occurring	Offer mutual support Say good-bye	Indicate goals have been met Say good-bye

safety does not develop, the group will not progress to the next stage.

During the working phase, the group openly addresses all kinds of feelings and concerns, positive and negative. Conflict and development of subgroups also need to be confronted and resolved. Tasks for members at this stage are to maintain trust, develop a sense of reliance on group members and then on oneself, and become responsible for group directions. The therapist's tasks are to model behaviors (such as listening intently), respond honestly, and support members as they expose their inner selves. The therapist keeps in mind that controlling activity is not therapeutic. Instead, she comments on the group process. She confronts unhealthy behaviors, such as monopolizing, putting oneself down, misinterpreting, assuming, and ignoring. The therapist does not give advice and insights from personal experience, even though sometimes it seems so obviously excellent. She also continually clarifies the work and goals of the group.

Termination can occur in three ways. In the closed group termination is planned by the group in advance and carried out on schedule. The second kind of termination is by the member who is unsuccessful in meeting his needs (in either a closed or open group). This person usually leaves abruptly without warning or eases out after a brief sojourn. Following are some reasons for premature termination:

EXTERNAL FACTORS	INTERNAL FACTORS
Moving away from the region	Not feeling accepted as a group member
Financial stressors	Not revealing needs to group
Acute physical disability or illness	Lacking trust or respect for leader or other group members
Obligations that conflict with sessions	Feeling overly pressured to participate actively
	Feeling that too much self-disclosure has occurred

The third kind of termination occurs in the open group when a member has achieved his goals. At first the individual tentatively signals that his goals have been accomplished. He may make statements about feeling good and having made changes. The leader may note that he is less active and more reflective. Others give feedback, stating how they view this member's progress. Sometimes the other members voice concerns (such as he still seems depressed), and the member may remain longer to do more individual work.

In many groups members are asked to remain for two or three sessions after making the decision to terminate to deal with the departure adequately. Ambivalent feelings, both sadness and happiness, in anticipation of the future are discussed. Other members also have mixed feelings about the termination, that is, sadness, envy, or anger. Usually everyone has a sense of loss.

In this final stage of the group, the therapist is more a resource person than an active leader. Group members are able to take care of their own needs and to give support to each other. Individual decision making is encouraged; however, the therapist continues to share her perceptions about what is occurring.

Regardless of the reasons for membership, the desired outcome is that the individual has a realistic self-perception, feels good about himself and others, and is ready to be responsible for himself in all areas of living.

Group Dynamics

Group dynamics involves all that takes place in a group from inception to termination, including group content and group process. *Group content* is the specific problems and tasks addressed, or the work of the group. *Group process* is the continuous interaction among members. Both process and content are equally important and occur simultaneously. The novice leader may recognize and work with content and ignore the process, even when it is disruptive. For example, the leader may be so intent on what one member is saying, she will not notice that two other members are whispering to each other. The constant nonverbal behaviors of group members are valuable clues to what is occurring inside each individual. As members become part of a group, they begin to reveal their usual patterns of behaving and relating. The leader and the other members scrutinize behaviors to identify possible areas for change.

Process refers to the many factors that help or hinder growth of group members. Among the important factors are *role behaviors*, behaviors used repeatedly by members. Role behaviors are divided into three major categories, outlined in Table 28-6.

Bales[4] used these groupings to categorize behaviors that affect process (Figure 28-2). Section *A* lists behaviors most conducive to implementing group process. Sections *B* and *C* are behaviors related to group task roles. Section *D* is behaviors that meet individual needs that may also hinder group process.

The Bales categorization is useful in identifying pro-

▼ TABLE 28-6   Role Behaviors

Type of Role	Effect on Group	Examples
Group task roles	Related to completing tasks or goals for which the group convened (group content)	Initiator, coordinator, evaluator, elaborator
Group building or maintenance roles	Related to building group cohesion and maintaining the group itself	Encourager, harmonizer, compromiser
Personal or individual roles	Related to needs of individual group members that do not assist the group task, building and maintenance roles	Aggressor, recognition seeker, dominator, blocker

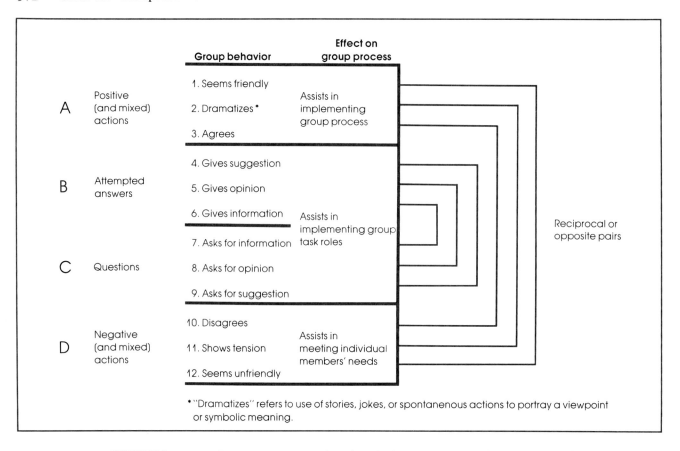

		Group behavior	Effect on group process		
A	Positive (and mixed) actions	1. Seems friendly 2. Dramatizes * 3. Agrees	Assists in implementing group process		Reciprocal or opposite pairs
B	Attempted answers	4. Gives suggestion 5. Gives opinion 6. Gives information	Assists in implementing group task roles		
C	Questions	7. Asks for information 8. Asks for opinion 9. Asks for suggestion			
D	Negative (and mixed) actions	10. Disagrees 11. Shows tension 12. Seems unfriendly	Assists in meeting individual members' needs		

* "Dramatizes" refers to use of stories, jokes, or spontanenous actions to portray a viewpoint or symbolic meaning.

FIGURE 28-2 Categories for interaction process analysis. *(Modified from Bales RF: Personality and interpersonal behavior, New York, 1970, Holt, Rinehart and Winston. Reprinted by permission of Holt, Rinehart and Winston.)*

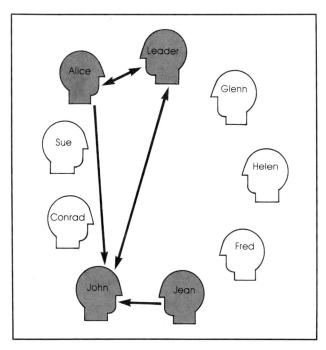

FIGURE 28-3 Process occurring during first 15 minutes of group therapy.

cesses in groups. While one co-leader leads the group, the other can act as recorder, using this scale to identify roles of the different members. The recorder checks the number of times each of the listed behaviors is used by each of the members. Obviously, this scale does not reveal the content of the communication, nor does it show the intensity of each behavior.

A method of identifying who talks to whom in a group is to have the therapist draw diagrams, or sociograms, of the group in time sequence immediately after the session ends. For each group there is a series of diagrams, which are accompanied by written capsules of the content of the interactions.

Figure 28-3 illustrates the process during the first 15 minutes of a therapy session. During this time the leader confronts John about his coming 20 minutes late to group 2 weeks in a row. John is apologetic, explaining that he had to drop off mail at the post office on the way and traffic was heavy. Alice sympathizes with John, saying that parking problems can also make it hard to be on time. The leader tells Alice that she is not helping John look at his behavior. Alice breaks into tears, stating that she likes John and was feeling sorry for him. Jean tells John that she feels annoyed with his lateness and excuse making.

Another useful tool for learning how group members interact is the Johari window (see Chapter 6). This tool can help members become aware of how much of the self

TABLE 28-7   Group Decision-making Procedures

Positive Process	Negative Process
Majority decision: More than half of the group come to agreement, but some disagree or compromise. *Consensus* (ideal): All group members come to agreement, with concern for both task achievement and persons involved; input is encouraged from all participants.	A *"plop":* A suggestion is given and it falls flat, usually causing the giver to withdraw. *Self-authorization:* One member makes a decision and expects it to be carried out regardless of group feelings. *Hand clasping:* Two group members support each other in decision making. *Minority decision:* A decision is made by less than half of the group by vocal and aggressive behaviors. *Rotten democracy:* A decision has already been made by the leader, but the decision-making procedure is carried out anyway. *"Group think"*[23]*:* Group pressure is imposed on members to be totally united in decision making regardless of individual concerns. Diversity of thought is discouraged.

is made available to others. The leader can also identify levels of risk taking as members ask for and give feedback.

Audiotapes of group sessions help the leader assess group interaction. Voice volume, tone qualities, rapidity and pitch of speech, pauses, and word emphasis give clues to underlying emotions. Videotaping gives the extra dimension of direct observation of participants and their nonverbal communication.

Members should be informed about any form of taping during the group, and their written permission should be obtained. The leader reassures members that only she and possibly other professionals learning about group therapy will review the tapes and that confidentiality will not be broken. Sometimes tapes are used in the sessions to review or clarify important incidents. In addition, members may review tapes to gain insight about their group interaction.

Decision making is both a group task and part of group process. Various means are used to make decisions, depending on type of leadership, degree of risk taking, sensitivity of the group to needs and wants of individuals and amount of trust. Table 28-7 identifies some helpful and unhelpful methods of decision making.

NURSING PROCESS

Assessment

Physical dimension When group members have obvious physical problems, such as disfigurement, obesity, or loss of a limb, the relationship to total body image is important to recognize and is appropriate for group focus. For example, the leader may notice that a young woman who is scarred or obese silently compares herself with someone who is attractive or slender. This client may lash out at the other member or avoid focus on herself. She may attempt to compensate by being overly helpful to other group members (being ingratiating in manner, smiling habitually, and saying and doing what she feels the others want) to avoid negative confrontation.

The nurse needs to assess how openly individual members acknowledge physical deficits or disabilities. The nurse assesses how members interact with individuals who put

themselves down or use ingratiating behavior because of unresolved feelings about real or perceived physical problems. She also assesses the impact of long-term or life-threatening illnesses, with responses of anxiety, anger, or depression.

Emotional dimension All the emotions felt by group members become part of the group process. Individuals in a group bring their fears, hopes, sadness, anger, and joy with them. These and their multiple attendant feelings create a unique mix in any group. The nurse assesses emotions experienced and expressed by members and the response of the others. The nurse also assesses feeling tones of the whole group. Sometimes a sense of sadness, lethargy, anger, or tension prevails. All are valuable messages about the process.

During group therapy anxiety is exhibited in a variety of behaviors. A member may be late, absent, or simply quiet. Anxiety may be triggered by many things, especially confrontation from other group members.

Anger is a component of group process. Some members are afraid of it, having been taught as children that anger is wrong. The therapist notes which members repress anger and cannot recognize it. She also notes which members attempt to be peacemakers or avoid angry participants. When anger is escalating, the nurse determines the degree that can be safely handled in the group and then decides how to deal with it constructively.

The nurse assesses guilt feelings in the group. She observes which members have themes of wrongdoing, making mistakes, neglecting to do things expected of them, or doing something displeasing to others.

Sometimes group members are despondent. They may withdraw, have poor personal grooming and hygiene, feel helpless and hopeless, or say that life is meaningless. Such behaviors frequently dampen the spirits of the entire group. The nurse notes the group's energy level. If she becomes aware of despondence in herself during group process, and it is not from personal concerns, she assesses where it is coming from in the group.

Intellectual dimension To benefit from group therapy and contribute to the work of the group, individuals must be able to verbalize well enough to be understood by the others and to think abstractly to deal with the ideas and feelings expressed. Usually, the acutely ill are not functional group members. A disoriented person is unable to receive accurate messages from others. An extremely egocentric person may attempt to monopolize the discussion. Membership is postponed until the client is able to both benefit and contribute.

The nurse is aware of how group members communicate with each other. Do they listen, interrupt, belittle, monopolize, use humor? What is the content of messages? Are some unclear and confusing? Are there repetitive themes? Are there distortions in thinking, such as viewing the therapist as an all-knowing, completely wise and good parent? Perhaps a member views the therapist or another group member as a person from his past, a parent, sibling, or spouse. If so, feelings of resentment, affection, or competition may emerge. These phenomena are important because they indicate unresolved conflicts.

Change in thinking may be gradual and subtle in expression. The group therapist looks for clues such as the client's more active participation in the group; asking for feedback from others; less rigid thinking, indicated by more receptiveness to reasons for behaviors of self and others; giving direct and honest responses instead of devious ones; and improvement in problem solving.

Social dimension The leader needs to be aware of individual behaviors and their effect on the group. Which members are chronic helpers, busying themselves with arranging the furniture or preparing coffee? Who are touchers, and who avoid touch? In each session the leader notes where people sit. Do they sit in the same location each time (territoriality)? Are they usually next to specific people? Are they near to or distant from the therapist? Do some attempt to sit apart from the group?

People in newly formed groups are reluctant to reveal sensitive aspects of themselves because trust has not yet been established. The therapist observes carefully who interacts with whom and how. As members learn to relate effectively with each other, they can learn to relate to an extended number of people outside of the group.

The nurse notes when individuals in the group are taking risks by exposing hidden parts of themselves and assesses whether others respond by being accepting and supportive. She considers all interactions among members. A monopolizer unchecked keeps others from having time to express their needs. A withdrawn member may feel cheated if not recognized and encouraged to participate. Some may attempt to draw attention away from troubling issues because of their own anxieties. Others may act seductively, condescendingly, or dependently. All of these reactions are clues to the members' responses outside the group.

Some members actively address needs and concerns of others but are unwilling to share personal thoughts and feelings. In some cultures, however, people do not readily reveal personal feelings or publicly display affection or other feelings. For example, African-American members in the presence of a white therapist may hide their feelings because of lack of trust. They may be ingratiating and attempt to second guess the therapist.[21] Latinos and Greeks often favor somatic complaints over emotional symptoms and are often reluctant to participate in "talking therapy."[13,48] Native American clients may be close to family members in private and diffident to people in public.[33] Mexican and Greek women may be very passive in a group, especially with men, and may perceive the therapist as having magical abilities.[13,48] Minority members in group therapy may also be much less expressive of feelings and thoughts when their native language is not used, even when they are fluent in the second language.[40,45] These generalizations are only guidelines and do not apply in all cases.

Spiritual dimension The group therapist needs to continually assess possible conflicts in values and beliefs that may interfere with group functioning. How, for example, does the group respond to differences in political, sexual, or religious stances? Does the group accept members who are economically, educationally, or socially different? Do such members feel rejected?

At times in the life of a group, important questions such as "Who and what am I?," "Where am I going?," and "How will I get there?" are addressed. Many persons have adopted values and beliefs from parents and others without much thought. The therapist notes if the group encourages the examination of these values, especially when the seeker's conclusions differ greatly from others in the group. Is there trust, inclusion, and group cohesiveness despite member differences? What is the client's sense of self-worth?

Analysis
Nursing diagnosis

The behavior of individual members and the total membership is analyzed, and group nursing diagnoses are formulated. To date, the North American Nursing Diagnoses Association (NANDA) has not dealt with diagnoses relating to group therapy. The following are examples of diagnoses that could relate to group or group member concerns as the nurse analyzes behaviors:

1. Lack of cohesiveness related to unwillingness of members to compromise
2. Increased anxiety related to perceived unsafe environment
3. Impaired group functioning related to need of member to monopolize
4. Unachieved group goals related to hostile member behaviors that are not confronted
5. Unwillingness to trust related to lack of confidence in the leader
6. Increased group anxiety related to confronting behaviors

Planning

As in other therapeutic methods, plans are made in group therapy to help promote the client's well-being. The nursing care plan provides some long- and short-term goals, outcome criteria, interventions, and rationales related to group therapy and are examples of the planning stage in the nursing process (Table 28-8). Each member is encouraged to set goals for himself and discuss how the group can help him achieve those goals. The goals of the group depend on the type of group and the needs of individual members.

Implementation

Physical dimension The nurse arranges to use a quiet room away from traffic flow so that she and group members can hear each other. Neutral or subdued room colors for most adolescent and adult groups are best. Bright colors are preferred for groups of regressed or older clients, who respond best to bright posters or other wall decorations and warm-colored furnishings. A floor-length mirror is useful in many groups for checking grooming and physical appearance. Simple and comfortable furnishings are provided, with chairs placed in a circle. When there are co-leaders, they may sit opposite each other to better observe all clients. Restrooms are always available.

Clients who are disfigured or disabled are encouraged to talk about themselves when comfortable enough. They may need a chance to share their feelings and are given time to grieve for what is missing or lost. They also may want to find out whether they are perceived as lovable despite deficits.

A major task for all group members is to learn how to take better care of themselves physically and emotionally. This task includes achieving a healthy life-style, with a balance of work, rest, and play. Each group member plans how to attain this healthy balance and is expected to enact it. The group gives support as changes are made. The nurse recognizes the improved appearance, increase in energy, and zest for living that accompanies feeling good.

Emotional dimension In group therapy the universality of negative feelings, such as anxiety, anger, guilt, and despair, is recognized. Expressing negative feelings can be healing. The chance to express these feelings with emotional support from others can allow emotional growth.

People need to face distressing emotional aspects of themselves instead of repressing or circumventing them. For example, group members are encouraged to experience their anxiety—to recall it in detail, relive it, and then, with help from the others, to deal with it. Ways of coping with anxiety include risk taking in the group, revealing feelings about group interactions, and asking for what is needed and wanted.

The angry group member is encouraged to verbally express the anger when it occurs and to direct it (verbally) to the person with whom he is angry. Members are also encouraged to hear angry messages from others when receiving feedback about behaviors or activities. These responses are useful in developing insight and constructively changing hurtful aspects of the self.

The client who feels guilt is encouraged to carefully assess the situations that trigger the feeling. If realistic amends need to be made, he is encouraged to make them. If relationships have been left hanging or activities are uncompleted, the nurse encourages the client with group support to find ways to bring about healthy resolutions. When no known situation causes the guilt, the person is encouraged to look at his past. Past messages may foster the need to feel guilty.

Depressed group members need caring from the others. These members are invited to contact both the therapist and others in the group between sessions if they need support (particularly if self-destruction is a possibility). They are strongly encouraged to attend group meetings even when disinclined and to take an active part. Assignments may be given for life outside of the group—tasks involving physical activity or doing a favor for someone else. Members report the results at the following session.

Depressed people typically focus on what they perceive as negative aspects of themselves and seek criticism from others. The nurse encourages them to accept nurturing from others (compliments and positive messages) as valid. Sometimes when the individual has been deprived of touch or when he feels withdrawn or out of contact with others, hugging or holding is especially healing.

Two messages are central to nearly all forms of group therapy. The first is that all people have a mix of all kinds of feelings, both positive and negative. All feelings are valuable parts of each person; no attempt to eliminate them is made. Group members learn to be in charge of these feelings, instead of being ruled by them. Each is encouraged to use feelings appropriate to the situation to become a more authentic and congruent individual.

The second message is to learn how to recognize and value the goodness in oneself. The nurse may use exercises such as telling the others what one likes about oneself and hearing positive messages from others. Fun and play are important for developing positive feelings, and members are encouraged to find many things to enjoy. As people learn to feel good about themselves, they will feel good about others.

Group therapy emphasizes that each person accept responsibility for emotions that are experienced. In the following example the therapist attempts to help group members become aware of this:

Therapist: No one can make you feel sad or glad or anxious or angry. You do this for yourself. These are your ways of experiencing and responding to what is happening in your life, inside and outside of yourself.

In all groups an important goal is to learn to feel good about oneself and to express negative feelings constructively.

Intellectual dimension When negative or rigid thinking is encountered during sessions, the therapist encourages clients to acknowledge it, to look at all sides of issues, and to select new patterns of behavior that will enhance interaction with others and give greater enjoyment (see Chapter 15).

Clients who have difficulty distinguishing fantasy from reality may benefit from group awareness exercises. These exercises focus on present reality and assessing the outer environment and one's own physical and emotional responses. Following is an example of an awareness exercise in which an individual alternates between focusing on outer environment and inner feelings.

Group member: I see (in the room) John smiling at me and leaning forward in his chair. . . . I feel scared, being the center of this attention. I hear people laughing a little. . . . My heart is pounding and my face feels flushed. . . . I see the yellow flowers on the table. . . .

This exercise continues until the client is better oriented to self, others, and environment and is relaxed.

Many group members may perceive the therapist as able to read their thoughts and solve their problems if only she were willing. Some even think she has magical abilities to perform miracles in their lives. These beliefs need to be confronted. The nurse verbalizes these perceptions of her omniscience and invites the group to share them with her. Simple denial of owning special powers may also be helpful and may need to be stated many times.

Social dimension One important goal of group therapy is to create a climate in which a client is truly free to address any concern. This cannot occur unless trust has been established; the therapist needs to provide an environment of trust and respect. The group rule on confidentiality keeps intimate knowledge about members in the group, thus creating a safe place in which to share such knowledge and work on behavioral changes.

When a member relates to the therapist or another member as someone else from his life experience, transference is taking place (e.g., when a member says to the therapist, "You remind me of a teacher I had once."). The nurse identifies this phenomenon and deals with the unresolved basic feelings. Sometimes the therapist relates to a group member as someone from personal life experience (e.g., an elderly uncle) (countertransference); she needs to recognize this so that her responses in the group are valid for that member.

The therapist confronts avoidance behaviors, and support is given by all for self-disclosure. The therapist can discourage avoidance and encourage disclosure by refusing to be authoritative in leading the group, modeling self-confidence and assertiveness, and supporting group members who reveal inner parts of themselves.

▼ **TABLE 28-8   NURSING CARE PLAN**

GOALS	OUTCOME CRITERIA	INTERVENTIONS	RATIONALE
NURSING DIAGNOSIS: Self-concept disturbance: low self-esteem related to unwillingness to compete in school with sister who is "brilliant" and successful			
LONG TERM			
To make vocational plans that mesh with own needs, abilities, and desires	Joins in group discussions that focus on future vocations and careers		
To feel good about self and sister	Statements and behavior reflect good feelings about self and sister		
SHORT TERM			
To join group discussion that focuses on future vocations and careers	Joins discussion group with focus on vocations and careers	Inform client of available discussion groups	Information gained on vocations and careers helps client feel comfortable relating to others with similar problems
		Encourage client to participate in group discussion by being attentive, reflecting before responding, asking for clarification, sharing thoughts and feelings, listening to others, paraphrasing what others have said	Listening and sharing thoughts and feelings helps to clarify thinking and learn problem solving
		Help client evaluate progress made through group discussion	Participation in evaluation process enhances decision making skills and self-esteem
To exchange positive messages with others in group	Exchanges positive messages with others in group	Teach listening and communication skills	Positive interactions with others facilitate good feelings about self
		Help client increase self-esteem by looking directly at other person, thanking the other person, telling others what is liked about them, describing things liked about self	Good feelings about self help client like/accept self with strengths/limitations and like/accept sister as different with strengths/limitations

▼ **TABLE 28-9** Indicators of a Positive Group Experience

Dimension	Indicator
Physical	Feeling good about one's body image; demonstrating respect for one's physical well-being by improving life-style (eating habits, exercise, rest, work, and recreation)
Emotional	Accepting caring messages from others; being in charge of one's feelings and accepting all kinds of feelings as part of self; feeling good about self and others
Intellectual	Asking for feedback about behaviors; being reality oriented; having expanded awareness of self, others, and environment
Social	Being willing to risk trusting others; sharing self and reaching out to others
Spiritual	Having a sense of being a valued part of the human race

Closeness is fostered in the group when members are allowed to know one another by being open and honest with each other. Members are vulnerable when they relate without their protective facade; the therapist gives support and positive recognition. This technique encourages other members to risk sharing more of themselves.

Willingness to expose oneself fosters not only a healthier integration of self but also the ability to be intimate with chosen individuals. True intimacy is a common need of group members; in the group, then, people practice intimacy by choosing moments when they disclose the most sensitive parts of their lives. They learn that intimacy leaves one vulnerable to being loved or rejected, is therefore risky, and yet gives intensity and meaning to life.

Spiritual dimension Group members support the sorting of values and beliefs by the following: (1) recognizing individual uniqueness as well as shared commonalities, (2) learning more about themselves through experiencing and interacting with other members, and (3) maintaining and enlarging personal identities while appreciating and accepting differences in others.

As group members share their experiences, the tragedies and pathos inevitable in life may bring tears, whereas the recognition of shared foolishness and awareness of the world may evoke laughter. Sometimes members experience deep joy as feelings of love are shared, along with the message that no one is alone if he is willing to reach out to others. Individuals also learn that they are vulnerable to life's stressors, yet can be fully in charge of their responses as they are guided by their chosen values.

Evaluation

Subjectively, if group members feel good about themselves and others and have met their personal goals for group involvement, group therapy can be viewed as effective. Objectively, the nurse can evaluate clients who have recently completed their group therapy, noting the degree and nature of the change, the group experiences effecting that change, and the contributions of other factors in the

▼ **TABLE 28-10** Group Therapy Through the Life Cycle

Type	Purpose
CHILDREN	
Activity group therapy	For troubled children ages 7 to 12 to participate in creative and manual activities to increase self-esteem and gain acceptance from others
Activity-interview group psychotherapy	For discussing feelings generated by group interaction
Play group therapy	For disturbed children to increase play experiences and master drives and conflicts through verbal and nonverbal expression of feelings
ADOLESCENTS	
Peer groups	For increasing self-esteem and independence, affirming self-identity, and learning to relate to others
ADULTS	
Growth groups	For establishing interpersonal relationships and intimacy
Groups with a specific focus	For growing emotionaly, understanding self, and making behavioral changes
ELDERLY ADULTS	
Remotivation groups	For withdrawn, regressed persons for sensory and intellectual stimulation
Reality orientation groups	
Validation groups	
Reminiscence groups	For remembering past experiences
Expressive groups	For promoting expression of feelings

GROUP THERAPY THROUGH THE LIFE CYCLE

Table 28-10 outlines specific group therapies available for different age groups.

BRIEF REVIEW

Theoretical frameworks help determine the approach used in group therapy. Therapists choose theoretical frameworks in accordance with their personal belief systems and the goals of the group.

Groups are classified as (1) group therapy, (2) therapeutic groups, and (3) adjunctive groups. All groups progress in three phases. In the orientation phase anxiety is the dominant feeling and needs to be channeled so that trust can develop and members can identify with the group.

The major work of the group occurs during the working phase. Termination takes place when (1) the group reaches its scheduled end, (2) a member leaves the group without warning or planning, or (3) a member's goals have been reached.

Group dynamics involves all that takes place in a group from inception to termination. Group process and group content are the two equally important components of group dynamics.

Therapy is viewed as effective if group members feel good about themselves and others, have obtained their personal goals, and the achievement is validated by the group.

REFERENCES AND SUGGESTED READINGS

1. American Nurses Association, Division on Psychiatric–Mental Health Nursing: *Standards of psychiatric and mental health nursing practice,* Kansas City, 1982, ANA.
2. American Nurses Association, Division on Psychiatric–Mental Health Nursing: *Statement on psychiatric and mental health nursing practice,* Kansas City, 1976, ANA.
3. August I and others: Women's groups: a non-traditional method of mental health treatment, *Canadian Nurse* 81:26, 1985.
4. Bales R: *Personality and interpersonal behavior,* New York, 1970, Holt, Rinehart & Winston.
5. Birckhead I: The nurse as leader: group psychotherapy with psychotic patients, *Journal of Psychosocial Nursing* 22:24, 1984.
6. Brabender V and others: A study of curative factors in short-term group psychotherapy, *Hospital and Community Psychiatry* 34:643, 1983.
7. Bumagin S, Smith J: Beyond support: group psychotherapy with low income mothers, *International Journal of Group Psychotherapy* 35:279, 1985.
8. Cohn B: Keeping the group alive: dealing with resistance in a long term group of psychotic patients, *International Journal of Group Psychotherapy* 38:3, 1988.
9. Cox E, Lothstein L: Video self portraits: a novel approach to group psychotherapy with young adults, *International Journal of Group Psychotherapy* 39:2, 1989.
10. DeBosset F: Group psychotherapy in chronic psychiatric outpatients: a Toronto model, *International Journal of Group Psychotherapy* 41:1, 1991.
11. DeCarufel F, Piper W: Group psychotherapy or individual psychotherapy: patient characteristics as predictive factors, *International Journal of Group Psychotherapy* 38:2, 1988.
12. Delgado M: Hispanics and psychotherapeutic groups, *International Journal of Group Psychotherapy* 33:507, 1983.
13. Dunkas N, Nikelly A: Group psychotherapy with Greek immigrants, *International Journal of Group Psychotherapy* 25:402, 1975.
14. Durkin J, editor: *Living groups: group psychotherapy and general systems theory,* New York, 1981, Brunner/Mazel.
15. Echternacht M: Day treatment transition groups: helping outpatients stay out, *Journal of Psychosocial Nursing* 22:11, 1984.
16. Ettin M: Come on Jack, tell us about yourself. The growth spurt of group psychotherapy, *International Journal of Group Psychotherapy* 39:1, 1989.
17. Ettin M: By the crowd they have been broken, by the crowd they shall be healed: the advent of group psychotherapy, *International Journal of Group Psychotherapy* 38:2, 1988.
18. Gans J: Hostility in group psychotherapy, *International Journal of Group Psychotherapy* 39:4, 1989.
19. Grojahn M: *Handbook of group therapy,* New York, 1983, Van Nostrand Reinhold.
20. Hardy-Fanta C, Montana P: The Hispanic female adolescent: a group therapy model, *International Journal of Group Psychotherapy* 32:351, 1982.
21. Heckel R: Relationship problems: the white therapist treating blacks in the south, *International Journal of Group Psychotherapy* 25:421, 1975.
22. Hyland J and others: The impact of the death of a group member in a group of breast cancer patients, *International Journal of Group Psychotherapy* 34:617, 1984.
23. Janis I: Group think, *Psychology Today* 5:71, 1971.
24. Kahn E: The choice of therapist self disclosure in psychotherapy groups: contextual considerations, *Archives of Psychiatric Nursing* 1(1):62, 1987.
25. Kanas N, Stewart P, Haney K: Short term outpatient therapy groups for schizophrenics, *International Journal of Group Psychotherapy* 39:4, 1989.
26. Kaplan R: The dynamics of injury in encounter groups: power, splitting, and the mismanagement of resistance, *International Journal of Group Psychotherapy* 32:163, 1982.
27. King K: Reminiscing psychotherapy with aging people, *Journal of Psychosocial Nursing* 20(2):21, 1982.
28. Leszcz M and others: A mens' group: psychotherapy of elderly men, *International Journal of Group Psychotherapy* 35:177, 1985.
29. Lieberman M, Bliwise N: Comparisons among peer and professionally directed groups for the elderly: implications for the development of self help groups, *International Journal of Group Psychotherapy* 35:155, 1985.
30. Lieberman M: Understanding how groups work: a study of homogeneous peer group failures, *International Journal of Group Psychotherapy* 40:1, 1990.
31. Lieberman M: A group therapist perspective on self help groups, *International Journal of Group Psychotherapy* 40:3, 1990.
32. Marcovitz R, Smith J: Patients perceptions of curative factors in short term group, *International Journal of Group Psychotherapy* 33:21, 1983.
33. McGoldrick M, Pearce J, Giordano J, editors: *Ethnicity and family therapy,* New York, 1982, The Guilford Press.
34. McIntosh D, Stone W, Grace M: The flexible boundaried group: format, techniques, and patients' perceptions, *International Journal of Group Psychotherapy* 41:1, 1991.
35. Moss N: Child therapy groups in the real world, *Journal of Psychosocial Nursing* 22:43, 1984.
36. Newton G: Self help groups, *Journal of Psychosocial Nursing* 22:27, 1984.
37. Ormont L: The leader's role in resolving resistance to intimacy in the group, *International Journal of Group Psychotherapy* 38:1, 1988.
38. Perls F: *The Gestalt approach and eye witness to therapy,* Palo Alto, Calif, 1974, Science & Behavior Books.
39. Rogers C: *Carl Rogers on encounter groups,* New York, 1970, Harper & Row.
40. Ruiz P: Group therapy with minority group patients, *International Journal of Group Psychotherapy* 25:389, 1975.
41. Rutan J, Alonso A, Groves J: Understanding defenses in group psychotherapy, *International Journal of Group Psychotherapy* 38:4, 1988.
42. Soldz S and others: Patient activity and outcome in group psychotherapy: new findings, *International Journal of Group Psychotherapy* 40:1, 1990.
43. Stone W: Treatment of the chronically mentally ill: an opportunity for the group therapist, *International Journal of Group Psychotherapy* 41:1, 1991.
44. Sullivan HS: *The interpersonal theory of psychiatry,* New York, 1953, WW Norton.
45. Tylim I: Group psychotherapy with Hispanic patients: the psychodynamics of idealization, *International Journal of Group Psychotherapy* 32:339, 1982.

46. Weiner M: Group therapy in a public sector psychiatric clinic, *International Journal of Group Psychotherapy* 38:3, 1988.

47. Weiner M: *Techniques of group psychotherapy,* Washington, DC, 1984, American Psychiatric Press.

48. Werben J, Hynes K: Transference and culture in a Latino therapy group, *International Journal of Group Psychotherapy* 25:396, 1975.

49. Yalom I: *The theory and practice of group psychotherapy,* ed 3, New York, 1985, Basic Books.

50. Yalom I: *Inpatient group psychotherapy,* New York, 1983, Basic Books.

ANNOTATED BIBLIOGRAPHY

Ettin M: By the crowd they have been broken, by the crowd they shall be healed: the advent of group psychotherapy, *International Journal of Group Psychotherapy* 38:2, 1988.

A detailed and careful study of the evolution of group psychotherapy from the psychoeducation of Pratt in the early 1900s to the founding of the American Group Psychotherapy Association (AGPA) in 1942 by Slavson.

McGoldrick M, Pearce J, Giordano J, editors: *Ethnicity and family therapy,* New York, 1982, The Guilford Press.

An excellent resource for understanding cultural nuances in group as well as in family therapy. Twenty-four paradigms are included, with focus on cultural values and implications for therapy.

Weiner M: *Techniques of group psychotherapy,* Washington, DC, 1984, American Psychiatric Press.

Written for all mental health professionals, the book emphasizes ways to individualize techniques to specific treatment settings, patient populations, and individual patients. It also discusses institutional, legal, and research issues of group therapy.

Weiner M: Group therapy in a public sector psychiatric clinic, *International Journal of Group Psychotherapy* 38:3, 1988.

Addresses different approaches to group therapy with public sector clients, including advice giving, emotional support, concrete forms of social support, modeling, and direct teaching.

Yalom I: *Inpatient group psychotherapy,* New York, 1983, Basic Books.

A much needed focus on modifications from traditional group therapy for work with this population is presented. In the inpatient setting autonomy is often lacking when the administrative staff takes on many of the task functions of the therapist. In addition, group therapy is but one of several modalities used for client treatment. By necessity it will be of short duration. Yalom suggests in this setting that therapists be active, always supportive, and use a variety of techniques that facilitate the construction of a safe, trusting environment. One should have a here-and-now focus, and high- and low-functioning clients should be in separate groups. A readable and valuable resource for all nurses in institutional settings who are providing group experiences for their clients.

Yalom I: *The theory and practice of group psychotherapy,* ed 3, New York, 1985, Basic Books.

Definitive, classical writing relating to all aspects of group therapy. If the reader could have only one source for understanding group therapy, this would be the choice.

CHAPTER

29 Family Therapy

Susan H McCrone
Anne H Shealy

After studying this chapter, the student will be able to:

- Identify historical events related to family therapy
- Describe the psychopathology of the medical diagnoses, other specified family circumstances, and phase of life problem or other life circumstance problem as described in DSM-III-R
- Discuss selected theoretical frameworks of family therapy
- Describe characteristics of a family therapist
- Discuss characteristics of family therapy
- Apply the nursing process to clients who are seen for family therapy
- Identify current research findings relevant to family therapy

The definition of what constitutes a family has changed greatly in the last decade. The concept of the traditional two-parent family has been expanded to include the concepts of single-parent families, blended families, and often nontraditional families. The family can be more broadly defined today as people who are linked together by blood, affection, loyalty, and/or time and who see their lives as interconnected.

The family unit occupies a position between the individual and society. Its functions are twofold: (1) to meet the needs of the individuals in it, and (2) to meet the needs of the society of which it is a part. For the adult members, the family stabilizes their lives—meeting their affectional, socioeconomic, and sexual needs. For the children, the family provides physical and emotional care and directs personality development. The family is the primary early learning context for the individual's behavior, thoughts, and feelings. For society, the family, through its procreation and socialization of new members, fills a vital need. It is a group of individuals that society treats as a unit.

Family therapy is that branch of psychiatry that sees an individual's psychiatric symptoms as inseparably related to the family in which he lives. Different theories of family therapy incorporating the idea of the family as the focus of treatment have evolved over the last 50 years. They serve as a framework for assessing and intervening in family problems. Today, most family theorists identify the individual's problems as a symptom of trouble within the family.

After a discussion of DSM-III-R diagnoses, this chapter presents the historical development of family therapy as a treatment modality. It briefly describes several selected the-

oretical approaches to family therapy and discusses characteristics of the therapist and the clients who benefit from this type of therapy. Finally, the nursing process within the context of family therapy is discussed.

DSM-III-R DIAGNOSES

The diagnostic categories that relate to family therapy are classified as V codes. V codes are used for conditions not attributable to a mental disorder that are a focus for treatment. Clients in family therapy may have major mental disorders, but the focus of treatment is the family as a unit. Two DSM-III-R classifications apply to family therapy. *Other*

▶ DIAGNOSES Related to Family Therapy

MEDICAL DIAGNOSES	NURSING DIAGNOSES
Other specified family circumstances	**NANDA**
Phase of life problem or other life circumstance problem	Altered family processes
	Family coping: potential for growth
	Ineffective family coping: compromised
	Ineffective family coping: disabling
	PMH
	Impaired family role

HISTORICAL OVERVIEW

DATES	EVENTS
World War II	War led to increased concern over treatment of the family as a whole.
1954	Bowen, one of the pioneers in family therapy, began to hospitalize and observe the schizophrenic child and the entire family.
1957	Midelfort's work, *The Family in Psychotherapy*, emphasized the importance of the family's involvement in the therapy of the psychotic member.
1958	Ackerman contributed an important milestone in the development of psychoanalytical family therapy with publication of *The Psychodynamics of Family Life.*
1959	Family therapy became nationally known. Jackson formed the Mental Health Research Institute (MHRI), which served as an arena for research on family problems. Satir joined Jackson at MHRI as the first female family therapist.
Early 1960s	Minuchin began a research project to study the families of delinquent boys.
1961	Many books and journals on family therapy were published; among these was *Family process,* authored by Ackerman and Jackson.
1965	Ackerman founded the Family Institute (later named the Ackerman Family Institute).
1966	Ackerman's publication, *Treating the Troubled Family,* made the greatest early contribution to family therapy as treatment of the whole family.
	Committee on the Family of the Group for the Advancement of Psychiatry (known as of 1970 as the Group for the Advancement of Psychiatry) distributed a questionnaire and learned that many theorists were interested in family therapy.
1967	First joint meeting of family therapy clinicians and researchers.
Late 1960s to early 1970s	Family therapy included as an aspect of the curriculum of master's specialization in psychiatric–mental health nursing.
1970s-1980s	Psychiatric–mental health nurses publish articles and books on family therapy. The family is one of the clients for whom the psychiatric–mental health nurse provides treatment.
1979	Beginning of a bridge between child therapy and family therapy.
1990s	Families are targeted for intervention around the issues of violence (abuse, neglect, incest), codependence (adult children of alcoholics), and caregiving.
Future	Families will be broadly defined and preventive family therapy used to prevent crises.

specified family circumstances is a classification that can be used when a family's difficulties are not due to a parent-child or marital problem. Interpersonal problems with an aged in-law or sibling rivalry are examples of the focus of treatment. The second classification, *phase of life problem or other life circumstance problem,* can be used when the focus of treatment is related to a problem with the family's developmental life cycle.

THEORETICAL APPROACHES

The term family therapy refers to a wide variety of methods and techniques that includes many different theoretical approaches. When family therapy was first identified as a special type of therapy, it was generally defined as the treatment of the whole family group in joint interviews. As family thinking developed and as family therapists gained experience, family therapy has become a new orientation toward psychiatric problems. It is no longer defined by the number of bodies present in the room with a therapist.

Family therapy today is not a treatment method in the usual sense of the word; it is a way of conceiving problems. There are no generally agreed-upon set of procedures that practitioners who consider themselves family therapists follow. What these practitioners from different theoretical orientations have in common is the belief that problems in an individual may be expressions of family problems. They share the conviction that seeing members of a family together offers advantages over seeing individual family members alone in individual psychotherapy. Even if they see an individual, they view the family as the basic unit of treatment. From these basic views, various methods of assessment and interventions have emerged, all of them considered theoretical orientations to family therapy.

Psychoanalytical

With the development of psychoanalytical family therapy, Ackerman departed from the ideas of traditional psychoanalytical therapy, which focused on the individual, to a view that identified the family as the primary focus and the individual members as a secondary focus. However, he still identified the client's problems from an individual and intrapsychic (arising within the self) viewpoint.

After an initial psychosocial evaluation of the whole family was completed, Ackerman thought the therapy should focus on restoring the internal balance of the forces in the individual's personality. Therapy should be oriented "to the specific dynamic relations of personality and family role and to the balance between intrapsychic (internal) conflict and family (interpersonal) conflict."[1] Change was thought to occur as a result of a corrective relationship with the therapist, not through change among the family members. As this change occurred, however, emotional health in the individual's relations with the family group would occur spontaneously.

Ackerman identified several main principles in the psychotherapy of a family group[1]:
1. The illness of one member of the family, both diagnosis and symptoms, is a reflection of the emotional problems of the entire family.
2. The individual who is referred for therapy is either the scapegoat or a replacement for a more disturbed family member.
3. Often the illness and accompanying defense patterns are passed from one generation to the next.
4. Illness results from the conflict between the need to be connected to the family and the need to establish a self-identity.
5. In disturbed families, many people have psychiatric disorders.

To bring about change within the individual and the family, Ackerman believed that the therapist needed to enter the family in the role of a parent figure. This technique would enable the therapist to provide support, control interpersonal danger, and provide the emotional elements that the family was lacking. The therapist identified defense mechanisms within the individual, thus allowing intrapsychic conflicts to be expressed as interpersonal interaction. This process is achieved through a mechanism Ackerman identified as *tickling the defenses,* a confrontive technique in which the therapist points out the contradiction between conscious attitudes and patterns of action. The therapist acts as a facilitator for efforts of the family members to balance sameness and differences, togetherness and individuation. Finally, the therapist serves as an educator of healthy family functioning. By combining these roles of supporter, interpreter, confronter, and educator, the therapist shakes up the usual functioning of the family and opens the way for a healthier realignment of family relationships.

Psychoanalytical theory, as it applies to families, moved the focus from purely individual to looking at the impact of intrapsychic conflict in the individual on the interpersonal environment of the family.

Systems Theory

Many family therapy theoretical approaches use ideas from general systems theory. All family members are part of the family system and everything outside of the family system is the environment. Some important characteristics of a system apply to the family.
1. One part is interdependent on the other. If there is a change in one part, there is a change in the whole system. When one family member changes, the whole family changes.
2. The system has organization of some kind; everything is related. Each family has a unique structure of organization.
3. A system is greater than the sum of its parts. The family is not the mere sum of its individual members.
4. A system strives to maintain balance, often referred to as homeostasis or steady state. Families are trying to achieve a balance and resist change.
5. The more energy it takes to operate the system, the less is available for growth. Each system moves around energy. If it takes a large amount of energy to maintain balance in the family system, there is little left for growth.
6. The same elements are parts of more than one system. Families are part of larger systems such as church, school, and work.

With these characteristics in mind, two models of family therapy that incorporate system's ideas are discussed.

Structural family therapy

Minuchin[35] was the first theorist to describe structural family therapy. Based on this approach, the family with a problem is seen as a system that is in dysfunction. The problem in the system is sustained by the underlying structure of the family. Minuchin believed that families reveal dysfunctional structures through their interactions. The role of the therapist is to join the family in a position of leadership, identify and evaluate the family structure, and then create situations that allow the structure to change. Structural therapists are not interested in the origin of the problem as are the psychoanalytical family therapists; instead they focus on the problem as it exists in the present. The goal is to find and change the underlying family structure that supports the problem's existence.

The three most important concepts noted in the assessment phase of structural family therapy are boundaries, alignments, and power. The idea of boundaries is taken from general systems theory. Minuchin identifies the boundaries of subsystems within the larger family system. Frequently, the siblings are defined as one subsystem and the parents as another. Other subsystems such as the older and younger children or boys and girls may exist. Minuchin uses the subsystems to change the structure of the family.

Boundaries are further described as rigid or diffuse. Rigid boundaries lead to a distance between the family and the environment, which may promote emotional isolation and hamper communication. These families can be described as *disengaged,* a term meaning apathetic, unresponsive, and lacking in relationships or connections among members. Boundaries described as diffuse offer warmth and support from the family but may not allow for autonomy and individuality. These families can be identified as *enmeshed,* meaning that interactions are intense and focus on power conflicts rather than affection.

Alignment is a concept that describes who takes sides with whom. In assessing a family, the structural family therapist may draw a map as a shorthand method of identifying membership in subgroups, boundaries, and alignments. The therapist uses the map only as a guide for herself or as a tool to teach families these concepts. Figure 29-1 illustrates this type of map. In this family, a diffuse boundary exists between Susan, Mother, and Grandmother. In other words, Mother and Grandmother are both trying to parent Susan instead of each generation accepting its own role. Cindy is clearly in conflict with Mother with a rigid boundary, and Grandmother is staying out of that relationship. Sam is shown on the family map as having clear boundaries between the female members of the family and himself.

The concept of power within the family is significant to assessment and treatment in structural family therapy. Min-uchin found that the symptomatic person in the family was often in the position of power even if that person was a child. The therapeutic goal in these cases was to "join" the family to change the relative power positions.

The structural family therapist intervenes actively to modify the structure of the family. Whether the therapist joins by taking sides with the weak parent to provide support in the discipline of a child or directs the child from the sidelines to interact directly with the father without going through the mother, the therapist is in the middle of the family.

The therapist's next task is to restructure the situation so that the dysfunctional structure is replaced by a more functional one. In the situation described by the map, Mother may be joined by the therapist to empower her to tell Grandmother to let her parent Susan. This returns the power to parental subsystem and changes the boundaries in the system.

Three techniques unique to structural family therapy are well known: system recomposition, symptom focusing, and structural modification. An example of *system recomposition* is the removal of the grandmother in the relationship between the mother and Susan. With this extraction, the mother and daughter have an opportunity to interact within their designated roles.

Symptom focusing is probably one of the better known techniques in structural family therapy. The therapist em-

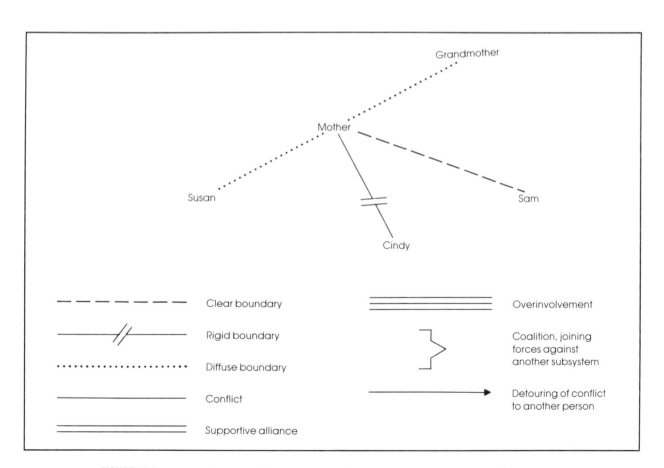

FIGURE 29-1 Mapping. *(From Minuchin S: Families and family therapy, Cambridge, Mass, 1974, Harvard University Press.)*

phasizes the symptom by encouraging the client to increase it. In this way, the therapist takes control of the system. For example, the client who acts depressed and withdrawn is told to become more depressed and withdrawn. He is told to increase the amount of time that he is miserable by setting aside numerous, specific times each day to dwell on and magnify his condition. The client is willing to follow the therapist's prescription to get better, and the family is less upset than before because the therapist has prescribed the behavior. The client finds that having to be depressed and withdrawn more of the time is tiresome, which encourages him to seek out alternative ways to get attention from the family.

In the third technique, *structural modification,* the therapist may ask family members to move physically during a session to create this modification. For instance, a therapist may observe an overly close alliance between mother and son, conflict between father and son, and a problematic marriage. The therapist may use structural modification in the session by separating the son from his mother's side and sending him to sit with his siblings, and then telling the father to move and sit beside his wife. Modifying the structure during a therapy session presents appropriate generational boundaries physically in the seating arrangement.

While joining the family, the therapist is able to maintain enough objectivity to effect change. The therapist gives directions to the family and continually assesses the effectiveness of the interventions based on the family's response. Although most often therapists work with the nuclear family, others such as teachers, clergy, and friends may be included if they are relevant to the problem.

Bowen theory

As with structural family therapy, Bowen theory derives many of its concepts from general systems theory. The family is considered the unit of treatment. The individual family member, whom the family identifies as the patient, is seen as reflecting the disturbances and anxieties of the family itself. The family system is considered the most intense system with which any person is involved. It has the most consistent, on-going influence in the development of a person's capacity to deal with other people. People learn patterns of behavior in their families. Although there are eight basic concepts of family systems theory,[6] six can be used easily in working with families. These concepts apply to all families, functional or dysfunctional.

The first and most fundamental concept of the Bowen theory is the *triangle.* The triangle is the basic emotional unit in the family system. A two-person system is smaller but unstable; the triangle is the smallest stable relationship system. It is a three-person system with relationship patterns that repeat in periods of calm and stress. For example, in a family with a teenaged daughter, if there is conflict between the mother and daughter over curfew time, the daughter may bring the father into the issue to support her. If this maneuver is successful, this triangle is repeated. Triangles are patterned ways of dealing with intense anxiety and of avoiding dealing directly with a problem or issue in a relationship, in this case the mother-daughter relationship. The family has been described as a series of interlocking triangles.

The second concept is the *undifferentiated family ego mass* or *nuclear family emotional system.* This concept is similar to Minuchin's enmeshment. Members of families do not see themselves as separate from each other. What happens to one person is seen as happening to the whole family. It is a stick-togetherness or "emotional oneness." Examples of comments that indicate the existence of an undifferentiated family ego mass are family members saying they know what someone in the family is going to do before he does it, or saying that they know what someone is going to say before he says it. All families have some undifferentiated ego mass. To the extent that individual members can draw on this shared self when needed yet differentiate their individual self, the family becomes more mature, stronger, flexible, and capable of dealing with the environment.

These ideas of undifferentiated ego mass lead to the third concept of *differentiation of self.* Individuals in the family will differ in the amount of their involvement in this family ego mass. This concept corresponds roughly with emotional maturity. Differentiation involves the degree to which someone's thinking and feeling are separated from each other. Bowen saw differentiation as determined by the degree to which one's self fuses or merges into another self in a close emotional relationship. The more differentiated a person is, the more he functions from a thinking rather than a feeling system.

Bowen developed a scale of differentiation from 0 at the lower end to 100 at the upper end (Figure 29-2). In reality, no one is totally emotionally mature (differentiated) or immature (undifferentiated). Persons on the lower end of the scale are so ruled by their emotions that decisions are made on the spur of the moment and are not well thought out. Theoretically, these persons experience the greatest frequency of psychiatric, social, and physical problems. An undifferentiated person may commit to support a proposal before a meeting, but seeing that his friends are voting against the proposal, he votes against it. In explaining his position, he says, "I wouldn't have supported the proposal before the meeting if you had told me my friends were voting against it."

Individuals on the upper end of the differentiation scale base their decisions on thoughts (Figure 29-3). They function more independently and as a result have fewer problems. People in the midrange have enough basic differentiation for thinking and feeling systems to function side by side. When anxiety gets high, however, feelings tend to predominate thinking. A more differentiated person votes

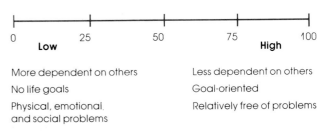

FIGURE 29-2 Differentiation-of-self scale.

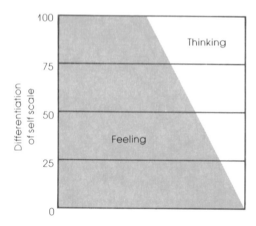

FIGURE 29-3 Conception of balance between thinking and emotional systems as it relates to differentiation-of-self scale. *(Diagram created by Anne H Shealy.)*

his beliefs no matter what his friends vote. His response to his friends may be, "It's all right if you cannot accept me. This is the way I am."

Individuals in a family who are lower on the differentiation scale will experience more anxiety and hence a greater fear of fusion. Bowen suggests that the family use four major mechanisms to deal with the anxiety caused by the fear of fusing.

1. *Emotional distance:* The most universal mechanism. People gain distance from each other by activities such as watching TV, playing golf, going to school, having affairs, or moving across the country.
2. *Marital conflict:* In this form each spouse fights, either verbally or physically, for an equal share of family ego mass.
3. *Dysfunction in one spouse:* The two selves come together and form a "shared self." One of the partners uses this shared self so much that the other partner is left with so little self that he becomes dysfunctional.
4. *Transmission of the problem to the child:* Once a child joins the marital dyad a triangle occurs. The parents transfer the anxiety about their own relationship and fusion onto the child and focus their attention on the child. The child becomes symptomatic and expresses the conflict for the family. This is called the *family projection process.*

These four mechanisms operate in *all* families, not just in dysfunctional ones. Most normal families use all of them at various times rather than using one and excluding the others.

The *family projection process,* the fourth concept, is the way in which the anxiety of the parents is passed onto a child. There is no way to predict which child will receive the focus of this parental intensity, but it is often related to the level of differentiation each spouse brought into the marriage and to the circumstances surrounding a child's conception and birth. For instance, a child who is born on a beloved grandfather's birthday may become the child who is the focus of parental intensity, or a child with physical handicaps may become the projected child.

When the family projection process goes through successive generations, it is called the *multigenerational transmission process.* This fifth concept describes the projected child as usually having a higher degree of anxiety and a lower level of differentiation. That child grows up and marries a person with a similar level of differentiation, and the multigenerational transmission process continues into the next generation. Just as a genetic predisposition for diabetes can be traced through the use of a genogram, anxiety can be traced in families through the use of multigenerational transmission.

The final concept is *sibling position.* This idea was borrowed from the work of Walter Toman.[13] Toman found that the sibling positions and family configurations predict certain behavior trends, personality traits, and social inclinations and are determined by the sexes and age ranks of all the persons in the immediate family. For instance, an older brother of brothers would have different characteristics than an older brother of sisters.

The three generational genogram (Figure 29-4) is used to discover how the system has worked over time and how it is working currently. Through the construction of the genogram, triangles are identified, mechanisms for dealing with anxiety are illustrated, and sibling position can be determined. A triangle can actually be drawn on the genogram with the indication of the close and conflictual legs of the triangle. By pointing out patterns of biological as well as emotional transmission of traits such as heart disease or anxiety from one generation to the next, the therapist can identify patterns of multigenerational transmission. The family system, not an individual person, is the focus of treatment.

Bowen stresses that the therapist must not enter the family's emotional system and must be able to recognize attempts to pull her into the system. For instance, in the genogram (Figure 29-4), both the mother, Martha, and the daughter, Jane, may try to triangle the therapist into joining their side in their conflictual relationship with each other. Bowen also stresses that the therapist must remain in emotional contact without taking sides.

One goal of family therapy, based on the Bowen theory is to identify and modify important, usually fixed triangles. The therapist gets the two main people in the triangle together, and the therapist becomes the third member of the triangle. In this way, the therapist reacts and responds differently from the person who usually is in the triangle. This approach keeps the conflict where it belongs, between the two key people. By remaining neutral, the therapist forces the couple to deal with each other and to clarify issues between themselves. For example, a couple is referred for family therapy because of recurring depression in the husband, which prevents him from working. His mother has been aiding the family by caring for the husband and children while the wife now works two jobs. Because the wife cannot express her anger at her "sick" husband or unselfish mother-in-law, she, too, is becoming depressed. The therapist sees the couple together and is able, by not taking sides, to get the couple to think about the situation and express their thoughts to each other. In this way, she removes the mother-in-law from the triangle, and provides a neutral third leg. Emotional systems in families are automatic. People in them cannot see them easily. For family members to see how they operate with each other, the therapist must interrupt the cycle.

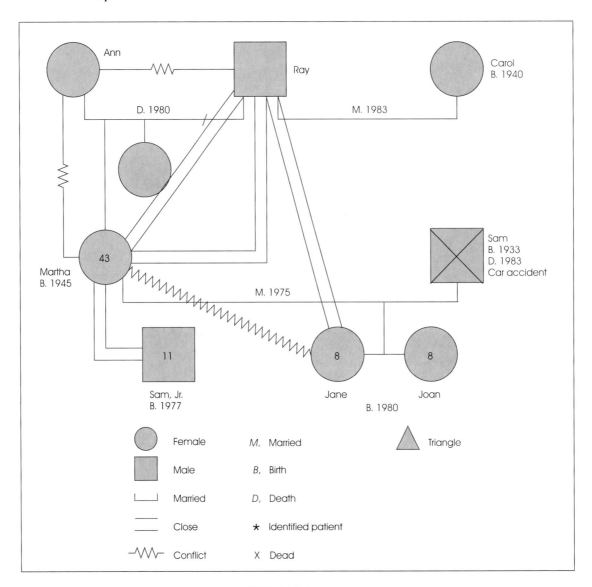

FIGURE 29-4 Genogram.

Unlike the structural family therapist who joins the family, the therapist using Bowen theory remains an observer, educator, and coach. To maintain this neutrality, it is important for the therapist to have undertaken work on her own family of origin. Unless she gains direct knowledge of the process of differentiation in her own family, the therapist cannot be useful to the client family. A second requirement is ongoing supervision. Without an objective outside opinion, the therapist is at risk of getting triangled into the family.

Humanistic

Communication

Virginia Satir conceptualized treating dysfunctional families from a group therapy framework.[40] She intentionally focused on communication among family members as the area in the family that needs the therapist's attention. The goal of therapy is to improve communication, making it clear, accurate, and meaningful to the family.[22]

The therapist who supports a communication framework accepts several principles.[39] First is the assumption that there is no way not to communicate because communication occurs on a behavioral and emotional level even when someone is silent. Second is the assumption that communication is an exchange of information in a family that becomes repetitive and predictable and is governed by unspoken family rules about what is to be discussed and by whom. Because the family is seldom aware of their unspoken rules of communication, the therapist observes the behavior that supports the rule and verbalizes it for the family to consider. For example, if Susan asks Mother for money for a new dress, Mother may tell her that Father says the money is not available. The rules may be that Mother protects the children from Father. The therapist may comment on this rule, allowing family members the option of dealing with each other more directly.

Another aspect of Satir's communication theory in dealing with troubled families examines how a person's style of nonverbal communication fits with his self-esteem. She stated that the postures of the placater, the blamer, and the computer identify how he feels about himself.

For example, the placater is always trying to please someone else, and his posture looks as if he were begging for the merest crumb of acknowledgment or recognition.[10] The placater's words are full of agreement, and his goal seems to be to constantly please his audience because he sees his own opinion as worthless.

On the other end of the scale is the blamer. The blamer's stance complements that of the placater. The blamer is always criticizing everyone and has a tight facial expression and pointing finger to go with this blaming stance. The blamer acts superior but inside is actually feeling scared, lonely, and probably unsuccessful.

The computer appears ultrareasonable, as if everything is under control. His posture is reserved, cool, and collected; and he reveals no emotion through facial expression. He uses big words in a drawn-out monotone, attempting to impress others with his vocabulary and intelligence. The person who maintains a computer stance is like someone with a steel rod down his back, who cannot move his head and who must talk slowly to keep from making a mistake.

Satir suggested that the family therapist structure at least the first two sessions of therapy by taking a family life chronology, which involves a series of questions to identify the history of the family.

From a Satir communication theory approach, the therapist has several goals: (1) helping the family make implicit rules explicit, (2) helping each family member become aware of his posture and how it communicates messages to others on a nonverbal level, and (3) helping family members begin to see that other members are not malicious or full of ill intentions but that their communications are not clear.[22] To accomplish these goals, the therapist does not enter the family system, but acts as a corrective feedback mechanism to disturb the present dysfunctional communication[24] and as a role model of clearer, more congruent communication.

Sociocultural

Duvall,[14] who addresses a family life-cycle perspective, identifies eight core developmental tasks common to most families:

1. Providing shelter, food, clothing, and health care
2. Meeting costs and allocating resources
3. Assigning tasks of support and management of the home and its members
4. Ensuring socialization
5. Establishing interaction within norms of society
6. Bearing and rearing children
7. Relating to society
8. Maintaining morale and motivation

From this early work, other authors have addressed the life cycle and changing life cycle of the American family.[11]

The family life cycle perspective views symptoms and dysfunctions within the family in relation to normal functioning over time. It views therapy as reestablishing the family's developmental momentum. Because family stresses are likely to occur around life cycle transition points, it is important for the family therapist to identify chronologi-

---

▼ **TABLE 29-1** Summary of Theoretical Approaches

Theory	Theorist	Goal	Role	Focus of Treatment
Psychoanalytical	Ackerman[1]	Corrective relationship with the therapist	Neutral; nondirective; makes interpretations of individual and family behavior	Specific dynamics of the individual's personality and role in the family; the perceptual distortion between family members
Humanistic Communication	Satir[10]	Assists family to make explicit rules, to become aware of their nonverbal communication, and to recognize that ill feelings in the family are due to unclear communication	Intervenes in dysfunctional communication by acting as a corrective feedback mechanism (to role model clear and congruent communication)	Communication among family members
Systems				
Structural	Minuchin[35]	To change the underlying structure of the family organization that maintains dysfunctional family interaction	Actively joins family; directs and realigns family interaction	Family boundaries, alignment, power, and coalitions
Bowenian	Bowen[6]	Self-differentiation of each member from family of origin	Neutral; coaches and teaches the family how to become differentiated and detriangulated	The entire family system over several generations; may work with one partner for a period of time
Sociocultural	Duvall[14]	Reestablish family's developmental momentum	Identifies chronologically dates and occurrences of stressors	Family stress that occurs around normal life-cycle transition points

cally dates and occurrences of stressors. Recent changes in the composition of the "normal" family has modified the description of the cycle of the "intact middle class American family life cycle" to identify the definition of the "major variations in the family life cycle."[11]

Within the intact family are included the stages of leaving home (the launching of the single young adult); the joining of families through marriage (the couple); families with young children; families with adolescents; launching children and moving on; and families in later life. Major variations occur in families with divorce and remarriage, poverty, and/or cultural factors such as the effects of ethnicity and religion. Table 29-1 presents a summary of the theoretical approaches.

CHARACTERISTICS OF THE FAMILY THERAPIST

Qualifications

Currently no universally accepted training is required to become a family therapist, but all therapists have preparation at least at the graduate level in the mental health field, with family theory classes and clinical supervision of practice. Although some psychiatrists practice family therapy, most often they have been exposed primarily to a medical model of psychiatric illness that supports dealing with the family in a limited way. Psychologists, psychiatric social workers, and psychiatric nurses have completed graduate programs in family therapy and supervision, although psychiatric social workers and psychiatric nurses often have had a broader base in this area because of their frequent family contacts.

The primary skill for a family therapist, as in all areas of psychiatric intervention and treatment, is self-awareness. The ability to observe one's own thinking, feeling, and behaving is a prerequisite to being able to help a family deal with a problem. A second requirement is ongoing supervision. Maintaining a stance that is objective enough to get a different perspective on the family is difficult without ongoing peer support and feedback.

Roles

The specific roles of the family therapist depend on that therapist's way of conceptualizing the family's problems, as presented in the preceding discussion of theoretical approaches. Some therapists intentionally "join" the family (Minuchin) whereas others maintain a more objective distance (Bowen). In general, any family therapist may function as a role model, an educator, or as a feedback mechanism, depending on the therapist's theoretical orientation. Some schools of family therapy regard the family's gaining insight into the problem as essential (psychoanalytical), whereas others focus on the change in the family structure to remove the presenting symptom (structural).

CHARACTERISTICS OF FAMILY THERAPY

Client Selection

The family may refer itself for therapy. It is not uncommon for self-referral to occur in response to a problem with a child in the family. Families may be referred for treatment by agencies such as the school system, welfare board, parole officers, and judges. The family may not agree that a problem exists and may feel coerced into therapy. For example, when abuse has taken place, the judge may order parents to enter family therapy as a condition for leaving the child in the home. Some families are referred for therapy from emergency room psychiatric services after a visit caused by a crisis in the family such as a drug overdose. On discharge from a psychiatric hospital, a client and his family may be referred for family therapy. Ministers, private physicians, and families who are familiar with family therapy may make referrals.

Family therapy is the treatment of choice when there is a marital problem or sibling conflict. Situational crises such as the sudden death of a family member and maturational crises such as the birth of the first child may cause sufficient stress to warrant family therapy. When there is fusion or overcloseness of family members, family therapy may be beneficial. Family therapy may also be indicated when problems are caused by using one child as the scapegoat.

Types of Family Therapy

The therapist may help the family in several ways. The type of therapy is usually determined by the therapist's training. The therapist may be comfortable with several approaches and decide after the first interview with the family which method is best suited for that particular family.

Individual family therapy

With individual family therapy each family member has a single therapist. The whole family may meet occasionally with one or two of the therapists to see how the members are relating to one another and work out specific issues that have been defined by individual members. This model works well with individual growth and the development of the individuality of each family member who is in therapy. Direct effect on the family system to facilitate the interactional and connective process with the unit as a whole is minimal. The family becomes the reference point for what is happening and is not the primary focus of the process.

Conjoint family therapy

The most common type of family therapy is the single-family group, or conjoint family therapy. The nuclear family is seen, and the issues and problems raised by the family are the ones addressed by the therapist. The way in which the family interacts is observed and becomes a focus of therapy. The therapist helps the family deal more effectively with problems as they arise and are defined. Both the family and the therapist define the goals, which change as the problems are redefined. The integrity of the family system and its individual members is supported. Communication patterns are continually addressed to facilitate more effective relationships among family members.

Couples therapy

Couples are often seen by the therapist together. The couple may be planning to marry and may want to examine and strengthen their relationship. Because they are experiencing difficulties in their marriage, couples in therapy may begin to work together to seek resolution or to facilitate a separation. Family patterns; interaction and communication styles; and each partner's goals, hopes, and expectations of each other are examined in therapy. This examination enables the couple to find a common ground for resolving conflicts by recognizing and respecting each other's similarities and differences. Couples therapy is discussed in detail in Chapter 30.

Multiple family group therapy

In multiple family group therapy, four or five families meet weekly to confront and deal with problems or issues they have in common. Ability or inability to function well in the home and community, fear of talking to or relating to others, abuse, anger, neglect, the development of social skills, and responsibility for oneself are some of the issues on which these groups focus. All of the families in these groups have problems coping with change. Most of the families in these groups are isolated and have difficulty forming relationships outside their nuclear family.

Because four or five families make up the group, a larger and different social network is formed. These families begin or further develop the skills needed for more effective communication. Over time, the level of fear in these families is reduced. Often family members in these groups have lived in constant crisis because of the feeling that they were alone and no one was there for support. These feelings change in the groups. The multiple family group becomes the support for all the families. Although crises continue to occur and overwhelm these families, the number of crises is significantly reduced because these families form a sustaining network that in many cases is transferred to the home. The network also encourages each person to reach out and form new relationships outside the group. These families become more effective in dealing with change as their need for adaptation increases.

Multiple impact therapy

Therapists can also bring families together for intensive work, usually over a 3-day weekend or weeklong encounter. In multiple impact therapy, several therapists come together with the families in a community setting. They live together and deal with pertinent issues for each family member within the context of the group. Multiple impact therapy is similar to multiple family group therapy except that it is more intense and time limited. Like multiple family group therapy, it focuses on developing skills of working together as a family and with other families.

Multiple impact therapy groups are goal oriented and always deal with immediate issues of problem solving. Reactions, feelings, and confrontation are important aspects of this type of therapeutic encounter. Because of the intensity of the encounter, this approach is not used in families with a psychotic member.

Network therapy

Network therapy is conducted in people's homes. All persons interested or invested in a problem or crisis that a particular person or persons in a family are experiencing take part. This gathering includes family, friends, neighbors, professional groups or persons, and anyone in the community who has an investment in the outcome of the current crisis. People who form the network generally know each other and interact on a regular basis in each other's lives.

The network group is called together by its members under the guidance of the therapy team. The team enters the home to assist the network in solving the immediate problem. A network may include as many as 40 to 60 people, all of whom are interested in and invested in making things better for the person or family in crisis.

The rewards are great when all persons involved mobilize energy and management of the problem. The power is in the network itself. The answers to each problem come from the network and how people in the network decide to manage each issue as it arises. The therapists serve as guides to clarify issues, manage the process of each major network meeting, reinforce the importance of and need for the network toward its members collectively and individually, and assist in the development and effective management in the evolution of the problem resolution.

The network determines how often it meets. Generally, it meets formally with the network team only three to six times before its goals are accomplished. In the intervals between the formally called meetings, network members often encounter one another informally. Issues and problems are dealt with realistically as they occur. This method is very powerful. It supports people's strengths and abilities to help themselves. They are much less dependent on professionals to continually give them answers about issues that arise. The network members must come up with their own answers.

Because of the familiarity, intimacy, and interest this group has and continues to have in each other's lives, a renewal of the concept of community and home is discovered by all who participate in the network.

NURSING PROCESS
Assessment

Depending on the theoretical approach of the therapist, different tools may be used to obtain information about the dimensions of the family. For instance, with structural family therapy, the therapist may use a map to describe boundaries and coalitions. Using a Bowen theory approach, the therapist may collaborate with the family to draw a genogram (family diagram), and, from a communication approach, the therapist may use a family life chronology. Because Duvall[14] identifies stressors affecting the life cycle, the Family Stress Index[32] and the Family Coping-Coherence Scale[32] may be administered by the nurse to assess family functioning within these realms. Use of these tools is well described in the research highlight on p. 590. With any of these methods, information about the physical, social, emotional, intellectual, and spiritual functioning of the family can be obtained.

Physical dimension A dysfunctional family may encounter problems meeting the physical needs of its members: sufficient food, shelter, or protection from common physical dangers. The adults may fail to meet the family's needs because of limited finances, lack of knowledge, disinterest, or for other reasons. The nurse may observe

RESEARCH HIGHLIGHT

Families of Children with Development Disabilities: An Examination of Family Hardiness
• S Failla and LC Jones

PURPOSE

Family hardiness may play an important role in the adaptation process used by families of children with special health care needs. The majority of hardiness research has previously focused on the individual, rather than the family. The purpose of this study was to examine relationships between family hardiness and family stressors, family appraisal, social support, parental coping, and family adaptation in families of children with developmental disabilities.

SAMPLE

The sample consisted of 57 mothers who had one developmentally disabled child, 6 years of age or younger. For the purpose of the study, a child was considered developmentally disabled if there was a cognitive and/or physical impairment. The mother from each family was recruited from a government program that offered health care to handicapped children with developmental disabilities.

METHODOLOGY

The Family Hardiness Index was used to measure hardiness.[32] The Family Stress Index was used to measure stress

Based on data from *Research in Nursing and Health,* 14(1):41, 1991.

in the family.[32] Social support was measured by the Norbeck Social Support Questionnaire. Family use of appraisal skills as they cope with stressful life situations was measured by the Family Coping-Coherence scale. The Coping Health Inventory for Parents was used to measure coping, and the Feetham Family Functioning Survey was used to measure family functioning. The measures were compared by a multiple regression analysis to determine which variables predicted satisfaction with family functioning.

FINDINGS

Over 42% of the ability to predict satisfaction with family functioning was explained by four variables: family hardiness, total functional support, family stressors, and age of the parent.

IMPLICATIONS

Family hardiness acts as a resistance resource that diminishes the effects of stress, increases the use of social support, and facilitates adaptation. In this study, higher levels of family hardiness were associated with the use of coping behaviors that strengthen family relationships. Families with a high level of hardiness perceived stressful life events as challenges not burdens.

---

indications of physical neglect, incest, and physical abuse. Spouse and child abuse are common occurrences in some troubled families. The nurse observes for physical signs, such as bruises, that may indicate abuse. She also notes the family members' response to arguments because abuse may follow arguments.

When performing an assessment, the nurse may learn that various members of the family have physical problems in response to family conflict. As the nurse collects a thorough history of the family's physical functioning, she may learn that this pattern is repeated over generations. Physical illnesses, such as gastric ulcers or asthma, may be present as patterns in some families.

One method of tracking physical health is by using a genogram often used within the Bowen framework (Figure 29-4). The entire family's physical complaints and illnesses are placed on the genogram, usually clearly demonstrating that the person with the identified complaint is not the only person experiencing distress. By including dates, the genogram also helps the therapist and the family observe that acting out often follows or coincides with a significant physical diagnosis in the family. For example, an adolescent may be expelled from school for fighting on the same day his grandmother is scheduled for a radical mastectomy for cancer. If the only focus of treatment is this disruptive youngster, the whole family's anxiety and pain about grandmother's cancer can easily be overlooked.

Emotional dimension Using Duvall's theory, the nurse assesses the family's ability to change. The dysfunctional family is likely to be inflexible and unable to shift roles and levels of responsibility.[14] The family may seek therapy because of the members' inability to deal with developmental changes in the family, such as the birth of children, departure of children to school, and young adults leaving (empty nest syndrome). Some families cope well with certain stages of the family's development; however, during a period of considerable change in family rules and roles, the family may become dysfunctional. As indicated in the research highlight, in families with a child who is developmentally disabled, family hardiness, support, stressors and the age of the parent were the variables predictive of satisfaction with family functioning. It is important for nurses to assess these variables to predict family functioning.

Some families' emotional response to stress is not evident. The nurse discerns these feelings by observing the family's response to stress-related words such as guilty, angry, or upset. She also listens for accounts of experiences associated with feelings, for example, "I was worried when..." Encouraging the family members to engage in storytelling about illness or other stressful experiences provides valuable information about anxiety, guilt, or other feelings. The nurse may learn about the family's true emotions by attending to their attempts to gain sympathy or emphasize negative experiences.

The focus of family problems may be losses: illness, death, job, or home by fire or natural disaster. Such losses may be sufficient to shift the delicate balance in a functional family and motivate them to seek therapy. The family's ability to grieve in response to the losses needs to be assessed. The family as a whole may be unable to express grief and they may disallow a specific member from doing so by blocking any discussion of feelings about the loss.

Family members may experience guilt when a member resents assuming additional responsibility because of the illness of another member or because a member does not carry his share of responsibility for tasks. A child in the family may experience guilt when told his behavior is the cause of the family's problems. This reaction is an example of scapegoating in which the focus needs to be taken off the child and replaced by a focus on the family. Feelings of inadequacy in a situation, for example, caring for a new baby, may give rise to feelings of guilt. The guilt that one member experiences affects the whole family system. The family may be aware of the guilt and use secrecy in an effort to conceal the feeling from the nurse. The nurse listens for indications of a need for punishment, overly apologetic behavior, and scapegoating. The absence of a reasonable expression of anger may be an indication of guilt (see Chapter 12).

Anger and hostility may be the presenting emotions of the family and may be expressed as verbal hostility or physical abuse. In the case of physical abuse, the safety of the individual family members is the first area for assessment. In assessing verbal hostility, the nurse looks for conflictual relationships either between spouses in the form of marital conflict or hostility directed toward a child as the scapegoat. It is important for the therapist to help the family identify the circumstances surrounding the expressions of hostility. Bowen refers to these as "toxic" issues. Frequently, as anxiety increases in the family, more anger is expressed. Psychoanalytically oriented family therapy identifies the origins of the current conflicts as unconscious and unresolved issues in the early mother-child relationship. Assessment using this approach involves dream analysis and free association.

The nurse may note a problem in the expression of any feelings between family members. It is important to identify the degree and quality of the emotional involvement that family members have in each other's needs, interests, and activities. The emotional expression may be too intense or too little; excessive emotional closeness prevents the family members from developing the autonomy they need. Minuchin refers to this phenomenon as enmeshment and Bowen as fusion or lack of differentiation. When the family is emotionally distant, members may not receive sufficient emotional support.

The therapist also identifies triangles as described by Bowen during the assessment phase. Pivotal family issues that often lead to potential conflict and triangling are discipline, sex, money, religion, and in-law relationships. Each family has its own "toxic" issues that prompt emotionality, conflict, and triangulation. Identifying and observing triangles in the family show the nurse which family members are the closest and which issues cause the most distance and conflict.

Intellectual dimension Within the Bowen framework, the nurse assesses the intellectual dimension of the whole family as she observes the family's ability to separate thinking and feeling. Some families may appear to be intellectually duller than they are because of the long-term effects of chronic anxiety. An elderly family member with disorientation or confusion may be viewed as the cause of the problem. The nurse, after many questions, may be able to ascertain that the "confusion" is primarily a problem when certain toxic issues are addressed, or that the "disorientation" is much more apparent with some family members than with others. These kinds of findings during a family assessment may indicate that the intellectual functioning (confusion) of the elderly family member is more related to family problems than to organic brain changes.

The family may have myths that conflict with reality. *Family myth* refers to a family's beliefs about their family that are fairly well integrated and shared by all members.[15] These myths concern each family member and his position or role in the family. Well-functioning families have myths that are changeable and explicit. Dysfunctional families have myths that conflict with reality. For example, the family believes, "we would be okay if people didn't pick on us." In reality, the son is a bully and the father often picks a fight with the neighbor after a few drinks. Such myths deny the problems in the family and make it difficult for family members to assess realistically their own behavior and to be responsible for it. These beliefs are not challenged by family members because they are not identified as myths by the family.

The nurse may learn that the dysfunctional family does not know how to problem solve. Their handling of problems is based on reaction rather than on a constructive approach. Or, they may reduce complex problems to simple solutions. Ineffective problem-solving abilities may be evident when family members quarrel without identifying the basis for the argument or offering an alternative solution to verbal fighting.

Many families who come for therapy have problems in verbal and nonverbal communication. The nurse attends to the family's communication pattern to determine whether their pattern is functional or dysfunctional because breakdown in communication is a clue to trouble in the family. Communicative behaviors such as poor eye contact, interruptions, changing the subject, and speaking for one another are indications that the family has a communication problem.

The family's communication may be insufficient to provide family members with enough information to function well as a family. Because of vague or ambiguous communication, family members may not get a clear message as they communicate.

Double-bind communication,[5] conflicting messages given simultaneously, may be the predominant communication pattern in a dysfunctional family. An example of double-bind communication is a daughter who is away at camp and whose mother visits. The daughter is glad to see her mother and impulsively hugs her, whereupon the mother stiffens. The daughter withdraws her arm and the mother asks, "Don't you love me anymore?" The daughter blushes, and the mother says, "Honey, you must not be so easily embarrassed." Conditions necessary to produce a double-bind include the following:

1. Two persons, one of whom is the victim (in this case, the daughter)
2. A repeated experience, so that a double-bind becomes the expected mode of communication
3. A primary negative response (the mother stiffens)
4. A secondary response conflicting with the first, but at a more abstract level, also threatening punishment ("Don't you love me anymore?")
5. A third negative response prohibiting the victim from escaping ("You must not be so easily embarrassed.")

The nurse determines whether communication is direct or indirect. Dysfunctional families tend to use indirect communication, in which the family members may send messages to the intended member by another family member and sometimes members outside the home, rather than direct communication, in which the message is sent to the intended family member. Indirect communication leads to misunderstanding, mistrust, and greater distortion of communication in the family.

Social dimension Communication patterns provide information about relationships in the family. Often the way family members sit in the session provides nonverbal information about their relationships. For example, a member may sit across from the person from whom he seeks validation for his ideas. As family members interact, the nurse notices who talks to whom, who interrupts, and who gives help and confirms what another member says. This information provides clues to who is close to whom and the dyads and triads in the family. It also provides information about family roles, which Satir would describe as placater, blamer, and computer.

According to Minuchin, the power between the husband and wife frequently is not balanced in a troubled family, and this may lead to conflict that affects the family system. The nurse assesses the power in the family by noting who makes the decisions in the family. The nurse can ask family members directly who makes decisions and how they are made. This information helps the nurse determine who has the power in the family system and whether decisions are made impulsively, with little thought, or with so much thought that indecision results. The nurse may learn that the power for decision making has changed during the life of the family, for example, the husband made decisions early in the marriage and now the wife does. Other means for assessing who makes decisions include observing the interaction between spouses, between parents and children, or between siblings and the family as a whole; self-reporting; and asking questions such as, "Who has the last say about important issues?" and "Who wins when there is disagreement?"

Satir believes that a family's rules are often rigid and do not allow flexibility. Although the rules are likely to be implicit, family members assume that the rules are known and understood by all members.

The family that seeks therapy is likely to have problems in performing their roles. Roles may not be clearly defined or there may be a lack of agreement as to who fulfills certain roles. Frequently, the dysfunctional family has never openly identified roles and discussed who performs them. The roles may be rigid, and the family members may be unable to shift roles to meet the needs of the family members. The nurse inquires about the roles the various members are assuming and whether they meet the needs of the family members.

In an effort to deal with stress, the family members may unconsciously assign the role of *scapegoat* to one of its members.[12] A scapegoat is one who bears the blame for the family problem. This member, usually a child, shows symptoms of the family disturbance and thus keeps the family from focusing on the problem as a family problem. The scapegoat serves the function of keeping the rest of the family united. Often this focus on the scapegoat is the only thing the family can be united about. When doing an assessment the nurse may note that the family presents the scapegoat as the identified client.

The nurse may observe the role of "parental child" in the family. In this role the older child is given parental responsibilities for younger children and sometimes the parent. For example, a father may not fulfill aspects of his role because of alcoholism or another problem, and the mother may place the oldest boy in the role of "man of the house."

Within a system's perspective, the family system may be closed, have little interaction with the community, and rely entirely on family members for emotional sustenance. A family that functions as a tightly closed system is in a precarious position because it does not have outside sources of support. When a crisis occurs, the family members in a closed system are more reactive and more easily become dysfunctional physically, emotionally, or socially because of limited emotional resources.

An open family system allows and encourages contact outside the family and is less vulnerable. Crises occur in all families, but the family members in an open family system are able to rely on people outside their family and therefore have more emotional support during crises.

Spiritual dimension It is useful to inquire about the family's spiritual beliefs, as well as how differences about spiritual beliefs are handled. Differences may produce tension. In some instances the children are in conflict when the parents have different religious affiliations and each parent wants the child to practice his or her faith. A dysfunctional family may disallow a discussion of ethical and religious issues and values. Some families are very antagonistic toward someone who married "outside the faith" or toward someone who espouses religious beliefs but behaves in an immoral way. Other families are unconcerned about these issues, but it is useful for the therapist to know not only what the spiritual beliefs are, but also how and in what context religion is an issue in the family.

In dysfunctional families value systems may be rigid and chaotic. The family members may adhere to their values so rigidly that they become preoccupied with religion or a supreme being. The family may not participate in therapy because of their belief that a supreme being will solve their problems, if it is his will.

Analysis
Nursing diagnosis

Altered family processes, family coping: potential for growth, ineffective family coping: compromised, and ineffective family coping: disabling, are nursing diagnoses ap-

▼ ALTERED FAMILY PROCESSES

DEFINITION

The state in which a family that normally functions effectively experiences a dysfunction.

DEFINING CHARACTERISTICS

- **Physical dimension**

  Family system unable to meet physical needs of its members

  Inappropriate level and direction of energy

- **Emotional dimension**

  Family system unable to meet emotional needs of its members

  Inability to express or accept wide range of feelings

  Inability to express or accept feelings of members

- **Intellectual dimension**

  Parents do not demonstrate respect for each other's views on child-rearing practices

  Inability to accept or receive help appropriately

  Rigidity in function and roles

  Family does not demonstrate respect for individuality and autonomy of its members

Family unable to adapt to change or deal with traumatic experience constructively

Ineffective family decision-making process

Failure to send and receive clear messages

Inappropriate or poorly communicated family rules, rituals, symbols

Unexamined family myths

- **Social dimension**

  Family unable to meet security needs of its members

  Inability of family members to relate to each other for mutual growth and maturation

  Family uninvolved in community activities

  Family fails to accomplish current or past developmental tasks

- **Spiritual dimension**

  Family unable to meet spiritual needs of its members

Modified from Kim MA, McFarland GK, McLane AM, editors: *Pocket guide to nursing diagnoses,* ed 5, St Louis, 1993, Mosby–Year Book.

▼ INEFFECTIVE FAMILY COPING, DISABLING

DEFINITION

Behavior of significant person (family member or other primary person) that disables his or her own capacities and the client's capacities to effectively address tasks essential to either person's adaptation to the health challenge

DEFINING CHARACTERISTICS

- **Physical dimension**

  Neglectful care of client in regard to basic human needs and/or illness treatment

  Psychosomatic tendency

  Taking on illness signs of client

- **Emotional dimension**

  Agitation

  Depression

  Aggression

  Hostility

- **Intellectual dimension**

  Distortion of reality regarding client's health problem, including extreme denial about its existence or severity

Decisions and actions by family members that are detrimental to economic or social well-being

Intolerance

Carrying on usual routines; disregarding client's needs

Prolonged overconcern for client

- **Social dimension**

  Rejection

  Abandonment

  Desertion

  Neglectful relationships with other family members

  Helpful, inactive dependence of client

- **Spiritual dimension**

  Impaired restructuring of a meaningful life for self

  Impaired individualization

Modified from Kim MA, McFarland GK, McLane AM, editors: *Pocket guide to nursing diagnoses,* ed 5, St Louis, 1993, Mosby–Year Book.

proved by NANDA that apply to family therapy. The defining characteristics of altered family processes are listed in the box on p. 593. The following case example illustrates characteristics of altered family processes.

▼ Case Example

Mrs. Randle was referred to the nurse for family therapy because she felt that her home life had fallen apart since her husband's death 4 months earlier. She has a 16-year-old son and a 13-year-old daughter. The daughter was very close to her father and has become increasingly withdrawn since his death. The son was supportive of the mother shortly after his father's death. Now the son is spending most of his time away from home; he no longer does chores unless his mother tells him to do so and then he rebels. Mrs. Randle has developed various physical complaints since her husband's death and feels overwhelmed with family responsibilities and the financial crisis she faces now that the family's savings are gone. She admits to difficulty managing the children and her physical health. With much encouragement she agreed to attend family therapy.

The defining characteristics of ineffective family coping, disabling, are listed in the box on p. 593.

The following case example illustrates characteristics of ineffective family coping, disabling.

▼ Case Example

The Barnes family came to the mental health center because of Mrs. Barnes' concerns about her 12-year-old son's failing performance in school and her inability to discipline him. Other members of the family are Mr. Barnes, a 13-year-old son, and two daughters, aged 9 and 7 years. Mr. Barnes is frequently out of work and the family is on welfare. Often the children do not have adequate food and clothing because the money the family receives is used to pay the rent. When Mr. Barnes earns a small amount of money, it is not unusual for him to spend it on gambling or alcohol. During the interview, Mr. Barnes was loud and aggressive and the rest of the family seemed fearful of him. It was disclosed that he sometimes physically abuses the children, especially the boys, in an effort to discipline them. It was also noted that he sometimes hits Mrs. Barnes. The 12-year-old son is blamed for the family problems; the other children are considered "good kids."

Planning

Table 29-2 provides a nursing care plan with some long- and short-term goals and interventions and rationales for family therapy that are examples of the planning stage in the nursing process.

Implementation

Physical dimension The nurse recommends that all family members undergo complete physical examinations if physical problems are present. She emphasizes the importance of adhering to their medical and nursing regimens. If the nurse determines that the family finances are insufficient for proper food and shelter, she refers them to social services. The nurse secures a protective environment for any abused member in the family and discusses the abusive behavior in the family session (see Chapter 34). It is important for the nurse to identify genetic predispositions for certain disorders, such as alcoholism and affec-

tive disorders, to alert the family to an occurrence of this problem in successive generations and perhaps lead to early detection and treatment. Within the Bowen theoretical framework, the nurse educates the family about the problem, using the genogram to explain to the family how family problems may be passed down through each generation.

Emotional dimension The nurse assists the family in resolving grief without distancing the grieving member or members from the rest of the family. There are four stages for family grief work: family announcement, family acknowledgment, family mourning, and family renewal.[18] See Table 29-3 for the characteristics of these stages. In family announcement, the nurse makes certain that each member participates, asking each member to share his thoughts about the loss and the family's emotional response. If the family uses denial during family acknowledgment, the nurse intervenes by asking each member to share his experience of the death and its meaning to him.

The nurse respects the family's need to experience guilt. She guides the family to elaborate and explore their feelings. It is helpful for the nurse to respond neutrally as a family describes feelings of guilt. With knowledge of what is causing the guilt, for example, feelings of inadequacy in a new role, the nurse explores with the family member realistic expectations without negating the member's feelings.

It is important for the nurse to explore the use of anger in the family. Anger may be the only emotion that some families are comfortable expressing. The nurse helps the family enlarge their number of expressed emotions, as anger may be covering guilt and/or fear. She also helps families identify other ways to express anger besides physical punishment (see Chapter 11).

Intellectual dimension One intervention strategy based on Bowen theory is to assist the family members to distinguish between the processes of thinking and feeling. Thinking is a necessary component to solve problems and to effect change. The therapist asks specifically for the person's thoughts about the situation and gets the person to distinguish these thoughts from feelings.

To enable each person in the family to begin to define a more differentiated self, the therapist models "I" positions, that is, statements about what the therapist is and is not willing to do. For example, in the case example of the Randle family, the mother may attempt to involve the therapist in aiding her to get the children to assume more responsibility for the chores around the house. The therapist might say, "I will not participate in your determination of appropriate household tasks for the children, but I will help you separate your thoughts and feelings on the issues." The more the therapist is able to state beliefs and convictions, the easier it is for the family to begin this process with each other. Efforts to differentiate are often met by one family member asking another to revert to the old behaviors. If the differentiating person can remain calm in the face of the other family member's increasing anxiety, both family members can move toward a higher level of differentiation. Throughout the therapy, when anxiety is lower, the therapist is teaching the family how emotional systems operate.

Within Satir's framework, role playing can be useful when the family handles the problems on an intellectual level. For example, the family may be asked to act out what

▼ **TABLE 29-2   NURSING CARE PLAN**

GOALS	OUTCOME CRITERIA	INTERVENTIONS	RATIONALES
NURSING DIAGNOSIS: Powerlessness related to difficulty in making decisions that affect family functioning			
LONG TERM To recognize the effect of decision making on feelings of power	Verbalizes knowledge of relationship between decision making and power	Guide client in a discussion of the relationship between decision making and power	Increases knowledge for effective decision making
	Identifies feelings related to decision making	Assist to identify feelings of power and powerlessness related to decision making	Increases self-awareness
	Examines the effects of decisions made on family and self	Explore with client the specific effects of his decisions on family members and himself	Increases the ability to analyze actions
SHORT TERM To become comfortable making decisions that affect family functioning	Appears more at ease when making decisions	Teach client ways to deal with discomfort when making decisions	Decreases anxiety and increases confidence in ability to make decisions
	Shows willingness to make decisions	Support client's efforts to make decisions	Increases confidence and encourages client to continue the behavior
	Tolerates family's lack of agreement with decisions	Encourage to accept some disagreement with decisions	Increases ability to withstand conflict
	Uses different approaches to decision making	Teach various approaches to decision making	Increases repertoire of decision-making strategies
NURSING DIAGNOSIS: Impaired verbal communication related to sharing of insufficient information			
LONG TERM To recognize factors that interfere with effective communication	Initiates and accepts feedback from family about nature of communication	Encourage client to discuss nature of communication with family	Increases effectiveness of communication
	Notes own and family's nonverbal behavior while communicating	Assist client to identify nonverbal factors that influence communication	Client learns that nonverbal communication influences verbal communication
	Verbalizes knowledge of deterrents to effective communication	Facilitate client's identification of obstacles to effective communication	Provides information for changing behavior
SHORT TERM To increase ability to share adequate information	Shares information spontaneously	Promote sharing by giving positive feedback	Increases self-confidence in sharing information
	Verbalizes willingness to share sufficient information	Assist to use strategies that promote sharing sufficient information	Helps to learn means for sharing sufficient information
	Seeks feedback from others	Encourage client to seek feedback from others	Decreases anxiety about feedback
	Determines what is sufficient information for a given situation	Encourage client to ask if he has shared sufficient information for the situation	Increases knowledge about effective communication

▼ **TABLE 29-3**   **Stages for Family Grief Work**

Stage	Characteristics
Family announcement	Family members relive the emotional aspects of their experience related to the loss.
Family acknowledgment	Realization by all family members that the loss has occurred and cannot be changed.
	With acknowledgment, the family can enter the stage of mourning.
Family mourning	Each family member directly shares and manifests his feelings.
	Family members recognize similarities of their expression, empathize with each other, and recognize their mutual pain.
	Family members learn about each other and can transfer this knowledge to future family problems.
Family renewal	Family members find alternative means for meeting the psychosocial needs that were previously met by the deceased.
	If the family was able to share feelings and experiences during the preceding stages, they may now function at a higher level than before the death.

happens when the mother asks them to do household chores, if this has been a problem. The nurse begins the role playing with a simple, nonthreatening situation. Role playing brings the reality of the family's life into the family session and provides the nurse with a concrete tool.

Social dimension Using Minuchin's framework, the nurse uses clarification as a technique for intervention in the family's dysfunctional communication. Clarification allows the family to recognize discrepancies between (1) what they are saying and what others are hearing, (2) what they are hearing and what others are saying, and (3) what both the individual and others mean but are not saying in a clear and congruent way.

Using Bowen's theory, the nurse redirects the family's indirect communication through her behavior. For example, when a family member talks to her about another family member, she directs the message to the intended family member. She tells the family member of the expectation that they will talk to one another and then actively directs them to do so. The nurse gives the family homework based on the expectation that they practice talking directly to each other in the home; they discuss how well they achieved this goal at a subsequent family session.

Satir's framework stresses the importance of the nurse

intervening in problems in roles by labeling the roles or having the family members label them, with assistance from the nurse. Then the nurse develops a plan for changing nonfunctional roles. For example, if the father is uninvolved in the care of the children and family activities, the nurse may actively bring him into a discussion of these matters during a family therapy session and have the whole family share thoughts about ways he can become involved. The nurse can also give the father homework that requires his active family participation.

Also included within the Satir framework is changing the role of scapegoat. This task is difficult and lengthy. The family is made aware of their behavior regarding this family member. As the family works toward resolving their problem, the role of scapegoat will no longer be needed to maintain the family's stability.

Spiritual dimension It is important for the nurse to help families identify a philosophical belief that guides their life. These beliefs may not be the same for each member. Although all members may not share the same concept of religion, often a common ideal is the belief in a higher being and the translation of this belief into religious practices.

Evaluation

Evaluation of the outcome of therapy is seen primarily from the family's perspective. Often what the therapist sees as minor improvement may be beneficial from the family's point of view. Because it is the family and not the therapist who has to live with the problem and the outcome, the ideal outcome becomes one that is seen as satisfactory by the family.

BRIEF REVIEW

The field of family therapy is relatively new to psychiatry. Initial interest and research with families began in separate parts of the United States as therapists either became frustrated in attempting traditional psychoanalytical therapy with schizophrenics or came in contact with dysfunctional families through the problems of an emotionally disturbed child.

Psychoanalytical, systems, and humanistic schools of family therapy are some of many theoretical approaches to family therapy. The family therapist gathers data and plans interventions according to the chosen theoretical framework. The goals of treatment and the role of the therapist depend on what the therapist and family believe is the cause of the problem. Identifying and dealing with the issues in the therapist's own family and ongoing supervision are essential for the professional practice of family therapy.

REFERENCES AND SUGGESTED READINGS

1. Ackerman N: *The psychodynamics of family life,* New York, 1958, Basic Books.
2. Ackerman N: *Treating the troubled family,* New York, 1966, Basic Books.
3. American Psychiatric Association: *Diagnostic and statistical manual of mental disorders (DSM-III-R),* Washington, DC, 1987, The Association.
4. Aponte HJ, Van Deusen JM: Structural family therapy. In Gur-

man AS, Kniskern DP, editors: *Handbook of family therapy*, New York, 1981, Brunner Mazel.

5. Bateson G and others: Toward a theory of schizophrenia. In Howell JG, editor: *Theory and practice of family psychiatry*, New York, 1978, Brunner Mazel.

6. Bowen M: *Family therapy in clinical practice*, New York, 1978, Jason Aronson.

7. Bowen M: Theory in the practice of psychotherapy. In Guerin PJ Jr, editor: *Family therapy, theory and practice*, New York, 1976, Gardner Press.

8. Bright MA: Therapeutic rituals: helping families grow, *Journal of Psychosocial Nursing and Mental Health Services* 28(12):24, 1990.

9. Cain AD: Family therapy: one role of the clinical specialist in psychiatric nursing, *Nursing Clinics of North America* 21(3):483, 1986.

10. Campbell DW: Family paradigm theory and family rituals: implications for child and family health, *Nurse Practitioner* 16(2):22, 1991.

11. Carter EA, McGoldrick M: *The changing family life cycle*, New York, 1988, Gardner Press.

12. Collison CR, Miller SL: The role of family re-enactment in group psychotherapy, *Perspectives in Psychiatric Care* 23(2):74, 1985.

13. Committee on the Family: *The field of family therapy*, vol VII, Report No. 78, New York, 1970, Group for the Advancement of Psychiatry.

14. Duvall EM: *Marriage and family development*, Philadelphia, 1977, JB Lippincott.

15. Ferreira A: Family myths and homeostasis, *Archives General Psychiatry* 9:457, 1963.

16. Forisha B, Grothaus K, Luscombe R: Dinner conversation: meal therapy to differentiate eating behavior from family process, *Journal of Psychosocial Nursing and Mental Health Services* 28(11):12, 1990.

17. Freidemann M: An instrument to evaluate effectiveness in family functioning, *Western Journal of Nursing Research* 13(2):220, 1991.

18. Greenberg L: Therapeutic griefwork with children, *Social Casework* 56:396, 1975.

19. Goldstein MZ: *Family involvement in the treatment of schizophrenia*, Washington, DC, 1986, American Psychiatric Press.

20. Guerin PJ Jr, editor: *Family therapy, theory and practice*, New York, 1976, Gardner Press.

21. Gurman AS, Kniskern DP: *Handbook of family therapy*, New York, 1981, Brunner Mazel.

22. Hansen JC, editor: *Health promotion in family therapy*, Rockville, Md, 1985, Aspen Systems Corp.

23. Jones S: Techniques of family therapy. In Lego S, editor: *The American handbook of psychiatric/mental health nursing*, Philadelphia, 1984, JB Lippincott.

24. Jones S: Family therapy as a psychiatric nursing intervention, *Advances in Psychiatric Mental Health Nursing* 1:1, 1982.

25. Jones S, Dimond D: Family theory and therapy models: comparative review with implications for nursing practice, *Journal of Psychiatric Nursing and Mental Health Services* 20:12, 1982.

26. Kaye LW, Jeffrey S, Applegate D: Men as elder caregivers: a response to changing families, *American Journal of Orthopsychiatry* 60(1):86, 1990.

27. Kerr M, Bowen M: *Family evaluation*, New York, 1988, WW Norton.

28. King J, Reid S, McSwain K: A nursing family assessment program, *Canadian Journal of Psychiatric Nursing* 27(3):12, 1986.

29. Koontz E, Cox D, Hastings S: Implementing a short-term family support group, *Journal of Psychiatric Nursing and Mental Health Services* 29(5):5, 1991.

30. Lansky MR: *Family approaches to major psychiatric disorders*, Washington, DC, 1986, American Psychiatric Press.

31. Lasky P and others: Symposium: development of a research group—developing an instrument for the assessment of family dynamics, *Western Journal of Nursing Research* 7(1):40, 1985.

32. McCubbin HI: FIRA-G family index of regenerativity and adaptation-general. In McCubbin HI, Thompson AI, editors: *Family assessment inventories for research and practice*, Madison, Wis, 1987, University of Wisconsin.

33. Midelfort CF: *The family in psychotherapy*, New York, 1957, McGraw-Hill.

34. Miller JR, Janosik EH: *Family-focused care*, New York, 1980, McGraw-Hill.

35. Minuchin S: *Families and family therapy*, Cambridge, Mass, 1974, Harvard University Press.

36. Minuchin S: *Family kaleidoscope*, Cambridge, Mass, 1984, Harvard University Press.

37. Oliveri ME, Reiss D: Family concepts and their measurement: things are seldom what they seem, *Family Process* 23(1):33, 1984.

38. Papero DV: *Bowen family sytems theory*, Boston, 1990, Allyn and Bacon.

39. Phipps LB: Theoretical frameworks applicable to family care. In Miller JR, Janosik EH, editors: *Family-focused care*, New York, 1980, McGraw-Hill.

40. Satir V: *Conjoint family therapy*, Palo Alto, Calif, 1967, Science and Behavior Books.

41. Sebastian L: Use of multi-family therapy groups in nursing, *Kansas Nurse* 61(12):1, 1986.

42. Siegel E: Scapegoating: manifestations and intervention, *Journal of Psychiatric Nursing* 19:11, 1981.

43. Toman W: *Family constellation*, New York, 1969, Springer.

44. Whall AL: In search of holistic family assessment: an investigation of a clinical instrument . . . Watzawick's structural family interview (SFI), *Issues in Mental Health Nursing* 6:105, 1984.

45. Whall AL, editor: *Family therapy theory for nursing: four approaches*, New York, 1986, Appleton-Century-Crofts.

46. Whitley CG, Reiss D: Altered parenting and the reconstituted family, *Journal of Child and Adolescent Psychology of Mental Health Nursing* 4(2):72, 1991.

47. Williams P: Family feeling, *Community Outlook* 1:9, 1987.

48. Wright LM, Leakey M: *Nurses and families*, Philadelphia, 1984, FA Davis.

ANNOTATED BIBLIOGRAPHY

Kaslow FW: *Voices in family psychology*, Newbury Park, Calif, 1990, Sage Publication.

The two volumes offer an historical account of the field of family psychology. Each chapter describes the work of a contributing family psychologist.

Papero DV: *Bowen family systems theory*, Boston, 1990, Allyn and Bacon.

This book emphasizes family as a new theory as well as a new method of therapy. It provides a unique presentation of a broad perspective on human emotional function and behavior in a concise way.

CHAPTER

30 Couples Therapy

Benni S Ogden
Sophronia R Williams

After studying this chapter, the student will be able to:

- State factors that have influenced the historical development of couples therapy
- Discuss marital problem and sexual disorders as described in the DSM-III-R
- Describe the concepts of three major theorists in the field of marital therapy

- Use the nursing process to provide care to clients in marital/couples therapy
- Identify current research relevant to marital/couples therapy

Couples therapy is a mental health service for married or unmarried couples who have difficulties in their relationship. Clinicians have practiced family and marital therapy for years, but the development and practice of couples therapy has recently emerged from the field of marital therapy. Couples therapy is unique and important in today's society.

The couple may or may not be married or even living together. The couple may not be a traditional heterosexual couple. The couple may seek therapy before marriage to resolve conflicts and decide whether marriage is a workable option. Some couples choosing to divorce seek therapy not to save their marriage, but to resolve conflicts that cause problems during and after the divorce.

The goal of therapy is to resolve the couple's problem. The therapist considers various psychodynamic, sexual, ethical, and economic aspects of the couple's lives. Couples are seen individually or together.

At times conflicts in couples also include problems in a child of the parents and cause them to seek help. If the assessment indicates that the child's problems arise from those of the adults, couples therapy will be recommended.

Serious prolonged physical health problems in either partner significantly affect the other partner and the relationship. Problems may be expressed as physical or emotional symptoms. Therapy can help such partners cope with the stressors resulting from these health problems. Treatment may be unsuccessful and the symptoms may not disappear until both partners particpate in therapy.

DSM-III-R DIAGNOSES

One of the diagnoses described in the DSM-III-R that applies to marital/couples therapy is marital problem. No defining features or manifestations exist for this disorder. The nurse uses this diagnosis when the marital/couple's problem is not caused by a mental disorder, for example, a conflict related to infidelity or divorce.

Many of the sexual disorders described in the DSM-III-R may be significant for marital/couple therapy because a major complication of sexual problems is disrupted marital or sexual relationship. On the other hand, disruptions in the couple's relationship may lead to some type of sexual problem.

Two groups of sexual disorders are described in the DSM-III-R: sexual dysfunctions and the paraphilias. Sexual dysfunctions are characterized by inhibitions in sexual desire or the psychophysiological changes that characterize the sexual response cycle. The phases of the sexual re-

---

▶ **DIAGNOSES Related to Couples Therapy**

MEDICAL DIAGNOSES	NURSING DIAGNOSES
Marital problem	**NANDA**
Sexual disorders	Altered sexuality pattern
	Sexual dysfunction
	PMH
	Altered sexuality processes

HISTORICAL OVERVIEW

DATES	EVENTS
1890	Social workers are providing counseling to married couples.
1910	Adler[1] and Jung[41] recognize the effect of the marital pair on the children's development in their writings on socially rooted theories in psychodynamics.
1924	Earnest R Groves teaches a noncredit course on marriage at Boston University.[28]
1930	Marriage counseling centers are started in Los Angeles by Paul Popenoe and in New York by Abraham and Hannah Stone.
1938	Psychoanalytically oriented therapists do advanced work in examining the nature of marriage and marital dysfunction. Marital therapy begins as a specialized professional approach.
1939	*Marriage and Family Living* begins as the official organ of the National Council of Family Relations.
1942	Family life educators, counselors, and a social hygienist first discuss forming a professional organization of marriage counselors.
1945	The American Association of Marriage Counselors is established.
1947	Fifteen nationally recognized centers for marriage counseling are operating in the United States.[28]
1956	Three accredited training centers are recognized in the United States.
1959	Don Jackson coins the term *conjoint therapy* to describe a therapist meeting with both husband and wife.
1960s	Professional disciplines publish works on marital therapy in journals of their primary professions.
1963	California becomes the first state to pass a licensing law for marriage and family counselors.
1970s	The name of the American Association of Marriage Counselors is changed to American Association of Marriage and Family Counselors (AAMFC). Psychiatrists gradually increase the use of conjoint therapy instead of individual therapy with marital pairs.
1975	*The Journal of Marriage and Family Counseling* is initiated by AAMFC.
1978	The name of AAMFC is changed to American Association for Marriage and Family Therapy (AAMFT).
1979	The name of the association's journal is changed to *Journal of Marriage and Family Therapy*.
1980	The Commission on Accreditation for Marriage and Family Therapy Education of the AAMFT is approved for inclusion on the list of recognized accrediting agencies by the US Department of Health, Education, and Welfare.[3]
1990s	The term *couples therapy* emerged to include nontraditional relationships.
Future	As more nontraditional couples seek therapy the practice of couples therapy will increase.

sponse cycle are listed in Table 30-1. Inhibitions in the response cycle may occur at one or more of the phases in the cycle, although inhibition in the resolution is rarely sufficient to warrant counseling. In most instances, when there are problems, the subjective sense of pleasure or desire and objective performance are disturbed.

The sexual dysfunction may be only psychogenic or psy-chogenic and biogenic, lifelong or acquired (developing after a period of normal functioning), and generalized or situational (limited to certain situations or with certain partners). The dysfunction may be expressed as a vague sense of not living up to what the person views as normal expectations. The person may have complaints such as depression, anxiety, guilt, shame, frustration, and somatic

▼ **TABLE 30-1** **Sexual Response Cycle**

Phase	Characteristics
Appetitive	Fantasies about sexual activity and a desire to have sexual activity
Excitement	Subjective sense of sexual pleasure and accompanying physiological changes
Orgasm	A peaking of sexual pleasure, with release of sexual tension and rhythm of perineal muscle and pelvic reproductive organs
Resolution	A sense of general relaxation, well-being and muscular relaxation

▼ **TABLE 30-2** **Types and Definitions of Paraphilias**

Paraphilia	Definition
Exhibitionism	Repeated acts of exposing the genitals to unsuspecting stranger to achieve sexual excitement
Fetishism	Repeated use of inanimate objects to achieve sexual excitement
Frotteurism	Sexual excitement achieved by touching or rubbing against a nonconsenting person
Pedophilia	Act or fantasy of engaging in sexual activity with prepubertal children
Sexual masochism	Sexual excitement produced by being humiliated, bound, beaten, or made to suffer
Sexual sadism	Infliction on another of physical or psychological suffering to achieve sexual satisfaction
Transvestic fetishism	Recurrent cross-dressing by a heterosexual male to achieve excitement
Voyeurism	Repeated observation of unsuspecting persons who are naked, in the act of disrobing, or engaging in sexual activity

symptoms. It is common for the person to express a fear of failure, develop a "spectator" attitude (self-monitoring), and be extremely sensitive to the reaction of the partner. These experiences may lead to greater impairment of sexual performance and satisfaction and then to secondary avoidance of sexual activity and problematic communication with the sexual partner.

Sexual dysfunctions generally begin in early adulthood, with clinical presentation in the late 20s and early 30s, a few years after establishment of a sustained sexual relationship. Factors that may predispose an individual to sexual dysfunction are anxiety, excessively high self-imposed expectations for sexual performance, and real or imagined rejection by a sexual partner. A person with a negative attitude toward sexuality due to life experiences, internal conflicts, or adherence to rigid culture values may also develop sexual dysfunctions.

The second group of sexual disorders, the paraphilias, are characterized by arousal in response to sexual objects or situations that are not a part of normal arousal-activity patterns and that may interfere with the capacity for reciprocal, affectionate sexual activity. The paraphilias are also characterized by recurrent, intense sexually arousing fantasies generally involving (1) nonhuman objects, (2) the suffering or humiliation of oneself or one's partner, or (3) children or other nonconsenting persons. The types of paraphilias are described in Table 30-2.

Other sexual disorders that may lead to problems in the marital/couple's relationship are (1) sexual desire disorders, (2) orgasm disorders, and (3) sexual pain disorders. The characteristics of these disorders are presented in Table 30-3.

THEORETICAL APPROACHES

Psychoanalytical

The use of psychoanalytical theory in couples therapy assumes that unconscious factors influence all aspects of the relationship: choice of partner, the problems in the relationship, and how the problems are resolved. The ther-

▼ **TABLE 30-3** **Sexual Dysfunctions**

Dysfunction	Definition
Hypoactive sexual desire disorder	Persistent, pervasive inhibition of sexual desire; age, sex, health, intensity and frequency of sexual desire, and environment considered
Sexual aversion disorder	Persistent and extreme aversion to and avoidance of almost all genital sexual contact with a sexual partner
Female sexual arousal disorder	Persistent failure to attain the lubrication swelling response of sexual excitement or a lack of pleasure during sexual activity
Male erectile disorder	Persistent failure to attain or maintain an erection until completion of the sexual activity
Inhibited female orgasm	Recurrent, persistent inhibition of female orgasm, manifested by delay or absence of orgasm
Inhibited male orgasm	Recurrent, persistent inhibition of male orgasm, manifested by delay or absence of ejaculation
Premature ejaculation	Ejaculation with minimal sexual stimulation sooner than desired
Dyspareunia	Intercourse associated with persistent genital pain
Vaginismus	Recurrent, persistent involuntary spasm of the musculature of the outer third of the vagina, which interferes with intercourse

apy focuses on *transference neurosis* that evolves from past and present unconscious infantile and childhood conflicts. The goal is to bring about personality changes. Some psychoanalysts see the partners alone; others see them alone and then together. The focus of treatment is likely to be the partner who has symptoms, the identified client. Usually the treatment is lengthy.

The aspect of psychoanalytical theory that is particularly useful in marital functioning and therapy is *object relations*. This aspect focuses on the link between the marital object and the couple's early object relations in the family of origin. Object relations refer to the emotional bonds between two persons. To achieve a healthy adult level of object relations, the individuals must separate from early, infantile object relations. This separation is referred to as *separation-individuation* or *differentiation*. It begins in infancy and is refined throughout adolescence. When this process has occurred, the marital relationship consists of spouses who have reached a level of maturity and are fully differentiated individuals.[7]

When the process of separation-individuation does not occur or is incomplete, the individual carries an impaired sense of self into adult life. Such adults have either a pattern of depending on others to tell them what to do and how to do it or a pattern of depending on others to express their feelings. The person with an impaired sense of self may use one and then the other pattern, depending on the situation. This process influences mate selection, the marital relationship, and parenting as the person tries to act as an adult but relates to the object on an infantile level. Relating to a marital partner on an infantile level involves *collusion*. Using this process, each mate unconsciously chooses a partner based on unmet infantile needs, expecting that the partner will meet the needs.[19] Each partner unconsciously forms an understood but unspoken *contract* to meet the mate's unfulfilled infantile needs.

Object-relations theory assumes that children develop a heterosexual sense of reality or family image as a part of normal development.[57] This development involves three processes that later affect the marital relationship.
1. Children recognize that they are part of an internal triangle that includes the parental dyad (the parents) as an object organism.[57]
2. Over time children identify each parent's roles as marriage partners and as parents; children realize they may experience these roles as adults.
3. Children become increasingly aware of their role, their separateness, and their lack of genital fulfillment in relation to the parental dyad.

A marital partner who has not mastered these developmental processes may idealize the partner early in the marriage and later discount and blame the partner. The blaming often results in conflict, and the couple may decide to seek therapy or separate.

Self-distortion may occur in persons in couples therapy. For example, partners who mistrust each other without reason project their distrust of another person to that partner. Such a projection is unconscious and can be resolved when insight is gained into this projection.

Sager[52] uses the term *contract* to refer to the partners' separate, unspoken, unconscious understanding of their expectations within the relationship. Problems arise as each

▼ **REMINDER LIST FOR MARRIAGE OR COUPLE CONTRACTS**

Each "Contract" Involves Three Levels of Awareness:
1. *Verbalized:* You and your partner discuss these parts of your contract with each other, although the one listening does not always hear what is being said.
2. *Conscious but not verbalized:* You are aware of these parts of your contract but do not verbalize them to your partner because you fear anger, disapproval, or embarrassment.
3. *Beyond awareness or unconscious:* These aspects are beyond your usual awareness, although you may have an idea of them. You often experience them as a warning light in your head or a fleeting feeling of concern that is pushed aside.

Modified from Sager CJ: In Gurman AS, Kniskern DP, editors: *Handbook of family therapy,* New York, 1981, Brunner/Mazel.

partner relates to the other as though both consciously know and have agreed on the terms of the contract; but because this is not true, each partner is disappointed when the contract is not fulfilled.

Sager supports *conjoint therapy* (seeing both partners) with couples so that both the conscious and the unconscious aspects of each partner's contract can be explored and revealed. Then the contracts are available so that the couple can negotiate a single, unified contract. During negotiations the couple becomes more aware of the contract's interactional component. This component includes the conscious and unconscious ways in which they cooperate with or sabotage each other as they attempt to fulfill the terms of their separate contracts.

Sager recognizes that the couple's complaints brought to therapy are symptoms. The therapist seeks the underlying difficulties in the partner's relationship expectations or in their biological and psychological parameters. In Sager's theory the therapist's role is to teach partners how to negotiate because the terms of their contract and the goals of their relationship vary to reflect changes in their life situation. The levels of awareness in each contract are outlined in the reminder list for marriage or couple contracts (see accompanying box).

Behavioral

Jacobson's behavioral marital therapy (BMT)[34,38] is more complex than changing problem behaviors through new learning. Jacobson gives credit to behavioral theory evolving from operant conditioning with children. However, he recognizes that the different conditions between partners require them to negotiate.[38] Therefore he adds communication and problem-solving skills to operant programs. Successful couples adapt effectively to the requirements of day-to-day intimacy. In particular they influence each other's actions by acknowledging desired behaviors in new rewarding ways.[34]

BMT assumes that a successful relationship depends primarily on the characteristics of the partners' exchanges and on environmental forces rather than on predetermined personality characteristics. Satisfaction in the relationship is thought to be directly related to partners' abilities to maximize individual rewards and minimize individual costs in their ongoing interactions. A proper balance between rewards given and received over time is related to a greater satisfaction in their relationship.

The therapist's role in BMT is to assess the problems and to select appropriate behavioral interventions. The therapy is directive and involves teaching as a major tool. The therapist uses a variety of assessment methods and selects behavior models that the couple can learn. Usually the goals are to minimize conflict and to direct the couple in establishing a better balance between individual rewards and punishments than the couple has experienced before therapy.

Systems

Bowen[12,13] is one of the first theorists to relate systems concepts to marital therapy. This theory can be applied to unmarried couples as well. The couple is perceived not only as a nuclear family, but also as a couple linked through various systems to the families of origin and the extended families for many generations.

Central to Bowen's theory[13] is the *emotional system,* the emotional chain reactions among family members that directly tie one member's emotional functioning to that of another. Awareness of the couple's emotional system is essential to understanding the development and course of their symptoms and whether they are symptoms of physical illness, mental illness, or social acting-out behavior.

Another important aspect of the emotional system is that it can exist in a state of equilibrium or disequilibrium. Increasing anxiety drives a balanced system toward imbalance. Short-term symptoms can have a balancing effect, but long-term symptoms can cause severe disequilibrium. Bowen[13] identifies two primary life forces that counterbalance each other in the emotional system: a force toward individuality, or differentiation, and a force toward togetherness, or fusion (undifferentiation). A disturbance in the balance of these forces can cause anxiety and lead to symptom development. The characteristics of these forces within persons, families, and other groups vary greatly. What constitutes imbalance in one circumstance may be balance in another. A person who grows up in a family in which the balance is strongly toward togetherness may be programmed only for fusion[22] and thus poorly differentiated.

The process of fusion (undifferentiation) is shown in Figure 30-1, in which the square represents the male and the circle the female. In fusion each partner blends some identity with the other. The adult who was fused to a parent

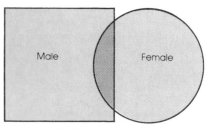

FIGURE 30-1 Fusion.

as a child carries the characteristic of fusion into relationships outside the family, including the couple's relationship. The fused person is likely to select a partner who is at the same level of differentiation (individuality). When the intensity of the fusion becomes too great to tolerate, emotional distance is used to cope with the increased anxiety. In Figure 30-2 the space and the line with a slash represent the emotional distance or the partners' effort to move away from each other. Fusion and distancing are two sides of the same coin. Emotional conflict allows intense relating to the partner and maintaining emotional distance at the same time.[42]

The term *fusion exclusion* describes a third compensatory mechanism in the emotional system. Bowen originally used the term *triangle* to refer to this emotional process.[22] The fusion-exclusion mechanism is shown in Figure 30-3. The wavy line denotes conflict, the straight line denotes closeness, and the straight line with a slash, cutoff. The emotional process symbolized is fusion in the couple's subsystem. This is balanced by conflict between the partners. The example pictures a married couple with a son. The wife and son are close to each other, and the husband and son are cut off from each other. Through this mechanism two people can stay in close contact with each other and avoid fusion-generated anxiety either by excluding a third person from their relationship or by focusing their energies on a third person, sometimes a child.

In a fourth mechanism for balancing the emotional system, *pseudoposition,* the spouses assume "pretend," directly opposite positions, for example, dominant-submissive, overresponsible-underresponsible, and overadequate-inadequate. One person acts and feels strong, and the other acts and feels weak.

These four mechanisms help couples maintain equilibrium in their relationships. Problems occur when additional stress strains the couple's few remaining coping reserves. In a further effort to maintain equilibrium, one partner develops symptoms, which replace the direct expression

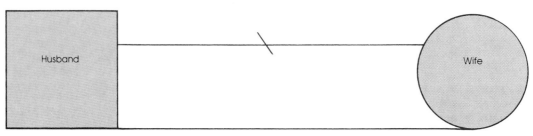

FIGURE 30-2 Distancing.

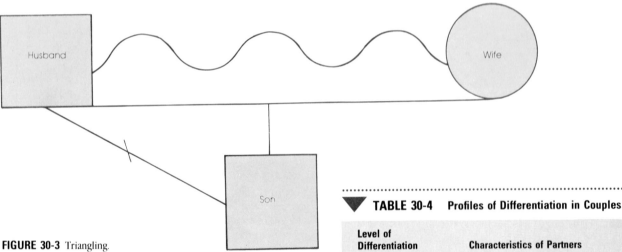

FIGURE 30-3 Triangling.

Based on data from Bowen M. In Olson D, editor: *Treating relationships,* Lake Mills, Iowa, 1976, Graphic Publishing Co.

of emotions. Alcoholism, obesity, physical illness, mental illness, and even criminal behavior at their extremes are symptoms that reflect a significant lack of differentiation.[12] Better-differentiated persons and couples can have the same problems, but they are likely to be in a milder form. These illness patterns can be seen in several generations, with the more fused generations having the more severe problems.

The therapist's role in Bowen's theory is (1) to assess the partner's needs, (2) to estimate each spouses' differentiation, and (3) to work with the couple as members of a multigenerational family system so that each person reaches a higher level of differentiation. Any profile of persons at various levels of differentiation is more hypothetical than real. Thus the profiles of differentiation given in Table 30-4 are for guidance only and should be used cautiously.

According to Bowen,[13] three main clinical approaches have been effective when the client's goal is differentiation of self: (1) psychotherapy with both partners, (2) psychotherapy with one family member, and (3) psychotherapy with one partner in preparation for a long-term effort with both partners. Usually the therapist meets with the client or clients monthly, thus giving them time to work on the problems between sessions. The therapist adjusts the focus from feelings to thinking and consistently implies that the couple "owns" the problems and thus are the ones who must solve them.

In the first approach the therapist listens to one partner while the other partner listens. The therapist asks many questions about the problems and about what each spouse has been thinking. The therapist detriangles situations as they arise, often by confronting the phenomenon and questioning its value to each spouse. The genogram is used during this process (Figure 30-4).

Using the genogram, the therapist points out the relationships across the generations. The couple is assigned to study the patterns of their extended families and of themselves and then to identify what they want to change or retain. The therapist coaches the clients as they take steps to change their relationships with selected family members.

Frequently, the couples are pleasantly surprised at the quality of their mate's thinking. The therapist supports each

▼ **TABLE 30-4** Profiles of Differentiation in Couples

Level of Differentiation	Characteristics of Partners
Moderate to good	Emotional and intellectual systems function cooperatively
	Use factual knowledge to make decisions that can overrule the emotional system in situations of anxiety and panic
	Can live freely with emotional system using logical reasoning when need arises
	Able to follow independent life goals
	Marriage is a functioning partnership
	Are responsible for selves
Pseudoself	Some beginning differentiation of emotional and intellectual systems
	Life guided by emotional system
	If anxiety is low, functioning resembles moderately differentiated self
	Life energy directed to winning friends and approval
	Self-esteem dependent on others
	Lack solid self-convictions; refer to authority
	Personal lives in chaos
	May be conforming disciples or rebels
	Have intense versions of overt feeling
	Develop high percentage of human problems, such as physical illness, social dysfunction, and emotional illness
Low	Dysfunctional
	Anxious
	Live in a feeling-dominated world
	Do not distinguish feeling from fact
	Totally relationship oriented
	No energy for life-directed goals
	Seek approval; often experience failure to have approval, leading to withdrawal or fighting in the relationship system.

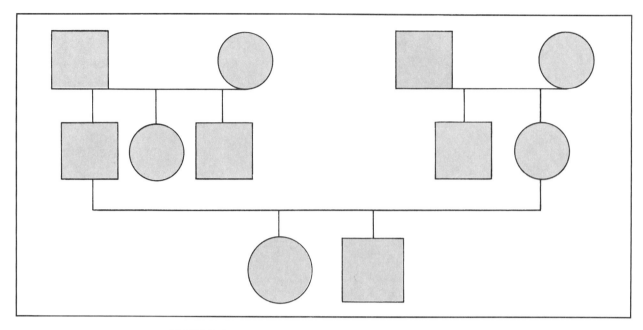

FIGURE 30-4 Family map, or genogram. *Squares,* males; *circles,* females.

person's expression of thoughts while differentiating thoughts from feelings. The therapist encourages each client to listen to the other's expressed thoughts, to think about the thoughts, and to respond with related ideas. The goal is to calm the anxiety in the relationship.

The teaching aspect of Bowen's therapy occurs when the couple's tension is reduced. At this point the couple can listen. The therapist makes comments from the "I" position; for example, "I have had some experience with other couples that may be useful for you to know or may not suit you. I do not want you to adopt it as it's described; but, if you want to use it, you can adapt it to your own situation." The therapist uses coaching to share ideas that may be useful. This method engages the clients in dialogue about alternative actions while leaving the choice to them.

In the second approach using systems theory when only one partner is present because the other dislikes the image of psychotherapy, the therapist proceeds as for one family member. In the third approach, eventually the other partner is impressed with the changes made by the one receiving therapy and may ask to join the sessions. At this point therapy proceeds as for couples together.

Existential

Whitaker's approach to marital therapy[65,66] is known as existential marital therapy and is a subsystem of existential family therapy. This approach can be adapted for nonmarried couples. The therapy advocates three values—experience, reality, and growth—and relies on the total, immediate experience of the moment. Emphasis is on reality and the facts of life. The aim of therapy is helping people grow, in contrast to helping people adapt.[66]

Whitaker[65] addresses premarital and marital myths. An example of a premarital myth is the expectation of receiving unconditional positive regard, which does not occur after

infancy. An example of a marital myth based on Whitaker's theory is "If you're going to run around with somebody else, don't tell me." Infidelity always involves a triangle, and usually both partners preplan and want it, according to Whitaker. The "someone else" may be a lover, money, school, or a house.

Whitaker points out two processes in a marriage, the legal commitment and the feeling experience, or the binding and the bonding. The feeling level is unstable and, as each partner grows, always changing, with peaks of love and hate. Each partner behaves in a way to maintain balance. The more one or both get stuck in a fixed role, the more each loses his or her humanness.

The couple is most likely to change at crisis points such as the honeymoon, pregnancy, birth, extramarital affairs, absences, and reentries. A noteworthy phenomenon is the 10-year impasse (deadlock) syndrome, when the couple has an opportunity to establish a wholehearted relationship or to provoke hostility.

The therapist uses Whitaker's typology of marriage as a guide to observe and evaluate the couple's behavior in the session and to understand their descriptions of their ongoing interactions:

1. Stable and dead, with the relationship frozen into pseudomutual politeness or hostility
2. Unstable and growthful, which can provide optimal conditions for continual individual and marital growth
3. Stalemated chaos, in which the system lacks well-defined limits; partners are locked into nongrowth-producing interactions

Whitaker recognizes the multigenerational system and its influence on the marital dyad. When necessary he directs one spouse to arrange for parents or siblings to attend the session. Whitaker accepts no excuses and does not hold the session until the other family members are present. Thus many multigenerational problems are solved, freeing

▼ **TABLE 30-5**   **Summary of Theoretical Approaches to Marital/Couples Therapy**

Theory	Theorist	Goal	Role
Psychoanalytical	Sager[52]	Separation-individuation (to achieve separation from early infantile object relations)	To assist partners to achieve a healthy adult level of object relations
		To determine the conscious and unconscious aspect of each spouse's contract (expectations in the marriage)	To teach partners how to negotiate a single, unified contract
Behavioral	Jacobson[34,38]	To minimize marital conflict and to direct the couple to achieve a better balance between reward and punishment	To assess the marital problems and to select appropriate behavioral interventions
Systems	Bowen[13]	To assist the couple to reach a higher level of differentiation (individuality)	To teach, coach, and assess the couple's needs; to estimate their level of differentiation; and to work with their multigenerational system
Existential	Whitaker[66]	To observe, evaluate, and understand the couple's behavior in the session	To free the couple from the multigenerational system so that they can proceed with the growth and development of their marital relationship

the couple to proceed with their own growth and the development of their relationship. Table 30-5 summarizes the four theoretical approaches to therapy.

CHARACTERISTICS OF THE MARITAL/COUPLES THERAPIST

Qualifications

Some states require that marital/couples therapists be licensed and define their qualifications. Most states apply the standards of the American Association for Marriage and Family Therapy (AAMFT). The AAMFT standards set minimal requirements as a master's degree in either marital and family therapy from an accredited institution or a master's degree in an allied mental health profession. In addition, the therapist must have 1500 hours of clinical experience (defined as face-to-face contact) in marriage and family therapy, with 200 of those hours supervised.

Marital/couples therapist must be persons of integrity with high ethical standards, as they are working with vulnerable persons who are often in great need of objective assistance and support. The therapists' training ideally has enabled them to differentiate their own biases from those of their clients.

Role

The therapist's role is defined largely by the theoretical framework used. Specific roles are presented in the previous discussion of theories. All couples therapy involves

a certain amount of teaching. The therapist makes recommendations for action based on theoretical knowledge and the couple's goal. In some therapy (for example, behavioral), teaching is a major goal.

Therapists use a certain level of activity appropriate for their theoretical orientation. Some therapists are active and use a directive approach in guiding the couple to resolve the conflict. Often therapists are nondirective while listening attentively to what each client has to share. With the latter approach, which is more typical of psychoanalytical therapy, the therapist believes the couple needs to make decisions based on their own conscious and unconscious motivations.

Some therapists work alone and others work in teams. Some advocate a male-female co-therapy team to avoid the appearance or occurrence of biased alliances that cause hostility and deadlock. Others advocate a coupled pair as therapists, believing that therapists' resolution of their own problems serves as a role model and a continuing demonstration of problem solving in a couple.[2]

Haley[29] believes that co-therapists complicate therapeutic efforts and that the most effective interventions can be made directly by one therapist. For persons training in strategic therapy (the problem-solving therapy developed by Haley), the supervisor is behind a one-way mirror and readily available to the trainee.

The choice of one therapist or co-therapists is often based on economic considerations. Co-therapy may be affordable in facilities with training programs, such as hospitals and clinics. In addition, co-therapy offers the opportunity for real life training. Many nurses are employed in settings where co-therapy may be used in the training program; thus they can serve as advisers to couples therapy trainees. In private practice or in other settings where funds are limited, co-therapy may be too expensive.

Goals

The goals of the therapist depend on the therapist's theoretical orientation, as discussed under theories of couples therapy. In addition, the goals may be to treat pathological disorders, to enable the partners to solve specific problems, and to foster satisfaction within the relationship.

CHARACTERISTICS OF MARITAL/COUPLES THERAPY

Client Selection

Crises may create a need for couples therapy. Many clients seek help because of the conflict or distance that troubles one or both partners. Some clients are self-referrals, and others are referred by social service agencies, attorneys, clergy, or physicians from whom they initially sought guidance. Marital/couples therapy is the treatment of choice when conflicts lead to spouse or child abuse. Often these couples are referred for therapy by the local police or a treatment service for victims of abuse.

The age range of clients is from the middle teens (15 to 16 years of age) to the 70s, with most couples in their late 20s to early 40s. Suitable candidates for marital or couples therapy generally are ambulatory and are sufficiently in touch with reality to participate actively in the session and report their problems. Some therapists provide couples therapy for clients with a diagnosed psychotic disorder.

Some therapists think an appropriate time for couples therapy is when clients need assistance in getting a separation or divorce. Others reject couples for therapy when the relationship is beyond repair and separation or divorce is imminent.

Stages

Marital/couples therapy has three stages: beginning, middle, and termination. At the beginning the therapy is aimed at relieving each partner's stress related to the problems and symptoms. The therapeutic interventions and the clients' behavioral and other changes help to relieve their anxiety so that each can think more clearly about options and solutions to their problems.

During the middle phase the therapy moves more slowly. A recurrence of past behavior accompanies each change as the partners struggle to use the learning from the sessions in daily life. Personal change and system change occur at a deeper level than in the beginning stage. The therapist relates the partners' tension expressed in the sessions to their families of origin and early experiences. The therapist coaches each partner about alternative ways to relate to family members and to each other.

During the termination stage the couple continues to practice their changed thinking, feeling, and behaving developed throughout therapy. They use termination time to consolidate their gains and to obtain the therapist's assistance in polishing their skills at problem solving and improving relationships.

NURSING PROCESS

Assessment

Physical dimension Throughout couples therapy the nurse monitors physical conditions and complaints. The nurse collects data about the health history, including current health problems, medications prescribed, and use and abuse of over-the-counter drugs as well as addictive substances such as alcohol and illegal drugs. Decreased satisfaction may result when the couple invests much time, energy, and money on chronic medical problems. Often the medical problem becomes the focus of their lives, making their interpersonal problem secondary. When either or both partners are receiving medication, the nurse considers the therapeutic effects and side effects in assessing behavior and symptoms. Discord often occurs when drug or alcohol dependency is a factor. The nurse determines if one or both partners used chemical substances before or in response to the conflict.

The relationship may have become dysfunctional after the birth of a child with a genetic defect. Each partner may blame the other for the child's problem and be unable to discuss the problem openly.

Changes in either partner's body image as a result of disfiguring surgery, hysterectomy, mastectomy, pregnancy, or weight gain may strain the relationship. Often persons are reluctant to discuss their thoughts on these subjects. During the assessment the nurse notes changes in sexual activity that result from physical health problems, such as cardiovascular disease or diabetes. When collecting sexual data the nurse starts with the less personal subjects and proceeds to sexual problems.

A complete physical examination after a thorough history may reveal physiological dysfunctions. The examination focuses on dysfunctions in the reproductive system that may interfere with sexual functioning.

Many physical factors affect sexual functioning: stress and fatigue and health problems, such as diabetes, debilitating illnesses, hepatic disease, or neurological disease (for example, multiple sclerosis and spinal cord injury). The nurse assesses medications that the client is taking. Some medications known to affect sexual functioning fall in the following classifications:
* Antihypertensives
* Antidepressants
* Antihistamines
* Antispasmodics and anticholinergics
* Antipsychotics
* Oral contraceptives
* Narcotics
* Chemotherapeutic agents
* Estrogen
* Diuretics

Signs of physical abuse may be evident during the assessment. Regardless of education, occupation, or social status, some couples have arguments that end in spouse or child abuse.

Emotional dimension The nurse closely observes the couple's emotions, including difficulties in expressing emotion. Sometimes one partner holds back feelings until provoked to express accumulated feelings and then may explode and become violent. The nurse uses the therapy session to look for positive feelings between the partners. Most couples have some positive feelings for each other; as they express and share these feelings, their outlook becomes more optimistic.

The couple's presence in the therapeutic setting may indicate that they care enough about each other to try to resolve the conflict. When assessing the couple, however, the nurse may learn that the caring is masked by strong emotions such as anger, anxiety, hate, fear, and depression. Many couples in therapy have a history of unresolved anger and anxiety. Strong negative emotions, for example, anger, guilt, and depression, disrupt sexual arousal and may lead to dysfunction.

Anger is a major cause of relationship failure. Anger may be in response to a partner's unconscious or unspoken infantile expectations for need satisfaction. Anger may also result from humiliation and the fear of further hurt. Over time the anger becomes so intense that it disrupts the relationship (see the accompanying research highlight).

The anxiety that the nurse observes during the first few sessions may reflect partners' discomfort in the therapy situation. However, uncertainty about the future if their relationship fails can also cause anxiety. In addition, either partner may experience anxiety about the other's complaining, blaming, and emotional distance. Anxiety, a major contributor to sexual dysfunction, may lead to impotence in men.

The nurse's assessment includes determining how the partners feel about seeking therapy. Sometimes one threatens separation if the other does not attend therapy. The threatened partner may respond with anger and remain detached from the process. If the problems are not resolved, the partner who initiated the therapy may feel guilty. One or both partners may experience guilt because each feels responsible for the dysfunctional relationship. A partner who has a secret, such as infidelity, may think this decreases the therapy's effectiveness and may feel guilt as well.

In the assessment the nurse is alert to symptoms of despair, depression, and potential suicide. Because depression typically occurs with relationship problems, the nurse needs to ask directly if either partner or any member of the immediate family has attempted or thought about suicide. Any major change may trigger depression and the potential for suicide: illness, death of a significant other, geographical relocation, job instability, or possible divorce or separation. Depression results in decreased sexual interest and frequently sexual functioning is impaired.

Temporary absences and reentries occur in some relationships, due to a job or military assignment. A crisis may occur when the partner reenters the couples system, when the imbalance in the system is sufficient to create discord,

RESEARCH HIGHLIGHT

The Unforgivable Humiliation: A Dilemma in Couple's Treatment
• W Vogel and A Lazare

PURPOSE

The purpose of this study was to determine ways to resolve conflict in partners who are unable to communicate due to incidents where one partner has been humiliated by the other and cannot express to the offending partner the nature of the insult in such a way that it is comprehended and accepted.

The hypothesis is that the disaffected partner has experienced humiliation at the hand of their partner. The study also outlines a plan for treatment citing case examples.

SAMPLE

Seven case examples of experiences where humiliation led to disruption of long-term stable relationships were studied.

METHODOLOGY

A qualitative study compared the case examples to identify common elements responsible for disruption of long-term relationships.

FINDINGS

Common elements in all seven case examples were the following:
1. All of the "humiliated" persons suffered from a sense of profound betrayal, which resulted in a breakdown of communication of their feelings to the partners.
2. This lack of communication made therapy difficult.
3. The extreme social behaviors exhibited by each of the humiliated persons led to diagnostic difficulties.
4. There was an imbalance of power between the principals in each case.

IMPLICATIONS

All cases of unforgivable humiliation do not have to end in dissolution of the relationship. There are steps in which a therapist can help couples resolve situations where humiliation has occurred.

Both parties must acknowledge the experience and see how the disaffected partner came to feel this humiliation. The therapist must help normalize the situation so that neither partner sees the disaffected partner response as pathological. The therapist must help negotiate restitution for the insult. The three elements included in the restitution are apology, compensation, and trust.

Based on data from *Contemporary Family Therapy* 12(2):139, 1990.

and when one or both partners experience anxiety and depression.

Intellectual dimension The therapist often assesses the clients' intellectual dimension in couples therapy by drawing conclusions from their vocabularies, levels of education, and socioeconomic status. Their feedback about understanding their therapist's information also provides clues. The nurse especially notes consistent and inconsistent elements in the couple's intellectual functioning as partners.

Clients may not have a sound knowledge of sexuality. Myths may lead to fear and anxiety about sex. The therapist gathers information about the client's knowledge about sexuality as well as the source of the information. Ignorance and misunderstanding may lead to fear and avoidance of sex.

The nurse assesses the clients' educational level to determine the appropriate type of intervention. People with less education may need a more direct and active approach. For example, the clients may request direct answers instead of a problem-solving approach. A difference in partners' educational level may be a problem, even when the couples discuss the differences in education before becoming involved. Sometimes feelings of inadequacy or superiority may lead to conflict.

One of the first problems mentioned by most couples who seek therapy is lack of effective communication. The nurse may hear the following complaints about communicating[27]:

1. A narcissistic partner who is self-centered instead of committed to the relationship
2. Indifference, in which the partner shows lack of concern through a negative approach toward the mate's feelings, needs, and wishes
3. Inability to reinforce and support the partner
4. Inflexibility, as evidenced by rigid attitudes and values
5. Inexperience in positive and meaningful relationships
6. Crossed transactions that reflect a poor link between verbal and nonverbal communication
7. Avoidance maneuvers, in which the mate communicates rejection by withdrawing
8. Distortion, in which messages are sent to the partner but not received

The nurse also determines the reason for blocked communication in therapy. The most common reason is a secret that causes the partner to anticipate rejection by the nurse.[45] The four most frequent secrets that impede communication between clients and the therapist are extramarital affairs, homosexuality, an incestuous experience, and racial or religious prejudices.

The expressiveness of each partner is another important function to assess. Inadequate, incomplete, and misperceived communications often cause discord. In response to the statement, "I know that you heard what I said, but do you know what I mean?" too many couples would say, "No." The assessment of expressiveness is a continual process during therapy.

The therapist also assesses each partner in terms of flexibility and rigidity of thinking and behavior. For some, rigid adherence to rules and their established values is essential and flexibility is perceived as weakness.

▼ Case Example

Bruce has a rigid requirement that established table manners be scrupulously observed at the dinner table. Sandra believes that the dinner table is a place for relaxed, informal visiting. When either of her sons, 10 and 12 years old, breaks a rule, Bruce reprimands them. Sandra says nothing at the time but is offended and adds this act to her grievance collection about Bruce. In therapy Bruce is emphatic that he will not modify his behavior. His rigidity and Sandra's flexibility are both areas of disagreement in their relationship.

One or both partners often use projection and displacement to deal with distress. The clients may state that the problem is entirely caused by the other partner. Some clients anticipate rejection if they share their problems, feelings, and secrets and may use denial, which is often accompanied by resistance. The couple may manifest this resistance by missing sessions, arriving late, and being silent for long periods during the session. These behaviors are an attempt to deal with some threat and are necessary for coping.

Because of anxiety, fear, lack of experience, or disagreement about the problem or what approach to use, a couple may be unable to use effective problem-solving skills. During the assessment the nurse may observe that the couple attempts to change behavior by coercion instead of the problem-solving method suggested by Jacobson and thus is aggravating the conflict.

Social dimension The nurse assesses the degree of dependence-independence in the couple's relationship by asking them about their styles of relating and by listening to their communication patterns, such as speaking for the other or looking to the other before replying. According to Bowen, assessment of this behavior helps determine the partners' level of differentiation (individuality). Both partners may complain of being frustrated at unmet dependence needs. The nurse may observe that each client has the conscious or unconscious expectation that dependence needs will be met by the other. Often the dependence needs of couples who seek therapy are at an infantile level and thus maladaptive. When such needs are not met to the partner's satisfaction, the question of the mate's fidelity may arise.

The nurse assesses the level of trust between the partners as well as between each partner and the nurse. Often this aspect is revealed directly as they interact in the session. Candor or guarded statements, expressions of suspicion, and periods of silence can all be clues to the couple's level of trust-mistrust. Mistrust may be in response to a family secret.

The couple's self-esteem and self-respect may be damaged by the time they come for therapy. The nurse listens for statements clients make about each other and themselves to assess their self-esteem.

Both partners are highly vulnerable to decreased self-esteem because of masculine and feminine stereotypes. One partner may reveal a sexual bias by belittling the other. For example, some men believe that women are inferior physically and intellectually. The nurse assesses how closely the couple adheres to the traditional relationship expectations of the man as breadwinner and woman as housewife and mother. If both partners work outside the home, the nurse is alert for clues to role conflict. For example, does the man expect the woman to manage the home, or does he share the chores? If the man assists the woman with what are traditionally considered female responsibilities does she discredit his efforts?

The couple may request assistance in resolving conflicts related to sexual adjustment. During the initial interview the nurse inquires about when the problem began and the nature of the sexual dysfunction. Sometimes the sexual maladjustment caused the conflict; at other times the sexual problem resulted from the distressed relationship. The two problems frequently are interrelated, as partners unconsciously displace other tensions into the sexual area. As the couple describe their distress, the nurse may learn that they really have a sexual relationship problem. Some couples will not talk directly about sexual concerns, but the nurse may suspect problems when a couple mentions sleeping in separate beds and bedrooms or allowing children to sleep with them. When a relationship problem is suspected, the nurse will explore the client's depth of commitment and trust.

The nurse assesses the effects of dependence and independence in the couple's relationship on their sexual functioning. Long-lasting relationships may generate dependence and the partners may begin to magnify each other's flaws, creating sexual problems. Increased independence of one partner may create sexual difficulties when the couple fails to communicate needs and desires and takes the relationship for granted. A balance of dependence and independence is important so that one partner does not have unmet sexual needs due to the couple's failure to communicate clearly.

The environment is an essential element to assess when exploring the sexual relationship. Does the environment afford privacy necessary for sexual activity and allow for private communication between partners? The nurse explores learned sexual behavior and each partner's perception of sex roles. The cultural norms of the individual strongly affects the couple's sexual relationship. Examples are preferred position for sexual intercourse, whether the woman plays an active or passive role, and the length and type of foreplay. For example, kissing is accepted in western countries, but some societies believe it is unsanitary.

Typically, a couple who marries expect that their social relationships will endure. This expectation increases the pressure to have mutually satisfying interactions. When assessing the couple's social interaction, the nurse may observe that they have limited or no other social relationships and thus relate to each other intensively. This situation may be a factor in one partner distancing and the other becoming dysfunctional; it may also lead to conflict followed by physical abuse. Distancing may be a response to personal space needs.

On the other hand, the nurse may learn that the conflict is triggered by one or both partners spending increasing time away from the other. Examples of "rival" interests are a job, a favorite sport, community activities, alcohol, drugs, or care of an aged parent. The woman is more likely than the man to be involved in community activities. This may be her attempt to show her partner that she does not need him, especially if he spends much time with his job. On

examining the woman's community work, the nurse may find that even though active the woman is isolated and lonely.[56]

The nurse may pick up clues that an extramarital relationship decreases the couple's time together. According to surveys, infidelity ranks third as the cause of marital conflict; one half of clients who seek marital therapy have a problem involving infidelity.[51] More men than women seek intimate companionship outside the family. A woman may accuse her partner of infidelity after a vasectomy, and the man may do the same after the woman has a hysterectomy because each procedure eliminates the risk of pregnancy. Infidelity does not necessarily mean the partner no longer loves the mate. Boredom, revenge, and testing sex appeal are some of the reasons for affairs. If an affair is the present problem, the couple may be more candid if the nurse interviews them separately and promises confidentiality.

At times a partner may be creative and feel an intense need to be free to make choices. When the mate supports the creativity and freedom, the relationship is helped to flourish. Likewise, when restrictions are placed on the creative partner's freedom, the person may become dysfunctional, distance himself or herself from the other, or rebel and generate conflict.

Spiritual dimension The nurse considers the following when assessing the couple's spiritual dimension. What are each partner's beliefs about marriage and cohabitating and about "right" and "wrong" in sexuality? Are their beliefs in agreement or in conflict? Does each partner's philosophy of life include commitment to the relationship and to the other? When it does, it may be a powerful motivator to solve relationship problems.

According to Whitaker's existential theory, the spiritually healthy partner has the inner resources to transform relationship stresses into growth experiences. Those with limited spiritual health face threatening questions about the meaning of their lives. A woman may say, "If our life together is over, it's the end of me!"

Many modern couples have a firm faith in God or a supreme being and find that their shared faith assists them in tolerating the irritations of their life together. Others, who may have had religious education and participated in appropriate rituals, may drop out of organized religion. They may retain some faith in a supreme being or a higher power, but the belief may have limited influence on their life-styles. Such couples may be wed in a civil ceremony. Later, when conflict occurs, instead of having a strong desire to solve the problems, they may choose to dissolve the marriage.

Some clients with strict religious upbringings have rigid attitudes that cause anxiety and guilt about sex. Some religions teach that masturbation is a sin and forbid premarital sex. Those who experiment sexually may feel guilty and later develop sexual dysfunction. The couple's religious beliefs also influence other decisions. Some faiths perceive children as the purpose of a marital union and permit no efforts to limit family size. Other faiths allow various contraceptive measures and abortion. As long as the couple's practices reflect their religious beliefs and their beliefs are in harmony, conflict may not occur. When discord is present, however, serious problems may result. Strongly held, incompatible beliefs may support increased distance and blaming as in the following case example.

▼ Case Example

Mamie was reared in a particular religious faith, was a devout follower, and wanted her two children to attend worship services with her. Roland, her husband, had a very strong faith in a different religious belief that taught him that only those faithful to that belief could achieve salvation. Roland insisted that their children attend worship services with him and was extremely disapproving of Mamie because she would not convert. Mamie complained of feeling deeply depressed most of the time.

Analysis
Nursing diagnosis

Altered sexuality patterns and sexual dysfunction are nursing diagnoses approved by NANDA that apply to couples therapy. The defining characteristics of these nursing diagnoses are listed in the accompanying boxes.

The following case example demonstrates the characteristics of altered sexuality patterns.

▼ Case Example

Mary, a mother of two children, is a full-time housewife. Her husband, Joe, is an executive officer in a large corporation that demands more and more time away from the family. As a result of his absence and because Mary must assume responsibility for the household decisions without input from her husband, social distancing has occurred, and sexual functioning is affected. Mary feels trapped in a relationship that she cannot discuss with her very busy husband. The conflict continues to grow. She turns her full attention to the children and her social life without him.

The following case example illustrates the nursing diagnosis sexual dysfunction.

▼ Case Example

A 32-year-old man who was having difficulty having sexual intercourse with his second wife presented for therapy complaining of impotence. His first wife divorced him 1 year ago. The client viewed the divorce as rejection and believed the wife divorced him because he was sexually inadequate. In the present marriage he is preoccupied with the fear that he may be a failure during lovemaking. He engages in constant self-harassment and "spectator" behavior, assuring that he will be unsuccessful in having sexual intercourse. His behavior created marital difficulty and the couple agreed to participate in therapy.

The following list provides examples of NANDA-accepted nursing diagnoses with causative statements that apply to marital/couples therapy:
1. Impaired verbal communication related to failure to listen
2. Ineffective individual coping: anger related to marital discord
3. Sexual dysfunction related to extramarital affair
4. Impaired social interaction related to overinvolvement in community activities

Planning

Table 30-6 provides a nursing care plan with long- and short-term goals, outcome criteria interventions, and rationales related to couples therapy, all of which are examples of the planning stage of the nursing process.

Implementation

Physical dimension When the couple is experiencing discord in the relationship related to chronic medical problems, the nurse refers them to a physician and then to social services if the problem is financial. A community health nurse may be another useful source for services. The couple is informed that physical problems sometimes mask

---

▼ ALTERED SEXUALITY PATTERNS

DEFINITION
The state in which an individual expresses concern regarding his/her sexuality.

DEFINING CHARACTERISTICS
- **Social dimension**
  Reported difficulties, limitations, or changes in sexual behavior or activities

Modified from Kim MJ, McFarland GK, McLane AM, editors: *Pocket guide to nursing diagnoses,* ed 5, St Louis, 1993, Mosby–Year Book.

▼ SEXUAL DYSFUNCTION

DEFINITION
The state in which an individual experiences a change in sexual function that is viewed as unsatisfying, unrewarding, or inadequate.

DEFINING CHARACTERISTICS
- **Physical dimension**
  Actual or perceived limitation imposed by disease and/or therapy

- **Intellectual dimension**
  Verbalization of problem

- **Social dimension**
  Alteration in achieving perceived sex role
  Conflicts involving values
  Alteration in sexual satisfaction
  Seeking confirmation of desirability
  Alteration in relationship with significant other
  Change in interest in self and other

Modified from Kim MJ, McFarland GK, McLane AM, editors: *Pocket guide to nursing diagnoses,* ed 5, St Louis, 1993, Mosby–Year Book.

▼ **TABLE 30-6   NURSING CARE PLAN**

GOALS	OUTCOME CRITERIA	INTERVENTIONS	RATIONALES
NURSING DIAGNOSIS: Altered sexual pattern related to partner's excessive drinking			
LONG TERM			
To decide whether to continue the relationship	Both partners make a commitment to the decision	Encourage couples therapy	Provides a structured, safe environment to discuss reasons for and against continuing the relationship
To establish satifactory sexual activity	Performs sexually in a satisfactory manner	Introduce AA and group therapy to enhance sobriety, thus improving sexual functioning	Sobriety is essential to satisfactory sexual performance
SHORT TERM			
To deal constructively with negative feelings about drinking	Identifies causes of negative feelings	Allow for an expression of negative feelings	Client can express feeling in a nonthreatening environment
To discontinue drinking	Recognizes problems that drinking brings	Encourage AA and other therapies that offer support	Support is essential to continued sobriety

interpersonal difficulties. Resolving the medical problems releases energy to work on the factors causing stress. If one or both partners have a chemical dependence problem, the nurse refers them to Alcoholics Anonymous, Al-Anon, or a drug treatment program. The nurse also establishes ground rules at the first meeting that neither partner can attend the therapy session while under the influence of alcohol or illegal drugs.

Genetic counseling may be indicated if the couple has a child with a genetic defect. The couple needs to discuss thoughts and feelings related to the child in the therapy sessions.

The nurse provides an opportunity for the couple to discuss changes in body image and physical illnesses that have affected their relationship, including sexual functioning. The nurse may need to teach them ways to increase mutual satisfaction and explore alternative methods for sexual gratification. New positions for intercourse may be helpful, or new areas of erotic sensations may be developed.

The nurse assists the client with body image distortions after surgery or trauma to foster a more positive self-image. Focusing on the client's strengths and positive qualities may lessen the pain of having only one breast or being unable to reach orgasm. Clients can adapt to changes in sexual functioning by accepting lovemaking techniques that enhance rather than negate their body image.

◣ **Emotional dimension** Early in therapy the nurse shares observations of and reinforces the couple's positive feelings for each other. This intervention may increase their awareness of feelings they thought no longer existed. If the negative feelings are not overwhelming, the nurse may encourage each couple to share a positive feeling he or she has for the other.

Clients are assisted to deal with strong negative emotions such as anger, hostility, and resentment. The couple

needs to know early that beneath the anger may be unresolved hurt and that once the anger is resolved, they may experience increased intimacy. L'Abate and L'Abate[44] describe five guidelines for couples to deal with anger:

1. When there is anger, recognize that there is also hurt.
2. Address these hurt feelings and express them to your partner in terms of "I feel . . ." or "It hurt me when you . . . ."
3. Avoid projecting feelings onto your partner and assume responsibility for your own hurt.
4. Forgive yourself for trying to be perfect and invulnerable by trying to deny your hurt feelings.
5. Redefine yourself in terms of errors and weaknesses, as human, not "crazy." Do not demand invulnerability (superman, superwoman) from yourself.

With guidance from the nurse, the couple uses these guidelines to examine and resolve anger and hurt. The nurse helps the couple realize how negative emotions inhibit sexual functioning. Reducing performance anxiety is a primary treatment focus related to such emotions.

The nurse instructs the couple to keep a separate written record of any situation or behavior that causes anger or anxiety. The nurse asks them to keep the information confidential until they get to the session so that they can share and compare similarities and differences in their experience.[27]

It is important that the nurse allow the couple to ventilate feelings and experience some relief at the first session. The nurse emphasizes that physical violence is not allowed. This rule may help lessen the couple's fear that they will lose control of their emotions, especially anger.

By having both partners identify and label feelings, the nurse assists them to become responsible for learning means to cope with the feeling. Once feelings are expressed constructively, guilt may decrease. Fears of rejection, abandonment, and guilt often promote overconcern for a partner and impair sexual functioning resulting in depression. Depression may lift as the couple begins resolving the conflict.

Intellectual dimension The nurse guides the couple to recognize and examine their defense mechanisms. The nurse uses confrontation to help them face reality. A moderately directive approach may be used to provide information learned from the assessment about their problem.

The couple is guided to explore what is interfering with their ability to solve problems. They are taught the problem-solving process. The nurse discusses the steps in the process sometimes assigning homework. The couple reach an agreement about a problem and discuss their problem-solving approach at the next session. The nurse assists them to negotiate a contract using Sager's theory as a framework in conflict resolution.

Once a secret is revealed, the nurse lets the partner decide whether to share it with the other partner. Revealing a secret can clear the air, and therapeutic work can continue.[27]

Initially the nurse intervenes in dysfunctional communication by concentrating on the communication process between the partners. After they establish a positive two-way process, the nurse focuses on the content of the couple's messages. The nurse guides the couple to rephrase, restate, and clarify issues. The nurse also teaches and models appropriate and open communication. The couple may use role playing to share their perception of the dysfunctional communication and learn new ways to communicate their needs. They are guided to listen, make eye contact, and speak one at a time.

The nurse discusses the role playing and helps the partners to recognize each other's contributions to the problem. The partners learn to take responsibility for accuracy in their communication by using "I" statements. The couple also learn to make statements instead of asking questions. Gradually, each partner assumes responsibility for the communication problem and learns to communicate more clearly and accurately.

Social dimension Because sexual difficulties result from couple's interactions, the nurse may refer to sexual therapy to build and maintain a healthy relationship. The therapist identifies transferences, promotes feelings of trust, analyzes power struggles, and examines contracts to resolve conflicts in the relationship. When the partners spend too little time together, the nurse has them discuss their favorite activities with each other and arrange to alternate choosing the activities they enjoy together. The nurse encourages couples with limited social contacts to seek social opportunities and make new friends.

Spiritual dimension When the couple views their spirituality as a source of strength, the nurse reinforces their belief and helps them explore ways this strength may be used to resolve conflict. The couple discusses similarities and differences in their religious beliefs; when conflicts arise, the nurse guides them to explore compromises. If the couple did not previously seek counseling from their religious leader, the nurse refers them to that person. This intervention may be especially helpful when the couple is considering separation or divorce against their religious

teaching. Referral to a religious leader may also be appropriate when the partners' values about contraception are in conflict.

Evaluation

When the therapeutic experience is effective, the partners have improved their coping skills, communicate with each other effectively, and feel confident about their problem solving. Often their feelings for each other are warmer, and they are more effective in expressing tenderness and affection. They have found ways to appreciate each other's values, to exchange ideas objectively, and to share joy as well as sadness and disappointment. The couple can recognize the need for and seek assistance in the future before problems become overwhelming.

BRIEF REVIEW

Marital/couples therapy is a treatment modality directed toward improving or resolving couple's problems regardless of their marital status. Theoretical approaches to couples therapy include psychoanalytical, behavioral, systems, and existential. Object relations is the aspect of psychoanalytical theory that can be most effectively applied to couples therapy.

The therapist's specific role and goals are dictated by the therapist's theoretical orientation. All couples therapists assume the role of teacher and educator. The use of co-therapists can have positive and negative aspects. Clients for couples therapy are primarily self-referred; however, they may be referred by the court or persons such as ministers, lawyers, and teachers. In the treatment of couples the nurse selects interventions appropriate to the clients and their life circumstances.

REFERENCES AND SUGGESTED READINGS

1. Adler A: *The neurotic constitution,* New York, 1917, Moffat, Yard, and Co. (Translated by B Blueck and JE Lind.)
2. Alger T: Multiple couple therapy. In Guerin PJ, Jr, editor: *Family therapy,* New York, 1976, Gardner Press.
3. American Association for Marriage and Family Therapy Commission on Accreditation receives Department of Education approval, *AAMFT Newsletter* 12:1, 1981.
4. American Psychiatric Association: *Diagnostic and statistical manual of mental disorders,* Washington, DC, 1987, The Association.
5. American Psychiatric Association: *A psychiatric glossary,* ed 5, Boston, 1980, Little, Brown.
6. Ball JD, Henning LH: Rational suggestions for premarital counseling, *Journal of Marriage and Family Therapy* 7(1):69, 1981.
7. Baruth LG, Huber CH: *An introduction to marital therapy and theory,* Monterey, Calif, 1984, Brook/Cole Publishing Co.
8. Beck RL: The couple's assessment outline; a tracking tool for psychiatric training, *Clinical Supervisor* 1(1):5, 1983.
9. Berglund A, Fugelmeyer K: Sexual problems in women with urinary incontinence: a retrospective study of medical records, *Scandinavian Journal of Caring Science* 5(17):13, 1991.
10. Bjorksten OJW: *New clinical concepts in marital therapy,* Washington, DC, 1985, American Psychiatric Press.
11. Bloom BL and others: A preventive intervention program for the newly separated: final evaluations, *American Journal of Orthopsychiatry* 55(1):9, 1985.

12. Bowen M: Family therapy and family group therapy. In Olson D, editor: *Treating relationships,* Lake Mills, Iowa, 1976, Graphic Publishing Co.

13. Bowen M: *Family therapy in clinical practice,* New York, 1978, Jason Aronson.

14. Broderick B, Schrader SS: History of professional marriage and family therapy. In Gurman AS, Kniskern DP, editors: *Handbook of family therapy,* New York, 1981, Brunner/Mazel.

15. Campbell JC: Women's response to sexual abuse in intimate relationships, *Health of Women International* 10(4):335, 1989.

16. Christensen A, Shenk JL: Communicating conflict and psychological distance in nondistressed, clinic, and divorcing couples, *Journal of Consulting and Clinical Psychology* 59(3):458, 1991.

17. Coche J, Coche E: *Couples group psychotherapy: a clinical practice model,* New York, 1990, Brunner/Mazel.

18. De Santamaria MC: Couples therapy: analysis of a "praxis" with a Freirian perspective, *Family Process* 29(2):119, 1990.

19. Dicks H: *Marital tensions,* New York, 1967, Basic Books.

20. Fish RC, Fish LS: Quid pro quo revisited: the basis of marital therapy, *American Journal of Orthopsychiatry* 56(3):371, 1986.

21. Fogarty TF: Marital crisis. In Guerin PJ, Jr, editor: *Family therapy,* New York, 1976, Gardner Press.

22. Fogarty TF: Fusion, *The Family* 4(2):49, 1977.

23. Frank D: Sexual counseling with a developmentally disabled couple: a case study, *Perspectives in Psychiatric Care* 27(1):30, 1991.

24. Frank DI, Lang AR: Disturbance in sexual role performance of chronic alcoholics: an analysis using Roy's adaptation model, *Issues in Mental Health Nursing* 11(3):243, 1990.

25. Gottman JM, Krokoff LJ: Marital interaction and satisfaction: a longitudinal view, *Journal of Consulting and Clinical Psychology* 57(1):47, 1989.

26. Gray C, Koopman E, Hunt J: The emotional phases of marital separation: an empirical investigation, *American Journal of Orthopsychiatry* 61(1):138, 1991.

27. Greene BL: *A clinical approach to marital problems: diagnosis, prevention, and treatment,* ed 2, Springfield, Ill, 1981, Charles C Thomas.

28. Grover ER, Grover GH: *The contemporary American family,* Chicago, 1947, JB Lippincott.

29. Haley J: *Problem-solving therapy,* San Franscico, 1976, Jossey-Bass.

30. Hoskins CN: Activation—a predictor of need fulfillment in couples, *Research in Nursing and Health* 12(6):365, 1989.

31. Humphrey FG: *Marital therapy,* Englewood Cliffs, NJ, 1983, Prentice Hall.

32. Im W, Wilner RS, Breit M: Jealousy: interventions in couples therapy, *Family Process* 22(2):211, 1983.

33. Jacobs P and others: Sexual needs of the schizophrenic patient, *Perspectives in Psychiatric Care* 27(1):15, 1991.

34. Jacobson NS: Behavior marital therapy. In Gurman AS, Kniskern DP, editors: *Handbook of family therapy,* New York, 1991, Brunner/Mazel.

35. Jacobson NS: Behavioral versus insight oriented marital therapy: labels can be misleading, *Journal of Consulting and Clinical Psychology* 59(1):142, 1991.

36. Jacobson NS, Gurman AS, editors: *Clinical handbook of marital therapy,* New York, 1986, The Guilford Press.

37. Jacobson NS and others: Marital therapy as treatment for depression, *Journal of Consulting and Clinical Psychology* 59(4):547, 1991.

38. Jacobson NS, Weiss RL: Behavioral marriage therapy. III. The contents of Gurman and others. may be hazardous to your health, *Family Process* 17:149, 1978.

39. Jones SL, associate editor: Family, marital, and couples therapy:

40. Jones SL: Don't throw the individual out of couples therapy, *Archives of Psychiatric Nursing* 5(4):191, 1991.

41. Jung C: The association method, *American Journal of Psychology* 21:219, 1910.

42. Kerr M: Bowen theory and therapy. In Sholevar GP, editor: *The handbook of marriage and marital therapy,* Jamaica, NY, 1981, Spectrum Publications.

43. Kim M, McFarland G, McLane AM: *Pocket guide to nursing diagnoses,* ed 4, St Louis, 1991, Mosby–Year Book.

44. L'Abate L, L'Abate BL: The paradoxes of intimacy, *Family Therapy* 6:175, 1979.

45. L'Abate L, McHenry S, editors: *Handbook of marital interventions,* New York, 1983, Grune & Stratton.

46. Lieberman EJ: Couples group psychotherapy. In Simpkinson CH and others, editors: *Synopsis of the first annual Maryland/District of Columbia/Virginia Network Symposium,* Olney, Md, 1978, Family Therapy Practice Network.

47. McGoldrick M, Preto NG: Ethnic intermarriage: implications for therapy, *Family Process* 23(3):347, 1984.

48. Mikesell R: Therapy with couples living together. In Simpkinson CH and others, editors: *Synopsis of the first annual Maryland/District of Columbia/Virginia Network Symposium,* Olney, Md., 1978, Family Therapy Practice Network.

49. Morofka V: Marital therapy from a systems approach, *Perspectives in Psychiatric Care* 22(4):145, 1984.

50. Papp P: Staging reciprocal metaphors in a couples group, *Family Process* 21(4):453, 1982.

51. Price-Bonham S, Murphy DC: Dual career marriages: implications for the clinician, *Journal of Marriage and Family Therapy* 6(2):181, 1980.

52. Sager CJ: *Marriage contracts and couple therapy: hidden forces in intimate relationships,* New York, 1976, Brunner/Mazel.

53. Schaefer MT, Olson DH: Assessing intimacy: the PAIR inventory, *Journal of Marriage and Family Therapy* 7(1):47, 1981.

54. Smith DA and others: Longitudinal prediction of marital discord from premarital expression of affect, *Journal of Consulting and Clinical Psychology* 58(6):790, 1990.

55. Smolowe J and others: Can't we talk this over? Therapists encourage troubled couples to stay together, *Time* 137(1):77, 1991.

56. Snyder DK and others: Long-term effectiveness of behavioral versus insight-oriented marital therapy: a 4-year follow-up study, *Journal of Consulting and Clinical Psychology* 59(1):138, 1991.

57. Sonne JC, Swirsky D: Self-object considerations in marriage and marital therapy. In Sholevar GP, editor: *The handbook of marriage and marital therapy,* Jamaica, NY, 1981, Spectrum Publications.

58. Spark GM: Marriage is a family affair: an intergenerational approach to marital therapy. In Sholevar GP, editor: *The handbook of marriage and marital therapy,* Jamaica, NY, 1981, Spectrum Publications.

59. Stanton MD: Marital therapy from a structural/strategic viewpoint. In Sholevar GP, editor: *The handbook of marriage and marital therapy,* Jamaica, NY, 1981, Spectrum Publications.

60. Steinglass P, Tislenko L, Reiss D: Stability/instability in the alcoholic marriage: the interrelationships between course of alcoholism, family process, and marital outcome, *Family Process* 24(3):365, 1985.

61. Watson WL, Bell JM: Who are we? Low self-esteem and marital identity, *Journal of Psychosocial Nursing and Mental Health Services* 28(4):15, 1990.

62. Vogel W, Lazare A: The unforgivable humiliation: a dilemma in couples' treatment, *Contemporary Family Therapy An International Journal* 12(2):139, 1990.

a comparison, *Archives of Psychiatric Nursing* 4(3):145, 1990.

63. Weinstein RK: Bowen's family systems theory as exemplified in Bergman's "Scenes from Marriage," *Perspectives in Psychiatric Care* 19:157, 1981.

64. Wells RA, Giannetti VJ: Individual marital therapy: a critical reappraisal, *Family Process* 25(1):43, 1986.

65. Whitaker CA: *Making marriage work,* Chicago, 1970, Instructional Dynamics (Ten cassette audiotapes).

66. Whitaker CA, Greenberg A, Greenberg MI: Existential marital therapy: a synthesis, a subsystem of existential family therapy. In Sholevar GP, editor: *A handbook of marriage and marital therapy,* Jamaica, NY, 1981, Spectrum Publications.

67. Willi J: The concept of collusion: a combined systemic-psychodynamic approach to marital therapy, *Family Process* 23(2):177, 1984.

68. Williams AM, Miller WR: Evaluation and research on marital therapy. In Sholevar GP, editor: *The handbook of marriage and marital therapy,* Jamaica, NY, 1981, Spectrum Publications.

69. Woody EZ, Costanzo PR: Does marital agony precede marital ecstasy? A comment on Gottman and Krokoff's "Marital interaction and satisfaction: A longitudinal view," *Journal of Consulting and Clinical Psychology* 58(4):499, 1990.

ANNOTATED BIBLIOGRAPHY

Coche J, Coche E: *Couples group psychotherapy: a clinical practice model,* New York, 1990, Brunner/Mazel.

The text is a model of a closed ended group of four couples with an 11-month contract. The principles and concepts for structuring the model are outlined with emphasis on the importance of assessment before treatment. The combination of style, clinical sensitivity, scientific rigor, and respect for structure shows how integration of these elements fosters effective treatment. Clinical vignettes present strategies and exercises that when used appropriately can be very effective.

Polonsky D, Nadelson C: An integrative approach to couples therapy. In Bjorksten O, editor: *New clinical concepts in marital therapy,* Washington, DC, 1985, American Psychiatric Press.

The author stresses the importances of understanding unconscious collusions and the reenactments of early object relationships. Flexible therapeutic approaches are vital in helping the couple recreate aspects of their relationships with the family of origin. An attempt has been made to provide a link between a theoretical understanding of marital dynamics and a variety of technical approaches.

Sager CJ: Couples therapy and marriage contracts. In Gurman AS, Kniskern DP, editors: *Handbook of family therapy,* New York, 1981, Brunner/Mazel.

The author asserts that individual intrapsychic factors determine the system and in turn are affected by the interaction in the couple's system. The therapist should consider determinants of interactions. The text includes a typology of marriages with seven profiles and uses an eclectic therapeutic approach. Individual contracts are verbalized and conscious. The parameters may be based on the expectations of marriage, on intrapsychic and biological needs, or on external foci.

CHAPTER
31
Therapy for Clients with Eating Disorders

Rauda Salkauskas Gelazis
Alice R Kempe

After studying this chapter, the student will be able to:

- Define obesity, anorexia nervosa, and bulimia nervosa
- Discuss historical perspectives of eating disorders
- Discuss the psychopathology of obesity, anorexia nervosa, and bulimia nervosa as described in the DSM-III-R

- Describe theoretical bases for eating disorders
- Apply the nursing process to clients with eating disorders
- Discuss special issues related to eating
- Identify current research findings on eating disorders

Nutrition is crucial to growth and development throughout the life cycle. Food and fulfillment of needs are linked in infancy. As a person matures, eating behaviors take on new meanings and significance. Meanings that stem from family and culture influence the individual's self-concept. Problems in family relationships and interaction patterns and in one's self-concept can result in eating disorders.

Eating disorders are gross disturbances in eating behaviors. Three types of disorders are discussed in this chapter: obesity, anorexia nervosa, and bulimia nervosa. Also included are brief discussions of fasting, low-calorie diets, drug and hormone use, and the effects of vitamin deficiencies on mental health.

OBESITY

Obesity, a major health problem in the United States, is defined as weight 15% to 20% more than one's ideal body weight, as determined by the Metropolitan Life Insurance Standards and as an excessive proportion of fat or adipose tissue in the body mass. About 60 million Americans (one in five) are obese. Many emotional factors are associated with obesity, but studies fail to differentiate clearly between those related to the development of obesity and those caused by being obese.[53]

DSM-III-R Diagnoses

Generally, obesity is not associated with any distinct emotional or behavioral syndrome. However, when evidence suggests that emotional factors are important in the cause or course of obesity, it is discussed as a psychological factor affecting physical condition (see Chapter 19).

Theoretical Approaches
Biological

Obesity often begins early in life. Generally, 10% to 15% of an infant's body is adipose tissue. In the first year of life,

> ► **DIAGNOSES Related to Eating Disorders**

MEDICAL DIAGNOSES	**NURSING DIAGNOSES**
Anorexia nervosa	**NANDA**
Bulimia nervosa	Altered nutrition:
Eating disorders not otherwise noted	more than body requirement
	Altered nutrition:
	less than body requirement
	PMH
	Altered nutrition processes:
	more than body requirement
	less than body requirement
	Altered eating processes:
	anorexia

HISTORICAL OVERVIEW

DATES	EVENTS
1800s	Being overweight is considered healthier than being thin, which is associated with malnutrition. Excess weight is valued and considered beautiful.
1850	Florence Nightingale documents the importance of a sound diet for health in *Notes on Nursing*, with recommendations for foods and fluids to be included in one's daily diet.
1873	Anorexia nervosa is first described in the literature by two physicians, Sir William Gull and Dr. E. Laseque.
1890s	Freud observes that nutrition affects neuroses by influencing energy levels and promoting healthier brain cell functioning.
1900s	Worldwide interest in health and nutrition grows in the early twentieth century. Chemists and physiologists in Europe and the United States identify the need for proteins, minerals, vitamins, hormones, enzymes, and fatty acids to ensure digestion and metabolism for maximal health.
1930s	The League of Nations establishes standards for adequate nutrition.
1950s	The National Nutritional Conference sets up committees in every state to promote better nutrition. Recommended dietary allowances for various age and sex categories are established.
1960s	Studies to look at the effects of food intake on behavior and emotions show that schizophrenia and depression are affected by chemical imbalances and nutritional deficits.
1980s	Americans value thinness, especially for women. Billions of dollars are spent on diets and the pursuit of thinness. However, treatment strategies have had only limited success.
1990s	American interest in nutrition and exercise continues. To meet desire for better information about nutritional content of foods, many food companies supply nutritional information on packaging.
Future	Professional nurses will be challenged to educate the public about nutrition and to treat individuals with eating disorders to improve quality of life and longevity.

a definite increase occurs in adipose cell size but not cell number. In puberty and late adolescence the number of adult adipose cells stabilizes. Evidence suggests that adipose tissue usually does not decrease during the life cycle.

Cellular hypertrophy results from increased food intake and decreased energy expenditure. This suggests that obesity is not a disease but a symptom of an imbalance between caloric ingestion and energy use. Obese individuals tend to be less active than nonobese persons. One study concluded that heredity is involved in obesity but that environmental factors may have a greater influence. Genetic studies indicate that 60% of obese subjects have one or both obese parent(s). Studies of environmental factors affecting obesity suggest that infant's eating habits are a result of caregivers' feeding behaviors. If the caregiver ignores the children's cues, feeds them when the caregiver thinks they are hungry, and insists that they eat everything on the plate, children learn to ignore physical cues of hunger as a basis for eating or not eating.

Other biological theories suggest that endocrine disease, altered metabolism, and thyroid dysfunction may contribute to obesity.

Psychoanalytical

Psychoanalytical theorists view obesity as an expression of some intrapsychic conflict that occurred during the oral stage of psychosexual development. Obesity is seen as regression to the infant oral stage to fulfill unmet needs. Overeating is explained as a way to accomplish the following:

1. Decrease anxiety, insecurity, worry, frustration, or monotony
2. Express hostility or rebellion against authority or assert independence
3. Express anger at oneself
4. Punish oneself
5. Avoid competition in life
6. Compensate for lack of love, affection, and friends
7. Justify interpersonal or career failures
8. Achieve greatness by becoming bigger and stronger than others
9. Modify depression
10. Destroy oneself

Cognitive

Ellis and Harper[17] stated that irrational thinking may contribute to continued obesity. Obese persons may describe themselves as fat and unable to do anything about it. Because they may have unsuccessfully tried to lose weight in the past, they may fear another failure. The irrational assumption that nothing can be done about obesity prevents people from altering their eating behaviors.

Sociocultural

Eating is a socializing experience. Through the family the child learns the social customs, values, and mores of eating behaviors. Eating experiences in adulthood can symbolize childhood. Each eating experience expresses a relationship of giving and receiving. For example, the mother makes a meal for the family, who in turn receives the food. Rejection of the food may be seen as rejection of the mother. Mealtimes can become arenas where the give and take of relationships have lifelong effects.

In studying family influence on obesity, Orbach[45] relates obesity to the parent-child relationship. Ambivalence and conflicts are played out in feeding and eating behavior. For example, a child in a hostile environment of marital conflict who is used as a scapegoat for one or both parents may become obese.

Culture also strongly influences the development of feelings, attitudes, and preferences about food and eating built into the personality. Every culture has food preferences, habits, taboos, and variations in methods of eating. Some cultures focus on food, whereas others deemphasize it. The United States encompasses many cultural food value systems and many foods that represent or symbolize a person's ethnic roots. Leininger,[37] founder of transcultural nursing, emphasizes the importance of discovering and including cultural values and patterns of clients when giving professional nursing care. Knowing the eating patterns in different cultural groups is an important aspect of giving culturally congruent professional nursing care. Therefore it is important that a transcultural holistic perspective about food uses, beliefs, and practices be included in professional nursing care given to clients of diverse cultures.

Investigations of social influences on eating patterns indicate differences between obese persons and persons of normal weight. Both groups are influenced by the eating habits of the people with whom they eat. Some families spend considerable time conversing while eating, prolonging the meal and discussing events of the day. Others eat quickly with little or no interaction.

Learning

Learning theory focuses on overeating as learned behavior resulting from environmental cues and states of emotional arousal. An obese individual learns to respond to various emotions such as anger, loneliness, boredom, or stress by eating. Parents' use of food to deal with these emotions teaches the child that eating is a way of receiving attention or reward and that feelings do not have to be dealt with directly and appropriately. Food becomes associated with feelings; later those feelings elicit eating. Table 31-1 summarizes the theories of obesity.

Nursing Process
Assessment

Physical dimension The physical dimension encompasses all the effects and ramifications of obesity on the physiological functioning of the body, particularly the cardiovascular and respiratory systems. Symptoms include elevated blood pressure, shortness of breath, heart palpitations on exertion, and feeling warm even on cold days or with minimal activity. The nurse assesses the client's

▼ **TABLE 31-1** **Summary of Theories of Obesity**

Theory	Dynamic
Biological	An imbalance exists between calorie ingestion and energy use. There is a genetic tendency toward obesity. Endocrine disease, altered metabolism, or thyroid deficiency may cause obesity.
Psychoanalytical	Obesity is an expression or an intrapsychic conflict that occurred during the oral stage of psychosexual development.
Cognitive	Irrational assumptions about food, weight, and body contribute to continued obesity.
Sociocultural	Family and cultural values, customs, and mores strongly influence the development of feelings, attitudes, and preferences about food and eating behaviors.
Learning	Overeating is a learned behavior related to environmental cues and emotional states.

activity level, physical limitations, and exercise program and compares the client's weight to his ideal weight according to the Metropolitan Life Insurance standards (Tables 31-2 and 31-3).

A thorough nutritional assessment is needed. Obtaining a dietary intake for several days to identify eating patterns is helpful. Because clients may skip meals or eat several meals a day with numerous snacks, they may have trouble accurately describing usual dietary intake and daily food requirements. Obese clients often underestimate the amount of food they eat and the size of the portions. A person of normal weight eats when hungry; an obese client eats if food is available.

It is important to obtain information about the client's perception of body image and sexuality. The nurse questions views of physical self and thoughts and feelings about his body (its functioning and size). Obese clients typically do not like their bodies. They avoid looking in mirrors and may try to mask their size by wearing loose clothing. Figure 31-1 depicts an obese client.

The nurse also assesses the clients medications that may influence weight. Birth control pills and antipsychotics such as chlorpromazine (Thorazine) cause weight gain.

Emotional dimension Feelings of anxiety, anger, guilt, boredom, hopelessness, loneliness, frustration, unattractiveness, and depression induce overeating. Feelings are often difficult for overweight people. For example, when an overweight individual feels strong anger, he tends to turn to food because he is unable to express the feeling of anger toward the appropriate person. Over time the individual develops the pattern of turning to food rather than facing his true feelings and dealing appropriately with them. Many obese clients feel hopeless about changing their weight. Guilt frequently follows a deviation from a weight

▼ **TABLE 31-2** Desirable Weights for Men 25 Years of Age and Over (in indoor clothing)

Height				
Feet	Inches	Small Frame	Medium Frame	Large Frame
5	2	128-134	131-141	138-150
5	3	130-136	133-143	140-153
5	4	132-138	135-145	142-156
5	5	134-140	137-148	144-160
5	6	136-142	139-151	146-164
5	7	138-145	142-154	149-168
5	8	140-148	145-157	152-172
5	9	142-151	148-160	155-176
5	10	144-154	151-163	158-180
5	11	146-157	154-166	161-184
6	0	149-160	157-170	164-188
6	1	152-164	160-174	168-192
6	2	155-168	164-178	172-197
6	3	158-172	167-182	176-202
6	4	162-176	171-187	181-207

Courtesy Metropolitan Life Insurance Co, New York, Revised 1983.

▼ **TABLE 31-3** Desirable Weights for Women 25 Years of Age and Over (in indoor clothing)

Height				
Feet	Inches	Small Frame	Medium Frame	Large Frame
4	10	102-111	109-121	118-131
4	11	103-113	111-123	120-134
5	0	104-115	113-126	122-137
5	1	106-118	115-129	125-140
5	2	108-121	118-132	128-143
5	3	111-124	121-135	131-147
5	4	114-127	124-138	134-151
5	5	117-130	127-141	137-155
5	6	120-133	130-144	140-159
5	7	123-126	133-147	143-163
5	8	126-139	136-150	146-167
5	9	129-142	139-153	149-170
5	10	132-145	142-156	152-173
5	11	135-148	145-159	155-176
6	0	135-151	148-162	158-179

Courtesy Metropolitan Life Insurance Co, New York, Revised 1983.

loss diet. Depression often occurs in obese clients. See Chapter 14 for further information on assessment of depression.

Intellectual dimension The nurse determines whether the client's thoughts about being obese are rational. Statements such as, "I can't control my eating," demonstrate irrational thinking. The client's self-control and motivation for changing eating habits are assessed. It is important to assess the client's use of defense mechanisms. Some of the defense mechanisms include denial, overcompensation, substitution, and rationalization. An example of the use of rationalization as a defense mechanism can be seen in the client who excuses overeating with statements such as, "It's Christmas; everyone eats too much." Knowledge of nutri-

tion and healthy eating behaviors are assessed; many obese clients do not have an adequate knowledge of basic nutrition.

Social dimension Cultural background and ethnicity strongly influence dietary intake and the value placed on food. This influence is so strong that changes are slow and difficult to maintain over time. Patterns of eating are developed early in life based on family traditions and beliefs. Some nurse theorists such as Leininger base nursing care on a thorough knowledge of a clients' culture. It is important, for example, for the nurse to determine the cultural background of the client, the meaning of food in that culture, the client's food preferences and habits, and his food taboos (see the research highlight on the next page).

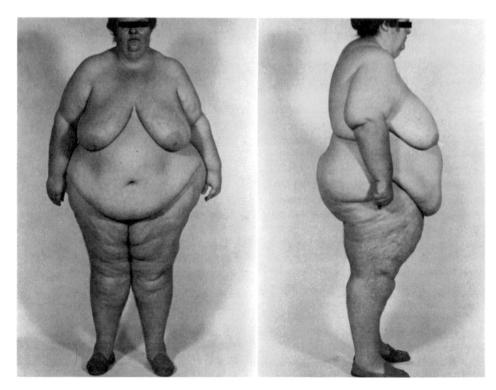

FIGURE 31-1 Obese client.

RESEARCH HIGHLIGHT

Women Who Successfully Manage Their Weight
• JD Allen

PURPOSE

The purpose of this study was to explore the characteristics of women who successfully manage their weight. The research questions were as follows: What methods for weight management are used by women who successfully manage their weight? What factors influence the selection of particular methods?

SAMPLE

The sample consisted of 21 white middle and working class women between the ages of 30 and 55 years of age who were given in-depth interviews.

METHODOLOGY

A naturalistic study design involving ethnographical interviewing methods was used. Data were collected over 7 months through the use of semistructured interviews lasting a mean of 4 hours. Data were analyzed by means of content analysis of each transcript.

Based on data from *Western Journal of Nursing Research* 11(6):657, 1989.

FINDINGS

Informants noted two methods for managing their weight: "dieting" or "changing one's whole life." Women who were most successful at weight loss and maintenance were motivated by self-focused reasons and viewed weight loss as part of a process in changing their life-styles in various ways, such as increasing exercise. Those unsuccessful at weight loss were interested in losing weight for others, "dieted," and tended to regain weight.

IMPLICATIONS

The results of the study imply that nurses in clinical practice may recommend use of multiple methods for weight loss. Eliciting reasons for wanting to lose weight may allow the nurse to predict long-term success.

The nurse also considers the client's support system. If family relationships are disturbed, the client may eat to compensate. Studies show that clients who have a partner's cooperation lose significantly more weight than those with an uncooperative partner.[10,23] A partner who is critical and negative toward the client's eating behavior may even sabotage a weight loss program. Fearing that the client's loss of weight may create a loss of bargaining power in arguments or promote infidelity, the partner may offer or talk about food. After a successful weight loss program, clients may have more control and independence in relationships.

For some persons food is more important than relationships. Obese clients see food as an important part of social activities. Sometimes a client's report of a social event focuses on what food was served rather than time spent relating to others.

Because the obese client's self-esteem is generally lowered, the nurse should assess this variable. Clients are self-conscious and may lack confidence in themselves and their achievements.

Spiritual dimension The nurse assesses the meaning and significance of food in the client's life. People eat for many reasons: to socialize, to meet basic needs, to cope with stress and disturbed relationships, to adhere to religious and cultural values, to demonstrate economic status and personal achievement, and to reward oneself. Obesity is also a self-destructive behavior; continuous overeating may be hastening the client's own death, although the client is generally unaware of this risk.

Clients may devalue themselves, believing that they are weak willed for being obese. Such a belief system increases

....

▼
ALTERED NUTRITION: MORE THAN BODY REQUIREMENTS

....

DEFINITION
The individual experiences an intake of nutrients that exceed metabolic needs.

DEFINING CHARACTERISTICS
- **Physical dimension**
  Overweight (10% over ideal weight for height and frame)
  Obese (20% over ideal weight for height and frame)
  Triceps skin fold greater than 15 mm in men and 25 mm in women
  Pairing food with other activities
  Concentrating food intake at end of day
  Sedentary activity patterns

- **Emotional dimension**
  Eating in response to internal cues other than hunger (e.g., anxiety)

- **Social dimension**
  Eating in response to external cues (e.g., time of day, social situation)

....

Modified from Kim MJ, McFarland GK, McLane AM, editors: *Pocket guide to nursing diagnoses*, ed 5, St Louis, 1993, Mosby—Year Book.

guilt and anxiety and leads to further overeating and hopelessness. The nurse determines the client's beliefs about personal worth and ability to change eating habits.

Analysis

Nursing Diagnosis Altered nutrition: more than body requirements is a NANDA diagnosis that applies to an obese person. The defining characteristics of this diagnosis are listed in the accompanying box.

The following case example illustrates the characteristics of this nursing diagnosis.

▼ Case Example

Jane, a 58-year-old housewife of Italian heritage, has been overweight since age 40. Her husband is a successful business man of normal weight. He is the decision maker for the family. Jane reports that her three children are all independent. In the last few years she has noticed that she is less active and lacks interest in exercise or new experiences. She states that she feels "bored and useless" much of the time. Her husband has begun to remind her frequently of her 25-pound weight gain this past year. She has attempted to lose weight by various fad diets but becomes easily frustrated and does not stay with them for more than a few days. Most recently she has begun to use diet pills to suppress her appetite. At her last physical examination her blood pressure was elevated. She was instructed to stop her diet pills, and her physician advised her to lose weight.

Planning

Table 31-4 presents a nursing care plan with examples of long- and short-term goals, outcome criteria interventions, and rationales related to obesity, which are examples of the planning stage in the nursing process.

Implementation

Physical dimension The nurse helps the client plan and incorporate a realistic weight loss program to reach ideal weight based on height and body frame. The client can monitor weight and food intake by keeping a diary of all foods eaten daily to describe more accurately the amount, type, and portions of food eaten and when they are eaten. The client can modify rate and amount of food eaten by putting utensils down between bites, talking between bites to increase the social pleasure of eating, chewing food more thoroughly, and designating only one place for eating.

Together the nurse and client establish an exercise program compatible with the client's interests. The information in the box on p. 622 can be used to help clients change their activity and exercise routines. For example, the client can see that he will need to walk at a leisurely pace for 60 minutes in order to use up 300 calories.

Emotional dimension The nurse helps the client identify feelings and determine how they relate to eating behaviors, particularly those that trigger overeating. Facilitating the expression of anger, guilt, anxiety, depression, and hopelessness is an initial step in becoming aware of the relationship between feelings and eating. Relaxation, exercise, sports, art (including writing and music), and assertive behaviors are appropriate ways to express feelings. Developing new strategies for dealing with feelings may help eliminate the need to overeat.

▼ **TABLE 31-4   NURSING CARE PLAN Related to Obesity**

GOALS	OUTCOME CRITERIA	INTERVENTIONS	RATIONALES
NURSING DIAGNOSIS: Altered nutrition: more than body requirements related to sedentary life-style			
LONG TERM			
To limit daily food intake to an amount that is nutritionally balanced and desirable for body build and energy expenditure	Stays within planned daily food intake	Assist client to develop a plan for recording daily intake that includes time and place for eating and the amount eaten	Provides baseline data about eating habits Increases client's awareness of food intake
	Identifies cues associated with food intake	Explore with client thoughts and feelings associated with eating	Helps client see the relationship between eating and thoughts and feelings Client recognizes how food may be used to cope with stress
	Limits daily food intake to 1000 to 1500 calories including each of the basic four groups	Assist to develop a diet from the food pyramid that does not exceed 1500 calories	Provides support and information about a nutritionally balanced diet
SHORT TERM			
To participate in planned energy expending activities at least 3 times per week	Exercises 30 minutes 3 days per week	Assist to develop a realistic exercise plan Encourage to implement plan and give positive feedback when client exercises	Client is more likely to adhere to a realistic plan With encouragement may follow through with plan Feedback reinforces desired behavior
	Participates in enjoyable active hobbies	Explore with client hobbies he enjoys at least three times a week	May not be aware of activities other than food that are enjoyable
	Rewards self for adherence to activities program	Teach appropriate nonfood rewards	To learn alternative means to experience satisfaction

Intellectual dimension Obese clients hold many irrational beliefs. The nurse may first confront clients with the irrational thought, then work out a more rational response with them. For example, if a client thinks, "I can control my eating," he tends to act on this belief and will try to follow the eating program. Irrational beliefs such as, "I've always been overweight," can be replaced by rational thoughts such as, "I can change my eating behaviors." Breaking down behavior patterns into small workable steps is useful in the change process. For example, the nurse can have the client focus on one meal at a time and limit his intake for that meal rather than think of the entire day. Specific ways of limiting intake can be outlined with each client. Some clients find it helpful to look at themselves in a full length mirror each time they are tempted to eat. Others may find it useful to call a friend before they indulge in snacking behaviors or overeating. By helping the client realize he can control his own behavior in various ways throughout each day, he may be able to control his eating behaviors. The client then begins to feel more confident that he has some control in his life.

Cognitive restructuring is essential for obese clients. As they become aware of the negative ways they view themselves, clients begin to develop more positive thinking and move toward positive self-regard. The nurse facilitates change in thoughts and feelings from negative to positive by the following:

1. Explaining the overall change desired
2. Identifying client's typical thoughts about being fat
3. Introducing new, rational thoughts
4. Helping the client practice positive thinking and self-talk
5. Encouraging rational thinking in daily life and following up with discussions of its effectiveness.

Social dimension Mobilizing social support for the obese client is an important aspect of care. A partner can assist by pointing out the positive aspects of change. A social network of significant others reinforces support

ENERGY EXPENDITURE FOR SELECTED ACTIVITIES

	Calories/Minute		Calories/Minute
Walking		**Mowing**	
3 mph (leisurely)	5	Riding	3
4 mph	7	Pushing power mower	5
5 mph	8	Pushing hand mower	8
Downstairs	7		
Upstairs	14	**Paddleball**	10
Uphill (3.5 mph)	11	**Painting**	5
Downhill (2.5 mph)	4	**Ping-pong**	6
Hiking with 40 lb pack	7	**Playing musical instruments**	4
		Raking leaves	6
Badminton (singles)	6	**Rope skipping**	
Baseball or softball	5	Leisurely	5
Basketball	6	Vigorously	13
Boating		**Running**	
Rowing	8	5 mph (jogging)	10
Sailing	5	7 mph (moderate)	15
Bowling	4	10 mph (very fast)	21
Calisthenics		Upstairs	17
Light	6	**Sawing hardwood**	20
Heavy	10	**Shoveling snow**	9
Cycling		**Shuffleboard**	4
5 mph	4	**Skating (ice or roller)**	
10 mph	7	Leisurely	7
13 mph	11	Rapidly	12
Croquet	4	**Skiing**	
Dancing		Snow downhill	8
Slow foxtrot	6	Cross country	
Fast step	9	4 mph	10
Square dancing	9	8 mph	17
Modern	5	Water	8
Fishing (From pier or boat)	4	**Snowshoeing**	10
Football (while active)	11	**Soccer**	13
Gardening	6	**Squash (Competitive)**	11
Handball (competitive)	6	**Swimming (Crawl)**	9
Horseback riding		**Tennis**	
Slow	4	Doubles	6
Trot	6	Singles	8
Hunting	8	**Volleyball**	7
Karate or Judo	12		
Mountain climbing	10		

during the weight loss process. It also discourages eating when lonely or bored, as others can be called on to fill the void. Support groups, such as Weight Watchers, Overeaters Anonymous, and Take Off Pounds Sensibly (TOPS), are useful for weight loss and maintenance. They decrease feelings of helplessness and hopelessness; increase feelings of confidence, control, power, esteem, and sexual attractiveness; and offer rewards for positive change. To maintain ideal weight, the client uses a variety of environmental supports, such as co-workers, who can be a powerful adjunct to treatment.

Praising any amount of weight loss and ignoring slight deviations from the prescribed diet are helpful. Nagging and criticism by significant others is detrimental. The nurse assists the client to develop a system that provides rewards for a successful week, such as a special movie or weekend activity. The nurse promotes the client's participating in pleasurable activities other than those involved in eating. When family relationships are disturbed, the client may be referred to family or couples therapy (see Chapters 29 and 30).

The nurse assists clients to accept responsibility for eating behaviors. Only clients can change their eating habits. A client cannot change others' behaviors toward his weight problem, and others may not be helpful or tolerate the client's continued emphasis on dieting.

The nurse is careful to promote activities in accordance with the client's family, culture, and ethnic traditions. New behaviors for special holidays can be established such as focusing on socialization rather than food, cutting down on daily calorie intake before the holiday, eating small portions of low-calorie foods, and limiting alcohol intake.

Spiritual dimension The nurse helps clients to value themselves as unique and special persons of worth, even though they are obese. Focusing on positive attributes, skills, and personal strengths counteracts the client's devaluing and negative belief system. Promoting better communication through assertiveness skills helps the client establish meaningful relationships with others and experience the give and take of loving, caring relationships.

The nurse offers hope to counteract depression and hopelessness by accepting lack of progress in weight reduction and by continuing work with the client who refuses treatment. She helps the client describe the meaning and significance of food and eating in his life and to incorporate this information into a life-style that balances gratification from eating with gratification from other sources.

Evaluation

Nursing intervention is successful when the client eats a balanced diet taken from the food pyramid; maintains optimal physical functioning; exercises adequately; and has increased self-esteem, feelings of control, and awareness of feelings that trigger eating.

ANOREXIA NERVOSA AND BULIMIA NERVOSA
DSM-III-R Diagnoses

Anorexia nervosa and bulimia nervosa are two eating disturbances described in the DSM-III-R. These disorders typically begin during adolescence or early adulthood. Clients with anorexia nervosa are predominantly female (95%). As many as 1 in 250 girls between 12 and 18 years of age develop the disorder. The most obvious symptom is extreme weight loss, up to as much as 15% of the client's body weight. Amenorrhea may precede or accompany the weight loss. Hypothermia, bradycardia, hypotension, edema, lanugo (neonatal-like hair), and various metabolic changes may accompany extreme weight loss. The person has an exaggerated interest in food, coupled with refusal to eat, and denies hunger because of intense fear of becoming obese. Individuals may prepare elaborate meals for others but limit themselves to a small amount of low-calorie food. They may hoard, conceal, or throw away food.

A distorted body image is a characteristic feature of anorexia nervosa. (See the research highlight on p. 628.) The disturbance in body image is manifested by the person's perception of body weight, size, and shape. The person says she is fat when in reality she is underweight or even emaciated. There is a preoccupation with one's body size and dissatisfaction with some aspect of one's physical appearance. The case example describes a client with anorexia nervosa.

▼ Case Example

Sharon, a 17-year-old high school senior, has become increasingly secretive about her eating for the past 2 months. Her parents are concerned about her recent weight loss of 20 lb and her preoccupation with thinness and diets. After school, rather than do her homework, she focuses on food. She frequently cooks the family dinners but eats only salad, carrot sticks, and celery. Sharon reads about nutrition and preparation of foods. She cooks many desserts and high-calorie foods but does not eat them.

Sharon is an excellent student but believes she has not done well enough. She is interested in sports and exercises at least 2 hours a day. It is not unusual to find her jogging early in the morning and again in the evening.

At the beginning of the school year, during the school annual physical examination, the physician was unable to obtain Sharon's blood for routine laboratory work. Extreme emaciation and anemia were noted, and her parents were advised to seek further medical help for Sharon. Her mother wanted to handle the problem on her own by insisting that Sharon begin to eat more, which resulted in continual struggles for control. When the nurse saw Sharon, Sharon weighed only 80 lb (she is 5'6" tall), and had fainted during gym class. She was hospitalized on the recommendation of the school nurse. At the hospital Sharon refused to eat and did not communicate with anyone.

Some people have eating binges followed by vomiting (purging). Binge eating, rapid consumption of a large amount of food in a discrete period of time, usually less than 2 hours, is characteristic of bulimia nervosa. The disorder usually occurs in females and begins during adolescence. Bulimia nervosa is six times more common than anorexia nervosa.

The bulimic person is unaware that the eating pattern is abnormal and fears not being able to stop eating voluntarily. She may consume two to three times the amount of an average meal. The intake of a large amount of food is characteristically followed by self-induced vomiting. The vomiting and other behaviors, such as the use of laxatives or diuretics, strict dieting or fasting, or vigorous exercises, are used to prevent weight gain. Generally, the person's weight is within normal range. Some people may be slightly underweight, and others may be overweight. The alternating binges and fasts lead to frequent fluctuations in weight greater than 10 lb.

The individual may plan the binges and gobble down food quite rapidly and as inconspicuously and secretly as possible. Once the person begins eating, she has difficulty controlling the amount she consumes. The binge is usually terminated by abdominal pain, sleep, social interruption, or self-induced vomiting. Electrolyte imbalance and dehydration and eventually death are complications of binge eating and vomiting.

After a period of binging and purging the client may become "hooked" on its tranquilizing effects. Many learn to vomit by reflex action. The bulimic client usually falls into a cycle of depression, guilt, self-criticism, and devastating isolation as seen in the following case example.

▼ Case Example

Jean, a 19-year-old college freshman, came to the hospital for abdominal pain after taking 30 Dulcolax tablets. Jean gave a history of having tried many diets for weight loss without success. She began to respond to stress by compulsive binge-purge behaviors. She talked readily about herself and described the development of her eating disorder in great detail. She was fixated on achieving thinness at any cost and became more and more frustrated, guilty, and depressed with each binge. She used induced vomiting when she was alone but turned to laxative use to enhance weight loss. Many times this behavior made her very weak; it was almost impossible for her to function at school, despite past scholastic success. The last binge episode convinced her to increase her laxative use, which resulted in a fluid-electrolyte imbalance requiring hospitalization. Her physical condition was quickly stabilized, but Jean continued to show signs of depression and guilt about the cost of the hospitalization and exposure of her eating disorder to her family.

Theoretical Approaches

The theoretical approaches for anorexia nervosa and bulimia nervosa are presented together because of the similarity of their dynamics.

Biological

The disease process of anorexia nervosa usually begins with the client deciding to lose weight. As she loses weight, she feels great satisfaction from the suppression of hunger. She fears regaining the weight and becomes preoccupied with remaining thin, although she looks emaciated (Figure 31-2). The need for exercise becomes exaggerated, at times obsessional. Physical activity, frequently to the point of collapse, is used to distract attention from hunger. Instead of getting satisfaction from the suppression of hunger, the bulimic client satisfies her hunger by binging, followed by self-induced vomiting.

Psychoanalytical

Theorists with a psychoanalytical orientation view eating disorders as regression to prepuberty. Generally, persons who develop eating disorders are experiencing diffi-

culties in coping with life, their feelings, or the transition into adolescence. They feel anxious and out of control. There seems to be a resistance to growing up and maturing. Anorexia nervosa and bulimia nervosa most often appear at puberty and are accompanied by amenorrhea, which leads theorists to believe that the disorder is related to sexual problems or to denial of sexuality.

Cognitive

Cognitive theorists see disturbances in perception as contributing to anorexia nervosa and bulimia nervosa. The client with a distorted body image may perceive herself as fat. She may draw her body as large but depict others in correct proportion. The client may have irrational beliefs and thoughts; she may be obsessed with the idea that she needs to exercise after eating or drinking even small amounts. She may spend all day thinking about and preparing food while being preoccupied with thinness.

Sociocultural

Bruch[6] believes the central factor in anorexia is the overly rigid parental expectations for the anorectic child. She described families who are educated and happy but who implicitly or explicitly burden their children with living up to their ideal. These children are usually described as exceptionally "good" but seem to lack the ability to set their own goals. Without clear goals of their own, they become overly compliant. Bruch[6] suggests that these children may have skipped the period of resistance in early childhood or adolescent development. Anorectic clients seem to remain convinced of their parents' perfection and feel an obligation to obey them. Thus anorexia nervosa is

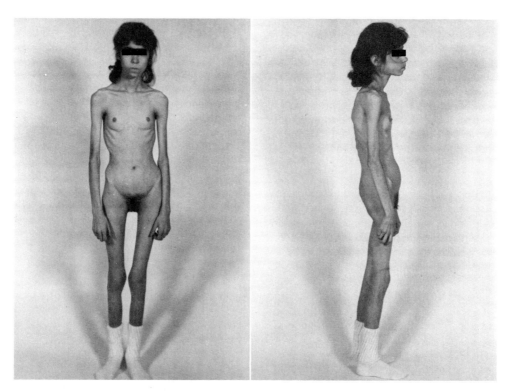

FIGURE 31-2 Girl with anorexia nervosa.

▼ **TABLE 31-5** **Summary of Theories of Anorexia Nervosa and Bulimia Nervosa**

Theory	Dynamics
Biological	The disease process begins with attempts to lose weight and an intense fear of gaining weight. Research is being conducted about the role of hypothalamus dysfunction and neuroendocrine imbalance as a cause of these disorders.[27]
Psychoanalytical	Eating disorders result from difficulties in coping with life, feelings, or the transition to adulthood with regression to the prepubertal stage.
Cognitive	Irrational thoughts and beliefs and distorted body image contribute to eating disorders.
Sociocultural	Family conflicts involving high parental expectations, controlling parents, and a resistant, dependent daughter contribute to eating disorders. Cultural overemphasis and value on thinness contribute to eating disorders.

an internal conflict between feeling enslaved and exploited and wanting to lead an independent life.

Parental concern is often expressed in overprotection and hypervigilance. The anorectic client is enmeshed in a family system with overly close family relationships. Parents and others find it more and more difficult to empathize with the anorectic person, who seems to focus only on weight and eating.

The family places a high value on appearance, conformity, and obedience. The typical anorectic client is intelligent and performs well in school. The client's accomplishments are not for herself, however, but an effort to gain family approval. The client is fearful of embarrassing the family in any way. She is generally very dependent on them; any independent activity is difficult for her. Believing she has little control in her environment, she finds that she can control her body and thereby manipulate her family. The struggle over food intake is an emotional struggle for autonomy and self-control.

The anorectic client has difficulty in developing relationships with peers. Although the client can adopt a normal facade, her difficulty with independent self-expression impairs her ability to form peer relationships.

Anorexia nervosa and bulimia nervosa start as a diet and continue as a weight maintenance technique until it becomes life threatening. Table 31-5 summarizes the theories of these disorders.

Nursing Process
Assessment: Anorexia Nervosa

Physical dimension The client's physical appearance is notable. Usually she appears emaciated, with a hollow face and sunken eyes. The client's skin may have a yellow

tinge from eating many carrots. The hair is usually dry and may fall out excessively. Lanugo (fine body hair), a possible reaction to prolonged malnutrition, is seen. Deterioration of mucous membranes and teeth, brittle nails and hair, amenorrhea, and loss of muscle mass also may occur. To make weight loss less apparent, the anorectic client often wears loose clothing.

The anorectic client avoids high carbohydrate foods but may allow herself substantial amounts of bulky low-calorie foods, such as celery, crisp breads, or cottage cheese. She usually avoids eating with others at conventional mealtimes to maintain abstinence in the face of hunger.

After collecting data about physical appearance and eating patterns, the nurse notes the client's activity level; daily caloric intake; physical signs and symptoms of malnutrition; and results of diagnostic studies, such as serum electrolyte studies, urinalysis, and hormone studies. She compares the results of these studies to normal values.

Emotional dimension According to psychoanalytical theory, the nurse assesses the client's feelings. Anorectic clients are often cold, indifferent, stubborn, angry, depressed, anxious, and withdrawn. Their fear of loss of control results in a hostile, overcontrolled affect. They may be out of touch with their emotions, reporting feeling good when they are physically ill or feeling angry with no apparent justification. According to psychoanalytical theory, the client fears sexual maturity; her emotional development may not have kept pace with her physical development. The adolescent stage of development requires skills or strengths that she may not have. She feels incompetent, helpless, and ineffective in dealing with a changing body and new social and emotional requirements.

Intellectual dimension The anorectic client is often negative about herself and her achievements and is critical of her body. When using cognitive therapy, the nurse explores irrational beliefs, such as the following: (1) It is important to be perfect in everything; (2) it is necessary to have love and approval at all times; and (3) happiness is achieved by being thin.

The nurse discusses the client's preoccupation with food, eating, thinness, and exercise. The client has usually been a high achiever in school, with grades gradually declining as she places increasing emphasis on weight loss and control. The nurse assesses the client's usual coping mechanisms (other than food and starvation). Because the client tries to be controlled in all aspects of her life, she may resist the nurse, who is an authority figure.

Social dimension Many anorectic clients have low self-esteem. The nurse therefore determines issues important to the anorectic client that can be used to build success into the plan of care to increase self-esteem.

The nurse looks for signs of overly close, enmeshed family dynamics. Clues include a parent who speaks for the client; a parent who sits extremely close to the client while the other parent is detached and further away; and communication patterns that do not include all members. Focus of attention and blame may be placed on the anorectic client. Seen as a model child, the client shows evidence of trying to conform to parental demands, goals, and expectations. Frequently, the client drives herself mercilessly to meet the high expectations of herself and her family. In some cases she may withdraw from family and peers.

Spiritual dimension Since the client and family may not come for treatment until significant trauma has occurred, the nurse may find that family members may have considerable hopelessness about altering behaviors. The nurse assesses the meaning of life for the client and family, especially if there have been suicidal thoughts and/or suicidal attempts.

Because of the client's poor physical condition, her motivation for emotional health and growth is constricted. Her preoccupation with food and thinness leaves little time to reflect on a purpose or direction for her life. Isolation and alienation from significant others further reduces her ability to receive pleasure. Assessment of the client's beliefs about health and illness reveals erroneous ideas about thinness based on distorted perceptions. She is unable to accept herself or her weaknesses; she believes she has little value.

Assessment: Bulimia Nervosa

Physical dimension The bulimic client reports frequent, recurrent episodes of binge eating, an awareness of abnormal eating patterns, frequent fluctuations in weight of more than 10 lb because of alternating binges and fasts, self-induced vomiting after binging, abdominal pain, and use of cathartics or diuretics. The nurse further assesses this client for severe physical signs and symptoms of malnutrition and pathophysiological changes.

The bulimic client often has a history of attempting to adhere to fad diets with little success in controlling eating behaviors. The client continues to eat large amounts of food, even though she is attempting to follow a restricted diet. When the client acknowledges her lack of success with low-calorie diets, she resorts to vomiting and/or use of cathartics to maintain her weight. The vomiting and amount of cathartics gradually increase as the client fails to lose weight.

The nurse questions the client about weight gain and loss patterns. The bulimic client may report weight gain (20 to 30 lb) or weight loss within a short time span. When vomiting or laxative use helps her lose weight, the bulimic client tries to regulate her binges so that her actual weight at the nurse's assessment may be within 10 to 15 lb of normal, thus giving her a false-normal appearance.

Only after a lengthy binge-purge pattern does the client begin to show physical signs and symptoms other than abdominal aches and feelings of fullness. Other symptoms include severe constipation, vitamin and mineral deficiencies from lack of absorption (as a result of vomiting), and ulceration and/or possible perforation of the gastrointestinal tract from irritation associated with vomiting and laxative abuse. Binging may also result in acute dilation of the stomach, menstrual problems, and salivary gland disturbances. Self-induced vomiting may produce metabolic disturbances (especially hypokalemia), cardiac dysrhythmias, renal damage, tetany and peripheral paresthesias, dehydration, epileptic seizures, erosion of dental enamel (perimolysis), chronic hoarseness, and gastrointestinal reflux. The purgative abuse may lead to steatorrhea and finger clubbing from rebound water retention.[20]

The bulimic client is not extremely overweight and is usually within 10 lb of ideal weight. Laboratory and radiological studies, such as blood work, urinalysis, and barium studies, usually reveal few abnormal findings, although the client often describes abnormal bowel patterns and many other physical symptoms in great detail.

Emotional dimension When the nurse assesses the emotional status of the bulimic client, she is aware that the client often has strong feelings and emotions associated with the binge-purge pattern. The nurse observes the client's verbal and nonverbal responses carefully for signs of anxiety, helplessness, anger, depression, and frustration and feelings of futility, inability to meet others' expectations, or even elation or joy. These feelings typically are experienced before binging. Feelings often reported during and after the binge-purge behaviors are guilt, repulsion, self-disgust, or the opposite extremes— excitement and increased energy. Frequently, bulimic clients report that tension drives them to food and that the binging and purging relieves it, producing a high or release similar to an orgasm, followed by calmness and a sense of relaxation. The bulimic client often hides binge-purge behaviors from family and significant others; this secrecy adds to the excitement. The excitement and frenzy of binging are frequently reported. Often the binge-purge behaviors result in sleep.

Intellectual dimension Manipulating body size and food intake may be an attempt to hide inner stress or adjustment difficulties. In making her assessment of the bulimic client, the nurse is alert to clues that lead to uncovering the sources of stress. This approach may be difficult, as the client (and family) may be locked into a pattern of denying underlying emotional causes of the eating disorder. The client makes an attempt to appear normal, except for the binge-purge behaviors. The nurse's attempts to identify problems can be met with hostility and anger, as the client's anxiety is increased by any remote hint of breaking through the denial system.

Social dimension Weight loss from techniques such as vomiting and laxative and diuretic abuse tends to decrease an already low self-esteem. Assessing the client's current level of self-esteem assists the nurse to identify ways to aid the client in building positive feelings about herself. Self-esteem tends to grow as relationships with significant others improve.

The nurse must assess the client's support system. The family may include overweight members, and the client may have identified with the family's established pattern of overeating. The client may describe a dominating, controlling mother and a distant, powerful father. Few clients describe positive relationships with their fathers. The nurse observes the family dynamics, watching for signs of power struggles, dominance, dependence, and enmeshment.

Bulimic clients may also have other impulsive behaviors. They may have a history of shoplifting, alcohol or drug abuse, suicide attempts, and self-mutilation. The nurse is alert to signs of the pathological behaviors and considers them in her assessment.

Spiritual dimension The interaction of all the dimensions affects the client's spiritual dimension. Her generally poor physical health, guilt, depression, self-disgust, self-criticism, irrational fears, and preoccupation with weight constrict the quality of her life and prevent her from giving and receiving many pleasures. Although the disorder is not as life threatening as anorexia nervosa, the condition may become chronic. Without treatment the client feels a sense of hopelessness about herself and her life.

Analysis

Nursing Diagnosis The defining characteristics of the nursing diagnosis, altered nutrition: less than body requirements, are listed in the accompanying box.

The following list provides examples of NANDA-accepted diagnoses related to anorexia nervosa and bulimic nervosa with causative statements:

1. Altered nutrition: less than body requirements related to self-induced vomiting
2. Altered bowel elimination: constipation related to insufficient food and fluid intake
3. Fluid volume deficit related to self-induced vomiting
4. Ineffective individual coping related to denial of hunger
5. Sexuality patterns, altered related to ineffective coping

Planning

Table 31-6 presents a nursing care plan with examples of long- and short-term goals, outcome criteria, interventions and rationales related to anorexia nervosa, which are examples of the planning stage in the nursing process.

Implementation: Anorexia Nervosa

Physical dimension The immediate goal of nursing intervention is to restore the anorectic client's nutritional state to normal. Nutritional rehabilitation occurs most efficiently and rapidly in the hospital. The severely ill client requires daily monitoring of weight, fluid, calorie intake, and urine output. Clients are usually fearful of var-

---

▼ ALTERED NUTRITION: LESS THAN BODY REQUIREMENTS

DEFINITION

The state in which the individual experiences an intake of nutrients insufficient to meet metabolic needs.

DEFINING CHARACTERISTICS

- **Physical dimension**

  Loss of weight with adequate food intake

  Body weight 20% or more under ideal for height and frame

  Weakness of muscles required for swallowing or mastication

  Aversion to eating

  Satiety immediately after ingesting food

  Abdominal pain with or without pathological conditions

  Sore, inflamed buccal cavity

- **Intellectual dimension**

  Reported inadequate food intake less than Recommended Daily Allowance

  Reported or evidence of lack of food

  Lack of interest in food

  Reported altered taste sensation

Modified from Kim MJ, McFarland GK, McLane AM, editors: *Pocket guide to nursing diagnoses,* ed 5, St Louis, 1993, Mosby—Year Book.

▼ TABLE 31-6   NURSING CARE PLAN Related to Anorexia Nervosa

GOALS	OUTCOME CRITERIA	INTERVENTIONS	RATIONALES
NURSING DIAGNOSIS: Altered nutrition: less than body requirements related to fear of gaining weight			
LONG TERM			
To restore nutritional status to normal	Establishes a pattern of eating that includes foods high in calories, protein, and complex carbohydrates	Assist client to select foods of choice that are high in calories, protein, and complex carbohydrate	Allows for smoother transition to normal eating patterns
		Assist client to develop a plan for regularly eating meals that includes the basic food groups	Client may learn to value and enjoy a healthy, nutritious diet
To stabilize weight and gradually increase to 10% greater than ideal weight	Engages in self-monitoring to maintain ideal weight	In collaboration with client, define realistic target weight	Helps to reduce anxiety and fear about weight
		Have client weigh self daily	Allows client to assume responsibility for maintaining weight
SHORT TERM			
To replace irrational fear about gaining weight with rational thinking	Verbalizes fewer fears about weight gain	Assist client to explore the irrational nature of the fears about gaining weight	Helps client develop new ways of thinking
		Teach client the connection between the fear and the eating disorder	Awareness of the connection decreases irrational thinking

ious types of foods, especially high-calorie foods, so the nutritional formula of vitamins, minerals, fatty acids, and carbohydrates given may be blended so the client cannot discard any item. If the client still fails to eat, lifesaving physical interventions, such as a gastrostomy tube, can be used.

The nurse defines a target weight for the client based on average weight tables. If the client has been ill for years, it may be appropriate to agree on weight that is lower than average.

Initially, the nurse monitors the client 24 hours a day and provides one-to-one supervision. It may be helpful to encourage the client to weigh herself daily and set a realistic goal for weight maintenance. This approach helps reduce the client's anxiety and fear about weight gain. Gradually, the nurse moves the client away from the preoccupation with weight. As the client gains weight, the staff can relax the controls. During the weight restoration period, the client may be allowed to select her own foods, which allows a smoother transition to normal eating patterns, and to practice maintaining her target weight with less aid from the nursing staff. Daily exercise is included in the client's activities. The type and amount is clearly specified to discourage overactivity.

Emotional dimension When the client seems unconcerned about the seriousness of her eating problem, the nurse attempts to help the client gain insight into its effect on her physical health through individual and group therapy. The client needs some awareness of her need to control the environment with her maladaptive eating patterns. It is also important to help the client deal with her fears: becoming fat, losing control, maturing sexually, fail-

ure, becoming independent from her family, and accepting adult responsibilities. The nurse assists the client to deal with these feelings by exploring them and helping the client to separate feelings from irrational thoughts.

Intellectual dimension Cognitive restructuring is useful to help the client replace irrational thinking and distorted perceptions about her body and eating (see the research highlight below). Cognitive restructuring involves ways to challenge and change the irrational belief system that the client uses to maintain the eating disorder.

The nurse helps the client substitute her preoccupation with being a perfect person with a more realistic perception of herself by being a role model of an adult, rational thinker. The nurse shows that the client is human, capable of making mistakes and accepting responsibility for them. The nurse also helps the client value her abilities and be more accepting of her limitations.

A difficult task facing the nurse is to help the client who does not accept her eating problem. The nurse is aware of the client's defenses (denial) and helps reduce the client's anxiety by discussing and exploring possible causes of her anxiety, thus lessening the need for the strong defenses.

Social dimension Behavior modification is the treatment of choice for anorectic clients. Reinforcers include physical activity, visiting privileges, and social activities, contingent on weight gain. Negative reinforcements, such as bed rest, isolation, and tube feeding, are also used at times, especially if the client is severely physically ill.

Most eating disorder programs include family therapy in the treatment regimen. The nurse needs to help both the client and the family recognize the importance of total family involvement in treatment. Often family members

---

RESEARCH HIGHLIGHT

Disturbed Body Image in Patients with Eating Disorders
• RL Horne, JC VanVactor, and S Emerson

PURPOSE

The purpose of the study was to determine whether patients with eating disorders experience more distortions in body image than individuals without eating disorders.

SAMPLE

The sample consisted of 214 women from an inpatient eating disorders program: 87 with anorexia nervosa alone, 72 with both anorexia and bulimia nervosa, and 55 with bulimia nervosa alone. A comparison group consisted of 61 female university students.

METHODOLOGY

Each subject used a three-dimensional measure to rate her body size. The subject stated her desired body size at seven points on her body. Then subject's measurements at each of these points were taken. Distortion in body image was calculated as the subject's perceived body size divided by her actual body size. All subjects were also given tests of intelligence, skill, and memory.

Based on data from *American Journal of Psychiatry* 148:2, 1991.

FINDINGS

All three patients groups differed significantly from the comparison group in distortions in body image. Most, but not all patients with eating disorders, had distortions in their body image.

IMPLICATIONS

These findings suggest that diagnostic criteria regarding disturbance of body image for both anorexia and bulimia need to be revised, provided that further research of body image is conducted.

think the client has "the problem" and resist coming to therapy sessions. The client, who is usually searching for approval from family and peers, is helped develop less dependence on others. The nurse can help the client progress toward more mature, independent, and interdependent actions by exploring the client's perceptions about her current status. The nurse helps her become more assertive by allowing her to try out independent actions (see Chapter 16). The family also needs help in understanding the changes in the client's behavior and in allowing the client to separate from the family.

Some clients are withdrawn and want to spend considerable time alone in their rooms. The nurse establishes a one-to-one relationship with the client and gradually encourages her to tolerate and eventually enjoy other people. This type of client isolates herself, particularly at mealtime. The nurse intervenes by helping the client gradually increase her tolerance to allow another person to be present at mealtimes. Diversional or recreational social activities are therapeutic. The nurse encourages the client's full participation in activities and recreational therapies, such as occupational therapy and school-related activities (if appropriate).

Therapy is most successful when a multidisciplinary approach is used. Usually a combination of group, individual, behavioral, pharmacotherapy, family, hypnotherapy, and nutritional therapy is required. Self-help groups and eating disorder clinics are growing in popularity. A complete list of self-help organizations for person with eating disorders may be obtained from the National Anorexic Aid Society, PO Box 29461, Columbus, Ohio 43229.

Spiritual dimension A primary goal in the spiritual dimension is to offer the client hope, thereby decreasing her feelings of despair. The nurse's confidence that the client can control her pathological eating patterns and the nurse's acceptance of the client as a worthwhile and valuable person are ways of offering hope. Promoting meaningful relationships with others and pleasurable activities can increase the client's feelings of worth and value. In addition, it is important to help the client accept herself as a person with potential for achievements and with some limitations.

It is essential to help the client examine reasons for her existence, because eating disorders are self-destructive behaviors. (See Chapter 14 for specific interventions for suicide and self-destructive behavior.)

Implementation: Bulimia Nervosa

Physical dimension Because the client may attempt to vomit in secret, limits are set and close observation is needed, especially after meals. A contract is made with the client to stop laxative and diuretic use and vomiting. The bulimic client usually feels desperate at this point and is open to a new approach. Reinforcement to learn controls is important. The nurse also emphasizes mouth care (frequent vomiting erodes dental enamel and may ulcerate the mucous membrane of the mouth), checks electrolyte studies, and monitors weight.

Emotional dimension The nurse recognizes the client's feelings of helplessness, anxiety, anger, frustration, guilt, and depression associated with her eating problem. In addition, she fears that she will not be able to stop eating

voluntarily. The nurse helps the client get in touch with these feelings by observing and acknowledging them. Helping the client identify feelings as she experiences them, discussing their possible causes, and exploring other ways of responding to situations that evoke these feelings are important. For example, because stress and tension often initiate a binge, the nurse explores with the client the cause of the stress and tension and discusses alternative ways to cope with them.

Intellectual dimension The client is aware that her eating is abnormal but cannot control her eating habits. The nurse explores with the client her impulses, needs, and feelings. This learning about herself helps repair some of her perceptual difficulties and promotes more realistic thinking. Examining her perceptions about her body and weight also assists in promoting realistic thinking and lessens self-criticism and self-disgust. The nurse does not argue or set unrealistic limits in response to the client's lack of progress.

A cognitive-behavioral approach works well with bulimic clients. Keeping a record of meals and binge episodes helps them become aware of their eating behavior. Self-monitoring is followed by a contract to restrict the client's eating to three or four planned meals a day. Self-control is emphasized. Gradually, the client learns to identify circumstances leading to the loss of control and to explore adaptive ways of coping.

Social dimension It is essential that the nurse help the client improve her self-concept. Participating in activities that are pleasant for the client, achieving success in tasks or projects, learning new skills, having meaningful relationships with others, giving positive statements to herself, and receiving positive statements from others all enhance self-concept.

Because the bulimic client may be involved in impulsive, acting-out behaviors, such as sexual promiscuity, stealing, lying, or drug abuse, the nurse needs to intervene in these behaviors as well. Setting and adhering to agreed-on limits for the client's behavior are important. The nurse also needs to help this client recognize her feelings and express them in a socially acceptable way. The need to act on feelings is eventually replaced by appropriate ventilation and expression. The nurse examines the sociocultural influences on binge-purge behaviors. Although society places great value on thinness and the mass media bombards the public with more and more foods to consume, the client can learn to ignore the temptations and control her impulse to eat.

The client may attend groups with other bulimic clients to receive peer support and to begin to reach out to others, which lessens her preoccupation with her own problem. She may also enjoy the humor and light-heartedness often found in groups of young people and begin to experience satisfaction in relationships with others.

Spiritual dimension The nurse helps the client deal with feelings of hopelessness by displaying confidence and encouragement. By offering hope that the client can control her impulse to binge, the nurse helps the client view life less pessimistically. The nurse helps the client find enjoyment, either in activities with others or in those performed alone. The nurse also encourages a sense of humor because bulimic clients tend to take themselves too seriously. The nurse models a light-hearted attitude and makes humorous

▼ **TABLE 31-7** **Comparison of Anorexia Nervosa and Bulimia**

Features	Anorexia Nervosa	Bulimia
Similar		Fear of fatness
		Pursuit of weight loss
		Fear of loss of control of eating
		Distortion of body image
Contrasting	Severely restricted food intake	Loss of control of intake leading to binges
	Diuretic laxative abuse	Abuse of laxative, diuretics or both
	No vomiting	Vomiting
	Younger	Older
	Obsessional, perfectionistic	Histrionic, antisocial, with loss of impulse control
	Denies hunger	Experiences hunger
	Severe weight loss	Variable weight loss
	Introverted	More extroverted
	Eating behavior a source of pride	Eating behavior source of shame
	Less sexually active	Sexually active
	Amenorrhea, loss of sex drive	Variable amenorrhea and change in sex drive
	Death from starvation or suicide	Death from hypokalemia or suicide
	"Model" child	May have behavioral problems

comments in appropriate situations. New activities, meaningful relationships, and decreased depressive symptoms increase the client's feelings of value and worth, restore a healthy balance to life, and help to decrease obsession with food and weight.

Table 31-7 provides a comparison of features of anorexia nervosa and bulimia nervosa.

Evaluation

The nurse uses the outcome criteria for each goal that she and the client have established to evaluate the nursing care plan's effectiveness. Treatment for clients with eating disorders is effective when the client maintains an appropriate weight over time according to her height and frame. The client's overall general health improves. She is in touch with her feelings and uses new adaptive skills to meet her needs rather than relying on food (or the lack of food). She has a realistic perception of herself and her body, and irrational beliefs are replaced with more authentic ones. Her self-concept is positive. Family relationships improve, and the client moves toward greater independence. In general the client experiences more satisfaction and pleasure when there is less focus on thinness and more emphasis on relationships and pleasurable activities that lead to a balanced and productive life.

Special Issues
Fasting

Fasting is complete abstinence from food for 24 hours to several weeks. It results in protein loss and severe nitrogen imbalance. About one third of the weight lost in a 24-hour fast is fluid and body mass. Persons fasting show progressive reduction of intestinal activity, which changes the overall physiological and biochemical activities of the gastrointestinal tract. Potassium, sodium bicarbonate, and multivitamin and mineral supplements are important. Therefore persons should fast only when under close med-

ical supervision. Complications associated with fasting are muscle wasting, severe postural hypotension, hyperuricemia, acidosis, mineral loss, hepatic and renal impairment, nausea and dizziness, increased uric acid levels, and dehydration.

Low-calorie diets

One popular low-calorie diet consists of liquid mixtures of protein, carbohydrates, and mineral fat and powdered minerals and vitamins. The powder is mixed with water, club soda, or other noncaloric beverage or fruit juice. The daily caloric content of such a diet ranges from 300 to 800 calories. Serious, sometimes fatal complications have been attributed to these diets. Potential complications are headache, nausea and vomiting, diarrhea or constipation, lethargy and lack of stamina, worsening gout, mineral and electrolyte deficiencies, gum disease from lack of chewing, and cardiac dysrhythmias. However, very low-calorie diets administered under careful medical supervision can be effective, particularly for the moderately obese (41% to 100% overweight) and the severely obese (100% overweight). Programs typically last up to 3 months and can be repeated if needed. An adequate diet provides at least 45 g of protein and 50 mEq of potassium/day. Persons on the diet are examined by health care professionals at least every 2 weeks so that health parameters can be monitored, including electrocardiograms and blood tests.

Other popular diets also have dangerous complications or at best do not meet their claims. The grapefruit diet, for example, claims to help burn off excess calories. On this diet a grapefruit is eaten with each meal, allegedly to increase metabolism. None of the claims of this diet can be substantiated. Weight loss results not from the grapefruit, but from the reduced calories consumed by the dieter. Another diet, the Zen macrobiotic diet, is a semistarvation regimen that can lead to nutrient (such as vitamin C) deficiencies, anemia, hypocalcemia, hypoproteinemia, and decreased renal function.

Appetite suppressants and thyroid hormone use

Many people turn to pills and injections to lose weight. Anorectic agents help an individual lose only a small amount of weight (about 0.23 kg/week), and efforts at weight loss using appetite suppressants may last only 6 weeks.[4] Appetite suppressants are generally amphetamine derivatives. Appetite suppressants and thyroid hormones have different methods of action, but both increase thermogenesis or depress appetite.

The common belief that obese persons have a hypothyroid or other thyroid problem is not true. Less than 1% of overweight persons actually have abnormal thyroid function. Complications associated with the use of thyroid hormones include palpitations and sweating and increased heart rate, systolic blood pressure, and urine calcium excretion.[4]

Vitamin and mineral deficiencies

A lack of vitamins and minerals affects a person's health. Behavioral changes can result from deficiencies in required nutrients. Much controversy today surrounds the biochemical effect of various nutrients on the brain and thereby on behavior and emotions. Some symptoms of vitamin and mineral deficiencies mimic mental illness. Table 31-8 lists behavioral effects of some vitamin deficiencies.[41]

▼ **TABLE 31-8   Behavioral Effects of Vitamin Deficiencies**

Vitamin	Behavioral Effect
Thiamine (B_1)	Wernicke's encephalopathy
	Memory loss
	Depression
	Apathy
	Irritability
	Korsakoff's psychosis
Riboflavin (B_2)	Change in body perception with severe physical symptoms
Niacin (B_3)	Organic dementia
	Delirium
	Memory deficits
	Apathy
	Depression
	Anxiety
	Hyperirritability
	Mania
Pyridoxine, pyridoxal, pyridoxamine (B_6)	Poor concentration
	Memory impairment
	Depression
	Nervous irritability
	Hyperacusis
Pantothenic acid	Poor concentration
	Restlessness
	Irritability
	Fatigue
	Depression
Biotin (H)	Lassitude
	Depression
Cyanocobalamin (B_{12})	Confusion
	Irritability
	Memory loss
	Hallucinations
	Delusions
	Paranoia
Folic acid	Forgetfulness
	Apathy
	Irritability
	Depression
	Psychosis
	Delirium
	Dementia
Ascorbic acid (C)	Lassitude
	Hypochondriasis
	Depression
	Hysteria

Modified from Mahan L, Rees J: *Nutrition in adolescence,* St Louis, 1984, Mosby–Year Book.

BRIEF REVIEW

Obesity is a severe eating disorder affecting not only the client but also the family and society. Overweight persons spend millions of dollars annually trying new methods for weight loss. Anorexia nervosa and bulimia nervosa are reaching epidemic proportions as young people seek to lose weight and thus severely impair their physical health by self-induced starvation and binging and purging.

Theoretical explanations for eating disorders are excessive dieting and exercising, rejection of female sexual development, a learned response to emotional arousal, irrational beliefs about thinness, a negative self-concept, family conflicts (especially between mother and daughter), and family and cultural influences about food and eating.

The components of the nursing process are described as they relate specifically to obesity, anorexia nervosa, and bulimia nervosa. Fasting, low-calorie diets, and the effects of vitamin and mineral deficiencies on behavior are also discussed.

REFERENCES AND SUGGESTED READINGS

1. Allan JD: Women who successfully manage their weight, *Western Journal of Nursing Research* 11:657, 1989.
2. American Psychiatric Association: Diagnostic and statistical manual of mental disorders (DSM-III-R). Washington, DC, 1987, American Psychiatric Association.
3. Anderson A: Anorexia nervosa and bulimia, *Journal of Adolescent Health Care* 4:15, 1983.
4. Blackburn G, Pavlov K: Fad reducing diets: separating fads from facts, *Journal of Dentistry for Children* 84:382, 1984.
5. Brownell K: Obesity: understanding and treating a serious, prevalent, and refractory disorder, *Journal of Consulting and Clinical Psychology* 50:820, 1982.
6. Bruch H: *The golden cage: the enigma of anorexia nervosa,* Cambridge, 1978, Harvard University Press.
7. Carpenito L: *Nursing diagnosis: application to clinical practice,* Philadelphia, 1989, JB Lippincott.
8. Cauwells J: *Bulimia,* New York, 1983, Doubleday.
9. Ciseaux A: Anorexia nervosa: a view from the mirror, *American Journal of Nursing* 80:1468, 1980.
10. Colliver J, Frank S, Frank A: Similarity of obesity indices in clinical studies of obese adults: a factor analytic study, *American Journal of Clinical Nutrition* 38:640, 1983.
11. Cosens R: Obesity in the aged, *Nursing Clinics of North America* 17:227, 1982.
12. Crisp AH: *Anorexia nervosa: let me be,* Orlando, Fla, 1980, Grune & Stratton.
13. Crocker K, Gerber F, Shearer J: Metabolism of carbohydrate, protein, and fat, *Nursing Clinics of North America* 18:3, 1983.

14. Daniels A: Obesity in adolescence. In Wolaman B, editor: *Psychological aspects of obesity,* New York, 1982, Van Nostrand Reinhold.

15. Deering C: Developing a therapeutic alliance with an anorexia nervosa client, *Journal of Psychosocial Nursing and Mental Health Services* 25(3):10, 1987.

16. DeJong W: The stigma of obesity: the consequences of naive assumptions concerning the causes of physical deviance, *Journal of Health and Social Behavior* 21:75, 1980.

17. Ellis R, Harper R: *A new guide to rational living,* North Hollywood, Calif, 1975, Wilshire Book Co.

18. Falk J, Halmi K, Tryon W: Activity measures in anorexia nervosa, *Archives of General Psychiatry* 42:811, 1985.

19. Fisher J, Nadler A, Whitcher-Alagna S: Recipient reactions to aid, *Psychological Bulletin* 91:27, 1982.

20. Flood M: Addictive eating disorders, *Nursing Clinics of North America* 24(1):43, 1989.

21. Forish B, Grothaus K, Luscombe R: Dinner conversation: meal therapy to differentiate eating behavior from family process, *Journal of Psychosocial Nursing and Mental Health Services* 28(11):12, 1990.

22. Garner D, Garfinkel P, editors: *Handbook of psychotherapy for anorexia nervosa and bulimia,* New York, 1985, The Guilford Press.

23. Gierszewski S: The relationship of weight loss, locus of control, and social support, *Nursing Research* 32:43, 1983.

24. Greary MC: A review of treatment models for eating disorders: toward a holistic model, *Holistic Nursing Practice* 3(1):39, 1988.

25. Hagenbuch V: Obesity and the school-age child, *Nursing Clinics of North America* 17:207, 1982.

26. Hawkins R, Frenmoow W, Clement P: *The binge-purge syndrome,* New York, 1984, Springer Publishing.

27. Horne RL, VanVactor JC, Emerson S: Disturbed body image in patients with eating disorders, *American Journal of Psychiatry* 148(2):211, 1991.

28. Hudson J, Laffer P, Pope H: Bulimia related to affective disorder by family history and response to the dexamethasone suppression test, *American Journal of Psychiatry* 139:685, 1982.

29. Jaffe ES: Working with troubled teens, *RN* 54(2):58, 1991.

30. Jarvis W: Food fads, fallacies, and frauds, *CDA Journal* 12:24, 1984.

31. Johnson P: Getting enough to grow on, *American Journal of Nursing* 84:336, 1984.

32. Kaye W, Gwirtsman H: *A comprehensive approach to the treatment of normal weight bulimia,* Washington, DC, 1985, American Psychiatric Association.

33. Keltner N: Bulimia: controlling compulsive eating, *Journal of Psychosocial Nursing and Mental Health Services* 22:24, 1984.

34. Kempe A, Gelazis R: Rational emotive techniques for overweight adults: a cognitive-behavioral group approach. In *Abstracts of Research Day,* Little Rock, Ark, 1984, The University of Arkansas for Medical Sciences.

35. Kruse M, Mahan L: *Food, nutrition and diet therapy,* Philadelphia, 1984, WB Saunders.

36. Lasky P, Eichelberger K: Implications, considerations, and nursing interventions of obesity in neonatal and preschool patients, *Nursing Clinics of North America* 17:199, 1982.

37. Leininger MM: Transcultural eating patterns and nutrition: transcultural nursing and anthropological perspectives, *Holistic Nursing Practice* 3(1):16, 1988.

38. Leon GR: Personality and behavioral correlates of obesity. In Wolman B, editor: *Psychological aspects of obesity: a handbook,* New York, 1982, Van Nostrand Reinhold.

39. Lukert B: Biology of obesity. In Wolman B, editor: *Psychological aspects of obesity: a handbook,* New York, 1982, Van Nostrand Reinhold.

40. MacKenzie JR, LaBan MM, Sackey AH: The prevalence of peripheral neuropathy in patients with anorexia nervosa, *Archives of Physical Medicine and Rehabilitation* 70(12):827, 1989.

41. Mahan L, Rees J: *Nutrition in adolescence,* St Louis, 1984, Mosby–Year Book.

42. Minuchin S, Rosman BL, Baker L: *Psychosomatic families: anorexia nervosa in context,* Cambridge, 1978, Harvard University Press.

43. Myers K, Smith M: Psychogenic polydipsia in a patient with anorexia nervosa, *Journal of Adolescent Health Care* 6:404, 1985.

44. Nightingale F: *Notes on nursing: what it is and what it is not,* Mineola, NY, 1960, Dover Publications.

45. Orbach S: *Fat is a feminist issue: the anti-diet guide to permanent weight loss,* New York, 1982, Jason Aronson.

46. Plehn KW: Anorexia nervosa and bulimia: incidence and diagnosis, *Nurse Practitioner* 15(4):22, 1990.

47. Pope H, Hudson J: *New hope for binge eaters,* New York, 1984, Harper and Row.

48. Rand C, Stunkard A: Obesity and psychoanalysis: treatment and four-year follow-up, *American Journal of Psychiatry* 140:1140, 1983.

49. Reed G, Sech E: Bulimia: a conceptual model for group treatment, *Journal of Psychosocial Nursing and Mental Health Services* 23:16, 1985.

50. Russ C: Fat diets for treatment of obesity, *CDC Journal* 12:60, 1984.

51. Staples NR, Schwartz M: Anorexia nervosa support group: providing transitional support, *Journal of Psychosocial Nursing and Mental Health Services* 28(2):6, 1990.

52. Stunkard A, Stellar E: Eating and its disorders, New York, 1984, Raven Press.

53. White J: An overview of obesity: its significance to nursing, *Nursing Clinics of North America* 17:191, 1982.

54. Williams S: *Basic nutrition and diet therapy,* ed 8, St Louis, 1988, Mosby–Year Book.

55. Wilson P, editor: *Fear of being fat,* New York, 1983, Jason Aronson.

ANNOTATED BIBLIOGRAPHY

Carino C, Chmelko P: Disorders of eating in adolescence: anorexia nervosa and bulimia, *Nursing Clinics of North America* 18:343, 1983.

This article suggests a holistic approach to nursing care for the anorectic client provides helpful suggestions for therapy, including ways to involve not only the client but also significant others. It also clearly defines the disorders and underlying theoretical premises.

Flood M: Addictive eating disorders, *Nursing Clinics of North America* 24:(1):45, 1989.

Anorexia and bulimia are described as other addictive patterns and diseases. Ideas are presented for helping such clients toward their own personal growth and recovery.

Leininger MM: Transcultural eating patterns and nutrition: transcultural nursing and anthropological perspectives, *Holistic Nursing Practice* 3(1):16, 1988.

This article presents a thorough discussion of culture and its influence on eating patterns. General principles are given that are helpful to nurses attempting to understand cultural influences and patterns.

After studying this chapter, the student will be able to:

- Describe the development of the current political, social, and legal status of the chronically mentally ill client
- Discuss theories related to chronically mentally ill clients
- Discuss how an individual develops the life of a chronically mentally ill client, according to symbolic interactionism

- List the characteristics and role of the nurse when working with chronically mentally ill clients
- Discuss application of the nursing process to provide care to chronically mentally ill clients
- Identify current research findings relevant to chronically mentally ill clients

The roots of what we now call deinstitutionalization are firmly lodged in a cyclical tradition of institutional reform. Each reform flourishes briefly, is implemented and becomes routine, then is forgotten and neglected by its creator and the general public until a kind of institutional rot sets in, whereupon another reform movement replaces it.[19]

Chronically mentally ill individuals are all around us. They are those individuals who remain "unhelped" by the health care system. Many of these persons are cared for in state hospitals, community mental health centers, board and care homes, and in families. Many are uncared for on our city streets, i.e., the homeless mentally ill. It is estimated that 200,000 to 3 million people are homeless, of that number, 30% to 40% have a diagnosed chronic mental disorder.[9] All chronically mentally ill clients share certain characteristics including a tendency to feel isolated from society.

According to Bachrach there are three criteria for the designation of chronic mental illness, *diagnosis, duration,* and *disability.*[2,3] It is not clear which of the "3-Ds" is most important. There is also no agreement about a common descriptive phrase that captures the essence of this chronicity. Some professionals find the word *chronic* demeaning and connoting irreversibility,[22] so they prefer terms such as *serious, prolonged,* or *persistent.* We use the term *chronic mental illness* for clarity intending neither to demean nor connote hopelessness.

A chronically mentally ill client depends to a great extent on the mental health system or a supportive network of family or friends. This dependency is the result of troublesome behaviors, maladaptive coping patterns, or disturbed patterns of thought that interfere with the client's self-care

and useful role in society. These clients may or may not appear different from other people. Some conform to the stereotypical image of the "mental patient," such as a street person with rambling speech, a "bag lady" with strange mannerisms, or the bizarrely dressed, ill-groomed man or woman. Others are not stereotypical in appearance or behavior.

After years of hospitalization, some clients have adapted to the life-style of the institution (institutionalization). Some have never learned to function on the "outside," whereas others have spent little time in the hospital and appear to function at a higher level. The appearance usually is deceptive as they have managed to avoid societally imposed relationships, responsibilities, and realities by constantly traveling. These individuals may work only enough to stay alive and keep moving. Hospitalization occurs only

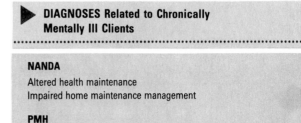

▶ **DIAGNOSES Related to Chronically Mentally Ill Clients**

NANDA

Altered health maintenance
Impaired home maintenance management

PMH

Altered health maintenance
Altered home maintenance

HISTORICAL OVERVIEW

DATES	EVENTS
Pre-1950	The chronically mentally ill client is institutionalized in long-term treatment facilities and receives primarily custodial care.
1950s	With the introduction of chlorpromazine the chronically mentally ill client with a poor prognosis is differentiated from the acutely disturbed client with a good prognosis.
1960s	Because of drug therapy, some psychotic clients are able to leave the hospital permanently.
	The image of the mental patient changes as hope and sophisticated therapies begin to replace blanket labeling and custodial care.
	An examination of all state mental health facilities by a presidential committee results in a directive to reduce the population of state hospitals and to limit admission to these facilities to clients posing an imminent danger to themselves and others.
	The presidential directive calls for community-based outpatient mental health facilities for treatment of chronically mentally ill clients.
	Chronically mentally ill clients become a target population for care and are viewed as unable or unwilling to learn necessary skills for survival out of the hospital.
	Nurses are given more independence in their work with chronically mentally ill persons.
1970s	A new group of chronically mentally ill clients, composed of individuals born in the 1950s and first hospitalized after the deinstitutionalization movement, is identified.
	The President's Commission on Mental Health (1978) recommends a national plan for defining the chronically mentally ill population and evaluating their needs and problems. This plan is to be implemented through national study and research as well as state level tracking of persons entering and leaving state mental health facilities.
	The term *deinstitutionalization* begins to be used to describe the exodus of patients from the state hospital system.
1980s	Professionals of all disciplines are seeing the importance of assigning experienced nurses to work with chronically distressed clients.
	The state public hospital population has dropped from a high of over 500,000 in 1955 to just over 100,000 by the late 1980s.
	Homelessness becomes a major focus of national attention as many homeless people are found to suffer from a diagnosable mental disorder.
	With increased focus on the needs of chronically mentally ill clients, nurses are more involved in planning nursing care for these clients.
1990s	As rumors of economic depression fill the headlines, the needs of the chronically mentally ill are relegated to a lower status.
Future	As the hospital based care of the chronically mentally ill continues to be brief, nurses need to develop creative strategies for meeting clients' needs in community based facilities.

when they get into conflicts involving the police.

Chronically mentally ill clients who have families to offer them emotional and financial support are rarely hospitalized in the larger public facilities but may enter private hospitals for brief stays several times a year. These clients may have much trouble negotiating with society at large, but manage quite well at home around less demanding friends and families. Their social skills remain intact except during acute episodes of psychosis.

Some chronically mentally ill clients, although rarely hospitalized, may routinely use outpatient departments for therapy and medication checks. During periods of acute psychosis they may attend daily. With support and guidance these individuals can care for themselves, work, marry, and have children.

Chronically mentally ill clients can function at a high level, perhaps for several years, then phase into a period of chaos during which they pass in and out of the hospital, cannot care for themselves, and overtax the coping capacities of their caregivers. Friends and family first blame themselves and then become angry with the disorganized client for these erratic changes. Many families struggle to keep the person at home but eventually come to the end of their rope and just want to be rid of the disruptive individual. Friends and family members need ongoing support to cope with all the crises, trials, and anxieties.

DSM-III-R DIAGNOSES

The DSM-III-R diagnostic categories associated with chronic mental illness are the schizophrenic disorders, delusional disorders, and other psychotic disorders. Many individuals who are diagnosed as psychotic, however, do not demonstrate the pervasive life disruption of the chronically mentally ill client.

THEORETICAL APPROACHES

Sociocultural Theory

Sociocultural theories explain chronicity as a product of sociocultural influence. For example, schizophrenia in third world countries is typically briefer, less likely to recur, and is not as intense as that in North America.[22]

Sociocultural theorists see chronicity as a side effect of American society—a product of a professional belief system that views the disintegration of the self as devastating and, perhaps, permanent. The individual is forced by society into a chronic role. Society then reinforces the role, the individual internalizes the role, and the stage is set for a chronic life-style of mental illness. Because of the paradigm through which society views this person, new behaviors are either not recognized or are interpreted as characteristic of the mental illness. The individual's character is seen only in the context of mental illness, and healthier aspects are ignored or extinguished. Two major sociocultural theories, symbolic interactionism and needs differentiation, are described here.

Symbolic Interactionism

Symbolic interactionism explains the role of society, social learning, cognition, and choice in the development of a chronic mental illness. This theory asserts that individuals interact through a series of roles that they choose according to their perceptions of the environment, their understanding of other people's expectations of them, and their understanding of available roles. If people are flexible and adaptive, they pass quickly through many roles according to their perceptions of the environment. If they are inner directed they maintain an inner view of self based on role successes and failures. People who are not flexible may strain a role to accommodate an environmental change. They may cling to a role and treat it as a complete identity, ignoring environmental cues to develop a new role. A rigid person may assume a role and make few adaptations despite others' expectations.

According to symbolic interactionism, the development of chronic mental illness is preceded by an initial period of a healthy self. Biological or early life influences result in behaviors that society considers characteristic of mentally ill persons. For a time, referred to as the *acute illness state,* the unhealthy behaviors (the role) create the person's primary identity as mentally ill. The hospital's therapeutic environment helps the client develop more adaptive behaviors and assume more acceptable roles in society.

After leaving the therapeutic environment, the client may find that many people behave as if he were still mentally ill. People around the "ex-mental patient" may respond to the person's behavior on their understanding of the mental patient role. The individual may find it difficult to reassume a healthy identity. The easiest, most acceptable role to choose is that of a mentally ill person.

The individual forming a new role uses information from the environment. The person forms a self-concept based on how others seem to perceive him. People may verbalize their support for an independent life-style, but their behavior indicates that they expect the individual to assume the role of a chronically mentally ill person. The person internalizes these expectations and accepts this role. The individual is now labeled.[16] Society sees the person as a "mental patient" and will observe only those characteristics appropriate for that image. In turn, the individual expects the characteristics of a "mental patient" to be his primary behaviors.

In this manner the individual has chosen the life of a chronically mentally ill client. The person views future goals as well as current realities from this perspective and expects to be dependent on the health care system. Fighting this role means exposure to uncertainties and new experiences that have failed in the past. Others' perceptions and expectations have reinforced the person's initial suspicion of being chronically mentally ill. To challenge these perceptions and expectations is to challenge an entire power structure. Besides, according to symbolic interactionism, the individual has already internalized society's pessimistic view of mental illness. The individual now expects only the life of a chronically mentally ill person and, in many ways, shapes life to fulfill these expectations.

The person learns the chronically mentally ill role from society and then refines it through interactions with others in the same role. These people create a subculture or perhaps several subcultures within society. These subcultures are probably complete, with their own mores, values, and nonverbal communication signals. One can easily identify these groups in the population of a large state hospital.

The process by which an individual develops the life of a chronically mentally ill client is summarized in the box on p. 636.

Needs Differentiation Theory

Several theorists have conceptualized a model to explain the needs of a new large group of chronically mentally ill individuals, persons between 25 and 45 years old.[29,32] Members from the baby boom era of the 1950s and later represent a group of clients who were not exposed to the influences of long-term institutionalization and custodial care. Sheets and others[32] hypothetically subdivided this population into three groups to show the distinct categories of their needs.

One group, "low energy, low demand," is characterized by passivity and low motivation. They depend on the mental health system, and, despite their lack of years of experience in the large state hospitals, they are well socialized into the client role.

Another group, "high energy, high demand," also depends somewhat on mental health workers but is also aggressively demanding, impulsive, and impatient with counselors and case managers. They push away those who try

▼
STEPS IN DEVELOPING CHRONIC MENTAL ILLNESS ACCORDING TO SYMBOLIC INTERACTIONISM

1. The self is born healthy, with genetic and/or environmental predispositions for the development of a mental illness.
2. Environmental and/or organic stressors occur.
3. The individual develops behaviors that society has labeled as representing the role of the mentally ill person.
4. The individual is identified as unsafe in society and placed in a therapeutic environment.
5. Maladaptive behaviors are controlled or extinguished, and the individual is returned to society.
6. If the person can be properly supported to reenter the normal role of a competent individual, the cycle is interrupted.
7. If society behaves as if the person were still mentally ill, the cycle continues.
8. Others interpret the individual's behavior as if he were still mentally ill.
9. The individual cannot reassume a "healthy identity."
10. The person chooses the easiest and most acceptable role, that of a mental patient.
11. People say they support adoption of a "normal" role, but behave as if they expect the person to assume the mentally ill role.
12. The person internalizes these expectations of society.
13. The individual is stigmatized.

14. The individual and society see the individual primarily according to the "mental illness" aspect of his personality.
15. The person and society observe only those behaviors characteristic of a mentally ill individual.
16. All the individual's behaviors are seen in the context of mental illness.
17. The person sees goals and current realities within the perspective of chronic mental illness.
18. The individual expects to be dependent on the health care system, as part of the mentally ill role.
19. The individual is afraid to challenge this self-perception because of uncertainty and negative reactions by others.
20. The person internalizes society's pessimistic view of mental illness: "once mentally ill, always mentally ill."
21. The individual shapes life to fulfill society's negative expectations.
22. The individual sees other people in various treatment centers who are also labeled chronically mentally ill.
23. These people represent a subculture with unique values, mores, and systems of nonverbal communication.
24. Interactions within this subculture strengthen the person's sick role and widen the gap between the individual and the norm.

to help them and often move from place to place, float in and out of jobs and public assistance, and go through sexual relationships quickly and dramatically. They are characterized by their high energy and their expectations of self-reliance, which are often frustrated. This group also includes the eccentric street people and the "revolving-door" clients (clients who are hospitalized over and over) who seek hospitalization when times are hard.

A final group, "high functioning, high aspiration," tends to function usually quite well and sometimes appear much healthier than they are. They may also be better educated and come from higher-income families than those of the other groups. They frequently consider traditional mental health activities to be unappealing and avoid anything that leads anyone to label them mentally ill. They wish to blend smoothly in society and have well-established goals for success.[6]

These groups are not official classifications, but they do help point out the variety of needs and problems seen in the population considered chronically mentally ill. The needs of younger psychiatric clients are also inherently different because of societal changes, including greater overall mobility, general loosening of family ties, increased availability of street drugs, and changes in the approach to rehabilitation of mental illness.

Table 32-1 lists treatment strategies for chronically mentally ill clients. Table 32-2 summarizes the theoretical approaches.

CHARACTERISTICS OF THE THERAPIST

Many nurses view the chronically mentally ill client as a substantial challenge. They must be patient and have realistic expectations to be effective. They avoid imposing their personal goals on the client or promising the client more nurturance than they can realistically provide in a professional role. The effective nurse:

• Has knowledge of general psychodynamics, psychopathology, and personality development and counseling skills
• Understands the nature of chronic problems and identifies the person's abilities and strengths
• Views the client as an individual and is not overwhelmed by chronicity
• Recognizes the cyclic nature of mental illness and the stressors that influence exacerbation
• Maintains hope for an optimal level of development while not superimposing societal time frames
• Maintains a patient, honest presence while awaiting the client to develop trust, test limits, and finally accept the relationship with the nurse
• Is clear, consistent, and concrete in her communication
• Uses clearly defined social skills and serves as a role model
• Is creative in both accepting and assisting the client, i.e., sharing oneself while maintaining a professional role and awareness of one's own limitations.

Roles

Generally, the nurse's role is to help the chronically mentally ill client accept and thus live more successfully. Thus the nurse focuses on everyday tasks by assisting the client to approach life and daily problems in a more realistic, responsible, and task-oriented manner. The nurse's problem-solving skills assist the client to function better, and it is hoped the client will learn these skills for more independent living.

The nurse maintains a variety of professional roles, depending on the client's needs. In the *surrogate mother* role the nurse assists the regressed client to reach out and begin

▼ **TABLE 32-1**   **Determination of Treatments for Chronically Mentally Ill Clients According to Level of Functioning**

Level of Functioning	Description	Setting for Treatment	Individual Treatment Strategies	Group Strategies	Family Strategies	Couple Strategies
Low	1. Shows obvious residual signs of mental illness 2. Depends on all or most personal care	1. Day hospital 2. Inpatient 3. Day activity program	1. Behavioral approaches 2. Supportive problem solving 3. Skills training	1. Clinician-led group 2. Skills training 3. Reality groups	1. Support 2. Teaching	1. Support 2. Information
Moderate	1. Requires consistent support to maintain motivation to complete personal care 2. Unable to live independently but requires only supportive assistance	1. Brief hospitalizations 2. Outpatient therapy	1. Consultant/peer approach 2. Individual therapy to strengthen healthy defense	1. Social network group 2. Peer-led group	1. Support 2. Communication therapy 3. Supporting boundary	1. Communication therapy 2. Supporting boundary
Independent	1. Able to live independently much of the time 2. Demonstrates basic skills of differentiating thoughts and feelings 3. Recognizes personal responsibilities in some situations 4. Is able to formulate own problem list and treatment plan with assistance (The nurse clinician offers insight-oriented and/or confrontive approaches if the client requests to work on issues about early life or changing life patterns. If the client does not request such work, the nurse plays a more passive role as consultant.)	1. Self-help programs 2. Liaison with outpatient programs 3. Outpatient clinics	1. More in-depth, insight oriented approaches 2. Consultant/peer approach	1. Peer-led group 2. Therapy groups 3. Insight oriented	1. More in-depth, "uncovering" therapy 2. Insight oriented	1. Uncovering 2. Insight oriented

▼ **TABLE 32-2** **Summary of the Theoretical Approaches to Chronically Mentally Ill Clients**

Theory	Theorist	Dynamics
Sociocultural (Symbolic interactionism)	Goffman[16]	The formerly mentally ill person internalizes and assumes a role that society perceives and reinforces as that of a mentally ill person.
Needs differentiation	Sheets[32] and others	The three groups of young adult, chronically distressed clients are low energy, low demand; high energy, high demand; and high functioning, high aspiration.

to trust. As the surrogate mother the nurse also accepts the client's dependence but still looks for growth cues. These are signs in the client's behavior that alert the nurse to encourage more responsibility or more individuation without risking imbalance or withdrawal. The nurse supports growth cues when the client is intimidated by trials and mistakes.

If a beginning level of trust and individuation is stabilized, the nurse assumes a role closer to that of *teacher* by instructing the client about adaptive behavior. The client frequently accepts the nurse as a role model and may temporarily mimic or at least adopt superficial habits of the nurse.

As the chronically distressed client progresses in goal attainment, the nurse may recognize temporarily stable behavior. At such times the most therapeutic role may be that of a *peer or partner* in problem solving. The client may better accept the nurse's assistance if it is offered as suggestion rather than directives, limits, or advice.

During periods of remission or adaptation, the client still faces the stigma of chronic mental illness in an increasingly complex society. Armed with appropriate skills and habits, the chronically mentally ill client may still need an *advocate*. This person assists the client to understand social systems, societal boundaries, and how to move smoothly within society.

Goals

The chronically mentally ill person has many basic problems; therefore multiple, simple goals are the norm. Six basic goals of therapy follow. Although other goals are helpful and may enrich the therapeutic climate, these six goals are almost always appropriate. For instance, the average citizen often fears the mentally ill person, investing them with superhuman power housed in an impulsive-driven body. Usually, these fears are not warranted, but enough

aggressive behavior (both to self and to others) does occur so that to dismiss the possibility of such behavior is to do the citizen a disservice. Consequently, an important therapeutic goal for many individuals is to control impulsive behavior and to do no harm to self or others.

Isolative tendencies are another behavior pattern characteristic of the chronically mentally ill person. Symbolic interactionism explains isolation as being a function of multiple social cues that have led a person to believe that he is not normal. A subsequent drifting away from these daily reminders culminates in a preference for aloneness. An appropriate goal of therapy is for the client to develop social skills and to engage himself socially.

Another life-style problem associated with chronicity is the inability for adequate problem solving. This inability manifests itself in multiple scenarios on a daily basis. Sautter and others[31] developed a problem-solving therapy approach at Tulane University that addresses this inability. Their goal is to help hospitalized clients develop an ability to problem solve in order to negotiate the give-and-take of daily life.

Hallucinations, a common perceptual distortion among the chronically mentally ill, can be both discomforting to the individual and frightening to those around him. An appropriate goal of therapy is to restore a sense of realness and to eliminate or minimize the discomfort cause by perceptual distortions.

A principal symptom of psychosis is disordered thinking. Disordered thinking can take many forms, from thought blocking to runaway thoughts. A major goal of therapy is the restoration of ordered, sequential thinking. Many clinicians believe that biological influences are responsible for these symptoms and attempt to modify those influences by the use of psychotropic medications.

Finally, the chronically mentally ill person may have somatic signs and symptoms that make his life more difficult and put him at odds with family, friends, and significant people in his life. For instance, insomnia, eating difficulties or peculiarities, hygienic practices, and burdensome hypochondriasis create their own set of problems and may exacerbate other problems (for example, poor hygiene can add to isolative behavior). A goal of therapy is to restore the client's physical well-being.

There are several basic goals for therapy. Yet goals are basic because the deficits experienced by the client are basic. The nurse should memorize these goals to be able to make an informed decision about activities and experiences that will help the client achieve them.

CHARACTERISTICS OF THERAPY

The therapeutic needs of chronically mentally ill clients are different from those of clients with acute, short-term problems. To some extent this difference results from chronicity itself. Long-term clients usually have deeply rooted dysfunctional patterns that have become integral parts of their personality.

To confront such patterns directly is asking the client to give up too much. Because these patterns are defensive, the nurse offers something with which to replace them. Therefore the nurse frequently varies therapeutic modalities, focusing on the positive goals mentioned earlier without directly addressing dysfunctional behaviors. The nurse works to create an environment or experience in which the client sees a clear personal advantage in giving up a dysfunctional pattern. Compounding these therapeutic efforts is the phenomenon of being "therapy wise." Many chronically mentally ill persons have heard the right words so long that they can fool even experienced nurses into believing that real learning is occurring.

Behavioral Approaches

Many individuals respond better to behavioral approaches than to those that emphasize communication skills. Behavioral approaches offer clearly defined expectations and foster reality orientation. Such approaches may be as complex as a token economy system (earning tokens in order to buy privileges) or as simple as time out (isolating a person who is not behaving) and social reinforcement (commenting on good appearances). All behavioral approaches are carried out with respect and acceptance.

Therapeutic Nurse-Client Relationship

The therapeutic relationship with the chronically mentally ill client is usually long term. The nurse may have followed the client through periods of hospitalization, stabilization, regression, and rehospitalization. The nurse keeps a healthy perspective by understanding that over time the client has varied and changing needs. The nurse stays flexible and encourages the client to maintain hope while assisting him to recognize realistic limitations.

Consultant Approach

Another individual therapy that frequently is helpful for the chronically mentally ill client is the *consultant* or *peer* approach. This approach is best used with the client who is stabilized and has learned to meet basic needs consistently but benefits from positive reinforcement and problem-solving assistance. The nurse avoids authoritative or parental roles while offering the client feedback in a nonjudgmental manner. This matter-of-fact consultant approach avoids confronting or challenging the client's reality while assisting him to trust and accept therapeutic assistance.

Insight-Oriented Approach

Insight-oriented approaches are generally least helpful. The focus with these clients is on building and reinforcing healthy defenses, not breaking down unhealthy ones.

Group Therapy Approach

Group therapy approaches are usually effective with chronically mentally ill clients. Such groups focus on problem solving, skill building, and support rather than on a confrontive or insight-oriented approach. The skilled nurse creates a learning environment for such clients by offering structure, encouraging but not requiring verbal participation, and modeling social skills. The nurse seeks to make the group experience enjoyable without drawing attention away from serious therapeutic goals.

After positive therapist-led group experiences, the motivated clients may prefer to participate in *peer-led* groups, i.e., support groups or skills training groups. Support groups offer the client a method of finding a family or "we group," a group of people who understand because "they've been there." The "we group" offers the client support and peer guidance while reinforcing a positive identity, a belief in the self as worthy and lovable.[12]

Family Therapy Approach

Family therapy is necessary to ensure the family's continued support of the chronically mentally ill client. As with other approaches, the family therapist avoids confrontation or even family restructuring unless the family and client are prepared and strong enough emotionally. Instead, the therapist may offer information and support to family members who are attempting to support the client. The therapist also teaches the family members and the client how to give and receive support among themselves. Other topics, as in any family therapy, include boundaries, communication, and family roles.

Couples Therapy Approach

When one partner is a chronically mentally ill client, couples or marital therapy may focus on giving support and information to the client's spouse or partner. The client in an intimate relationship often requires much support as well as assistance in clarifying boundaries. The client may also require support in bearing the pain associated with any intimate relationship. Maintaining clear communication is an important goal.

Psychopharmacological Approach

A major treatment approach in the care of the chronically mentally ill person is the use of psychotropic medications. The agents used most often are the antipsychotic agents. Chlorpromazine (Thorazine), the first antipsychotic drug, was introduced into the public mental hospital in the early 1950s. The most recent antipsychotic drug to be developed is clozapine, which was approved by the FDA in 1990. Clinical trials by Meltzer[26] indicate that as many as 68% of formerly treatment-resistant psychotic people are helped by this new drug. Clozapine not only holds much promise for chronically mentally ill individual but also is associated with a relative lack of extrapyramidal side effects (EPSEs), whereas other antipsychotic agents may cause a 70% rate of EPSE.[7] Other commonly used antipsychotic drugs are thioridazine (Mellaril) and haloperidol (Haldol). See Chapter 24 for additional information about these drugs.

NURSING PROCESS
Assessment

The assessment process with chronically mentally ill clients is important because assumptions are based on the client's current state rather than on past assessment data.

The client may be fairly hardened to the assessment

process. The nurse may face responses such as "It's in my old charts" and "You know all this stuff anyway." The nurse may gather historical information from past records and may decide to spread the assessment over several sessions to avoid overwhelming the client.

 Physical dimension If the client is an outpatient, the best place for the assessment is his home. In a residential treatment center a visit to the client's room is most informative. Caregivers, such as family or regular staff members, can provide valuable assessment data. The establishment of norms is essential for the nurse to determine the severity of the client's distress and to set more reasonable goals. A checklist that assesses how the client copes in the environment is a convenient tool for assessing important parameters of self-care (see the accompanying box).

Other common assessment concerns include current physical health (pain or chronic discomfort), adequacy of rest, family history of chronic distress, body image, and sexual image. An understanding of biochemical theory facilitates assessment. For example, a very specific and important piece of assessment data is fluidity of movement and bowel and bladder function. Because the anticholin-

ergic effects of many antipsychotic and antidepressant drugs slow peristaltic movement, constipation is a common problem.[8] Slowed movement (bradykinesia) and urinary hesitancy can also be triggered by the dopamine-blocking activity of antipsychotic drugs.

The chronically mentally ill client's income is generally low, and the nurse assesses skills the client may use to earn more money. The nurse notes the client's ability to prepare and follow a budget and use coupons and food stamps. The nurse assesses the client's ability to launder and repair clothes and to store and prepare foods.

Emotional dimension When assessing the emotional dimension, the nurse first observes the client's primary emotion. Emotions to assess include anxiety, anger, grief, despair, guilt, fear, joy, and hope. Clients may be unsophisticated about emotions and may not know what is meant by anxiety or even anger. They may deny the experience of an emotion because they believe it is too painful, too difficult to control, or too shameful to admit. Limited trust early in the nurse-client relationship may prevent clients from revealing information about their emotions during the assessment process.

The nurse assesses how intensely the client experiences various emotions and how the current affective state differs from the client's usual one. Also important to assess are the client's ability to control emotions and the degree of consistency between the client's emotional reaction and the type of situation provoking the reaction. Chronically mentally ill clients may express one emotion while experiencing another. The nurse clarifies what emotion the client is experiencing, any stimulus for the reaction, and the emotional intensity displayed. The nurse also assesses the client's general degree of emotional or affective liability.

Needs differentiation theory most clearly explains the rationale for assessing the emotional dimension for "younger" chronic clients. Emotions among this group range from apathy to frustration and anger caused by failure to meet role expectations. Being sensitive to individuals who fail to meet high aspirations is important when assessing the emotional state.

Intellectual dimension Assessment of the intellectual dimension usually reveals variations in a client's abilities between periods of regression and higher functioning. It is helpful to know the client's basic, healthy intellectual capacity rather than rely on assessments made during acute episodes. Formal testing during such an acute period may be of little assistance, but the nurse assesses the client's current intellectual capacity through the mental status examination and general observation.

During an acute period the client may also exhibit unusual thought content, such as bizarre thoughts or inability to control thoughts. The nurse determines whether these problems are also present during periods of higher functioning. The nurse assesses the client's flow of thought, observing for thought blocking and disruptions caused by hallucinations or delusions. The nurse also needs to differentiate disrupted or emotion-laded speech from abnormal thought. Chronically mentally ill clients may or may not accurately represent their thoughts in ordinary speech. They may use grandiose or unusual speech because of heightened emotions or illogical thinking. The nurse may try to help the client focus thoughts and clarify vague or

---

▼···

SAMPLE CHECKLIST OF ACTIVITIES OF DAILY LIVING TASKS

Personal Hygiene
Brushes teeth daily
Combs hair
Bathes daily
Shampoos hair three times weekly
Uses deodorant daily
Wears clean clothing
Keeps nails clean and trimmed
Dresses appropriately for activity and weather

Housekeeping and Food Management
Keeps kitchen clean and properly disposes of garbage
Does laundry as needed
Keeps bathroom clean
Keeps living areas clean and straightened
Prepares adequate, nutritious meals
Varies daily menus
Stores and cares for food properly
Keeps refrigerator and cupboards free of spoiled foods
Keeps entire area smelling fresh

Money Management
Budgets money for the month
Plans all expenditures; makes lists before shopping
Uses food stamps and coupons as much as possible
Pays bills on time and with checks or money orders
Keeps receipt of bills paid
Looks for bargains for major expenditures

Health Care
Has basic first aid supplies and uses them when needed
Keeps prescriptions renewed and filled as needed
Keeps schedule for all daily and weekly medications
Keeps schedule of regular health care appointments and makes additional ones as needed
Cares for minor illnesses appropriately
Asks for assistance or advice when needed

unusual speech to further assess intellectual function.

The nurse needs to assess how the client perceives the environment. How is the client responding to ordinary physical sensations, such as fatigue, warmth or cold, and bright or dim light? How do these perceptions differ from the norm for that client? In-depth assessment to differentiate long-standing from acute delusional systems helps the nurse plan more appropriate interventions.

The client's ability to retain and recall both recent and past information is assessed and compared to the client's normal abilities. This information helps the nurse determine the client's ability to benefit from various types of therapeutic interventions. When possible, the nurse uses observations rather than direct questions for such assessments. This approach is used because chronically mentally ill clients in an acute or regressed period become easily irritated and confused in response to direct mental status questions.

The chronically mentally ill client may have enough compensatory social skills to mask cognitive dysfunction. Thus the nurse needs to assess abstract and concrete thinking directly, such as by asking the client to interpret a proverb. Also, the nurse cannot assume orientation from conversation but rather assess it through direct questioning. Such direct questions may be less offensive if introduced in a nonthreatening manner. For example, the nurse may say, "I'm going to ask you some questions now that will sound pretty silly but are important so I can know how you think."

Many chronically mentally ill clients are rigid in their thinking. Such rigidity may be reflected in a simplistic right-wrong or good-bad view of the world. In contrast to the client with extremely rigid thinking, the client with a weak ego structure is characterized by overflexibility. This client may follow any lead, may adopt the mannerisms and values of others quite readily, and may be overly distractible. Again, it is essential to assess this behavior against the client's usual behavior.

Another intellectual variation is reflected in abnormally fast or slow speech. The nurse ascertains whether the client's rate of speech is slower or faster than the rate of thinking. The client may also exhibit overwatchfulness or unusually detailed thought and speech. Focusing on details prevents a client from perceiving the whole picture.

Chronically mentally ill clients may have little or no insight, lack appropriate judgment, and possess limited knowledge about the world and current events. The nurse assesses such information during the general interview. Questioning may focus on the client's understanding of his illness and need for assistance. The nurse may also ask how the client handles emergency needs. Casual conversation about current events seen widely in the newspaper and on television helps the nurse assess the client's general knowledge.

When assessing the client's speech, the nurse may observe aberrations such as bizarre speech, word salad, use of rhyme, and unusual voice tones. The chronically mentally ill client's nonverbal and verbal communication may be idiosyncratic during periods of higher functioning and frankly bizarre during periods of regression. For example, the client may normally use rhyme, a singsong voice, or head nodding and shrugging.

In all these areas the nurse assesses how and to what degree unusual patterns of thought and behavior affect the client's ability to function in the world. The behavior may be troublesome to others but otherwise does not interfere in the client's quest for independence. An example may be an unusual need for constant reassurance and direction. The client may know what to do but be afraid to proceed. Another example is muttering or making clicking noises. Such behaviors may need to be addressed to ensure employment but do not indicate inability to function appropriately.

The nurse also assesses vocational skills. Bachrach[1] suggests that at least six principles should be present for a successful vocational program. Principles include variety, support and back-up, realistic expectations, compensation, and acknowledgment of economic and political conditions.

Social dimension It often seems that chronically mentally ill individuals are not able to integrate their social knowledge into everyday living. Sloppy eating habits, inappropriate communication patterns, body language that frightens or repels, and disrespect for the personal space of another violate social rules of conduct. The chronically mentally ill person often breaks these rules and in the process drives away other people. The aforementioned overfocused behavior can be a causative factor as can preoccupation, distractibility, apathy, and the inability to read social cues. Symbolic interactionist theory is a helpful tool because with it the nurse can assess the extent to which the client can correctly decipher the cues of others. It is those cues that enable anyone to meet role expectations and thus develop and maintain rewarding social relationships. To the extent that we cannot read the social cues of others we tend to alienate ourselves from them.

The nurse also assesses the dynamics of family communication. Several patterns of faulty communication have been noted among families, and it can be argued that they have a more pronounced effect on this population. Communicative styles that include double messages, invalidating comments ("You screw everything up!"), lack of emotion, or high emotional content exacerbate problems among the chronically mentally ill population.

Other areas to assess include the client's level of self-esteem, the degree to which he has adopted the mental illness role, and his standing on the dependence-independence continuum. Self-esteem is an ongoing problem and is both causative and a product of chronic mental illness. That is, low self-esteem erodes therapeutic gains and hope, thus *causing* problems. The disordered state itself is a *product* of chronicity as the person is constantly reminded by life events that he is less than he "should" be. Viewing mental illness as a role, as described by symbolic interactionists, is appropriate because individuals become socialized and reinforced to act in certain ways. It is believed that the stronger the client identifies with the mental illness role the more resistant he becomes to therapeutic intervention. Assessment of dependence versus independence goes hand in hand with the assessment of self-esteem and role identification. The more dependent the client the more likely the presence of low self-esteem and strong role identification. Strategies to increase independence can be used to build self-esteem and healthier role behaviors.

As the nurse assesses these dimensions, an appropriate

plan of care can be developed to bolster social deficits. Socially acceptable behavior leading to meaningful social relationships, health-enhancing communication styles within the family leading to nurturing family dialogue, and care plans aimed at increasing independent behaviors are gained from accurate assessment data.

Spiritual dimension Chronically mentally ill clients may have difficulty with questions about their values, how they learned them, and how they make moral and ethical decisions. This difficulty results from concrete, overly abstract, or dichotomized thinking (seeing the world as only good or bad). The nurse asks questions about a belief in a higher power, in an organized religion, and in a purpose for life in general because psychiatry and religion unavoidably overlap.[10] Some elements of human brokenness are primarily spiritual.[10] As the client has the opportunity to discuss his thoughts and feelings with an objective person, the nurse is better able to assess the degree of spiritual influences on current problems.

Analysis
Nursing diagnosis

Impaired home maintenance management and altered health maintenance are examples of NANDA-approved nursing diagnoses that apply to chronically distressed clients. The defining characteristics of these nursing diagnoses are listed in the accompanying boxes.

The following case example illustrates the defining characteristics of altered health maintenance.

▼ Case Example

Mrs. S, a 60-year-old woman, has suffered from chronic mental illness for 25 years. Over the years she has been in and out of psychiatric hospitals. During her early adulthood, although having more difficulty with daily affairs than most, she managed to marry, have three children, and work outside the home. She was never able to keep a job for long, however, because of her inability to get along with co-workers and a suspiciousness that eventually alienated peers and supervisors. In 1965 Mrs. S had a "nervous breakdown" and was hospitalized in a state hospital for 3 months. Although the history of events after this point is sketchy, it is known that she has been divorced for some time, lives in a board and care facility, and has only brief, infrequent contact with her children. When she reaches the emergency room, the client is rigid and drooling and has a slightly elevated temperature. The board and care operator admitted that Mrs. S has not been eating. Mrs. S is unkempt and dirty and she has an offensive odor. The initial nursing diagnosis is altered health maintenance related to EPS manifested by inability (rigidity) to perform self-care (i.e., feeding, toileting, dressing, etc.).

The following case example illustrates the defining characteristics of impaired home maintenance management.

▼ Case Example

Mrs. L is a 50-year-old Hispanic woman with diabetes who lives alone in a run-down part of the city. She has a history of schizophrenia but has not required hospitalization because she is dangerous neither to self nor to others. The home health nurse finds the home to be overwhelmingly foul-smelling. There is dog feces all over the floors, the cluttered nature of the home makes movement difficult, and there is no clear place to sit or place her

---

▼ ALTERED HEALTH MAINTENANCE

DEFINITION

Inability to identify, manage, and/or seek help to maintain health.

DEFINING CHARACTERISTICS
- **Physical dimension**

  Lack of equipment

- **Intellectual dimension**

  Lack of knowledge about basic health practices
  Lack of adaptive behaviors to internal or external environmental changes
  Inability to take responsibility for meeting basic health practices in any or all functional patterns areas
  Expressed interest in improving health behaviors

- **Social dimension**

  Lack of health-seeking behavior
  Lack of financial or other resources
  Impairment of personal support system

Modified from Kim MJ, McFarland GK, McLane AM, editors: *Pocket guide to nursing diagnoses*, ed 5, St. Louis, 1993, Mosby–Year Book.

▼ IMPAIRED HOME MAINTENANCE MANAGEMENT

DEFINITION

Inability to independently maintain a safe growth-producing immediate environment.

DEFINING CHARACTERISTICS
- **Physical dimension**

  Disorderly surroundings
  Household members express difficulty in maintaining their home in a comfortable fashion
  Unwashed or unavailable cooking equipment, clothes, or linen
  Accumulation of dirt, food wastes, or hygienic wastes
  Offensive odors
  Inappropriate household temperature
  Lack of necessary equipment or aids
  Presence of vermin or rodents
  Repeated hygienic disorders, infestations, or infections

- **Emotional dimension**

  Overtaxed family members (e.g., exhausted, anxious family members)

- **Intellectual dimension**

  Household members request assistance with home maintenance

- **Social dimension**

  Household members describe outstanding debts or financial crises

Modified from Kim MJ, McFarland GK, McLane AM, editors: *Pocket guide to nursing diagnoses*, ed 5, St. Louis, 1993, Mosby–Year Book.

equipment. With a heavy accent Mrs. L states that the neighbors are always trying to break in and that she is afraid to go outside. The nurse is unclear as to whether Mrs. L is delusional. The nurse finds almost no food in the house and when the nurse asked to see Mrs. L's medication the nurse is shown a whole shoe box full of medications. Mrs. L is not clear what she is taking, why she is taking it, or when she should take it. The initial nursing diagnosis is impaired home maintenance management related to cognitive dysfunction manifested by unhealthy living environment (filthy home, no food, poor compliance to medications).

The following list provides examples of other nursing diagnoses with causative statements appropriate for the chronically mentally ill client:
1. Impaired decision making related to cognitive dysfunction
2. Impaired social interaction related to withdrawal from external world
3. Altered thought processes: delusion related to inability to evaluate reality
4. Social isolation related to withdrawal from others
5. Powerlessness related to low self-esteem

Planning

Table 32-3 presents a nursing care plan with long- and short-term goals, interventions, outcome criteria, and rationales related to therapy with the chronically mentally client, which are examples of the planning stage in the nursing process.

Implementation

Physical dimension The nurse provides clients who have lost bowel and bladder control with a toileting schedule. Punitive measures or any type of subtle confrontation in this area is counterproductive. The client responds best to regularity and consistency and a calm approach. For individuals who are constipated due to the anticholinergic effect of drugs, the nurse teaches the importance of adequate fluids and dietary roughage. Urinary hesitancy can be relieved by running warm water over the perineum.

Mr. T, a 67-year-old white man, has been hospitalized many times due to his schizophrenic behavior. He is taking Haldol, 5 mg bid. He is complaining of inability to void. The nurse assesses for bladder distention.

The nurse encourages improved body image by helping clients focus more on their bodies. A mirror may be used on an inpatient ward during supervised time to allow clients to assess themselves physically. Exercise programs often help clients relate more realistically to their physical functioning. Making clear, matter-of-fact comments about positive physical attributes gives the client useful feedback.

When assisting the client to learn hygiene skills, a concrete behavioral approach may be of greatest help. The nurse starts with very basic behaviors such as teaching the client to comb hair, brush teeth, or button a shirt. The nurse reviews these skills and has the client perform them. Next, the nurse tells the client when these behaviors are expected. A chart placed in the client's room is usually a helpful reminder. The client at first may require supervision and then only a reminder. After completion of each behav-

ior, the nurse praises the client. Comments about improved appearance are rewarding feedback. Eating habits may be shaped through a similar behavioral program. Nondisruptive mealtime behavior may be rewarded with nutritional treats or special privileges.

Bill R, a 40-year-old chronically mentally ill client, has an offensive body odor and is wearing dirty clothes. The nurse announces to Mr. R, "Your shower is ready. We have clean clothes for you to wear."

Chronically mentally ill clients usually have a higher level of functioning in all dimensions when they take medications properly. The nurse's first task may be to help the client recognize differences in personal function when taking and not taking medication. Clients may be impressed by before-and-after photographs; audiotapes; or feedback from family, friends, and staff. The client is helped to accept the necessity of the medication regimen as a current reality. The client who experiences more freedom and success while taking medication may be motivated by support and reminders to continue.

Chronically mentally ill clients usually display cues before they lose control or begin acting out. When cues of impending loss of control are observed, the client is removed to a less stimulating environment. The nurse avoids confrontations when the client is losing behavioral control. Nurses need to avoid entering into power struggles with the client who may be losing control. The nurse sets only limits necessary for the client's safety, ignores minor infractions, and uses extra care to enforce limits matter-of-factly and nonintrusively. It is safest for such clients to remain in their room or alone in a quiet room. Staff members check on the client frequently to make their presence known. In general the physical presence of alert staff serves as external control and reduces acting-out episodes.

The client's physical environment may be unstimulating, chaotic, or otherwise nonconducive to health. The nurse may wish to suggest or assist in improvements. Any cooperation or improvement is praised. The nurse may suggest changes in the environment that would better reflect the client's desires.

Eating and sleeping are made more pleasant to the client and are thus encouraged. The client is assisted to relax before meals or bedtime. Areas for dining or sleeping are used only for these purposes and are made attractive and comfortable. Clients with high levels of anxiety may require reassurance and support to relax enough to eat or sleep.

Emotional dimension Interventions in the emotional dimension begin with helping clients understand that they can bear uncomfortable experiences. With support and patience the nurse teaches the client how to tolerate higher levels of anxiety and greater sadness, as well as more intense anger.

Such emotional tolerance develops after the therapeutic relationship is established, when the client trusts the nurse sufficiently to discuss difficult emotions. When the client experiences intense emotions, the nurse reassures the client and suggests safe methods of decreasing anxiety. The nurse assists the client to defuse the situation by focusing on thoughts instead of feelings. The nurse accepts the client's emotional outbursts, sets time limits to prevent harmful escalation, and allows the client to return to activ-

GOALS	OUTCOME CRITERIA	INTERVENTIONS	RATIONALES
NURSING DIAGNOSIS: Altered health maintenance related to inability to use sound judgment			
LONG TERM			
To recognize early changes in health state and to take appropriate action	Gets more rest and increases fluid intake when client has a cold.	Teach client adequate amount of rest and fluid needed when he has a cold.	Awareness of what is adequate may motivate the client to meet the need for rest and fluid.
	Recognizes signs of a fever, takes temperature appropriately, and reports any elevation to visiting nurse.	Teach client to read a thermometer and know when temperature is elevated.	Enables client to make a decision about when to report to visiting nurse.
	Makes appointment to see physician if health disruption persists or worsens.	Provide name and telephone number of physician.	It is easier to contact the physician when client has name and telephone number.
SHORT TERM			
To take medications as ordered	Makes lists of medications with scheduled times.	Assist client in developing a list of prescribed medications with schedule for taking them.	Gives client a sense of participation and increases compliance.
	Pays attention to direction of taking medication before or after meals, or any other specific directions, and includes these with time schedule.	Discuss with client specific directions for taking medications.	Increases chances client will take medications as prescribed.
	Reminds physician when prescription renewals are needed.	Have client record name of physician and when prescription needs to be renewed on a calendar.	The visual aid serves as a useful reminder to renew prescriptions.
	Keeps prescriptions filled so that no doses are missed.		
NURSING DIAGNOSIS: Impaired home maintenance management related to lack of knowledge			
LONG TERM			
To recognize in advance and plan for needed home maintenance work	Recognizes slowed drainage in sink and notifies landlord.	Describe slowed drainage and how to notify landlord.	Provides client with information needed to notify landlord.
	Keeps sidewalks and outdoor stairs free of ice and snow for safe walking.	Assist client to develop a plan for keeping sidewalks and outdoor stairs safe for walking.	Prepares client to take action as soon as need arises.
	Investigates faucet drips and toilet leaks when possible, and notifies landlord if problem is complicated.	Teach client how to check faucet drips and toilet leaks and know when to notify landlord.	Gives client a feeling of responsibility.
SHORT TERM			
To keep home free of clutter, clean, and odor free	Does laundry frequently to avoid piles of dirty clothes.	Encourage to do laundry each week.	With a scheduled time for doing laundry, may follow through.
	Does dishes after every meal.	Explain importance of doing dishes after each meal.	Knowledge of importance may motivate client to do dishes after meals.
	Cleans bathroom fixtures weekly.	Show client how to clean bathroom fixtures.	Demonstration provides a clear, concrete example of what is expected.

ities without guilt or shame when behavior is under control.

Clients first learn the relationship between their physiological experiences and thoughts and behavior. The nurse assists the client in recognizing how the emotional experience relates to the situation or problem that resulted in such intense emotions. For example, clients learn how their body feels when they are angry. The nurse guides the client to examine the thoughts that accompany anger, such as "That person was unfair to me," "That person did not listen to me and acted as if I weren't there," or "I need to get even with that person." The client then learns that the stimulus was the perception of being ignored or overlooked by another person. The client's perception may have been inaccurate; the person involved may not have seen or heard the client. Even if the client is not motivated enough to understand why certain situations result in such strong reactions, he learns to minimize acting-out behaviors in response to intense emotion by learning that the intense emotions are not always cues to action and to think through the situation before acting.

With time, experience, and support the client frequently learns to understand the experience of intense emotions. These emotions may serve as cues that indicate a need to seek therapeutic assistance, resume taking psychotropic medications, or otherwise reduce stress and seek support. The client may also learn to decrease emotional reactions to hallucinations, delusions, or bizarre thoughts. Even if such experiences continue, they need not interfere with the client's functioning.

The nurse uses well-timed feedback, reassurance, modeling, and instructional information to teach the client new attitudes about emotions. The client learns that unpleasant emotions can be accepted and that they will not overwhelm the client or the nurse.

Intellectual dimension The nurse addresses motivation with the chronically mentally ill client. How can the client be helped to see a change of behavior as desirable? Staff approval or attention does not usually contribute to long-term change because clients tend to "act nice" for specific staff members rather than for themselves or their goals. With some clients a specific reward, such as a nutritional snack or a favorite activity, is helpful in maintaining progress. As their self-esteem and self-image grow, clients may wish to change simply to please themselves. However, clients frequently regress when goal attainment is in sight because of their anxiety about changing and assuming new roles and responsibilities.

Reaching a goal, such as independent placement or a job, may mean that the client's image to others and self will change. New expectations will be placed on the client. A total rearrangement of plans and goals may be necessary if the client really did not expect to attain the goal. Carrying a self-image of "helpless" or "incompetent" may not be pleasant, but it is at least familiar. Changes in self-image and behavior are closely supported and constantly reinforced by the nurse. The client may be discouraged easily if accepting the change in status means increased frustration. At such times the nurse strongly encourages the client to continue in the effort; too much confrontation shifts ownership of the goal to the nurse rather than to the clients and results in withdrawal, anger, or both. The nurse works *with* the client, not for or on the client. The motivation is ultimately the client's.

The client learns to accept the nature of delusions and hallucinations. Clients usually cannot accept such perceptions as false, but they may be able to accept them as meaningless, harmless, and unworthy of attention. The client may learn through a trusting relationship with the nurse that the hallucinations and delusions are not reality to other people. The client may also learn how to avoid revealing to others that he experiences perceptions that others do not. The nurse teaches this skill in a way that avoids shaming the client. The client needs to recognize that the nurse honestly accepts these perceptions as very real to the client.

Chronically mentally ill clients sometimes exhibit negative patterns of communication. Such clients complain constantly of being unable to do everything from opening their eyes to walking. A behavioral approach to this problem is to politely ignore such statements when they are repeated. The nurse diverts the client's attention through a firm, casual change of topic or directive. If the client says, "I can't walk," the nurse might say, "Take my hand and we'll walk down the hall." The nurse avoids trying to reason with chronically mentally ill clients; they may continue in their negativity even after their behavior has improved. As the client acquires more pleasant thoughts, such statements decrease.

The client's ability to communicate can be improved through the nurse's clear, consistent, and repeated feedback. The nurse asks the client to clarify general, confused, or bizarre communications when she observes that the client can tolerate such confrontations. During acute states the nurse may need to request clarification, but only to facilitate basic communication.

The nurse may assist the client in focusing the conversation. The nurse also asks the client to verbalize his understanding of what the nurse has said. The nurse does the same in response to the client's communications. These checks for distortions of perception also emphasize for the client the importance of clear communication between people.

The client can develop orientation, memory, and basic cognitive skills within a growth-promoting therapeutic relationship. Time is set aside daily for the nurse to orient the client. Games, storytelling, current events groups, and general conversation stimulate the client intellectually and eventually help improve cognitive function. As cognition improves, the client may find it easier to focus attention more on reality and goal setting and less on hallucinations or delusions. This approach will not extinguish dysfunctional perception, but it may allow the client to focus on something else.

Judgment generally improves with life experiences, especially successful ones. Chronically mentally ill clients tend to gain such maturity slowly and at great costs. They may never achieve real insight. A reasonable goal in this area is for clients to accept their own limitations, needs, and abilities. The clients, as well as the health care providers, may never know why such limitations exist. Motivation to achieve any insight probably comes from a supportive relationship, a realistic role model, and a consistent, client approach.

Social dimension The chronically mentally ill client is likely to require external motivation to develop new social behaviors. The nurse finds motivators for the client's specific interest; that is, food preference can be manipulated into a social context. The client probably will not be affected by a simple plea to display socially acceptable behavior. The client may not desire closeness with others or a supportive relationship and may therefore lack the ordinary motivators to adopt socially appropriate behavior. At the same time, social skills ultimately determine the client's chance for independence.

For many reasons the chronically mentally ill client is frequently not motivated to carry out socially accepted behaviors that may increase self-esteem. However, the client may learn self-understanding and self-acceptance if the nurse expresses understanding and acceptance of the client. If the nurse can genuinely accept the client's unpredictable disease, occasionally disruptive behavior, and sometimes bizarre communication and appearance, the client may accept experiences and behaviors and see how to make realistic changes. The research highlight describes a social learning approach to develop social skills.

The client frequently regresses after an initial period of increased responsiveness because of anxiety about change. However, a skillful nurse can effectively use the honeymoon period by encouraging as many new activities as the client can tolerate. The nurse hopes that during this responsive period the client is exposed to an activity or interaction that becomes an internal source of motivation. The nurse may find the client unusually open to feedback regarding hygiene habits or social skills. If other people praise the client's newly formed skills or improved habits, such behaviors may continue. The goal is for the client to find more

satisfaction in displaying socially acceptable behavior than withdrawn or regressed behavior.

A client experiencing severe regression responds best to consistent, one-to-one interactions with the nurse. Initially, the honeymoon effect of increased attention from another person will improve behavior. This effect occurs most often in clients who have not been previously involved in a therapeutic relationship. The client ideally views the relationship as a means of solving all problems, as if the acceptance and warmth alone can motivate any necessary change. The client may begin to mimic the nurse's behaviors. The nurse becomes a powerful role model in teaching social skills.

The nurse assists the clients to examine self-image and self-esteem. The nurse's support allows the client to evaluate self-image for its accuracy. The client also examines the degree of self-liking and the unfairness or harm of self-dislike. The nurse discusses self-image and self-esteem using reflection and active listening, thus making apparently social conversation a therapeutic measure. The chronically distressed client may respond better to social interactions than to analytical, confrontive, or otherwise professional interactions. The nurse maintains a professional role, but it may be more human, less objective, and less removed.

Appropriate sexual behaviors may be more difficult for nurses to foster because of their own discomfort with the subject. Again, specific behavioral expectations are clarified with the client. The nurse allows the client to express his feelings about sexual issues and offers sincere understand-

---

RESEARCH HIGHLIGHT

Teaching Chronic Psychiatric Inpatients to Use Differential Attention to Change Each Other's Behavior

- LP Baenninger and W Tang

PURPOSE

This study was designed to investigate the effectiveness of differentiated attention as a significant therapeutic modality.

SAMPLE

The subjects were clients in the Adaptive Living Program, a 26-bed coed unit in a state hospital. Nine men and four women patients were included and their improvement on 21 targeted behaviors was examined. Ages ranged from 19 to 37 years. Eight clients were white and five were black; none were married, and all were diagnosed as having some form of schizophrenia.

METHODOLOGY

A multiple baseline design was used. Target behaviors that could normally be observed between 8 and 9 AM were chosen. All clients were included in twice-a-week, half-hour classes in which they were taught differentiated attention. They were taught to praise targeted behaviors and to withdraw attention from unwanted behaviors. Interobserver agreement averaged 90.8.

From *Hospital and Community Psychiatry* 41:425, 1990.

FINDINGS

Targeted desired behaviors doubled in frequency. Peer-initiated target behavior improved more than self-initiated behaviors. Target behaviors included self-care and adaptive and social skills.

IMPLICATIONS

Clients who can perform self-care are better able to live outside the hospital. Clients who develop adaptive skills, that is, patients who can respond positively to the attention of others and to screen out criticisms, are less likely to experience relapse. Clients who develop social skills become more tolerable to others and are better suited to community living than they were before learning these skills.

ing of the client's problems in controlling behavior. The nurse helps the client understand possible consequences of sexual acting out. The nurse does not criticize the client's value system or moral character. Decisions about sexual behavior, especially when the client is viewed as competent, are ultimately left to the client. For example, a client may choose to begin a sexual relationship with another client in an outpatient therapy program. Unless the program prohibits such action, this decision should be left to the two clients involved. Another example is the client who has a homosexual relationship. This may seem inappropriate to some staff but may be the client's choice. Most inpatient settings do not permit sexual activity among clients, but it may still occur, especially when the clients are off the premises. The nurse may intervene only to offer information or to aid in decision making that would reduce the likelihood of harm to the client or others. In inpatient settings, calm, matter-of-fact vigilance by staff will generally prevent sexual acting-out behaviors.

Struggles concerning dependence and independence may be the nurse's greatest challenge. The nurse offers needed support and nurturance. As the client progresses, however, the nurse takes a more supportive role. Slowly, in response to cues of growth, the nurse becomes more of a peer consultant and helps the client find additional and appropriate means of meeting dependence needs. Decreasing dependence on the nurse is a frightening process for many chronically mentally ill clients; they may regress when faced with real independence, such as separation from the nurse. The nurse anticipates the regression and offers support and acceptance but always focuses on the goal of independence.

Throughout all these struggles, the client occasionally tests the nurse. Such testing continues throughout relationships with chronically mentally ill clients because trust is difficult for them. The nurse cannot expect rapid or complete trust; the client may have a lifetime of evidence indicating that trust is impossible or unwise. The nurse respects the client's need to test. During testing, the nurse uses an intellectual or rational approach to the client, as emotional approaches may be too threatening. See Chapter 17 for approaches to developing trust.

Clients progressing toward independence frequently benefit most from interactions with their peers. Group interactions may offer structured opportunities to try new social behaviors. Support groups help chronically mentally ill clients examine their past, current, and future roles as members of society. Such conversation helps clients reaffirm the reality of their perceptions, thoughts, and feelings while conveying a sense of shared experiences. Clients may discuss society's influence in labeling clients as mentally ill; they may even talk about institutionalization. Such discussion offers an opportunity to express anger in an appropriate context. The nurse encourages the client to find a supportive "we group."

Board and care homes provide an alternative to hospitalization. The client often enters a board and care facility not knowing a person in the home. Sharing a room, a relative lack of privacy and security for possessions, and structured times for meals and sleep all present challenges in the social dimension and create a measure of dependency. Board and care homes are a needed resource in our communities and, due to governmental control, are becoming more therapeutic environments.

Spiritual dimension The client who can think abstractly and concretely and maintain a realistic view of life may benefit from conversations with the nurse about the client's belief system, values, morals, and ethics. Chronically mentally ill clients may have been unable to integrate such information during adolescence because of disturbed behavior or cognition. These clients need an opportunity to explore concepts of values and personal ethics as part of the process of differentiation and individuation. Concepts of hope and faith assist clients to withstand society's pessimism regarding their goals and aspirations. Spiritual inquiries can aid clients in understanding that all people have struggles, thus reducing their isolation and alienation.

Some chronically mentally ill clients have problems with abstract and concrete thinking. They misinterpret the intent of spiritual discussions and cannot approach spirituality realistically or meaningfully. If clients have delusions about religious rituals or mysticism, the staff instructs them to avoid religious topics as a means of controlling psychotic thinking.

The nurse ascertains the client's ability to benefit from discussions of spirituality before entering into them. If such discussions occur, the nurse clarifies personal beliefs and biases so as not to adversely affect the client's thinking. The nurse also is careful not to influence the development of the client's belief system away from natural inclinations.

Evaluation

The chronically mentally ill client frequently offers the greatest challenge to the nurse's creativity. Evaluation conferences may reveal that the client has made little progress. In this case, more beneficial approaches are attempted.

The client may be more comfortable if close friends or family are present for a conference. These individuals are also useful sources of evaluation data and are integral to the client's treatment because they form the necessary support system. Staff should listen to family and friends regarding their impressions of the client's progress. The client may hide much of which the family is aware from staff members. The family also can better appraise whether the changes in the client will last.

PATIENTS' RIGHTS

Patients' rights, especially those of the severely dysfunctional, chronically mentally ill client, will require more attention in the future. Chronically mentally ill clients have the right to accept or reject assistance and to make their own decisions, even if their decisions do not seem to be based on sound judgment. Only if clients seem dangerous to themselves or others can interventions be made without their consent.

Although many chronically mentally ill clients probably will not benefit from any treatment approaches, some still have treatment forced on them. Some clients do respond to legally forced treatment and are released to pursue their usual, hazardous, marginal life-styles, refusing therapeutic services. Many clients recognize that they have to "get along" with the mental health system to survive and maintain what independence they have. They frequently feel bitter after receiving legally forced treatment and believe their rights and bodies were violated. Such treatment may destroy therapeutic goals of trust and goodwill.

The problem is complex. Chronically mentally ill clients may "look normal" but be dangerous to society or themselves. On the other hand, they may fit the stereotype of a psychotic person and be perfectly capable of caring for themselves and perhaps even nurturing others. These clients may distance health care professionals so that they are unable to assess their clients. Clients have the right to choose this distance if they desire.

BRIEF REVIEW

Chronic mental illness is the major mental health issue of the 1990s. Our city streets, board and care homes, public mental hospitals, and psychiatric units in general hospitals are among the many places where the chronically mentally ill currently live. These individuals are not homogeneous but vary widely in ability to function, maintain relationships, and communicate. The nurse is concerned with five dimensions of care: physical, emotional, intellectual, social, and spiritual. Through assessing and then implementing a plan of care in each dimension, the nurse provides a balanced approach to treating the chronically mentally ill client.

REFERENCES AND SUGGESTED READINGS

1. Andreason NC: Brain imaging application in psychiatry, *Science* 239:381, 1988.
2. Bachrach L: Dimensions of disability in the chronic mentally ill, *Hospital and Community Psychiatry* 37(10):981, 1986.
3. Bachrach L: Defining mental illness: a concept paper, *Hospital and Community Psychiatry* 39:383, 1988.
4. Bachrach LL: Perspectives on work and rehabilitation, *Hospital and Community Psychiatry* 42(9):890, 1991.
5. Baenninger LP, Tang W: Teaching chronic psychiatric inpatients to use differential attention to change each other's behavior, *Hospital and Community Psychiatry* 41:425, 1990.
6. Baier M: Case management with the chronically mentally ill, *Journal of Psychosocial Nursing and Mental Health Services* 25(6):17, 1987.
7. Barrett N, Ormistom S, Molyneux V: Clozapine: a new drug for schizophrenia, *Journal of Psychosocial Nursing and Mental Health Services* 28:24, 1990.
8. Batey RS: Schizophrenic disorders. In Di Piro JT, Talbert RL, Hayes PE, editors: *Pharmacotherapy: a pathological approach,* New York, 1989, Elsevier.
9. Bawden EL: Reaching out to the chronically mentally ill homeless, *Journal of Psychosocial Nursing and Mental Health Services* 28(3):6, 1990.
10. Browning DS, Jobe T, Evison JS: *Religion and ethical factors in psychiatric practice,* Chicago, 1990, Nelson-Hall.
11. Carlson C, Blackwell B: *Behavioral concepts and nursing intervention,* ed 2, Philadelphia, 1978, JB Lippincott.
12. deCangas JPC: Exploring expressed emotion: does it contribute to chronic mental illness? *Journal of Psychosocial Nursing and Mental Health Services* 28(2):31, 1990.
13. Dzurec LC: How do they see themselves? Self-perception and functioning for people with chronic schizophrenia, *Journal of Psychosocial Nursing* 28(8):10, 1990.
14. Flaskerud JH: Profile of chronically mentally ill psychotic patients in four community mental health centers, *Issues in Mental Health Nursing* 8(2):155, 1986.
15. Gallop R, Wynn F: Difficult young adult chronic patients: re-evaluating short-term clinical management, *Journal of Psychosocial Nursing and Mental Health Services* 24(3):29, 1986.
16. Goffman E: *Stigma,* Englewood Cliffs, NJ, 1963, Prentice-Hall.
17. Gold Award: A network of services for homeless chronic mentally ill, *Hospital and Community Psychiatry* 37(11):1148, 1986.
18. Goldman H, Gattozzi J, Taube C: Defining and counting the chronically mentally ill, *Hospital and Community Psychiatry* 32(1):21, 1981.
19. Johnson AB: *Out of Bedlam: the truth about deinstitutionalization,* New York, 1990, Basic Books.
20. Keltner NL, Schwecke L, Bostram C: *Psychiatric nursing: a psychotherapeutic management approach,* St Louis, 1991, Mosby–Year Book.
21. Koyanagi C, Goldman HH: The quiet success of the national plan for the chronically mentally ill, *Hospital and Community Psychiatry* 42(9):899, 1991.
22. Lefley HP: Culture and chronic mental illness, *Hospital and Community Psychiatry* 41:277, 1990.
23. Liberman RP, DeRisi WJ, Mueser KT: *Social skills training for psychiatric patients,* New York, 1989, Pergamon.
24. McCausland MP: Deinstitutionalization of the mentally ill: oversimplification of complex issues, *Advances in Nursing Science* 9(3):24, 1987.
25. Meddaugh DI: Reactions: understanding aggressive behavior in long-term care, *Journal of Psychosocial Nursing* 28(4):28, 1990.
26. Meltzer HY: Duration of clozapine treatment in neuroleptic-resistant schizophrenia, *Archives of General Psychiatry* 46:672, 1989.
27. Miller JF: Inspiring hope, *American Journal of Nursing* 85(1):22, 1985.
28. Norwind B: Developing an enforceable "right to treatment" therapy for the chronically mentally disabled in the community, *Schizophrenia Bulletin* 8:4, 1982.
29. Pepper B, Kirshner MC, Ryglewicz H: The young adult chronic patient: overview of a population, *Hospital and Community Psychiatry* 32:463, 1982.
30. Puryear DA, Lovitt R, Miller DA: Characteristics of elderly persons seen in an urban psychiatric emergency room, *Hospital and Community Psychiatry* 42(8):802, 1991.
31. Sautter FJ, Heaney C, O'Neill P: A problem-solving approach to group psychotherapy in the inpatient milieu, *Hospital and Community Psychiatry* 42(8):814, 1991.
32. Sheets JL, Prevost JA, Reihman J: The young adult chronic patient: three hypothesized subgroups, *New Directions for Mental Health Services* 14:15, 1982.

ANNOTATED BIBLIOGRAPHY

Koyanagi C, Goldman HH: The quiet success of the national plan for the chronically mentally ill, *Hospital and Community Psychiatry* 42(9):899, 1991.

Koyanagi and Goldman describe the 1978 national plan, the restraining forces that kept changes from occurring, and the "quiet" implementation of four major dimensions of the plan. An analysis of each dimension coupled with a good news–bad news evaluation provides informative reading. They conclude with recommendations for the future.

Johnson AB: *Out of Bedlam: the truth about deinstitutionalization,* New York, 1990, Basic Books.

Johnson thoroughly reviews the historical changes in American society that led to the evacuation of state hospitals and the consequent rise in homelessness. Johnson debunks a series of myths: that deinstitutionalization was planned, that it saves money, that drugs can cure mental illness, that the mentally ill are better off in the community, and that most of the homeless are ex-mental patients.

Therapy with Clients with Dementia

Judith R Lentz

After studying this chapter, the student will be able to:

- Discuss the historical development of ideas related to dementia
- Identify major theories related to the etiology of dementia
- Implement the nursing process with clients with dementia
- Discuss the psychopathology of dementia as described in the DSM-III-R
- Discuss research related to clients with dementia

Dementia is characterized by an observable disturbance in previously unimpaired mental functioning. It results from environmental, physical, or emotional impairments of brain functioning and causes disturbances in an individual's behavior, judgment, and intellect. Dementia often comes to the attention of caregivers when the family can no longer cope with an individual's deteriorating behavior and judgment.[29,71]

Dementia constitutes a major public health problem and a major mental health problem among the elderly. Dementia is by no means inevitable with aging, but the elderly are more vulnerable to it. Chronic illness, diminished hearing and sight, poor nutrition, social isolation, and drug reactions not only complicate but cause cerebral impairments. Physical illnesses, especially multiple conditions typical of older, more gravely ill clients, also seem to predispose to the development of dementia.[47,63]

Client management problems are common. Individuals overreact, become agitated and confused, wander off, or become unusually anxious or depressed and often disrupt usual social and interpersonal relationships. Caregivers are often overwhelmed trying to meet the individual's needs as well as compensate for his unmet roles and responsibilities. Caring for a seriously impaired individual is not only physically and emotionally demanding but often socially isolating and unrewarding.

DSM-III-R DIAGNOSES

Dementia is classified in the DSM-III-R under Organic Mental Disorders. The essential feature of dementia is impairment in short- and long-term memory. Impairment in abstract thinking, judgment, and disturbances in higher cortical functioning or personality change is also exhibited. The disturbances involve psychological or behavioral ab-

normalities and are associated with a brain dysfunction. No single description characterizes dementia. The differences in clinical presentation reflect differences in the location, mode of onset, progression, duration, and nature of the underlying pathophysiological process. The diagnosis of dementia is made when loss of intellectual functioning is sufficiently severe to interfere with social or occupational functioning.

Dementia may be progressive, static, or remitting. The reversibility of dementia is a function of the underlying pathology and the availability of effective treatment.

A wide variety of emotional, motivational, and behavioral abnormalities are associated with dementia, with memory impairment being the most common symptom initially. Severe emotional disturbances may accompany cognitive impairment including anxiety, depression, irritability, and shame. Paranoid attitudes and delusions may be exhibited. Decreased impulse control and social judgment often accompany the impaired cognitive functioning.

▶ **DIAGNOSES Related to Dementia**

MEDICAL DIAGNOSES	NURSING DIAGNOSES
Dementias arising during the senium and presenium	Altered thought processes
Psychoactive substance-induced organic mental disorders	
Organic mental disorders associated with Axis III physical disorders	

DATES	EVENTS
1500	Rene Descartes provides the conceptual basis for perceiving the mind as separate from the body.
1700-1800	The idea that psychological functions have a specific location and biological correlates is elaborated.
Late 1800s	Huling Jackson disputed the locational theory, which viewed cerebral organization and psychological functioning as determined by location, and advocated a holistic, integrated theory of brain organization and function.
1900s	Psychology and neurology become separate medical specialties.
1940s	Goldstein and Luria document the effects of brain damage on personality and social adjustment.
1950s	Luria documents that a lesion in a circumscribed area of the brain leads to complete loss of a function. He proposes that neurological organization is based on a vertical hierarchy of neurological function.
1960s	Extensive psychobiological research provides a scientific basis for overcoming the mind-body dichotomy. Technological advances give researchers and physicians a new view of the brain.
1970s-1980s	Neurobiological aspects of psychological functions are better defined, reopening old questions about brain and mind and about nature and nurture. Lipowski among others have further documented the physiological and psychological changes associated with delirium. Sociopsychological factors are increasingly implicated in the roles of cerebral/organization.
1990s	Increased emphasis on human consciousness and how various cultural artifacts, such as dependency on alphabetic writing systems, change the consciousness of social groups and how dreams, music, poetry, meditation (or prayer), and exercise change the consciousness of individuals.
Future	Neurological and psychological impairments are likely to be less clearly differentiated as both are increasingly described as changes in consciousness. As consciousness becomes a more important theoretical concept, researchers in both the neurological and psychological sciences are likely to look to Eastern philosophy and religions (Buddhism) or to modern physics (particle physics) for theoretical models that better explain the phenomenon of complex, organic relationships. As people live longer and various neurological diseases/injuries become less incompatible with life, nurses in all areas of practice can expect to identify and care for clients with a variety of limitations secondary to neurological impairment or damage.

Categories of dementia according to severity include the following:

Mild	Impaired work or social functioning Ability for independent living Adequate personal hygiene
Moderate	Independent living is hazardous Some supervision required
Severe	Continual supervision required because of impaired activities of daily living

Medical diagnoses related to dementia include those arising during the senium and presenium, those that are substance induced, and those associated with Axis III physical disorders.

Senium and Presenium Dementia

Dementias arising during the senium and presenium include primary degenerative dementia, Alzheimer type, and multiinfarct dementia.

Primary degenerative dementia, Alzheimer type

The essential feature of this condition is its insidious onset and a deteriorating course with loss of intellectual abilities and changes in personality. Onset is more common after age 65.

Multiinfarct dementia

The essential feature of this disorder is a dementia due to cerebrovascular disease. Patchy deterioration in intellectual functioning occurs, leaving some areas of intellect intact. Neurological signs and symptoms such as weakness in limbs, reflex asymmetries, and small-stepped gait are present.

Psychoactive Substance-Induced Organic Mental Disorders

This diagnosis is made when the ingestion of psychoactive substances directly affects the nervous system. The DSM-III-R lists 11 classes of nonmedical substances that are commonly taken to alter mood or behavior: alcohol, amphetamines, caffeine, cannabis, cocaine, hallucinogens, inhalants, nicotine, opioids, phencyclidine (PCP), and sedatives. These disorders are distinguished from psychoactive substance use disorders, which refer to the maladaptive behaviors associated with taking the substance. Frequently, people with a psychoactive substance use disorder also have a psychoactive substance-induced organic mental disorder.

Organic Mental Disorder Associated with Axis III

Specific organic mental disorders associated with physical conditions include the following:

1. Delirium	Reduced ability to maintain attention to stimuli, disorganized thinking, reduced level of consciousness, disorientation, memory impairment
2. Dementia	Impairment in short- and long-term memory
3. Amnesic disorder	Impairment of short- and long-term memory with remote events remembered better than recent events
4. Organic delusional disorder	Presence of delusions
5. Organic hallucinosis	Presence of hallucinations
6. Organic mood disorder	Persistent depressed or elevated mood
7. Organic anxiety disorder	Recurrent panic attacks
8. Organic personality disorders	Persistent personality disturbance, either lifelong or representing a change in a previous trait

(Each has an identifiable organic factor that contributes to the condition.)

THEORETICAL APPROACHES

Biological

Dementia is a chronic, progressive, and usually nonpsychotic deterioration in mental functioning. The onset of symptoms is often insidious, typically including progressive impairment of intellect. The nature and extent of intellectual impairment depends primarily on which brain and/or vascular structures are diseased.

Dementia is more common after age 65 and affects 20% of people over age 80.[58] Deterioration in intellectual functioning is recognized as a clinical syndrome when occupational or social performance becomes problematic. The amount of physical change necessary to cause observable or measurable deterioration in intellectual function is relative, depending on physical and emotional stress, preexisting knowledge and skills, and the complexity of the task at hand. Clients with dementia have increasingly less tolerance for any stress and less ability to recover from its physical and emotional effects. Their condition makes them susceptible to drug reactions, dramatic complications from minor physical symptoms such as constipation, and minor emotional or social disruptions. In time the progression of the disease affects the individual's ability to perform the most basic tasks.[58] Some become totally dependent, noncommunicative, and bedridden before death.

The most common dementia is senile dementia of the Alzheimer type. Alzheimer-type diseases are characterized by the appearance of abnormal structures such as senile plaques, neurofibrillary tangles, and granulovascular structures in the cerebral cortex and limbic system (hippocampus). These cortical dementias are characterized by impaired cognition, amnesia, aphasia without impaired speech, social inhibition, apathy, and normal motor function (until late stages).

Cortical Alzheimer-type dementias need to be differentiated from subcortical dementias, which involve lower brain structures (basal ganglia, thalamus, brain stem) and are often more amenable to treatment with surgery or drugs.[60] Common causes of subcortical dementia include Huntington's disease, hydrocephalus, chronic toxic metabolic disturbances, and Parkinson's disease. Unlike cortical dementias, these diseases are often characterized by depressed mood, speech dysarthria, and movement disorders.[53] The key to identifying, understanding, and managing the client with cortical dementia lies in recognizing and interpreting changing patterns of expression and behavior. Initially, the intellectual deterioration is often subtle; recognizing the diminished client's ability to make judgments and discriminations depends on the astute observations of family member or co-worker. As the dementia progresses, the client's problems with judgment, abstract reasoning, short-term memory, and time become more evident. Moderate dementia is usually characterized by increasing but not global disorientation, further deterioration of memory, concrete thinking, increasing dependence on environmental and social structure for knowing how to behave and by increasing psychological rigidity and emotional lability. The final stages are typically characterized by poverty of thought/speech, overt and global disorientation, marked susceptibility to catastrophic anxiety, and inability to cooperate with even the closest caregivers.

Korsakoff's syndrome is a particular type of dementia associated with chronic alcoholism and attributed to thiamine deficiency. This syndrome is characterized by the inability to form new memories but a more or less intact memory for past events and ability to recall previously learned facts and skills. Because similar memory defects result from lesions in midbrain and limbic structures (Figure 33-1), it appears that these structures play an important role in selective retention and in the recall of immediate sensory impressions and experiences.

Relatively mild lesions of the deep medial zones tend to be evident only when a client is required to retain and recall a complex series of information such as random numbers. The client does not have trouble recalling organized information such as sentences or stories. The client with massive lesions is unable to retain information or stimuli. His deficit is not so much in initial comprehension as in retrieval memory of other stimuli. However, traces of the "forgotten" information can suddenly reappear in another setting. The client may appear to remember when and what he wants to remember. Careful assessment, however, often reveals that specific memories are evoked spontaneously by environmental stimuli and that the client has lost voluntary access to and control of memories.

NURSING PROCESS

Assessment

Physical dimension Dementia is characterized by deterioration in the client's intellectual ability, emotional flexibility, and in the quality and quantity of social interaction. These changes are caused by conditions such

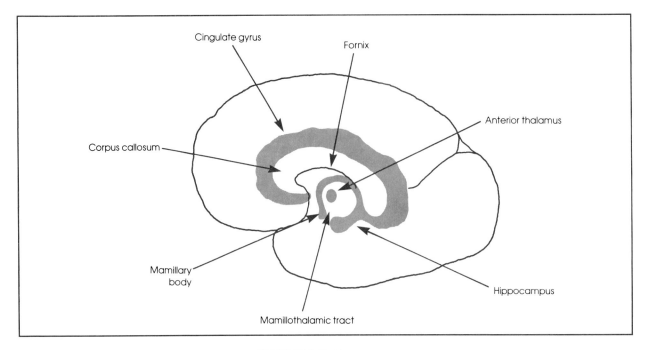

FIGURE 33-1 Limbic system.

COMMON CAUSES OF DEMENTIA

Degenerative Disorders

Alzheimer's disease
Pick's disease
Huntington's chorea
Idiopathic cortical atrophy

Mechanical Disorders

Trauma*
Normal pressure hydrocephalus
Subdural hematoma

Metabolic Disorders

Hypothyroidism
Hyponatremia
Hypercalcemia
Hypoglycemia
Porphyria
Hypoxia
Wilson's disease
Chronic anoxia
Uremia
Hepatic coma
Carbon dioxide narcosis
Disturbed protein metabolism
Electrolyte disorders

Exogenous Poisons

Heavy metals (lead, arsenic, thallium)
Bromides
Alcohol
Belladonna alkaloids
Organic phosphates
Hallucinogens
Idiosyncratic drug reactions

Vascular Disorders

Arteriosclerosis
Cerebrovascular accidents
Aneurysm
Collagen disease

Neoplastic Disorders

Gliomas
Meningiomas

Infections

Abscess
Chronic meningitis
Subacute encephalitis
Creutzfeldt-Jakob disease
Syphilis

Vitamin Deficiencies

B₁
B₆
B₁₂
Niacin
Folate

*Potentially reversible, at least to some degree, with medical or surgical treatment.

as arteriovascular disease, which impairs the normal functioning of nervous tissue, or by diseases such as Alzheimer's or syphilis, which destroy nervous tissues (see the accompanying box). Usually, symptoms that mark the onset of a dementia are subtle, and individuals, if they seek health care at this time, are likely to complain of anxiety or malaise or be preoccupied with particular bodily functions. As the disease process causing the depression worsens, the client's complaints often center around disconcerting feelings of fatigue, forgetfulness, or difficulty concentrating. Throughout the early stages, the individual often attempts to attribute these symptoms to familiar physical problems or to stressful interpersonal situations. Before seeking professional diagnosis and treatment, most clients have attempted to treat themselves with various home remedies, including alcohol and over-the-counter drugs.

By the time professional help is sought, it is not unusual for the client with progressive dementia to have diminished physical energy and a deteriorated physical condition. Clients are unable to complete tasks and often doze off during extended social encounters. They may be exhausted by the activities of daily living, so they are often poorly groomed. Nutritional deficits, anemia, and dehydration are common, along with other signs of neglect such as leg ulcers, cellulitis, and chronic diarrhea.

Physical tolerance for any type of extreme temperature is significantly diminished. Thermostat settings are constantly changed and complaints about being too hot or too cold become more frequent. Susceptibility to heat stroke or heat exhaustion without exertion can also indicate reduced physical tolerance.

Changes from an established baseline are especially important to the assessment. When physical changes occur slowly, as in the case of a slow-growing tumor, the body adjusts or adapts to its altered metabolic state. Only under

▼ **TABLE 33-1   History Format for Clients with Dementia**

Data Collection	Description
Past medical history	History of trauma, severe infections, seizures, chronic illness, violent or uncontrolled behavior, learning disabilities, fighting when intoxicated, hyperactivity, frequent auto accidents or traffic violations, and sexual or physical assaults; list of previous physicians and hospitalizations and their phone numbers and addresses
Medication	Use and patterns of use of any medication or drugs
	Use and patterns of use of alcohol
	Type and amount of drugs used in the past 24 to 72 hours, noting any change from usual patterns of consumption
	Use of herbs or folk remedies
	Use of mind-altering drugs or techniques (for example, yoga, spiritual experiences, or meditation)
Infection	Exposure to individuals known to have had an infection or contact with the blood, brain, or organs of an infected individual
	Travel, especially outside the United States, Canada, or Western Europe
	Recent symptoms of illness, such as rash, fever, vomiting, diarrhea, respiratory congestion, or pain
Toxic substances	Work responsibilities and environment—toxic chemicals or metals
	Home environment—peeling paint, toxic building insulation, environmental pollution or toxic waste products; new hobbies
	Air pollution, especially prolonged periods of stagnation or smog
Nutrition	Usual diet and dietary habits
	History of diarrhea, vomiting, skin rashes or eruptions, burns, or bleeding gums
	Food allergies
	Diet and dietary restrictions
	History of indications of fasting or binge eating
	Food cravings or excessive thirst—if so, what and when?
Onset of symptoms	What does the individual think is wrong, how do the client and family members describe the problem(s); to what do they attribute them?
	Has the individual undergone surgery or extensive medical tests or treatments? What were the effects on the body systems, length of procedure, exposure to anesthesia, complications, and other effects?
	When did the individual first feel sick? When was the illness or change of behavior apparent to others? Describe. What was the progression of symptoms?
	Has the individual ever acted or felt like this previously? If so, describe circumstances and symptoms in detail.
	What other things was the individual doing?
	Describe especially new or unusual activities, associations, or personal or environmental events.
	How have the current symptoms affected the individual's capacity and ability to engage in usual activities, responsibilities, and relationships?

stress do the symptoms of physical or emotional impairments become evident. Consequently, individuals with nonspecific symptoms at their initial visit need to have a physical evaluation. Table 33-1 suggests a format for taking a history of a client with dementia.

Emotional dimension The individual has trouble controlling the meaningful expression of emotion. Clients experiencing emotional lability also have difficulty interpreting other's emotional experiences or understanding the emotions they evoke in others. Loss of emotional control varies from barely recognizable to dramatic. Individuals generally have difficulty initiating an emotional response, but, once the response begins, the individual is less able to either modulate or terminate it. Consequently, the client may appear to overreact or to be insensitive.

The mood of the individual is frequently fearful; the attitude is suspicious if not overtly paranoid. As a result, caregivers are often perceived as dangerous and malevolent

(for example, agents of CIA, Mafia hit men). The care, particularly when it is painful, is resisted, perceived as harmful or as torture rather than an attempt to care or to heal. The client may attempt to flee or to resist treatment, pulling out tubes, removing dressings and monitors, or lashing out physically at nurses and physicians. There is little capacity to comprehend the long-term goals of or even the need for medical treatment; preoccupied with the discomforts and irritation, the client often appears resistant and noncompliant. The problem, however, is not one of compliance but an inability to cooperate with caregivers because of impaired mental processes and distortions of perceptual stimuli. Their tolerance for discomfort is minimal; physiological urges and drives require immediate satisfaction. And, if the nurse is unable to relieve the client's frustration, the irritability can quickly become a tirade of criticism and abuse. The client may often seem impatient, demanding, insensitive, and even crude.

Particular mood disturbances are often influenced by the following interrelated factors:

1. Premorbid personality
2. Nature and cerebral location of the specific disease process
3. Environmental stimuli
4. Understanding of environmental stimuli and the social relationships involved

One of the hallmarks of dementia is the client's ease of recovery from expressing strong feelings. Sobbing or convulsive laughter is often not the expression of felt emotion but the result of the individual's inability to modulate his emotional expression. Instead of being able to express sadness, anger, anxiety, or pleasure in degrees of more or less, the person characteristically expresses these feeling states in terms of all or nothing. The more severe the organic impairment, the more likely the individual is to experience euphoria, rage, morose depression, panic, or catastrophic anxiety. Removal from the interpersonal environment or problematic situation often results in an almost immediate behavioral change. Clients seldom exhibit residual happiness, anger, sadness or anxiety; but they may be slow to recover, become less responsive, fail to accomplish routine tasks, and resist the people, activities, or situations that evoked their overwhelming feelings.[31]

When dementia progresses to a moderate or severe stage, emotional expression is increasingly characterized by the absence of spontaneous emotion and subsequently by lability of emotional expressions. To the casual observer, the client may appear depressed. Facial expressions may be absent; and the client may appear to have a blank, empty gaze, directed purposelessly into space. If asked about sadness or depression, he is most often mystified by the suggestion. Some clients report that they do not feel anything; and the nurse, physician, or family members often conjecture that the individual is engaging in the protective mechanism of denial.

Once a feeling state is elicited, however, its expression tends to be overwhelming. Even a client who is moderately impaired may progress suddenly from a rather normal verbal expression of sadness to a state of uncontrolled sobbing. The observer usually notices that the individual is overreacting, but frequently tries to rationalize the response. The nurse may underestimate the importance of a particular issue, or the client's response may be out of proportion. This determination is not an easy one to make; however, significant insight can be obtained by asking the following questions:

1. How would I expect someone of the same sex, age, and sociocultural background to react to the same or similar comment or situation? What is an expected and appropriate response?
2. Are there any data to suggest that the client may have organic mental disorder? Is or has he been sick?
3. How has this client responded to similar situations or comments in the past? Do family members or close friends find his emotional responses unusual, exaggerated, or disturbing?
4. How quickly and under what circumstances does the client recover from apparent dramatic expressions of emotions? Does he cry easily, but once distracted, does he seem as if he had not cried at all? Does the individual seem mystified or confused when asked later about feeling so sad?

As the dementia worsens, the client has more trouble handling anxiety. In the unimpaired individual, moderate levels of anxiety tend to improve motivation and performance; clients with dementia are further impaired by even low levels of anxiety. These clients have lost the capacity for abstract thought; they are confined to the present, and they are unable to react selectively or sequentially to particular aspects of an experience. A common example of this total undifferentiated response in an adult is catastrophic anxiety. Individuals with this response show signs of physical collapse as well as overwhelming emotional distress.[65]

Anxiety is inherent in many routine aspects of living; therefore, *catastrophic reactions* are common in the organically impaired. Diminished physical and intellectual capabilities increase the probability of catastrophic anxiety. The individual may initially appear calm, pleasant, cooperative, and competent. However, when confronted with a task (such as putting on a shirt or shoes, cutting meat, or answering a question) that he cannot accomplish, mood and behavior change drastically. He may appear dazed, become agitated, fumble, and become hostile, assaultive, or evasive. His reactions are not only inadequate but also disordered and inconsistent.

The conditions that produce catastrophic reactions are neither fully predictable nor consistent. Those who work or live with the predisposed individual need to be aware of the possibility and signs of an impending catastrophic reaction. Common indicators include sudden and profound deterioration in mood, resistance or stubborness, and increased agitation. After a catastrophic reaction, the individual is even more vulnerable and less competent. Caregivers need to assess for deficits and attend to more basic needs so that the exhausted individual is not neglected or endangered.

Intellectual dimension The intellectual changes commonly associated with dementia include attention deficits, memory impairment, and misperceptions or misinterpretations of environmental stimuli (illusions and delusions). These deficits lead to secondary symptoms such as poor recall of recent information, incoherent communication, lack of judgment, misunderstandings, inability to make common associations, and diminished ability to organize personal possessions or behavior. Noncompliance with medical regimens or hospital policy or blatantly poor decisions often attract professional attention to the condition.[33,63]

Further assessment of the intellectual deficits usually reveals additional deficits that parallel the client's premorbid compulsive habits and cognitive vulnerabilities. Impaired clients who have smoked habitually, even compulsively, or shopped indiscriminately are more likely to engage in these activities, even if it clearly jeopardized their immediate health, safety, and security. More marginal areas of intellectual functioning, such as calculations, are obvious signs of deterioration and incompetency. Learning, especially in strange environments or of new material, is likely to be significantly impaired because it depends on the ability to attend to a situation selectively and commit relevant aspects of new information to memory.

Agnosia, apraxia, and aphasia usually result from disruption in any of the cerebral lobes; the location of the lesion determines the specific deficit or impairment. Lesions in the left frontal lobe are most likely to interfere with the expression of speech, whereas a similar lesion in the right lobe is more likely to interfere with the understanding of speech. The following list of cognitive functions is associated with the left and right cerebral hemispheres:

LEFT CEREBRAL HEMISPHERE	RIGHT CEREBRAL HEMISPHERE
Logic	Intuition
Symbols	Experience
Scheduling	Free
Language	Simultaneous
Structuring	Pictures
Planning	Timeless
Numbers	Imaginative
Specifics	Patterns
	Whole

Agnosia, apraxia, and aphasia are not always pathological. They are exaggerations of common interruptions of thought, movement, or expression. Everyone occasionally has difficulty finding the right words, naming an object, or understanding how pieces of a pattern fit together. Measurable differences in performance occur when one is anxious, distracted, frightened, or confused. These deficits usually become pathological when they are consistently more severe or more frequent, both of which are often best assessed individually. The distinction between normal and abnormal is not absolute. Consequently, change in the frequency and severity of symptomatic behaviors may be more significant than the behaviors themselves. For some individuals, something as subtle as hesitancy or erratic performance may be more significant than consistent, overt errors; therefore it is usually important to know about an individual's past performance and to observe the individual in many situations to determine the significance or implications of a particular behavior or symptom.

The confusion associated with dementia arises more from diminished understanding of stimuli than from diminished perception. The two functions are intimately associated, so dysfunction in one area creates problems in the other. As dementia progresses, the individual is only able to understand objects and events in the most concrete, personalized way.

One of the unrecognized effects of aging is that the brain becomes more sensitive to its internal (metabolic) environment. As a result, almost any disorder or substance that alters the body's homeostasis may mimic dementia. In the elderly, common causes of *pseudodementia* (reversible impaired intellectual functioning) include diuretics, digitalis, oral antidiabetic drugs, analgesics, antiinflammatory agents, sedatives, and psychopharmacological agents. Pseudodementia may also be present in clients who develop cardiac, pulmonary, renal, or hepatic failure; endocrine disorders; fluid and electrolyte disturbances; depression; anoxia; anemia; disruption of circadian rhythms; infections; nutritional deficiencies; hypothermia or hyperthermia; and increased intracranial pressure or intercranial lesion.[32,44]

Alzheimer's disease, hardening of the arteries, and multiple cerebral infarcts account for more than 80% of the dementia among the elderly.[44,65] Unlike the intellectual and functional changes, which typically occur as a normal con-

sequence of aging, Eslinger and others[17] found that those suffering from dementia were more likely to experience difficulty when an activity required temporal orientation, logical (rational) memory, or the retention of visual stimuli. These types of deficits reflect the client's fundamental impairment in abstract reasoning. As a result, clients have difficulty using ideas and concepts (i.e., clock time, calendars, institutional routines, principles of wellness) to order their lives (i.e., use bureaucratic hierarchies such as channels of communication, job descriptions, social roles). Increasingly dependent on immediate experience and sensations (i.e., pain, hunger, tiredness, and darkness to know when to eat, sleep, or wash or toilet). These clients' personalities and life-styles are altered radically as their intellectual ability deteriorates.

Not surprisingly, clients who are highly educated and intellectually oriented are more likely to be impaired by and impaired sooner by dementia than those who are illiterate, have unskilled jobs, or generally rely on less conceptual means for knowing about and functioning in the world.[48] Aberrations in short-term memory and disorientation to time and place are the most obvious intellectual symptoms. The client may appear to comprehend and may accurately repeat requests or instructions. However, behavior a short time later is contradictory. Behavior tends to be an automatic response to need, and conscious thought is diminished, if not obliterated. Judgment and discrimination are impaired, and the meanings of all events and phenomena are personalized.

Impairment in the individual's recent memory can approximate the time of disease onset. Memory disturbances that involve past memories, particularly the remote past, indicate an extensive disease process and an unfavorable prognosis.[24,43] In addition, the nature and extent of memory loss infrequently provide clues to both the origin and the location of a lesion or tumor.

Assessment of memory loss is seldom as straightforward as is often believed. Past and present memories are highly variable categories; the individual's observable behavior and responses seldom reflect only one category of memory. The more mundane aspects of day-to-day living are essentially automatic and based on remote memories. Not until familiar ways of doing things become impossible or nonadaptable is there undeniable evidence that an individual is not adequately incorporating new experience, stimuli, or information. Therefore individuals who live in a stable, secure, predictable environment, despite significant impairment of memory, are able to cope and compensate automatically and effectively. So long as the interpersonal and social environment remains stable and supportive, the individual's generic descriptions and generalizations are sufficiently understood and do not disrupt patterns of communication or social action.

Indications of memory loss are initially subtle and are frequently undetected. Nurses need to control their desire to fill in the details. Careful observation of the individual in novel situations and his responses to new people and to familiar people in new social roles are particularly revealing. Besides the usual memory-related questions on the mental status examination, the nurse may ask some of the following questions or make some of the following observations:

1. Does the client resist going to new places or resist new activities? Is this characteristic, or is there any indication of increased resistance?
2. Does he have difficulty accepting a new individual or role? Difficulties are commonly related to issues of authority and responsibility. Those that are frequently problematic involve a transfer of authority or responsibility from the client to a previous subordinate.
3. Is the individual using a known title, such as nurse, doctor, lawyer, pastor, or Father, to address recently introduced individuals rather than their names?
4. Is the conversation of the individual becoming increasingly historical? Does the client talk about current affectual states by recounting previous situations that elicited the current feelings and conflicts?
5. Is the individual's conversation becoming repetitive, less spontaneous, or less descriptive? Does the individual tend to fall asleep (doze off) when the topic no longer specifically concerns him or involved others are no longer seeking his input?
6. Is the client relying on cliches rather than description to explain or is he inviting the interviewer to fill in the description by saying such things as "You know"?
7. Does the individual have trouble telling a story sequentially or putting thoughts together in an orderly manner so that they are comprehensible for the interviewer?
8. Is the individual's ability to communicate either orally or in writing impaired? Are responses often restatements of another's statement or letter? Is there a notable absence of adjectives and adverbs and, for well-educated individuals, an absence of complex sentences and appropriate use of dependent clauses?

Individuals with dementia have decreased capacity for learning and therefore are considered to have lost intelligence. However, unlike the lack of intellectual endowment in the mentally retarded individual, the problem focuses around the loss of intellectual capacities. Recent observations of those suffering from dementia, especially Alzheimer's disease,[37,42] suggest that performance in intellectually demanding tasks or judgment in socially sensitive situations is initially compromised. In most instances the individual can successfully hide cognitive impairment.

In the early phases of dementia, the impaired individual is still capable of learning and to some degree can compensate for deteriorating skills,[59] particularly if the new learning involves less complex strategies and the use of preexisting social or psychomotor skills. However, the ability to learn is closely associated with the individual's memory capacity or impairment.

Because judgment is such a complex intellectual phenomenon, it is also the most susceptible to impairment in dementia, especially those forms that result from a general toxic condition or generalized deterioration of cortical tissue. In fact, deterioration in judgment is often one of the first indications of dementia. Once an individual's memory is impaired, he is less able to learn from current experiences. The meanings of all events and phenomena are personalized. The degree to which his past memory is impaired provides a crude measure of the individual's ability to use previous knowledge and experience as the basis for guiding his behavior.

As the individual's capacity for abstract thinking deteriorates, he is less able to see similarity or likeness in present and past experiences. Consequently, the individual's responses become increasingly situation specific; every situation is increasingly isolated. Although the client's learning is not totally impaired, he may be unable to transfer learning from one situation to another.

The inability to recognize new forms of old stimuli is also a common manifestation of a decreased ability to think abstractly. If magazines or newspapers change their covers, they are likely to be left unread or discarded. The impaired individual is even likely to make vehement protests that he did not get the goods or services he ordered or wonder why he is receiving "this junk."

Language disorders are particularly common manifestations of dementia. Dementia is characterized by a *poverty of speech*. The vocabularies for speaking, reading, or writing become progressively restricted. The client in the early stages of dementia may preserve a facade of normality, but only as long as the individual is not under emotional, physiological, or social stress. The individual relies on stock words and phrases, especially for conversational purposes, and may start sentences and allow the listener to finish them. He may have difficulty finding words; although he does not always hesitate to apply a term to an object, the term may be inappropriately applied or the term may be a neologism. If asked for examples of a generic class such as dogs, cats, cheeses, or wines, he may be unable to respond or give only limited examples, which have personal relevance. The capacity for symbolic language, one measure of the ability to think abstractly, is impaired. This impairment may range from mild to severe.

Telegraphic speech patterns are another language disturbance commonly experienced by individuals with dementia. Replies to questions may be relevant, but with little elaboration. Speech is less spontaneous, characterized by less descriptive words and fewer examples. As capacity for language decreases, the individual is less likely to be able or willing to make declarations or propositions unless there is some immediate bodily need.[8] Even then, the individual is likely to resort to exclamations and demands. Perseveration is also common.

The individual is less able to make subtle social discriminations and judgments, and the social behavior deteriorates. Inappropriate and sexually explicit jokes often seem to be the total humorous repertoire. Less able to differentiate one situation from another, other individual's or group's sensitivities, or the self from the group, the impaired individual places personal needs above the more obvious or immediate needs of others. Jokes are often told for their immediate effect or attention, and people in the environment are evaluated in terms of their willingness or ability to satisfy needs. Disagreement, however honest and understandable, is often interpreted as disloyalty and in some instances emotional abandonment. Jokes, compliments, promised rewards, and punishments become ways to distract others from one's deficits and for avoiding confrontations with one's own disabilities.

Poor judgment is evident in the individual's apparent need for immediate gratification. Bodily needs become paramount and tend to increasingly dominate the individual's relations with the environment and other people. The body needs may be primary, such as hunger, thirst, sex, rest, or elimination, but they may also include addictions or cravings, such as for alcohol, sugar, or tobacco. There is an increased sense of urgency. Requests become demands when the client cannot obtain what he wants. Less sensitive to the time, place, or manner in which the requests are made, the client may demand to return to his room to rest in the middle of a meal or church service. If cigarettes are not immediately available, the organically impaired individual may prowl the halls pestering others for cigarettes or resort to smoking butts of other's cigarettes.

The impaired individual is frequently thought to be rude, inconsiderate, dangerous, or thievish, particularly when requests to cease such behaviors are not heeded. However, the client perceives most strongly immediate needs and has little capacity for insight into how his behavior affects others. He does not necessarily realize he is functioning less appropriately or less effectively. Consequently, as the dementia progresses, the client can be expected to experience more interpersonal and social difficulty unless his environment and relationships are appropriately limited and structured.

Personality changes are commonly associated with dementia. However, the individual's personality does not become so much different as it becomes increasingly rigid. Existing personality traits or characteristics are exaggerated. If the individual was prone to suspiciousness, compulsivity, passivity, or frankness, these traits become more pronounced, are less easily modified, and are more likely to evoke negative responses from others.

The maturation process perfects and adds to an individual's adaptive skills; cerebral dementia depletes it. The client has only the coping skills that he knows best. Loss of flexibility often causes inappropriate responses, especially in novel or stressful situations. Defense mechanisms such as sublimation, repression, and denial give way to regression and projection. The impaired client often assumes a paranoid or passive attitude that makes it increasingly difficult for him to cooperate with others or his environment. The use of projection also tends to increase the angry responses the client elicits from others.

In advanced dementia, most clients can no longer effectively communicate with others, interact purposely with the environment, or willfully control their bodily functions. Unable to anticipate needs or manipulate their environment, clients are likely to experience repeated episodes of catastrophic reactions and to be perceived as inappropriate or disruptive. Clients can live for several years with advanced dementia; only when stupor or coma develops is death imminent.

Along with observation and interviewing, the mental status examination and psychometric testing are frequently used to assess a client's intellectual capacities (see Chapter 8).

Social dimension Increased dependence is common in organically impaired individuals. The nature of this change is determined by the severity and nature of the cortical impairments and the usual responsibilities and expectations of the client. An individual can suffer significant cortical damage while living much as before. Other family members may routinely have cooked, cleaned, or shopped for the client, so inability or difficulty in performing these tasks may go unnoticed. On the other hand, if the individual is unable to perform competently in an expected manner, the other family members will feel the burden of increased responsibilities and duties.

The burden that families assume varies a great deal and their perceptions of the manageability of this burden depend on many factors. Following are some factors that play a part in determining whether a family can successfully cope without additional input or assistance:
1. The ability and willingness of the family to identify its own needs and those that the impaired individual met but can no longer or only partially meet.
2. The ability and willingness of another family member to assume the functions of the impaired individual.
3. The number and ages of family members available for sharing the additional tasks and responsibilities.
4. The extent of the family members' existing responsibilities and commitments.
5. The care or direct supervision that the impaired family member requires.

The nature of care and the extent of direct supervision are important factors in determining whether clients can remain in their own homes or can be cared for adequately in the homes of their adult children. Dangerous or socially disruptive individuals are difficult to care for at home. When the individual does not perceive his limitations, ordinary activities such as cooking or taking a walk can become problems. Forgetting the stove is on results not only in burned food but also in fires; forgetting where one was going and how to get home can result in the individual's becoming lost. If the behavior of the impaired individual endangers others, the need to supervise him can become the predominant factor for organizing the family's relationships and activities.

Care-related responsibilities and hardships are especially dramatic if only a few members can share or are willing to assume these additional responsibilities. If the family can obtain assistance from the community or extended family and friends, an otherwise intolerable situation may be made manageable. Financial, personal, and interpersonal resources available to care for the client are important factors in determining where the client will live. Neglected clients and angry, exhausted family members often suggest that available resources are inadequate and that the family is overwhelmed. A family's decision to institutionalize the client, however, is most likely to occur after a physician confirms that the client's condition is irreversible and suggests placement. Neglected clients and sick or exhausted family members are the consequences of overtaxed, overwhelmed families.

The amount of physical care required by an impaired individual is another important consideration. Infirm or paralyzed clients require frequent care or assistance to meet basic needs such as toileting, eating, bathing, moving, and socializing. When these needs are substantial, meeting them is time consuming because the client needs the constant presence of another person. Planning more than a few minutes or hours ahead may be impossible because the demands for toileting or comfort are largely unpredictable.

Interpersonal conflict tends to exacerbate, particularly in the case of progressive generalized deterioration. Unable to perceive errors in reason or judgment, some individuals insist on performing their usual activities and making their usual decisions. Attempts to frustrate these behaviors, particularly in a previously aggressive or determined person, can lead to physical resistance and angry outbursts. If the individual's premorbid personality was dependent, passive, or congenital, he is less likely to oppose increased supervision and control. For these individuals, the increased attention is likely to be perceived as love and caring. However, if his independent domains of functioning, such as driving, cooking, cleaning, enjoying hobbies, and caring for himself are limited, he, too, is likely to become resistive and defensive.

Other family members often receive a disproportionate share of the client's paranoid attitude and defensive behavior. Children who assume responsibilities for a parent can be particularly problematic if they have never established an adult relationship with the parent. In such a relationship, the significantly impaired parent is unlikely to see the child as more competent than he or be willing to be supervised or controlled by his offspring, especially if the parent is physically unimpaired and unable to perceive his increasing deficits.

Attempts by the family or significant others to point out the client's disabilities may change the nature of the relationship and be unsuccessful. The family's inexperience and ineptness with their new tasks and roles may only compound the problem. Even to a skilled observer, the client may appear to be victimized, displaced, and able to perform his role better than those who are overtaking it. Consequently, the client may succeed in gaining outsiders' support, thereby validating his suspicions about his family and co-workers. Conflict can subsequently escalate, and open

verbal battles frequently occur between opposing factions; the issue of the client's incompetence or illness becomes secondary. People who need to work together and share their information and efforts on the client's behalf may be irrevocably split. Anger, hostility, and hurt feelings are common and may be reflected in behaviors that sever the troublesome relationships; friendships are terminated, wills are changed, family members may be ostracized, and the client may ultimately be abandoned.

Sometimes attempts to displace or redelegate the individual's authority, responsibilities, and duties are threatening to the client. In dramatic cases he may become certain that others are out to get him or take his job, money, or even family. Not unexpectedly, the client may use his resources to prevent this perceived assault. Verbal assaults, physical defenses, employment of detectives to scout out the culprits, reports to the police, and repeated changes in phone numbers or complaints about tapped lines are among the more common defensive moves. Less common, but potentially disastrous, is the growing tendency of clients to arm themselves or booby-trap their home and property to ward off the expected threat.

Often what begins as social or interpersonal conflict ends in familial conflict, as family members either try to control the aberrant behavior or are embarrassed, disgusted, or even ostracized because of it.

Consequently, by the time a family seeks professional help, they are discouraged and tired. They have tried everything they can imagine and judged all to have failed. The medical help they seek is often some combination of a rest and a miracle. If neither is forthcoming, family members

---

RESEARCH HIGHLIGHT

The Long Haul: The Effects of Home Care on the Caregiver
• SE Gaynor

PURPOSE

The purposes of this study were to describe the effects of long-term caregiving at home for a medically disabled relative on the physical and mental health of elderly women and to examine patterns of illness symptoms in elderly female caregivers and the relationship of those symptoms to both age and the caregiving role.

SAMPLE

The sample consisted of three groups: 87 long-term caregivers, 38 short-term caregivers, and 30 noncaregivers. The groups were matched according to marital status, husband's age, and site of discharge destination from hospital.

METHODOLOGY

A case control design was chosen to examine the differences between caregivers and noncaregivers. Questionnaires were mailed to the three groups of women with written explanations of the study. Three instruments were used for hypothesis testing; The Zarit Burden of Care Scale, the Linn and Linn Self-Evaluation of Life Function Scale, and Liang's Model of Self-Reported Physical Health.

From *Image: Journal of Nursing Scholarship* 22(4):208, 1990.

FINDINGS

The burden scores were lowest during the first 2 years of home care. Highly significant differences were found between the long-term caregivers and the other groups on the number of physician visits made, both for the caregiver's health and the husband's health, suggesting that as the years of caregiving continue, there is an increase of stressful aspects of home caregiving for a frail or disabled spouse.

IMPLICATIONS

The study implies that while caring for a frail or disabled family member may be a family choice, it may be detrimental to the overall emotional and physical health of the caregiver. If caregivers are to extend their home services, supportive services must be developed and provided, especially at the critical 2- to 4-year period when stress levels are highest.

may become angry, overtly hostile, or withdrawn. Other effects on the caregiver are described in the research highlight.

The behavior of tired, discouraged families and that of uncaring, uninterested, unsupportive families often looks similar to the observer. Professional efforts to care and plan for the client can impose additional burdens if the nature and needs of the particular family are not considered. This approach almost certainly causes resistance, and even the most skillfully designed arrangements may be destined to fail for the client, the family, or both. Careful attention to and assessment of the condition of both the family and the client enable the family to remain supportive. The ongoing assessment of the family's ability to cope with stress is facilitated if the nurse regularly asks the following questions:

1. What types of trouble or embarrassment has the client caused his family and individual members of his family? Is the family exhausted, discouraged, angry, and depressed?
2. What was the nature and quality of the relationship before the recent problem? What new interpersonal problems have developed? What problems have been exacerbated?
3. When did the family become suspicious that the client was having problems? When and how did they become involved? What is different? What does or does not happen now that is different?
4. What has the family tried to do? What were the results of their efforts? What was the final incident or observation that made them seek help?
5. What does the family want and expect to happen? Are these expectations realistic in regard to (a) the client's condition and prognosis, (b) the client's financial resources, (c) community resources and services, and (d) available technology?
6. Is the family able to mourn the loss of their previous relationships with the client?
7. Can family members assume the roles and responsibilities that the client can no longer fill?
8. Can the family allow the client a new, still valuable role within the family, one based on being rather than doing?
9. Does the family have resources to help them learn and assume new tasks and roles? Are there untapped resources, neighbors, friends, extended family, or community agencies? Do people need help finding the resources and learning how to appropriately use them?

Spiritual dimension   Variation in the expression of symptoms and in how these symptoms affect the process of life and living continually make assessment and treatment for clients with dementia difficult. Generally, understanding how organic impairment affects an individual's sense of himself and his purpose for living depends on the interaction of numerous factors, including the following:

1. The individual's philosophy of life, his beliefs and values, and what life and living have meant to him and his significant others
2. The nature and extent of cortical impairment, the individual's perception of that impairment, and the personal meaning ascribed to his particular disabilities
3. The socially and culturally ascribed meaning of personhood: How are personal and social competence defined

and judged? What social or cultural meanings are ascribed to the individual's deficits?
4. The ability of the client to establish meaningful relationships and to participate in the living environment.

The organically impaired individual is less able to participate in the activities he values. The more his deficits conflict with his values, the more dramatic the impact. If a person is no longer able to engage in the activities and relationships that were central to his social acceptability, feelings of hopelessness and despair may occur. In addition, the individual's ability to receive another's caring gestures may be diminished by feelings of unworthiness and failure or loss of ability to perceive the symbolic expressions of others.

As an individual becomes increasingly impaired, particularly by processes that diminish intellectual capacity, he is unable to engage successfully in activities or maintain the attitudes prescribed by his values. Unlike persons whose incapacities are predominantly physical, those who have significant intellectual deficits also have diminished capacity to adapt and change. Thus they are less likely to learn new things and to engage in alternative but valued activities. Therefore it is essential that the client's ordinary living environment be adapted to their ability(s) rather than attempting to modify the clients' behaviors.

The maintenance or self-worth becomes particularly problematic when the individual's worth is determined by the values of progress, achievement, individualism, and activism. Investing time, energy, and love in the care of a person who may never again be independent, achieve goals, or show progress may seem unproductive. Rational thought provides little support or motivation; values of kinship, loyalty, obligation, belonging, and mutual dependence effectively convey unconditional acceptance of the client. The degree to which family and caregivers can accept the impaired individual provides important clues about their ability to make necessary adjustments in their expectations and attitudes and to meet and sustain the client's spiritual needs.

Measurement Tools

Table 33-2 lists some of the more common instruments used to measure dementia.

Analysis
Nursing diagnosis

Altered thought processes is the most common nursing diagnosis approved by NANDA that applies to dementia. The defining characteristics of this nursing diagnosis are listed in the box on p. 660. A case example illustrating the characteristics of the nursing diagnosis altered thought processes follows.

▼ Case Example

James, a 25-year-old single white man, was admitted for the fifth time to the psychiatric unit of a general hospital. As during the other times he had been admitted, James was intoxicated. He had not taken his phenytoin (Dilantin) for some time, and as he began to withdraw from the alcohol, he experienced convulsions. After his neurological condition was stabilized, James was trans-

▼ **TABLE 33-2   Instruments to Measure Dementia**

Instrument	Measures
Bexler-Maudley Automated Psychological Screening Maps (BMaps)*	Assess psychological defects relating to organic brain damage
Mini-Mental Exam[19]	A shortened form for assessing mental status
Global Deterioration Scale[54]	Assess the severity of dementia
Kendrick Battery for Detection of Dementia in the Elderly*	Assess demented function of the elderly
Wechler Adult Intelligence Scale (WAIS)*	Assess the intellectual abilities of the adult
Wide Range Intelligence and Personality Test*	Assess abilities as well as behavior in individuals

*Conoley J, Kramer J, editors: *The tenth mental measurements yearbook,* Lincoln, Neb, 1989, The University of Nebraska Press.

ferred to the psychiatric unit for treatment for alcohol addiction. A review of James' medical history revealed that he had sustained a closed head injury in a car accident 3 years earlier. Since the accident James had not been able to hold a job, even though he had experience as a house painter. James' problems with drinking began about 3 months after he had resumed independent living. Observations of his behavior on the unit revealed a rather passive but agreeable young man who tended to get lost if he had to find his way in new settings and would follow his impulses and the suggestions of his peers without any apparent awareness of possible consequences. Psychological testing revealed that James had some impairment of short-term memory and judgment and discrimination and could not effectively sequence events or objects. James could not effectively anticipate trouble or analyze a situation or plan; rather he reacted more or less stereotypically. It became evident that James' alcohol problems were not separate from his problems from his cognitive deficits. James lived alone above a bar and his friends were the bar's regular patrons. Unable to separate himself from his physical and social environment, treating James' addiction involved arranging for him to have a chemical-free environment to continue his recovery. James agreed to go to a half-way house for recovering alcoholics and addicts; 6 months later, he continues to be sober.

Numerous NANDA nursing diagnoses can apply to clients with dementias. Although nature and severity are the two most significant factors in determining the type of problems that a client will have, most experience some problems with memory and coping. Impaired clients can be expected to experience at least some disorientation and confusion. Hence several NANDA nursing diagnoses are usually applied in the care of the organically impaired client. The following list provides examples of additional NANDA-approved nursing diagnoses.
1. Social isolation related to poverty of speech
2. Altered thought processes related to impaired memory
3. Self-care deficit related to physical impairments
4. Fear related to memory loss
5. Sensory/perceptual alterations related to hearing voices
6. Altered nutrition; less than body requirements related to inability to feed self

▼ **ALTERED THOUGHT PROCESSES**

DEFINITION
A state in which an individual experiences a disruption in cognitive operations and activities.

DEFINING CHARACTERISTICS
- **Physical dimension**
  Altered sleep pattern
  Hyperactivity

- **Emotional dimension**
  Inappropriate/labile affect

- **Intellectual dimension**
  Altered states of consciousness
  Disorientation to time, place, person
  Impaired memory, recent and remote
  Confabulation
  Distractability
  Disturbed thought flow (e.g., circumstantial, tangential, neologism, flight of ideas, loose associations, word salad, blocking)
  Disturbed thought content (e.g., delusions, obsessions, preoccupations, phobias)
  Impaired problem solving
  Impaired judgment
  Inability to follow conversation
  Alteration in perception (e.g., hallucinations, illusions)
  Cognitive dissonance
  Suicidal/homicidal ideation
  Attention deficit
  Egocentricity
  Inappropriate/nonreality based thinking

Modified from McFarland G, McFarland E: *Nursing diagnosis and intervention: planning for patient care,* ed 2, St Louis, 1993, Mosby–Year Book.

Planning

The nursing care plan (Table 33-3) provides some long- and short-term goals, outcome criteria, interventions, and rationales related to dementia, which serve as examples of the planning stage in the nursing process.

Implementation

Physical dimension Professionals or family members often need to supervise the administration of medication and take measures that decrease the risk of physically complicating conditions. Health care providers and family members need to adjust their expectations of the client to reflect the individual's capacity to function. This approach helps ensure that the client is neither unduly restricted nor pushed to assume tasks and responsibilities before he is physically able.

Generally, the more ordinary and routine the activity has been for the client, the less judgment and discrimination he needs to perform it competently. Therefore when a client does not comply satisfactorily with treatment, does not meet the expectations of his family, or appears to be socially insensitive or inept, his higher intellectual functions

▼ **TABLE 33-3 NURSING CARE PLAN**

GOALS	OUTCOME CRITERIA	INTERVENTIONS	RATIONALES
NURSING DIAGNOSIS: Altered thought processes related to increased disorientation and confusion at night as evidenced by sun-downing			
LONG TERM			
To maintain orientation to place and person at night and distinguish between day and night activities	Establishes a regular nighttime routine and bedtime	Assist with bedtime routine: have toilet articles in same place, a regular bedtime hour, and same caregiver if possible	To prevent anxiety and lessen confusion
	Sleeps at least 5 hours during nighttime hours	Monitor sleep patterns	To ensure adequate sleep
	Knows own room and bed	Assist to locate own room and bed by using colored bedspread, pictures on door	To promote confidence in self; to lessen confusion
	Recognizes caregivers and calls appropriate persons for assistance	Teach names of caregivers	To know who can be depended on for help
SHORT TERM			
To feel safe and secure with immediate environment	Does not experience episodes of catastrophic anxiety	Show genuine care and concern; plan a structured day time routine	To let client know he is cared about; to prevent undue anxiety
To interact positively in/with the treatment environment	Recognizes own belongings and wears own clothes	Have client wear own clothes	To reinforce self-identity
	Responds to being called by name	Call by name at each interaction	To maintain self-identity
	Can be redirected when behavior becomes disoriented or confused	Present reality when confused or disoriented	To maintain contact with reality
	Does not become aggressive toward caregivers or become verbally disruptive	Observe for aggression or disruptive behavior	To prevent negative consequences from escalating behavior
	Can participate in own care and meet own ADL in the treatment environment	Assist with ADL when client needs help	To show caring, to foster self-esteem
	Maintains continence	Help to establish bowel and bladder control	To prevent incontinence, embarrassment
	Dresses in clean, appropriate, nonrestrictive clothing	Assist with dressing and grooming	To maintain self-respect
	Receives direction and support necessary to care for self or to participate with caregivers	Give positive reinforcement for self-care or cooperation with caregiver	To foster appropriate behavior

need to be reassessed and treatment and expectations realigned accordingly. Accusing the client of being disgusting or unmotivated is rarely effective in changing unacceptable behaviors. Because the offending observable behaviors are more often a result of the client's being unable to do something (rather than unwilling), it is often more effective to simplify or change the task than to try to alter the client's attitude.

As the impairment worsens, the individual becomes less able to attend to his physical needs without direct supervision or intervention. Interventions that reduce demands on the individual's energies often are most helpful. Providing Meals-on-Wheels, housekeeping services, shopping assistance, laundry services, and occasional haircutting or grooming facilitate the client's accomplishing a few things more adequately. Secondarily, these direct services help prevent complications. The individual is less likely to experience anemia from not eating, accidents from cluttered or poorly repaired homes, and loneliness due to unacceptable personal and environmental odors and appearances.

Once an individual becomes severely demented, his ability to perceive and to meet his own physical needs is minimal. The ability to cooperate or interact constructively with one's environment is severely decreased. At this time, others must assume responsibility for the individual's physical care, which may include washing, dressing, toileting, and feeding. On the other hand, a client who is physically capable of feeding or dressing himself may need step-by-step directions about what to do and how to do it. If left alone to eat, the client will not eat, will wander off, or will report that he is not hungry and does not like the food. The nurse or caretaker needs to remember that the client cannot, rather than will not, do these things for himself.

Measures to stabilize the client's internal and external environment are important because of his diminished tolerance for either internal or external physical stress. Maintaining a stable temperature, a familiar environment, and adequate nutrition and preventing infections and injuries, particularly immobilizing injury, are important nursing interventions.

With severe dementia, physical safety for the client and those around him becomes more of a problem. The client needs continual supervision, which means not being left alone for even brief periods. Locking doors and windows may be necessary. Even then, disoriented clients seem to somehow slip away. Authorities, co-workers, and neighbors need to be alerted immediately about the client's disappearance. One never assumes that the impaired individual will or can return on his own. A search needs to begin immediately. The subject matter of the client's most recent conversations and fondly remembered places often provide clues for the search. However, the impaired individual may become easily distracted and forget his destination. Consequently, he is likely to become frightened and wander randomly trying to find a familiar place; he could go anywhere. Radio and television announcements and distributing a description are sometimes necessary and helpful for finding the lost individual.

Modern appliances become hazardous when used inappropriately or when they are abandoned without being turned off or disconnected. Because even the moderately organically impaired individual is easily distracted, coffeepots, stove burners, and heating pads are often left operating unattended. Setting a bag of groceries or the mail on a hot stove burner can quickly cause a fire, potentially a tragic situation and one that the individual cannot be expected to respond to appropriately.

Enforcing common safety regulations frequently involves removing problematic appliances or supervising their use. Requests for cigarettes and matches and requests to borrow small or personal appliances are often accommodated almost automatically. However, the danger such common objects pose needs to be explained to some clients. Involving family or other responsible adults in the supervision of the client while he smokes, shaves, or makes coffee often provides a satisfactory alternative for maintaining social contact and expressing interpersonal caring.

Other problems include the use of flammable items such as cleaning fluids, cigarettes, gasoline, or firewood. The client's inability to identify dangerous environmental factors and to anticipate the consequences of his method of handling dangerous materials make some situations potentially explosive.

Cigarette smoking is no doubt the most common source of fire. Dangerous smoking habits such as indiscriminately flicking the hot ash, forgetting and abandoning half-smoked cigarettes, and smoking in bed or while dealing with gasoline are responsible for innumerable fires and injuries.

Because smoking is often a response to physiological and emotional urges, the client often needs to meet this immediate urge more than to comply with social norms. Once the urge is satisfied, the client may abandon the cigarette without further concern about it. Consequently, smoking often needs to be controlled or supervised. Control may include removing the cigarettes from the client or restricting cigarette smoking to specific supervised situations and environments.

Emotional dimension Because the client is increasingly unable to manage his own emotional expression, someone may have to assist him. The assisting person needs to understand that the degree of expression is not an accurate assessment of the initial feeling. The intensity of the feeling may be judged better by the situation within which it originates. Unless the caregiver can establish an accurate sense of proportion, either of two responses is likely to occur: (1) The caregiver does not take any part of the individual's expression as valid and withdraws, ignoring the client as well as the disturbing behavior; or (2) the caregiver overevaluates the seriousness of the emotion and begins to consider ways to provide extraordinary support instead of trying to understand and manage the individual's behavior.

Generally, interventions seek to control the expression of emotion. Being aware of the client's escalating behavior may allow both time and opportunity to withdraw the client either emotionally (change the subject, distract him) or physically (remove him to another location) before the response is totally out of control.

Once it is clear that certain types of situations or subjects are prone to elicit either catastrophic anxiety or severe emotional lability, it is often helpful to avoid these situations. By keeping the environment stimulating but calm and routine, avoiding conflict and confrontation, many catastrophic responses can be prevented.

The client's lack of control of emotional expression does not imply that he does not experience emotions. Although his expression may become distorted, his emotions can be interpreted. Again, attention to context, theme, and particularly action is often more revealing than verbalizations or facial expressions. Clients who are only mildly or moderately impaired often use biographical stories as a means of dealing with a particular emotion. If the client is experiencing personal loss, the stories often focus on other incidences of personal loss. Concern about abandonment may be expressed by talking about people leaving or dying. The nurse may only need to listen, state simply that she understands, or just stay quietly until the end of the story. At this point the client may begin to relax and move on to other things.

In the early stages of dementia, many clients have some awareness of their diminishing capabilities and loss of personal control. Grieving the loss of the previous self may be necessary before adaption and rehabilitation are possible. Feelings of sadness and anger often occur and may be more disabling than the dementia itself. Recognizing and treating

RESEARCH HIGHLIGHT

A Comparison Between the Care of Vocally Disruptive Patients and Other Residents at Psychogeriatric Wards

• I Hallberg, A Norberg, and S Eriksson

PURPOSE

This Swedish study explores the relationship between the occurrence of vocally disruptive behavior and the routine nursing management of clients suffering from dementia. Unlike other studies that typically focus on the evaluation of techniques for controlling disturbing behaviors, this study attempted to identify why such disruptive behavior occurs. Specifically, the study focused on identifying significant factors that differentiate the vocally disruptive patient from those who are not. In addition, the study attempts to reveal the meaning of or reasons for the disruptive behavior.

SAMPLE

In the absence of an accepted definition of vocally disruptive, the term was operationally defined as behavior that was regularly noisy for an extended time and was characterized by the repetition of words, sentences, or sounds. A group of 37 vocally disruptive patients were identified from an institutional population of 264 clients on the basis of their behavior during the two weeks before the study. A control group of 37 clients matched for sex and ward were selected from the hospital population. Significantly, more than one-half of the clients in both groups were diagnosed with dementia of the Alzheimer type, had spent at least 2 continuous years in the hospital, were markedly disoriented, and were dependent on nursing staff for their activities of daily living (ADL)—bathing, dressing, toileting, eating.

METHODOLOGY

Semistructured observations of all subjects were performed between the usual waking hours of 7:00 AM and 10:00 PM, for a total of 15 hours of observation. These observations were spread out over 2 to 4 week days and divided into five 3-hour intervals. The focus of the observations were activities, behaviors, and the interactions between clients and between client and nurse. Subsequently, the observations were analyzed according to type, amount, and frequency of activities; interactions initiated by the nurses were differentiated from those initiated by the client.

From Hallberg I, Norberg A, Eriksson S: *Journal of Advanced Nursing* 15:410, 1990.

FINDINGS

Analysis of the client observations revealed that the vocally disruptive clients were more physically dependent and more psychologically impaired than their nondisruptive counterparts. The disruptive clients tended to be more confused and to be more likely to exhibit psychotic reactions. The researchers also noted that environmental factors such as restricted mobility, extended periods of idleness, limited visual and auditory stimulation, and infrequent contact with others were thought to lead to sensory deprivation. It appeared that the pattern of short functional interactions may, in fact, increase the number of confused reactions because the more severely impaired clients were not given enough time to fully comprehend what was happening or enough support to participate meaningfully in the activity. In addition, staff interactions with the disruptive patients tended to be more corrective and therefore more likely to evoke anxious or fearful responses.

IMPLICATIONS

Because the environment was not adequately adapted to the client's needs, the environment appears to increase severely impaired client's disturbed behaviors. It appears that vocally disruptive patients had specific needs because of their physical dependence, disorientation, and confusion. These needs, in part, might be met by explicit and slow interactions and care activities and by a continuous close interpersonal relationship. It also appears that these clients continue to need social interactions and variations in their daily lives. The challenge for nurses is to (1) recognize that failure to meet client needs for meaningful participation and supportive interpersonal relationships may in fact maintain the patient's disruptive behaviors, (2) discover realistic ways to balance these clients' needs for solitude and social interactions, and (3) enable these clients to participate in their care and their environment.

---

the accompanying depression may facilitate the client's independence and productivity for several months or years.

As a dementia progresses, however, it becomes necessary to shift the therapeutic focus from trying to accommodate the client to the environment to accommodating the environment to the client. Attempts to orient the client to time, place, and person are somewhat helpful at least until the disease is advanced and the deterioration is profound. As the deterioration progresses, successful interventions elicit the client's participation in a simple, common activity such as eating, walking, bathing, clapping to music, or playing with a toy. Participation as a therapeutic technique makes contact with others in the environment meaningful and offers stimulation that the client can comprehend, thereby decreasing the incidences of catastrophic anxiety, aggressive behavior, and disruptive vocalization (see the research highlight above).

Intellectual dimension Organically impaired individuals depend particularly on external cues for knowing what to do, how to behave, or what others expect from them. Simple things such as familiar tablecloths and table settings remind the client to eat in a socially acceptable manner. Wearing his own pajamas and robe can help the client to stay in bed or at least rest, curtailing the urge to wander. Familiar furnishings and possessions often help remind the individual that he is at home, he belongs here, and that this is his room. These surroundings and routines are reassuring and also facilitate the maximal level of independent function.

The following strategies compensate for the individual's decreased intellectual capacities:

1. Give the client specific, personalized written and verbal instructions for things such as diet, medication, and treatment.
2. Minimize the complexity of new information.
3. Adapt diet, care, and medication schedules to existing patterns and schedules.
4. Plan for additional time and instruction to accomplish new learning; learning is facilitated by teaching in the client's usual environment and with the equipment that the client is expected to use.
5. Use more than one sense to help the client to see changes in his environment and relationships.
6. Use many sensory approaches to assist the individual with learning; for example, taste, feel, and look at new medication.
7. Use visual cues such as picture charts to help the individual make necessary associations.
8. Encourage the simplifying and structuring of the client's interpersonal relationships, financial responsibilities, and occupational obligations and tasks.
9. Use existing knowledge, old learning, and habitual strategies to deal with new situations and expectations.
10. Elicit desired behaviors and responses by evoking them rather than requesting them. Begin the activity (for example, hum or sing a few bars of a familiar song or gently put the spoon or toothbrush to the client's mouth) and then let the client take over; remain close by in case the client forgets or is distracted.

Because problems with intellectual function are all interrelated, management takes into consideration all deficits that the individual is experiencing. The interventions in Table 33-4 are often helpful in assisting the client and family to cope. Success in working with the severely impaired individual often involves changes in the caregiver's own attitude and expectations.

As the client becomes more intellectually impaired, verbal communication becomes more limited and self-centered. Frustration, a common consequence of the client's attempts to communicate verbally, leads to acting-out behaviors. The client's concrete thinking and impaired memory make it difficult, if not impossible, for the client to think of alternative ways to say things to obtain attention or fulfill needs.

Throwing things, yelling, cursing, pushing, soiling, or spitting are often the client's means of communication. Such socially aberrant behavior often indicates that the client's immediate needs are not being met or that he has been confronted by his deficits. These outbursts are often avoidable if the nurse can anticipate the client's needs and control the physical and social environment. Careful attention to the theme, environmental context, and emotional tone of the client's story often provides more information than the actual words he speaks. Standing in the bathroom may mean the client needs help to toilet himself. Recounting previous incidences of being left alone or expressing

anger at those who left may mean that the individual is lonely or concerned that the nurse will not stay with him.

Clients with significant disturbances in verbal communication have trouble not only expressing themselves but also understanding what others mean. Simplifying language is an important strategy for communicating effectively with the severely impaired client. Ideally, only one idea is communicated at a time.

Verbal communications are best understood when they are kept simple and direct. Single words and short sentences facilitate understanding. However, verbal communication often needs to be supplemented with visual clues, pictures, or pointing. The client who has difficulty finding the right word also has difficulty remembering the meaning of words. Although the word may sound familiar, association with the object can be problematic. Even more difficult for the severely impaired client is remembering how to use objects and tools. Pictures of the needed object or desired activity help the client remember to perform a task.

If telling a client what to do next does not elicit the desired behavior, the behavior may be demonstrated or initiated. Physically guiding movements often helps him understand more effectively than verbal directions. Touch is a concrete, direct way to express care and concern, and it is often understood long after verbal directions have deteriorated. When words confuse or agitate, a hug, firm grip, or guiding arm communicates presence and attentiveness; sitting quietly beside an individual often provides more security and relief than words.

These strategies may allow effective communication with a severely aphasic client. Those with limited disorders often benefit from intensive therapy, either relearning speech skills or learning alternative symbolic methods of communication such as sign language. For those who have more generalized disease, more iconic methods, particularly the use of pictures and gestures, are often successful. Singing and listening to music rather than talking may still be possible and provide an avenue for communication as well as an alternative source of pleasure. It is also important to remember that clients who are no longer able to readily comprehend verbal communications often become more attuned to the nonverbal aspects of others' communication, enabling them to comprehend some or all of messages. The inability to effectively comprehend words paradoxically makes the aphasic individual more sensitive to falsehood, malice, or equivocal intention.

Sensory deprivation that results from environmentally imposed idleness and immobility is a severe problem among those with advanced dementia, especially for those who are cared for in hospitals and nursing homes. Because the intellectual impairment is so obvious and profound, caregivers have erroneously assumed that such clients have no intellectual needs, often leaving them to sit alone in a geriatric chair for extended periods. One study (see the research highlight on p. 666) suggests that severely impaired clients continue to have needs for intellectual stimulation and that those needs can be met partially by providing the clients with toys they can manipulate.

Social dimension New physical and social environments are often disorienting because it is difficult for the marginally oriented to adapt their knowledge and skills to new environments. When the client is confronted with

TABLE 33-4   Interventions for Clients with Dementia

Problem	Intervention
Impairment of short-term memory	Simplify new procedures Adapt treatment regimens to establish habits and preferences Limit new information to the essentials Expect incomplete and/or erratic compliance Use memory aids—calendars, reminders, notes
More global memory impairment	Adapt the environment to the clients' needs and abilities Attempt to evoke memory by doing rather than telling Place client in situation where desired response is most likely to occur "naturally" Do not expect the clients to perform or complete an activity on their own—stay with them, support their efforts
Concrete thinking and impaired judgment	Use recognized authority rather than logical explanations when clients' compliance is essential Continue supervision of clients' use of medication and performance of ADLS by way of a supportive family member and/or community agency Avoid confronting the clients with decisions and judgments they are unable to make Have others assume increased responsibility for financial, legal affairs and the performance of critical community and occupational responsibilities as dementia progresses Suggest power of attorney and guardianship if the client is no longer capable of giving informed consent Limit the client's choices—alternative ways of accomplishing the same goal can be unnecesarily confusing Make expectations clear; give simple, clear directions; use short sentences Say *exactly* what you mean—avoid interferences, metaphors, or allegories—show rather than tell if possible Do not expect the client to generalize—teach a skill in the context the clients need to perform it and with the equipment they will be using Avoid changes in medication, diet, or treatment as a client is being discharged to a less structured or protective environment
Intensification of personality traits and increased reliance on primitive defense mechanisms—projection	Anticipate and prepare family members for less flexibility of attitude and more stereotypical reactions Avoid scolding or punishing; expect the clients to assume less responsibility for the consequences of their behavior Structure the environment and interpersonal situations to ensure success Avoid conflict and threatening situations—do not confront the client; help him withdraw gracefully
Disorientation and confusion	Provide a predictable treatment environment and consistent caregiver Avoid changing the client's room and bed Accompany the clients if they leave their immediate living environment Use color rather than numbers to help the client identify his room and bed Allow the client to have a particular chair in the dining room or community area if possible Use client's personal belongings to personalize the environment Have clients wear their own clothes—encourage families to bring familiar rather than new clothing for the patients to wear
Sensory deprivation	Provide for physical activity and mobility Encourage activities in which previous skills and memories might be evoked (dancing, singing familiar songs, watching old movies) Encourage and facilitate regular visits from family and friends Encourage visits from children and pets Structure the environment so that if clients wander, they are unlikely to get lost Avoid cold, constipation, excessive heat, hunger, thirst, tight clothes; clients should be physically comfortable Use mechanical restraints only as a last resort and only so long as the client is immediately endangering himself or others Help client to correctly identify environmental stimuli Avoid the use of central nervous system depressants and observe closely for medication reactions Provide clear verbal and visual indicators of time—clock, open curtains, seasonably appropriate decorations, looking out the windows; state length of time between events Avoid activities that follow detailed rigid sequencing Avoid competitive activities and large group activities Encourage parallel activity, dyads, and simple physical responses Provide care so that the client can participate Provide foods that are safe but appealing to the client Be sure client has appropriate dentures, hearing aids, glasses, and mobility aids Avoid confining clients to bed, geriatric chairs for extended time

RESEARCH HIGHLIGHT

The Play Project: Use of Stimulus Objects with Demented Patients
- K Mayers and M Griffin

PURPOSE

Demented patients need to interact with their environment. When denied the opportunity to move, interact, or explore objects in their environment, these patients' functional abilities and behavior deteriorate. Because of their serious intellectual deficits and functional limitations, the nurse must often take extraordinary measures to help these patients experience meaningful interactions with the people and objects in their environment. This study observed demented patients' interest in and response to selected toys and stimulus objects.

SAMPLE

A sample of nine male patients was selected from the available population of demented patients hospitalized on a geropsychiatric medical unit in a state psychiatric hospital. Five of the patients were diagnosed as having Alzheimer's disease; four were diagnosed as having dementia secondary to chronic alcohol abuse. All patients were 66 years or older and have exhibited assaultive or agitated behaviors.

METHODOLOGY

Ten preselected stimulus objects, including a stuffed dog, a dressed doll, fabric book, keys, toy cars, busy boxes (3), and transformers (2) were provided to the patients over a 2-week period. The procedure was repeated again in 3 months with the five Alzheimer patients. Each patient was presented with a different toy each day (10 days, 10 objects) for a 10-minute period. The patient's response to the object was then observed and recorded.

From Mayers K, Griffin M: *Journal of Gerontological Nursing* 16(1):32, 1990.

FINDINGS

Although interest patterns varied greatly from session to session, patients exhibited substantial interest in most of the toys. The only toy that failed to interest was the cloth book. Otherwise, the amount of interest in any toy depended, in part, on the patient's ability to discover how to play with it. Patients were interested in the toy dog, but they were content to just hold it; the busy boxes stimulated the most active interaction. One of the transformers was determined to be too complex; patients did not figure out how to make it work and their interest quickly waned. Generally, the optimal stimulus objects were toys that were normally selected for infants and preschoolers.

IMPLICATIONS

Environmentally imposed idleness and sensory deprivation are common but underappreciated problems for the institutionalized demented patients. Toys originally designed for young children appear to be a readily available means for these patients to continue to engage safely and adaptively in stimulus seeking and exploring behavior despite their obvious cognitive impairments. Even though the size and scope of the study was severely limited, it appears that the act of playing with toys might help the patient organize their thoughts and behaviors. By appropriately increasing the environmental stimulation and interaction, it might be possible to decrease the incidence and severity of aggressive and disruptive behaviors among the severely demented. If in fact this is the case, then toys might be an alternative to restraining and medicating these patients to prevent disruptive and destructive episodes.

---

the impersonal and unfamiliar routines of a hospital or a nursing home, his behavior often deteriorates quickly. New environments and unfamiliar routines render him more dependent, often on strangers. Because these changes often create the potential for hazardous situations, every attempt needs to be made to support the efforts of customary caregivers and to maintain the client in a familiar environment.

As the dementia becomes more severe, the individual's sense of self becomes more restricted and his needs more self-centered. This does not mean that those clients need less social contact, only that they can no longer gain approval through their achievements. They can receive only unqualified acceptance. Social acceptability is often fundamental to meeting the client's needs for human contact and support. Families, friends, and even professional caregivers are more likely to care for, visit, or just sit with the client if they are not overwhelmed by offensive behaviors, appearances, or odors.

Successful maintenance or reestablishment of family relationships is important to the client's well-being. If the family is unable to cope with the client or renegotiate their

own roles and relationships, the family not only becomes less cohesive but also may be in danger of disintegration. This possibility significantly increases the likelihood that the client will be abandoned or neglected either physically or emotionally. Providing for necessary and timely help to the family is often the most significant way to ensure immediate and future support for the client. Some families may need assistance to identify the meaning of their loss and to redefine their roles and responsibilities. These are appropriate issues for short-term family therapy.

In addition, most families benefit from professional interventions that help them maintain a physically and emotionally safe environment. Fundamental to the achievement of this goal is support for the primary caregiver(s). Zarit and Zarit[71] suggest the following interventions for maintaining continuity of caregivers and of the physical and social environment:

1. Provide caregivers information that helps them understand what is happening to the client; support their efforts to anticipate and plan for present and future needs.
2. Assist caregivers to understand the effects of cognitive

deterioration on the individual's behavior. Sometimes health care professionals can help by acknowledging the caregivers' frustrations and explaining that the client with severe memory loss cannot remember that he cannot remember.

3. Encourage caregivers to slow down, to make only one request or give one instruction at a time. This approach facilitates maximum independent performance by the client and minimizes the emotional and physical demands of the responsible caregiver.

4. Encourage and assist caregivers in their efforts to solve problems as the individual's cognitive status deteriorates and/or new dilemmas arise. Health care professionals can often help by reminding caregivers that there is no "right" approach and by encouraging them to try different attitudes, approaches, and responses and to use the one that is most successful.

5. Encourage caregivers to attend to their own needs and to plan for periods of relief from their caretaking responsibilities. Caregivers may schedule intermittent breaks before tensions get too emotionally or physically exhausting. This technique often involves helping family members, particularly spouses, to accept help for some of their ongoing responsibilities. Before these alternatives can be explored, however, primary caregivers may need an opportunity to share their pain, frustration, conflicts, and grief.

6. Present alternative ways of getting help. For the professional health care provider, this means not only knowing about and suggesting available community resources (respite care, Meals-on-Wheels, homemaker services, home care by nurses or physicians, day care centers, activity programs, sitters) but serving as an advocate for the development of support services.

Generally, environmental disruptions are best avoided; however, if they become unavoidable the event needs to be treated as having the potential for immense emotional crisis. If the client's increased dependence is unrecognized and no additional support is provided, he typically becomes more anxious and his behavior more intolerable and unmanageable. When home management is no longer feasible, special consideration is given to admitting a cognitively impaired person to an institution. Clients can be expected to become less anxious and less confused in circumstances that require them to make the fewest changes in their routines. It is particularly helpful if institutional care is individualized to accommodate the client's habits and capitalize on existing memories and use retrievable memories. Restraint, however well intentioned or rationalized, tends to cause significant stress for clients with dementia and may cause increased disorientation, agitation, constipation, incontinence, and falls. Currently, caregivers are being urged to find alternatives to restraints. Hollywood beds and rubber padded rugs can reduce the risk of injury if the client falls out of bed. Positional alarms attached comfortably to the thigh alert patient and staff alike to impending danger, and door alarms alert staff to the impending departure of a wandering patient. In addition, the availability of meaningful activity and interactions in a structured daily routine have been identified as a practical alternative to reliance on chemical and mechanical restraints.

Hospitalization or change in clients' usual living arrangements often confront them with new social norms and expectations. New social norms can also be confusing and provoke anxiety for clients. When old memories are inadequate or provide inappropriate prescriptions for behavior, the individual is likely to become withdrawn, disoriented, or dependent or to behave inappropriately. Interactions with those who hold differing personal, social, ethnic, and religious beliefs can be as confusing and disorienting to a severely impaired client as moving him to a totally new neighborhood or city. Confrontations and challenges can occur when such interactions are forced.

Provisions for social and environmental stability also enhance the individual's perception of being cared for, as well as the nurse's ability to care about the clients. Caring is probably the most culturally determined aspect of human expression. Teasing, arguing, embracing, or closeness is understood differently depending on one's social and cultural background. Teasing can be an expression of affection in one case and an expression of hostility in another. Food, gifts, and visitors also have their cultural specificity; favorite foods or the giving of food is, for some, essential to the expression of love and concern. Rules or conditions that inhibit such usual exchanges effectively restrict both the expression and reception of human caring. The client needs to be successful in his social interactions. Sensitive, perceptive nursing interventions can ensure that success.

Spiritual dimension Despite significant cognitive deterioration, an individual is still capable of having religious feelings and beliefs. Because of their diminished intellectual capacities, however, organically impaired clients depend on their families and caregivers to evoke spiritual or religious memories and to communicate associated attitudes of love, dignity, peace, and belonging. Attitudes of peace and belonging are often communicated through the caregivers' own sense of accountability to a high spirituality or deep sense of commitment to their fellow humans. The presence of the client's Supreme Being, the integration of the universe, and the meaning of life are often evoked through continued participation in familiar religious rituals and ceremonies.

Given the present lack of scientific understanding of clients with dementia and the limited technological resources for intervention, interpersonal relations that communicate love and acceptance are the nurse's primary means for imparting hope to these clients. Hope may be generated whenever people realize that other people care about them and will rally to their needs when they are afflicted.

Religious rituals are usually part of one's lifelong experiences. Imbedded in these rituals are prescriptions for attitudes, behaviors, and relationships. Participation in familiar religious services is often most beneficial because the service remains familiar and recognizable. In Catholic and orthodox denominations, regular attendance is often sufficient because the services have been ritualized and are familiar. In Protestant and other heterodox religious traditions that are not highly structured, it may be more important for the individual to attend a familiar church or join in the singing of familiar hymns to recognize and to participate meaningfully in the service. To the degree that the religious service remains familiar, the experience is capable of evoking the associated attitudes and behaviors.

The totality of the experience may give the client a sense of wholeness or completeness, which has become increasingly rare in his incomprehensibly fragmented everyday life. For example, the director of a Jewish nursing and retirement home described marked changes in behavior in clients with some of the home's most severely regressive cases of Alzheimer's disease during Passover services.[32] Many of these clients were able to participate in the Seder; many others sat quietly and responded appropriately throughout the entire pre-Seder service. With some amazement, the director noted that these same residents were incapable of attending to even their most basic personal needs and had been wandering the halls aimlessly just before the services.

Although nurses rarely have a direct role in the organization or conduct of religious or spiritual services, they may facilitate these activities and experiences by following some of the measures listed here:

1. Alter institutional routines and schedules to facilitate attendance at services.
2. Welcome clergy and religious leaders in the care facilities and help them understand the problems of the impaired clients so they can adapt their care and services accordingly.
3. Encourage families to continue to include even the most impaired member in important religious occasions (holy days and religious rituals and ceremonies—marriages, communion, bar or bat mitzvah).
4. Participate with clients in spiritual activities held in the institution if able to do so sincerely and comfortably.

Table 33-3 is a sample nursing care plan for a client with dementia. A summary of key interventions for clients with dementia is presented in Table 33-4.

Evaluation

Evaluating the care of a client with dementia is highly individualized but generally focuses on identification of the organic impairment and management of the resulting symptoms. It is essential to preserve the client's maximal level of functioning and independence, while ensuring that his basic physical, emotional, intellectual, social, and spiritual needs are met. Success is not particularly objective or measurable, nor does it necessarily involve a cure. Rather, successful nursing care sustains individuals and their families. Salient parameters of evaluation include the provision of quality relationships and meaningful experiences for the clients and the personal and professional growth of caregivers. Care can generally be considered effective if secondary complications do not occur or, in the case of the more severely impaired individual, an optimal level of functioning is maintained.

BRIEF REVIEW

Dementia involves disturbances in every dimension of functioning. Disturbances in the physical dimension include the client's inability to care for himself. Disruptions in the emotional dimension are seen in the client's emotional lability and inappropriateness of emotional expression. Impairments in the intellectual dimension include

false perceptions such as delusions and difficulty communicating, understanding, remembering, and making judgments. In the social dimension, disruptions in relationships with family members and other caregivers are seen. Because of the numerous disruptions, clients with dementia frequently are unable to accept and understand their illness or to develop a philosophy about life that promotes hope and spiritual contentment.

Relating to clients with dementia requires patience, tolerance, and a belief that care makes a difference in the quality of the client's life. Those who successfully care for the organically impaired client often gain appreciation for the less objective and less material aspects of life, as well as their own humanity and that of others. The warmth, patience, tolerance, and understanding acquired through caring for clients with dementia are often transferred to other aspects of the caregivers' lives.

The nursing process provides a systematic way of caring for clients with dementia by assessing disturbances and impairments within the five dimensions and analyzing the data to form nursing diagnoses. Planning and interventions focus on maintaining the client at his highest level of functioning. Evaluation is based on the successful management of symptoms.

REFERENCES AND SUGGESTED READINGS

1. Beam I: Helping families survive, *American Journal of Nursing* 84:229, 1984.
2. Berndt R, Mitchem C, Price T: Short-term memory and sentence comprehension—an investigation of a patient with crossed aphasia, *Brain* 114:263, 1991.
3. Blakeslee J and others: Making the transition to restraint-free care, *Journal of Gerontological Nursing* 17:4, 1991.
4. Bower T: The alternatives to restraints, *Journal of Gerontological Nursing* 17:18, 1991.
5. Burnside I: *Working with the elderly*, ed 2, Monterey, Calif, 1984, Wadsworth.
6. Cahel C, Arana G: Navigating neuroleptic malignant syndrome, *American Journal of Nursing* 86:671, 1986.
7. Colston L: The handicapped. In Wicks R, Parson R, Capps D, editors: *Clinical handbook of pastoral counseling*, New York, 1985, Paulist Press.
8. Coyle MK: Organic illness mimicking psychiatric episodes, *Journal of Gerontological Nursing* 13(1), 73, 1987.
9. Critchley M: *The divine banquet of the brain*, New York, 1979, Raven Press.
10. Cummings J: Dementia: neuropathological correlates of intellectual deterioration in the elderly. In Vlatowska H, editor: *The aging brain: communication in the elderly*, San Diego, 1985, College Hill Press.
11. Dacey R and others: Relative effects of brain and nonbrain injuries on neuropsychological and psychosocial outcomes, *Journal of Trauma* 31(2):217, 1991.
12. Davidhegar R, Gunden E, Wehlage D: Recognizing and caring for the delirious patient, *Journal of Psychiatric Nursing and Mental Health Services* 16:38, 1978.
13. Detmer W, Lu F: Neuropsychiatric complications of AIDS: a literature review, *International Journal of Psychiatry in Medicine* 16:21, 1986.
14. Devaul R, Hall R: Hallucinations. In Hall R, editor: *Psychiatric presentations of medical illness*, Jamaica, NY, 1980, Spectrum Publications.
15. Donahue E: Reality orientation: a review of the literature. In Burnside I, editor: *Working with the elderly*, Monterey, Calif, 1984, Wadsworth.

16. Ellenberger H: Psychiatry from ancient to modern times. In Arieti S, editor: *American handbook of psychiatry,* vol 1, New York, 1984, Basic Books.

17. Eslinger P and others: Neuropsychologic detection of abnormal mental decline in older persons, *Journal of American Medical Association* 253:670, 1985.

18. Fischer R and others: Reversed lateralization of cognitive functions in right handers, *Brain* 114:245, 1991.

19. Folstein M, Folstein S, McHugh P: Mini-mental state: a practical method for grading the cognitive state of patients for the clinician, *Journal of Psychiatric Research* 12:189, 1975.

20. Freeman A: Delusions, depersonalization and unusual psychopathological symptoms. In Hall R, editor: *Psychiatric presentations of medical illness,* Jamaica, NY, 1980, Spectrum Publications.

21. Frommelt P and others: Familial Alzheimer disease: a large, multigeneration of German kindred, *Alzheimer Diseases and Associated Disorders* 5(1):36, 1991.

22. Guynn R: Psychiatric presentations of cardiovascular disease. In Hall R, editor: *Psychiatric presentations of medical illness,* Jamaica, NY, 1980, Spectrum Publications.

23. Gwyther L, Matteson M: Care for the caregivers, *Journal of Gerontological Nursing* 9:92, 1983.

24. Hall R: Anxiety. In Hall R, editor: *Psychiatric presentations of medical illness,* Jamaica, NY, 1980, Spectrum Publications.

25. Hallberg I, Norberg A, Eriksson S: A comparison between the care of vocally disruptive patients and that of other residents at psychogeriatric wards, *Journal of Advanced Nursing* 15:410, 1990.

26. Harrington L: Depression and hypoxia in post-myocardial infarction patients, *Cardiovascular Nursing* 25(6):31, 1989.

27. Jahnigen D: Delirium in the elderly hospitalized patient, *Hospital Practice* 25(8):135, 1990.

28. Jeste DV, editor: *Neuropsychiatric dementias: current perspectives,* Washington, D.C., 1986, American Psychiatric Press, Inc.

29. Johnson C, Johnson F: A micro-analysis of senility: the response of the family and the health professionals, *Culture, Medicine and Psychiatry* 7:77, 1983.

30. Katzman R: Dementia in the context of the teaching nursing home. In Schneider EL and others, editors: *The teaching nursing home,* New York, 1985, The Beverly Foundation Raven Press.

31. Lezak M: *Neuropsychological assessment,* New York, 1976, Oxford University Press.

32. Lipowski J: A new look at organic brain syndromes, *American Journal of Psychiatry* 137:674, 1980.

33. Lipowski Z: Transient cognitive disorders (delirium, acute confusional states) in the elderly, *American Journal of Psychiatry* 140:1426, 1983.

34. Lucus M, Steele C, Bognanni A: Recognition of psychiatric symptoms in dementia, *Journal of Gerontological Nursing* 12:11, 1986.

35. Luria AR: *The man with a shattered world,* New York, 1972, Basic Books.

36. Luria A: *The working brain,* New York, 1973, Basic Books.

37. Luria A: *Higher cortical functions in man,* ed 2, New York, 1980, Basic Books.

38. MacDonald E: Personal communication, 1986.

39. Mackey A: OBS and nursing care, *Journal of Gerontological Nursing* 9:74, 1983.

40. Mayers K, Griffin M: The play project: use of stimulus objects with demented patients, *Journal of Gerontological Nursing* 16(1):82, 1990.

41. McKean K: Memory, *Discover* 4:10, 1983.

42. Mesulan M: Dementia, its definition, differential diagnosis and subtypes (editorial), *Journal of the American Medical Association* 253:2559, 1985.

43. Morgan A, Morgan M: *Manual of primary mental health care,* Philadelphia, 1980, JB Lippincott.

44. National Institute on Aging Task Force: Senility reconsidered, *Journal of the American Medical Association* 244:259, 1980.

45. National Interfaith Coalition on Aging, Inc: *Spiritual well-being: a definition,* Washington, DC, 1985, National Retired Teachers Association—American Association of Retired Persons.

46. Pajik M: Alzheimer's disease inpatient care, *American Journal of Nursing* 84:216, 1984.

47. Palmateer L, McCartney J: Do nurses know when patients have cognitive deficits? *Journal of Gerontological Nursing* 11:6, 1985.

48. Palmer M: Alzheimer's disease and critical care, *Journal of Gerontological Nursing* 9:86, 1983.

49. Parva J: Sundown syndrome, *RN* 53(7):46, 1990.

50. Pincus J, Tucker G: *Behavioral neurology,* ed 2, New York, 1978, Oxford University Press.

51. Price W, Forejt J: Neuropsychiatric aspects of AIDS: a case report, *General Hospital Psychiatry* 8:7, 1986.

52. Rader J: Modifying the environment to decrease use of restraints, *Journal of Gerontological Nursing* 17(2):9, 1991.

53. Reisberg B: Stages of cognitive decline, *American Journal of Nursing* 84:225, 1984.

54. Reisberg B, Ferris S, De Leon M: The global deterioration scale for assessment of primary degenerative dementia, *American Journal of Psychiatry* 139:1136, 1982.

55. Richerson K: Right brain—left brain: the nurse consultant and behavior change following stroke, *Journal of Psychiatric Nursing and Mental Health Services* 20(5):37, 1980.

56. Richardson K: Hope and flexibility: your keys to helping OBS patients, *Nursing 82,* 12:64, 1982.

57. Sacks O: *The man who mistook his wife for a hat,* New York, 1985, Summit Books.

58. Schwab M, Radar J, Doan J: Relieving the anxiety and fear in dementia, *Journal of Gerontological Nursing* 11:8, 1985.

59. Shamoian CA, editor: *Biology and treatment of dementia in the elderly,* Washington, DC, 1984, American Psychiatric Press.

60. Shapira J, Schlesinger R, Cummings J: Distinguishing dementias, *American Journal of Nursing* 86:698, 1986.

61. Swanson B, Cronin-Stubbs D, Colletti J: Dementia and depression in persons with AIDS: causes and care, *Journal of Psychosocial Nursing* 28(10):33, 1990.

62. Taft L, Barkin R: Drug abuse? Use and misuse of psychotropic drugs in Alzheimer's care, *Journal of Gerontological Nursing* 16(8): 4, 1990.

63. Trzepacz P, Teague G, Lipowski Z: Delirium and other organic mental disorders in a general hospital, *General Hospital Psychiatry* 7:101, 1985.

64. Walsh K: *Neuropsychology: a clinical approach,* Edinburgh, 1978, Churchill Livingstone.

65. Weddington W Jr: The mortality of delirium: an underappreciated problem? *Psychosomatics* 23:1232, 1982.

66. Weiler K, Buckwalter K: Care of the demented client, *Journal of Gerontological Nursing* 14(7):26, 1988.

67. Wolanin M: Physiologic aspects of confusion, *Journal of Gerontological Nursing* 7:236, 1981.

68. Wood F, Novack T, Long C: Post-concussion symptoms: cognitive, emotional and environmental aspects, *International Journal of Psychiatry in Medicine* 14:277, 1984.

69. Zarit S, Cole K, Guider R: Memory training strategies and subjective complaints of memory in the aged, *Gerontologist* 21:158, 1981.

70. Zarit S, Miller N, Kahn R: Brain function, intellectual impairment and education in the aged, *Journal of the American Geriatrics Society* 26:58, 1978.

71. Zarit S, Zarit J: Cognitive impairment. In Lewinsohn P, Teri L,

editors: *Clinical geropsychology,* New York, 1983, Pergamon Press.

ANNOTATED BIBLIOGRAPHY

Luria AR: *The man with a shattered world,* New York, 1972, Basic Books.

This book is based on the life experiences of a Russian soldier who received a bullet wound that destroyed part of his brain. It incorporates material from his journals, which provide first-person memories. Particularly interesting are the descriptions of his attempt to use these memories to participate in the activities of living. How a brain injury makes the familiar strange and the simple complicated is conveyed through this soldier's accounts of determining right from left, taking a train home, and attempting to repair a barn door. The soldier's accounts are supplemented by Luria's discussion of neurophysiology and neuroanatomy.

Sacks O: *The man who mistook his wife for a hat,* New York, 1985, Summit Books.

Currently available in the popular press, this collection of clinical cases for the professional and laymen provides numerous, sometimes amusing, examples of what it might mean to have a neurological disease. The author describes the problems of neurological disease and how individuals consciously and unconsciously attempt to adapt to their altered circumstances. The star of this book is not the physician but his patients; from each one he learns something more about human determination and capability.

Brower HT: The alternatives to restraints, *Journal of Gerontological Nursing* 17(2):18, 1991.

This article provides the historical context that makes present attitudes about restraints understandable and provides initial strategies for making the necessary changes in organizational policy, nursing care, structural alterations and educational programs. Other articles in this issue deal more specifically with how to make the transition to restraint-free care and how to modify and to effectively use the environment as a therapeutic tool.

Taft L, Barkin R: Drug abuse? Use and misuse of psychotropic drugs in Alzheimer's care, *Journal of Gerotological Nursing* 16(8):4, 1990.

This article discusses the use of particular classes of drugs in the various stages of Alzheimer's disease and presents a proposed set of guidelines to be used by caregivers when administering psychotropic drugs.

Therapy with Victims of Abuse

Ruth Parmelee Rawlins
Virginia K Drake

After studying this chapter, the student will be able to:

- Discuss historical perspectives related to victims of abuse
- Define and identify major types of abuse and neglect
- Discuss theoretical approaches to abusive situations
- Describe characteristics of individuals at risk for being a victim or perpetrator of abuse

- Review common myths and beliefs about victims and perpetrators of abuse
- Implement the nursing process to provide care for clients at risk for or involved in abusive situations
- Identify current research findings related to victims of abuse

Types of abuse include child abuse, sexual abuse, spouse abuse, elder abuse, and rape. These types of abuse occur irrespective of age, race, religious, socioeconomic, occupational, educational, cultural, or other boundaries. Each of these forms of violence is a serious concern to society and to health care professionals.

The following definitions are used in this chapter:

- *Physical abuse* is an intentional injury, harmful deed, or destructive act inflicted by a parent, spouse, guardian, mature child, or caregiver on another person with whom an interpersonal or advocacy relationship is shared.
- *Physical neglect* is the volitional deprivation of the care necessary to sustain life, growth, and development. Neglect may ensue from acts of omission in securing the essential physical care or through failure to provide a safe environment.
- *Emotional abuse* is the use of implicit or explicit threats, verbal assaults, or acts of degradation that injure or damage an individual's sense of self-worth. Verbal or nonverbal actions intended to provoke suffering or disrupt another's psychological equilibrium constitute emotional abuse.
- *Emotional neglect* is the lack of maintaining an interpersonal atmosphere conducive to psychosocial growth and development of personal worth and well-being. Healthy psychological maturation is stifled and thwarted, resulting in varying degrees of emotional crippling.
- *Material abuse,* primarily perpetrated on the elderly, is the theft or misuse of an individual's property or money.

- *Violation of rights* is a form of elderly abuse occurring when an individual is forced from his home or coerced unnecessarily into a nursing home.

Definitions of child abuse, sexual abuse, spouse abuse, elderly abuse, and rape are provided as these specific topics are discussed in the chapter.

THEORETICAL APPROACHES

Social Learning Theory

In general, social learning theorists agree that violence in the family begets violence. Children learn behavior by imitating or modeling the behavior of family and friends. Physical punishment by a parent can teach a child some unintended lessons. They learn that the persons who love them the most are the ones who strike them. They also learn that violence may be used to obtain a desirable result, which implicitly sanctions the use of violence as a means to an end. Because most parents do not use physical pun-

---

 DIAGNOSIS Related to Victims of Abuse

NURSING DIAGNOSIS
Rape trauma syndrome

HISTORICAL OVERVIEW

DATES	EVENTS
1800s	British common law permitted husbands to discipline their wives as long as the "rod" was no thicker than the husband's thumb.
Mid-1800s	The Society for the Prevention of Cruelty to Animals interceded on behalf of a child discovered in New York City who was suffering from malnutrition and severe beatings inflicted by her adoptive parents.
Late 1800s	US laws gave men implicit and explicit permission to beat their wives.
1871	The Society for the Prevention of Cruelty to Children was established in New York City.
1886	A bill proposed in Pennsylvania to make wife beating a crime failed.
1962	The phrase *battered child syndrome* was originated by Kempe to emphasize the malevolent actions perpetrated on children by their parents or other adults.
1968	All states had developed legal mandates to report child abuse.
1973	The Child Abuse Prevention and Treatment Act advanced the legal responsibilities of nurses and other health care providers encountering child abuse or neglect.
1975	The label *battered child syndrome* was replaced by the term *child abuse and neglect*.
Late 1970s to Early 1980s	Recognition of elderly abuse expanded, and nurses began to write about their role in responding to the problem.
1980s	Legislation affording women protection from their husbands' physical assaults emerged; at least 43 states enable abused spouses to obtain civil protection orders without initiating divorce proceedings, as previously required.
1985	Approximately half of the states recognized marital rape as a criminal offense.
	A U.S. Surgeon General's report stated that health care professionals must take the lead in preventing and protecting individuals against family violence.
	Only eight states had legally abolished corporal punishment in schools.
1990s	With the number of elderly people expected to double in the next 50 years, it is highly probable that the incidence of elder abuse will increase. Other types of family violence will probably be affected by a refocusing of family values brought about by the AIDS epidemic.
Future	Nurses, because of the variety of work settings, are in a position to detect and assist victims of abuse. However, they will need adequate education and preparation to effectively counsel abuse victims.
	As society comes to accept rape as a crime of violence, additional resources will be allocated for responding to the needs of the victim as well as finding solutions to the problem.

ishment until all else has failed, the child may learn violence as a solution when other methods have been unsuccessful. Children become violence-prone adults or potentially vulnerable victims of violence.

Mounting evidence suggests that the dynamics of abuse within a family are essentially the same whether a child or adult is the object of the attack. The perpetrator of the assault responds to a perceived threat from the victim with aggressive behavior. At the time one individual is subordinated by the other's use of force. Exposure to violence within a family affects every member of the household, even those not directly involved.

Straus, Gelles, and Steinmetz[39a] found a positive corre-

lation between the amount of physical punishment a child experiences and the rate of spouse abuse. Each form of abuse increases in relation to the other: "The people who experienced the most punishment as teen-agers have a rate of wife-beating and husband-beating that is four times greater than those whose parents did not hit them." The lowest rate of conjugal violence is among individuals who were not struck by their parents as teenagers.

Stress management is a skill lacking in abusive families. Their inability to handle stress contributes to problems of abuse or neglect. Increased stress generates greater frustrations. Poor impulse control, a characteristic of abusers, causes them to react without benefit of problem solving.

Victims tend to blame themselves for the chaos the family is experiencing. No one in the family feels good, each member feels pulled in many directions, and support for one another is minimal or nonexistent.

THE CYCLE OF VIOLENCE

Similarities in the cyclical nature of family violence exist regardless of the age, sex, or role status of the victim. Walker[11] has identified three phases in the cycle of violence: tension building phase, explosion phase, and honeymoon phase (Figure 34-1).

Phase I of the cycle of violence is the tension-building phase. During this time of minor assaults, perpetrators may push or throw things at their victims, inflict contusions, subject them to verbal assaults and threats, or humiliate and harm them in other ways. Initially, victims may attempt to comply with demands of their mates in an effort to squelch their anger and hostility. In so doing the victims become unwitting accomplices by implicitly accepting partial responsibility for the abusive situation. Batterers become increasingly oppressive and possessive to maintain control over their victims. This approach is usually effective. Women take extraordinary measures to maintain the precarious equilibrium. Fearing that the aggression may be unleashed on others close to them, battered women distance the couple from supportive persons such as grown children, parents, siblings, and close friends. This isolation gives batterers even greater leverage and control, further jeopardizing the women's safety. As the delicate balance becomes more difficult to maintain because of escalating tension, coping mechanisms begin to disintegrate. Mounting tension can no longer be contained, and phase II erupts.

Phase II is ushered in by an incident of major trauma. It is characterized by a volatile discharge of aggression by the offender, lack of control, and destructiveness. During this time some batterers are so consumed by rage that they lose conscious control of their behavior. Lack of predictability and total lack of control characterize phase II, which lasts approximately 2 to 24 hours. Only the batterers can interrupt this stage. Victims can do little more than try to protect themselves or find a safe place to hide. Acute battering ceases when perpetrators become so physically and emotionally drained that they collapse.

Shock and disbelief follow these attacks. To minimize their fear, victims attempt to ignore or understate the severity of their injuries. The gravity of the injuries usually determines when and if battered women seek medical care.

The cycle concludes with phase III, the honeymoon phase, a period of tenderness, love, contrition, or truce, which is a respite for the couple from the viciousness of phase II. The calm characteristic of phase III follows almost immediately on the heels of the storm of phase II. Victims yearn to believe that love will prevail and that the last attack will be the final one. Phase III lasts longer than phase II but is briefer than phase I as the cycle begins again.

Chronic cycles of violence are often shortened into two phases: tension buildup and violent eruption. Periods of respite become shorter and the truce more uneasy.

CHARACTERISTICS OF VICTIMS

Victims of abuse share common characteristics regardless of age or sex. They are dependent, helpless, and powerless or suffer crippling feelings of dependence, helplessness, or powerlessness (see the research highlight on p. 674). Feelings of terror, anger, and heightened anxiety, numerous physical complaints, and health problems mark the victim profile. Individuals feel responsible for the abuse or neglect inflicted on them, accepting blame or blaming themselves for the perpetrator's actions. The victims are unclear about their reasons for feeling guilty; they assume they must cause the offender to behave the way he does. Victims will recite a litany of explanations for the perpetrator's actions.

Victims also exhibit low self-esteem and depression. They question that they are worthy to be loved and treated with respect. If they are worthy, victims wonder, why then do they suffer at the hands of those who profess to love them? When blamed by perpetrators for their malevolent behavior, victims readily accept the idea. Emotional damage persists long after physical health is restored, but permanent scars from physical trauma are not uncommon to victims of abuse.

In both child and spouse abuse, the response of victims is to "try harder." They believe that if they can only do better in the future, the abuse will cease. Batterers readily support this fallacious logic to shift the blame for their offenses. Victims are doomed to fail because they can never fulfill the unrealistic needs and expectations of the offenders.

CHARACTERISTICS OF PERSONS WHO ABUSE

Perpetrators of abuse exhibit a frightening lack of control over the aggressive impulses discharged through explosive behavior. Many similarities exist among spouse, child, and elder abusers. The offenders explain their assaultive behavior as attempts at disciplinary action that "got

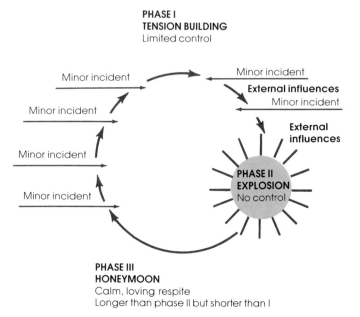

PHASE I
TENSION BUILDING
Limited control

Minor incident

Minor incident

Minor incident

Minor incident

Minor incident

Minor incident

External influences

Minor incident

External
influences

PHASE II
EXPLOSION
No control

PHASE III
HONEYMOON
Calm, loving respite
Longer than phase II but shorter than I

FIGURE 34-1 Walker's cycle theory of battering.

RESEARCH HIGHLIGHT

Comparison of Long-term Effects of Child Abuse by Type of Abuse and by Relationship of the Offender to the Victim

• L Feinauer

PURPOSE

The purpose of this study was to demonstrate differences in emotional distress experienced by childhood victims of sexual abuse when abused by relatives, friends, or strangers.

SAMPLE

Three hundred fifty client files were randomly selected from the 1982 to 1985 files of a nonprofit, university-affiliated clinic specializing in marriage and family therapy.

METHODOLOGY

Each subject completed the Derogatis Symptom Checklist-Revised Edition (SLC-90R). The SLC-90R was used to measure distressed vs denial syndromes, which tend to reflect the global distress index. Distressed clients tend to respond with higher scores on depression, hostility, and somatization items. Denying clients tend to score low or deny distress on anxiety and obsessive items.

Based on data from the *American Journal of Family Therapy* 17(1):48, 1989.

FINDINGS

A higher level of depression was found in women who were abused repeatedly, and greater distress resulted when the offender was considered to be a known and trusted person.

IMPLICATIONS

The increase in emotional distress seen in victims who were abused by a person who was known to and trusted by them supports the clinical finding that sexually abused women may have difficulty in the intimate relationships that occur during marriage and parenting. If the victim trusted and then felt betrayed, choosing to trust again will be the essential focus of therapy. To become intimately involved with another person requires experiences in risk taking, testing, and gaining an ability to trust within the context of a relationship. Attempts to gain intimacy indicate that the client is ready to deal with past events.

---

out of hand." They protest their innocence as abusers with spurious explanations.

Abusers experience low self-esteem and project the blame for their shortcomings on others. They are easily frustrated and unable to control their feelings of frustration constructively.

Emotional immaturity characterizes the perpetrators. They are unable to favorably process reality. As their levels of tension and anxiety escalate, these individuals finally erupt, striking out at the most accessible, vulnerable person in their environment.

The deficit in their emotional maturity is characterized by narcissism. The abusers' self-centeredness prevents them from engaging in meaningful adult relationships. Abusers are too preoccupied with self-gain to invest any substantial quality of themselves in others. Their egocentricity interferes with their ability to recognize other's needs. These narcissistic, emotionally immature adults perceive others as objects responsible for meeting their needs.

Persons who abuse tend to be suspicious of everyone—family, friends, business associates, and strangers. An obvious explanation for their suspicion is fear of being exposed. The fact that individuals who batter usually become violent within the confines of their own homes lends credibility to the speculation that they are aware of their transgressions against the norms of western society.

Distrust of others compels those who abuse to isolate their families. The spouse and children are discouraged from having friends and attending activities unaccompanied by the abuser. The omnipresent fear is that someone will discover the abuse. Children are urged not to answer questions or talk to persons outside the nuclear family. Even

the nuclear family becomes distanced from the extended family to preclude discovery of the abusive pattern. The one who abuses often goes to extraordinary lengths to protect the cover-up. The family's social network becomes minimal.

Ordinarily, the person who abuses possesses greater physical strength than the victim, which may be one reason more women than men are abused during cohabitation. In elder abuse, gender may not be a dominant factor.

Physical size, strength, and power do not play as important a role in child abuse. Clearly both parents are stronger, larger, and more powerful than their children until adolescence.

Persons not familiar with characteristics of abusive situations are misled if they expect the participants in violence to appear abnormal, mentally ill, or mentally incompetent. Individuals who abuse are difficult to detect in a social or business setting. Some may exhibit overt symptoms of emotional dysfunction; however, the nurse cannot rely on overt psychopathological features to identify perpetrators of abuse and neglect.

NURSING PROCESS

One individual should be responsible for conducting the in-depth interview in each treatment setting so that detailed interviews are not repeated by every person requiring information.

The victim's interview must be private. Someone remains with the victim at all times to provide emotional support and ensure the client's safety. In general, the victim needs to be interviewed separately from other individuals providing data. This arrangement provides an opportunity to evaluate the reliability and consistency of interview data. If abuse has occurred, this separate arrangement may meet with resistance from the perpetrator. In some agencies, one staff member interviews the victim while others interview the people who accompanied the victim to the treatment setting.

Interviews are approached matter-of-factly and nonthreateningly. Vocal tones and inflections are carefully controlled. A nonjudgmental attitude is crucial, and establishing trust is essential. Histories of assault are accepted as being truthful unless concrete evidence to the contrary is uncovered. Victims are more likely to deny assault than to fabricate it.

The interview is best structured by initially asking general, less-threatening questions. For example, the nurse may begin with, "What can I do to help you today?" rather than focusing immediately on obvious injuries. This communicates the nurse's personal willingness to assist the client and her readiness to listen. Some victims experience a sense of urgency to discuss their abuse or crisis, as if waiting will prevent them from admitting the truth. Other victims may test the nurse before revealing intimate information they think will reflect on them unfavorably.

When abuse is suspected, the nurse needs to question the client about it directly. For example, the nurse may say, "Your injuries are like those of another woman (or child) I cared for. That person had been beaten (assaulted, attacked, or raped). I am wondering if the same thing happened to you. We are prepared to help people in those circumstances." The victim needs to know that if abuse is revealed, she will be afforded some protection. Frequently, the victim's assailant is the person who accompanies her to the health care agency. Offers for assistance that cannot be provided are never extended to the victim.

The nurse needs to exercise extreme caution in her contact with suspected batterers. They expect to encounter hostility and skepticism and to have their statements attacked. If so, their expectations that no one understands or will help them are confirmed, and they are lost as allies in the nursing process. Cooperation from the alleged batterer will benefit the victim's treatment. A stalemate or negative relationship between the nurse and suspected batterer is destructive to treatment. Although it is difficult for others to understand, the nurse needs to remember that most victims continue to love their abuser.

Abusers and victims may choose alternate treatment settings to avoid arousing suspicion. If they are not known or familiar to any specific caregivers, they avoid establishing an obvious or traceable pattern of repetitious injuries.

The nurse involved in cases of abuse may be called to testify in court. The nurse's assessment is recorded carefully, comprehensively, and explicitly. Verbatim statements are used whenever possible. A tape-recorded statement or interview is more useful. Clear, precise statements about observations, supplemented by examples when possible, are necessary. The nurse's notes need to be decisive. Terminology such as "Client *appears* to have a contusion on left upper arm" is avoided. Either a contusion is present or it is not. When the nurse cannot be certain about an observation, she should note what was observed or heard that contributed to the conclusions.

▼ **ASSESSMENT GUIDELINES FOR ABUSED VICTIMS**

Assess:

Nonverbal communication between client and parent, partner, or caregiver

Verbal communication between client and partner or parent

Nonverbal communication between client and nurse and parent, partner, or caregiver

Body language of client and parent, partner, or caregiver

Balance of communication among interviewer, client, and parent, partner, or caregiver

Dominant or submissive behavior of client and parent, partner, or caregiver

Ineffectual responses to interview material

Ability to answer directly versus subject changes and evasive, tangential, or irrelevant answers

Comfort levels of individuals during interview

Basic psychiatric nursing principles are required to provide optimal care for victims of abuse, even though these individuals are not usually seen by psychiatric nurses. Commonly, victims are assessed for their physical injuries in emergency rooms, private physicians' offices, and other facilities. When hospitalization is required, the client is usually admitted to a unit specializing in care for the victim's type of physical injuries. Whenever possible a psychiatric nurse is consulted for input to the care plan, even when she will not be the primary care provider. Keen observation of the interactions and behavior of the individuals being interviewed can yield a wealth of information. The box above outlines some general guidelines for the assessment interview with the abused client.

CHILD ABUSE

Child abuse or neglect is the physical or mental injury, sexual abuse, negligent treatment, or maltreatment of a child under the age of 18 years by a person who is responsible for the child's welfare under circumstances that indicate that the child's health or welfare is harmed or threatened. Because all states have mandatory reporting laws for confirmed or suspected child abuse, failure to report these cases puts the nurse in direct violation of the law.

Assessment

Physical dimension Their almost total dependence on caregivers places infants, toddlers, and preschool children at particularly high risk for abuse. Unrefined cognitive, motor, and verbal skills keep children from comprehending their predicament, defending themselves, or articulating their plight. Still more vulnerable are children with handicaps and special needs or problems. Although the probability of physical abuse decreases with age, incest and sexual abuse become more likely.

An important feature of child abuse is the cyclical, repetitious nature of the act. Previous trauma may have left the child with permanent physical impairment or other telltale signs, such as scarring.

A detailed history focusing on the injury is obtained from the parents. The child is interviewed in a manner suitable to his age and physical and emotional status. The interviewer proceeds with extreme caution to mitigate defensiveness in the parents and child. Age-appropriate explanations are given to the child as the examination proceeds.

All external signs of trauma are observed and precisely recorded for appearance, size, location, color, and shape. Evidence of scarring is recorded. Head injury is the major cause of death and permanent disability in children under 2 years of age; therefore special attention is given to internal ear and ophthalmoscopic examinations. All body orifices are inspected carefully for indications of trauma. Bones and joints are manipulated for tenderness and range of motion.

Sleep patterns are explored with child and parent. Evidence of *night terrors, somnambulism, somniloquy, enuresis, insomnia, excessive sleeping, chronic fatigue*, or any other change is probed. Eating patterns are also investigated. Failure to thrive and malnourishment are common manifestations of child abuse. The child's height, weight, and head circumference are compared to the norm. Excessive weight gain or loss may signify interpersonal problems. Difficulty swallowing or chewing may result from head or neck trauma. Because head injuries are so prevalent among battered children, neurological function is carefully evaluated. Mastery of age-appropriate developmental tasks is assessed and deficiencies recorded. The current status of immunizations and dental care is evaluated because they are usually unmet in children suffering from abuse or neglect.

Individuals unfamiliar with child abuse find it difficult to comprehend the severity and atrocity of inflicted trauma. No form of torture can be ruled out. Health care providers need to avoid appearing shocked and disbelieving when hearing histories of abused children. Those who work with child abuse are familiar with cases of infants being placed in hot frying pans on the stove; submerged in scalding water; or burned with cigarettes, electric cords, or electric cattle prods. Common injuries resulting from battering of children are listed in the accompanying box.

Any delay in obtaining medical attention alerts the nurse to the possibility of child abuse. Parents who inflict injury on a child postpone seeking treatment for the victim. Victims of child abuse are often dead on arrival at the health care agency.

Radiological studies need to be conducted in every case of suspected abuse of children under age 5 years. Decisions on older children are made consistent with initial signs and symptoms. Frequently, multiple bone injuries in various stages of healing are demonstrated in abused children.

If death results from an assault, the case automatically becomes a police matter. The nurse needs to scrupulously avoid disturbing any possible evidence. The body is not to be handled without permission. Nothing is discarded or cleaned until clearance has been granted.

Identification or suspicion of child abuse immediately evokes the question of sexual abuse. If a vaginal examination is required, all persons involved need to know proper protocol. Evidence that meets legal criteria is collected during the course of the examination. Specimens for sexually transmitted diseases are collected if there is evidence of genitourinary trauma.

COMMON INJURIES OF BATTERED CHILDREN

Head injuries
Internal injuries
Multiple fractures
Soft tissue trauma
Facial trauma (for example, black eyes, gag burns, nose injuries, damaged or missing teeth)
Contusions over entire body
Marks on neck suggestive of strangulation
Burn marks from cigarettes, stove burners, or radiators
Rope burns on wrists and ankles
Lacerations from belt buckles or coat hangers, especially on back or buttocks
Hematomas
Blisters or burns from scalding water
Human bite marks
Bald spots on head from which hair has been pulled
Trauma to genitalia
Injuries in various stages of healing
Evidence of scarring and healed fractures

Emotional dimension The emotional reactions to abuse may be expressed through a variety of behaviors. A child who has been maltreated by those who should love him the most finds it difficult, if not impossible, to trust. Efforts to "give to" the child will precipitate suspicious feelings. The child will find it difficult to accept that strangers want to give him what his parents will not. Emotional responses to note are fear, sadness, hopelessness, helplessness, depression, suspicion, withdrawal, flat or blunted affect, unusual aggressiveness, hostility, mood swings, inappropriate affect, or other erratic behavior. Any child may experience any of these responses for other reasons. It is the nurse's responsibility to make some sense out of the child's emotional response or consult with someone about the meaning of the child's behavior.

Fear in the presence of parents is an especially revealing clue to child abuse. The child may avoid looking at his parents, or his eyes may dart back and forth nervously. The youngster may appear to shrink away from his parents or to hide from one parent behind the other. In strange or frightening situations, most children look to their parents for comfort and reassurance; the abused child may not seek them out.

Lack of age-appropriate anxiety in the presence of strangers is characteristic of abused infants; instead of experiencing the separation anxiety normally seen in infants 9 to 12 months of age, abused babies may relate to anyone. Decreased discrimination may continue for several years and may be misinterpreted as evidence of a well-adjusted baby. Older children may be too intimidated and frightened of adults to interact comfortably with anyone. The environment of victimized youngsters is a terrifying place.

Inappropriate interaction between parents and child warrants exploration by the nurse. The parents may hover too closely about the child or may be preoccupied with themselves. Some adults and children demonstrate unusual affects in times of stress. Unusual affect is not necessarily evidence of child abuse; however its significance to the total assessment needs to be noted.

Intellectual dimension Delayed speech and limited vocabulary are not uncommon in abused children. Academic achievement may decline or classroom performance may be poor for no reason obvious to educators. The cognitive skills usually present in children who are of like age, developmental stage, and intellect may be lacking in young victims of abuse. These youngsters may display decreased attention spans or memory impairments.

Social dimension Observation of parent-child interaction is a fertile area for cues indicating difficulty. The following questions assist with the assessment:

1. Do the parents appear overly solicitous or protective of the child?
2. Will the parents allow the child to answer questions directed toward him, or do they interrupt and try to answer instead?
3. Are the parents unwilling or reluctant to leave the child alone with the nurse or other health care providers?

The parents may be afraid of what the child will say if asked how the injury occurred. They want to control or "interpret" anything the child says. If the parents demand to be in the room when the nurse is talking to the child, the nurse firmly reminds the parents that the question or comment was directed to the child. The case example below illustrates inappropriate parental behavior.

▼ **Case Example**

A 9-year-old girl was admitted to an emergency room on an extremely hot day in July after having sustained third-degree burns over 60% of her body. The mother explained that the girl had been playing with matches and "caught on fire." The girl corroborated the mother's explanation of the fire. This mother demonstrated behaviors characteristic of an abusive parent. The nurse noticed the mother was wearing a coat and chain smoking. When the nurse suggested that the mother remove her coat, she became very defensive, verbally assaulting the nurse. The mother maintained she was extremely cold. Later, when it became necessary for the mother to remove her coat, her clothes beneath reeked of gasoline. The mother had drenched her daughter in gasoline and set her afire. The girl was unable to admit the truth until she had established a trusting relationship with one of the nurses after being hospitalized for several weeks.

The child's school attendance record is explored in cases of suspected abuse. School nurses and teachers are potential sources of information. Their observations about classroom attendance and behavior may be useful to the assessment. Abused children may have a pattern of visits to the school health clinic with vague complaints or problems from their injuries. Recurrent physical illnesses caused by inadequate health care or physical trauma may keep the child out of school. The child may lack adequate clothing or supplies, and it is not uncommon for parents to keep older children out of school to care for younger siblings or perform household chores. Distancing the child from school is another way to socially isolate the youngster from inquisitive people.

Abused children may not be allowed to establish relationships with peers, or they may be reluctant to do so. Being a "loner" provides some protection from questions about visible injuries. Deficient social skills may interfere with the victim's ability to establish or maintain peer relationships. The more isolated the victim's social network, the less likely the abuse will be uncovered.

Spiritual dimension The child may question the existence of a benevolent Superior Being who allows his life to be so miserable and painful. The child may decide on the basis of his maltreatment that he is unlovable or bad. Parents may tell the child he is being beaten to ward off or drive out evil spirits. Some parents view this form of "discipline" as their religious duty. These practices are more common in strict, fundamentalist religions.

Analysis
Nursing diagnosis

The following list provides examples of NANDA-accepted nursing diagnoses:

1. Altered parenting related to having been abused as a child
2. Ineffective family coping related to secrecy about abusive situation
3. Fear related to child abuse
4. Anxiety related to parent's abusive behavior
5. Self-esteem disturbance related to repeated abuse by mother
6. Sleep pattern disturbance related to fear of being abused

Planning

The nursing care plan (Table 34-1) provides some long- and short-term goals, outcome criteria interventions, and rationales related to child abuse, which are examples of the planning stage in the nursing process.

Implementation

Physical dimension When abuse is suspected or confirmed, immediate intervention is directed toward protecting the child from additional trauma and treating his current injuries. Hospitalization may be indicated for temporary protection, and an in-depth diagnostic workup may allow time to outline long-term treatment strategies.

Laboratory and x-ray procedures ordered by the physician are carefully explained to the parent by the nurse, who remains with the child for support. Depending on the injuries, a tetanus booster may be indicated and other immunizations updated. Special diets are provided for nutritional deficiencies or excesses. Classes in nutrition can be offered for parents who lack the knowledge to provide adequate nourishment. Subsidized meal programs may be available at school to provide for children nutritionally neglected in low-income homes.

If a child experiences sleep disturbances, the nurse plans extra time with the youngster at bedtime for a story, back rub, or other activity to promote sleep. Medication for rest or pain can be administered when ordered. The nurse anticipates the needs of battered children, who, unaccustomed to having their needs met by others, are unlikely to make requests.

Emotional dimension Therapeutic experiences for the abused child permit him to explore his feelings about his family and a society that allows him to be mistreated. Intensive psychotherapy is critical for resolving the conflicts and negative feelings of battered children. Lifelong emotional consequences are not uncommon for victims of

▼ **TABLE 34-1   NURSING CARE PLAN**

GOALS	OUTCOME CRITERIA	INTERVENTIONS	RATIONALES
NURSING DIAGNOSIS: Fear related to abuse			
LONG TERM			
To reduce fear of interacting with adults	Demonstrates ability to interact with adults without fear		
SHORT TERM			
To express feelings of fear	Expresses feelings of fear	Assist to express fear by writing, talking, drawing, crying	Identifying feelings, and expressing them helps to acknowledge them as normal and appropriate
		Help client to evaluate safe/unsafe relationships	Not all adults are abusive nor does abuse in a relationship preclude caring
To name resources for help when/if abuse occurs	Names resources	Give information: telephone number, location, person to contact	Provides a sense of control, increases confidence and ability to manage situation

child abuse because their ability to form trusting, interpersonal relationships is damaged.

The nurse encourages the abused youngster to express his feelings by reassuring him that he is safe in the health care environment and will not be punished for verbalizing anger and hostility. Abused children need to be taught acceptable ways of expressing their feelings. Many find it difficult to modify behaviors they have adopted for protection. The nurse explains when, where, how, and with whom it is safe to express negative feelings.

Behaviors useful for decreasing victims' fears and anxiety include the following:
1. Moving slowly around the child
2. Using night lights and avoiding loud noises
3. Giving frequent explanations and reality orientation
4. Administering oral medication instead of injections when possible
5. Keeping the child near the center of activity
6. Placing oneself at eye level to the child instead of above him

To reduce feelings of helplessness, the child is encouraged to participate as much as possible in decisions about his care.

Few if any demands are placed on the victim. The nurse invites him to share feelings and thoughts or participate in activities, but does not insist. Victims often think that nonvictims do not have negative thoughts and feelings. The nurse may stimulate discussion by sharing a comment; for example, the nurse can say, "I really get scared (or angry) when people do mean things to me," or "My feelings are hurt when I try hard to do things right and someone yells at me or calls me stupid," or "I've been punished for things that were not my fault, and I remember feeling confused because I didn't understand why I was punished." Responding to a child's mood swings, withdrawal, apathy, slow progress, and erratic behaviors requires abundant patience.

Intellectual dimension Interventions in the intellectual dimension focus on teaching the child and family to cope with hostility and frustration. If rage behavior is learned from punitive parents, as many theorists believe, abusive families can be taught nonviolent coping mechanisms. The cycle of abuse and violence is broken only by teaching victims and offenders healthy behavior to substitute for unhealthy behavior. Parent Effectiveness Training (PET) is offered in most communities. Nurses teach problem-solving skills that enable parents to identify healthy alternatives to violence and expand their repertoire of coping mechanisms.

Maltreatment resulting from parental ignorance can be resolved by eliminating specific knowledge deficits. In cases of educational neglect, efforts are made to secure appropriate educational opportunities for the child. A tutor is arranged for the child absent from school for a long time as a result of his injuries. The public school system must provide appropriate educational opportunities for children unable to attend school, which is paid for by taxpayers and appropriated from the school budget. These teachers are secured by consulting the child's school and following the policy prescribed by the school system. Preschool-aged children who are educationally disadvantaged in the home can be referred to an educational program to compensate for deficiencies. The abusive family may be too disorganized or unaware of available resources to implement useful suggestions; therefore the nurse provides specific information and assistance. Battered children may lack certain skills for daily living because they have not been taught. Lessons for managing these activities can bolster the child's self-confidence.

Even young children can be taught basic survival tactics. They can learn to get out of the house until the crisis fades if they sense a battering may be imminent. Some victims are very perceptive in identifying warning signs of violence.

For example, if the parent is intoxicated and usually batters when in that state, victims can be instructed to leave the home. They are reminded frequently to tell someone if they are being battered or neglected. They can learn the appropriate people to contact about their situation.

Some children who may be inclined to tell someone about their abuse fail to do so because they do not know how to find assistance. The nurse can teach them how to dial the emergency telephone number for child protective services, a health care provider, police, or 911 if available. Used selectively, this strategy can save a youngster's life, but, it needs to be very carefully planned on an individual basis. The nurse needs to explore the responsiveness and attention given to a call from a child in the community before suggesting that the child call a particular number for help. She can have practice help sessions with her client, in which she teaches him how to call and what to say. The primary message to the child is to tell someone as quickly as possible when abuse occurs.

Social dimension The role of the nurse is not to "rescue" the child from his parents. The nurse hopes that, with adequate treatment for the child and his family, they can be reunited and violence ended. Nurses are careful not to criticize the parents. As difficult as it is for others to understand, victims and perpetrators of child abuse generally do love each other. The battered child is reassured that he is loved and lovable and is not responsible for his parents' behavior. Unquestionably, the nurse is the child's advocate, but a working relationship with the parents is essential to treatment.

Recognizing the child's input as important may help him begin to build or renew a positive sense of self-esteem. Activities to encourage positive feelings about himself are planned around the child's interests and preferences. Initially, the activities need to be short term to provide immediate gratification. Occupational therapy can assist the child's success with selected projects. Self-esteem can be enhanced by acknowledging behaviors that would be effortless for others but are taxing for battered children. For example, attending or participating actively or passively in group activity, initiating or responding to conversation, requesting something for himself, or saying *no* can represent major advances for the maltreated child.

Nursing interventions also include assisting abusive family members to expand their interactions with society. Families are encouraged to develop support systems and social networks.

Battering parents are referred to Parents Anonymous, a group similar to Alcoholics Anonymous. Interaction with other perpetrators of abuse allows parents to learn that their abusive behavior is not unique. Another parent who has learned not to abuse is assigned as an advocate for the batterer to contact when feeling stressed. Reformed abusers can serve as role models for active batterers. Parents Anonymous groups provide a perspective that abusers cannot find elsewhere.

Parents are referred to all appropriate social and community service programs. The nurse gives written numbers of these programs to the offenders during their first contact. Trained volunteers working 24-hour hotlines are available to talk with offenders. Crisis hotlines provide immediate and continuous availability. It is useful for the nurse to help

the batterer establish this contact before he leaves the treatment setting.

Poverty is not a prerequisite for child abuse; however socioeconomic conditions contribute to the problem. Subsidized programs to alleviate hardships caused by these stressors may decrease the incidence of battering in a family. Housing assistance, food programs, temporary child care, unemployment compensation, employment counseling, and medical care programs are useful services for many abusive families. Battered women who abuse their children can be economically strained and in need of temporary assistance during times of separation or divorce.

Intervention with the parents is necessary for the child's welfare. Both parents need treatment if the family is to stay together. Siblings need to have the opportunity for therapy as well. The nurse decides the most appropriate treatment modality, for example, individual or family therapy. Role conflicts, guilt, and frustrations of parenting are explored. As parents learn to meet their own needs, they become better able to meet the needs of their children.

The nurse helps maltreated children develop peer relationships. This process can begin in the hospital if other children are there. Otherwise the nurse can role play meeting other children and practice communication skills with the child. Interactions with sensitive, empathic adults allow the youthful victim to experience healthy, nontraumatic relationships. Gradually, these experiences may allow the abused child to begin to trust.

Spiritual dimension When a child has been told by his parents that his beatings are punishment from God because he is not a good child, the nurse is cautious in disagreeing. The nurse comments matter of factly that some people do not believe God punishes children. However, the nurse does not criticize the parents' belief. The child is reassured that he is not a bad person. The nurse helps the child strengthen his inner resources by emphasizing his self-worth and inherent value as a human being.

Pastoral counseling is available in many health care agencies. A member of the clergy needs to be included on the family violence interdisciplinary team. For hospitals without a task force, the nurse may find a member of pastoral counseling a willing ally to lobby for the formation of a task force.

Nurses can facilitate the requests of children who request clergy. The nurse can offer to listen to a child's prayers or may say one with him. A child accustomed to attending church or Sunday school may profit from a visit to the hospital chapel. The pastoral counseling member of the family violence team can be enlisted for input to meet the child's spiritual needs. Table 34-1 is a nursing care plan for

KEY INTERVENTIONS FOR CHILD ABUSE

Treat the injuries
Protect from additional trauma
Help child feel safe in the health care environment
Facilitate sharing thoughts and feelings
Teach child survival tactics
Give child name of safe person to contact when/if abuse occurs
Restore child's self-esteem
Refer parents to Parents Anonymous

an abused client. Key interventions for the abused child are listed in the box on p. 679.

SEXUAL ABUSE AND INCEST

Sexual abuse is the engagement of dependent children or developmentally immature individuals in exploitative or physically intimate sexual activity (see the research highlight). Activities include fondling, masturbation, unclothing, oral and/or genital contact, and the use of objects for the purpose of physical stimulation. Sexual abuse may be violent or nonviolent. In nonabusive situations sexual partners are able to comprehend the significance of the intimate activity and grant informed consent. Comprehension and consent are not part of abusive sexual activity.

Incest is a particular form of sexual abuse. The National Center on Child Abuse and Neglect views incest as sexual activity performed "on a child by a member of the child's family group," not limited to sexual intercourse but including any action performed to sexually stimulate the child or use the child to stimulate others.[43]

Assessment

Physical dimension Children or adolescents of either sex discovered with injuries of the perineum and/or genitourinary system are probably victims of some type of sexual assault. Health care providers are obligated to vigorously pursue this possibility until a definite diagnosis has been established. Trauma of this type rarely results from other causes. Contusions, hematomas, genital edema, vaginal or rectal bleeding, genitourinary infections, or burns on the genitalia strongly suggest sexual abuse. Venereal disease in children is almost conclusive evidence of sexual abuse. Incestuous relationships may be limited to being forced to fondle, fondling, exhibitionism, or other forms of sexual interaction not including intercourse.

Pregnant adolescents are questioned about a history of incest or sexual abuse, especially if they are vague about boyfriends or other voluntary sexual activity. Pregnant teenagers are often defensive, evasive, fearful, or anxious when questioned about the paternity of the fetus. Their verbal and nonverbal responses to inquiries about incest or sexual assault need to be carefully evaluated. Younger pregnant girls may heighten suspicions of incest, although age is not the major clue to the presence of these crimes.

Emotional dimension Despite the absence of conspicuous evidence of emotional trauma, child sexual abuse has the potential to completely shatter the victim in later life. Sexual molestation without intercourse can be as emotionally destructive as assault including intercourse.

Most victims display symptoms of emotional distress although the cause may be unclear or concealed. The omnipresent need to keep their molestation secret generates substantial fear for victims. Molesters use intimidation, threats, bribes, and manipulation. They endear themselves to the victim and use their dominant positions to secure the victims' cooperation for the sexual activity and silence. Victims are convinced by the perpetrator that no one will believe them if they tell. Some victims may be persuaded to think that these sexual activities are acceptable.

RESEARCH HIGHLIGHT

Sexual Victimization of Child and Adolescent Patients
• V Newbern

PURPOSE

The purpose of this study was to determine whether patient abuse occurred and if so, in what form and with what frequency, where it occurred, which patients were most likely to be abused, and which caregivers were most likely to inflict abuse.

SAMPLE

The sample consisted of 272 caregivers from six caregiver categories who practiced in a variety of settings including acute care institutions, nursing homes, and state institutions.

METHODOLOGY

The Patient Abuse Questionnaire was administered. The questionnaire asked subjects to indicate for each of the three categories of abuse (physical, psychological, and socially acceptable abuse) abusive behaviors observed, the frequency observed, and the caregiver title. Demographical information was also obtained to provide information on discipline and number of years of experience.

Based on data from *Image: Journal of Nursing Scholarship* 21(1):10, 1989.

FINDINGS

Responses to the questionnaires indicated that patient abuse is pervasive in health care settings. The frequency most often reported was one or more times a week. Women, the elderly, patients perceived as aggressive, and those with chronic conditions were most vulnerable to abuse.

IMPLICATIONS

Findings were consistent with the literature; girls were the most frequent victims, men were most often the perpetrators. Because of the perpetrator's strength and power, children and adolescents are at risk for victimization. Being in a health care setting makes them even more vulnerable to victimization. This study provides a basis for larger studies that document abuse and offer ways to end abuse to children and adolescents in health care settings.

Responses to child sexual abuse include immobilizing anxiety, depression, guilt, shame, substance abuse, suicide attempts, and other forms of self-destructive behavior. Young victims, especially girls, who show these behaviors alert health care providers to consider incest or sexual abuse. A history of sexual exploitation may be uncovered for the first time in adult women initially seen with symptoms of emotional disequilibrium. Cases of child molestation or incest may be repressed for many years.

Intellectual dimension Adolescents victimized by incest or sexual abuse can find themselves so emotionally drained and preoccupied with concealing the secret that their academic performance suffers. These youngsters may respond with increased absences from school or by quitting school.

Young children describe their symptoms in rudimentary language. For example, during a physical examination the child may say, "It hurts down there," or "He hurt me down there," or "He put something inside of me." The child may use sexually explicit terminology too advanced for his age. Such comments must never be ignored! Children do not fabricate sexual experiences. They lack the information and background to articulate such events unless they occurred. Children whose attempts to tell their mothers have been rejected are unlikely to tell others. If a mother expresses disbelief, victims presume strangers will not believe them either.

Social dimension The burden of keeping the secret of incest prevents sexually exploited youngsters from forming close peer relationships. As these children mature, they fear physical and emotional intimacy with others. Superficial relationships and social isolation characterize these victims.

Role confusion and ambivalence are major features of the father-daughter incest victim profile. The victims experience intense rage toward the offender from whom they expected nurturing, guidance, and love. Many children risk parental rejection if they attempt to reveal their secret. The mother may respond with hostility, disbelief, and punishment. She may blame the victim for initiating the intimacy, leaving the victim without an advocate or protector in the family.

Commonly, missing children or runaways are victims of sexual abuse. The parents may profess not to know why their child would leave. Rarely does an incestuous relationship exist without the mother's knowledge. Mothers may remain passive and uninvolved for reasons that meet their own needs.

Some teenagers will remain in their abusive situation to "save" younger siblings from the same fate. It is not unusual for fathers to victimize all of their daughters when the girls reach a certain age. Some fathers claim they believe it their duty to teach their daughters about sex through incestuous relations.

Spiritual dimension Victims may feel spiritually unclean after they have been sexually violated. They may distance themselves from their spiritual support system as a result of these feelings or a perceived need for secrecy. Older victims may feel they have been unfaithful to religious teachings, promoting a greater sense of isolation. Sexually exploited youngsters may emerge with a developmentally distorted sense of values and morality.

Analysis and Planning

Because sexual abuse and incest are types of child abuse, the reader is referred to Table 34-1 for examples of long- and short-term goals, outcome criteria, interventions, and rationales related to child abuse.

Implementation

Physical dimension Prenatal care for the pregnant adolescent addresses the higher risks incurred by the younger obstetrical client. Venereal diseases must be reported, and the client needs to be questioned about her sexual partners. The nurse remains with the client during the interview to provide support.

Emotional dimension The most significant contribution to the victim's emotional well-being is early case finding to interrupt patterns of chronic sexual abuse. The earlier the incest victim is treated the greater the chance to prevent or resolve major emotional trauma. The prognosis for full emotional recovery without permanent emotional scarring becomes graver the longer the abuse continues.

Nurses assist victims by responding to them in a nonjudgmental, supportive manner. Victims are repeatedly reassured that they are not to blame for the sexual offenses. Opportunities to experience a safe closeness, with the potential for interpersonal trust, are provided. The nurse recognizes that a pregnancy conceived under these circumstances may generate ambivalent or hostile feelings. The nurse encourages expression of these feelings and makes herself available to listen. Assistance is provided so the victim can make a mutually beneficial, informed decision about her pregnancy.

Victims are encouraged to join groups specifically for incest and sexual abuse. These groups allow victims to confront their fears and rage with support from other victims. They begin to see themselves as survivors rather than helpless victims. Individual therapy also promotes emotional healing.

Intellectual dimension Children are taught that their bodies are private. They need to understand that it is permissible to say "no" to any adult urging intimate contact. Activities that involve close body contact and cause youngsters to feel uncomfortable probably have incestuous overtones. Numerous booklets addressing sexual abuse of children are available.

Sex education that includes a discussion of healthy sexual attitudes and age-appropriate sexual activities is provided for victims. Negative feelings and confusion about sexual function need to be addressed. Teachers comfortable with their own sexuality can facilitate candid discussion about sexual concerns.

Youngsters are instructed to inform their parents or another responsible adult if they are sexually exploited. They are urged to keep telling until they find someone who believes them and agrees to help. The child's dilemma is identifying a safe person with whom to communicate. This task requires children to be assertive in a difficult situation. Role playing can give children practice in telling.

Social dimension Suspected or confirmed cases of incest or sexual exploitation are reported to authorities in accordance with state laws. Health care providers are in violation of the law if they do not report these cases.

Interventions are designed to assist victims to develop peer relationships and expand social networks. The nurse helps them identify activities that may lead to meeting people their own age with similar interests (for example, church groups, scouting, special interest groups at school, YWCA programs, community education programs, or volunteer programs). Nursing intervention can help the victim understand that everyone has events in their lives they prefer not to reveal. Positive interpersonal interactions promote self-confidence and decrease fear of intimacy with other persons.

Child protective services (CPS) are notified to assist in protecting the victim. The nurse collaborates with CPS in the youngster's care. CPS attends to the family, including other siblings at risk in the home. This strategy relieves the victim of the burden of protecting and caring for her siblings while she is struggling to maintain her own equilibrium. Public health nurses may follow a pregnant adolescent through her pregnancy and provide postpartum care.

Teenagers are encouraged to remain in or return to school. The nurse collaborates with the school nurse to discuss a general treatment plan. She helps the school personnel to understand the feelings and problems experienced by victims of sexual exploitation. Adult dropouts are given information about obtaining a high school equivalency diploma, which may improve their feelings of accomplishment and self-worth.

Spiritual dimension The nurse can locate clergy of various religions in the community who are particularly sensitive to counseling victims with spiritual problems resulting from sexual abuse. In many hospitals, nurses are good resources for those who need assistance in this area. Key interventions for sexual abuse are listed below.

SPOUSE ABUSE

Spouse abuse is the battery of an *emancipated* minor aged 18 years or older who is the victim of an intentional act of physical violence occurring during the course of an intimate, interpersonal relationship with a spouse or partner.

There are no uniform laws to mandate reporting of suspected or confirmed spouse battery.

Assessment

Physical dimension Spouse abuse is seriously considered a problem for any woman who has injuries that appear to be trauma induced. Frequently, the first incident of battering will occur during a pregnancy. Caregivers need to consider the possibility of battering in pregnant women with any type of injury.

Common injuries incurred by battered women are listed in the accompanying box.

Women can be pushed down the stairs and thrown out of moving cars and have their hands purposely slammed in doors. The cruelty of these acts can strain the boundaries of believability.

Battered women are reluctant to reveal the cause of their injuries, preferring spurious explanations such as falling down the stairs, automobile accidents, stumbling over objects, or bumping into things. When the victim's statement about the cause of her trauma is incongruent with her injuries, abuse should be suspected. Spouse abuse is suggested by the way the victim responds to the history taking and physical examination. If the woman fails to acknowledge her situation, the nurse who suspects abuse directly asks her if she was battered.

The unrelenting emotional trauma caused by battering precipitates many alterations in victims' health. Women living in an atmosphere of escalating tension before the acute battering episode are afraid to go to sleep, fearing they will be attacked in bed. These women may be unable to obtain proper sleep for weeks. When they do get sleep, it is fitful and restless. They may experience eating disturbances (especially anorexia), insomnia, fatigue, unremitting headaches, gastrointestinal disorders, hypertension, palpitations, hyperventilation, and dermatitis.

Emotional dimension Emotional problems often follow an acute battering episode, for example, depression, malaise, withdrawal, feelings of despair and helplessness, suicidal thoughts, guilt, shame, blunted or inappropriate affect, increased anxiety, and hostility. Fear permeates the battered woman's existence. Rarely does she feel safe from the impulsive rage of her abuser, even when they are not together. She is afraid the batterer will return or find her wherever she may be and beat her again.

Intellectual dimension The intellectual abilities of abused women may be compromised because of the adversity they face. Physical and emotional impairments interfere with ego functioning. The victim may stutter, ex-

KEY INTERVENTIONS FOR SEXUAL ABUSE

Assess for disease (STD, AIDS), pregnancy
Respond in nonjudgmental, supportive manner
Reassure that victim is not to blame for sexual offense
Teach healthy sexual attitudes and age-appropriate sexual activities
Encourage victim to tell responsible person when/if exploited
Report exploitation to authorities
Encourage victim to remain in school and to develop peer friendships
Refer to support group

COMMON INJURIES OF BATTERED WOMEN

Facial injuries (such as black eyes, missing, chipped, or loose teeth, fractures of the nose or jaw, and hematomas or lacerations of the lips and mouth)
Head injuries (such as concussions, bald spots from which hair has been pulled, and blurred vision or tinnitus)
Fractures of the upper extremities incurred by raising the arms to ward off blows
Joint tenderness from the perpetrator grabbing or twisting the arms
Contusions or other strangulation marks on the neck
Contusions and hematomas of the abdomen in pregnant women
Cigarette burns
Spontaneous abortion
Damage to the fetus
Human bite marks, especially on the breasts
Trauma to the genitalia

hibit halting speech, or grope for words. Memory may be impaired by physical or emotional difficulties. Battered women use many different coping mechanisms. Rationalization, projection, displacement, denial, suppression, repression, and regression are common. They may try to minimize or deny the event. Some women experience periods of dissociation.

Not uncommonly, victims articulate intellectual comprehension of their plight, yet experience behavioral immobilization. Battered women characteristically report feeling "trapped" or being "under mind control." External locus of control is characteristic of battered women. Furthermore, there is no relationship between intelligence level and the ability to think and act rationally while being abused or to evaluate the abusive situation. The victim's terror is so extensive and denial so pervasive that rational assessment eludes them.

The nurse gathers data about the couple's behavior during times of disagreement and methods they use to solve arguments. There is a high correlation between verbal aggression and physical violence. Recurrent verbal disputes within a relationship increase a couple's risk for physical abuse.

Social dimension Abused women are also victimized by a society that tolerates comments implying lack of intelligence or placing the blame on battered women. "She should have sense enough to leave," "You'd think she'd be smart enough to get out," "She must like it to put up with it," and "I'd never let someone do that to me" are recurring themes.

Social isolation prevails among abused women for several reasons. Societal attitudes contribute to their perceived need to isolate themselves. Perpetrators use social isolation to increase their control over the victims' lives and reduce threats of exposure. Support systems are weak or absent because of the victims' withdrawal. Fearing the batterer will vent his rage on others, victims distance themselves from extended family members and friends. Some women remain in their homes for days after a severe beating to avoid embarrassing questions and detection. Tinted glasses may be worn to cover eye injuries. The nurse evaluates patterns of socialization in victims of trauma and looks for changes in patterns of social activity that denote increasing isolation.

The less the victim interacts with others, the less opportunity she has to develop support systems and maintain social skills. Isolation contributes to self-doubt and thwarts efforts to validate behaviors in the relationships of her peers. Many women are genuinely surprised to learn that all women are not battered on occasion during the course of marriage or an intense relationship, especially if violence existed in their family as children. Victims are commonly blamed by their extended families for the conjugal violence. Family members pressure the victim to resolve the conflicts. The nurse assesses the potential availability of support from extended family members.

Spiritual dimension Although spouse battering can occur in individuals of all religious denominations, lack of religious affiliation in both partners correlates with the highest rate of conjugal violence.

The woman's value system and religious beliefs influence her responses to the abusive situation. Religion may be a dominant factor in determining the victim's alternatives to an abusive marriage. She may feel it would be morally reprehensible to expose the father of her children. Her commitment to keep her family together at any cost may be an extension of her religious beliefs. On the other hand, religious commitment can support victims who are contemplating committing suicide or killing their attacker.

To a battered woman, religion may be viewed as a support or cause for punishment. The battered woman may think she has been victimized for not adhering to her faith or attending church regularly. She may see the abuse as her punishment for failure as a wife or for infidelity or other indiscretions. Unmarried women may link abuse to involvement in a legally unsanctioned intimate relationship.

Analysis
Nursing diagnosis

The following list provides examples of NANDA-accepted nursing diagnoses.
1. Anxiety related to anticipation of next abusive episode
2. Pain related to trauma of physical abuse
3. Ineffective family coping related to poor use of support system to bring relief from abuse
4. Ineffective individual coping related to inability to leave abusive situation
5. Disturbance in self-concept related to continual derogatory statements by spouse
6. Social isolation related to embarrassment about physical scars from abuse
7. Altered thought processes related to extreme fear of being beaten
8. Sleep pattern disturbance related to fear of abuse

Planning

Table 34-2 provides some long- and short-term goals, outcome criteria, interventions, and rationales related to spouse abuse, which are examples of the planning stage of the nursing process.

Implementation

Physical dimension In the cycle of violence, women are most likely to seek care for their battering during the brief interval after the explosion phase. Their vulnerability at this time makes them particularly receptive to intervention. Trauma has been inflicted, and the victims are in pain or worried about their injuries. Caregivers who fail to identify abuse at this time usually have to wait until the cycle of violence repeats itself for another opportunity to help.

Victims are often in a state of shock after the assault and may be unaware of the severity of their injuries. Intervention may include hospitalization for observation and full evaluation. Nursing care appropriate to specific injuries is implemented.

A signed permit from the victim allows photographs of her injuries at the time of treatment. The client's name, the time, date, place, and the name of person taking the photos are noted on the film. If the client decides to prosecute, these photos are valuable evidence. The nurse reminds the

▼ **TABLE 34-2   NURSING CARE PLAN**

GOALS	OUTCOME CRITERIA	INTERVENTIONS	RATIONALES
NURSING DIAGNOSIS: Fear related to conjugal violence			
LONG TERM			
To establish a safe environment	Client resides with her family without being assaulted.		
	Family does not participate in family violence.		
To use support systems to alleviate stress	Client identifies potential stressful situations.		
	Client uses support systems before violence erupts.		
	Client identifies alternate approaches to avoid being victimized.		
SHORT TERM			
To find a safe shelter for temporary residence	Client resides in a safe setting.	Provide telephone number, location, person to contact for shelter.	Giving information promotes a sense of control that increases confidence and self-esteem.
	Client makes decisions about future living arrangements.		
To make decisions that promote safety	Client makes decisions that ensure her safety.	Teach problem solving.	Helps client to weigh risks and benefits of decisions and make responsible choices.
		Encourage client to attend support group.	To share thoughts and feelings and to reduce isolation.

client to get additional color photos in the next few days, if possible, because soft tissue injuries become more apparent with time.

Care for victims' other health problems, such as sleep and nutritional deficits, is also planned. Warm soaks, heating pads, extra pillows for support, massages, and muscle relaxants or pain medication are therapeutic interventions for general body soreness and pain. Pain reduction promotes restful sleep, and many muscle relaxants produce drowsiness. Oral hygiene may be needed as a result of trauma to the jaw, mouth, or teeth. These injuries may also necessitate a special diet.

If the victim is pregnant, interventions are planned to protect the fetus. Possible pregnancy is ruled out before completing orders for x-ray studies. Medications are used cautiously in pregnant victims. Head injuries may preclude the use of medication until a definitive medical diagnosis has been established. A tetanus booster may be required for women with bites, burns, puncture wounds, or lacerations.

Emotional dimension The nurse may find crisis intervention techniques useful during initial contact to reduce the client's anxiety level (see Chapter 27).

After an acute episode of battering, the victim needs to recover emotionally and physically. During the initial 24 to 72 hours after the battering, victims are helped to rest and to reduce stress levels. The nurse acts as a facilitator to relieve the victim of child care and housekeeping chores.

Battered women are encouraged to verbalize their feelings of ambivalence, hostility, and guilt. The nurse's attitude facilitates communication. Victims find it difficult to understand why they love a man who treats them so cruelly. Although most interventions in the emotional dimension require extended nurse-client contact, therapeutic principles of basic psychiatric nursing are equally essential in short-term encounters. Each positive interaction has the potential to demonstrate to the victim that she deserves to be treated with dignity and respect.

Intellectual dimension Women with injuries that suggest battering are given written information about available health, social, and legal services. If the victim feels that the information may jeopardize her safety if the abuser finds it, she is given instructions about how to conceal the information. The victim may tape the phone number of a shelter or crisis hotline to the bottom of a drawer. A preferable alternative for some women is to show them where the numbers are listed in the telephone book; however, in times of crisis it is more difficult to find the numbers.

The strong relationship between external locus of control and greater severity of physical and nonphysical abuse indicates that victims may profit by learning to be responsible for controlling or influencing the outcome of events in their lives. The client learns to accept that she cannot control the batterer, only her responses to the batterer and to her situation. Battered women are informed that the frequency and severity of abuse increase the longer the abusive relationship lasts, which puts them in increasingly greater danger. Interventions focus on the difficulties that make the victim unable to disengage from a destructive relationship. The nurse helps the client identify her options in response to the abuse. The client learns problem-solving skills and then demonstrates them by assessing and discussing alternatives related to one of her problems.

The victim needs to make her own decision regarding the abuse. If she chooses to leave the abusive situation, books that focus on learning to leave can be helpful. Victims who leave precipitously usually take only the clothes they are wearing. By the time they get assistance, the batterer has cleared any mutual bank accounts of all funds, terminated the woman's access to charge accounts, changed the door locks, and prevented the victim from getting her belongings. Victims are encouraged to plan leaving to their own advantage and not to leave abruptly except to protect themselves and their children. Once the client has made a decision, the nurse supports her in that decision whether or not the nurse agrees.

Social dimension Efforts are aimed toward assisting the victim to increase her self-concept. A trusting relationship between the nurse and client is the foundation for the client to be more receptive to positive statements about herself. Groups are valuable resources and can provide support and feedback. Consistent positive responses from other persons can slowly reduce negative feelings.

The victim is assisted to identify her strengths and capitalize on them. With the caregiver's help, the victim develops realistic awareness of liabilities and ways to overcome them.

Legal options such as protective orders and prosecution are discussed with the woman. Sources to contact include the League of Women Voters, the state bar association, and the state central office for domestic violence. Community services are now available to battered women. Shelters for battered women and their children are located in almost every community.

Crisis hotlines offer a wide variety of services to abused women. They are good resources for women or caregivers who need information about available services. The nurse may want to coordinate her care plan with the services offered through the hotline. Many communities provide support for the woman choosing to prosecute.

KEY INTERVENTIONS FOR SPOUSE ABUSE

Treat injuries
Offer protection from additional injuries
Obtain consent to photograph injuries
Decrease stress level by relieving victim of child care responsibilities
Help victim express feelings of ambivalence, guilt, anger
Give information about available health care, social and legal services, and crisis hotlines
Teach problem-solving skills and demonstrate use of them with one problem
Help victim make own decisions, e.g., to stay or leave situation
Support victim's decision
Increase self-concept
Refer to support group
Refer to vocational rehabilitation or employment counseling

Lack of education and job skills narrows some victims' options. Clients who are unable to secure employment to support themselves and their children can be referred to vocational rehabilitation or employment counseling programs.

Spiritual dimension Interventions are personal and are guided by the client's values and beliefs. The nurse can help arrange spiritual counseling if the client desires. Victims contemplating divorce or other actions resulting in separation of the family unit may profit from pastoral counseling. This strategy is most effective if the clergyman has had specialized training in working with the problems of family violence. Table 34-2 is a sample nursing care plan. Key interventions for spouse abuse are listed in the accompanying box.

ELDER ABUSE

Elder abuse is any willful or negligent act that results in malnutrition, physical assault or battery, or physical or psychological injury of an elderly person by other than accidental means, including failure to provide necessary treatment, rehabilitation, care, sustenance, clothing, shelter, supervision, or medical services. Many states have laws that mandate the reporting of elder abuse. Colorado, Wisconsin, Iowa, and Wyoming have voluntary reporting laws.

Assessment

Physical dimension As with other types of abuse, a thorough history and physical examination need to be performed. The client is observed for signs of striking, shoving, beating, or restraining injuries such as those described for physically abused women and children. The client is asked if he has been shaken, shoved, hit, restrained, burned, locked up, or left unattended inappropriately.

Medication abuses include excessive, missed, or withheld medicines. The nurse explores the possibility of these types of abuse by questioning the client and caregiver. Some older persons require assistance with their personal hygiene. Omitting or refusing required assistance can lead to multiple physical problems. Clients inappropriately dressed for the environment also evoke concern.

Malnutrition is one of the most common forms of elder abuse. Clients are carefully questioned about any weight loss. They may not be receiving an adequate amount of food, or their diet may be grossly unbalanced. Some older people need assistance to eat. Inattention to oral hygiene and dental care affect abilities to eat properly.

Contusions, hematomas, and fractures can be attributed to conditions such as circulatory impairments, osteoporosis, failing vision, or skin changes caused by aging. Similarly, changes that interfere with the perception of extremes of hot or cold can delay reflex responses and result in injury. Thus the nurse is cautious in assessing the origins of the injuries and in interpreting the explanation provided by the caregiver and client. Adequate consideration is given to possibilities of injuries occurring in nonabusive situations in the aged client.

Emotional dimension Abused elderly individuals share many responses to abuse common to other victims. They fear retaliation from the perpetrator if they complain or report the abuse. Their fear may be reflected in vigilant attention to the caregiver's actions, distancing themselves from the caregiver, and dodging or ducking when their caregiver moves. This fear needs to be distinguished from paranoid behavior or confusion.

The older person may experience guilt and shame for raising children who abuse him. Shame can be as powerful as fear of retaliation in keeping the client from revealing his abuse. The control the caregiver exercises may promote feelings of helplessness and hopelessness, which can lead to depression and withdrawal.

The caregiver is observed for hostile, secretive, insulting, threatening, destructive, or aggressive behavior. The caregiver may also show little concern for the elderly person and appear withdrawn, passive, or disinterested in the nurse's suggestions. On the other hand, the caregiver may demonstrate exaggerated concern or defensiveness, indicating guilt or an effort at disguise.

Caregivers' feelings about maintaining or losing control of their own behavior and the older person's are important because those who abuse are often obsessed with their fear of losing control.

Intellectual dimension Because of the stereotype of elderly individuals as "forgetful" or "confused," their credibility may be questioned when they report abuse. Thus it is crucial to assess the elderly person's clarity of thinking and memory. Nurses need to know that loss of recent memory and focus on remote events can be normal for an elderly person. Ample time is allowed to respond to questions during assessment. A client who feels pressured to respond quickly may experience increased anxiety, which impairs cognition.

The caregiver's knowledge of the client's medical condition and necessary care is assessed. What looks like neglect or abuse may be the caregiver's inadequate knowledge about providing care.

Social dimension Elderly abuse is more likely to be committed by those who have been victims of or witnesses to familial abuse as children. The client is questioned about theft or misuse of finances, property, or possessions by the caregiver. He may believe that his caregivers are entitled to make all decisions about disposition of his material goods, or he may be forced to forfeit control of his material possessions.

The roles and relationships, past and present, of all family members are evaluated for their actual or potential contribution to an abusive situation. For example, an adult child with unresolved negative feelings toward his parents may consciously or unconsciously reverse roles with the elderly parent and enact some of these negative feelings through abuse.

The family's cohesiveness, its social isolation or alienation, and its available support systems are other important considerations. The amount of contact outside the home indicates the client's level of social isolation and the caregiver's role in facilitating or controlling this contact. Such control is common when others need to be kept out of the home to maintain the secrecy of the abuse.

The degree of the client's dependence on caregivers for financial and physical support is assessed. Knowing who assists the client with daily living needs provides data about the degree of stress on the family. It is important to assess

whether the caregiver's own dependent needs have been met, as it is more difficult for the caregiver to accept the dependent needs of the aged person if his own needs for dependence have not been met.

The elderly person's role expectations of himself and the caregiver, as well as the caregiver's expectations of his own role and the aged person's role, need to be explored. Data from this assessment can assist the nurse in determining whether these experiences are realistic or unrealistic and in identifying role conflict or role reversal.

Spiritual dimension The values of both the aged person and the caregiver affect their reactions in situations with potential for abuse. If the spiritual values of the elderly person and the caregiver include a deep respect for another person's life and a sense of caring that transcends problems imposed on the losses of aging and the resulting responsibilities taken on by the caregivers, there is a strong force against potential abuse. On the other hand, if the individual's spiritual values do not help them accept the losses experienced in aging and the necessity of the caregiver's role in support of the elderly person, those involved may more readily find an abusive situation justifiable.

Other aspects of the assessment of the spiritual dimension are the resources for support for both the elderly person and the caregivers from the religious affiliations and activities.

Analysis
Nursing diagnosis

The following list provides examples of NANDA-accepted nursing diagnoses:
1. Altered health maintenance related to caregiving responsibilities
2. Fear related to maltreatment by caregiver
3. Altered family processes related to grandparent moving into home
4. Ineffective family coping related to acting-out behavior of older adult

Planning

The nursing care plan (Table 34-3) provides some long- and short-term goals, outcome criteria, interventions, and rationales related to elderly abuse, which are examples of the planning stage of the nursing process.

Implementation

Physical dimension Adequate physical care to meet the victim's health needs is provided, which includes a diet tailored to the individual's requirements. The client is given foods that he can manage. To promote his independence, the client is encouraged to do as much as possible for himself. Caregivers supplement care as warranted by the person's condition.

Emotional dimension Frequently a feeling of helplessness discourages older people from trying to stop their abuse. They may need assistance in restoring feelings of control and hopefulness about their situation. Fear of retaliation by the caregiver or fear of losing a preferred living situation may also be present. The nurse can assist

▼ **TABLE 34-3 NURSING CARE PLAN**

GOALS	OUTCOME CRITERIA	INTERVENTIONS	RATIONALES
NURSING DIAGNOSIS: Ineffective individual coping related to caregiver's increased responsibilities			
LONG TERM			
To establish a caring, co-operative relationship between the caregiver and the elderly person	Elderly person experiences satisfaction with the care given him.		
	Caregiver experiences satisfaction with role as caregiver.		
To use adequate support systems for the caregiver when responsibilities become unmanageable	Caregiver can identify family and community resources available for assistance in caregiving responsibilities.		
SHORT TERM			
To realistically balance job and caregiver responsibilities	Caregiver sets realistic limits on her responsibilities.	Have caregiver list activities for which she is responsible.	Determine activities she can realistically carry out and those that can be delegated to others
	Caregiver recognizes her needs and responsibility for her own health.	Have caregiver list activities others can do.	
		Encourage caregiver to identify others who can assist with caregiving responsibilities occasionally and on a regular basis.	Provide relief from caregiving responsibilities
		Encourage caregiver to take time off from responsibilities to pursue own pleasures.	Maintain physical and emotional health and to enrich own life

the older person in exploring and working through the fear by providing a relationship in which the older person feels comfortable enough to express his fear.

The caregiver can discuss guilt and frustration with the nurse. Group therapy, such as Children Anonymous groups, provides middle-aged children a forum in which to explore together their feelings and the difficulties in caring for an elderly parent. They can then use each others' experiences to identify ways to cope.

◢ **Intellectual dimension** The client is provided with as much information about his care as he can understand. Explaining realistic care expectations enables clients to recognize abuse or neglect when it occurs.

Preventive interventions include teaching nonviolent behavior early in life and educating the family about the normal aging process. Managers of senior centers or nutrition sites, as well as community "gatekeepers," such as postal workers or grocery clerks, may suspect abuse and neglect but not know what to do. Training can focus on signs of abuse, available services, and reporting procedures. Health care professionals need to tell gatekeepers that it is all right to be suspicious and also to reinforce their reporting and other forms of involvement. Programs such as the Gatekeeper Project in Philadelphia have been successful in promoting the detection of abuse.[10] Nurses can also teach self-care to elderly clients or appropriate care to caregivers.

◢ **Social dimension** Most interventions involve ways to promote relief from the caregiver's often continual responsibilities. Interventions may include using a home health aide for personal care or an adult day care center. An alternate living arrangement, such as a nursing home or an adult foster home, may be necessary. Hospitals have begun to form Adult Protection Teams (APT). These teams employ interdisciplinary groups of professionals to implement care for families involved in elderly abuse.

Family counseling to clarify role expectations is a useful intervention. When role conflicts are identified, expectations about the needed roles can be clarified, the family member's ability to enact the new roles can be strengthened, and families can be assisted in performing the new roles.

Families need to be encouraged to develop extended kinship networks. Because older people are often more likely to bring their problems to friends in the neighborhood than to formal agencies, nurses need to encourage a mutual help model in communities that emphasizes a reciprocal exchange of services and "watching out for each other." For example, a neighborhood block home for the elderly can be identified as a place where families turn for

KEY INTERVENTIONS IN ELDER ABUSE

Provide physical care if victim is unable to do it.
Help victim express fears, guilt, frustration.
Discuss realistic care expectations with victim and caregiver.
Offer services to caregiver for relief from responsibilities, e.g., day care, home health aide, neighbor or family member sitter.
Teach community service personnel to be alert to abuse, e.g., postal workers, senior citizen sites.
Refer to support group for caregivers.

assistance, or a neighborhood elderly sitting pool could be established. Shelters for battered women can also develop support groups for aged women who have left abusive situations.

Spiritual dimension Actions by the nurse that display a valuing of older people and a concern for the quality of their existence serve as an example for families who may be discouraged in their caregiving efforts. At the same time, the degree of love and concern displayed by many families caring for older people in the most difficult of situations is often an inspiration to the nurse and extends the nurse's knowledge about ways to assist families who are not able to cope successfully in similar situations.

Frequently, church or synagogue members provide a variety of supports to families of the elderly, including participation in the care and an affirmation of the family's spiritual beliefs regarding their important role in providing for the older family member. Counseling may also be part of the church's or synagogue's ministry to its members. Table 34-3 is a sample nursing care plan. Key interventions for elder abuse are listed in the accompanying box above.

RAPE

Rape is the legal term for an act of engaging another person in unlawful sexual intercourse through the use of force and without valid consent of the sexual partner.

Statutory rape is a legal term for the act of sexual intercourse with a person under the age of consent determined by state law. Sexual intercourse with a minor person is considered unlawful even with consent of the minor to the sexual act.

Acquaintance rapes are committed by men known to the victim. College women are more vulnerable to rape by someone they know than by a stranger. As many as 77% of the reported cases of sexual assault have occurred while on a date.[37] It is believed that the American dating system contributes to rape, with studies of male sex aggression supporting this belief. According to the Center for Women Policy Studies, many date rapes are due to misunderstandings between men and women. Communications between the sexes during foreplay frequently leads to misunderstandings that contribute to date rape. Men often interpret unresisted, progressive sexual foreplay (particularly when the man is allowed to fondle the female's genitals) as an invitation to intercourse, whereas the woman may not have had this intent. Many men are deficient in understanding women and misinterpret their behavior and likewise, many women are deficient in understanding men and misinter-

pret their behavior. A lack of communication between both sexes confounds the issue.

Nurses and other health care providers are not required to report rape or sexual assault to authorities in most states. In the absence of a legal mandate, health care providers must have permission from the client before notifying the authorities.

Assessment

Physical dimension Physical assessment of sexual assault victims includes the standard history and physical examination outlined in professional protocols. For sexual assault victims, special attention is given to menstrual, sexual, and obstetric history. Date of the last menstrual period, present form of birth control, current use of medications, and last act of coitus before the assault are recorded. The necessity for candid disclosure of this information is explained to the victim. The assault needs to be described and recorded in minute detail.

Specific data are obtained about penile penetration, orifices violated, duration of intercourse, use of a condom, occurrence and/or site of assailant's orgasm, and physical activities since the assault. The victim is asked whether she has bathed, showered, douched, urinated, defecated, vomited, cleansed her mouth, or changed clothes.

The total body is examined for any contusions, abrasions, lacerations, hematomas, burns, scars, or other anomalies. The victim's clothing is examined and retained, with her approval, for use as evidence. All body orifices are carefully inspected for signs of trauma. Swabs of body cavities are taken as deemed necessary. The pelvic examination includes procedures to detect sexually transmitted diseases and the presence of semen. The woman's pregnancy status is determined by laboratory tests. Pubic hair samples and fingernail scrapings are obtained. With the victim's consent, photographs are taken for additional documentation of injuries. Evidence is sealed, labeled, dated, and signed by the collector and the receiver. Nurses need to be aware of the importance of adhering to strict protocol for evidence collection. A breach of protocol could make evidence inadmissible in court if the woman prosecutes.

A variety of somatic responses follow forced sexual contact. Sleep disturbances, increased motor activity, sobbing, crying, headaches, oropharyngeal trauma from oral sex, disrupted eating patterns, musculoskeletal discomfort, gastrointestinal difficulties, genitourinary problems, sexual dysfunction, nausea, vomiting, and malaise are some of the more common problems.

Emotional dimension Rape victims display a vast array of emotional responses. Personality structure, previous coping strategies, and life circumstances at the time of the attack all contribute to the victim's reaction.

The prevailing initial response to sexual assault is extreme fear. The unexpectedness of the attack, coupled with loss of control and threats from the assailant, explain the victim's overwhelming fear. Some women feel grateful to have escaped with their lives, whereas others feel guilty for having survived. Victims report being frightened of physical injury, mutilation, and death during the attack. Fear prevents them from leaving their homes or being alone.

Other emotional responses to sexual assault are feelings

of acute stress, persistent uncleanliness, guilt, shame, embarrassment, humiliation, shock, disbelief, phobias, night terrors, anxiety, vulnerability, and depression. These feelings may be intermittent or prolonged. Alcohol or drug use, not uncommon after a sexual attack, is used in an effort to numb the pain.

Intellectual dimension The psychic energy required by the victim to prevent further emotional trauma is depleted, leaving little energy for cognitive tasks. Disorientation and disorganized thought processes are common immediately after sexual assault and may continue for some time. Decision-making and problem-solving skills may be weakened or disrupted. Some sexual acts are so repulsive to the victim that she may suppress or repress their occurrence or feel too ashamed to report them. Some victims dwell on the experience and are preoccupied with thinking about what they could have done differently to prevent or change the outcome of the assault. Other victims may focus on their work to avoid thinking about the rape.

The victim has to make many decisions during this time, when she is least prepared to make them—decisions about seeking health care, preserving physical evidence, notifying the police, providing for her own security, telling the family, caring for children, and other practical matters of daily living. The victim's basic intellectual capacity affects her ability to comprehend the significance of the event and make decisions about necessary arrangements.

Social dimension One major problem confronting victims of sexual assault is what, when, and how to inform the family or significant others. These persons are usually the frontline support system for loved ones in crisis. In cases of sexual assault family members are, in a sense, victimized as well. Reports have indicated that husbands and significant others often respond to the victim's rape with divorce, terminating the relationship, or blaming the victims. Such reactions further intensify the victim's trauma.

Husbands, fathers, or significant others, usual sources of support for victims during crises, may find themselves unable to meet the victim's needs because they are dealing with their own feelings and needs. Men may distance themselves sexually and emotionally from their mates. For others, the implicit or explicit question is whether the victim provoked her attack. Family members may pressure the victim not to prosecute or notify authorities because they do not want to risk publicity. This lack of support is another way the family communicates its shame or embarrassment to the victim. Victims may express reluctance to reveal their attack because they are concerned about the impact on their family. Relationships are also threatened if the assailant is an employer, family friend, relative, or neighbor.

Social isolation is common after a rape. Victims are uncomfortable being with other people, even close friends. Fear, suspicion, and other emotional responses prevent victims from wanting to leave their homes.

Spiritual dimension Religious beliefs, faith, and moral values may be highly significant for the rape victim. She may be confronted with very difficult decisions if she becomes pregnant. Some women are unable to cope with a pregnancy resulting from rape yet would experience extraordinary guilt consenting to an abortion. Pregnancy prevention therapy may conflict with the victim's religious beliefs. Children conceived as a result of rape may not be accepted by the victim, her husband, or other family members. Relinquishing a child, even though fathered by a rapist, may provoke guilt for the victim. The victim may find herself forced to choose from a list of undesirable alternatives.

Rape victims who believe in God may question their faith, feel angry at God, or feel they have been punished by God. Victims may experience guilt if they are unable to forgive their assailant. Religious faith may be a victim's greatest source of comfort during times of stress.

▼ **RAPE TRAUMA SYNDROME**

DEFINITION

Forced, violent sexual penetration against the victim's will and consent. The trauma syndrome that develops from this attack or attempted attack includes an acute phase or disorganization of the victim's life-style and a long-term process of reorganization of life-style.

DEFINING CHARACTERISTICS

- **Physical dimension**

    General soreness/bruising
    Gastrointestinal irritability
    Genitourinary discomfort
    Muscle tension
    Sleep pattern disturbance
    Reactivated symptoms of previous physical illnesses or psychiatric illnesses (compound reaction)
    Reliance on alcohol and/or drugs (compound reaction)
    Increase in nightmares (silent reaction)
    Pronounced changes in sexual behavior (silent reaction)

- **Emotional dimension**

    Anger
    Depression
    Embarrassment
    Fear of physical violence and death
    Humiliation
    Dealing with repetitive nightmares and phobias
    Increased anxiety during interview (silent reaction)
    Sudden onset of phobic reactions (silent reaction)

- **Intellectual dimension**

    No verbalization of the occurrence of rape (silent reaction)
    Drop in academic performance
    Self-blame
    Age-inappropriate sexual vocabulary
    Intrusive thoughts/day dreams

- **Social dimension**

    Revenge
    Changes in residence
    Seeking family support
    Seeking social network support
    Abrupt changes in relationships with men (silent reaction)

Modified from McFarland G, McFarlane E: *Nursing diagnosis and intervention: planning for patient care,* ed 2, St Louis, 1993, Mosby–Year Book.

Analysis

Nursing diagnosis

The defining characteristics of the NANDA-accepted nursing diagnosis of rape trauma syndrome are presented in the box, p. 689. This syndrome includes three subcomponents: rape trauma, compound reaction, and silent reaction. Those characteristics unique to the compound reaction or the silent reaction are indicated in parentheses.

The following case example illustrates characteristics of the nursing diagnosis of rape trauma syndrome.

▼ Case Example

Beth, a 34-year-old divorced mother of two, was brought to the emergency room by her neighbor. The neighbor found Beth, clothed in a nightgown, rocking back and forth in a chair and crying. Her children, a daughter age 12 and a son age 10, reported their mother was "acting funny." Beth reported she had been raped by a man wearing a ski mask who surprised her on the way to her car the previous evening after work. Although Beth had several contusions on her face and arms and signs of perineal trauma, she expressed concern that perhaps she had not fought off her attacker vigorously enough. "I was afraid he would kill me if I screamed or fought him anymore. At least, that's what he told me he would do." Beth had stayed home from work because she did not want anyone to see how bad she looked. She had not notified the police because she feared her fiance would learn she had been attacked. He had cautioned her not to go to her car alone after dark. She believed he would break their engagement because she had been assaulted. Beth worried she could not be a "real wife" to her prospective husband.

Planning

The nursing care plan (Table 34-4) provides some long- and short-term goals, outcome criteria, interventions, and rationales related to rape. These serve as examples of the planning stage of the nursing process.

Implementation

Physical dimension Ideally, the client is treated initially in a designated sexual assault treatment center. These facilities are best equipped to provide comprehensive care for rape victims because they follow a detailed protocol to maximize treatment. If the victim makes telephone contact before being seen by a professional caregiver, she is encouraged not to shower, bathe, douche, or change clothing and to seek health care as soon as possible.

Evidence is collected according to strict legal guidelines, even if the client has not decided whether to notify the police. Initially, the victim may feel overwhelmed and unable to make that decision. Properly collected evidence preserves the victim's option to press charges.

The way the victim's needs are met during initial contact has major implications for her prognosis and recovery. Many facilities provide female nurse practitioners or female physicians to take the history and perform the physical examination of the rape victim. A detailed, verbatim account of the sexual attack is included in the client's record. The examination proceeds slowly, with clear explanations provided before every procedure. The victim is not touched without being told first and asked for her permission. The victim is made as physically comfortable as possible because she is likely to be in great pain from her ordeal. Short rests may be necessary if the victim expresses fatigue or undue discomfort. The victim may appreciate being offered a beverage at some point during the treatment process unless this is contraindicated by incomplete laboratory work or specific injury. The victim will want to wash out her mouth as soon as possible if she had oral contact with her assailant. Anything that helps the victim clean up will benefit her physically and emotionally.

Pregnancy prevention measures are discussed with the client if the rape occurred within the previous 72 hours. All options are explained, including the benefits and risks of each alternative. The possibility of sexually transmitted diseases is addressed. Some agencies implement prophylactic antibiotic therapy, appropriate for specific venereal diseases, during the initial visit. Other agencies administer treatment only after a sexually transmitted disease is diagnosed. A third alternative is to treat only those victims deemed to be high risks to not receive follow-up care.

Victims are given medication for sleep or pain if needed. They are encouraged to contact the health care provider if pain or sleep disturbances continue.

Emotional dimension The priority for intervention in the emotional dimension is to establish trust with the victim. Ideally, the client is seen as quickly as possible by a rape counselor. Initial contact with the rape counselor may occur by telephone or in an emergency room, outpatient unit of a hospital, counseling center, crisis center, physician's office, victim's home, or police station.

Nursing intervention focuses on reducing the victim's fear. The nurse understands that her client's temporary fear about a repeat attack is real and not immediately amenable to logic. Repeated reassurance of the victim's safety is offered. The client is urged to focus on measures enacted for her protection. The nurse assists the client in concentrating on increased security measures such as new window and door locks, police surveillance, someone to stay with her, or someone to accompany her outside her home. If the fear continues after a few weeks and shows no signs of abating, psychotherapy is considered. Crisis intervention techniques are also useful after a sexual assault (see Chapter 27).

During sexual assault the victim is controlled by someone else. She has been degraded and humiliated. It is important for the victim to regain control. Well-intentioned persons may try to take charge of the victim's life and do everything for her. However, she needs to be given as many opportunities as possible to make decisions for herself. Consulting the victim about who she prefers to have with her, her daily schedule, and her follow-up treatment are examples of giving her control.

Treatment choices are the victim's decision. Once the victim makes a decision, that decision is supported. Others may not agree with her decisions; however, it is important that their values are not imposed on her.

The nurse assists the victim in resolving feelings of self-blame. Victims are not responsible for their assaults. They are urged not to accept the responsibility for another's behavior or the projections of other's feelings onto them.

Intellectual dimension Intellectual disorganization and disorientation may mean the victim needs assistance with problem solving and decision making immediately af-

▼ **TABLE 34-4   NURSING CARE PLAN**

GOALS	OUTCOME CRITERIA	INTERVENTIONS	RATIONALES
NURSING DIAGNOSIS: Rape trauma syndrome related to recent rape experience			
LONG TERM			
To resume prerape activities	Demonstrates ability to resume full range of activities of daily living		
To resume prerape level of functioning	Feels comfortable without antianxiety medication		
	Demonstrates understanding of her role as a victim by discussing the incident calmly and rationally		
SHORT TERM			
To decrease anxiety	Identifies and discusses factors that increase her anxiety level	Encourage client to talk about the assault.	Talking with an empathic person reduces anxiety and promotes emotional healing
	Demonstrates reduced anxiety	Assist to identify factors that increase anxiety.	Promotes insight and leads to preventive measures or ways to manage anxiety
		Identify ways to reduce anxiety.	Promotes emotional health
		Provide information about rape, crime of violence; client is not to blame self.	Reduces anxiety and clears up myths/misperceptions about rape
To identify members of her support system and accept their assistance	Informs family/friends of sexual assault	Have client name persons that can be supportive.	Support persons help to reduce the trauma and increase the victim's sense of worth significance
	Accepts assistance from friends and others trained to provide postrape interventions		
	Contacts rape crisis unit		
To obtain necessary medical care	Permits physical examination	Help client seek medical care.	Promotes physical and emotional health and prevents symptoms from occurring at a later date
	Complies with medical treatment recommendations		

ter the rape. The nurse helps the client identify options for situations requiring decisions.

Finding the assailant, preserving evidence, and successful prosecution hinge on prompt notification of the authorities. The victim is not pressured into the decision during a period of vulnerability, but she needs to be aware of the reasons for a quick decision. The victim or family members need to be reminded not to clean the scene of the crime if police involvement is anticipated. As the shock, disbelief, fear, and anxiety levels subside, the victim will have more energy for cognitive functions.

Information about available treatments and services is given in language the victim understands. Medical and anatomical jargon is avoided. Communication is on the client's level, with statements such as, "I am going to have to ask you some difficult questions," or "Some things may be difficult for you to discuss. We can take it slowly, but there are things that need to be discussed as soon as possible."

Apparent reluctance to discuss the sexual assault may not be directly related to the attack, but to other information that would be revealed. For example, girls whose parents don't know they are sexually active or women using birth control without their husbands' knowledge may be hesitant to report the incident to the police, knowing that their secrets may surface during an investigation. Victims are not questioned in front of family members unless they ask that the family member be present for support.

Written instructions for home care, signs and symptoms to report, follow-up care, appointments, and medication information are given to the client because victims are unlikely to remember verbal instructions under stressful circumstances. Classes in self-defense for women, often taught by local police departments, may help decrease a woman's feelings of vulnerability.

Social dimension Rape victims are given privacy in a quiet room. Someone trained to handle rape crisis stays with the victim. The number of personnel attending

▼
KEY INTERVENTIONS FOR RAPE

Encourage victim not to shower, bathe, douche, or change clothing
Preserve all evidence
Treat the physical injuries
Reduce fear, reassure that victim is safe in the health care setting
Allow victim to make own decisions about moving, door locks, pressing charges
Support decision, even if you do not agree with it
Help victim refrain from self-blame, guilt
Offer information on available resources for health care, legal aid, crisis intervention
Refer to self-defense groups
Have supportive person stay with victim; do not allow victim to return home alone
Refer to support group

to the victim is kept to a minimum. Required tasks may be shared to keep personnel involved to a minimum; for example, the nurse or physician may collect blood samples rather than an unfamiliar laboratory technician.

National registers provide information about the nearest victim assistance program. Services are listed in telephone directories under terms such as *rape, abuse,* or *battering.* Some provide transportation services, accompany the victim to court, bring clothes to the hospital if the victim's are held as evidence, or see the victim in her home to provide support. The victim is given information about rape support groups and services. She is urged to use those services, which are usually free.

Many areas have support groups for husbands, fathers, or significant others. These groups help the men resolve their feelings about the assault and teach them ways to provide support for the victim. The nurse refers these men to a treatment service.

The nurse assists the victim to identify ways to inform others about the assault. Role playing lets her practice telling others. The victim may decide not to tell others, but plans are made in case the need arises.

 Spiritual dimension Pastoral counseling is appropriate for the victim of a sexual assault. Victims may desire pastoral counseling about pregnancy prevention; abortion; prosecuting her assailant; disclosing the rape to her fiance or husband; and the implications of her hatred, vindictiveness, and rage toward the rapist. The nurse offers to contact clergy of the victim's choice. Table 34-4 is a sample nursing care plan. Key interventions for victims of rape are listed in the accompanying box above.

Evaluation

Progress in preventing family violence and helping families and health care providers in dealing with abusive situations is extrinsically tied to society's attitudes toward abuse and rape, as well as its willingness to recognize and give attention to the problem. When society can better accept that abuse and rape respect no boundaries, additional resources will be allocated to find solutions.

The success of the nursing process with abused clients and their families is measured by the cessation of the abuse

through interruption of the cycle of violence and, on a more long-term basis, by the ability of the victim to resolve the abuse. Other indicators of goal attainment are learning impulse control and problem solving by the abuser and the ability of the family to learn less destructive methods of handling their negative emotions.

BRIEF REVIEW

Abuse is a dynamic, interactive process involving two or more persons. Clients seeking treatment for physical injuries are asked directly if they are victims of abuse unless there is concrete evidence to the contrary. Every health history contains questions designed to elicit information about possible abuse. Case finding of any victim enters an entire family into the health care system.

Failure to identify abused clients remains an important issue in prevention and treatment of health problems resulting from abuse. Informed nurses increase the probability of identifying abusive situations. Their knowledge, skills, and expertise can be used to raise the consciousness of and educate other health care providers about the problems experieced by victims of abuse. All nurses will encounter victims of abuse. Early diagnosis and treatment provide the best opportunity for rehabilitation and improved prognosis.

REFERENCES AND SUGGESTED READINGS

1. Attorney General's Task Force: *Family violence,* Washington, DC, 1984, Department of Justice.
2. Beck CM, Ferguson D: Aged abuse, *Journal of Gerontological Nursing* 7:333, 1981.
3. Beck CM, Phillips LR: Abuse of the elderly, *Journal of Gerontological Nursing* 9(2):97, 1983.
4. Bergman AB, Larsen RM, Mueller BA: Changing spectrum of serious child abuse, *Pediatrics* 77:113, 1986.
5. Bragg DF, Kimsey LR, Tarbox AR: Abuse of the elderly: the hidden agenda. II. Future research and remediation, *Journal of the American Geriatrics Society* 29:503, 1981.
6. Brendtro M, Bowker H: Battered women: How nurses can help, *Issues in Mental Health Nursing* 10:169, 1989.
7. Briere J, Runtz M: The trauma syndrome checklist (TSC-33) early data on a new scale, *Journal of Interpersonal Violence* 4(2):151, 1989.
8. Browne A: *When battered women kill,* New York, 1987, The Free Press.
9. Campbell J: A test of two explanatory models of women's responses to battering, *Nursing Research* 38:18, 1989.
10. Campbell J, Sheridan D: Emergency nursing interventions with battered women, *Journal of Emergency Nursing* 15(1):12, 1989.
11. Champlin L: The battered elderly, *Geriatrics* 37(7):115, 1982.
12. Conte J, Scheurman J: The effects of sexual abuse on children, *Journal of Interpersonal Violence* 2:380, 1988.
13. Dobash RE, Dobash RP: Research as social action: the struggle for battered women. In Yllo K, Bogard M, editors: *Feminist perspectives on wife abuse,* Newbury Park, CA, 1988, Sage Publications, Inc.
14. Drake VK: Battered women: a health care problem in disguise, *Image* 14(2):40, 1982.
15. Drake VK: *An investigation of the relationships among locus of control, self-concept, duration of the intimate relationship, and severity of physical and nonphysical abuse of battered women,* Ann Arbor, Mich, 1985, University Microfilms International.
16. Drake VK, Steinmetz C: *Spouse abuse: dynamics and inter-*

vention strategies—Training Key No. 352. Gaithersburg, Md, 1985, International Association of Chiefs of Police.

17. Dutton D: *The domestic assault of women,* Newton, Mass, 1988, Allyn & Bacon.

18. Falcioni D: Assessing the abused elderly, *Journal of Gerontological Nursing* 8:208, 1982.

19. Faller K: The myth of the "collusive" mother, *Journal of Interpersonal Violence,* 3:190, 1988.

20. Federal Bureau of Investigation: *Crime in the United States,* Washington, DC, 1984, Department of Justice.

21. Feinauer L: Comparison of long-term effects of child abuse by type of abuse and by relationship of the offender to the victim, *American Journal of Family Therapy* 17(1):48, 1989.

22. Finkelhor D, Pillemer K: The prevalence of elder abuse: a random sample survey, *Gerontological Society of America* 28(1):51, 1988.

23. Fulmer T: The hidden victim, *Aging and Leisure Living* 3(5):9, 1980.

24. Giarretto H: Humanistic treatment of father-daughter incest. In Helfer RE, Kempe CH, editors: *Child abuse and neglect: the family and the community,* Cambridge, Mass, 1976, Ballinger Publishing Co.

25. Gondolf E: The effect of batterer counseling on shelter outcome, *Journal of Interpersonal Violence* 3(3):275, 1988.

26. Hickey T, Douglas RL: Mistreatment of the elderly in the domestic setting: an exploratory study, *American Journal of Public Health* 71:500, 1981.

27. Hickey T, Douglas RL: Neglect and abuse of older family members: professionals' perspectives and case experiences, *Gerontologist* 21(2):171, 1981.

27a. Jehu D: Mood disturbances among women clients sexually abused in childhood, *Journal of Interpersonal Violence* 4(2):164, 1989.

28. Kelly L: How women define their experiencs of violence. In Yllo K, Bograd M, editors: *Feminist perspectives on wife abuse,* Newbury Park, Calif, 1989, Sage Publications.

29. Kimsey LR, Tarbox AR, Bragg DF: Abuse of the elderly: the hidden agenda. I. The caretakers and the categories of abuse, *Journal of the American Geriatrics Society* 29:465, 1981.

30. King M, Ryan J: Abused women: dispelling myths and encouraging interventions, *Nurse Practitioner* 14(5):47, 1989.

30a. Koop CE: Introduction to workshop on violence and public health, *National Organization For Victim Assistance Newsletter.* 9:11, 1985.

31. Landenburger K: Conflicting realities of women in abusive relationships, *Communicating Nursing Research* 21:15, 1988.

32. Landenburger K: A process of entrapment in and recovery from an abusive relationship, *Issues in Mental Health Nursing* 10:209, 1989.

33. Newbern V: Sexual victimization in children and adolescent patients, *Image* 21(1):10, 1989.

34. O'Reilly J: Wife beating: the silent crime, *Time,* September 1983, p 23.

35. Rew L: Long-term effects of childhood sexual exploitation, *Issues in Mental Health Nursing,* 10:229, 1989.

36. Rubinelli J: Incest: its' time we face reality, *Journal of Pyschiatric Nursing and Mental Health Services* 18(4):17, 1980.

37. Schultz L, DeSavage J: Rape and rape attitudes on a college campus. In Schultz E, editor: *Rape victimology,* Springfield, Ill, Charles C Thomas.

38. Select Committee on Aging: *Elder abuse: an examination of a hidden problem,* US House of Representatives, Comm Publ No 97-277, Washington, DC, 1981, US Government Printing Office.

39. Steinmetz S: *Elder abuse: Aging* 135-136:6, 1981.

39a. Straus MA, Gelles RJ, Steinmetz SK: *Behind closed doors: violence in the American family,* Garden City, NJ, 1980, Anchor Books.

40. Stuart E, Campbell J: Assessment of patterns of dangerousness with battered women, *Issues in Mental Health Nursing* 10:245, 1989.

41. Thobaben M, Anderson L: Reporting elder abuse: it's the law, *American Journal of Nursing* 85(4):371, 1985.

42. US Department of Health and Human Services: *Elder abuse,* Washington, DC, Administration on Aging, DHHS Publ No (OHDS) 81-20152, Washington, DC, 1980, US Government Printing Office.

43. US Department of Health and Human Services: *Executive summary: National study of the incidence and severity of child abuse and neglect,* DHHS Publ No (OHDS) 81-30329, Washington, DC, 1982, US Government Printing Office.

44. Walker LE: *The battered woman,* New York, 1979, Harper & Row.

45. Walsh D, Liddy R: *Surviving sexual abuse,* Dublin, 1989, Attic Press.

ANNOTATED BIBLIOGRAPHY

Campbell J, Alford P: The dark side of marital rape, *American Journal of Nursing* 89:946, 1989.

This article discusses marital rape, its effects on women's health, and how the authors' concern for the victim changed state laws.

Cornman J: Group treatment for female sexual abuse victims, *Issues in Mental Health Nursing* 10:261, 1989.

This article describes the wide range of symptoms seen in sexually abused adolescents. The dynamics of sexual abuse, using Finklehor and Browne's framework, and the application of these dynamics in group interventions strategies is discussed.

Dutton D: *The domestic assault of wives,* Newton, Mass, 1988, Allyn & Bacon.

This book presents an overview of current research on batterers and treatment programs for batterers.

Gondolf E, Fisher E: *Battered women as survivors,* Lexington, Mass, 1988, Heath & Co.

This book is based on research with survivors of abuse. Challenges surrounding assumptions about abused women are presented. Also discussed are help-seeking measures that survivors use as well as descriptions of the abuser.

Walsh D, Liddy R: *Surviving sexual abuse,* Dublin, 1989, Attic Press.

Written for survivors of childhood sexual abuse, this book summarizes types of assaults, common responses to assault, and strategies for healing. Case studies are also presented.

PART IV

Life-Cycle Phases

From conception to death, each person continues to evolve and change while undergoing a series of alternating periods of stability and transition. At each stage in the life cycle, individuals have distinct developmental tasks to achieve, and they encounter stressors that are specific to that stage. To enhance understanding of the discrete stages in the life cycle, the following artificial age delineations were chosen for this text: the infant (birth to 1 year), the child (1 to 11 years), the adolescent (12 to 21 years), the young adult (22 to 45 years), the middle-aged adult (46 to 65 years), and the aged adult (over 65). Although the dissection of the life cycle into discrete stages is necessary for purposes of discussion, the mental health–psychiatric nurse best applies the knowledge gained from this discussion by looking at all ages and stages as they intermingle.

Each chapter in Part IV discusses the process of mental health–psychiatric nursing with clients at a specific stage in the life cycle. Theories that explain the individual's physical, emotional, intellectual, social, and spiritual development are examined. The process of mental health–psychiatric nursing with individuals at each stage in the life cycle is presented with emphasis on developmental tasks and stressors unique to each age. A holistic assessment tool in each chapter contains assessment information specific to each stage in the life cycle. The focus of Chapter 35 is development during the first year of life. In Chapter 36 the childhood years are divided into several stages, and the unique patterns of growth within each are discussed. During the adolescent years, the individual is growing out of childhood into adulthood. This transition stage is the subject of Chapter 37. The three adult phases of the life cycle are presented in Chapter 38 through 40.

CHAPTER

35 The Infant

Sarah M Powell

Eva Hester Lin

After studying this chapter, the student will be able to:

- Discuss significant historical contributions to the development of infant psychiatry
- Discuss the psychopathology of reactive attachment, ruminations, and autism in infants as described in the DSM-III-R
- Describe the major developmental theories of infant mental health and illness

- Describe the unique nature of the therapeutic relationship with the infant
- Apply the nursing process to the mental health care of infants
- Describe current research findings on infant mental health and illness

Infancy, beginning with birth and ending with the emergence of language and ambulation, is the most dependent phase of human development. For many years the infant was considered a totally passive organism, little more than a bundle of undifferentiated reactions and responses. Healthy physical and mental development of the infant was believed to depend almost completely on the mother's nurturing. The evolving relationship between the infant and caregiver is still viewed as a basic determinant of mental health, but the focus now is on its reciprocal nature and includes the prenatal period.

The infant today is seen as an active, striving individual, who not only seeks and elicits stimulation from the environment, but also influences parental attitudes and behaviors.[53] Knowledge of normal mental health development in infancy has expanded rapidly in the past decade and continues to grow. Researchers are working to integrate theoretical frameworks, from genetics to psychology, to address the complexity of infant development. Equipped with new insights, health care professionals are able to detect and treat anomalies early in the infant's life. In addition, they are able to identify and treat infants at risk for developing mental health problems at increasingly earlier ages. Early intervention is therapeutic and preventive. Behaviors and relationships are easier to redirect during infancy than in later life, when maladaptive coping strategies may have become more entrenched.

Nurses, currently active in settings that emphasize primary prevention such as well-baby clinics, pediatric units, or other settings for the newborn, are also taking on expanded roles as educators and counselors to family members. A clear understanding of the dynamic nature of the first 18 months and an appreciation of this phase's challenging tasks are requisite for examining infant mental health. Awareness of general developmental trends allows for early intervention and prevention of long-term problems. The main objectives of infant mental health are prevention of maladaptive behavior and promotion of normal development. Knowledge of DSM-III-R disorders relevant to infancy enables the nurse to assist family members to deal with the impact of these disorders in an adaptive manner. This chapter discusses three disorders: reactive attachment disorder of infancy, rumination disorder of infancy, and autistic disorder.

DSM-III-R DIAGNOSES

Three infant pathological conditions identified in the DSM-III-R include reactive attachment disorder, autistic disorder, and rumination disorder. The etiology, age of onset, and essential features according to the DSM-III-R are listed

DIAGNOSES Related to Infants

MEDICAL DIAGNOSES
Reactive attachment disorder
Rumination disorder
Autistic disorder

HISTORICAL OVERVIEW

DATES	EVENTS
1905	Publication of Freud's *Three Essays on the Theory of Sexuality* highlighted the significance of infantile sexuality in personality development and adult mental health.
1940	Arnold Gesell's publication of *The First Five Years* presented new observational data on early behavior patterns of infants.
1943	Article on *Infantile Autism* by Leo Kanner was a milestone in identifying early psychopathological conditions.
1945	Rene Spitz published his findings on the profoundly pathogenic effect of institutionalization and hospitalization on infants.
1951	John Bowlby in *Maternal Care and Mental Health* identified mother-child attachment as the core of the infant's emotional life.
1954	Graduate nursing programs in child psychiatry were created, providing a professional psychiatric nursing corps for infants and children.
1972	Advocates for child psychiatric nursing formed a nationwide professional nursing organization to promote research in this field. Annual scientific meetings were initiated.
1974	American Academy of Child Psychiatry established a Committee on the Psychiatric Dimensions of Infancy that meets annually.
1976	*Infant Psychiatry* (Rexford, Sanders, and Shapiro), a book of articles by experts in child psychiatry and child development synthesizing researrch and clinical observations, was published.
1977	National Center for Clinical Infant Programs was formed to improve and support professional work in infant mental health and development.
1981	National Institute of Mental Health established a Center for Study of Child and Adolescent Psychopathology.
1985	*Guidelines for Health Supervision,* which identifies emotional milestones to help pediatricians assess the emotional (as well as physical) well-being of infants, was published by the American Academy of Pediatrics.
1990s	More psychiatric nurses are needed to identify infants at risk for psychiatric problems, to work with problem infants, and to help families alter unhealthy child-rearing practices.
Future	As increasing numbers of infants are born with fetal alcohol syndrome and AIDS, nurses will be challenged to change existing attitudes and to develop innovative methods for caring for these tiny victims in their own community and nationally and worldwide.

along with guidelines for disease prevention and health promotion. See the boxes accompanying each disorder.

Reactive Attachment Disorder

Grossly pathogenic care preceding the onset of the disturbance is thought to be the cause of this disorder. Clear evidence of such care is required before the diagnosis can be made. These infants often do not receive well-baby care; they are most often identified by a pediatrician who sees the child for a complicating physical illness, i.e., infection, injury, or feeding problem, associated with failure to thrive physically.

Pathogenic care may include neglect or abuse of the child. The caregiver may consistently ignore the child's basic physical and emotional needs including failure to feed the child; protect the child from physical danger; or provide the child with comfort, affection, and stimulation. Emotional abuse may be noted in a caregiver who is too harsh with the child; physical and/or sexual abuse may also be seen.

Factors that interfere with the emotional attachment of the child to a primary caregiver are thought to predispose to the development of this disorder. From the caregiver's perspective, these factors may include obsessions of infanticide that prompt the caregiver to stay away from the infant, a history of severe neglect or abuse in the caregiver's own childhood, isolation and lack of support systems, and severe depression. From the infant's perspective, factors may include the absence of bonding between the infant and the primary caregiver during the first weeks of life (e.g., prolonged confinement of the infant in intensive care without body-to-body contact between the infant and the primary caregiver) or special care requirements of some infants (e.g., infants with physical or mental handicaps whose special needs may excessively frustrate the caregiver, thus discouraging appropriate caregiver behavior). In addition, frequent and repeated change of the primary caregiver may serve as a causative factor, as it prevents the development of a stable attachment between infant and caregiver.

The disorder occurs before the age of 5 years and can be diagnosed as early as within the first month of life. After that age children respond differently to grossly pathogenic care and thus present a different clinical picture. The essential features include the following:
- Notable disturbance of social relatedness that begins before age 5
- Weight loss or failure to gain weight
- Poor muscle tone
- Hypomobility
- Weak rooting and grasping in response to feeding attempts
- Weak cry
- Excessive sleep
- Lack of interest in the environment
- Excessive familiarity with relative strangers
- Lack of visual tracking of eyes and face by 2 months of age
- Lack of visual reciprocity by 2 months of age
- Lack of smiling in response to faces by 2 months of age
- Lack of alerting and turning toward caregiver's voice by 4 months of age
- Lack of vocal reciprocity with caregiver by 5 months of age
- Lack of participation in playful games with the caregiver by 5 months of age

········▼·······································

GUIDELINES FOR DISEASE PREVENTION AND HEALTH PROMOTION FOR REACTIVE ATTACHMENT DISORDERS

Evaluate cause of pathogenic care
Refer caregiver for treatment as indicated
Evaluate parenting skills and provide intervention as needed
Provide family education regarding the disorder and ways to cope
Facilitate bonding and nurturing between infant and primary caregiver
Teach the primary caregiver to spend quality time with the infant on a daily basis
Educate primary caregiver and family regarding normal growth and development of the infant and child
Advocate routine health care visits to facilitate health maintenance and illness prevention
Encourage and support primary caregiver as needed
Promote family support of primary caregiver
Assist primary caregiver and family to identify community support systems
Promote family planning and parenting education in high schools
Identify infants at risk and intervene as indicated
Make referrals as needed
Educate community agencies regarding the need for stable placement of infants and young children

- Failure to reach spontaneously for caregiver by 6 to 10 months of age
- Failure to initiate vocal or visual communication with caregiver by 6 to 10 months of age
- Grossly pathogenic care by caregiver
- Overly harsh treatment of child
- Consistently ignoring the child
- Failure to protect the child from physical danger
- Failure to adequately feed the child
- Failure to protect the child from assault including sexual abuse
- Consistent disregard of the child's basic emotional needs for affection, comfort, and stimulation
- Repeated change of primary caregiver

Autistic Disorder

Various prenatal, perinatal, and postnatal conditions leading to brain dysfunction may predispose infants and children to develop autistic disorder. Conditions associated with the disorder include untreated phenylketonuria, anoxia during birth, infantile spasms, and encephalitis. The disorder seems to occur more often in siblings of children who have the disorder than in the general population and is more commonly seen in males than in females. The diagnosis of mental retardation often accompanies the disorder.

Onset of the disorder is generally reported to be before the age of 3 years; however, some cases occur after the ages of 5 or 6 years. It is noted that the age of onset is sometimes difficult to determine retrospectively due to the lack of accurate information from the primary caregiver regarding the child's development of sociability, play, and language. Manifestations of the disorder are more subtle in infancy and thus difficult to identify before the age of 2 years. In addition, parents of an only child may not notice the problem until they are able to observe the child with other children, such as when the child enters school for the first time.

In extremely rare cases, the disorder is manifested after an initial period of apparently normal development followed by a rapid onset of the characteristic features of the disorder. The essential features include the following:
- Impairment in social interaction
    Lack of interest in other people
    Pervasive lack of response to others
    Failure to cuddle
    Lack of eye contact and facial responsiveness
    Indifference or aversion to affection or physical contact
    Failure to develop normal attachment behavior
    Abnormal social play
- Impairment in development of communication skills (verbal and nonverbal) and imaginative activity
    Deficits in language development (echolalia, metaphorical language)
    Inability to name objects
    Total absence of language (in some situations)
    Absence of fantasy or symbolic play with toys
    Lack of play acting of adult roles
    Imaginative activity ("pretend" play) restrictive in content and repetitive and stereotyped in form

▼ **GUIDELINES FOR DISEASE PREVENTION AND HEALTH PROMOTION FOR AUTISTIC DISORDERS**

Provide family education regarding the disorder and ways to cope

Educate primary caregiver and family regarding normal growth and development of the infant and child

Evaluate parenting skills and provide intervention as needed

Encourage and support primary caregiver and family as indicated

Advocate support within the family system

Promote the use of sign language with the infant to increase communication

Advocate the use of special education facilities and day care centers early in the infant's development

Teach family that long-term treatment will be required

Assist the family in exploring treatment options

Advocate routine health care visits to facilitate health maintenance and illness prevention

Assist primary caregiver and family to identify community support systems

Make referrals for treatment and community support as indicated

Suggest genetic counseling when indicated

Promote family planning and parenting education in high schools

Advocate good prenatal, perinatal, and postnatal care

▼ **GUIDELINES FOR DISEASE PREVENTION AND HEALTH PROMOTION FOR RUMINATION DISORDERS**

Encourage small frequent feedings to prevent distention and subsequent vomiting

Promote frequent mouth care

Suggest changing infant's clothing often to control noxious odor

Facilitate bonding and nurturing between infant and primary caregiver during feedings

Encourage and support primary caregiver as needed

Promote family support of primary caregiver

Provide family education regarding the disorder and ways to cope

Evaluate parenting skills and provide intervention as indicated

Educate primary caregiver and family regarding normal growth and development of the infant and child

Advocate routine health care visits to facilitate health maintenance and illness prevention

Assist primary caregiver and family to identify community support systems

Make referrals as needed

Promote family planning and parenting education in high schools

---

- Impairment in repertoire of activities and interests
    Bizarre responses to minor environmental changes
    Labile moods
    Stereotyped body movements
    Fascination with movement (staring at fans, spinning objects)
    Preoccupation with parts of objects

Rumination Disorder

Rumination disorder generally occurs between the ages of 3 and 12 months. However, the disorder may occasionally begin at a later age in children with mental retardation. Presently there is no information regarding the etiology of this rare disorder.

The essential feature of this disorder is repeated regurgitation in the absence of congenital anomalies or gastrointestinal illness for a period of at least 1 month after normal functioning. Other characteristics include the following:
- Repeated regurgitation of food without retching, nausea, disgust, or gastrointestinal illness
- Holding head back, arching the back and straining
- Spit out or chewed and reswallowed regurgitated food
- Sucking movements made with tongue and satisfied appearance from regurgitation
- Irritability and hunger between episodes
- Avoidance of caregiver caused by infant's noxious odor
- Understimulation of infant caused by avoidance
- Loss of weight or failure to gain weight as expected
- Regurgitation immediately after eating
- Malnutrition
- Developmental delays
- Discouraged caregiver due to failure to feed child successfully
- Alienation from caregiver
- Spontaneous remissions common

THEORETICAL APPROACHES

The infant development theories of Gesell, Greenspan, Erikson, and Piaget share some basic assumptions: that there is a reciprocal relationship between the infant's biological makeup and social environment and experiences (nature and nurture); that the personality emerges in an orderly, sequential, gradual, and progressive pattern; and that infant personality is linked to a consideration of the physical self and the caregiver. The merging of the self with the world, of body with mind, is the bedrock of infant experience. Thus it is particularly crucial to evaluate the infant within a holistic framework, that is, examining all areas of the infant's life and the relationships among those areas, and a family framework, that is, evaluating the relationships within the family system.

Biological

Gesell's studies of infant behavior were linked to a careful, detailed analysis of physical maturation. He believed that behavior is a function of structure; that is, the body that one inherits determines the way one behaves. In the first year of life, the rapid development of the infant's central nervous system (CNS) provides the organic pathway for personality development. The sequence of development, with increasingly complete behavior emerging, is continuous and the same for all, although the rate varies. Thus all infants sit before they walk, but they sit and walk at different ages.[19] Infant development is closely tied to the maturation of the nervous system: No amount of encouragement can make an infant sit without support until the nervous system is ready for it.

Gesell and Amatruda[19] focused on four major behavioral areas: motor, adaptive, language, and personal-social. Using data from extensive observational studies, they identified norms of behavior in these areas at successive stages in infancy. They perceived infancy as a dynamic period of progressive development in all spheres of behavior based on increasing neuromuscular maturity. In the earliest phase basic physiological regulation is achieved. Most of the infant's energy is then consumed by growth. The physical aspects of nurturing are primary; the infant can survive only under carefully controlled conditions. Social interaction between the infant and caregiver increases with the achievement of physiological homeostasis. As the infant's initiative and power grow, he develops a more active role in the family's life. Sensory stimulation and social experience then become important "nutrients" for further development.[31]

Psychoanalytical

Erikson emphasized how the personality develops within the web of its particular social fabric in a sequence of psychosocial critical tasks. Infancy's challenge is establishing a capacity for basic trust.[13,14] The caregiver's responsiveness to the completely helpless infant, dominated by body needs and impulses, determines the outcome of this task. Earliest needs are physiological but satisfied in a social context. If babies can eat, sleep, and achieve a sense of physical comfort with relative ease during the period in which they need others to manage these functions, they learn to feel that life is sufficiently consistent and reliable, and they develop a sense of security. Because the boundary between the self and the outer world is not clear in infancy, the infant's feelings about the environment and self are one and the same. If the world is perceived as predictable, caring, and responsive, infants also establish a basic trust in themselves, their physiological processes, and their self-image. The blending of these physiological and psychological experiences serves as a pattern for the infant's future social world. A sense of inner certainty and outer predictability, which forms basic trust by the end of infancy, also provides the hope necessary for the next developmental step. The infant can then reach out for new experiences with confidence. With a firm foundation of basic trust, the child's energy can be used to accept new challenges. Once

achieved, this basic trust remains throughout life as the core of self-confidence and trust in others; this crucial task affects the whole of emotional life and all social relations.

Interactional

Greenspan[23] described the sequential stages of emotional development of infants and young children. To him, emotions play a critical role in developing the infant's self-concept. Through sensations and feelings the infant gradually learns to discriminate, differentiate, and organize experiences. Intellectual and emotional functions merge in this process, and consequently their respective development cannot be separated. The child's capacity for organizing experiences depends on the infant's social experiences and CNS maturity. Thus emotions are the result of the interaction among the child's neurological, cognitive, social, and expressive functions. Each infant has a unique constitution and temperament, but each passes through predictable stages of emotional growth. Greenspan[20] identified six stages in emotional development, four in the first 18 months of life (Table 35-1).

Cognitive

Piaget focused on intellectual development in infants and children. He emphasized the role of adaptation in the organism-environment relationship. Piaget noted that development occurs in invariant stages, each building on previous ones. All infants pass through the same sequence of development but at different rates. Intelligence evolves from the interplay between infant and environment. Thus environmental understimulation slows the rate and hinders the complexity of learning.

Piaget viewed intellectual development as one aspect of general adaptation to the world. He believed that intellectual development occurs in four stages. Only one of these stages, the sensorimotor stage, occurs in infancy. Babies are born with reflexes and reflexlike behavior that enable them to interact with and make discoveries in the environment.

▼ **TABLE 35-1**   **Summary of Greenspan's Stages of Emotional Development**

Stage	Stage-Specific Task	Stage-Specific Behaviors and Accomplishments
Achievement of homeostasis (birth to 3 months)	Self-regulation and interest in the world	The infant begins to control or regulate attentional states by focusing on sensory experiences.
Attachment (2 to 7 months)	"Falls in love" with primary caregiver	The infant's interest in external environment progresses and becomes more selective. Vocalizations of the primary caregiver induce a response.
Intentional communication (3 to 10 months)	Purposeful signaling	The infant's communications become more interactive; emotions are expressed in response to specific situations. Through the process of affecting others by emotional reactions, the infant learns cause and effect.
Behavioral organization (9 to 18 months)	Development of conceptual philosophy about world	The infant begins to reason about the world, as newly developed physical abilities (crawling, standing, walking) are integrated with previously acquired emotional skills (self as causal agent, intentional communication). The infant becomes a unique person, demonstrating complex and innovative behaviors.

Through their senses—mouth, eyes, ears, nose, and skin—infants incorporate experiences of their motor activities, from objects with which they have contact, i.e., mother's body, bottle, crib. Behaviors such as sucking, biting, touching, grasping, and kicking provide bits of experience that gradually assume meaning. Thus mental functions are ultimately derived from the effects of the infant's motor actions on concrete objects. The growth of intelligence can be seen as the progressive transformation of these motor patterns into thought patterns.[39,40]

The original reflexlike behavior of the newborn is gradually modified by contact with the world into more complex motor coordinations. They became aware of occasional discrepancies between previous experience and new stimuli. This tension creates curiosity, which leads to further extension of behavior beyond the body to the perception of the effect of personal actions on objects. The beginning of intentional behavior lies in this increasing exploration, which displaces earlier random activity. Purposeful behavior enables infants to accommodate their actions to real circumstances. They reach out toward an increasingly interesting and ever expanding world. Increasing cognitive development occurs with the development of memory and object constancy (the ability to represent an object internally, which enables infants to perceive the object as externally existent). Babies learn that other people exist independently of themselves and their actions. The magical omnipotence of infancy is gradually reduced, leading to the beginning of a more objective and accurate appraisal of reality.

At the end of the sensorimotor stage, infants are far more competent in getting what they want through their actions. The emergence of goal-directed behavior, which signals the end of infancy and the beginning of the preconceptual stage of development, is the hallmark of intelligence and a landmark achievement. The infant's simple need to repeat inborn reflexes has evolved into the complex, purposeful activity characteristic of all intelligent action.[39,40]

Social Learning

Ainsworth and others[1] believed that social attachment is achieved in four stages, three of which occur in the first 18 months of life. In the first 3 months the infant learns to identify the individual characteristics of the primary caregiver. Through reflexes (sucking, rooting, grasping, cuddling, smiling) and sensory experiences (visual tracking, gazing, vocalization) the infant is able to seek closeness with the caregiver. In the second stage (at 3 to 6 months of age) the infant begins to show preference for familiar people by smiling more and showing more excitement.

In the third stage (at 7 to 18 months) large motor competencies (crawling and walking) emerge and enable babies to seek physical closeness with the object of attachment. Such behavior is purposeful, with the intent to maintain or prolong physical contact. Two behaviors in this stage signify the development of *attachment: stranger anxiety* (at 6 to 9 months) and *separation anxiety* (at about 9 months). Stranger anxiety is an infant's wariness or discomfort with unfamiliar adults. Generally, infants demonstrate stranger anxiety through a variety of avoidance behaviors, including gaze aversion, tensing at a stranger's touch, or refusing to

▼ **TABLE 35-2 Summary of Theoretical Approaches**

Theory	Theorist	Dynamics
Biological	Gesell	Infant development is closely tied to CNS maturation. The sequence of development is similar for all; the rate varies.
Psycho-analyti-cal	Erikson	The caregiver's response to the helpless infant determines capacity for basic trust.
Interac-tional	Greenspan	Emotions result from the interaction among individual neurological, cognitive, social, and expressive functions and develop in sequential stages.
Cognitive	Piaget	Evolution of intelligence occurs in stages as the result of the interplay between infant and environment.
Social learn-ing	Ainsworth	The ability to discriminate between familiar and strange adults emerges from secure and intimate associations with a familiar adult.

be held by anyone but the primary caregiver.[28] Observable stranger anxiety is a good indication that the infant has developed an attachment to the primary caregiver. The ability to discriminate between familiar and strange adults emerges from the infant's secure and intimate association with a familiar adult.

Separation anxiety describes the fear and loss infants feel when separated from their primary attachment figure. Separation anxiety is believed to be a natural result of attachment[26]; the infant must have an investment in another person to notice her absence. The infant usually responds to separation in one of two ways. Separation may either stimulate attachment behaviors (the infant seeks to find the attachment figure and regain physical proximity) or evoke protest, despair, or detachment, depending on the duration of the separation. Initially, the anxiety occurs at the time of actual separation, but gradually the infant may experience it when separation is anticipated. The emergence of separation anxiety parallels the infant's development of *object permanence* (since now the infant is able to include the attachment figure in the imagination) at 8 to 10 months of age. In time infants become more adaptable and tolerant of separation, and eventually the anxiety diminishes almost totally.

Table 35-2 summarizes the major theories discussed.

NURSING PROCESS

Assessment

Physical dimension The integrity of the sensorimotor functions is critical to the infant's optimal development. Using Gesell's theory,[19] it would be important to assess the infant's physical structure and maturity. Physical maturity at birth varies widely. Several factors influence it: sex (on the average girls are about 2 weeks more mature than boys at birth in CNS and bone development), gestational age, and birth weight. Premature infants (those delivered before 37 weeks' gestation) often have serious physical problems that interfere with the early functions of breathing, digestion, sleeping, and waking. These difficulties often impair the infant's ability to adjust and adapt to the environment in ways that promote mental health.

Assessing the newborn's physical status begins immediately after delivery. The Apgar score is commonly used in the delivery room to evaluate cardiopulmonary and neurological integrity.[3] The Apgar scale also identifies gross CNS abnormalities.

In the first 28 days of extrauterine life, the infant makes a number of physiological adjustments to the world and begins to respond to internal and external stimulation. Life outside the womb requires dramatic adjustments. For example, before delivery infants live in a state of nutritional equilibrium. After birth infants' survival depends in part on their ability to recognize and convey feelings of hunger to their caregivers. Successful nourishment, then, depends in part on the integrity of an infant's physiological and sensory capacities (sensing hunger) and his expressive and motor capabilities (crying and sucking). Based on Erikson's theory,[13,14] it is crucial to assess how the caregiver meets this and other physiological needs.

Neonates' voluntary muscles are poorly controlled, but they come equipped with a variety of reflexes, including sucking, grasping, rooting, coughing, and stepping (the prancing movements of the legs when the infant is held upright with feet touching a table or crib). Many of these reflexes protect the infant against noxious stimuli. In addition, the newborn's sensory system functions at a much higher level than his motor functions. Optimal mental health development during the first year of life results from the successful melding of sensory experiences with motor activities,[20] as the following case example illustrates.

▼ Case Example

Maureen, age 3 months, one of a set of identical twins, was referred to an infant mental health specialist by her pediatrician, who could find no physiological cause for her recent weight loss, poor muscle tone, and withdrawn appearance. Her mother described Maureen as "the good one; she hardly ever cries and is content for hours just playing with her hands. She always goes right to sleep—sometimes I think she'd sleep all day if I didn't wake her up." Christine, Maureen's twin, was smaller at birth and had developed respiratory distress syndrome after delivery. She was described by the mother as "very difficult, very fussy. She's so demanding, just the opposite of Maureen."

Maureen's inability to elicit a response from her environment has placed her at both a physical and mental health risk. She shows signs of hypoarousal and appears sleepy and subdued. She shuts out sensory stimulation by ignoring it or falling asleep. She fails to recognize sensory experiences in the world and has a limited ability to communicate her needs to her mother. Her mother, stressed from attempting to nurture the difficult and possibly hyperaroused twin, believes that Maureen does not demand attention because

she does not need attention. Thus a potentially dangerous pattern of mother-infant interaction has been initiated.

Other areas the nurse considers when assessing the physical dimension are the infant's state of arousal or attention; the consolability of the baby; and feeding, elimination, and sleeping patterns. Before looking for problems in behavior or activities, however, the nurse needs a basic understanding of what is considered "normal." Pediatric texts will validate normal physical development. Ideally, an infant is able to use sensory experiences to prolong interest in the world. Thus the infant's level of attention is enhanced by the ability to taste, feel, smell, see, and hear. These experiences in turn provide a means of self-consolation. An infant who is relaxed and attentive while awake will also eat and sleep better than one who is tense and overwhelmed by sensations.

The infant's digestive processes (including feeding and elimination patterns) provide information about sensorimotor and expressive abilities. The caregiver's reciprocal behavior can provide valuable insight into his or her ability to read the baby's cues and signals of hunger and satiation (see the research highlight). Feeding and elimination change with age.

Sleeping difficulties are distressing for parents and may produce long-lasting maladaptive patterns of interaction. Sleeping problems also often accompany attentional or arousal problems, in which the infant is unable to "turn off" exciting environmental stimuli; in the opposite extreme, the infant uses sleep to escape from the world.

Emotional dimension Infants' emotional development evolves from the unique and highly individual blend of at least three basic ingredients: (1) the integrity of their cognitive and physical (sensorimotor) structures, (2) their basic behavioral style (temperament), and (3) the type and amount of social feedback received. Infants' ability to notice and react to the environment is crucial to their emotional development. Sensorimotor functions, discussed previously, enable the infant to experience the environment. Cognitive abilities, discussed in the next section, change with time. The gradual development of full emotional capability parallels the emergence of intellectual abilities, which enable the infant to organize and make sense of experiences and respond differentially.

An assessment of the infant's temperament provides important data. As any parent of more than one child knows, no two babies act alike. Some infants are born with a zest for life, a happy-go-lucky attitude that allows them to adapt gleefully to the world. Others respond to the world with intensity and chaos. Research by Thomas and Chess[50-52] identified three specific constellations of behavioral traits in neonates: the easy child, the difficult child, and the slow-to-warm-up child.

Temperamental individuality is well established by the time a baby is 2 to 3 months old and is thought to be influenced by genetic makeup and prenatal and early postnatal experiences. Studies by Plomin and others indicate that individual differences of emotionality (reactiveness), activity (including tempo and vigor), and sociability are influenced by heredity.[42-44]

Social feedback is the third element necessary for infant emotional development and an essential assessment factor. Emotions are critical to infant-caregiver communication.

RESEARCH HIGHLIGHT

Mothers' Working Models of Infant Feeding: Description and Influencing Factors
• K Pridham, C Knight, and G Stephenson

PURPOSE

The purpose of this study was to explore feeding models central to regulation for mothers of infants in their first 2 months and to examine their relation to mothers maternal experience, age, education, income, and feeding method.

SAMPLE

The sample included 123 mothers: 50 WIC clinic clients, 63 family practice clients, 5 mothers from Lamaze classes, and 5 mothers recruited from personal contact.

METHODOLOGY

Interviews were conducted using two instruments; (1) Information About You and Your Family and (2) How My Baby Feeds. Four aspects of a mother's model of infant feeding were examined: (1) infant behavior that cues feeding decisions, (2) infant self-regulative behavior, (3) importance of self-regulative behavior, and (4) maternal effort and value given to task-oriented and efficient feeding.

From *Journal of Advanced Nursing* 14:1051, 1989.

FINDINGS

Highest ratings were given to two items. The items included baby's fussing/crying as a sign of readiness to feed and baby's getting sleepy as a sign of being full. Other findings indicated that more primipara than multipara gave high ratings to the importance of the baby feeding long enough and that regular feedings were more often not as important to the multipara as to the primipara.

IMPLICATIONS

The findings indicate that some aspects of the models of infant feeding are a function of feeding method, maternal age, and income. The issue of maternal structuring of the infant's feeding to support the development of infant self-regulative capacity with specific mothers remains unknown. Although mothers are often encouraged to let the baby determine the initiation, pace, and termination of the feeding, they may not understand the role they play in recognizing the cues infants use to regulate the feeding and in giving the infant opportunities to exercise these cues.

Through feelings, expressions, and reactions babies become actively involved with others. Infants depend on others to stimulate and encourage their emotional behavior. According to Greenspan's theory, then, it is imperative that the nurse consider many areas of development when assessing the infant.[23] Consider the following case example.

▼ Case Example

Sammy, 10 months old, is playing by himself. He is having a good time banging two wooden blocks together. His mother dislikes the noise and comes toward him to take the blocks away. When Sammy sees his mother, his excitement builds and he squeals loudly and throws one of the blocks toward her, his way of "sharing" his joy and attempting to involve his mother in his play. However, his mother sees this behavior as disrespectful and mean; the block struck her painfully on the shin, and she is angry with Sammy. She reaches down, grabs the other block from him, shakes him by the shoulders, and yells, "No! You bad boy! Don't you ever hit me again!"

Sammy's mother has misinterpreted her son's intentions. She has projected her own ideas (that he was intentionally trying to hurt her) onto his behavior. She responded to his feelings of pain, fear, and anger. His feelings of joy and delight were neither reciprocated nor enhanced. If this pattern of interaction is repeated often, Sammy may begin to think that his feelings of joy and desire for his mother's company are bad and that he needs to be punished. Similarly, Sammy's mother (observing her son with a look of obvious delight on his face before throwing something at her) might begin to think that Sammy was happy because

he was about to do something he knew she would not like. This type of emotional misreading or miscommunication is detrimental to the development of optimal emotional health.

A gradual differentiation of emotions occurs during the first 12 months. Early emotional responses tend to involve the entire body. The hungry infant, for example, communicates this feeling by crying, stiffening the body, and clenching the fists. As infants mature, emotions are not tied as closely to their internal state, and they begin to react to things and events in the environment. Later emotional expression (between 6 and 12 months) is related to increasing awareness of the social context of events.[37] Feelings of hunger are expressed differently by the 6-month-old baby, who stops fussing and smiles at the parent who arrives with the bottle. Older infants (who have a better idea of where and when hunger is relieved) may become upset and cry when hungry but will also crawl toward the high chair and become ecstatic when the parent opens the refrigerator to begin meal preparations. A wide range of emotional responses emerge in a regular pattern. Specific emotions appear with age and depend on both cognitive and social development.[49]

An assessment tool to identify specific infant behavior patterns is shown in the box on p. 704.

◤ **Intellectual dimension** A mental health evaluation begins with an assessment of sensorimotor capabilities. Infants with serious sensory or motor problems often do not develop optimal intellectual functions. The nurse also assesses the infant's environment, which needs to allow safe and stimulating exploration and produce consistent, de-

ASSESSMENT OF SPECIFIC BEHAVIOR PATTERNS IN THE INFANT

I. Self-regulation and Interest in the World
Birth to 3 months
Increasingly (but still only sometimes):   YES   NO
—able to calm down
—sleeps regularly
—brightens to sights (by alerting and focusing on object)
—brightens to sounds (by alerting and focusing on your voice)
—enjoys touch
—enjoys movement in space (up and down, side to side)

II. Falling in Love
2 to 7 months
When wooed, increasingly (but still only sometimes):   YES   NO
—looks at you with a special, joyful smile
—gazes at you with great interest
—joyfully smiles at you in response to your vocalizations
—joyfully smiles at you in response to your interesting facial expressions
—vocalizes back as you vocalize

III. Developing Intentional Communication
3 to 10 months
Increasingly (but still only sometimes) responds to: YES   NO
—your gestures with gestures in return (you hand her a rattle and she takes it)
—your vocalizations with vocalizations
—your emotional expressions with an emotional response (a smile begets a smile)
—pleasure or joy with pleasure
—encouragement to explore with curiosity (reaches for interesting toy)
—interactions (expectantly looks for you to respond)
—joy and pleasure (woos you spontaneously)
—comforting (reaches up to be held)
—exploration and assertiveness (explores your face or examines a new toy)

IV. Emergence of an Organized Sense of Self
9 to 18 months
Increasingly (but still only sometimes)   YES   NO
—initiates a complex behavior pattern such as going to refrigerator and pointing to desired food, playing a chase game, rolling
   a ball back and forth with you
—uses complex behavior in order to establish closeness (pulls on your leg and reaches up to be picked up)
—uses complex behavior to explore and be assertive (reaches for toys, finds you in another room)
—plays in a focused, organized manner on own
—examines toys or other objects to see how they work
—responds to limits that you set with your voice or gestures
—recovers from anger after a few minutes
—able to use objects like a comb or telephone in semirealistic manner
—seems to know how to get you to react (which actions make you laugh, which make you angry)

From *First feelings—milestones in the emotional development of your baby and child,* by Stanley Greenspan, MD, and Nancy Thorndike Greenspan. Copyright Stanley Greenspan, MD, and Nancy Thorndike Greenspan, 1985. Reprinted by permission of Viking Penguin, Inc.

pendable responses. The nurse then examines the infant's patterns of vocalizations and (later) verbalizations, because language development is closely tied to cognition.

Infants' intellectual development depends on active experiences with the environment during the first year of life. This environmental involvement takes two forms: first, an organizing of basic rhythms, such as crying, sucking, breathing, and resting; second, an active and voluntary participation in the environment. Both provide opportunities for the infant to associate patterns of movement and sensation with specific environmental events and signal the beginning of intellectual development.[12] Each facet of environmental involvement needs to be assessed.

During the first 12 months intellectual abilities emerge sequentially. By repeating simple reflex activities the infant begins to differentiate between self and environment. In the beginning self is the cause of everything. When the hungry baby cries, milk arrives. Eventually, with repetition, different stimuli become associated. The angry baby learns to stop crying when the caregiver's voice is heard (since now the arrival of milk is anticipated). The infant begins to recognize objects in the environment as separate from self as well as the self's effect on these objects.[41]

This early notion of cause and effect is directly related to a beginning self-conception. Through repeated experiences, the infant begins to sense relationships between action and the stimulation of action. This awakening awareness of the part the infant plays in the action helps to further differentiate self from environment. Using Piaget's theory, then, the nurse assesses the infant's ability to separate self from the environment and the effect the separation has on the infant.[39,40]

Social dimension The infant, dependent on the social environment for optimal development, has a repertoire of capacities and characteristics designed to attract the caregiver. For example, from birth infants are drawn to the human voice and face. Their physical appearance (large eyes in proportion to the face; large head in proportion to the body; fuzzy hair; soft, smooth skin; and baby fat) entices most adults into some form of nurturing. Furthermore, infants are able to shape interactions by their abilities to communicate, or signal, their feelings. Infants' signals and responses enable them to become involved in reciprocal interactions with their caregivers. This interaction helps ensure survival during the long period of physical and emotional dependence.

Two important areas of social assessment are attachment and development of a sense of trust. Trust emerges from a strong primary attachment to the caregiver. Attachment is the specific positive emotional relationship that forms between infant and primary caregiver (Figure 35-1). Newman and Newman[37] list three indicators of formed social attachment: (1) the infant tries to maintain contact with the object of attachment, (2) the infant shows distress when the object of attachment is absent, and (3) the infant is more relaxed and comfortable with the object of attachment than with others.

According to Erikson,[14] developing a sense of trust is the main task of infancy. The infant's trust evolves from repeated experiences with a consistent and responsive caregiver. Caregiver response, however, is influenced in part by the infant's ability to communicate successfully. Ideally, the caregiver learns to interpret the infant's behavior appropriately. The infant begins to feel confident of the caregiver's ability to understand his needs, and mutual trust is established. The infant's ability to trust is critical for be-coming a successful member of a larger social network later. Thus, when assessing the strength of the social dimension of the infant, the nurse looks for signs of attachment and trust, such as separation and stranger anxieties.

Spiritual dimension Human spirituality may begin to develop at birth. There is no literature on infant spirituality, but one logical assumption is that the basis of spirituality is derived from the infant's earliest role models of nurturing authorities. Consequently, it is rooted in family experiences and closely related to the development of trust. The spiritual aspect, related to an understanding of the ultimate meaning and purpose of life, is linked to later cognitive and moral development. However, cognitive and emotional structures (which permit moral reasoning) begin to develop in infancy and at the very least serve as a foundation for full spiritual capabilities in later life. The ultimate development of an individual's spiritual dimension, then, at least partially depends on the integrity of the underlying intellectual, emotional, and social dimensions. Assessment of the infant's spirituality involves consideration of these three areas.

The following holistic assessment tool (pp. 706-707) contains assessment information specific to infants. It is to be used in conjunction with the assessment tool in Chapter 8 (The Nursing Process in Psychiatric Nursing).

Another simple screening tool, which provides a guide for data collection, was developed by Haslett.[24] It uses a mnemonic device, "SCREAM," to designate the six areas to address when assessing infant mental health.

S   Sensitivity. Are there unusual sensitivities to sound, light, touch, smell or taste? (To assess sensory integrity)

C   Cuddliness. What is the infant's reaction to being cuddled? (To assess attentional state and consolability)

R   Reactivity. What is the intensity of the infant's reaction? (To assess temperament)

E   Emotional maturity. What level of emotional maturity has the infant reached? (To assess the progression of the infant's ability to relate to other human beings)

A   Autonomic stability. Is there any evidence of autonomic nervous system instability? (To assess early CNS vulnerability)

M   Motor maturity. Is the infant progressing normally through the major motor phases? (To assess physical or motor development)

Other useful tools for assessment are growth charts and the instruments listed in Table 35-3.

Analysis
Nursing diagnosis

The following list provides examples of NANDA-accepted nursing diagnoses with causative statements:

1. Pain related to colic
2. Altered growth and development related to stimulation deficiencies
3. Altered nutrition: less than body requirements related to feeding problems
4. Sleep pattern disturbance related to colic
5. Sensory perceptual alteration related to hearing impairment
6. Impaired communication related to alteration in sensory perceptual state

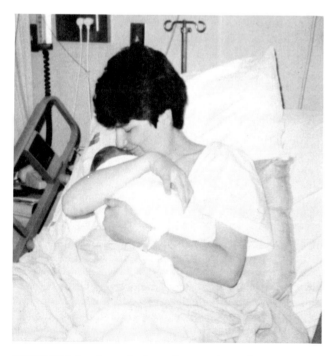

FIGURE 35-1 Attachment has begun between this mother and her newborn.

HOLISTIC ASSESSMENT TOOL: THE INFANT

Physical Dimension
Genetic history

Do any family members have a history of mental or emotional illnesses, such as depression, schizophrenia, or alcohol or drug addiction?
Are there any genetically linked conditions in the family that could affect the infant's growth and development (such as metabolic or neurological disorders)?

Prenatal history

Did the mother receive prenatal care?
Did the mother use alcohol or drugs or smoke during pregnancy?
Was there any maternal illness, unusual stress, or injury during pregnancy?

Neonatal history

Is this a high-risk infant (for example, premature, small for gestational age, one of a multiple birth, offspring of an adolescent mother)?
Were there any problems at birth that required medical treatment (for example, respiratory distress, jaundice)?
What were the infant's Apgar scores?

Physical examination

Has the infant had a complete physical examination by a physician or a certified pediatric nurse practitioner?
Have arrangements been made to obtain well-baby health supervision?
Have routine immunizations been initiated?
Is the infant in good physical condition?
Is growth and development progressing normally?
Does the infant have any health deficits?
Are all sensorimotor capabilities present?
Does the infant have any congenital anomalies?

Level of arousal

How does the primary caregiver describe the infant's temperament?
What does the primary caregiver think about the infant's sleeping and waking cycle?
Is the baby sleepier or more awake than expected?
How does the baby react to new situations and people?
How does the baby react to a sudden loud noice, such as a door slamming nearby?
Does the baby ever seem upset for no reason at all?

Consolability

Does the baby enjoy being held and cuddled?
How does the primary caregiver get the baby to stop crying?
Does the same method always work?
Does the baby ever stop crying without intervention?
Does the baby ever suck his thumb or fingers?
How does the baby fall asleep (for example, only while being held, while nursing or being fed, in crib alone)?
Is it hard for the baby to calm down once upset?

Feeding and elimination

How does the baby convey feelings of hunger?
Does the baby have any problems with feeding?
How does the baby respond to new foods and new textures when eating?
Does the baby have problems making bowel movements?

Sleeping

How many hours (in 24 hours) does the baby sleep?
Does the baby ever have trouble falling asleep?
Does the baby wake up frequently in the night?
Are there any specific positions the baby cannot tolerate (for example, on the back, tummy)?
Does the baby need help to fall asleep (for example, being swaddled, rocked, or walked)?
Does the baby ever engage in self-induced rhythmic activities, such as rocking or head banging?
Does the baby require a bottle to go to sleep?
Where does the baby sleep (for example, parents' bed, own crib)?

Emotional dimension

How does the primary caregiver characterize the infant's predominant style of behavior (for example, easy going, slow to warm up, irritable)?
Does the primary caregiver find the infant's temperament difficult to deal with?
How regular is the infant's schedule?
Does the infant seem to mind if this schedule is altered?
How would the infant react to delayed or interrupted feeding or naps?
Is the infant easily distracted during feeding?
How does the infant react to other people?
How does the infant react to being bathed?

---

7. Impaired communication related to caregiver's inability to adequately interpret infant cues or signals
8. Ineffective individual coping related to inconsolability
9. Anxiety related to stranger's presence
10. Anxiety related to separation from mother

Planning

Because the infant cannot be assessed or treated apart from the family and environment, plans include the entire family. Any plan that merely revolves around the baby is likely to fail because the infant has no existence apart from the caregiver and environment.

The nursing care plan (Table 35-4) lists some examples of long- and short-term goals, outcome criteria, interventions, and rationales for two selected nursing diagnoses, which provide a model for the planning stage in the nursing process.

Implementation

The nurse's interventions are directed primarily toward the caregiver, with specific plans to alter infant behavior or environmental factors. Consequently, the nurse will generally find the roles of consultant, role model, and teacher the most successful when implementing changes to foster infant mental health.

Specific suggestions and new information coupled with appropriate feedback are often sufficient to assist some caregivers to develop new patterns of interaction with their infants. In other situations the nurse may need to function as a role model for alternative behaviors. In these cases the nurse recognizes the caregiver's dependence need and supports this need long enough to permit the caregiver to internalize a sense of personal competence. The caregiver may feel threatened and defensive as new behaviors are demonstrated and encouraged and may test the strength of the therapeutic relationship through noncompliant and

▼ **HOLISTIC ASSESSMENT TOOL: THE INFANT—cont'd**

Intellectual Dimension
Intellectual activities

0 to 4 months of age
Does the infant show special interest in some sights and sounds?
Does the infant enjoy being moved up and down, side to side, through space?
Will the infant follow a slowly moving object or person a full 180 degrees?
Is the infant able to hold and briefly mouth two objects?

4 to 8 months of age
Does the baby enjoy playing with rattles?
Does the baby shake the toy to produce the rattling sound?
Will the baby reach out to the primary caregiver to be picked up (after caregiver initiates movement toward picking up the infant)?
Is the baby able to search for and find a partially hidden toy?

8 to 12 months of age
Does the baby engage in imaginative games, such as pat-a-cake and peek-aboo?
Is the baby able to discriminate strangers?
Does the baby cry or attempt to retreat when strangers are present?
Can the baby anticipate events from signs, such as when the caregiver puts on a coat before leaving the house?
Does the baby drop or throw objects intentionally?
Does the baby ever use objects according to their social significance (for example, hugging a doll or wearing a hat)?

Language skills

0 to 4 months of age
Does the baby coo and smile in response to another person's voice?
Does the baby cry in response to distress?
Is the baby able to repeat his or her own sounds?

4 to 8 months of age
Does the baby respond to his own name?
Does the baby ever babble repetitive syllables (for example, ba ba ba)?
Does the baby ever vocalize different emotional states, such as anger or happiness?

8 to 12 months of age
Is the baby able to initiate interactions through deliberate use of vocalizations?
Does the baby shake his head to show "no"?
Can the baby wave good-bye?
Can the baby say three or more words other than "mama" or "dada"?
Does the baby respond to simple requests (for example, "come here," "sit down")?
Does the baby respond to "no, no"?
Does the baby vocalize in response to the presence of a familiar person?

Social Dimension
Social skills

Does the infant exhibit prosocial behavior (for example, smiling, cooing, visual tracking, turning head to interesting sounds)?
Does the infant show a preference for the primary caregiver?
Does the infant imitate sounds or gestures?
Does the infant initiate interaction with the primary caregiver?
Does the infant engage in reciprocal social games, such as peekaboo?
Does the infant avoid new people? (If so, is it age appropriate?)
How does the infant react to separation from the primary caregiver? (Is this behavior age appropriate?)
Does the infant reach out for toys?
Does the infant initiate new behaviors by himself?
Can the primary caregiver generally figure out the infant's needs? For example, how does the caregiver determine whether the infant is crying from hunger as opposed to fatigue?
Does the infant every engage in gaze aversion? If so, with whom and when?

▼ **TABLE 35-3   Instruments for Assessing Infant Development**

Instrument	Reference	Description
Bayley's Scale of Infant Development	Bayley*	Intelligence test for children less than 3 years of age that evaluates cognitive and motor functioning and integration. Although measurements of infants are less reliable than those for older children, they can be predictive when scores are markedly subnormal or superior. This instrument is best used by developmental psychologists.
Brazelton Neonatal Assessment Scale	Brazelton[7]	Assessment of newborn behavior such as motor maturity, alertness, and consolability. This focus on individual infant behavior can be used to prepare parents for their baby's individual temperament. Neonatal nurses and physicians can use this in promoting better mother-infant relations.
Developmental Diagnostic Profile	A. Freud[18]	Comprehensive and dynamic evaluation of neuropsychiatric, intellectual, emotional, and social development, using psychoanalytical principles. For use by psychiatric professionals who work with infants and children.
Developmental Screening Inventory Scale	Knobloch and Pasamanick[29]	Detailed questionnaire for use with caregiver of infant. Determines achievement level of infant in five areas: adaptive, gross motor, fine motor, language, and personal-social. Based on Gesell's findings, this instrument can be used by nurses and physicians with pediatric knowledge and interviewing skills.
Denver Developmental Screening Test	Frankenburg and Dodds*	Objective screening test for development in four areas: personal-social, fine motor-adaptive, language, and gross motor. Based on Gesell's work establishing norms of development in these areas. Because this instrument is easy to administer and score and takes about 15 to 20 minutes to use, it is economical and widely used to screen for early abnormal development. Nonprofessionals and professionals can be trained to administer the test. It can be used in all settings that serve children's educational and health facilities.

*Conoley J, Kramer J, editors: *The tenth mental measurements yearbook,* Lincoln, Neb, 1989, The University of Nebraska Press.

▼ **TABLE 35-4** **NURSING CARE PLAN**

GOALS	OUTCOME CRITERIA	INTERVENTIONS	RATIONALES
NURSING DIAGNOSIS: Anxiety related to separation from attachment figure			
LONG TERM			
To develop normal human relationships with others	Infant demonstrates preferential response to attachment figure.	Instruct caregiver to observe infant closely to learn infant's individual behavioral style.	Encourages the development of a rich, rewarding relationship between infant and caregiver; relationship is then fostered by spending pleasurable time together at play.
	Infant differentiates caregiver from strangers.	Educate caregiver to spend pleasurable time at play with infant through use of activities such as gently moving infant through space while maintaining eye contact and cooing.	
To develop trust in others	Caregiver provides attachment: secure, consistent emotional base from which infant can explore.	Educate caregiver to accurately interpret infant's signals and to provide a consistent, responsive environment.	Facilitates the development of a trusting relationship.
	Caregiver demonstrates ability to allow infant to experience the environment and others (not overprotective).	Advocate that caregiver allow infant to experience, explore, and manipulate as much of the environment as safely as possible.	
SHORT TERM			
To reduce anxiety	Caregiver establishes methods to diminish infant's sense of abandonment: leaves doorways between rooms open so infant can see, caregiver responds verbally to infant when out of sight.	Encourage caregiver to increase distal modes of communication by keeping door open to allow infant to make visual contact with caregiver, calling to infant from other rooms.	A gradual separation diminishes infant's sense of abandonment, thus reducing anxiety.
	Infant responds verbally to caregiver when out of sight.	Instruct caregiver to play simple games with infant, such as peekaboo, "Where is it?," waving bye-bye.	Facilitates development of object permanence, which decreases anxiety.
To reduce attachment figure's anxiety	Caregiver accepts phase as normal and as a desired consequence of infant's ability for object permanence.	Interpret infant's separation anxiety as developmentally normal and desirable to caregiver.	Many parents find developmental guidance helpful to determine normal infant behavior.
To foster ability to separate	Caregiver provides consistent alternative caregiver.	Advocate that caregiver provide a consistent alternate caregiver.	A consistent, stable environment facilitates infant's ability to separate.
	Caregiver provides infant with transitional object, such as teddy bear or blanket.	Encourage caregiver to provide infant with transitional object, such as teddy bear or blanket.	

▼ TABLE 35-4   NURSING CARE PLAN —cont'd

GOALS	OUTCOME CRITERIA	INTERVENTIONS	RATIONALES
NURSING DIAGNOSIS: Sleep pattern disturbance related to colic			
LONG TERM			
To develop regular age-appropriate diurnal sleeping patterns	Caregiver establishes consistent night sleep patterns. Infant establishes day nap pattern. Infant falls asleep in crib instead of caregiver's arms.	Instruct caregiver to establish consistent night sleep patterns for infant, allow infant to establish day nap pattern, allow infant to fall asleep in crib instead of caregiver's arms.	Facilitates infant's self-regulating ability.
To provide gratification in activities of daily living	Adequate caregiver-infant interaction during the day. Caregiver spends time each day in pleasure-producing play with infant. Infant can comfortably spend time alone.	Encourage caregiver to spend adequate amounts of time interacting with infant each day, a portion of which is spent in pleasure-producing play; allow infant to spend time alone each day.	Establishes healthy and mutually gratifying patterns of care.
SHORT TERM			
To reduce anxiety	Caregiver understands infant's physiological needs: has expectations, reads infant's signals and cues accurately (recognizes distress crying), recognizes own response to infant, seeks and receives support and encouragement from others.	Educate caregiver to recognize infant's physiological needs, accurately respond to infant's needs, identify own response to infant, seek and receive support and encouragement from others.	Increases caregiver's self-confidence and facilitates development of trust relationship, thus reducing anxiety in caregiver and infant.
To establish realistic, reasonable limits	Caregiver establishes regular bedtime, maintains regular routines, and responds to continued crying (after 15 minutes) by providing comforting measures (no feeding or playing). Caregiver eliminates excessive stimulation before bedtime and maintains quiet nighttime environment.	Instruct caregiver to maintain regular routines, establish regular bedtime, eliminate stimulation before bedtime, maintain quiet nighttime environment, and respond to continued crying (after 15 minutes) by giving comforting measures only (no playing or feeding).	Provides consistent, responsive environment, facilitates development of self-consoling behaviors in infant; establishes realistic, reasonable limits.

provocative behavior. The nurse is prepared for such behavior, remaining consistent and supportive while helping the caregiver explore the meaning of the behavior. The nurse needs to recognize this behavior as part of the therapeutic process and not react emotionally to the caregiver's hostile attitude.

A wide variety of interventions is used in the helping relationship, depending on individual need. The duration, pattern, and methods of treatment depend on the parents' background, readiness, and insight. An eclectic approach helps determine individual plans. *The ultimate goal is the same: to promote mental health in infants through improved reciprocal caregiver-infant interactions.* Interac-

tions are described in the accompanying research highlight on p. 710.

Physical dimension Infants at risk for serious physical problems (such as premature and low-weight babies, babies with birth defects, and those born to alcoholic and drug-abusing mothers) need to be referred to medical experts for thorough evaluation and treatment.

Feeding and sleeping problems are major concerns in young infants. Many of these problems stem from the infant's inability to regulate his state of arousal, which is often caused by CNS immaturity and usually outgrown by the age of 3 months. Nurses can provide valuable assistance in teaching parents to facilitate their infant's self-regulating

RESEARCH HIGHLIGHT

Predicting Paternal Role Enactment

- J Rustia and D Abbott

PURPOSE

The purpose of this study was to investigate factors related to infant care behaviors over time by first time fathers. Specifically, the authors tested whether expectations and prior learning experiences about parenting were predictive of parental role performance across a 2-year period. Mothers' expectations of paternal involvement were also evaluated as possible predictors.

SAMPLE

The sample consisted of 53 mother-father subject dyads recruited from the postpartum units of three hospitals in two midwestern metropolitan cities. Subjects were married or cohabitating.

METHODOLOGY

Data were collected by trained interviewers at seven times during the first 2 years after birth. Standardized interview schedules were used. General demographical information and information on socialization experiences of the father were also collected.

FINDINGS

Fathers reported "doing almost as much as mothers" in playing with baby, cuddling, and holding. Fathers also reported that mothers did more diapering, bathing, and getting up at night. Fathers reported doing less than they said they would; however, their willingness and actual performance of infant care increased over time. Fathers' performance of infant care lags behind mother's expectations. However, over time, mothers lowered their expectations of fathers' performance. There was no relationship between fathers prior learning of the parental role and their paternal role performance.

IMPLICATIONS

Although fathers were not as involved in care taking tasks as mothers, they appeared to be moving in the direction of assuming greater responsibility for infant care. Findings also suggested that society's beliefs and norms about fathers' parental roles have changed more rapidly than fathers' actual performance. This discrepancy may lead to guilt in some fathers. Nurses are well situated to assist new fathers in acquiring new parenting behaviors. Anticipatory guidance can begin in prenatal classes and in the hospital before discharge.

From *Western Journal of Nursing Research* 12(2):145, 1990.

---

ability. However, early intervention is important, as first experiences are critical in establishing healthy and mutually gratifying patterns of care.

Early self-regulatory problems can often be alleviated through interventions that increase the baby's attention and help the baby learn self-consolation. Strategies include teaching the parents about the self-regulating capacities of the infant by stating that infants adapt to the world using different attentional states by which they demonstrate distinct behavioral differences. For example, an actively crying and kicking baby is effectively shutting out other stimuli, whereas a quiet baby sucking on a thumb may be attuned to visual and auditory events in the environment. Other strategies include encouraging self-consoling behaviors such as thumb sucking; providing simple sensory stimulation at an appropriate level for the baby; providing a consistent, calm atmosphere; and assisting the parents to accurately interpret the infant's signals.

Occasionally, self-regulation problems are related to specific sensory problems. In the case of sensory hyposensitivity or hypersensitivity, the nurse can offer strategies to decrease or increase specific sensory stimulation. For example, some babies are extremely sensitive to high-pitched noises and will disorganize quickly when exposed to such sounds. Caregivers can be taught to moderate their own voices to a pitch that is not painful and to control environmental noises as much as possible. Severe sensory problems, such as visual or hearing impairments, require interventions that provide increased stimulation through other intact senses.

Generally, an infant who is able to integrate sensory experiences and regulate attentional states will not develop major feeding or sleeping problems. Persistent feeding difficulties accompanied by vomiting, elimination problems, or weight loss may be due to a physical problem, and the nurse refers the parents and infant to a physician. Occasionally, a feeding problem may result from a temperamental mismatch between the infant and caregiver. An easily distracted, hyperalert baby will have difficulty settling down to nurse. Such behavior may cause the mother to feel tense and inadequate, which will further increase the infant's distraction. The nurse, through observation of the feeding process, can often suggest practical methods for promoting more rewarding feeding experiences. For example, a baby who feeds briefly, stops to look around frequently, and requires encouragement to return to the breast or bottle may need to be fed in a less stimulating environment, such as a darkened room. The caregiver's distraction or tension can produce a reciprocal tension in the infant. Encouraging a relaxed attitude, which will enhance a mutual responsiveness, is accomplished by exploring the caregiver's feelings about and behavior during feeding and by teaching relaxation techniques.

Persistent sleeping problems require interventions to increase the infant's deep sleep period. When infants first fall asleep, they enter the rapid eye movement (REM) state.

Later they enter the deep sleep stage, during which maturational processes occur in the body and CNS. The infant with a sleeping disturbance may be getting predominantly REM-stage sleep and as a consequence may remain neurologically immature. This immaturity makes it difficult for the infant to self-regulate, which inhibits the infant's ability to fall asleep without help. Thus instead of arousing slightly when moving to deeper sleeping levels, the infant completely awakens and never experiences the deeper levels of sleep. Interventions that promote sleep include giving adequate feeding, being warm and dry, reducing environmental stimuli, and having a relaxed caregiver.

Emotional dimension An infant's emotional problems result from his difficulty either experiencing the environment (sensorimotor problems) or integrating an interpreting the experiences accurately (intellectual problems). As an example, consider the fretful, tense, and inconsolable infant who cries easily and is often upset. The slightest change in the environment is enough to set off this infant; and normal sights, sounds, and tactile stimulation are irritating. Interventions in this case increase the infant's self-regulatory capacities. Likewise, the depressed or apathetic infant requires stimulation that is interesting and enticing yet modulated to allow the baby to become involved gradually. Stimulation and affection with such babies are provided in a gentle and unobtrusive way, as these infants become easily overwhelmed and "tune out." Nurses working with withdrawn infants offer low-key stimulation, approaching them with one sensory experience at a time (lightly stroking the infant's limbs *or* talking in a quiet voice, not both at once).

When an infant appears to have an emotional impairment that is not due to a sensorimotor problem or intellectual deficits, the nurse considers the influence of social feedback. If the problem resulted from inappropriate or inadequate caregiver behavior, interventions are aimed at improving the emotional reciprocity between caregiver and infant. The nurse focuses on improving the quality of the caregiver's nurturing activities. First, the nurse assesses the caregiver's level of child-rearing skills. When the caregiver is inexperienced and lacks knowledge of appropriate caregiving behaviors, the nurse intervenes by teaching the caregiver about the infant's individual emotional needs. Specifically, the nurse helps the caregiver to interpret accurately and respond to the baby's cues, points out the infant's selective responses to the caregiver, and encourages the caregiver to remain consistent and available and to engage in pleasurable activities with the infant. If the caregiver is not able to provide adequate nurturance because of emotional problems, the nurse refers the infant and caregiver to an appropriate resource.

Intellectual dimension When a severe intellectual deficit is suspected, the nurse refers the infant to a neurologist, pediatrician, or an infant mental health center for further evaluation and treatment.

Several nursing interventions foster optimal intellectual developments. The nurse encourages caregivers to allow their infants to become actively engaged in the environment, to manipulate and explore as much of the world as safely possible. Many parents find developmental guidance helpful. The nurse interprets as desired and normal the infant's seemingly meaningless repetitive activities for the parents. For example, the infant who continuously drops dishes, food, and silverware from the high chair is developing early recognition of a sequence of events, which is necessary for attaining the concepts of cause and effect. The nurse can also assist parents in understanding and facilitating the development of object permanence through simple games, such as peekaboo, "Where is it?," and waving bye-bye.

The related concepts of stranger and separation anxiety are also explained. Specific strategies to decrease separation anxiety are teaching parents to increase the use of distal communication; for example, calling to the infant from other rooms, keeping doors open to allow the infant to make visual contact with the parent; providing the infant with a transitional object, such as a teddy bear or security blanket; and maintaining consistent, sensitive responses that convey acceptance of the infant's feelings but do not reinforce the infant's fearfulness. For example, a quick hug of reassurance, coupled with a distraction to some other interesting toy or event, is better than prolonged soothing and intense physical contact, which exaggerates the infant's dependence on the caregiver and ultimately makes separation more difficult.

Language development depends partly on the integrity of intellectual foundations that enable intentional, receptive, and expressive functions. The infant's failure to meet age-expected vocalizations and verbalizations may necessitate referral for evaluation. Many community health centers and public schools have speech evaluation services. The nurse may also refer the infant directly to a speech pathologist.

Social dimension The infant experiencing a problem in the social dimension, such as an attachment disorder, may demonstrate behavior such as gaze aversion and withdrawal from human contact or may demonstrate insecure attachments through clinging and intense fearfulness on separation from the attachment figure. Early interventions educate caregivers about the process of attachment. Parents can help develop a trusting relationship by learning to interpret accurately their baby's signals and providing a consistent and responsive environment.

Because attachment to a primary caregiver is one of the most important developmental tasks of infancy to ensure optimal mental health, the nurse encourages caregivers to form a rich and rewarding relationship with the infant. This process can be facilitated by having parents observe their infants closely to get to know their individual behavioral style. Caregivers need to provide interesting experiences that allow the infant to experience multisensory stimuli. These experiences can be as simple as moving the infant gently through space, maintaining eye contact and offering warm expressions, and cooing or talking to the baby. Some infants require special wooing, a method to attract the infant's attention. Developing a sense of attachment first requires a relationship between caregiver and infant. The relationship is then fostered by spending pleasurable time together at play. Some parents may need to learn *how* to play. The nurse provides valuable assistance through demonstration, role modeling, and observation and feedback sessions. Because the process of attachment is thought to be central to the optimal development of mental health, the nurse needs to refer parents and infants for further evaluation and treatment when serious attachment problems are suspected. Referral to an infant mental health specialist is critical when the infant's physical growth and development are affected by the attachment disorder.

When working with a caregiver-infant dyad, the nurse is sensitive to the needs of the caregiver and is careful to offer assistance in nonjudgmental ways that will ultimately augment the caregiver's self-esteem. In one useful technique, the nurse interprets the infant's behavior and speaks for the nonverbal infant, either directly or indirectly. For example, in the direct approach the nurse who is enhancing the attachment process between caregiver and infant would point out the infant's preferential smile for the caregiver by saying, "See Mommy (or Daddy)? This is my special smile just for you. You make me feel so good, no one else is quite like you." In the indirect approach the nurse communicates the infant's needs and intentions by directing questions and comments to the infant in the presence of the listening caregiver. After observing and interpreting an infant's behavior, the nurse comments, "Are you sleepy? You always start to fuss and then you rub your eyes when you're tired. I think you're a sleepy baby." Both approaches help the caregiver accurately interpret the infant's behavior.

Many infant mental health centers provide programs that offer appropriate supportive environments for infants. Therapeutic daycare centers provide opportunities for caregivers to learn parenting skills in growth-enhancing environments. Other centers have therapeutic nurseries, which focus more on the direct care of infants who have special mental health care needs.

Spiritual dimension Interventions to ensure spiritual development in infancy enhance optimal emotional, social, and intellectual development, as it is believed that spirituality incorporates all these dimensions.

Evaluation

Evaluation of the nurse's interventions is a judgment of the extent to which the treatment goals and outcome criteria have been met. Because care focuses on the caregiver-infant relationship, the behavior of both is evaluated. The caregiver's perception about changes that have occurred and goals that have been met is important.

Various criteria can be used to evaluate both the process and the specific interventions.

1. *Adequacy.* Did the nursing interventions primarily involve relief of the infant's symptoms, and did they also include educating the caregiver and family? Did the caregiver and family education include normal infant development, how to accurately identify and meet infant needs, and ways to manage problem behaviors? If the caregiver was also experiencing problems, did interventions address these issues? Did these interventions focus on symptom relief, and did it also address ways for the caregiver to recognize and manage self-behavior?

2. *Appropriateness.* If the infant was in severe distress, was intervention started immediately and appropriate referrals made? Did interventions foster the development of a therapeutic alliance based on trust between the nurse and caregiver? Was the caregiver included in the setting of goals? Did the caregiver agree with established goals? Were the interventions relevant for the problems identified in each of the five dimensions?

3. *Effectiveness.* Did the goals and interventions specifically relate to the problems identified? To what degree were the problems alleviated, behaviors changed, symptoms relieved, and/or learning achieved?

4. *Efficiency.* Were the interventions for the infant and caregiver enough to alleviate the problems identified? Were support systems and community resources coordinated to impact further the problems identified?

In addition, continued periodic evaluations, along with anticipatory guidance and continuing parent education, are necessary for the promotion and maintenance of infant mental health. For these reasons, these activities should be emphasized and care taken to avoid premature termination of the infant relationship.

Although the caregiver's improved responsiveness, self-confidence, and competence and the achievement of normal developmental tasks indicate a readiness for termination, it may not be in the infant's best interest. Absolute termination of the helping relationship with an infant prevents ongoing monitoring and evaluation and is thus not desirable. Instead, termination is often restricted and relative. With the consent of the caregiver(s), frequent and regular meetings cease gradually, as in weaning. It is also advisable to include auxiliary care and availability in the termination agreement.

An explicit plan for reentry into treatment at times of extra stress, whether developmental, personal, or social, is essential. Predetermined, periodic meetings for careful, caring monitoring and evaluation of child rearing are imperative. These meetings, which constitute primary preventive care, are particularly useful at transitional stages of child development when reassessment and anticipatory guidance can be provided. Adherence to these guidelines provides a vehicle for continuous evaluation.

BRIEF REVIEW

In mental health–psychiatric nursing, the therapeutic relationship with the infant is unique. Parameters in the relationship are discovered through the nursing process, which includes data collection in all five dimensions during the prenatal, neonatal, and infancy period. Because the relationship between infant and caregiver is reciprocal, the nursing process is directed toward both.

Biological, interactional, cognitive, psychoanalytical, and learning theories provide understanding of infant growth and direct clinical actions. Knowledge about normal emotional development provides the nurse with standards to identify deviations from the norm and high-risk factors.

A number of measurement tools are available for assessing infant development, such as "SCREAM," Brazelton's Neonatal Assessment Scale, and the Developmental Screening Inventory Scale. These tools aid in assessing the infant in each dimension. Referral to another professional or agency may be necessary for more serious conditions, such as reactive attachment disorder, rumination disorder, or infantile autism.

The ultimate goal is improved mental health in infants through improved caregiver-infant interactions. The nurse can be a change agent to create an improved climate for the promotion of infant mental health.

REFERENCES AND SUGGESTED READINGS

1. Ainsworth MDS and others: *Patterns of attachment: a psychological study of the strange situation,* New York, 1978, John Wiley & Sons.
2. Anderson G: Risk in mother-infant separation postbirth, *Image: Journal of Nursing Scholarship* 21(4):196, 1989.
3. Apgar V: Proposal for a new method of evaluation of the newborn infant, *Anesthesia and Analgesia* 32:260, 1953.
4. Barrera ME, Maurer D: The perception of facial expression by the three-month-old, *Child Development* 52:203, 1981.
5. Benoit D, Zeanah C, Barton M: Maternal attachment disturbances in failure to thrive, *Infant Mental Health Journal* 10:185, 1989.
6. Bowlby J: *Attachment and loss,* vol 2, Anger, NY, 1973, Basic Books.
7. Brazelton TB: *Neonatal assessment scale,* Philadelphia, 1973, JB Lippincott.
8. Brazelton TB: Precursors for the development of emotions in early infancy. In Plutchik R, Kellerman H, editors: *Emotions in early development,* vol 2, New York, 1983, Academic Press.
9. Bromwich R: *Working with parents and infants,* Baltimore, 1981, University Park Press.
10. Call JD, Galenson E: *Frontiers of infant psychiatry,* New York, 1982, Basic Books.
11. Dalton S, Howell C: Autism: psychobiological perspectives, *Journal of Child and Adolescent Psychiatric and Mental Health Nursing* 2:92, 1989.
12. Elkind D: *Children and adolescents: interpretive essays on Jean Piaget,* New York, 1981, Oxford University Press.
13. Erikson E: *Childhood and society,* ed 2, New York, 1963, WW Norton.
14. Erikson E: *Insight and responsibility,* New York, 1964, WW Norton.
15. Field TM: *High-risk infants and children: adult and peer interactions,* New York, 1981, Academic Press.
16. Field TM: *Infants born at risk: behavior and development,* New York, 1979, SP Medical & Scientific Books.
17. Fraiberg S: *Clinical studies in infant mental health: the first year of life,* New York, 1980, Basic Books.
18. Freud A: *Normality and pathology in children: assessments of development,* New York, 1965, International Universities Press.
19. Gesell A, Amatruda CS: *Developmental diagnosis,* ed 2, New York, 1947, Paul B Hoebner.
20. Greenspan S: *Psychopathology and adaptation in infancy and early childhood,* New York, 1981, International Universities Press.
21. Greenspan S, Porges S: Psychopathology in infancy and early childhood: clinical perspectives on the organization of sensory and affective-thematic experience, *Child Development* 55:49, 1984.
22. Greenspan S, Greenspan N: *First feelings,* New York, 1985, Viking Penguin.
23. Greenspan SI: Emotional and developmental patterns in infancy. In Kestenbaum CJ, Williams DT, editors: *Handbook of clinical assessment of children and adolescents,* vol 1, New York, 1988, New York University Press.
24. Haslett NR: Treatment planning for children: a complete child psychiatry evaluation outline, *Journal of Continuing Education in Psychiatry* 11:21, 1977.
25. Holmes S: Planning for the best start in life, *Professional Nurse* 6(4):200, 1991.
26. Kandzari JH, Howard JR: *The well family: a developmental approach to assessment,* Boston, 1981, Little, Brown.
27. Keefe M: The impact of rooming-in on maternal sleep at night, *Journal of Obstetric, Gynocologic, and Neonatal Nursing* 17:122, 1988.
28. Kiltenbach K and others: Infant wariness toward strangers reconsidered: infants' and mothers' reactions to unfamiliar persons, *Child Development* 51:1197, 1980.
29. Knobloch H, Pasamanick B: *Gesell and Amatruda's developmental diagnosis,* ed 3, New York, 1974, Harper & Row.
30. Lemmer Sr C: Parental perceptions of caring following perinatal bereavement, *Western Journal of Nursing Research* 13(4):475, 1991.
31. Lindz T: *The person,* New York, 1968, Basic Books.
32. Lugo SO, Hershey GL: *Human development,* New York, 1974, Macmillian.
33. Mack JE, Ablon SL: *The development and sustenance of self-esteem in childhood,* New York, 1983, International Universities Press.
34. Mahler MS and others: *The psychological birth of the human infant,* New York, 1975, Basic Books.
35. McCormick L, Schiefelbusch R: *Early language intervention,* Columbus, Ohio, 1984, Charles E. Merrill.
36. Maier HW: *Three theories of child development,* New York, 1978, Harper & Row.
37. Newman B, Newman R: *Development through life,* Homewood, Ill, 1984, The Dorsey Press.
38. Peterson E, Alexander N, Moghissi K: A.I.D. and AIDS: too close for comfort, *Fertility and Sterility* 49(2):209, 1988.
39. Piaget J: *The origins of intelligence in children,* New York, 1952, International Universities Press.
40. Piaget J: *The construction of reality in the child,* New York, 1954, Basic Books.
41. Piaget J: *Psychology of the child,* New York, 1969, Basic Books.
42. Plomin R, Rowe DC: Genetic and environmental etiology of social behavior in infancy, *Developmental Psychology* 15:62, 1979.
43. Plomin R: Developmental behavioral genetics, *Child Development* 54:253, 1983.
44. Plomin R, DeFries JC: *Origins of individual differences in infancy,* New York, 1985, The Colorado Adoption Project Academic Press.
45. Pridham K, Chang A: Mothers' perceptions of problem solving competence for infant care, *Western Journal of Nursing Research* 13(2):164, 1991.
46. Rapoport JL, Ismond DR: *DSM-III-R training guide for diagnosis of childhood disorders,* New York, 1990, Brunner/Mazel.
47. Rubin N: Family rituals, *Parents Magazine* 64(3):105, 1989.
48. Stern D: *The first relationship, mother and infant,* Cambridge, Mass, 1977, Harvard University Press.
49. Stroufe AL: Socioemotional development. In Osofsky JD, editor: *The handbook of infant development,* New York, 1979, John Wiley & Sons.
50. Thomas A, Chess S: *Behavioral individuality in early childhood,* New York, 1963, New York University Press.
51. Thomas A, Chess S: *Temperament and behavior disorders in children,* New York, 1968, New York University Press.
52. Thomas A, Chess S: *Temperament and development,* New York, 1977, Brunner/Mazel.
53. Weaver R, Cranley M: An exploration of paternal-fetal attachment behavior, *Nursing Research* 32:2, 1983.
54. Winnicott DW: *Therapeutic consultations in child psychiatry,* New York, 1971, Basic Books.
55. Yarrow LJ: *Historical perspectives and future directions in infant development,* New York, 1979, John Wiley & Sons.

ANNOTATED BIBLIOGRAPHY

Dinkmeyer D, McKay G: *The parents handbook: systematic training for effective parenting,* Minnesota, 1989, American Guidance Service.

This is an essential teaching guide for parents. The authors describe basic skills for the beginning nurse in parenting styles, misbehavior, communication, and discipline through natural and logical consequences.

Ferber R: *Solve your child's sleep problems,* New York, 1985, Simon & Schuster.

This is an excellent and practical guide to understanding sleep mechanisms and requirements of infants and young children. Advice offered is based on sleep research at the Center for Pediatric Sleep Disorders at the Children's Hospital in Boston (the only sleep center in the country devoted to children). It is easy to read and suitable as a parent resource.

Fraiberg S: *Clinical studies in infant mental health: the first year of life,* New York, 1980, Basic Books.

This easy-to-read collection of case studies of therapeutic relationships with infants and mothers reflects Fraiberg's sensitive and empathic approach.

Greenspan SI, Greenspan NT: *First feelings: milestones in the emotional development of your baby and child from birth to age 4,* New York, 1985, Viking Penguin.

Written primarily for parents, this book is also informative to health professionals. The emotional milestones are related to the different developmental stages that make up Greenspan's developmental-structural framework, which emerged from research by Greenspan and colleagues at the National Institute of Mental Health. The book is punctuated with interesting and illuminating vignettes from the original study.

Lawhon G, Melzar A: Developmental care of the very low birth weight infant, *Journal of Perinatal Neonatal Nursing* 2(1):56, 1988.

This article challenges the nurse to become skilled at recognizing the very low birth weight infant. The nurse's role in assessing for stressors, reducing stress within the neonatal environment, and teaching parents to recognize and understand the infant is discussed.

Osofsky J: *Handbook of infant development,* New York, 1979, John Wiley & Sons.

This comprehensive collection of reviews on infant development covers cognitive, social, and emotional development and theoretical and clinical issues.

CHAPTER

36 The Child

Patricia Ann Clunn

After studying this chapter, the student will be able to:

- Discuss historical developments related to psychiatric nursing care of the child
- Discuss the psychopathology of the developmental disorders, separation anxiety, tic, elimination, and attention deficit hyperactive disorders as described in the DSM-III-R
- Discuss various theoretical approaches to child development
- Apply the nursing process to the mental health needs of children
- Identify current research findings relevant to the mental health care of children

Children under 18 years of age constitute one third of the population of the United States. Estimates are that 12% to 15% of these children are in need of some type of mental health or psychiatric services.[81] Children in need of mental health or psychiatric services are defined as children whose personality development is arrested or interfered with so that the child shows impairment in reasonable and accurate perceptions of the world, in impulse control, in learning, and in social relations with others. The magnitude of the problem is summarized as follows:

1. Approximately 1 million children are institutionalized for mental illness.
2. Drug abuse, including alcohol consumption, has increased remarkably among elementary school children.
3. Venereal disease is a major epidemic of childhood, with the largest incidence in children between the ages of 10 to 14 years.
4. Suicide has increased among children over 10 years of age, with the largest increase among children aged 5 to 14.
5. Many pediatric AIDS cases are infants with perinatal infection and live for several years with chronic illness.

Population projections indicate that between 1980 and 2005 there will be an increase in the population under 15 years of age. Statistical data on disruptions in society and the family, the essence of the child's environment, are alarming. The risk factors listed in the box on p. 717 mandate expansion of child psychiatric services.[80]

Children with mental health–psychiatric disorders have historically been an underserved population, with only sporadic attention given to their plight. During the last part of the 1980s, however, passage of several major national and international legislative policies suggest that child psychia-try is coming of age, with commitments toward future improvements in care, services, and funding for children's mental health. Growing national and international public awareness and research documenting relationships between the social problems plaguing contemporary society

▶ DIAGNOSES Related to the Child

NURSING DIAGNOSIS	MEDICAL DIAGNOSES
Altered growth and development	Developmental disorders
	Mental retardation
	Pervasive developmental disorders
	Autism
	Specific developmental disorders
	Developmental arithmetic disorder
	Developmental writing disorder
	Developmental reading disorder
	Developmental articulation disorder
	Developmental coordination disorder
	Separation anxiety disorders
	Tic disorders
	Elimination disorders
	Attention deficit hyperactivity disorder

HISTORICAL OVERVIEW

DATES	EVENTS
16th Century and Before	No distinction is made between "little" and "big" people; the same social expectations are held for all beyond the age of infancy.
Industrial Revolution	Childhood is recognized as a discrete life stage as industry becomes the framework for organizing society. "The century of the child" begins in France and spreads to America with passage of child labor and compulsory education laws. Education and learning became, and continue to be, the major work of children.
1850s	Compulsory school attendance brings large numbers of emotionally disturbed children needing services under the jurisdiction of public school officials and the Child Guidance movement begins with Children's courts, judges, social workers and school psychologists providing professional services through family laws and social services for children with problems.
1900s	Clifford Beers founds the Mental Hygiene Movement. Establishment of disciplines from which many theories of child psychiatry derived: developmental psychology, education, genetics, physiology, anthropology, pediatrics, adult psychiatry.
1920s	Recognition of child's play as vehicle of research and treatment, fosters Darwin, ethnologists. John Dewey introduces learning through play and discovery in child education.
1930	White House Conference on Children proclaims "play is the work of children," giving educators, psychologists official support to use play to foster child development, learning, socialization.
1933	American Psychiatric Associations recognition of child psychiatry as a unique subspecialty.
1954	First graduate education program in child psychiatric nursing is started at Boston University.
1963	Community mental health act is passed funding community mental health centers. Children recognized as individuals with unique needs and problems with special services provided.
1968	Child Psychiatric Nursing Educators Conference resolution supporting care of children in community outside custodial institutions.
1971	President's Commission on the Mental Health of Children cites children's mental health problems had reached crisis proportions. Advocates for Child Psychiatric Nursing is founded.
1973	Joint Commission on Mental Health of Children cite serious implications of unmet mental health and social service needs of children, need to change traditional training service delivery systems to preventive orientation.
1974	Fagin publishes the text, *Readings in Child and Adolescent Psychiatric Nursing.*
1975	US Public Law 94-142 is passed, proclaiming the right to equal education for all handicapped children.
1976	Pothier publishes the text, *Mental Health Counseling with Children.* Certification examinations with two levels of psychiatric nurses: generalists (C) and clinical specialists (CS) in Child and Adolescent Psychiatric Mental Health Nursing.
1979	UN sponsors Year of the Child, emphasized increased numbers of children with emotional problems, need for psychiatric services.
1980	Use of DSM-III-R in most psychiatric training programs results in social and professional peer consciousness raising, awareness, of child psychiatry.
1985	Revised Standards on child and adolescent psychiatric and mental health nursing practice (ANA) published and approved.

DATES	EVENTS
1986	Public Law 99-457, Education of the Handicapped Act is enacted, reauthorizing programs under EHA, strict agenda for improved services. Early interventions for eligible disabled infants from birth to 3 years of age; multidisciplinary evaluation of developmentally delayed infant and toddler, case management, development of Individualized Family Service plans.
1987	Surgeon General's Conference on Children with Special Health Care Needs is sponsored by the Maternal and Child Health Bureau and American Academy of Pediatrics.
1988	*Journal of Child and Adolescent Psychiatric Mental Health Nursing* begins publication.
1989	United Nations (UN) convention drafts Rights of Children, adopted by UN General Assembly, legally binding nations signing as a treaty, emphasizing the rights of children, progress toward human dignity.
1990	National Advisory Mental Health Council publishes National plan for research on child and adolescent mental disorders, a national research incentive to intensify work with youth with psychiatric disorders that will influence future service delivery and research.
Future	World Summit for Children: world declaration on the survival, protection and development of children with a plan of action with specified international goals for 1990-2000.[64]

and the alarming numbers of emotionally disturbed children supported legislation for public funding of programs for preschool and school-aged children. These laws protect the rights of children, ensuring early intervention services, and represent an effort on the part of the Federal government to ensure that early intervention services are provided to handicapped children and their families.

A national agenda has gradually emerged for providing care for children with special physical, mental health, and educational needs as a result of profound advances in medical technology and new psychological understandings for diagnosing and treating children with special health care needs. There has been an evolution in concepts of care: broadened diagnostic categories; comprehensive concern for the whole child; and coordinated services that are family centered, community based, and supported and advanced by congressional action and activities of U.S. Public Health Service.[60]

Increased parental participation and activism are the major components of recent legislation for children with spe-

cial health needs. Family support as a national public policy includes family-centered care, community-based services with coordinated case management, and a shift away from institutional care.[48] The emphasis is on prevention, defined as the identification and intervention in risk factors, which are situations in the child's environment that are potentially hazardous to the child's mental health.

On an international level, a World Summit Meeting for Children was held in September 1990. Goals included reducing by one-third infant death rates world wide; decreasing by one-half the incidence of malnutrition and numbers of women who die in childbirth; and assuring rights of access to adequate health care, education, child services, housing, and cultural activities, all by the year 2000.

DSM-III-R DIAGNOSES

The etiology and essential diagnostic features for the medical diagnoses of developmental disorders, separation anxiety disorders, tic disorders, elimination disorders, and attention deficit hyperactivity disorders presented in this chapter are briefly summarized in this section.

Developmental Disorders

Mental Retardation, Specific Developmental Disorders, and Pervasive Developmental Disorders are under the rubric of Developmental Disorders and are noted on Axis II in the DSM-III-R.[4] The major problems of children diagnosed in this group are disturbances in acquisition of cognitive, language, motor, or social skills. The disturbance may involve a general delay, as in Mental Retardation, a failure to progress in a specific area of skill acquisition, as in Specific Developmental Disorders, or in multiple areas in which there are qualitative distortions of normal development, as in Pervasive Developmental Disorders.

RISK FACTORS

1. Children of minority groups, particularly blacks and Hispanics, who are without access to mental health services and appropriate programs
2. Poverty and unemployment resulting in increasing numbers of runaway and homeless children
3. Child abuse and neglect leading to juvenile delinquency and criminality
4. Family dissolution (divorce and single parenting) with its ensuing economic, social, and psychological losses
5. Parental alcoholism resulting in conduct disorders, substance abuse, depression, and social inadequacy
6. Children with AIDS

Mental retardation

The essential features of mental retardation are (1) significantly subaverage general intellectual functioning, accompanied by (2) significant deficits or impairments in adaptive functioning, with (3) onset before the age of 18. The DSM-III-R states specific IQ score parameters for four levels: mild mental retardation (educable: IQ levels 50-70), moderate mental retardation (trainable: IQ 35-49), severe mental retardation (IQ 20-34), and profound mental retardation (IQ below 20).

The DSM-III-R uses the American Association on Mental Deficiency (AAMD) for mental retardation definition. Two diagnostic areas are emphasized: the child has to function on a retarded level intellectually and in adaptive functioning. Subaverage intellectual functioning refers to an IQ of 70 or below on an individually administered IQ test. Adaptive behavior refers to how effectively the child meets standards of personal independence and social responsibility expected for his or her chronological age and cultural group.[1] Children with mental retardation are not specifically addressed in this chapter. Assessment and treatment of mentally retarded children with psychiatric disorders are similar to those with children with normal intelligence. Nurses adjust care to the child's cognitive level.

Pervasive developmental disorders

Pervasive developmental disorders are characterized by impairment in the development of (1) social interactions, (2) verbal and nonverbal communication skills, and (3) imaginative activity. There often is a markedly restricted repertoire of activities and interests, which are stereotyped and repetitious. These disorders are frequently accompanied by other conditions such as distortions or delays in intellectual skills; language and speech; posture and movements; patterns of eating, drinking, or sleeping; and responses to sensory input. Pervasive developmental disorders are distinguished from mental retardation in that children with mental retardation are sociable and can communicate, even nonverbally, if they have no speech.

Autistic disorder is a type of pervasive developmental disorder. Children with this diagnosis demonstrate the preceding three characteristics during the first 36 months of life. Impaired social interactions include a lack of awareness of the existence or feelings of others (treats another person like a piece of furniture or does not notice anothers' distress), does not seek comfort in times of distress, does not imitate activities such as wave "bye-bye," prefers solitary play, and has no interest in peer friendships.

Impaired communication is manifested as no communication, babbling, or in abnormal nonverbal communication (stiffens when held, fixed stare, does not smile). Other manifestations include no imaginative activity such as play acting or fantasy characters; abnormalities in pitch, volume, or intonation of speech; and an inability to initiate or sustain a conversation.

Restricted repertoire of activities and interests are seen in stereotyped body movements such as head banging or spinning objects. The child may be preoccupied with parts of objects, demonstrate marked distress over trivial changes in the environment (moving a vase), or exhibit only one narrow interest (lining up objects).

Specific developmental disorders

Specific developmental disorders are characterized by inadequate development of specific academic, language, speech, and motor skills. All the specific developmental disorders are associated with impairment in academic functioning. Impairment is most marked when language is affected. If the child is not in school, there may be impairment in activities of daily living.

Academic skills disorders are specific areas of development, which include disorders in arithmetic, writing, reading, articulation, language, and coordination. The essential features of each of these disorders include marked impairment in the skill as measured by a standardized, individually administered test. The skills are markedly below the expected level, given the child's schooling and intellectual capacity. The essential features of developmental coordination disorder is a marked impairment in the development of motor coordination that is not due to mental retardation or a physical disorder.

Separation Anxiety Disorders

The essential feature of this disorder is excessive anxiety, for at least 2 weeks, concerning separation from those to whom the child is attached. When separation occurs, the child may experience anxiety to the point of panic. The reaction is beyond the child's developmental level. The onset may be as early as preschool age. The child may demonstrate behaviors such as persistent worry about possible harm to attachment figures, or that a calamity will separate the child from a major attachment figure. He may refuse to go to sleep or go to school for fear of separation. Complaints of physical symptoms are frequently heard such as headaches, stomach aches, nausea, and vomiting.

Tic Disorders

A tic is an involuntary, sudden, rapid, recurrent, non-rhythmical, stereotyped, motor movement or vocalization. Common motor tics include eye blinking, shoulder shrugging, or facial grimacing. Common vocal tics include coughing, throat clearing, or sniffing. Tics can be suppressed for varying periods of time. All tics are exacerbated by stress and decrease during some absorbing activities such as reading or sewing.

Tics are the essential feature of three disorders: chronic motor or vocal tic disorder, transient tic disorder, and Tourette's syndrome. Given the diagnosis of chronic motor or vocal tic disorder, either motor or vocal tics are present but not both. With transient tic disorder, single or multiple motor or vocal tics are present. They may occur many times a day, nearly every day, but for no longer than 12 consecutive months.

The essential feature of Tourette's syndrome is multiple motor or vocal tics. Motor tics typically involve the head, torso, or other limbs and may include touching, squatting, and retracing steps. Vocal tics include various sounds such as clicks, grunts, yelps, barks, coughs, or words. Vocal tics often include uttering obscenities.

Elimination Disorders

The essential feature of enuresis is repeated involuntary or intentional voiding of urine during the day or night in bed or clothes after an age at which continence is expected. The disorder is primary when the disturbance is not preceded by a period of urinary continence lasting for 1 year. The disorder is secondary when the disturbance is preceded by a period of urinary continence lasting for 1 year.

The essential feature of encopresis is repeated involuntary passage of feces in inappropriate places (clothing or floor). At least one such event occurs for at least 6 months. Encopresis is primary if it has not been preceded by a period of fecal continence lasting for 1 year and secondary if it has been preceded by a period of fecal continence lasting for 1 year.

Attention Deficit Hyperactivity Disorder (ADHD)

The essential features of this disorder are developmentally inappropriate degrees of inattention, impulsiveness, and hyperactivity. Children with this disorder generally display some disturbance in each of these areas, but to varying degrees. Manifestations of attention deficit hyperactivity disorder usually appear at home, in school, and in social situations. Symptoms typically worsen in situations requiring sustained attention such as listening to a teacher or completing classroom assignments or chores at home.

Other characteristics of children with ADHD include inability to complete tasks; blurting out answers to questions before they are completed; commenting out of turn; failing to wait one's turn; interrupting others; excessive restlessness, fidgeting, twisting, and wiggling; failing to follow rules of games; and engaging in dangerous activities without considering the consequences. The child may also demonstrate low self-esteem, mood lability, low frustration tolerance, and temper outbursts. The disorder may occur in as many as 3% of the population and is six to nine times more common in boys than girls.

THEORETICAL APPROACHES

Psychoanalytical

Freud's theory of human development emphasized six stages of psychosexual development. Development was seen as a series of crises that result from psychosexual conflicts that had to be resolved before the child could move on to the next stage (see Chapter 4). Although Freud did not treat children, his description of the developmental stages and parent-child relationships provide a useful base for assessing the child's social and emotional development.

The basic tenants of Anna Freud's theory of developmental lines followed Sigmund Freud's psychoanalytical theory, emphasizing that ego defenses available to the child depend on the child's maturation level.[35] Her theory was unique, however, in conceptualizing the role of defense mechanisms in assisting the child's developing personality to adapt and defend against stress and anxiety in the child's environment. Anna Freud adapted psychoanalytical concepts to children's play and fantasy activities to develop a play technique of psychoanalytical treatment of the child.

Klein[51] was one of the first theorists to describe attachment disorders in young children. She called the painful anxiety small children experience when they are first separated from their reassuring mother a "depressive position," which was a normal developmental stage during which the child learned to modify ambivalence and sustain periodic loss of the "good mother." Klein expanded and refined descriptions of *anaclitic depression* set forth by Spitz,[74] which described the failure to thrive and marasmus observed in young children who were prematurely separated from their parents during World War II and placed in orphanages. These theorists described symbiotic reactions as opposed to anaclitic depressions that occurred when children and their parents failed to negotiate the separation-individuation process. Because school attendance is the first enforced separation of mother and child, symbiotic reactions are usually manifested first in school phobias.

Bowlby[12] posited a three-stage "loss" process for children: protest, despair, and detachment. He suggested that when children lose a loved one, their initial feelings are ambivalent. This ambivalence is especially strong if the one lost is a parent or significant other who had disciplined or set limits on the child's behavior, thus angering the child by delaying immediate needs gratification. The stronger the child's ambivalence, the less difficult the loss experience. Negative ambivalent feelings help the child to deny or delay grief through idealization and reaction formation, defense mechanisms that allow the child to resolve guilt aroused by negative (wish fulfillment) feelings. It was believed that if children felt sadness and unhappiness, the feelings were brief and manifested in transient grief behaviors of restlessness and hyperactivity, thought to be signs that the mechanism of reaction formation was being established in the child's emotional structure.

Bowlby believed that trauma or loss during infancy and early childhood create a negative cognitive set that results in a vulnerability or "mental set" so that the child responds in the same negative way when they encounter similar experiences later in life. It is not the loss itself, according to Bowlby, but the lasting impairment to the child's self-system that is a consequence of the loss. The implications for clinical practice of these theoretical positions and research findings are that nurses need to be aware of continuity as well as discontinuity and change in the child's self-concept as the child's cognitive processes mature and include these changes in interactions with the child.

Erikson's theory of child development includes ages and stages based on psychoanalytical theory.[31] He believed that children's play provided the resolution of the conflict or developmental crisis being worked through.

Erikson described the intrinsic psychological reasons children use specific toys and games at various ages. For example, children ages 1 to 3 are in the anal-muscular stage in which developmental tasks focus on resolving conflict that centers around the basic sense of autonomy versus shame and doubt. These children prefer parallel play. Children aged 3 to 6 years old are in the genital-locomotion stage and the developmental tasks center on the basic sense of initiative versus guilt. They enjoy cooperative play, fantasy, and elaborate dramatic scenes and dramas through which they symbolically resolve many conflicts by imitating adults. Children ages 6 to 12 years are in the latency stage in which the developmental task is one of resolving the conflict of a basic sense of industry versus inferiority. These children perfer games governed by complex rules and regulations, such as chess and checkers.

Erikson's developmental theory (see Chapter 4) is based in psychoanalytical concepts and emphasizes that development is a lifelong series of psychosocial crises. At each stage, children encounter a developmental crisis that they must resolve by acquiring a new state of social interaction. Unsuccessful resolution of a psychosocial crisis impedes further development and can have a negative effect on the child's personality. Although his work is psychoanalytically based, Erikson puts more emphasis on socialization and the demands of society than other early developmental theorists. Erikson's work on developmental tasks is viewed as particularly useful in understanding the development of the school-aged child.

Other psychoanalytically oriented life span theorists have built on Erikson's theory. These life span theorists followed the basic assumptions and definitions of life events in describing the stages of the life cycle in an epigenic sequence. These researchers also used Erikson's definition of conflicts, for example, "life crisis," as times that adults or children are confronted by conflicting psychosocial tasks affecting ego development. As each task is mastered, a gain is made that adds a new ego quality and another dimension of personality strength. Recent extrapolations of these findings to child coping and vulnerability studies have resulted in the identification of type A behaviors in elementary school children, and suggestions for life-style changes designed to alter these patterns at an early age have been developed.

Cognitive

Piaget's theory of the development of intellect revolutionized traditional views of child development and established that children think differently from adults and that often children spontaneously learn on their own, without input from adults.[66] He defined development as a process governed by the child's activities that contributed to and resulted in an increasingly complex cognitive structure. Piaget claimed that his six stages were due to the child's intrinsic growth (see Chapter 4). His research verified that the first three stages applied to children of all cultures and changed at the stage of adolescence. It is only then, when the intellect matures to formal operational processes, that thinking is less individualized and influenced more by environmental factors and becomes similar to that of adults.

Piaget viewed the external environment as a source that provided stimulating, interesting, conflicting information, which, in turn, stimulates children's thinking and growth. Stimulation comes from the child's peers during play and conversations, and his theory of the child's growth of social thinking paralleled his theory of cognitive development. His study of moral reasoning verified that young children have a developmental inability to distinguish their perceptions from those of others. Young children cannot intellectually understand that rules, as in games and in life, can be changed until they reach adolescence.

Piaget's cognitive theory asserts that maturation, physical experience, social interaction, equilibration, and an internal self-regulating system combine to influence cognitive development. At different age/stage periods the type of information that can be processed and cognitive operations that can be performed vary. Cognitive development is a coherent, fixed sequence with certain cognitive abilities expected at certain ages. Piaget's theory guides child psychiatric nurses in selecting developmentally appropriate modes of interacting with the child and setting appropriate goals for cognitive development and change in the child. For example, children in the concrete operations stage solve problems using real or observable objects and have difficulty with problems that are hypothetical and entirely verbal. Verbally oriented, abstract counseling interventions would be inappropriate and counterproductive for children in this developmental stage.

Kohlberg[53] expanded Piaget's theory and created a theory of moral development, identifying specific stages of moral development. Kohlberg's theory attributed moral development to schemata within the child's cognitive structure that grows as the child interacts with others and from role taking skills that result from the child's participation in social activities, such as play and games (Table 36-1).

Kohlberg's research focused on the child's development of morality or what children believe would be the morally correct response to various problem situation. He defined moral judgment as an age-bound variable that develops in

▼ **TABLE 36-1**   **Kohlberg's Stages of Moral Development**

Level/Stage		Description
Level 1	Preconventional morality	A concrete level at which limits are set externally.
Stage 1	Punishment and obedience	The motivation is to confirm to those in authority.
Stage 2	Instrumental and hedonistic	Behavior is externally controlled, but the child manipulates the authority figure to fulfill needs.
Level 2	Conventional morality	External control gradually fades.
Stage 3	Good child morality	The child mimics what is perceived as the right thing to do, conforms to elicit approval from others.
Stage 4	Law and order	The child makes moral decisions based on the conventions of society rather than other individuals' approval.
Level 3	Postconventional morality	Morality is defined by principles that have been accepted by the individual.
Stage 5	Social contract and democratically accepted	The rigid adherence to one's own rights and laws becomes flexible and the rights of others are considered.
Stage 6	Morality of universal ethical principles	Morality is based on ideals, concepts, and abstractions.

the same way that cognition emanates. At different ages, children have certain beliefs about their reasons for displaying moral behavior, the values they attach to human life, and reasons they give for conforming to moral standards. Awareness of the stages of moral development provides child psychiatric nurses insights into the behavior of the child, as well as providing content for therapy sessions, and suggests that interventions be conducted at levels commensurate with the child's current moral development level.

Kagan[19] believed that moral development was interrelated with the emergence of a sense of self and contributes to biological maturation of the child; there is a specificity of some neurons that is intensified by exposure and reinforcement, whereas other neurons fade and are extinguished through disuse. Kagan states that between the ages of 18 and 24 months normal children, those with a biologically sound brain, first become aware that they have intentions and feelings and that they can act on them. This insight results from the interaction of the child's maturing brain and the child living in a world of interactions. According to Kagan, no matter how many interactions the child has before the middle of the second year, the sense of self cannot be experienced since the child's brain has not sufficiently matured biologically.

The child's developing sense of self can be observed in a simple rouge test. A dab of rouge is placed on the end of a child's nose and the child is placed in front of a mirror. Children 3 to 10 months of age with rouge on their nose will not reach up and touch their nose when looking at themselves in a mirror. They do not recognize that the face in the mirror is their face. However, by 18 to 20 months of age, children with rouge on their nose will reach up and touch their nose, indicating that their sense of self has matured.

Other behavioral signs of the emergence of a sense of self are the child's use of words as "I," "me," and "mine." Research with deaf children of deaf parents who are learning sign language to communicate make the sign for "I" and touch themselves at the same age/time that children with normal hearing touch their noses in rouge tests. This finding suggests a biologically unfolding time table in the development of a body precept of self.

Kagan's[49] theory holds that the second developmental milestone interrelated to the emergence of a sense of self is the development of a moral sense. When playing, children indicate concern and distress when they find something damaged or flawed, such as a broken toy, or a toy with paint chipped off. The child rejects the toy or object, saying it is "broken," "dirty," or "bad" and becomes upset, usually taking the toy to their mothers or caretakers. Kagan claims this "flawed toy" perception is also maturational, as children 12 to 15 months do not respond this way. The flawed toy response indicates the 18-month-old has a primitive understanding that there is an integrity to objects, and, if this integrity is violated, someone has done something wrong.

The sense of self and the moral sense are two qualities of mind programmed by biology that emerge during development. From this perspective, other qualities shown by the developing child emerge and fall in place. For example, within this cognitive developmental framework, the child of 2 years is not going through a normal period of stubbornness (the "terrible twos"); instead, this is a developmental period during which the child is trying to establish the difference between right and wrong and a time when the relationship between cognition and emotions becomes clear

Thus children cannot show separation or stranger anxiety or fear that their mother will leave them until they are cognitively mature enough to remember the past. Nor can children experience guilt until they are mature enough to recognize that they could have acted differently in a given situation. These newer theories assert that most of the profound emotions and conflicts children experience depend on cognitive maturation. The environment, including parenting, mesh with genes and the maturation of biological programming to sculpt the mind.

Recently, there has been a renewed interest in the "self-system." The central idea in the concept of the self-system is that children develop a set of beliefs about themselves and their environment that are influenced by the interaction of the various self-system qualities, such as self-esteem, self-efficacy, and locus of control. Social comparisons (e.g., how children define themselves in relation to others) are fostered by the reflected appraisals of parents, teachers, and peers. Self-regard is vitally affected by the child's social surroundings and much of childhood socialization through home and primary school education attempts to implant in children standards that may, thereafter, allow them to determine when and in what ways they are "good" or "bad" and when they are correct or right (valued) or incorrect or wrong (devalued). The more intensive the learning of such standards, the less susceptible the child may be to either reflected appraisals or comparisons in immediate situations. Unfortunately, such early learning may also reduce the child's capacity to adapt to new and changing circumstances.

Discrepancies and changes in children's self-concepts across childhood are also areas of concern of child developmentalists, and continuity and discontinuity in children's self-esteem have been the focus of numerous clinical studies and observations. Some experts emphasize the importance of the child's cognitive interpretation of their experiences and changes in these interpretations as the child's cognitive processing abilities mature.

Sociocultural

Social definitions of normality are especially important in child psychiatry because the family and significant others in the child's social environment make the initial referral and bring the child for care. Children are usually unaware that their behaviors are creating problems. This is the result of their immature and limited social perceptions, coupled by their limited verbal abilities due to age and development. Small children also depend on the adults with whom they have ongoing contact to learn social norms and roles.

Families label the child brought in for psychiatric care as the *identified patient* in psychosocial language, inferring that the family or social system has identified this person as the patient.

Labeling theories have been discussed considerably in recent psychiatric literature as the rationale for some clinician's objections to diagnosing (labeling) a child with

DSM-III-R disorders because of the societal stigma attached to psychiatric labels. For example, a child labeled as a juvenile delinquent may continue to carry that label throughout life. Thus many child clinicians have been reluctant to label the developing child with the more severe diagnoses group labels. The child's evolving and emerging developmental changes render the child's personality both fluid and in transition. Adjustment reactions have been the most popular psychiatric diagnoses for children and teenagers.

Bronfenbrenner[14] contends that child theorists need to give greater consideration to the larger social context in which children develop, a position strongly reinforced by their own research observations when studying children of other cultures. These observations have stimulated renewed scientific investigation, resulting in clinical interventions with the child's father, peers, friends, and siblings. This broadening of concerns for the child's social support has paved the way for the renewed regard for the study of the child as an anchor or root of his own social network and as a recipient of social support resources from others.

Children's support systems develop in ways that are congruent with the ecological contexts in which they live. The nature of the child's own social relationships also influences the kinds of opportunities and experiences they will have and the kinds of competence they will develop. There are universally recognized behaviors that children use to signal that help and support are needed or that they are being provided. Providing support and help is characterized by certain behaviors throughout the world, especially regarding children. These behaviors include affection, physical comfort, assistance in problem solving, offering food or other material resources, and protective interventions to prevent aggression or harm. These universal similarities may be due to a shared human capacity for recognizing signals of distress in others and for responding to offers for help. These shared human features for providing support may come from biosocial evolution and common social and functional requirements. Four support functions likely to be found everywhere in the world have been identified: tangible help, positive appraisal, self-esteem enhancement, and a sense of belonging.

Communication

Chomsky[20] developed a theory of language development that was a major scientific contribution to understanding the developing child and the child's ability to verbally communicate. Chomsky found that children learning to speak followed a developmental schedule that follows universal sequences comparable to the cognitive developmental theory of Piaget and that children learn an extensive language system on their own. They pick up language at home, at school, and from TV and then sort the overload of words into grammatical rules and structures to merge as language. There is a biological-maturational predisposition for the development of language and linguistic accomplishments because of an innate language acquisition device (LAD). The LAD helps the child establish rules and regularities in the use of words. Although rudimentary at birth, the LAD matures with the child's central nervous system and children's own activity and play fosters the use of words. Chomsky theorized that the LAD is sufficiently broad to accommodate the diverse languages of the world. Children from all cultures learn language in a standard sequence. Mastery proceeds from one word to two and progresses to working on syntactical rules of inflections, phrases, structures, and negatives in the same manner. Cognitive and linguistic structures have parallel development. The development of speech, thoughts (ideation, cognition), and locomotion (walking) foster the child's development in the emotional and social dimensions; the evolving of a self-concept allows the child to separate from the mother. Balance among these

▼ **TABLE 36-2**   **Summary of Theoretical Approaches**

Theory	Theorist	Dynamics
PSYCHOANALYTICAL	Anna Freud	The defense mechanisms used by the child depend on his maturational level.
	Spitz and Klein	Separation anxiety and anaclitic depression result from the normal negotiation of the separation-individuation process.
	Bowlby	Children generally experience ambivalent feelings on initial loss of a loved one.
	Erikson	There are intrinsic reasons why children use specific toys and games at various ages; children's play provides for the resolution of conflict and developmental crises.
COGNITIVE	Piaget	The process of development is governed by the child's activities and results in increasingly complex congitive structures.
	Kohlberg	Moral development proceeds in specific stages.
	Kagan	Moral development is interrelated with the emerging sense of self and contributes to the biological maturation of the child.
	Harter	Self-concept is influenced by self-esteem, self-efficacy, and locus of control.
SOCIOCULTURAL		
Labeling		Because of stigma, the child's evolving and emerging development precludes a diagnostic label.
Invulnerability		There is a shift from disease entities to a focus on healthy psychosocial capacities.
	Bronfenbrenner	Great concern is given to the larger societal context in which children develop.
COMMUNICATION	Chomsky	There is a biological-maturational predisposition for the development of language that occurs because of an innate LAD.

developmental lines is essential for mental health, and a lag in any of these interdependent systems can result in serious mental health problems.

Mastery of language is a major developmental task of childhood that emerges gradually. Most children express their needs primitively and nonverbally through the use of primary process and play, symbolic expressive activities, and games.

As children gain mastery in moving about independently, they begin to learn to control their emotions; perceptions, memory, and mobility combine to help distinguish self from the object world. First, children verbalize perceptions by naming or labeling, and gradually verbalize feelings or emotions. Naming objects and feelings reinforces the child's emerging sense of control of feelings. It helps the child distinguish what is real, providing a vehicle for testing reality by verbally validating names of objects and feelings with others. The development of language facilitates the process of reality testing, is basic to self-identity and differentiation, and spans all dimensions of the developing child.

Theoretical approaches are summarized in Table 36-2.

NURSING PROCESS

Assessment

Assessment includes evaluation of the child's total situation, the nature of the disorder being evaluated, and sources of information. The "four pillars of child assess-

ment" are structured interviews, observations, informal assessment and norm-referenced psychological tests.[72] Assessment consists of three segments: initial discussions with the child, parents and siblings, or adult(s) responsible for the child; an individual interview session with parents; and the mental status examination (MSE) of the child.

The most frequent reasons to refer children for mental health services are the following:

1. A family crisis, with accompanying changes in the child's capacity to cope, attend school, maintain peer relationships, learn, and play.
2. An acute physical illness, with concomitant depression, overactivity, and hyperactivity as manifestations of denial of illness.
3. Chronic physical illness, with the child showing gradual loss of adaptive functions, increased family conflicts, and a risk of family dissolution. The effects of repeated hospitalizations on parents is described in the research highlight below.
4. Depression in children.
5. General acute changes in the child's thinking, behavior and/or expressions of feelings, such as suicidal and/or acute rages and/or withdrawal in younger children, often with concurrent loss of speech.

Physical dimension The child's age is important because of the developmental changes that occur with time. However, development is the outcome of intrinsic and extrinsic factors, and the child's capacity for continued progress from one age/stage to the next is often as impor-

---

RESEARCH HIGHLIGHT

Hazardous Secrets and Reluctantly Taking Charge: Parenting a Child with Repeated Hospitalizations

• E Burke, E Kauffmann, E Costello, and M Dillon

PURPOSE

The purpose of this study was to gain an understanding of the stressful process for parents involved in repeated hospitalizations of children with chronic conditions.

SAMPLE

Theoretical sampling spanned 4 years and included a series of five groups of mothers and children. Each subject was selected to be representative of those who could answer the study question, "What is the nature of the stressful process surrounding the repeated hospitalization of a chronically ill child?"

METHODOLOGY

Grounded theory methods were used to describe the process. Group 1a, 30 mothers of disabled children, were interviewed twice in their homes and administered the Visual Life Events Schedule (VLES). Responses were contrasted with 30 sociodemographically matched mothers with healthy nondisabled children (Group 1b). Two theoretical samples were chosen to follow up the findings from the Group 1a and 1b mothers. Perceptions from both

From *Image: Journal of Nursing Scholarship* 23(1):39, 1991.

groups regarding the nature of parental stress were noted and presented to a group of 100 other parents of chronically ill children and to six nurses who cared for the children. Data were content analyzed and a general list of parental stressors categorized.

FINDINGS

Results indicated dominant patterns of stress: for parents, reluctantly taking charge; for the child, hazardous secrets. Hazardous secrets include negative information, gaps or omissions in information, and inexperienced health care workers performing invasive procedures. Reluctantly taking charge is the parents' response to the hazardous secrets and includes taking over, calling a halt, or tenaciously seeking help.

IMPLICATIONS

Hazardous secrets and reluctantly taking charge describe a process in which stressors and parental reactions are identified. Nurses can work to understand and support parental reactions or develop interventions with parents of repeatedly hospitalized children with chronic conditions.

tant as the child fitting within the age/stage framework. A child's physical developmental patterns may differ from the norms of other children in that age range but be consistent with familial patterns. For example, very short or very tall children may vary from the average, yet be "normal" for their family/genetic trait.

The motor activity and coordination component of the child's mental status assessment are related to observations suggesting hyperactivity. This behavior lacks clear-cut baseline normative data. It has not been established "how much" activity is excessive. Hyperactivity is attributed to environmental factors; developmental lag; and psychological, organic, or biological deficits. Conditional hyperactivity is due to factors in the external environment; development hyperactivity is due to maturation delays in functioning of the central nervous system; psychological hyperactivity is due to anxiety and/or faulty ego development and lack of impulse control; and organic hyperactivity is due to abnormalities in brain structure, function and/or biochemical processes. Thorough neurological examination provides the baseline data in these four areas of neurological/motor functioning. Because of the important relationship between neurological and both emotional and intellectual development, the neurological examination is an important part of assessment of the child. Play assessment is a useful way to gather neurological data because it includes play activities that most children know. These play adaptations of the neurological examination are less threatening and especially useful with children who are overly active, distractible, impulsive, and excitable. The following play activities are suggested in assessing the child's behavior.

1. *Cerebral functions.* Games such as hide-and-seek, Simon Says, Blindman's Bluff, and naming games can be adapted to assess specific areas of cerebral functioning. Hide-and-seek can be used to assess the child's *stereogenesis* by having the child identify objects with eyes closed. Simon Says is a useful game for assessing the child's temporal sequence because it requires following a series of commands.
2. *Reflexes.* Games such as Let's Take Turns and You Play Nurse help eliminate the child's fear of reflex hammers and other instruments used in a physical examination.
3. *Cerebellar functions.* Games such as Follow the Leader and Pin the Tail on the Donkey can be adapted to evaluate the child's coordination and balance. The child's ability to hop or stand on one foot, rapidly touch various body parts, and balance with his eyes closed contributes to this evaluation.
4. *Sensory functions.* Body tapping and tickling games before the assessment of the child's responses to touch, pain, vibration, and temperature may alleviate this sensitive aspect of assessment that involves body contact. It is suggested that this part of the neurological examination be left to the final assessment because children often become uncooperative, which may affect the ability to gather other data.
5. *Cranial nerves.* Following lights, whispering games, and playing dentist assist in assessing the child's visual acuity; visual fields; movement of eyeballs and jaws; sensations of taste; corneal reflexes; hearing; movement of the mouth, throat, and tongue; facial expressions; and sensations in the forehead, jaw, and cheeks.

The normal, expected findings in the neurological-perceptual examination of a 5- to 6-year-old child follow:

1. *Alternating movements.* The child can turn hands over rapidly or tap thumb and index finger.
2. *Associated movements.* When wooden sticks are placed between the fingers of each hand, the child will not drop more than five extra sticks in six trials.
3. *Eye-hand coordination.* When the peripheral visual field is stimulated by a moving finger, the child can point to the moving finger without looking from side to side.
4. *Eye movements.* The child can visually pursue an object without head movement.
5. *Choreoid movements.* When arms are extended and eyes closed, no choreiform movements are noted.
6. *Copying ability.* The child can copy a circle, cross, square, and triangle.
7. *Perceptual reversals.* When asked to copy the letters *B, P, D, Q,* or other letters, the child reproduces the letters without reversals, inversions, rotations, or mirror images.

Tomographical techniques are just beginning to be used for diagnostic clarification with children. Two main areas of brain imaging techniques are being developed. The first area focuses on brain anatomy and uses computerized tomography (CT) and magnetic resonance imaging (MRI). The second area focuses on the different brain functions: blood flow, metabolism, receptor status using positron emission tomography (PET), single photon emission computerized tomography (SPECT), and electrophysiology using computerized electroencephalography (CEEG). Brain imaging techniques examine the brain in different ways, and although additional studies are needed for conclusive statements, research evidence has challenged traditional theories of hyperactivity. Organic brain changes have been found in children and adolescents with obsessive-compulsive disorders contributing to more accurate diagnostic and treatment decisions. Similar brain structure and function abnormalities found support for biological explanations of dyslexia and learning disabilities in some children and adolescents. Differences in the brain structure and functioning have indicated a number of childhood disorders, such as autism, Gillesdela Tourette's syndrome, depression, and schizophrenia.

The child's body image is also assessed. The body schema begins at birth and unfolds through the maturing child's gradual differentiation of self. The progressive inclusion of body imagery in the child's mind can be measured by children's drawings. A specific measurement, the Goodenough-Harris Draw-A-Person (DAP) test, is based on the premise that a child's drawings are related to his developmental age. Norms for children's drawings have been established, and the child's neurological integrity, psychomotor skills, and graphomotor and fine motor development can be assessed through the DAP test. Figure 36-1 illustrates the progressive complexity of children's drawings. The mandala in children's art is of interest because it is a universal religious symbol spontaneously drawn by most children.

Emotional dimension The emotions of fear, anxiety, anger, guilt, hope, hopelessness, and depression, vary during childhood; and there are age appropriate expressions of these emotions for the developing child. Although childhood fears theoretically are related to cognitive-

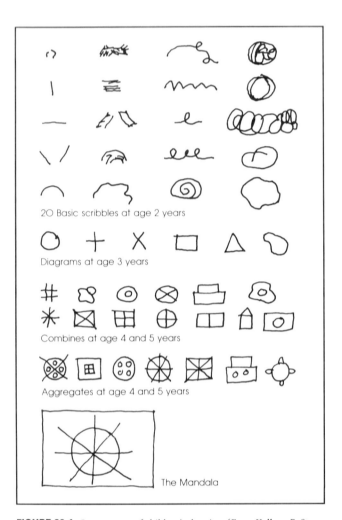

20 Basic scribbles at age 2 years

Diagrams at age 3 years

Combines at age 4 and 5 years

Aggregates at age 4 and 5 years

The Mandala

FIGURE 36-1 Components of children's drawing. (From Kellogg R: Stages of development of preschool art. In Lewis HP, editor: *Child art: the beginning of self-affirmation*, Berkeley, Calif, 1966, Diablo Press.)

perceptual development and anxieties to the emotional dimension, they are reviewed together here.

Children's fears become more realistic, varied, and global as the child matures. Normal fears of children 2 to 7 years of age include fear of falling and fear of animals, such as dogs, snakes, or tigers. Children aged 7 to 11 fear bodily injury, punishment, illness, death of parent, and failure in social situations, such as at school. Between the ages of 11 and 12, children express more global fears such as natural hazards, accidents, and nuclear explosions.

Many children have bedtime fears that are often related to fears of dreaming and being alone in the dark. Research on rapid eye movement (REM) sleep has led to a reevaluation of Freud's notion that repression is required for dreaming. It appears that infants and small children experience some form of dream activity that is different from the REM (dream) activity experienced by children who can use symbols for recall.

Because small children are unable to discern between dreams and reality, "night terrors" often occur in children under 5 years of age. Children's dreams are a product of interactions during development and thus their content contains the most pressing tasks that the child is experiencing at different developmental stages. Dreams play an important role in the child's development of language, cognition, and management of emotions.[67]

There are important distinctions between normal dreaming, daydreaming, fantasy, and the serious psychiatric disorders related to lack of contact with reality and reality orientation. Daydreams and fantasy are similar to the concepts of delusions, hallucinations, and loss of contact with reality; and the similarity in these behaviors concern parents. Many parents become distressed about their child's dreams, daydreaming, and fantasizing and consider them unacceptable, nonproductive activities. There is a great misunderstanding about the place of fantasy as in the small child's life. The nurse needs to clarify the place of fantasy for overanxious parents. Most children use fantasy, play, dreams, and daydreams to strengthen their contacts with the real world and reduce stress and anxiety. In contrast, emotionally disturbed children and children with physical illnesses do not use play to reduce their stress and anxieties. Usually the child's lack of play is the first sign parents perceive and report to clarify that "something is wrong" with the child. Conversely, parents usually report the child is improving when he or she resumes usual play behaviors.

Anxiety due to change seems to be a necessary component of growth, and most children negotiate developmental stage changes with a minimum of fear, anxiety, and crisis. The major sources of childhood anxiety have been identified, and knowledge of these characteristic behaviors provides nurses areas on which to focus for assessment, such as unstructured play sessions that identify anxieties and fears. In the preschool-aged child sources of anxiety are related to loss of parental love, evolving to anticipation of physical injury; loss of control; and expressions of dependency, aggression, and anger as the child develops independence. In the school-aged child, major sources of anxiety are related to concerns for failing to master socially valued skills, such as an inability to succeed in the classroom and failure to demonstrate accepted sex role behaviors.

Hospitalization for physical problems is a major source of both fear and anxiety during childhood. The major fears during early childhood are exaggerated when the child is vulnerable and physically in pain. In addition to observations, nurses use various projective picture tests that depict specific hospital situations and mutual story telling techniques to assess the child's anxiety. These story telling games include the nurse reading picture books and other illustrated child reading materials and "imagining" a story in response to these stimuli. Barton's Hospital Picture Test, widely used in pediatric settings, assists the nurse in identifying misperceptions as well as anxiety in younger hospitalized clients.

Depression is often masked by acting out behaviors, poor school performance, inability to study, isolation, somatic complaints, and proneness to accident. The potential of suicide and suicide attempts by children are generally underestimated. Parents tend to deny their child's sad or depressed feelings. Depressed children often have low self-esteem and feelings of helplessness with resulting angry feelings toward parents or authority figures. The child may feel rejected and act out angry feelings toward the parents, who in turn become angry with the child, setting up a destructive cycle that may include child abuse. The cycle intensifies as parents become more determined to "straighten the child out" when their authority is challenged.

Temper tantrums are violent, unpredictable outbursts of anger during which the child is out of control and screams, kicks, and strikes out at others. Children often throw things and may lose bladder and bowel control. These violent outbursts have been related to power struggles between children and parents or significant others, such as teachers or caretakers.

Children with antisocial behaviors often lack the necessary ego strength to control overt expressions of anger and aggressive impulses. Impulsivity and hyperactivity can also be related to minimal brain damage when impulses are acted out. Deficits or limitations in language create situations for the child in which words fail and action seems the only resource. As the child develops language skills, there is a decline in the hitting, shoving, and pushing of other children.

Expressions of anger and aggression in children also differ from those of adults. Through socialization children are expected to master impulse control and learn to delay gratification (Figure 36-2). Parental discipline provides external controls that the child gradually internalizes. As discussed earlier, small children are egocentric and tend to blame themselves for unpleasant happenings; thus they often have strong, unrealistic feelings of guilt and shame when they express their anger.

◥ **Intellectual dimension** An assessment of the child's use of language provides initial information about the child's development. At the age of 18 months the child uses and understands a limited number of single-word utterances which are rooted in action, such as "run," "walk," and "give," and the child's first verbal activity is an extension of the sensorimotor structure.[67] By the age of 2 years the child begins to put two words together to express relationships. The two-word association phase is a universal characteristic of all human language development.

Between the ages of 2 and 3 years children begin using words in subject-verb-object order. In addition to adding the suffix *-ing* to words, children learn to use "no." Between 3 and 6 years of age children begin to use "where, what, and why" questions and tags, which are little questions at the end of a sentence, such as "isn't it—can't we—doesn't it." Tags result from complex transformation operations originating in the child's tendency to solidify new capacities by overuse.

Between 5 and 7 years children master verbal intricacies as operational thought evolves. As logical links are grasped in the manipulation of the external world, the thought processes include more than "surface" phenomena. Despite a growing command of grammar, words acquire meaning only in concrete life situations. Separation of speech from action does not occur in children until the ages of 11 to 13 years, when the human brain reaches physical maturation. At that time the neuroanatomical and neurophysiological framework necessary for hypothetical and deductive thinking replaces pragmatic "here and now" thinking. When the stage of formal thinking is achieved, children express thoughts independently of immediate experience and initiate language about past, present, and future events. Language becomes abstract and implements thought.

The Mental Status Examination (MSE) provides essential information about the child's growth and development. The

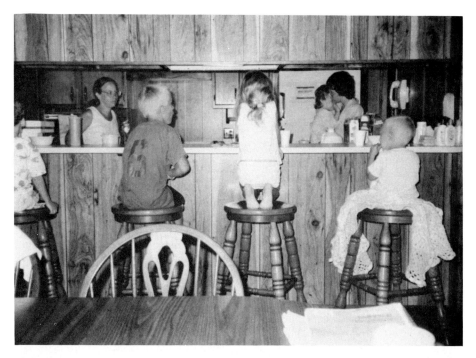

FIGURE 36-2 These children are enjoying social interactions while learning acceptable mealtime behaviors.

child's MSE is arrived at indirectly by observations of non-verbal behaviors. The MSE format organizes initial assessment data and usually covers the following areas:

1. Overall demeanor, attitude, orientation
2. Motor activity and coordination
3. Cognition: alertness, attention span, intelligence, ability to communicate
4. Emotions: mood, anxiety, anger, other feelings
5. Language: speech, formal characteristics of vocabulary, grammar, usage
6. Thoughts: associations, preoccupations, dreams, fantasies, wishes; richness or poverty of ideation, talent, hallucinations, delusions
7. Social interaction: eye contact, openness, shyness, cooperation, aggression
8. A brief statement of the reactions of the examiner to the child
9. Summary and diagnostic impression

A number of psychological tests are available to evaluate children whose assessment suggests the presence of more complex psychological situations, as when psychosis, suicide, loss of control, or aggressive acting out is suspected. Most psychological tests are norm referenced; that is, psychologists have identified norms of response for various ages and diagnostic groups. Most psychological tests require clinical psychologists to administer and interpret results. Nurses, however, need to be familiar with the tests generally used with children, the behaviors they measure, and the normal expectations. Some of the most widely used tests are listed in Table 36-3.

Social dimension The child's temperamental disposition, present at birth, provides a context for eliciting parents overall descriptions of child's developmental milestones. However, children's temperaments do not "fit" or follow norms or averages of other children at the same developmental level and are not age-stage specific. Temperament is defined as how the child behaves, in contrast to developmental theories that seek to explain why children behave in a certain way.[77]

The child's temperament is not related to the parents' temperament and disposition and is not biologically determined. Temperament is the child's unique, individual style of approaching people and situations that develops after birth and becomes a basic component of the child's personality. Temperament produces different social response styles that influence the child's developmental patterns, attachment behaviors, and development of psychopathology.[30]

Bender explains the application of the concept of temperament as representing a variety of predictable behavioral responses to various changes in the environment and a tendency to respond in a particular way. As noted earlier, some children respond to failure by "trying" harder, whereas other children "give up" and avoid trying again. A number of interacting aspects in task mastery have been attributed, in part, to the child's innate temperamental disposition, for example, the way the child characteristically behaves when approaching a task or a life experience. These aspects include the child's cognitive appraisal of the task or experience, the child's mental reaction to the appraisal, and the child's action, or how he deals with tasks and situations.[71]

Temperament issues are often prominent in the child's behavioral difficulties that cause parents to bring the child to the attention of the mental health worker. The "goodness of fit" between the child's and parent's temperaments is an important area to be evaluated and explored as possible sources or contributing factors to the child's presenting problem.

Chess, Thomas, and Hertzig[19] identified nine temperamental categories of a child's constitutional-temperamental endowment by age and stage. These categories are summarized in a checklist format in Table 36-4. The checklist is useful to collect assessment data from the parents and to use later during the clinical evaluation of the child's mental status and can be used as a diagnostic tracking format for identifying changes in temperamental qualities over the child's early age periods. For example, parents may

---

▼ **TABLE 36-3** **Psychological Tests for Children**

Type of Test	Name	Measures
Intelligence tests	Wechsler Intelligence Scale for Children	Measures intelligence
Personality/Projective tests	Thematic Apperception Test	Assesses child's psychological needs; self-esteem, defense mechanisms, coping skills
	Symonds Picture Test	
	Rorschach Test	Gives information about relationships, reality testing, imagination
	Incomplete sentences	Assesses stressors, coping skills, defenses
Personality inventories	Personality Inventory for Children	Measures personality traits
Psychiatric diagnoses	Diagnostic Interview Scale for Children	Provides diagnostic information
	Children's Version of the Schedule for Affective Disorders and Schizophrenia	
	Children's Depression Inventory Anxiety Scale	
Social adjustment	Vineland Social Maturity Scale	Measures social adjustment and maturity
	Children's Global Assessment Scale	Provides adaptive ratings
Developmental retardation	Denver Developmental Screening	To determine severity of developmental lag

▼ **TABLE 36-4** Temperamental Categories, Definitions, Assessment Questions, and Typical Parental Descriptions

Category	Definition
1. Activity level	The motor component of the child's functioning and diurnal proportion of active and inactive periods: motility during bathing, eating, playing, dressing, handling. Sleep-wake cycle, reaching, crawling and walking. Examples: *Infancy.* Parental statements and direct observations illustrating high activity levels, "Moves a great deal during sleep; kicks wildly during bath. Low activity illustrations: "Sleeps in same position; can turn over, but doesn't do it very much." *Toddler.* Parents reports of high activity, "Runs wildly when friends around. Low activity descriptions, "Prefers to sit quietly drawing or looking at a picture book." *Middle childhood.* Parent's high activity statements, "When comes home from school, outside immediately playing active games; when inside, constantly doing acrobatics, perpetually in motion." Low activity descriptions, "Gets involved in jigsaw puzzles, sits quietly working for hours."
2. Rhythmicity	Predictable and/or unpredictable regularity in time, analyzed by sleep-wake cycle, hunger, feeding, eating, and elimination patterns. *Infancy.* Regular pattern reports: "Nap time never changes, no matter where we are." Irregular pattern report: "Wouldn't know how to start toilet training, as his bowel movements come anytime, 1 to 3 times a day." *Toddler.* Parents reporting high rhythmicity, "Big meal at lunch, otherwise, just picks." Low rhythmicity descriptions, "Falls asleep right after dinner, or up until midnight." *Middle childhood.* Parent's high regularity statements, "Wakes up like clockwork at 6 every morning." Low regularity descriptions, "Continues to do homework until finished, never gets sleepy at the same time."
3. Approach/Withdrawal	Nature of initial responses, way child responds to new stimuli: toy, food, persons. Approach responses positive with smiling, reaching for, etc.; withdrawal reactions negative: crying, or motor activities: pushing away. *Infancy.* Parent high approach descriptions, "Smiles at strangers; loves new foods, new toys." High withdrawal descriptions, "Ignores new toys, spits out new foods." *Toddler.* High approach descriptions, "Plunges right in new group or activity." High withdrawal, "Remains outside of group and won't participate or talk to others for weeks." *Middle childhood.* Parent's high approach statements, "Came home from new school excited, knew everyone by name." High withdrawal, "When starting new school subject, gets all confused and upset."
4. Adaptability	Responses to new or altered situations, ease of modifying or altering directions. *Infancy.* Parent's statements and observations of high adaptability, "First rejects things, but in a few days, enjoys them." Low adaptability, "Every time I put on new clothes she screams, goes on for months." *Toddler.* Parent's reports of high adaptability, "When she got her new tricycle, she couldn't ride it, called it stupid. Then, practiced and mastered it, uses it all the time." Low adaptability descriptions, "Took all fall for him to contentedly go to nursery school and each time gets sick and is out for a few days, reluctant to go again." *Middle childhood.* High adaptability descriptions, "Attended tennis camp last summer, adjusted to new schedule and got involved the first week." Low adaptability descriptions, "Started new school with different teaching style; after 3 months, still gets confused."
5. Threshold of responsiveness	Intensity level of stimulation needed to evoke a discernible response, irrespective of form response takes or sensory modality affected. Reactions to sensory stimuli, environmental conditions and objects, and social contacts. *Infancy.* Parental descriptions of low threshold, "If a door closes, he's startled; he loves fruits, but add cereal and he refuses it." High threshold statements, "Can get a bump on his head and won't cry or stop what he was doing." "Can't tell if soiled by his actions, so have to check." *Toddler.* Parent's low threshold reports, "Will only eat eggs if they are fixed the same way." High threshold descriptions, "Won't complain of being cold, even though shivering and lips are blue" or "comfortable in any kind of clothes." *Middle childhood.* Parent's low threshold statements, "First one to notice an odor or changes in room temperature." High threshold descriptions, "Didn't notice blister on heel while playing ball," or "lights went out one evening, she didn't notice and kept on working."

Modified from Chess S, Thomas A: *Temperament in clinical practice,* New York, 1986, Guilford Press.

▼ **TABLE 36-4**   Temperamental Categories, Definitions, Assessment Questions, and Typical Parental Descriptions—cont'd

Category	Definition
6. Intensity of reaction	Energy of responses, irrespective of quality or direction. *Infancy.* Parental observations of high intensity, "When hungry, screams; if hears music, loud laughter and bounces in time to it." Low intensity descriptions, "Had ear infection and didn't notice it," or "ignores loud noises." *Toddler.* Parent's reports of high intensity, "Screams when can't complete a task." Low intensity, "If another child takes his toy, he grabs it back, but doesn't cry." *Middle childhood.* Parent's observations of high intensity: "Called a poor loser, he yells opponents cheated, throws things in anger." Low intensity, "I knew he was upset to fail the test, but he was deadpan about it."
7. Quality of mood	Amount of pleasant, friendly behavior, contrasted with unpleasant, unfriendly behaviors, as crying. Examples: *Infancy.* Parental statements and direct observations of negative mood, "When sees something he doesn't like, whines and fusses until its taken away," or "Cries when put to sleep for 5 to 10 minutes." Positive mood descriptions include, "If he isn't smiling, I know he's getting sick." *Toddler.* Parent's descriptions of negative mood, "Usually comes home from nursery school full of complaints." Positive mood descriptions, "When got new shoes, ran around with joy, showing everyone," or "It's a pleasure to take him to the grocery store, he's so pleasant and happy." *Middle childhood.* Parent's negative mood descriptions, "Only back in school a week, already has a list of grievances against the teacher." Positive descriptions, "Doesn't object to helping around the house, takes the garbage out willingly, does whatever asked pleasantly."
8. Distractibility	Effectiveness of extraneous environmental stimuli altering the direction of the child's ongoing behaviors. Examples: *Infancy.* Parental statements and direct observations of high distractibility, "If someone passes while she is nursing, she looks and stops sucking until the person is gone." Low distractibility: "She can't be sidetracked, keeps on doing something until it's mastered," or "When hungry and has to wait, can't get him involved in play; keeps crying until fed." *Toddler.* High distractibility, "Not a nagger; if she sees something she wants, she will ask, then accept a substitute," or "His room is strewn with toys; he scarcely begins one game when his attention is caught by something else and he forgets to put things away." Examples of low distractibility: "He got new blocks and wouldn't leave them even to play with a friend," or "If it's raining and she wants to go outside and play, she will fuss and not accept any substitute." *Middle childhood.* Parent's descriptions of high distractibility, "His homework takes so long because his attention is constantly sidetracked," or "She is constantly losing something, as she gets involved with something else and forgets it." Low distractibility shown by descriptions as, "If friends ask him to play when he's making a model airplane, they can't get him away," or "Once she starts to read, we can't get her to stop until she's finished a chapter."
9. Attention span and persistence	Includes two categories: the length of time a particular activity is pursued and persistence, the continuation of an activity in face of obstacles to maintenance of the activity direction. *Infancy.* Parental statements of high persistence, "Despite all our efforts to distract him, he returns to his task of poking in the electric outlet." Long attention span descriptions include, "If I give her a book, she will tear up paper for as long as an hour. Statements showing low persistence include, "If the bead doesn't go on the string immediately, she stops playing with it." Short attention span descriptions are, "While she loves her doll, she only plays with it for a few minutes." *Toddler.* Parental statements of high persistence, "If pushing a toy around and it gets stuck in the furniture, he yells until it moves or someone comes to help him; he doesn't give up." Long attention span descriptions include, "She can be engrossed in playing for almost an hour." Low persistence and low attention span descriptions examples are, "She asked to be taught to do something, but loses interest after the first try." *Middle childhood.* Parental statements of high persistence and a long attention span include, "She couldn't understand her homework at first, but stubbornly kept at it until she mastered it, even though it took several hours." Short attention span, with high persistence is illustrated by, "She wouldn't give up until she learned her part, but would work at it for about 15 minutes at a time. Statements indicating short attention span, but low persistence, are, "He decided to learn how to skate, after 5 minutes, gave up."

report changes in motor activity levels and adaptability after infancy when describing a child in the middle childhood years. Experts in this area claim that "what IQ has been to the understanding of cognition, temperament has become in the comprehension of personality development."[19]

Collecting data from parents provides opportunities to assess the parent-child relationship and the parents' strengths and limitations. The parents' child-rearing behaviors are carefully evaluated as they affect the child's trust and dependence-independence needs. Information about the child's peer relationships, caretakers, and school activities is also assessed.

Assessment of the child's parents begins with the initial interview, a structured process during which roles, confidentiality, and rationale for family and individual interviews are clarified. The reasons for the visit (for instance, clarification of the problem, duration of symptoms, the parents' perceptions of the problem, their concerns and efforts to solve the problem) are initial topics. If the child is referred by a teacher or physician, the reason for the referral needs clarification. It is important to identify how the parents and others, such as teachers, may want the child to change and what role parents see for themselves in the change process.

Information about the child's family constellation is best gathered by developing a genogram. Genograms facilitate the establishment of the therapeutic relationship, may take several sessions to complete, and provide the parents with a concrete exercise that alleviates initial anxiety. By viewing themselves and their child within a broad intergenerational context, parents often feel less guilty and will more readily discuss their relationships.

During the data collection the nurse observes and records both content and process. Process includes behaviors such as seating arrangements, verbal and nonverbal patterns of communication, and who speaks and when. Verbal themes, such as assuming responsibility for others' behavior, are noted and clarified during the interview.

Family and social considerations in assessing the child have become increasingly important in recent years because the major mental health problems now confronting children are psychosocial. The effects of social change on the child and assessment of the changes represent a small segment of the many aspects of social changes affecting the child that the nurse assesses and integrates into the data analysis and treatment plan.

The life event scales developed by Coddington provide systematic assessment tools for evaluating the amount of stress the child is experiencing as a result of social factors. The life event scales presented in Table 36-5 provide ranges of expectations for normal children. If the child is not progressing normally for his age the reaction is referred to as a *developmental crisis.*

The kinds of social changes children experience and the amount of stress that these changes cause in children are assigned life change units (LCUs). The standardized data on healthy children indicate that life stress increases with age; children in elementary school average 102.8 LCUs, and children in junior high school average 195.6 LCUs.[22] Also, as the assigned life change numerical values show, stress levels differ for children at different ages. For the preschooler the death of a parent has been assigned a weight of 89 LCUs, whereas the death of a parent of children ages

6 to 11 years has a higher life change value (109 LCUs).

The revised scale for children ages 6 to 11 years reflects changes in society since the life event scales were first developed. For example, on the 1972 life event scales a child becoming involved with drugs was assigned a weight of 38 LCUs; in 1983 stopping use of drugs was a new item and was assigned 23 LCUs. When the scale was developed most children ages 6 to 23 years did not have experiences of initiating and withdrawing from drug use. It is important that the nurse use the most recently available, updated editions of the life event scales because societal changes are reflected in the items. For example, the recession during the early 1980s and consequent parental unemployment affected children's stress and life change units.

Recently, efforts have been made to examine stressful events from the child's perspective rather than from the adult's.

Because more of the child's time is spent in daycare centers and schools, assessments by the teacher or care provider are extremely important for a comprehensive data base of the child's social behaviors. Many problems during childhood, such as drug abuse, result in the child exhibiting some signs and symptoms at home and other symptoms in school or other social contexts.

Spiritual dimension Moral development is one of the major tasks of the school-age child and includes development of the child's percepts of right and wrong, responsibilities in relation to others, and ability to understand the feelings of others. These data can be gained by assessing how the child relates to peers and adults.

Role taking, in Kohlberg's theory, refers to understanding what situations mean to another person.[53] Interpersonal perception includes the development of concepts of norms, social responsibility, and justice. As discussed earlier, there is a close relationship between intellectual and moral development. Children's verbalizations and actions, as well as teacher's and parents' reports of the child's social roles, provide guides to the child's level of moral development. Children who are socially popular and "leaders" generally have well-developed moral reasoning. Observation of the child playing with peers also provides data on the child's interpersonal awareness.

There are other opportunities for assessing the child's level of moral development in the nurse-child encounters. For example, as the assessment session begins the nurse carefully states the "rules" for behavior and confidetiality during the child-nurse relationship. School-aged children will usually request rules if they are not volunteered, indicating their reliance on rules and structured situations.

The holistic assessment tool in the box on p. 732 contains assessment information specific to the child. It is to be used in conjunction with the assessment tool in Chapter 8.

See Table 36-6 for assessment norms for children.

Analysis
Nursing diagnosis

The following list provides examples of NANDA-accepted diagnoses with causative statements:
1. Self-esteem disturbance related to disturbed relationships with peers

▼ **TABLE 36-5   Life Event Scale**

Life Event	Life Change Units	Life Event	Life Change Units
PRESCHOOL AGE*		**AGES 6 THROUGH 11***	
Beginning nursery school	42	Death of parent	109
Increase in number of arguments with parents	39	Death of brother or sister	86
		Divorce of parents	73
Change in parents' financial status	21	Marital separation of parents	66
Birth of brother or sister	50	Death of grandparent	56
Decrease in number of arguments between parents	21	Hospitalization of parent	52
		Marriage of parent to stepparent	53
Change of father's occupation requiring increased absence from home	39	Birth of brother or sister	50
		Hospitalization of brother or sister	47
Death of grandparent	30	Loss of job by parent	37
Outstanding personal achievement	23	Major increase in parents' income	28
Serious illness requiring hospitalization of parent	51	Major decrease in parents' income	29
		Start of new problem between parents	44
Brother or sister leaving home	39	End of problem between parents	27
Serious illness requiring hospitalization of brother or sister	37	Change of father's occupation requiring increased absence from home	39
Mother beginning to work outside home	47	New adult moving into home	41
		Mother beginning to work outside home	40
Change to new nursery school	33		
Change in child's acceptance by peers	38	Being told you are very attractive by friend	23
Decrease in number of arguments with parents	22	Beginning first grade	20
Increase in number of arguments between parents	44	Move to new school district	35
		Failing a grade in school	45
Serious illness requiring hospitalization of child	59	Suspension from school	30
		Start of new problem between you and your parents	43
Loss of job by parent	23	End of a problem between you and parents	34
Death of close friend	38		
Having visible congenital deformity	39	Recognition for excelling in sport or other activity	21
Addition of third adult to family	39		
Marital separation of parents	74	Appearance in juvenile court	33
Discovery of being adopted child	33	Failing to achieve something you really wanted	28
Jail sentence of parent for 30 days or less	34		
		Becoming adult member of church	21
Death of parent	89	Being invited to join social organization	15
Divorce of parents	78	Death of pet	40
Acquiring visible deformity	52	Being hospitalized for illness or injury	53
Death of brother or sister	59	Death of close friend	52
Marriage of parent to stepparent	62	Becoming involved with drugs	38
Jail sentence of parent for 1 year or more	67	Stopping use of drugs	23
		Finding an adult who really respects you	20
		Outstanding personal achievement (special prize)	34

From Coddington RD: The significance of life events as etiological factors in the diseases of children: a study of normal populations, *Journal of Psychosomatic Research* 16:205, 1972.
*The purpose of this form is to record events that occurred in the child's life during a 3-month period.

2. Sleep pattern disturbance related to anxiety over separation from parents
3. Impaired social interaction related to impulsive behavior
4. Dysfunctional grieving related to loss of sibling
5. Impaired adjustment related to academic problems
6. Altered growth and development related to chronic illness

Altered growth and development is a NANDA-approved nursing diagnosis that applies to the child. The defining characteristics are listed in the box at the bottom of p. 732 and described in the case example, which is also found on p. 732.

Planning

The nursing care plan (Table 36-8) provides long- and short-term goals, outcome criteria, interventions, and rationales related to childhood, which are examples of the planning stage of the nursing process.

▼
HOLISTIC ASSESSMENT TOOL: THE CHILD

Physical Dimension
Diet and elimination

Are the child's food preferences, eating patterns, and elimination patterns appropriate for his age group?

Exercise and activity

Are the child's play activities appropriate for his age group?

Sleep and rest

Are the child's patterns of sleep and rest appropriate for his age group?

Body image

What is the child's body image?

Sexuality

Is the child's curiosity in exploring his own sexuality appropriate?

Emotional Dimension

How appropriate is the child's mood to his experiences?

What is the child's ability to tolerate frustration, anger, sadness, and pleasure?

Has the child achieved the developmental tasks of his age group?

Intellectual Dimension

How appropriate is the child's attention span to his age group?

How appropriate is the child's memory capacity to his age group?

What, if any, difficulties does the child have in learning and in school performance?

Are the child's language skills and vocabulary appropriate to his developmental stage and chronological age?

What concerns does the child have?

What is the child's perception of his problems?

Social Dimension

What is the child's self-concept?

How age appropriate are the child's social interaction patterns?

How age appropriate is the child's attachment to and dependence on his parents?

How satisfied is the child with his friendships?

What is the child's temperament?

Spiritual Dimension

What are the child's concepts of right and wrong, good and bad?

What importance does religion, God, or a Supreme Being play in the child's life?

▼ **Case Example**

Seven-year-old Timmy requires constant supervision to keep him from disrupting the classroom. His teacher describes him as overactive, impulsive, excitable, inattentive, and unable to wait his turn. Timmy does not complete his school work and intrudes on the work of others in the classroom. His mother also describes him as unable to be still for any length of time and is constantly moving, jumping, running, or fiddling with something. He often wanders off by himself without letting anyone know where he is going. Timmy was diagnosed as having an attention deficit disorder with hyperactivity.

Implementation

Physical dimension Although most adults are watchful with small children, there is a need for increased vigilance with the child who has perceptual or neurological deficits. Rooms need to be uncluttered and well lit. Nightlights help control perceptual distortions that can stimulate fearful illusions.

Hyperactive children require environmental modifications. It is important to minimize sensory stimulation such as noise, light, and colors. Arrangements are made for the child to receive additional rest and sleep, and plans need to be made for the hyperactive school-aged child to rest during the day. Attention to the hyperactive child's diet is important because these children require a higher caloric intake than do less active children. Parents need to monitor the child's diet and eliminate foods that seem to contribute to the child's overstimulation, such as sweets.

Most small children spontaneously establish a variety of rituals, and parental reinforcement of these rituals helps provide structure for the child. This approach is especially important for activities of daily living such as mealtimes, bedtime, and bathing and for other physical care activities.

Play activities can be used to help the child master the physical environment by strengthening integration of physical-neurological processes. When counseling parents of emotionally disturbed children, the nurse can prescribe specific, developmentally related play activities that use the child's energies constructively. Activities that strengthen the emotionally disturbed child's control and mastery of the physical world and his self-control, such as games or

Text continued on p. 737.

▼ **ALTERED GROWTH AND DEVELOPMENT**

DEFINITION

A state in which an individual demonstrates deviations in norms from his or her age group.

DEFINING CHARACTERISTICS

• **Physical dimension**

Abnormal movement patterns
Decreased coordination and balance
Abnormal tone
Unable to perform age appropriately in activities of daily living

• **Intellectual dimension**

Deficient in expressive and receptive abilities
Deficient in following instructions

• **Social dimension**

Impaired adaptive functioning
Impaired ability to interact with others
Deficient in modulation behavior
Requires more care than most children

Modified from McFarland G, McFarlane E: *Nursing diagnosis and intervention: planning for patient care,* ed 2, St Louis, 1993, Mosby–Year Book.

TABLE 36-6 ▶ Assessment Norms for Children Ages 2 to 11 Years

		Dimension		
Physical	**Emotional**	**Intellectual**	**Social**	**Spiritual**	**Characteristic Play**
AGE 2 YEARS					
Runs, balances, throws and kicks balls	Graduation from infancy with beginning of "me" and "I" concepts	With mastery of sensorimotor period, child has an efficient, well-organized mechanism for dealing with immediate environment	Presocial; masters object permanency, that is, that objects are separate from self, leads to sense of self as separate object, beginning of self-concept	Preconventional morality; knows "good" and "bad"	Sensorimotor play predominates
Opens doors, turns the pages of a book	Anal stage			Has unquestioning obedience to authority; rules are absolute, coming from higher authority	Enjoys solitary play or play with other children nearby (parallel play)
Can build a six-tower structure with play cubes	Tasks of autonomy vs. shame and guilt, yet still needs confirmation of trust, with mother within reach or within sight	Uses symbols, including images and words, requiring child to reorganize thinking; throughout preoperational period (2-7 years) child's thinking is unsystematic and illogical[66]	Enjoys looking and being looked at	Begins to have self-judgment	Maternal, imitative play with dolls, relating to household things such as cleaning and cooking
Clumsy, falls often, ceaseless activity, curious			Egocentric, views things only from own perspective	Pain and pleasure help child conform to rules	Repetition pervades with little risk, no plot, some fantasies
Explores body	Volatile, has suggestible feelings, imitates others, reflects their actions, attitudes, moods	Uses animism, attributes life to physical objects; egocentricism, thinks things function as he does; views things from one perspective; oriented toward present	Requires constant supervision by adult		
Establishes hand preference			Indicates wants other than by crying; talkative, chatters to self, enjoys songs, uses three-word sentences ("me do it" typical), uses "no"		
Scribbles, makes zigzags and circles, holds crayons in fist guided by index fingers; copies horizontal stroke	Impulsive, functions on punishment-reward basis	Makes choices, uses projection and undoing as adaptive mechanisms	Requires routines, upset by unpredictability; needs constant, firm, gentle discipline		
Muscular maturation for sphincter control; important for autonomy, independence			Has egocentric perspective, knows others have thoughts and feelings, but cannot differentiate theirs from his; thoughts and feelings are responded to in physical terms or with egocentric wishes		
Needs 12 hours of sleep plus nap			Tests limits of authority, resents help, may use toilet training as a battleground to assert self and self-control		
Dreams are considered real, external events			Attention-seeking, self-assertive		
Distractable, short attention span					

Continued

▶ TABLE 36-6   Assessment Norms for Children Ages 2 to 11 Years — cont'd

	Dimension				
Physical	**Emotional**	**Intellectual**	**Social**	**Spiritual**	**Characteristic Play**
AGE 3 YEARS					
Nodal age in which previous processes of development culminate Domesticated; bladder and bowel training completed Names pictures in books, knows action depicted in pictures, knows a few nursery rhymes by heart Holds a crayon with fingers, draws incomplete person, copies circles Feeds and dresses himself Can walk a line, hand dominance established Has eye-hand coordination; perceptual development includes size, colors; can make curved and straight lines with crayon Alternates feet when going upstairs, can stand on one foot and balance well Has body image and directionality	Preoedipal stage Tasks of initiative vs. guilt Begins to use reality principle Concepts of social and physical reality emerging Can delay immediate gratification, is "in control," can stand alone, has impulse control Beginnings of initiative and self-control leading to self-esteem Needs things to be orderly and to have routines; will help pick up or clean up Self-protective stage	Represents thoughts through language, drawings, dreams, play Continues to be preoperational, bases conclusions on what he feels or would like to believe Continues to think out loud, talk to himself but uses correct syntax; language deals with concrete situations but asks rhetorical questions Dissociation of spoken word from associated body movements begins Uses gender words such as "he" and "she"; uses prepositions to denote a beginning of time concept formation Vocabulary of about 900 words, knows *up, down, over,* and action commands; uses three- to four-word sentences Sound-symbol relationships begin	Interested in events outside immediate home Has concept of "what's mine is mine" and is possessive; understands this by identification Status in family important Begins to understand social requirements, cultural norms, and expectations, wants to keep behaviors within family "norms" and acceptable bounds; often asks if behaviors are right; seeks approval; notices differences in home and others Knows sex differences, interested in gender, roles, abilities, feelings, thoughts; likes to please; identification prone, with emerging self-ideal	Uses rules to own advantage: "Don't get caught"; no longer totally dependent on external constraints, blames other people and things ("bad chair")	Recognizes others and otherness—takes turns Cooperative play is best with one or two others; plays with others in same activities with cross-references Dramatization and imagination enter into play; combines playthings such as dolls and cars Imitative, dramatic play, symbolic play to unburden guilt Rich fantasy life with difficulties telling what is real and what is pretend Imaginary companions
AGE 4 TO 6 YEARS					
Fine visual motor organization with form and symbol discrimination Ability to maintain balance (age 5)	Continued phallic oedipal stage Rivalry, jealous competition with parent of same sex	Continued preoperational level Thinking and reasoning begins replacing acting out Thinks in pairs, not wholes	Goes on errands outside home Friendships are strong, especially spurred on by rivalry, and competitive feelings evolve	Needs help with explanations of his behavior and conduct; time to talk to parents about ideas and value questions	Comparative, socialized, associative play; creative, uses props and infinite variety of roles, plots, family romance themes, settings; drama and risk involved

Right and left body orientation Can copy cross, triangle, square, tie knots in string Draws people with body parts Walks downstairs, one foot to step Can tell front from back Unilateral right-handed behavior predominates Draws square, stops at proper length to make a right angle	Intuitive thought; thinking more complex and elaborate Egocentricism replaced by social signs At age 4, formulates five- to six-word sentences; by age 5, 90% of language and words mastered (2,400 words); words used in thought Uses repression and identification; imitation very strong, especially as to behaviors, feelings, reactions More flexible in language use Begins to tell time by clock (6 to 7 years)	Subjective perspective; sees people as interpreting social events — e.g., "a friend is someone you play with" Cooperative but interested in winning Knows what is his but is willing to share, understands things can be used and returned Begins a value judgment system, traits and ideals of role models now become part of self-ideal, an inner standard of behavior one strives for (superego) Self-ideal becomes the direction for behavior, providing more self-assurance and independence; "should" system evolves Conformist phase: begins to identify own welfare with that of family; obeys rules because they are family rules, not for fear of punishment; traditional-directed conformity	Concepts of God include notion that He is responsible for everything, yet good and bad continue to be what parents approve and forbid	Plays in groups of two to five; likes to work on projects that are carried over, on and on Shares Play helps dissolve oedipal ties; development of followers, leaders; seeks adventure and accomplishment
AGE 6 TO 8 YEARS Continued neuromuscular growth Body image solidifies Prints name, defines concepts such as brave and nonsense Knows days of week Knows seasons Rides bicycle Muscles develop, energy and skill increase Practices to attain efficiency Learns value of money Orders, relates parts to whole	Latency stage Tasks of industry vs. inferiority Develops wholesome attitude about self Concrete operations Conceptual organization takes stability, coherence, and rationality Weight and volume viewed as consistent despite changes in size and shape (can conserve) Shift from inductive to deductive reasoning begins Uses reaction formation and rationalization to justify behavior	Sibling relationships important; needs many exchanges with peers and adults Develops hobbies Seeks companionship Interested in community leaders, teachers; has many role models and ego models Self-reflective perspective in which child understands reciprocity, that is, not only can people have feelings but also they can react to one another — thus growth in self-awareness and	Observes rules; develops conscience; conforms because conformity is itself a value Scale of values evolve	Cooperative play with peers, prefers members of same sex; rules, programs, rituals, organized play, shared fantasy, gangs, group alliances and activities

Continued.

▶ **TABLE 36-6** Assessment Norms for Children Ages 2 to 11 Years — cont'd

	Dimension			
Physical	Emotional	Intellectual	Social	Spiritual	Characteristic Play
AGE 6 TO 8 YEARS — cont'd			clearer definition of self begins; acknowledges one can have several perspectives, thus the potential for inner conflict Superficial, but experiences sympathy for others Other-directed conformity Wins recognition through productivity		
AGE 9 TO 11 YEARS Prelude to puberty; develops secondary sexual characteristics — breasts, pubic hair (girls about 1½ years ahead) Boys voice deepens, he develops facial hair Period of steady growth, one of the most healthy periods, pause between childhood and adult "Daring" years, most accident prone Absorbed interest in body changes — growth spurt Growth may seem disproportionate; may be clumsy, uncoordinated; increased interest in sports, athletics, "team" games Heterosexual interests and experiences (some); concerned about appeal to opposite sex	Continued tasks of identify vs. diffusion Fantasies of romantic love	Reaction formation and sublimation Intellectualization begins (11 to 12 years) Formal operational thought begins at about age 11 years; can now deal with world effectively, not only with immediate but also with possibilities, "as if" cognition is now of adult type, uses deductive reasoning, has ability to evaluate logic and quality of own thinking; ability for abstractions provides child with ability to deal with laws and principles Has capacity for insight Can adapt to another opinion or point of view Makes decisions based on stored knowledge Can define abstract terms	Peer in-groups and outgroups Emancipated from parents; makes inner-directed decisions, develops sexual identity, changes and experiments with roles, talks things over with peers Needs "best" friend Third-person perspective leads to ability to take view of disinterested spectator or "generalized other";[67] moves from reciprocity to mutual interest; people's attitudes become stereotyped because of limited discriminations Is self-aware Begins inner-directed conformity Has empathy for others Uses slang, group "jargons," peer culture language Prepares for vocational choice	Rules can change by mutual agreement Right and wrong are logically clear Follows peer group mores Conventional moral level oriented to authority, duty, law	Collaborates with groups in organized way Loyalty to "chum" may exceed loyalty to family

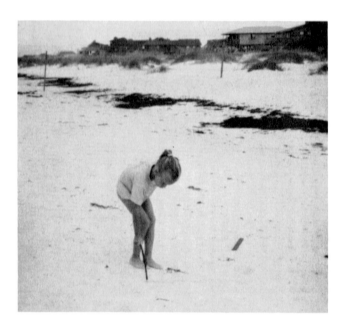

FIGURE 36-3 This 5-year-old is demonstrating self-assurance and independence as she explores a new environment.

sports, are major interventions. These interventions are critical in working with children who are hyperactive and distractible and who have short attention spans and reality distortions, regardless of the etiological factors underlying their psychopathology.

Physical activity is a prime aspect of child's play and a medium through which children develop physical skills and body confidence (Figure 36-3). The early explanations of play focused on its physical benefits such as expending "surplus energy." Gesell, Ilg, and Ames[38] stated that no one need teach a child how to play, that play is automatic and the result of intrinsic maturational forces that direct the child to "do what needs to be done" so that growth, maturation, and development are integrated and balanced. Most of children's spontaneous free play involves physical contact and closeness with one another; young children touch, hug, roll, and toss, whereas older children enjoy body contact sports and touching games.

Table 36-7 provides a schema for selecting age-appropriate developmental play activities. In this schema the "self" refers to physical actions relevant to the physical dimension, not the self-concept. Type I objects are play materials that can change shape and form when manipulated, such as paints, clay, sand, water, and unstructured art media. Type II objects are those that change shape and form when combined with similar or dissimilar objects, such as blocks and tinker toys. Type III objects are toys that do not change shape or form, such as dolls and trucks.

Emotional dimension The child's language and cognitive structures are not sufficiently developed to express concepts verbally. Developmentally children first express their feelings and desires through action, then through fantasy, and, finally, through language. Therefore the therapeutic use of play assists children to resolve internal, emotional problems, such as stress, anxiety, depression, and anger.

Interactions with a child 4 years of age or younger are limited to naming feelings, wishes, or fantasies relating to others and the child making simple requests of adults. The young child lacks the language and cognitive structures to discern relationships between events, and verbalizations need to be limited to words to which the young child can respond. The nurse needs to make simple statements by "naming" feelings and objects, and through these identifications the nurse adds to the child's language repertoire and provides the child a new option of behavior.

Although the 5-year-old child has learned syntax and grammar, the child's ease in using language to express feelings is still limited. Play materials provide familiar concrete objects and materials that stimulate the child to symbolically express areas of concern. Engaging the child in ongoing dialogue while he plays helps clarify the child's thought organization. Conversation stimulated through play may be the most important part of the intervention. The child is assisted by verbal interactions and clarification to organize experiences and fill in missing data. The nurse has the opportunity to identify and clarify the child's misinterpretations.

Children 9 to 12 years of age are usually very verbal, and their language and communication skills can be expanded and refined during therapeutic dialogues. Although the older child's language and cognitive concepts may be sufficient for expressing feeling, the older child may be inexperienced or uncomfortable discussing feelings and interpersonal situations. Focusing on play materials may help alleviate uncomfortable barriers that eye-to-eye interaction may stimulate. Older children are extremely sensitive to social and adult-child size differences, and these perceptions may impede free and open verbal expression. Children ages 9 to 12 years spend much time talking with peers, and group therapies with children in this age range may be indicated.

Children often need parental help in mastery of impulse control and angry feelings. Most children have outbursts of anger and frustration while learning to delay gratification, and behavior modification interventions often enforce limits and help both child and parent to be consistent.

Intellectual dimension When nursing interventions include teaching, the child's learning capacity and style can be determined from conferences with nursery or school teachers. It is important that teaching interventions in the nursing care plan are consistent with the child's learning capacities and experiences. The child's language development, reviewed earlier, is an important consideration in teaching plans and interventions with the emotionally disturbed child. This is especially true with children with delayed speech or expressive language problems, such as blocking or stuttering. It is important that the child have a complete evaluation by a speech therapist to rule out the possibility of neurological or organic sensory problems. Many children with emotional problems fail to maintain the eye contact that is basic to learning the mouth movements necessary for clear enunciation. Thus many speech problems in children disappear when the underlying emotional stress has been alleviated. The resolution of the language problem symptoms is often an indication of effective intervention within the emotional dimension of the child.

▼ **TABLE 36-7   Play Behaviors**

	2-3 Years	3-4 Years	4-5 Years	5-6 Years
HUMAN OBJECTS				
Parents	Asking to listen to same story, over and over without any change in wording	Not asking to hear same story word for word	Bragging, e.g., "I can do ____"; asking "why" questions, listening to stories—fairy tales	Asking "why" questions; wanting to know what to expect, wanting to listen to realistic stories as opposed to fairy tales
Peers	Parallel (playing alongside on same or different activity); fighting, pinching; defending play objects; taking objects from another	Parallel; beginning to take turns	Enjoys being with other children; sharing materials; bragging and name calling	Cooperative (two or more working on same project); wanting playmates; playing group games in which everyone has a turn—no competition; imaginative action—roles differentiated, e.g., one plays mother, one plays baby
Self	Practice of newly acquired motor skills, e.g., balancing, rolling	Identifying body with other people or things, e.g., I am a bear, I am a fireman—does not ask for costumes for such action, may have imaginary friends	May have imaginary friends	No play-specific information reported
NONHUMAN OBJECTS				
Type I	Emptying and filling containers, splashing (with water); making marks and using many sheets of paper (with paint or crayons); tasting, putting on self, squishing through fingers; patting; pulling apart; extending efforts beyond boundary of paper or surface; does not name product or ask to have it saved	Attending to results of efforts (e.g., "Look what I made," and naming of products); treating product as object itself and not a representation of object; likely to throw a clay ball	Intends to make something when begins although may end with different product; talking about what is being made; treating product as representation of object—not likely to throw clay ball—product does not have to be a realistic representation; wanting to put name on product and wanting it saved	Attempting to make realistic representation; definitely wanting products saved and displayed; putting name on products
Type II	Stringing beads, working puzzles, building vertically, placing in rows, building floorlike arrangement; making arch, transporting in containers	Working puzzles; building wall-like arrangement; floorlike arrangement, arch, or solid structure (a wall of several thicknesses), using the form built in; imaginative action	Naming what is being built although not intent on making product a realistic representation; wanting structures saved; collecting, e.g., variation of nature objects mainly	Constructing simple projects that can be completed within 20 minutes; projects must be useful (e.g., potholders)

6-7 Years	7-8 Years	8-9 Years	9-11 Years
In listening to stories, has greater tolerance for fairy tales in the form of magic	Asking to listen to heroes own age in setting he can recognize; opinions of group more important than opinions of parents; boys want some individual time with father; girls want individual time with mother	Rebelling against parents especially when group opinions conflict with parental ones	No play-specific information reported
Wants to be with a group although there is little cooperation; important to obey customs of group—must act, look, talk like others; may tattle; game action—unable to put rules of game above need to win; learning to work as team in relay races; imaginative action—includes more than one or two children and often depends on leader; details in costume	Group is very important—a for or against age in which one is in or out of group; game action—rules apply to everyone except him; group games in which everyone has a chance to play; trading of objects; imaginative action—each group has organization and leader; imitation of reality; separation of sexes, e.g., girls—house, boys—war	Group is very important—must compete with others and conform to code; secrecy of gang important; game action—rules can still apply to everyone except him; imaginative action—done in group and reflects events outside of home and school; scouts or cubs important; trading of objects	Group is very important—joins many groups; game action—more conscious about rules and obeys them; competition is strong and plays for personal and team glory at the same time; imaginative action is rare
No play-specific information reported	No play-specific information reported	No play-specific information reported	No play-specific information reported
Attempting realistic representation	In a hurry for results—prefers crayons to paint as does not want to wait for paint to dry; concerned with realistic representation	Paints and uses casein; concerned with realistic representation	Making projects (for example, clay modeling)
Has trouble finishing any simple project—gets bogged down in middle; very critical of self in work	Sampling age—tries many different crafts and explores use of tools in relation to them; in a hurry for results so does not use best workmanship	Makes things that move and work; constantly overreaching self in projects—needs someone to help get materials and show procedures; exploring many processes in crafts (e.g., potato carving)	Exploring many crafts (e.g., model making, weaving, woodworking, metalworking, working with leather, carving, making baskets, sewing); projects made need to be useful

Continued.

▼ **TABLE 36-7**   **Play Behaviors**—cont'd

	2-3 Years	3-4 Years	4-5 Years	5-6 Years
NONHUMAN OBJECTS—cont'd				
Type III	Looking at and playing with same object, manipulating parts: taking simple things apart or off; placing pegs in board; pushing and propelling over obstacles; kicking, climbing, imaginative action—ascribing action (e.g., making dolly eat, sleep, cry, making truck "start")	Fine motor action—hitting nail with hammer, dropping buttons through small openings; propelling over obstacles; imaginative action—ascribing action; identifying one object as another by speech before using in action (e.g., paper as blanket, shell as cup)	Fine motor action—cutting, sewing on cards; gross motor action—arranging perilous feats for self, e.g., jumping, climbing jungle gym; imaginative action—identifying body with other people, wanting a few elements of costume; sequences more complex, e.g., more than one event (feeding, bathing dolly), or expansion of one event	Fine motor action—making mosaics; gross motor action—leaving earth with ropes in jumping; imaginative action—identifies body with other people and wanting whole costume; using miniature objects to represent real ones; attempting to imitate others

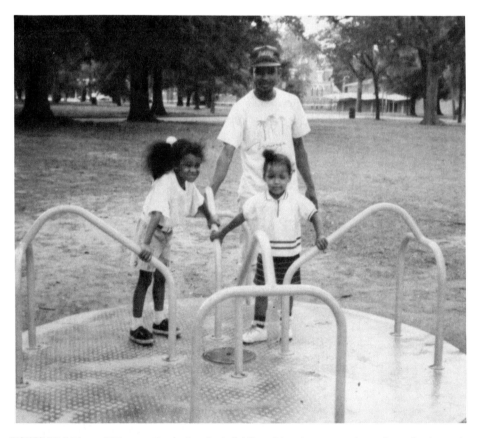

FIGURE 36-4 These children are developing physical skills and learning cooperation and coordination under the watchful eye of their dad.

6-7 Years	7-8 Years	8-9 Years	9-11 Years
Collecting items—quantity important—taking objects apart (e.g., clocks); speed important in sport activities (e.g., roller skating)	Beginning to collect only certain items; gross muscle action—speed important; trying to improve physical skills and sampling new skills (e.g., swimming, archery, riding, skiing)	Reads and chooses fairy tales and legends—stories about everyday people in everyday situations; gross muscle action—gross muscle sports of hopscotch, roller skating, kite flying, wrestling, not ready for fine precision sports (e.g., tennis, golf); collecting according to individual interests	Exploring a variety of books (e.g., adventure, fantasy, biography, mysteries, westerns, sports, animal, scientific); exploring a variety of sports, trying many and concentrating on a few and practicing those skills

Social dimension The stressors on children can be addressed with many of the same stress management techniques that are used with adults. Because children and parents with mental health problems often withdraw from social relationships, it is important to encourage peer relationships for both child and parents (Figure 36-4). As part of the evaluation of the therapeutic process, social relationships need to provide the social support networks on which families and children rely.

Implementing the child's treatment plan depends on the therapeutic alliance with the parents. By the time parents seek professional help for the child, they usually have tried many techniques of their own and have followed advice of family and friends. Sometimes parents are troubled, deny a problem exists, and seek support to prove others wrong. Thus it is important that the nurse help parents regain confidence in the parenting role. Sufficient time needs to be taken to allow the parents to identify and discuss their feelings, successes, frustrations, and anxieties.

The therapeutic relationship with the child's parents begins with the initial assessment of their roles and relationships with the child and the child's problems and includes ongoing strengthening of the parents' potential to help the child. The treatment goal of working with emotionally disturbed children and their families is the reestablishment of the normal child-parent relationships appropriate for the child's developmental level. The problems identified by parents often have little or no relationship to the child's subjective feelings of distress. It is important, however, to learn parents' concerns and resolve them concurrently with intervention with the child. The nurse is nonjudgmental while gathering the information, allowing each parent to give his or her point of view. The parents' trust is gained, and the therapeutic alliance is established if positive feedback, information, and reinforcement are provided. For example, the mother of a hyperactive child can be asked how she provides for her own well-being and restoration of

energies. The child's and parents' strengths are emphasized to provide the parents with hope.

Therapeutic interventions with the child's parents are based on a parallel process that strengthens the parents' potential to help the child. Table 36-8 is a sample nursing care plan. The parents' and child's developmental tasks in progress are set forth in Table 36-9 for the child from 18 months to 12 years of age. Table 36-10 gives psychopathological conditions of the child 18 months to 12 years of age and related behaviors of the parents. Tasks in process, acceptable behavioral characteristics, minimal psychopathology, and extreme psychopathology are important guides to the nurse during implementation as well as during evaluation of behavioral change.

Spiritual dimension Interventions in the spiritual dimension are so integrally related to the other dimensions for children that they are not addressed separately here. The box on p. 745 summarizes key interventions for the child.

Evaluation

Development is uneven, and not all children can be expected to change simultaneously. An important criterion is the child's developmental progress; children with mental health problems often seem "fixed" at a developmental stage. Positive evaluation reflects the child's productive return to the expected developmental stage. Materials used in assessment often provide useful guidelines to evaluate therapeutic outcomes, such as children's drawings compared before and after interventions.

Evaluation takes into consideration the parents' perceptions of the child's progress and changes in parent-child relationships. The research highlight on p. 723 indicates that the child's perceptions are of equal importance in the evaluation process. In many instances, parents are unaware of the child's worries and concerns.

▼ **TABLE 36-8   NURSING CARE PLAN**

GOALS	OUTCOME CRITERIA	INTERVENTIONS	RATIONALES
NURSING DIAGNOSIS: Altered growth and development related to hyperactivity			
LONG TERM			
To reduce level of activity so that social interactions and academic achievement are attained at the child's optimal level	Achieves optimal level of growth and development by controlling hyperactivity		
SHORT TERM			
To channel impulsiveness so that it can be controlled	Uses acceptable controls that delay or prevent impulsive actions	Reduce impulsiveness with negative reinforcement	Behaviors that are not rewarded (ignored, given time out) are less likely to be repeated
		Reward behaviors not acted on impulsively	To increase self-esteem. Behavior that is rewarded is likely to be repeated
To reduce responsiveness to environment	Sits still/concentrates for increasing periods of time	Provide activities child can complete in short periods of time	Attention span is short. Completion of a task increases self-esteem
To develop language skills through which frustration, anger can be expressed	Verbalizes feelings of anger and frustration	Assist with verbal skills that allow for expression of feelings	Reduces the need to act out
		Provide immediate feedback	So that child will know quickly how well he is doing
To participate in groups without distracting others	Requests permission to leave group if restless or becoming overresponsive	Supervise play with others	Child is impulsive and may need assistance in controlling his behavior
		Determine methods of limit setting and discipline	To help child know the boundaries of his behavior

▼ **TABLE 36-9   Developmental Tasks and Acceptable Behavioral Characteristics of the Child and Related Tasks and Behaviors of the Parents**

Tasks in Process		Acceptable Behavioral Characteristics	
Child	**Parents**	**Child**	**Parents**
18 MONTHS TO 5 YEARS OF AGE			
To reach physiologic plateaus (motor action, toilet training)	To promote training, habits, and physiologic progress	Gratification from exercise of neuromotor skills	Is moderate and flexible in training
To differentiate self and secure sense of autonomy	To aid in family and group socialization of child	Investigative, imitative imaginative play	Shows pleasure and praise for child's advances
To tolerate separations from mother	To encourage speech and other learning	Actions somewhat modulated by thought, memory good; animistic and original thinking	Encourages and participates with child in learning and in play
To develop conceptual understandings and "ethical" values	To reinforce child's sense of autonomy and identity	Exercises autonomy with body (sphincter control, eating)	Sets reasonable standards and controls
	To set a model for "ethical" conduct		Paces herself to child's capacities at a given time
	To delineate male and female roles		

From Senn MJE, Solnit AJ: *Problems in child behavior and development*, Philadelphia, 1968, Lea & Febiger.

TABLE 36-9   Developmental Tasks and Acceptable Behavioral Characteristics of the Child and Related Tasks and Behaviors of the Parents—cont'd

Tasks in Process		Acceptable Behavioral Characteristics	
Child	**Parents**	**Child**	**Parents**
18 MONTHS TO 5 YEARS OF AGE—cont'd			
To master instinctual impulses (oedipal, sexual, guilt, shame)		Feelings of dependence on mother and separation fears	Consistent in own behavior, conduct, and ethics
To assimilate and handle socialization and acculturation (aggression, relationships, activities, feelings)		Behavior identification with parents, siblings, peers	Provides emotional reassurance to child
To learn sex distinctions		Learns speech for communication	Promotes peer play and guided group activity
		Awareness of own motives, beginnings of conscience	Reinforces child's cognition of male and female roles
		Intense feelings of shame, guilt, joy, love, desire to please	
		Internalized standards of "bad," "good"; beginning of reality testing	
		Broader sex curiosity and differentiation	
		Ambivalence toward dependence and independence	
		Questions birth and death	
5 TO 12 YEARS OF AGE			
To master greater physical prowess	To help child's emancipation from parents	General good health, greater body competence, acute sensory perception	Ambivalent toward child's separation but encourage independence
To further establish self-identity and sex role	To reinforce self-identification and independence	Pride and self-confidence, less dependence on parents	Mixed feelings about parent surrogates but help child to accept them
To work toward greater independence from parents	To provide positive pattern of social and sex role behavior	Better impulse control	Encourage child to participate outside the home
To become aware of world at large	To facilitate learning, reasoning, communication, and experiencing	Ambivalence regarding dependency, separation, and new experiences	Set appropriate model of social and ethical behavior and standards
To develop peer and other relationships	To promote wholesome moral and ethical values	Accepts own sex role: psychosexual expression in play and fantasy	Take pleasure in child's developing skills and abilities
To acquire learning, new skills, and a sense of industry		Equates parents with peers and other adults	Understand and cope with child's behavior
		Aware of natural world (life, death, birth, science); subjective but realistic about world	Find other gratifications in life (activity, employment)
		Competitive but well organized in play; enjoys peer interaction	Are supportive toward child as required
		Regard for collective obedience to social laws, rules, and fair play	
		Explores environment; school and neighborhood basic to social-learning experience	
		Cognition advancing; intuitive thinking advancing to concrete operational level; responds to learning	
		Speech becomes reasoning and expressive tool; thinking still egocentric	

TABLE 36-10   Minimal and Extreme Psychopathological Conditions of the Child and Related Behaviors of the Parents

Minimal Psychopathology		Extreme Psychopathology	
Child	**Parents**	**Child**	**Parents**
18 MONTHS TO 5 YEARS OF AGE			
Poor motor coordination	Premature, coercive, or censuring training	Extreme lethargy, passivity, or hypermotility	Severely coercive and punitive
Persistent speech problems (stammering, loss of words)	Exacting standards above child's ability to conform	Little or no speech, noncommunicative	Totally critical and rejecting
Timidity toward people and experiences	Transmits anxiety and apprehension	No response or relationship to people, symbiotic clinging to mother	Overidentification with or overly submissive to child
Fears and night terrors	Unaccepting of child's efforts; intolerant toward failures	Somatic ills; vomiting, constipation, diarrhea, megacolon, rash, tics	Inability to accept child's sex; fosters opposite
Problems with eating, sleeping, elimination, toileting, weaning	Overreacts, overprotective, overanxious	Autism, childhood psychosis	Substitutes child for spouse; sexual expression via child
Irritability, crying, temper tantrums	Despondent, apathetic	Excessive enuresis, soiling, fears	Severe repression of child's need for gratification
Partial return to infantile manners		Completely infantile behavior	Deprivation of all stimulations, freedoms, and pleasures
Inability to leave mother without panic		Play inhibited and nonconceptualized; absence or excess of autoerotic activity	Extreme anger and displeasure with child
Fear of strangers		Obsessive-compulsive behavior; "ritual" bound mannerisms	Child assault and brutality
Breathholding spells		Impulsive destructive behavior	Severe depressions and withdrawal
Lack of interest in other children			
5 TO 12 YEARS OF AGE			
Anxiety and oversensitivity to new experiences (school, relationships, separation)	Disinclination to separate from child; or prematurely hastening separation	Extreme withdrawal, apathy, depression, grief, self-destructive tendencies	Extreme depression and withdrawal; rejection of child
Lack of attentiveness; learning difficulties; disinterest in learning	Signs of despondency, apathy, hostility	Complete failure to learn	Intense hostility; aggression toward child
Acting out; lying, stealing, temper outbursts, inappropriate social behavior	Foster fears, dependence, apprehension	Speech difficulty, especially stuttering	Uncontrollable fears, anxieties, guilts
Regressive behavior (wetting, soiling, crying, fears)	Disinterested in or rejecting of child	Extreme and uncontrollable antisocial behavior (aggression, destruction, chronic lying, stealing, intentional cruelty to animals)	Complete inability to function in family role
Appearance of compulsive mannerisms (tics, rituals)	Overly critical and censuring; undermine child's confidence	Severe obsessive-compulsive behavior (phobias, fantasies, rituals)	Severe moralistic prohibition of child's independent strivings
Somatic illness; eating and sleeping problems, aches, pains, digestive upsets	Inconsistent in discipline or control; erratic in behavior	Inability to distinguish reality from fantasy	
Fear of illness and body injury	Offer a restrictive, overly moralistic model	Excessive sexual exhibitionism, eroticism, sexual assaults on others	
Difficulties and rivalry with peers, siblings, adults; constant fighting		Extreme somatic illness: failure to thrive, anorexia, obesity, hypochondriasis, abnormal menses	
Destructive tendencies; strong temper tantrums		Complete absence or deterioration of personal and peer relationships	
Inability or unwillingness to do things for self			
Moodiness and withdrawal; few friends or personal relationships.			

From Senn MJE and Solnit AJ: *Problems in child behavior and development,* Philadelphia, 1968, Lea & Febiger.

▼ **KEY INTERVENTIONS FOR THE CHILD**

To manage tension	Accept delays in the child's development
	Use videotapes, modeling to foster parental attuning to child's arousal state
	Enhance secure relationships with parental figures
To strengthen attachment	Increase parental responsiveness
	Foster a positive sense of self in parental figures
	Be available and constant
	Provide parenting skills, support groups, and therapy for caregivers
To strengthen autonomy	Encourage child to deal with environment actively and adaptively with limits to provide safety
	Nurture child's trust
	Foster social and language skills and achievements
	Help parents to increase positive caretaking skills
To alter environment	Improve interactions by modeling
	Assist parents to accept and have positive feelings about an irritable, passive child
	Provide relief from caregiving responsibilities
To strengthen cognitive controls	Set limits
	Use behavior modification techniques
	Encourage age-appropriate speech and language skills
	Promote secure attachment relationships
To enhance school functioning	Meet basic needs; physiological, safety, love, belonging
	Provide positive adult models as social reinforcers
	Use Big Brothers, foster grandparent programs to provide multiple positive experiences with adults
To improve peer relations	Facilitate adaptive ways of dealing with emotional expression
	Use individual, peer, or play therapy
To strengthen interpersonal relationships	Use supportive peer culture
To enhance social skills	Increase social competence, coping skills, and adaptation
	Foster play and peer friendships
To promote adaptation to school	Facilitate competence in social and academic skills
	Promote peer interactions

SPECIFIC TREATMENT MODALITIES

Play Therapy

Children with neurotic problems usually have little insight and respond best to play therapies based on psychoanalytical theories. This approach uses play for working through or resolving conflicts through repetitive fantasy and make believe. The therapist's role is active in that the toys used in therapy are purposefully selected for their therapeutic value. The therapeutic communication with the child during play helps him develop abilities in interpretation and insight.

Erikson[31] expanded Freud's psychoanalytical theory of play to include social mastery, stating that the purpose of children's play is to master the specific areas of conflict involved in developmental crisis. In Erikson's play therapy methods, the therapist controls the play session by introducing toys and activities that facilitate the child's development and mastery, while recognizing at the same time that the child will spotnaneously choose materials and activities to alleviate conflicts and development crises.

Theraplay

The technique of *theraplay* differs from traditional forms of child treatment. Theraplay uses active physical contact and control of the child. Theraplay grew from the work of Hellendoorn[46] with autistic children, in which they forced the child to acknowledge their presence by insisting on eye contact, speaking loudly when the child "tuned them out," and aggressively insisting on interactions. Their interventions involved physical contact that forced the autistic, self-absorbed child to acknowledge their presence in the here and now. The theraplay techniques have been adapted to interventions with children with less severe psychopathological conditions and are of benefit to children with psychosocial retardation and benefit children having difficulties in elementary school settings.

BRIEF REVIEW

Nursing care of children with emotional problems requires an understanding of the development of the five dimensions of the child and the interrelatedness of the dimensions in the developmental process. Several theoretical models for understanding child development are discussed in this chapter including psychoanalytical, cognitive, sociocultural, and communication. The application of these models provides a framework for the nurse in her care of children.

A discussion of the DSM-III-R medical diagnoses—developmental disorders, separation anxiety, elimination disorders, and attention deficit disorders—provides the nurse with the basic knowledge for understanding and caring for children with these disorders. Treatment is based on the child's age/stage considerations. Play therapy, a specific treatment modality, can be structured with the focus on the content of the child's play or unstructured, providing a framework for learning, socializing, and limit setting.

Therapeutic communication with children focuses on communicating with the child at the appropriate age level of word usage and adding to the child's growing understanding of language. Therapeutic treatment of the child includes helping the child reach higher levels of development in all dimensions.

Because the relationship between the parent and child is reciprocal, the nursing process is directed toward both. Data are collected in all five dimensions. The analysis lists nursing diagnoses applicable to childhood behaviors. The immediate goals of intervention with children are to alleviate the child's distress and to help the child get back on the developmental tract. Long-range goals are to expand the child's coping strategies and to alter his environment so the problems do not recur. The goals include working with families or significant others so that the childs' uniqueness is understood, the developmental process and tasks are mastered, and changes are facilitated and supported.

A sample nursing care plan (Table 36-8) illustrates long- and short-term goals, nursing actions, and rationales for the nursing actions. Evaluation is based on the child's return to his expected developmental stage. Evaluation also considers the parents' perception of the child's progress and changes in the parent-child relationship.

REFERENCES AND SUGGESTED READINGS

1. Adams P, Fras H: *Beginning child psychiatry,* New York, 1988, Brunner Mazel.
2. Adkins AA: Helping your patient cope with Tourette syndrome, *Pediatric Nursing* 16:135, 1989.
3. American Nurses' Association: *Standards of child and adolescent psychiatric mental health nursing practice,* Kansas City, Mo, 1985. The American Nurses Association.
4. American Psychiatric Association: *Diagnostic and statistical manual of mental disorders,* ed 3, Revised, Washington, DC, 1987, The Association.
5. Barkley RA: Attention deficit disorder with hyperactivity. In Mash EJ, Terdal LG: *Behavioral assessment of childhood disorders,* ed 2, New York, 1988, Guilford Press.
6. Barkley RA: *Defiant children: a clinician's manual for parent training,* New York, 1987, Guilford Press.
7. Barker P: *Clinical interviews with children and adolescents,* New York, 1990, WW Norton.
8. Barkley RA: A review of child behavior rating scales and checklists for research in child psychopathology. In Ruter M, Tuma AH, Lann I, editors: *Assessment and diagnosis in child psychopathology,* New York, 1987, Guilford Press.
9. Bemporad JR, Schwab ME: The DSM-III and clinical child psychiatry. In Million T, Klernman GL, editors: *Contemporary directions in psychopathology: toward the DSM IV,* New York, 1986, Guilford Press.
10. Bender WN: Behavioral correlates of temperament and personality in the inactive learner, *Journal of Learning Disabilities* 20:5, 1987.
11. Berrigan LP, Stedman JM: Combined application of behavioral techniques and family therapy for the treatment of childhood encropresis: a strategic approach, *Family Therapy* 14:51, 1989.
12. Bowlby J: *Attachment and loss III: loss, sadness and depression,* New York, 1980, Basic Books.
13. Brody C, Forehand R: Maternal perceptions of child maladjustment as a function of the combined influence of child behavior and maternal depression, *Journal of Consulting and Clinical Psychology* 54:237, 1986.
14. Bronfenbrenner U: *The ecology of human development,* Cambridge, 1979, Harvard University Press.
15. Burke E and others: Hazardous secrets and reluctantly taking charge: parenting a child with repeated hospitalizations, *Image: The Journal of Nursing Scholarship* 23(1):39, 1991.
16. Campbell J: *The portable Jung,* RFC Hull, translation, New York, 1971, Viking Press.
17. Carlson GA, Cantwell DP: Unmasking masked depression in children and adolescents, *American Journal of Psychiatry* 137:445, 1980.
18. Chamberlain J: Challenges for child psychiatric—mental health nusing, *Journal of Child and Adolescent Psychiatric and Mental Health Nursing* 1:1, 1988.
19. Chess S, Thomas AS, Hertzig ME, editors: *Annual progress in child psychiatry and child development,* New York, 1988, Brunner/Mazel.
20. Chomsky N: *Reflections on language,* New York, 1975, Pantheon Books.
21. Chu JA, Dill DL: Dissociative symptoms in relation to childhood physical and sexual abuse, *American Journal of Psychiatry* 147:887, 1990.
22. Coddington R: The significance of life events as etiological factors in the diseases of children: a study of normal populatios, *Journal of Psychosomatic Research* 16:205, 1972.
23. Combrinck-Graham L: Family treatment of childhood anxiety disorder. In Combrinck-Graham L, editor: *Treating young children in family therapy,* Rockville, Md, 1987, Aspen Publishing.
24. Clunn PA, editor: *Child psychiatric nursing,* St Louis, 1991, Mosby—Year Book.
25. Coler MS: Diagnoses for child and adolescent psychiatric nursing: combining NANDA and DSM-III-R, *Journal of Child and Adolescent Psychiatric Nursing* 9:115, 1989.
26. Dalton ST, Howell CC: Autism: psychobiological perspectives, *Journal of Child and Adolescent Psychiatric and Mental Health Nursing* 2:5 1989.
27. Davis S, Schwartz M: *Children's rights and the law,* Lexington, Mass, 1987, DC Health.
28. de Leon Siantz ML: Issues facing child psychiatric nursing in the 1990s, *Journal of Child and Adolescent Psychiatric and Mental Health Nursing* 3:65, 1990.
29. Earls T: Application of DSM III in an epidemiologic differential study of preschool children, *American Journal of Psychiatry* 139:242, 1982.
30. Earls F, Jung KG: Temperament and home environment characteristics as causal factors in the early development of childhood psychopathology. In Ellis RB, Allen GN: *Traitor within: our suicide problem,* Garden City, NJ, 1961, Doubleday.
31. Erikson EH: *Childhood and society,* ed 2, New York, 1963, WW Norton.
32. Eth S, Pynoos RS, editors: *Posttraumatic stress disorder in children,* Washington, DC, 1985, American Psychiatric Press.
33. Fagin C, editor: *Readings in child and adolescent psychiatric nursing,* St Louis, 1974, Mosby—Year Book.
34. Fassler D and others: Children's perceptions of AIDS, *Journal of American Academy of Child and Adolescent Psychiatry* 29:459, 1990.
35. Freud A: *Normality and pathology in childhood: assessments of development, the writing of Anna Freud,* vol 6, New York, 1965, International Universities Press.
36. Freud A: *The psychanalytical treatment of children,* London, 1946, Image.
37. George C, Solomon J: Internal working models of caregiving and security of attachment at age six, *Infant Mental Health Journal* 3:222, 1989.

38. Gesell A, Ilg A, Ames L: *Infant and child in the culture of today,* New York, 1974, Harper & Row.

39. Ginott HG: The theory and practice of "therapeutic intervention" in child treatment, In Haworth MR, editor: *Child psychotherapy,* New York, 1964, Basic Books.

40. Glasser K: Suicide in children and adolescents. In Abt LE, Weissman SL, editors: *Acting out,* ed 2, Northvale, NJ, 1987, Jason Aronson.

41. Gomes-Schwartz B, Horowitz JM, Sauzier M: Severity of emotional distress among sexually abused preschool, school-age and adolescent children. *Hospital and Community Psychiatry* 36:503, 1985.

42. Goodman JD, Sours JA: *The child mental status examination,* ed 2, New York, 1988, Basic Books.

43. Greenspan SI: *The clinical interview of the child,* New York, 1981, McGraw-Hill.

44. Harnett NE: Conduct disorder in childhood and adolescence: an update, *Journal of Child and Adolescent Psychiatric and Mental Health Nursing,* 2:74, 1988.

45. Harter S: Developmental perspectives on the self-system. In Hetheringtron EM, editor: *Socialization, personality and social development,* vol 4, Mussen's Handbook of Child Psychology, ed 4, New York, 1983, John Wiley.

46. Hellendoorn J: Imaginative play techniques in psychotherapy with children. In Schaefer CE, editor: *Innovative interventions in child and adolescent therapy,* New York, 1988, John Wiley.

47. Hoyt LA and others: Anxiety and depression in young children of divorce, *Journal of Clinical Child Psychology* 19:26, 1990.

48. Hutchins VL, McPherson M: National Agenda for children with special health needs: special local policies for the 1990s through the 21st century, *American Psychologist* 46:141, 1991.

49. Kagan J: Development. In Restak R, editor: *The mind,* New York, 1990, Bantum Books.

50. Kemp VH: Mothers' perceptions of children's temperament and mother-child attachment, *Scholarly Inquiry for Nursing Practice* 1:51, 1987.

51. Klein, M: *The psychoanalysis of children,* London, 1949, Hogarth Press.

52. Knell SM, Moore DJ: Cognitive-behavioral play therapy in the treatment of encorpresis, *Journal of Clinical Child Psychology* 19:55, 1990.

53. Kohlberg L: *Recent research in moral development,* New York, 1971, Holt, Rinehart & Winston.

54. Laben J, McLean C: *Legal issues and guidelines for nurses who care for the mentally ill,* Owings Mills, Md, 1989, National Health Publishing.

55. Laufer MW, Denhoff E, Solomons G: Hyperkinetic impulse disorder in children's behavior problems, *Psychosomatic Medicine* 19:38, 1957.

56. Loeber R: Natural histories of conduct problems, delinquency and associated substance use. In Lahey BB, Lazdin AD, editors: *Advances in clinical child psychology,* vol 11, New York, 1988, Plenum Press.

57. Maziade M and others: Temperament and intellectual development: a longitudinal study from infancy to four years. In Chess S, Thomas A, Hertzig ME, editors: *Annual progress in child psychiatry and child development,* New York, 1989, Brunner/Mazel.

58. McBride A: Coming of age. Child psychiatric nursing, *Archives of Psychiatric Nursing* 2:57, 1988.

59. McFarland G, McFarlane E: *Nursing diagnosis and intervention: planning for patient care,* St Louis, 1989, Mosby–Year Book.

60. National Advisory Mental Health Counsel: *National plan for research on child and adolescent mental disorders,* Rockville, Md, 1990, US Department of Health and Human Services.

61. Neubauer PB: The many meanings of play, *The Psychological Study of the Child* 42:3, 1987.

62. Opie ND, Slater P: Mental health needs of children in school: role of the child psychiatric mental health nurse, *Journal of Child and Adolescent Psychiatric and Mental Health Nursing* 1:31, 1988.

63. Orzek AM: The child's cognitive processing of sexual abuse, *Journal of Child and Adolescent Psychotherapy* 2:110, 1985.

64. Pasamanick B: A world emancipation procamation for children and women, *Ameican Journal of Orthopsychiatry* 61:5, 1991.

65. Perlmutter IR and others: Childhood schizophrenia: theoretical and treatment issues, *Journal of the American Academy of Adolescent Psychiatry* 28:965, 1989.

66. Piaget J: *The growth of logical thinking from childhood to adolescence,* New York, 1958, Basic Books.

67. Piaget J: *The origins of intelligence in children,* New York, 1963, WW Norton.

68. Post CA: Play therapy with an abused child: a case study, *Journal of Child and Adolescent Psychiatric and Mental Health Nursing* 3:34, 1989.

69. Pothier PC: Child psychiatric nursing, *Journal of Psychosocial Nursing* 3:11, 1984.

70. Roberts RN and others: Family support in the home: programs, policy, and social change, *American Psychologist* 46:131, 1991.

71. Rutter M: The role of cognition in child development and disorder. In Chess S, Thomas A, Hertzig ME, editors: *Annual progress in child psychiatry and child development,* New York, 1988, Brunner/Mazel.

72. Sattler JM: *Assessment of children,* ed 3, San Diego, 1988, JM Sattler.

73. Shafii M and others: Psychological autopsy of completed suicide in children and adolescents, *American Journal of Psychiatry* 142:1061, 1985.

74. Spitz RA: Hospitalism: an inquiry into the genesis of psychiatric conditions in early childhood, *Psychoanalytic Study of the Child* 1:55, 1945.

75. Stoker D, Meadow A: Cultural differences in child guidance clinic patients, *International Journal of Social Psychiatry* 20:4, 1974.

76. Terr LC: Childhood trauma: an outline and overview, *American Journal of Psychiatry* 148:10, 1991.

77. Thomas A, Chess S: *Temperament and development,* New York, 1977, Brunner/Mazel.

78. Timmreck TC: Behavioral therapy for high bed wetting children with parents as therapists, *Journal of Psychosocial Nursing and Mental Health Services* 21:31, 1983.

79. Trad PV: *The preschool child: assessment, diagnosis and treatment,* New York, 1989, WW Norton.

80. Tuma J: Mental health services for children, *American Psychologist* 44:188, 1989.

81. U.S. Congress, Office of Technology Assessment: Children's mental health. problems and services—a background paper. OTA-PB-H-33, Washington, DC, 1986, US Printing Office.

82. Wallerstein JS: Children of divorce: preliminary report of a followup study of older children and adolescents, *Journal of the American Academy Child Psychiatry* 24:545, 1985.

ANNOTATED BIBLIOGRAPHY

Clunn P: *Child psychiatric nursing,* St Louis, 1991, Mosby–Year Book.

This book focuses on the mental and emotional needs of children and their families. The content spans the spectrum of children's problems including severe psychopathology. Also discussed are intervention strategies and suggestions for enhancing therapeutic treatment settings.

Dinkmeyer D, McKay G: *The parents' handbook: systematic training for effective parenting,* Minnesota, 1989, American Guidance Services.

This book provides the basic skills for the nurse working with children. Parenting styles, the meaning of misbehavior, and communication skills are described. An excellent teaching aid for parents.

Kestenbaum C, WIlliams D: *Handbook of clinical assessment of children and adolescents,* New York, 1988, New York University Press.

This book presents comprehensive content on diagnostic categories, syndromes, and other behavioral problems of children and adolescents.

Simeon J: Pediatric psychopharmacology, *Canadian Journal of Psychiatry* 34:115, 1989.

This book summarizes the current knowledge of pediatric psychopharmacology including diets used in the treatment of child psychiatric disorders.

Alice R Kempe
Ruth Parmelee Rawlins

- Discuss the historical development of mental health–psychiatric nursing related to the adolescent
- Describe theoretical approaches to understanding adolescence as a unique phase of development
- Discuss the psychopathology associated with disruptive behavior and adolescent antisocial disorder as described in the DSM-III-R

- Apply the nursing process to the mental health care of the adolescent
- Describe current research findings related to the adolescent
- Describe specific treatment modalities that can be used in meeting the mental health–psychiatric needs of the adolescent

Adolescent mental health–psychiatric nursing involves the care of adolescents, with particular emphasis on their emotional needs. Adolescence is a phase of development during the years of 12 to 20 when the individual experiences great surges of physical growth, engages in identity formation, and develops plans for the future. Adolescence is an accelerated age in which a sense of balance is needed but rarely achieved until adulthood. During the adolescent period the physical and emotional characteristics of adulthood emerge; and social, intellectual, and spiritual beginnings for the early years are sharpened, tested, and shaped for fuller use. Idealism, optimism, impatience, eagerness, and doubt characterize adolescence. Energies once turned outward to explore the world are now turned inward in introspection and self-analysis. The mind becomes capable of deep thoughts. Perceptual abilities broaden, and intellectual capabilities expand.

Adolescence serves several functions. Structurally, adolescence links childhood with adulthood. Although factors such as environment and training can intervene or be disruptive, development is usually characterized by continuity. Functionally, adolescence is a process within which physical, emotional, and intellectual growth prepares the individual for future roles: adult; sexual partner; parent; and responsible member of family, community, and society. As a process, adolescence unfolds systematically and, in spite of its chaotic appearance, occurs orderly and sequentially. When this sense of order is violated, the individual may require a health care professional to help restore order and

facilitate further growth and development of the disrupted process.

DSM-III-R DIAGNOSES

The DSM-III-R diagnoses related to pathological conditions in adolescence presented in this chapter include disruptive behavior and adolescent antisocial behavior. A discussion of the essential features of each of these pathological conditions follows.

Disruptive Behaviors

Disruptive behaviors are characterized by behavior that is socially disruptive and is often more distressing to others than to the person with the disorder. This classification of disorders includes conduct disorder and oppositional defiant disorder.

 DIAGNOSES Related to the Adolescent

MEDICAL DIAGNOSES
Disruptive behavior disorder
   Conduct disorders
   Oppositional defiant disorders
Adolescent antisocial disorder

DATES	EVENTS
Pre-1700s	Children and adolescents are treated as chattel and often used as slave labor. Harsh treatment is based on the biblical use of "spare the rod and spoil the child" and "children should be seen and not heard."
	The theological view of human nature encompasses ideas that humans and innate tendencies toward sinfulness, that people are basically bad, and that without severe discipline, they will become worse during the developmental years.
1700s	Stern discipline and moral rigidity are prevalent. People believe that children and adolescents are miniature adults.
	John Locke challenges the notion that adolescents are miniature adults and suggests that social conditions and environment influence the development of the adolescent's mind. He also sees adolescence as basically different from adulthood and as the period during which rational reasoning emerged.
	Rousseau emphasizes the adolescent's need to be free from the unnatural, strict discipline of the adult world and advocated treatment and education of adolescents as adolescents rather than as miniature adults.
1800s	Many families are moving to unexplored areas in the United States. Most adolescents marry during their teens and continue to be thought of as miniature adults. Before marriage many spend time working with their families in rural setting.
1835	A child labor law in Massachusetts requires that children attend school at least 3 months a year until they are 15.
	Manufacturers are not allowed to hire children to work in the mills for more than 9 months a year.
1900s	Children continue to be viewed as a cheap labor force and their use continues in factories.
1930	A White House Conference focuses on problem of child labor. Another such conference is held in 1950.
1970s	Nurse leaders contribute to changes in attitudes and clinical practice that focus specifically on adolescents: Claire Fagan (*Readings in Child and Psychiatric Nursing*, 1974), Shirley Smoyak (*The Psychiatric Nurse as a Family Therapist*, 1975), and Jeanne Howe (*Nursing Care of Adolescence*, 1980).
	Certification by the American Nurses' Association (ANA) recognize child and adolescent psychiatric–mental health nursing as a specialty area.
1980s	As society alters and expands its view and care of adolescents, nursing alters and expands its views of educational and clinical preparation of the professional nurse caring for adolescents. The increasing number of adolescent suicides today requires that nurses and other health professionals identify those adolescents at risk and that they intervene quickly with competence and confidence to prevent this tragic loss of life.
1990s	The problems associated with adolescence, such as alcoholism, drug abuse, pregnancy, sexuality, and bulimia, increase in number and severity and require more nurses with special knowledge, skills, and attitudes to work with both adolescents and their parents in this stage of development.
Future	Educational programs will continue to be developed and implemented, which may decrease the use of drugs and alcohol by adolescents.
	A family focus in providing nursing care to adolescents will become more prevalent as family nursing theories develop and their usefulness is identified.

Conduct disorder

The essential feature of conduct disorder is a persistent pattern of conduct in which the basic rights of others and age-appropriate societal norms are violated. The behavioral pattern is typically present in the home, at school, with peers, and in the community. Adolescents with this disorder are aggressive, may be physically cruel to others or to animals, and frequently destroy property. They may steal, mug, purse snatch, use extortion, or commit armed robbery. At older ages the violence may take the form of rape, assault, or homicide.

Stealing ranges from "borrowing" others' possessions, to shoplifting, forgery, and breaking and entering another's home or car. Lying and cheating in games and school work are common. Youngsters may be truant from school or run away from home. It is common for adolescents with this diagnosis to use tobacco, liquor, or nonprescribed drugs and to become sexually active earlier than their peers. In addition, they may have no concern for feelings and the well-being of others; behavior is callous, without feelings of guilt or remorse, and blame for misdeeds is placed on others.

Self-esteem is low, although adolescents may project an image of toughness. Other frequent characteristics include poor frustration tolerance, irritability, temper outbursts, and recklessness. Academic achievement often is below the expected level.

The criteria for severity of a conduct disorder include the following:

Mild	Demonstrates few conduct problems in excess of those required to make the diagnosis
Moderate	Demonstrates a number of conduct problems with mild to severe effect on other
Severe	Demonstrates many conduct problems in excess of those required to make the diagnosis or the conduct problems cause considerable harm to others (e.g., serious injury to victim, extensive vandalism, prolonged absence from home)

Conduct disorders may be of three types: (1) group type—behavior that occurs mainly in groups, (2) solitary aggressive type—involves physical aggression toward both peers and adults and initiated by the adolescent, and (3) undifferentiated type—a mixture of features that may be either the solitary or group type.

Oppositional defiant disorder

The essential feature of this disorder is a pattern of negativistic, hostile, and defiant behavior without the more serious violations of the basic rights of others that are seen in conduct disorder. The diagnosis is made only when oppositional and defiant behavior is much more common than that seen in others of the same mental age.

Characteristics commonly seen in this disorder include being argumentative with adults, frequently losing one's temper, swearing, resentful, and easily angered and annoyed by others. Adolescents may actively defy adult requests or rules and deliberately annoy others. They tend to blame others for their own mistakes. Evidence of the disorder is usually seen in the home and later extends into the community with peers or adults. The heavy use of tobacco and illegal psychoactive substances (alcohol, marijuana) is common.

Adolescent Antisocial Behavior

This diagnosis is made when the focus of treatment is antisocial behavior in an adolescent that is not due to a mental disorder such as conduct disorder. Examples include isolated antisocial acts that are not a pattern of behavior.

THEORETICAL APPROACHES

Biological

Hall[10] was the first psychologist to recognize adolescence as a unique developmental phase and to study it scientifically. He expanded Darwin's concept of biological evolution into a theory that included a four-stage division of development. Hall considered adolescence a period of "storm and stress," characterized by contradictory tendencies such as idealism versus selfishness, solitude versus friendship, and cooperation versus rebellion. Hall's theory of adolescence suggests that adolescence (1) is genetically determined and (2) occurs in a set pattern initiated by physiological factors. He underplayed the importance of cultural and environmental factors.

Psychoanalytical

Freud[9] proposed that psychosexual development occurs in genetically determined states that are independent of environmental factors. Sexual life begins not at puberty but earlier in life, with the first years being the most formative in terms of personality development and the later years being most formative in problem resolution. In this theory adolescence occurs between 13 and 18 years in the fifth, or genital, stage of development. During this stage sexual interest is reawakened because of physiological maturation, release of sex hormones, and sexual exploration. Two main developmental tasks are identified during this time: (1) the attainment of genital primacy, which includes detachment from the "incestuous object" (the parent) and forming an attachment with a nonincestuous object and (2) the establishment of a sense of balance between the self (ego), sexual drives (id), and parental and social mores (superego).

Erikson's eight developmental stages were modifications of Freud's emphasis on instinct.[6] According to Erikson, the main developmental task in the identity versus role diffusion phase is the acquisition of ego identify, during which the individual defines his ego identity. Self-concept, body image, sexual identity, vocation or career, and independence from parents are all facets of the adolescent's identity. Failure to develop ego identity results in role diffusion, creating trouble with sexual roles, social roles, choosing a career, separating from parents, and interpersonal relationships. An adolescent who enters young adulthood with a clear sense of identity can establish a mature relationship with a member of the opposite sex, choose a marital partner, and perform work and social roles.

Cognitive

Piaget focused on qualitative changes in intellectual structure from birth to maturity, with each structure being built on the previous one.[12] The integration of old into new provides continuity and development and leads to increasingly complex logical thought. During adolescence the individual is able to think abstractly, to reflect, and to use symbols in a variety of ways. The ability to reason increases, moral judgment is enhanced, and spiritual and religious beliefs are sought. As the adolescent increases his reasoning abilities, new understandings are considered. Problem solving and the ability to see a situation from more than one viewpoint becomes possible.

Sociocultural

Lewin[15] proposed that each person is surrounded by "life space," and the behavior within that life space is a function of the person within the space and the environment. Bio-

▼ **TABLE 37-1**   **Summary of Theories of Adolescence**

Theory	Theorist	Dynamics
Biological	Hall	Adolescence is genetically determined and occurs in patterned, universal stages regardless of environment.
Psychoanalytical	Freud	Adolescence occurs in the genital (psychosexual; predominately biological) stage of development, during which sexual interest is reawakened because of physical maturity.
	Erikson	The developmental stages of identity versus role diffusion occurs.
Cognitive	Piaget	By adolescence there is an ability to reason, to think abstractly, to reflect, and to use symbols in logical ways.
Sociocultural	Lewin	The task of adolescence is the transition from family group to peer group, from the child world to the adult world. Changes occur as a result of biological development and environmental influences.

logical, social, environmental, and emotional factors are interdependently related within the life space. The life space begins somewhat simply and develops complexity as these factors change. Adolescence is a period of transition when the life space becomes further differentiated. Lewin recognized that not only individual differences but also factors within the environment and within the social structure contribute to the life space changes. To understand an adolescent's behavior, the nurse must have some knowledge of the environment in which the behavior occurs. In Lewin's field theory,[15] the primary tasks of the adolescent include (1) transition of membership from family group to peer group; (2) transition of self-image as the body changes in unknown, unreliable, and unpredictable ways; and (3) transition from structured world of the child to the unstructured world of the adult. The transition consists mainly of changing membership from the child world to the adult world. During the time the adolescent straddles the border between the two worlds, the adolescent experiences a conflict in values, life-styles, and ideologies between the two worlds; experiences emotional and social tension; and has a readiness to take extreme positions and to change behavior radically and quickly, all of which are outgrowths of the differentiation and change within the life space.

Table 37-1 summarizes the theories of adolescence.

NURSING PROCESS

Assessment

Physical dimension According to Hall's biological theory, the early phase of adolescent development is often referred to as pubescence and is marked by physical changes in the male such as skeletal growth, enlargement of the testes, appearance of straight pigmented pubic hair, and early voice changes.[10] This stage is followed by the ability to ejaculate; kinky, pigmented pubic hair; maximum physical growth; the appearance of downy facial hair and axillary hair; and finally voice changes, coarse, pigmented hair, and chest hair. Although the age at which each of the body changes appears varies, the appearance of body changes represent the initial stages of adolescent devel-

opment. The sequential, orderly process of physical change is usually complete by the late teens or early twenties. Adolescent girls also undergo a similar orderly process of physical change: skeletal growth; breast development; and straight, pigmented pubic hair followed by maximal annual growth increment; kinky, pigmented pubic hair; menstruation; and the appearance of axillary hair.

According to Freud's psychoanalytical theory, adolescents, particularly boys, express both anxiety and curiosity about sexual development.[9] For example, masturbation, a minor interest in latent years, now increases. Although masturbation appears to be more prevalent in boys than girls, such activity is normal unless it is excessive, prohibits physical and social relations with others, or results in excessive guilt. Curiosity, experimentation, tension reduction, and pleasure all contribute to the adolescent's enhanced interest in sexual development. Discussion of penis size or breast development is common, with attempts made to equate virility and attractiveness with physical size and appearance.

Although adolescents are prone to comparing, rigid norms for physical development are difficult to establish because of the wide range of individual differences. This variability makes it difficult for the adolescent who develops earlier or later than his peers.

Regardless of the wide range of development, the nurse notes the adolescent's height, weight, system development, sexual development (breast buds, genital development, onset of menses), skin changes, and any anomalies that were previously undetected. Rapid growth may result in orthopedic problems, and absence of growth may signal endocrine deficits. A thorough family history of parents and siblings is needed to establish the family norm for growth and development. During the physical examination, the nurse can explore adolescent concerns about sexuality, school problems, peer pressure, or family difficulties.

In addition to history taking and physical examination, the nurse asks the adolescent information regarding a typical day. The day is described in detail for a 24-hour cycle, including number of hours slept, soundness of sleep, time of rising, breakfast, morning activities, after-school activities, return home, supper, evening activities (family, school, church), friends visited, games attended, and bedtime and associated activities such as bathing. One may need to compile activities of several days before a representative day is profiled. This information gives the nurse an overall picture of the adolescent's physical health practices. Alterations in patterns from the norm need to be investigated more fully.

Patterns that emerge in the adolescent's typical day are diagnostic in their deviation from the norm. The depressed or anxious adolescent may report uneasy sleep and early awakening. Eating patterns and meal habits often become bizarre in the adolescent, developing into anorexia or bulimia nervosa. Activity patterns are useful in diagnosing the socially withdrawn, isolated, or shy adolescent and the adolescent who is abusing drugs or alcohol. Adolescents use drugs and alcohol for reasons such as experimentation, boredom, curiosity, and most frequently peer pressure. They are often introduced to drugs and alcohol by an older sibling, parent, or older peer. Most adolescents use drugs and alcohol as a form of relaxation, occasionally for experimentation, or at parties. When drugs are used in excess, school performance, social relations, and family life are often harmed. The substance abusing adolescent often appears disinterested, lethargic, easily distracted, irritable, and moody. School performance and social relations hit highs and lows in relation to periods of substance abuse. Addiction to drugs or heavy reliance on alcohol may cause the adolescent to become abusive, hostile, and difficult to manage. The adolescent who abuses drugs and alcohol may be impulsive and self-destructive and often draws attention to himself through such acts.

The nurse asks herself, to what extent do the adolescent's habits and patterns seem to promote health, and to what extent do these patterns deviate from health. Patterns that reflect deviations often appear disorganized, are difficult to chart, and may vary widely. In contrast, healthy patterns present an overall consistent picture with a balance among sleep, exercise, eating, eliminating, and use of leisure time.

In assessing the physical dimension the nurse determines whether and to what extent the adolescent falls within the normal range of development as described by Erikson's developmental theory[6]; where the adolescent is within the sequential development of body changes; to what extent sexuality (masturbation, ejaculation, menstruation) is a concern; to what extent chronic health problems such as juvenile diabetes are affected by the onset of adolescence; to what extent physical changes or patterns are accompanied by alterations in mood; and to what extent overall patterns seem to promote and support healthy physical development.

Emotional dimension Emotionally, adolescence is a time of highs and lows. One day the adolescent may be happy and outgoing. Later, the adolescent may be crying and worried that he has no friends and is understood by no one (see the research highlight). One moment the adolescent may feel good about himself and the next moment express self-doubt and lack of self-confidence. According to Erikson's theory of development, the adolescent exists within a whirlwind of emotional change and unpredictability, particularly from ages 12 to 15 years.[6] After that time the emotions even out, the adolescent is more trusting of his feelings, and the periods of unpredictability are spaced further apart.

The physical aspects of adolescent development are difficult to separate fully from the emotional aspects because much of the emotional development is linked with physical and sexual changes. Body image, concern for physical appearance, ability to attract the opposite sex, and sensing oneself as appealing is integral to the adolescent's acceptance of himself as attractive (Figure 37-1). Skin blemishes,

RESEARCH HIGHLIGHT

Loneliness in Early Adolescence: An Empirical Test of Alternative Explanations

• N Mahon and A Yarcheski

PURPOSE

The purpose of this research was to study two explanations of loneliness, situational or characterological theory.

SAMPLE

Subjects included 112 boys and girls between the ages of 12 to 14 years of age.

METHODOLOGY

Subjects were asked to complete the Revised UCLA Loneliness Scale as well as instruments that measured the situational or the characterological explanations of loneliness.

FINDINGS

Results of this research study showed that situational loneliness (62%) is a more important variable than loneliness related to the characterological variable (33%).

IMPLICATIONS

The adolescent client experiencing loneliness and his family may need the assistance of the professional nurse to look at situational factors contributing to feelings of loneliness. For example, the adolescent who comes home every day to an empty house because both parents work may need to have scheduled activities immediately after school with peers, as well as have scheduled individual time with parents. The adolescent often expresses a desire to be more independent. As a result, the nurse can help the adolescent share feelings of loneliness with the parents so that they can plan to be more available.

From *Nursing Research* 37:330, 1988.

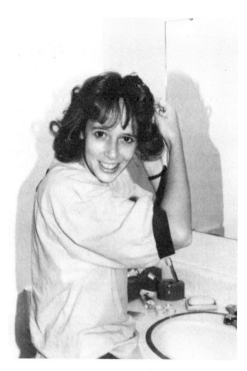

FIGURE 37-1 The adolescent's concern with physical attractiveness is related to emotional development and sexual changes.

uncoordinated body movements, and physiological functions that are unpredictable and beyond conscious control, such as erections or menstruation, induce anxiety. While the adolescent is struggling with emotional control, the body's demands require energy; the adolescent responds to physical changes with fear and anxiety. Anxiety can take many forms, ranging from an occasional sleepless night to excessive thinking and worrying about real as well as fantasized problems.

Anxiety often occurs around individual lags or extreme variations in growth and development. A year or two in the life of adults is a small segment of time; however, the same 2 years can seem much more important to adolescents, who may be worried and confused about their development. The adolescent often asks the question, "Am I normal?" Fears of not being normal, especially related to sexuality, can lead to anxiety and to acting out.

Emotional instability is indicated by a number of symptoms: inability to sleep; disrupted eating patterns (too much or too little); altered relations with friends and peers, especially withdrawal; increased and unexplained conflict with family members; preoccupation with body functions; abrupt and unexplained mood swings; and inability to gain control over impulses. The degree to which such changes are present indicates the severity of the emotional problem. For example, inability to sleep may indicate stress associated with an impending examination. When combined with other symptoms, an underlying depression may be suspected.

Clinical depression in the adolescent can manifest itself in a number of ways:

1. Withdrawal

2. Acting out
3. Angry outbursts
4. School problems
5. Sexual difficulties
6. Running away
7. Inability to pay attention
8. Flat affect
9. Lack of hope
10. Poor self-regard
11. Negative attitude
12. Loss of interest in usual activities
13. Changes in physical appearance
14. Mood changes
15. Appetite changes
16. Marked decrease or sudden increase in physical or social activities
17. Unpredictable patterns of behavior

When depression is related to a specific event, such as the death of a parent, it is normally considered a transitory adjustment problem resulting in unhappiness, tearfulness, nervousness, irritability, and possibly school problems. Such depression generally occurs from 3 to 9 months after the specific event and does not significantly affect family or social relationships.

Depression may also occur without any apparent link to a specific event, in which case a chronic pattern of low self-esteem, feelings of worthlessness, and a pervasive sense of failure may be triggered by some minor and unrelated situation. This type of depression is manifested by sleeplessness, loss of appetite, lack of interest in physical appearance, decreased productivity at home and school, and feelings of hopelessness and may result in excessive use of alcohol, drugs, or suicide attempts.

An anxious adolescent may experience some of the same symptoms as the depressed adolescent, such as distractibility, fears about the future, and irritability. However, the anxious adolescent does not experience symptoms to the extent exhibited in depression, does not experience muted or blunted affect, has sleepless nights only occasionally, and generally overcomes the problem in a shorter time.

Like depression, anxiety can result from direct changes in the adolescent's life such as frequent moves or parental discord. Anxiety, self-doubt, and identity confusion can also occur unrelated to any specific event. A 5-year critical incident survey is helpful. The survey compiles information about critical incidents or events, such as death of a grandparent, divorce of parents, or severe physical illness, that may require emotional adaptation and coping and determines the extent to which these events preceded the onset of symptoms or problems. Symptoms and the onset of problems can occur anywhere from 3 months to 2 years after such events. The survey can be taken with the adolescent and with family members, since the adolescent may not fully remember all events (see the box on p. 755).

The degree of change in overall functioning, including perception of and reaction to reality, differentiates the emotionally anxious from the more severely troubled adolescent. Adolescence has been described as a time of "natural craziness," when acting out and weirdness are typical teen behavior. However, when acting out occurs in more than transitory periods or when anxiety severely impedes the ability to function socially, academically, or in terms of

▼ ··

FIVE-YEAR CRITICAL INCIDENT SURVEY

Instructions

Try to recall the important things that happened to you or your family at 5-year intervals. Which events stand out in your mind as being the most significant? What do you remember most about these incidents?

Stages

Birth to 5 years:
6 to 10 years:
11 to 15 years:
16 to 20 years:

Problem

What is the relationship between the events or series of events and emotional problems that have developed? Did emotional problems appear within 3 months to 2 years of any one event?

---

personal care, the degree of disturbance is greater than typical teen behavior.

Assessment of the adolescent's emotional dimension involves developing an overall profile of emotional development. In regard to suspected emotional problems such as anxiety, angry and hostile behavior, or depression accompanied by feelings of worthlessness and hopelessness, the nurse determines the extent of the impairment and assesses the relationship between specific events that have occurred and the problems that the adolescent is experiencing.

Intellectual dimension Projection of one's own internal state onto others is most prevalent during adolescence. Adolescents find it difficult to trust others because they do not trust or understand their own feelings. This lack of trust and concerns is related to an uncertainty regarding the future and causes adolescents to project onto others a lack of understanding. "You don't understand me" is often a camouflaged way of saying that "I don't really understand myself; therefore how could you possibly understand me?" Just as uncertainty is associated with feeling states, actions that stem from these feelings are often considered by the adolescent to be unpredictable. The adolescent expressing his anger will say, "If I told my old man what I really thought, he'd knock my block off." Although the adolescent may be correctly predicting his father's response, a greater probability is that the adolescent fears that he himself will lose control, and reads this possibility into his father's behavior.

Using Piaget's theory, the adolescent develops an increased ability to think abstractly, to reason, and to understand at higher levels. Such heightened intellectual abilities compete with intense and distracting physical and emotional changes. The early years of adolescence are particularly troublesome because great surges of physical growth and sexual development and the increasing awareness of the self as a separate entity develop simultaneously. Lewin[15] describes the adolescent at this time as making the transition from his family group to his peer group. Success in this transition allows the adolescent to develop a separate identity from the family.

During this phase, the adolescent's energies are divided among the various facets of personality development. However, according to Piaget's cognitive theory, as adolescence progresses the ability to think critically, to reason rationally, to probe into unknown areas, and to engage in intellectual and philosophical debates increases.[12] The vigorous debates in which adolescents engage often seem pointless to the adult because of the adolescent's preoccupation with the debates themselves and overall lack of concern for any direct action based on the outcomes of the debates. This is a time of asking, "Why doesn't someone do something about the poor...the disabled...the elderly...foreign countries?" while saying, "I don't know why we have to go to Grandmother's house every Sunday. There isn't anything to do there." The adolescent can usually better cope with personal inconsistencies in behavior and thinking than adults, primarily because adolescents tend to ignore such inconsistencies. When an adult focuses attention on these inconsistencies, heated arguments tend to occur.

The best gauge of the adolescent's intellectual functioning is the overall academic record. One also assesses the home environment, the cultural background, and the role models available to the adolescent. Despite individual differences, however, the adolescent's grade point average, motivation, achievement, and classroom performance are often indicators not only of intelligence but also of emotional states. The troubled adolescent often signals a need by altering his patterns of classroom performance, acting out, picking fights, being tardy, demonstrating a loss of interest, and achieving lower grades.

Alterations in classroom behavior do not always signal acute or chronic episodes of mental illness; however, this is a critical time when previously undetected problems may appear. Classroom performance can signal many other problems, including use and abuse of alcohol or drugs; family problems; personal adjustment problems; fears or concerns about pregnancy, impotence, or venereal disease; unresolved grief process; or simply concerns regarding the future. Whatever the source of the problem, classroom behavior is a critical signal that requires further investigation by observing and interviewing the adolescent, the family, and when appropriate, school personnel and peers. Peers and peer group relations can provide valuable information about the adolescent. Changes in classroom behavior may be accompanied by changes in social relationships. Because the social clique often provides the adolescent with a sense of support and a testing ground for reality, any changes in these relationships are viewed with concern.

Social dimension A prevalent problem encountered in adolescence is the inability to answer the question, "Who am I?" The adolescent with an identity crisis or conflict has not been able to find a sense of self and experiences much uncertainty about future goals, friendships, sexual orientation, and spiritual beliefs. This adolescent may express a desire to pursue goals but is unable to undertake direct actions to achieve those goals.

The nurse may ask the following questions to confront adolescents experiencing identity problems.
- What are your fantasies about yourself?
- Where do you see yourself in 3 years?
- If you could be anything or anyone, who would you be and what would you be doing?

Power struggles with parents and other authority figures are an outgrowth of the search for identity, a need to test and experiment with the limits of power. In an attempt to experience themselves as adults or nearly adults, adolescents often overstep the limits of their own ability. The obedient, cooperative adolescent may become a rebellious, argumentative, disobedient person who refuses to abide by curfews, insists on driving at breakneck speeds, and loses any and all interest in being part of the family, particularly refusing to engage in family activities. Family life and the interactions between the adolescent and family members are significant to the adolescent's development of autonomy, independence, self-esteem, and ability to communicate consistently and congruently outside the family. Disturbance in these relationships and inability to get along with parents can both affect the adolescent's peer relations. Alterations in peer relations, running away, aggressive and hostile acts, and symptoms of anxiety and depression can be the outcome of parent-child conflict.

Parent-child conflict is more prevalent in families with economic problems, marital discord, chronic physical health problems, inadequate sexual identities, and poor communication skills. Parent-child conflict can be minor (disagreements, irritability, and lack of communication) or more severe (angry outbursts, loud screaming matches, failure to communicate, unreasonable and restrictive discipline measures, and physical or emotional abuse).

Increasing conflict often erupts between the adolescent and younger siblings who are suddenly a source of embarrassment and a constant reminder of that which the adolescent has just experienced (childhood). Sibling rivalry during the adolescent years can be intense and severe. At the same time, the adolescent can be loyal and supportive. Many of the adolescent's uncertainties are vented on siblings, yet rarely with the awareness of or intent to do harm.

Adolescents are often ambivalent about intimacy, wanting to be close but fearing the loss of self. They feel engulfed by their own emotional intensity but project the feeling of engulfment onto others, particularly close friends or members of the opposite sex. The need to nurture and be nurtured is strong in the adolescent; however, the fear of commitment and being "tied down" that accompany such feelings is also strong. Unable to work out a balance, the adolescent may engage in excessive sexual activity or may become socially withdrawn. Acting out or promiscuity is often evidence of strong, unmet emotional needs, just as shyness and social isolation can be evidence of the same unmet needs and require sensitive assessment.

Acting out is characterized in the early stages by conflict at school, for example, minor and repeated infractions of rules that result in the student's being sent to the principal or having to serve detentions. Acting out is also characterized by conflict with parents, usually resulting in fights over curfews or minor scrapes with community authority figures. At this stage the adolescent is considered to be engaging in antisocial behavior by minor infractions of social and family norms. The adolescent may progress from the antisocial stage of acting out to repeated and more severe forms of rule breaking such as shoplifting, drinking excessively, driving at excessive speeds, street fights, or burglary.

Adolescents who engage in repeated patterns of breaking social and legal rules are often manipulative, distort the truth, run in gangs, create problems with peers, and become hostile and aggressive when confronted by authority figures. Without help, these adolescents become chronic rule breakers and difficult to reach. In later years they may engage in more serious rule breaking and later criminal behavior.

In the early stages this behavior signals the need for professional help for either the adolescent or the family. More courts are assigning these adolescents and their families to therapy early in the process to prevent acting-out, antisocial behavior from becoming a more severe conduct disorder.

The adolescent does not have a fully developed sense of consequences. Without life experiences to fall back on, the adolescent engages in behavior that often seems dangerous and self-defeating, for example, having sex without birth control, driving down a main highway with the lights of the car turned off, and refusing to take examinations because "tests are all stupid anyway." Most adolescents engage in some risky behavior, but the adolescent who consistently engages in such behaviors is not only experiencing emotional turmoil but also losing control of it. The adolescent who constantly engages in dangerous and self-destructive behavior is asking for help to cope with changes that have gone beyond his control. The research highlight on p. 757 examines coping styles used by adolescents.

▼ Case Example

Don is 15 years old. For his birthday his parents gave him a motor bike, which he used to jump ditches and drive down railroad tracks.

Don is having trouble accepting the responsibility of the motorbike but is asking for help in controlling his behavior. In essence he says, "I'm a gambler. I'm out to see if I can beat life at its own game." Don has an unrealistic and self-destructive need to pit himself against powerful forces, probably hoping that someone will stop him and set the limits that he cannot set for himself.

Loneliness, fear of intimacy, and the strong need for comfort can lead to a number of problems, including obesity from oral attempts to be self-nurturing; sexual promiscuity in which sexual behavior is used to attain closeness; delinquency in a social attempt to gain recognition; and conflicts with authorities in an attempt to gain attention and even acceptance. Erikson says that a boy prefers to be a bad boy than no boy at all. By this he means that an adolescent seeks to establish an identity, even a negative identity, rather than think he is like no one at all, unnoticed and unrecognized. Lack of recognition and notice is often equated with lack of love by adolescents. Without recognition and the emotional support that comes with notice, the adolescent has trouble developing a positive, self-accepting identity.

The adolescent strives for a competent and stable sense of self. Through such development the adolescent experiences a wide range of feelings, on one hand, believing he is able, strong, and competent and, on the other hand, believing he is powerless, helpless, and vulnerable.

The adolescent strives to achieve balance among a number of competing forces, including physical change and emotional upheaval, identity development with internal fears of rejection, a need for autonomy, and a sense of

RESEARCH HIGHLIGHT

Adolescent Coping Styles and Behaviors: Conceptualization and Measurement

- J Patterson and H McCubbin

PURPOSE

The purpose of this study was to construct, develop, and test the validity of a tool measuring coping styles and behaviors of adolescents.

SAMPLE

Subjects included 709 adolescents and 509 families who were enrolled in a large health maintenance organization in the Midwest. Fifty-eight percent of the sample was 12 to 13 years old, 34% were 14 to 18 years old, and 8% were 11 years old.

FINDINGS

The 12 coping styles described by adolescents include ventilating feelings; seeking diversions; developing self-reliance and optimism; using social support; using spiritual support; solving family problems; seeking professional support; using humorous activities; demanding work activity; relaxing; and close friends. Boys tended to use humor more frequently than girls, whereas girls reported using social support, close friends, family, and developing self reliance more frequently than boys.

Based on data from the *Journal of Adolescence* 10:163, 1987.

IMPLICATIONS

The professional nurse can use this information on coping styles when assisting the adolescent to learn new ways to deal with problems or stressful experiences. The adolescent needs to build a wide variety of coping strategies, and discussing these commonly used ways of handling stress may assist the client to find new or more successful strategies that are better suited to his or her situation.

---

closeness. When the balance is achievable and reachable, the adolescent often maneuvers successfully toward a competent sense of self. When this is not possible, emotional problems may result.

One task the adolescent faces is the transition from family group to peer group, during which the adolescent strives for autonomy and a sense of individual freedom. This striving for individuality is a concern on one level; on another level, adolescents want very much to be like their peers. An 18-year-old client expressed such concern by saying, "All my parents ever wanted for me was to be different. All I ever wanted was to be like my friend." However, while striving for autonomy and associated freedom, the adolescent struggles with the need to be dependent on others. Following is a typical interview:

Client: My parents never give me any responsibility. I don't know how my parents expect me to make any decisions. I don't have any experience (pause). My parents don't trust me.

Nurse: I'm wondering what you have done to make them feel that way.

Client: Nothing. (pause). I got drunk and wrecked the family car, but that was 2 months ago.

The nurse needs to ask the question, "How autonomous can an adolescent realistically hope to be, given the particular individual ability and set of circumstances in which the adolescent lives?" One observation the nurse can make is of the family atmosphere regarding individual independence.

▼ Case Example

The Robinson family brought their 16-year-old daughter, Megan, for counseling. They are concerned that she is not demonstrating the "independence" required of her to go to college in 2 years. Megan is the youngest of three children (two older brothers) of parents in their mid-50s. The parents' expressed concern is that Megan needs to gain and demonstrate independence at home and in her social life to show that she is dependable before she can earn privileges. However, observations of and sessions with the family reveal a conflict. When Megan asks to date, her father refuses because the "boy is too old." When Megan wants to go shopping to buy a dress for the school dance, her mother tells her she is "too young to be picking out her own clothes." When Megan goes out after a football game on Friday night and doesn't come home until 1 AM (curfew is midnight), an older brother calls home from college the next day to ask Megan how she could be so "inconsiderate" and "worry" her parents.

Although the parents express concern that Megan lacks independence and cannot be trusted, their unexpressed fear is that she will become too independent, too self-sufficient. Their inconsistency is a barrier to her independence. The parents say that they want Megan to grow up; however, they are highly invested in keeping her a little girl. Both parents are indirectly threatened by Megan's increasing independence and undermine her every attempt to successfully break away from their domination.

In assessing the adolescent's striving for independence, the nurse examines the emotional tenor in the family. She looks for warmth, authentic expression of feelings, honest exchange and communication, unconditional positive regard for one another, a physical expression of affection, expectations appropriate for age and experience, encouragement and support for individual aims, and support or conflict in allowing and providing the disagreement and argument. Especially important is the congruence of communication, that is, a consistent pattern in which what is said is congruent with what is done and in which underlying messages are brought out in talk and action.

Within the peer group the adolescent practices being independent and works to resolve the quest for freedom with the need for intimacy. The peer group serves as an important testing ground. In a sense the peer group becomes a subculture. Members of the peer group compete, tease, and test one another. But they also share their confusion and fear associated with breaking away. The adolescent is extremely loyal and expects a sense of justice in the peer group.

An adolescent reared in an open family will have a greater opportunity to seek and establish an individual identity than will an adolescent reared in a rule-dominated family. The warm, supportive, accepting family fosters adolescent development that is outgoing, socially active, and independent, whereas the rule-dominated authoritarian family produces adolescents who lack self-confidence, experience low self-esteem, and express themselves in rebellious ways. Rebellious behavior, social withdrawal, poor school performance, and overall lack of adjustment may be manifestations of a rigid family atmosphere.

At the other extreme is the family with no rules and little if any interest in the children. Adolescents from such homes may develop strong identities in spite of such indifference but more often are poorly motivated, indifferent to others, confused, and lacking in self-worth. The formation of a positive identity and a sense of autonomy is difficult at best in either a family that is excessively rule oriented or one in which emotional indifference is the norm.

The peer group is a safety net, above which the adolescent can play out the drama of fantasized relationships, can establish intimate and nonintimate relationships, is able to experience the social aspects of the personality, and practices the sexual aspects of personality development.

Adolescents seem to spend an inordinate amount of time with one another, which leads some authors to label this period of time as *pseudohomosexuality* because adolescents often prefer the company of members of the same sex. The company of one another helps them to avoid the anxiety of establishing a relationship with a member of the opposite sex. On the other hand, adolescents spend a great amount of time in mixed groups. The pressure is great among adolescents to be sexual partners to justify spending time together, to have a date on Friday night, and to avoid the anxiety of being alone and lonely.

Although a sense of loyalty is great within the peer group, intimate relationships can be transitory and brief; best friends may exchange best friends. Some adolescents can remain friends through such exchanges, others cannot. It is a learning experience in the building and maintaining of relationships.

How adolescents select the peer group within which to build relationships is not well known. Adolescents can be attracted to someone similar to them in terms of family background, religion, and social status, just as they can be attracted to someone from differing family, class, and religious backgrounds. The importance of peer group relationships is that adolescents have a group with whom they can relate, be with someone they feel understands them, and have someone with whom they can practice testing reality. Without this source of support and reality testing, the adolescent may learn to rely on an untested, internal fantasy world.

Through peer relations, the adolescent examines and explores topics that parents find embarrassing, repulsive, silly, or frightening, such as sex, war, death, and divorce. Whereas parents often assume that adolescents are unaware of or turned off by what goes on around them, adolescents are deeply affected by social and political issues in a way that often influences their outlook on life. No topic is taboo.

The adolescent is intrigued by life and death and may even fantasize his own death. An adolescent may say that "I'm sure I won't live past 20." It is perhaps an unconscious recognition that the person before the age of 20 is not the same person after his twentieth birthday; a certain amount of grief needs to be resolved when one leaves adolescence, just as when one leaves childhood. The peer group also helps in this transition.

The peer group helps establish acceptable norms of behavior, provides an arena for testing new behaviors and exploring old ones, and aids in the development of healthy coping skills in managing the struggle for independence. Of parental conflict about independence, adolescents often say that "It's only a stage your parents are going through. They'll get over it by the time you're a senior." In the "us against them" attitude of the adolescent against the parent, the adolescent when pushed will often choose the friend over the family member. The friend is an extension of the self—the good self and the bad self—and the adolescent will go to great lengths to protect and defend this fragile projection of self.

The adolescent who fails to make the transition from the family group to the adolescent group will experience difficulty separating from family later and may exhibit signs of social isolation and lack social interactive skills. The loner, the adolescent who rejects and is rejected by his peer group, may experience difficulty in later establishing long-term intimate relationships because the "practice time" was lost during the adolescent peer group experimentation.

Suicide and attempted suicide are alarming problems that occur often among adolescents. Fear of failure, pressure to achieve, excessive concern for material gain, lack of acceptance among peers, and parent-child conflict all contribute to teenage suicide. The three most important factors that contribute to suicide are family disorganization and marital discord between parents, family history of emotional disturbance with attempted suicides, and adolescent use of and abuse of drugs and alcohol.

The suicidal adolescent may show previous symptoms of disturbance such as poor school performance; drunkenness; or incurring traffic fines, especially for excessive speed or reckless driving. The suicidal adolescent may make an apparently sudden and unexpected attempt at wrecking a car, drinking and driving, or physical recklessness with guns. Or the adolescent may engage in long-term self-destruction such as excessive use of drugs and alcohol, which

TABLE 37-2   Warning Signs of Suicide

Warning Sign	Example
Change in personality	From studious or withdrawn to the class clown; from an actively participating student to one who drops out of all activities
Sudden moods swings	Persistent ups and downs
Inability to concentrate, apathy	Declining grades, loss of interest in school
Loss of or dramatic change in friends	Dropping friends or becoming so obnoxious that friends drop him
Loss of important person or thing	Parents' divorce or death, remarriage of parent, loss of boyfriend or girlfriend, removed from team
Feelings of hopelessness	Inability to get pleasure from any activity; loss of interest in appearance, in opposite sex: "What's the use?" attitude
Obsession with death	Suicidal threats, taking big risks, frequent accidents
Completing personal or business affairs	Unusual display of affection or generosity; giving away favorite records or tapes; making a will

borders on social suicide but may go undetected until a more drastic step is taken that brings the adolescent professional help. Table 37-2 lists the warning signs that may alert the nurse to a possible suicide attempt by an adolescent.

In assessing the social aspect of development, the nurse determines the people with whom the adolescent spends time, the groups to which he belongs, the kind of part-time job at which he works, and the kinds of relationships he has formed outside the family. The nurse is also interested in the following:

1. The extent to which relationships are enduring or transitory
2. The amount and quality of time spent with friends
3. The extent to which the adolescent is sexually active and, if active, the extent to which birth control and venereal disease protection are maintained
4. How active or passive a role the adolescent takes in making friends, keeping friends, and changing relationships
5. The amount of conflict between adolescent and parents regarding friends and social activities in which the adolescent participates
6. The amount of peer pressure that the adolescent feels in terms of social, sexual, and other activities

Spiritual dimension Spiritually, the adolescent seeks to understand the meaning of life and uses this understanding to approach present and future decisions. This searching takes many forms such as questioning parental beliefs, rejecting institutionalized religion, sampling differ-

ing religious beliefs, comparing religious and philosophical beliefs of peers, and examining one's own beliefs. Adolescents often ask "What is life all about anyway?" This age is perhaps the first time in the life cycle that the individual realizes that life is not forever, that humans are mortal, and that, in adolescence, life is beginning to take on a new seriousness.

Several opposing and contradictory beliefs can be held simultaneously by the adolescent. For example, the adolescent may strongly believe that all people (particularly oneself) should have the right to think and act in a unique and personal way. However, teachers and classroom instructors are often made fun of in a way that reflects intolerance and insensitivity. The adolescent strives to develop a belief system by seeing the world in a "me" and "not me" framework. If the situation is one with which the adolescent can identify, then it makes sense. However, if the adolescent cannot identify with the situation, then the situation is viewed as irrelevant. This perception results from the adolescent's lack of experience and underdeveloped ability to see any position other than his own. Empathy and a view of the world that includes the other person's perspective come after many years of life experiences.

The adolescent develops philosophical beliefs through trial and error as life experiences are collected. It is the age of the ideal, of heroes, and of perfection. The adolescent looks for the perfect parent, mate, class, friend, religion, and sense of self. It is a time of periodic disappointment when the perfect friend, parent, or hero makes mistakes, disagrees with what the adolescent thinks or believes, or does something to make the adolescent feel let down. The adolescent may respond to such fallibility with transitory disappointment, in which case other heroes are found and other ideals sought. On the other hand, the adolescent may react with confusion, bitterness, despair, and caution about finding replacements.

The adolescent is often confused by others' inconsistent behavior, particularly when this behavior is an outgrowth of an underlying value, such as the parent who espouses honesty and intentionally fails to report income for tax purposes, the coach who instructs players in fairness and then pushes them to win at all costs, or the teacher who talks about equality but selects only a few favored students for recognition. The adolescent holds loyalty, fairness, and honesty important and looks for examples of how to implement these qualities in daily practice.

Most adults in the adolescent's environment become fair game to use as examples. Parents' lifelong beliefs and practices are questioned and tested, as are spiritual beliefs with which the adolescent has been reared. Part of the examination often results in temporary rejection of such beliefs, and the adolescent practices this rejection by attending services less often and questioning parental commitment to such practices. In later years the belief system of many adolescents will be similar to that of their parents despite protests and early rejections.

At the same time that the adolescent is challenging, testing, and perhaps rejecting social and religious norms, he holds firmly to a moral and peer-oriented code that guides behavior. This code can be identified as the nurse presents the adolescent with a set of hypothetical situations that are social, family, or peer oriented but that require a set of

▼ HOLISTIC ASSESSMENT TOOL FOR ADOLESCENTS

Physical Dimension
Genetic history

Who in your family has had any of the following mental or emotional illnesses?
depression
suicide
drug addiction
schizophrenia

Health history

What illnesses, injuries, hospitalizations, or surgeries, have you had?

Growth and development history

Describe your physical growth.
Describe your sexual growth.
Tell me about your experiences in kindergarten, elementary school, high school, college, or work.

Activities of daily living

Describe your typical day beginning with when you get up in the morning through the day until you go to bed at night.

Diet and elimination

What changes in your appetite and weight have occurred and over what period of time?
What problems are you having with elimination?

Exercise and activity

What kinds of activities do you participate in? How often? For how long?
What kinds of exercise do you participate in? How often? For how long?

Sleep and rest

How many hours of sleep do you get? Is it adequate?
What difficulties do you have going to sleep or staying asleep?

Tobacco, drugs, alcohol

How much do you smoke?
What drugs or medication do you take?
How much alcohol do you drink? What kinds of alcohol?
In what ways do drugs or alcohol interfere with your daily activities?

Leisure activities

What do you do for fun and recreation?

General appearance

The nurse notes any unusual physical characteristics, the style of dress, grooming, gait and posture, and general behavior.

Body image

Describe yourself physically.
What do you think about your body?
How do you feel about your body?
Do you see yourself as normal?
What would you change about your body if you could?

Sexuality

What are your worries, concerns about your sexual self?
What problems are you having with menstruation, birth control, erections, intercourse, or masturbation?
What is your sexual preference?

Emotional Dimension
Affect

What is the adolescent's affect?
How appropriate is his affect?

Mood

What is your predominant mood?
Do you have mood swings?
How well do you control your emotions?
How well do you express your feelings?
What are your fears and anxieties?
Are you depressed, suicidal, angry?
Do you feel hopeless?
What are your coping skills?

Intellectual Dimension
Sensation and perception

Do you see, hear, feel, smell, or taste things that others do not?
Do you believe that your actions are outside your control?
How realistically does he perceive events and situations?

Memory

Immediate: Ask adolescent to repeat a question you asked.
Recent: Ask for events leading up to the adolescent's seeking help.
Remote: Ask for descriptions of events in the adolescent's early childhood.

Cognition

Is the adolescent oriented to time, place, person?
What is his knowledge of current events?
How well is he functioning academically?

Judgment

How does the adolescent make decisions?

Insight

Does the adolescent recognize that he is ill and needs help?
How much does he blame others for his difficulties?
How much awareness does he have of the impact of his behavior on others?

Abstract thinking

What is the adolescent's style of thinking, concrete or abstract?

Attention

What is the adolescent's ability to listen and concentrate?

Communication

What is the rate of speech?
What is the tone of speech?
Does the adolescent have any speech impediments?
Is he verbally active?
Does he respond freely to questions?
Are his responses relevant?
How well organized are his thoughts?
Does he demonstrate blocking, circumstantially, tangentiality, flight of ideas, loose association, neologisms?

Flexibility-rigidity

How open to new ideas and alternatives is the adolescent?
How upset does he get when his routine is disrupted?

HOLISTIC ASSESSMENT TOOL FOR ADOLESCENTS—cont'd

Social Dimension

Self-concept

Describe yourself, including your strengths and limitations.
What kind of person would you like to be?

Interpersonal relations

Who is your best friend?
How do you get along with your parents, your brothers and sisters, your
    peers, and people at school, at work, and in the community?
How much time do you spend with your family?
Who is supportive for you?
How do you get along with authority figures?

Cultural factors

What traditions do you and your family observe?
What conflicts arise from these traditions?

Environmental factors

What situations or events are stressful for you?
In what risk-taking events do you participate?

Level of socialization

How conforming or nonconforming is the adolescent?
What evidence is there of legal difficulties?
How well does he accept responsibility?

Trust-mistrust

How suspicious is the adolescent?
How naive is the adolescent?

Dependence-independence

What evidence is there of dependence-independence conflicts?
In what areas does the adolescent demonstrate autonomy?
In what areas does he demonstrate dependence?

Spiritual Dimension

Philosophy of life

What is the purpose of life?
What is important about life to you?
Who is your hero?

Sense of transcendence

Are you an optimist or a pessimist?
Do you think life can be better?
What can you do to make it better?

Concept of deity

What is your view of God or a higher power?
How similar is it to your parents' or family's view?
How comforting is your relationship with God or a higher power?

Spiritual fulfillment

What is beautiful to you?
What are your creative abilities?
What do you believe about life and death?
Are you preoccupied with religion?
What conflicts arise from your religious beliefs?
How much do you question or reject your parents' beliefs?
How do you implement your own belief system?

---

values and beliefs to arrive at a solution, as in the following examples:

Richard, a 13-year-old boy, has been caught shoplifting. Should he (1) be kicked out of school, (2) be grounded for 6 weeks, (3) be lectured by his parents, or (4) be turned over to the police and let them handle it? What is the most important aspect of this solution?

Robert, a 15 year-old boy, has been smoking marijuana on the school grounds. Would you (1) ignore his behavior, (2) tell his older brother, (3) report it to the principal or a teacher, or (4) keep your mouth shut?

Patricia, a 14-year-old, is going steady with Bill, a senior in high school. He wants her to "go all the way" with him. If she refuses, Bill tells her he will find someone else. Should Patricia (1) have sex with Bill, (2) tell Bill no and accept the consequences, (3) get Bill's best friend to reason with him, or (4) ignore the situation and hope that Bill forgets about it? Why?

In listening to the adolescent's response to situations involving shoplifting, substance abuse, and sexual behavior, the nurse assesses the guiding belief or set of beliefs that compels the adolescent to select a particular option, the primary values that the adolescent is trying to uphold by acting in certain ways, and the compromises the adolescent is forced to make when the options are limited. An adolescent with strong religious beliefs about birth control and sex outside marriage may feel forced to choose between such beliefs and the strong need for intimacy and physical

closeness. The same adolescent who later becomes pregnant may be forced to choose again between the value that says that life must be preserved and the value that is critical of the unwed mother.

The nurse assesses themes of fairness, honesty, loyalty, sanctity of family, authority of parents, and peer pressure (resistance or acceptance) that appear and reappear in the solutions that the adolescent chooses. An adolescent's ability to resist peer pressure is often based on a set of beliefs and convictions that operate despite such pressure. It is frequently a conviction that has been debated, argued, challenged, and perhaps once rejected but finally accepted as workable. An adolescent who believes in "a healthy mind in a healthy body" may be able to resist peer pressure to experiment with mind-altering drugs and alcohol, not only to maintain good physical condition but also to remain consistent with beliefs.

Another mechanism for eliciting philosophical beliefs that guide the adolescent is to present the adolescent with a set of statements, such as the following, and to ask the adolescent to agree or disagree:

1. People are primarily responsible for what happens to them.
2. People can achieve anything if they try hard enough.
3. A persons' destiny is determined at birth, and nothing can be done about it.
4. Adolescents should be under the control and direction of their parents as long as they live in the parent's home.

5. Death is not a finality but a transformation of energy from one state to another.

Responses to such statements reveal underlying beliefs that guide the adolescent and indicate how much control the adolescent believes he has over life in general. Whereas adolescents experience uncertainty about the future and maybe even an occasional anxiety attack, the healthy adolescent maintains control over and believes he has some direction in his future, real or fantasized.

The nurse assesses that which the adolescent holds to be important, how the adolescent implements his belief system in setting priorities, how similar the adolescent's ideas and values are to those of the peer group, and how his beliefs contribute to overall functioning. Despite fluidity in thinking and expansion of personal and social space, the healthy adolescent works to develop consistent beliefs and practices. Regardless of his criticism of others, the adolescent maintains a sense of fairness, loyalty, honesty, and inner direction concerning present and future goals and can tolerate change in these goals. The unhealthy adolescent often cannot articulate a set of beliefs or has such a rigid set of beliefs that any change results in major emotional and social upset.

The holistic assessment tool (see the box on pp. 760-761) contains assessment information specific for adolescents.

Analysis
Nursing diagnosis

The following list provides examples of NANDA-accepted nursing diagnoses with causative statements:
1. Anxiety related to underdeveloped body
2. Ineffective individual coping related to abuse of alcohol
3. Ineffective individual coping related to depression associated with the feelings of worthlessness
4. Dysfunctional grieving related to loss of grandmother
5. High risk for violence to self related to anger associated with alienation from parents and peers
6. Altered nutrition: more than body requirements related to feeling unloved
7. Altered thought processes related to unrealistic body perception
8. Self-esteem disturbance related to lack of self-confidence
9. Sensory perceptual alteration related to hearing voices
10. High risk for violence to self related to overdose of drugs.

Planning

After determining appropriate nursing diagnoses from the data collected during the assessment phase of the nursing process, the nurse plans interventions that will improve the health of the adolescent. Interventions usually focus on school performance, social interactions, and family functioning. The plan is individualized and specific to the identified nursing diagnosis while including the least amount of restrictions possible. Through allowing the adolescent choices within a safe, accepting environment, growth is more likely to occur within a holistic perspective. Both the adolescent and parents are involved in the plan for success and movement toward health. The plan includes all dimensions of the individual including: physical, emotional, intellectual, social, and spiritual.

The nursing care plan (Table 37-3) lists examples of long- and short term goals, outcome criteria, interventions, and rationales related to adolescents, which are examples of the planning stage of the nursing process for the adolescent.

Implementation

Physical dimension Clinical intervention in the nursing care of the adolescent's physical needs occurs on two levels. One level is to focus on and intervene in the self-care habits, including eating, sleeping, exercise, and use of leisure time. The healthy adolescent is notoriously neglectful of self-care habits and often skips breakfast, eats junk food for lunch, has nachos and soda for snacks, hurries through supper, runs to activities immediately after school, falls asleep late, and rises early. Eventually the hectic pace catches up, however, and the adolescent adjusts to meet physical needs. The unhealthy adolescent may neglect self-care needs altogether.

On the other level, the nurse is interested in physical needs as they relate to emotional factors. The adolescent may not understand the relationship between emotional changes and physical responses. For example, in the obese adolescent, interventions focus on helping the adolescent understand the relationship between emotional factors, such as disappointment, and physical responses, such as overeating and obesity or undereating and anorexia nervosa.

On both levels, the adolescent is instructed in specifics such as diet and dietary needs related to individual requirements. When the nurse is not adequately prepared to counsel the adolescent on dietary needs, a nutritionist can assist in dietary instruction and planning. Adolescents are instructed in the relationship between physical activity and exercise and in the recognition of internal triggers, such as fear, anger, or cravings, and allergies that set off physical responses, such as destructive eating habits.

Adolescents are also instructed in recognizing external cues that set off patterns of self-neglect, self-abuse, or self-destructive tendencies. Overeating, going on food binges (bulimia), undereating (anorexia nervosa), anxiety attacks, substance abuse, or periods of depression may stem from externally triggered events or situations. Successful treatment of adolescents who are severely disturbed may include treatment of the family. Treatment for persons who abuse drugs and alcohol is discussed in Chapter 18.

To learn about the interrelationship between physical and external and internal cues, the adolescent is helped to develop self-monitoring skills, including the recognition that stress, fatigue, and physical illness alter the body's need for nurturance and rest. The adolescent's concern with body image may require help with physical appearance and establishing self-care habits that bolster self-esteem, for example, hair care, oral hygiene, or cleanliness. Discussing sexuality with the adolescent and instructing the adolescent about physical changes associated with development relieves anxiety.

▼ **TABLE 37-3**   **NURSING CARE PLAN**

GOALS	OUTCOME CRITERIA	INTERVENTIONS	RATIONALES
NURSING DIAGNOSIS: Potential for violence related to suicide attempt secondary to loss of grandmother			
LONG TERM			
To develop positive attitude about self and future	Statements and behavior reflect positive attitude about self and a will to live		
To resolve grief adaptively	Incorporates loss of grandmother into daily living		
To develop hope for future	Speaks in future terms with optimism		
SHORT TERM			
To eliminate self-destructive acts	Does not engage in self-destructive acts	Form a no-harm contract with client	Providing safety is a nursing responsibility. The nurse represents life during client's period of hopelessness.
		Observe and assess client for suicidal ideas/gestures/attempts	Close observation is essential for depressed suicidal clients to prevent impulsive acts.
To express sad, angry, hopeless feelings about loss of grandmother	Expresses feelings about loss of grandmother	Facilitate expression of feelings by listening, respecting, and using empathy	Expressing feelings helps to become aware of them, accept them as normal, consider ways to manage them, and begin the healing process
To focus on what client can hope to accomplish	Statements reflect strengths, abilities for achieving short-term goals	Help client define achievable short-term goals	Participating in planning care increases self-esteem, lessens feelings of helplessness. Feeling helpless prevents one from feeling hopeful.

Emotional dimension Through role modeling, the nurse demonstrates and supports attempts to put feelings into words. The nurse may ask the adolescent to "put words to your feelings so that I can understand what is going on inside you." The nurse accepts the adolescent's presentation of self, giving positive recognition for aspects that are appropriate and healthy and ignoring or confronting the adolescent on inconsistent, unhealthy, or inappropriate behavior. In giving positive recognition for healthy and appropriate actions, the nurse can say, "I like the way you stick up for yourself" (exhibiting self-confidence), "I appreciate your admitting that you made a mistake" (presenting self authentically), or "Thank you for coming. I learn something new about you each time you come" (saying by your coming that you think you are an important person).

The adolescent who experiences anxiety can be instructed in recognizing early symptoms such as rapid heart rate and in developing a self-monitoring program such as progressive relaxation, in which the adolescent gives himself quieting messages. The adolescent can be taught, after recognizing physical symptoms, to find a quiet place and practice relaxing, saying, "I am in control of what happens to me. I can sit here and safely relax. As I breathe deeply, I will let tension and fear slip away from me. I experience calmness, relaxation, and serenity." As the adolescent gains an appreciation for the interplay between mind and body, he gains confidence in controlling the interaction to some extent. Once physical control is mastered, the adolescent gains new insight into underlying emotional factors, for example, fear of death, loss, or separation that triggers anxiety attacks.

When the adolescent is depressed and a suicidal attempt is suspected, a few low-key questions such as "You haven't been yourself lately" or "You've been looking sad for the past few weeks. What is bothering you?" may help the adolescent to open up. Quite surprisingly, most suicidal adolescents honestly and openly discuss their thoughts about suicide once they are asked. Often the adolescent is relieved to have someone to talk to about his problems. Understanding and empathy are essential. Statements such as "You have had a lot of disappointments lately" or "Sometimes you wonder if it is worth it to keep struggling" are helpful and communicate understanding. Hospitalization is necessary when there is a suicide attempt.

Intellectual dimension The nurse provides for the intellectual needs of the adolescent who is experiencing a temporary crisis through maintaining continuity with formal learning settings. For more severe or extended problems, the nurse may be involved in providing for and assisting with learning needs.

Tutors, homebound teachers, and special education teachers are available for the hospitalized or homebound adolescent, enabling the student to continue his studies. These personnel are available from 1 or 2 weeks to an entire semester if necessary. Arrangements are made through the school system with either the school psychologist or the special education division at the district level. When the adolescent is hospitalized, the nurse coordinates time for study, tutorial visits, and tests or examinations with the hospital routine to alleviate disorder and to promote cooperation.

In preparing the tutor for the adolescent's problem, the nurse may arrange a conference time for mutual consultation. The nurse may educate the tutor about grief and its emotional requirements and impact on learning, about depression and its impact on attention spans, about anorexia nervosa and its effect, about divorce or parental separation and its impact on security and feelings about self, and about general emotional needs that detract from the ability to learn during periods of adolescent adjustment. The nurse may have to attend sessions with the tutor if the adolescent is severely depressed, suicidal, aggressive and hostile, or withdrawn.

Continuing study is important for the adolescent in terms of educational needs and the anchoring effect that school involvement has on the adolescent's overall adjustment. Attendance or continuing contact with these learning experiences is as important as accomplishing the work associated with such learning.

Length of educational sessions depends on the adolescent's emotional and physical states. Intellectual stimulation is geared to the adolescent's capacity at the given time to ensure some margin of success, especially for the adolescent experiencing an identity disorder. More difficult and complex material can be introduced as emotional problems or crises resolve.

When the adolescent exhibits undesirable or inappropriate behavior, the nurse intervenes to alter the behavior. For example, when the adolescent is seen talking to himself, the nurse may say, "Jack, I see you talking to yourself. I'd be willing to listen if you'd like to talk with me." In giving a choice of whether to respond, the nurse lets the adolescent know that he is not alone with his fears and fantasies. The relationship between the nurse and the troubled adolescent becomes an anchoring experience and provides contact with reality. Through the relationship, the adolescent may maintain control over fears and fantasies that contribute to confusion and disorientation and impede learning.

For the less-disturbed adolescent, the nurse works to maintain previous patterns of learning and assists the adolescent in coping with problems that are contributing to disruption in learning. The anxious adolescent may need

---

▼ **KEY INTERVENTIONS FOR AN ADOLESCENT EXPERIENCING AN ACADEMIC PROBLEM**

1. Encourage and support school attendance.
2. Use positive statements regarding attendance to succeed.
3. Discuss events and situations that impeded learning.
4. Recognize efforts to improve school work.
5. Explore with the adolescent thoughts and feelings about individual ability and parent-teacher expectations.
6. Coordinate health needs and goals of the learning environment.
7. Establish reasonable goals and priorities.

---

help controlling fear and running-away reactions. The unhappy adolescent may benefit from an altered program of learning that includes insight into events causing the unhappiness. The adolescent with low self-esteem needs small, achievable steps of success built into the learning program to bolster self-confidence and self-worth. Providing extensive work on developing coping skills enhances the adolescent's sense of self-control. Being able to recognize problems, engaging in work with other adolescents experiencing the same problem, talking about problems, and developing strategies for maintaining self-control are all intervention strategies aimed at bolstering the adolescent's problem-solving ability. Key interventions for the adolescent with an academic problem are listed in the accompanying box.

Social dimension The adolescent is encouraged to look for and identify options and to develop an internal sense of alternatives. Clinical interventions that focus on the social needs of the adolescent include helping the adolescent find answers to the question "Who am I?" The depressed or suicidal adolescent often replies to this question with "Nobody." Not only does the adolescent believe he is worthless, but also he thinks his options are limited. Interventions are geared toward restructuring the way the adolescent thinks about himself and the alternatives that grow from restructuring.

In developing a sense of identity using Erikson's theory, the adolescent may need assistance with developing a sense of ownership of behavior. For example, when the adolescent experiences anger, he must learn to discriminate his anger from the anger of others and to direct his anger in appropriate and productive ways. The adolescent is taught to recognize fear, sadness, and anger and to take responsibility for actions that stem from these feelings. The adolescent learns to share feelings with others but is often reluctant at first, particularly when the feelings are created by the person with whom the adolescent needs to share negative feelings. The adolescent is reluctant to reveal inner feelings primarily because of confusion in identifying these feelings and uncertainty about the outcomes of revealing the feelings. Participation in group therapy and other planned peer groups helps the adolescent learn to share his feelings with others in a safe environment.

Confronting the adolescent on unhealthy or inappropriate aspects of the self may include statements such as "I'm not going to let anyone push you around, but I'm not going to let you push anyone around either" (bullying);

▼ **KEY INTERVENTIONS FOR AN ADOLESCENT EXPERIENCING AN IDENTITY CRISIS**

1. Explore with the adolescent the question, "Who am I?"
2. Help the adolescent think in future terms:
   a. Where will you be in 5 years?
   b. What do you want to be like?
   c. Who is the ideal you?
   d. Who is the real you?
3. Explore intimacy needs and how best to meet them appropriately.
4. Instruct in recognizing emotional states and actions stemming from them.
5. Discuss sexuality.
6. Build self-esteem by recognizing the positive contribution of the adolescent to the therapy process.
7. Confront and eliminate inappropriate acts and self-degrading remarks.
8. Encourage positive "I" statements.

▼ **KEY INTERVENTIONS FOR AN ADOLESCENT WHO IS ACTING OUT**

1. Encourage the client to elicit feedback from peers regarding his behavior.
2. Teach consequences (social and legal) of the behavior.
3. Instruct on interactions in social situations, internal triggers, and external triggers that prompt or support lack of impulse control.
4. Establish impulse control through a program that positively recognizes attempts and ignores, confronts, or penalizes loss of control.

"We're not going to get anywhere if you just sit there and pout for the entire session" (withdrawing and controlling by silence); or "You say that you want to get better, but your behavior tells me that you would rather stay sick and be taken care of" (needing parenting and noncompliance). Key interventions for an adolescent with an identity crisis are listed in the accompanying box.

The adolescent is helped to gain a broadened perspective of himself and to be safe and confident in his abilities. For the adolescent to feel safe and engage in risk taking associated with self-examination, the nurse and staff provide a warm, accepting, and predictable environment. For example when possible, appointments are made at a regular time on a regular basis with consistent personnel. The plan of care is shared with and made available to the adolescent, who can then know about and prepare for daily activities. As the adolescent explores more and more the internal dimensions of self, such environmental consistencies are internalized by the adolescent as his own.

The nurse promotes ongoing relationships with peers and assists the adolescent to gain independence and autonomy from the family. The nurse-adolescent relationship is often a bridge for the adolescent to maneuver from family to social and peer relationships. As the nurse builds a bridge through communicating with the adolescent, the adolescent observes and practices similar bridge building with peers. As the adolescent experiences individuality and experiments with autonomy by making decisions and being independent, he has a basis for moving away from the family system.

Clinical strategies with the adolescent provide social skills that the adolescent lacks. Long-range clinical interventions focus on helping the adolescent develop successful and autonomous social relationships. Group exercises are geared toward teaching problem solving, sharing experiences, and developing networks to facilitate the transition from family to peer group relationships.

The adolescent who fails to develop these networks may exhibit acting-out behavior. The following interventions are intended for an adolescent who is acting out (see the accompanying box).

The withdrawn adolescent may experience a sense of worthlessness and abandonment because of perceived or fantasized losses. If the loss is real, clinical strategies aim toward interpreting the event and incorporating the lost person into the adolescent's life. The adolescent is helped to see the person as real and to avoid any idealization of the person. The adolescent is helped to express feelings of anger, resentment, and helplessness resulting from the person's leaving and from his inability to control life and death. When the loss is fantasized or potential, the adolescent is encouraged to view himself as independent from the other and capable of coping despite threats to integrity.

In addition to establishing a sense of options, encouraging the adolescent to experience and express feelings, and helping him to identify actions that stem from feeling states, the nurse assists the adolescent to meet and cope with intimacy needs. A sexually abused adolescent may have trouble establishing close relationships, especially if the perpetrator was a close family member or someone the adolescent trusted. The sexually or emotionally abused adolescent often thinks he is to blame and lacks self-confidence in seeing himself as attractive, acceptable, and lovable. "If I am such a good person," one abused adolescent asked, "then why has this horrible thing been done to me?" Placing blame and seeking appropriate peers and adults for intimate relationships are actions the adolescent often learns by trial and error.

When the adolescent seeks to meet intimacy needs inappropriately, as with staff members, the nurse sets limits and lets the adolescent know that staff members are not to be included in the search for relationships. The nurse may say, "It is important for you to make close friends with your peers. Staff members are here to help you and support you in making friends and in developing close relationships, but they are not here to become a part of an intimate relationship with clients." In this way, the nurse sets limits and lets the adolescent know that he is safe within the environment and that the nurse is willing to support and assist but not engage in intimate relationships with the adolescent. As the nurse acts as a role model for behavior appropriate to age and sex, the adolescent may imitate and practice healthy ways of interacting.

Spiritual dimension A crisis in beliefs often occurs in adolescence, and clinical interventions promote normalizing these experiences as much as possible. The adolescent who experiences a crisis in beliefs because of the death of a friend or family member often challenges religion, doubts God, and strikes out at family and friends. The adolescent may say, "If there was a God, he would not let my brother die."

The adolescent who believes that family or friends have let him down or disappointed him often confronts and challenges not only deep-seated beliefs but also others' practices. Churchgoing parents who profess sanctity of family and then separate or divorce are often perceived as hypocritical. Inconsistency between professed and practiced beliefs often causes despair, disappointment, and unhappiness. These experiences can lead the adolescent through periods of doubt, skepticism, and lack of trust in institutionalized religion. The deeply disturbed adolescent may incorporate religious symbols into distortions of reality. Clinical strategies assist in separating reality from fantasy.

The nurse recognizes the normality of doubting, searching, and denial of belief and facilitates the adolescent's acceptance of questioning as essential to the development of personal values, beliefs, and practices. Adolescents can be philosophical and probing in their search for meaning and can raise doubts and questions in the mind of the unprepared adult or nurse. Just as the nurse accepts the adolescent's doubts and questions, the nurse must be prepared to accept similar episodes of doubting in herself.

The nurse encourages the examination of life, its meaning, and the meaning it has for the adolescent. She also supports the adolescent in doubting and critically examining beliefs without fearing punishment or loss of control. The nurse helps the parents accept such searching as normal and desirable adolescent behavior and not as rebellion or parental disrespect. Clinical interventions promote the development in the adolescent of a lifelong pattern of questioning that incorporates an acceptable and workable set of spiritual beliefs that meets the needs of the particular adolescent. If the nurse believes she is unprepared or in need of support, religious and spiritual personnel such as priests, rabbis, ministers, and pastoral counselors are available for consultation. Clinical intervention strategies are geared toward assuring the client that thoughts, which may be confusing and frightening, are normal. Key interventions for an adolescent experiencing spiritual distress are listed in the accompanying box.

▼
KEY INTERVENTIONS FOR THE ADOLESCENT EXPERIENCING SPIRITUAL DISTRESS

1. Encourage doubting and questioning.
2. Support examination of beliefs.
3. Encourage testing of values.
4. Involve the client in group sessions.
5. Pose questions such as "What is meaningful in your life?"
6. Read and share philosophical writers such as Fromm, Frankl, and Jourard.
7. Discuss relationship of values, beliefs, and practices.
8. Use resources of various religions to examine spiritual beliefs and practices.
9. Examine differences between doubting and having no faith.
10. Discuss the disappointment associated with inconsistencies between stated beliefs and practices of significant others and oneself.

Evaluation

Expected and observed changes in the behavior of the adolescent include the following:

1. Demonstrating initiative
2. Taking responsibility for actions
3. Discussing thoughts and feelings without probing on the part of the nurse
4. Identifying and rectifying inconsistencies in communication
5. Taking risks and having positive regard for oneself
6. Accepting termination of the clinical relationship
7. Using "I" statements that indicate a more positive self-esteem
8. Participating in ongoing classroom work
9. Being oriented to time, person, and place
10. Being able to distinguish reality from fantasy
11. Establishing contact with peers
12. Being able to accept basic uncertainties in daily living and future planning.

The adolescent's progress and successful change reflect the extent to which a successful relationship of trust and collaboration has been established and reflect the appropriate use of intervention strategies.

Specific Treatment Modalities

Several treatment modalities can be used in treating the adolescent: (1) group therapy identified as YES (Youth Expression Sessions) in which the adolescent shares with other adolescents his concerns through discussions in sessions, and (2) group therapy sessions called EDIT (Example Describing Ideas Trying Out) in which the adolescent and his peers role play setting up and solving a problem with feedback from peers.

YES sessions led by an experienced therapist who encourages adolescents to think, talk, and exchange ideas and feelings. Groups are designed to convey a positive and accepting attitude and to encourage the adolescents' active participation in a group that meets 1 to 3 hours a week for 8 to 10 weeks. Membership is open, with joining along the way, to provide the experience of separation and termination of relationships within the framework of supportive peers. The meetings are held in homes, after school, or in a clinic. They are designed to provide an opportunity for the adolescent to bring up issues, raise questions, seek support, and learn about the dynamics of interpersonal exchanges. The adolescents take turns in leading the group, suggesting group activities, observing and making comments about the dynamics involved, and participating in exercises geared to teach decision making and conflict resolution. The group includes adolescents with a variety of backgrounds and experience and in various stages of doubt, confusion, fear, and identity development. Positive sharing helps the adolescent experience others as helpful and experience himself as contributing positively toward the growth of others.

The following are basic rules of the YES groups: (1) each adolescent speaks for himself; (2) each adolescent listens to others and lets others know that listening is taking place; (3) each adolescent gives at least one feedback comment per session; and (4) withdrawing, hostile, or destructive behavior is not accepted. Adolescents examine and discuss loneliness, depression, and divorce and experiment with new ideas. Adolescents learn to make connections between what happens at home and what happens at school. They learn the value of peer support and feedback for handling conflict or disagreement. YES groups, named to develop an adolescent's saying YES to life, are uniquely prepared for, co-led by, and carried out by adolescents in various states of emotional and social development. It is one of several treatment modalities geared toward healthy adolescent development.

Another example of a structured learning experience for adolescents is EDIT, which involves the following steps: (1) finding an example of a situation that the adolescent would like to change or understand, (2) describing the situation to the group with the peer group asking clarifying questions, (3) having the peer group generate ideas about the problem, and (4) having the adolescent, with peer help, try out suggested approaches and solutions through role playing. EDIT is essentially a semistructured role playing situation in which the adolescent actively participates in describing a problem, seeking solutions, obtaining support from others, and practicing a variety of solutions with feedback from peers. Such activity promotes problem solving while enhancing social networking with peers. The success of the adolescent in the peer experience often ripples into family and school relationships.

BRIEF REVIEW

Adolescence is a time of change. The adolescent experiences great surges of physical development that are accompanied by emotional, social, intellectual, and spiritual changes. In Lewin's terms the life space of the adolescent is expanding and becoming more complex. Throughout these changes, the adolescent experiences fluidity of ideas, attitudes, and emotions. When the changes and developing complexities result in imbalances in health, the adolescent may need the assistance of professional mental health–psychiatric personnel who establish treatment programs and intervention strategies to facilitate the resolution of problems and promote healthy development of the adolescent.

Throughout the treatment modalities, the nurse establishes a warm, supportive, intellectually stimulating, and emotionally honest atmosphere so that the adolescent can question, doubt, rebel, and try out new behaviors while feeling safe and accepted. The nurse sets limits when necessary and encourages the adolescent to establish and maintain self-imposed limits when possible. The relationship the nurse establishes with the adolescent is temporary yet permanent; that is, the nurse conveys to the adolescent, "You belong here, but you may not stay forever." The nurse encourages the reengagement of the adolescent with his peers and supports the adolescent in seeking growth potential outside the therapy process.

Through the establishment of a positive, growth-induced relationship, the mental health–psychiatric nurse encourages the adolescent to seek uniqueness. The adolescent learns to trust others and finally to rely on himself. The test of the success of the process comes in the adolescent's leaving the relationship; becoming a whole person in con-

tact with and aware of the physical, emotional, intellectual, social, and spiritual dimensions of himself; and recognizing that the unfolding of those dimensions is a lifelong process.

REFERENCES AND SUGGESTED READINGS

1. American Psychiatric Association: *Diagnostic and statistical manual of psychiatric disorders (DSM-III-R)*, Washington, DC, 1987, The Association.
2. Adams G, Montemayor R, Gullotta T: *Advances in adolescent development*, California, 1989, Sage Publications.
3. Beunen G, Malina R: Growth and physical performance relative to the timing of adolescent spurt, *Exercise and Sport Science Reviews* 16:503, 1988.
4. Burke P: Adolescents' motivation for sexual activity and pregnancy prevention, *Issues in Comprehensive Pediatric Nursing* 10:161, 1987.
5. Corr C, McNeil J: *Adolescence and death*, New York, 1986, Springer Publishing Co.
6. Erikson, EH: *Childhood and society*, ed 2, New York, 1964, WW Norton.
7. Falley G, Herbert F, Echardt L: *Handbook of child and adolescent psychiatric emergencies and crises*, New York, 1986, Medical Examiners Publishing Co.
8. Frankl V: *Man's search for meaning*, New York, 1969, Washington Square Press.
9. Freud S: *A general introduction to psychoanalysis*, New York, 1953, Permabooks. (Translated by J. Riviers.)
10. Hall G: *Adolescence*, vol 2, New York, 1916, D Appleton.
11. Howe C: Developmental theory and adolescent sexual behavior, *Nurse Practitioner* 11:65, 1986.
12. Inhelder B, Piaget J: *The growth of logical thinking*, New York, 1958, Basic Books. (Translated by A. Parsons and S. Milgram.)
13. Klerman G: *Suicide and depression among adolescents and young adults*, Washington, DC, 1986, American Psychiatric Association.
14. Leone P: *Understanding troubled and troubling youth*, California, 1990, Sage Publications.
15. Lewin K: *Field theory and social sciences*, New York, 1951, Harper and Brothers.
16. Lynam M: Adolescent communication: understanding its dynamics and fostering its development, *Nursing Papers* 18:67, 1986.
17. Mahon N, Yarcheski A: Loneliness in early adolescents: an empirical test of alternate explanations, *Nursing Research* 37:330, 1988.
18. Maslow A: *Motivation and personality*, New York, 1954, Harper and Brothers.
19. Montemayor R, Adams G, Gullota T: *From childhood to adolescence*, California, 1990, Sage Publications.
20. Millers D: Affective disorders and violence in adolescents, *Hospital and Community Psychiatry* 37:591, 1986.
21. Patterson J, McCubbin H: Adolescent coping style and behaviors: conceptualization and measurement, *Journal of Adolescence* 10:163, 1987.
22. Peplau HE: *Interpersonal relations in nursing*, New York, 1952, GP Putnam's Sons.
23. Petosa R: Achieving high level wellness, *Health-Values* 13:14, 1989.
24. Pfeffer C: *The suicidal child*, New York, 1986, Guilford Press.
25. Pond V: The angry adolescent, *Journal of Psychosocial Nursing* 26:15, 1988.
26. Robinson D, Greene J: The adolescent alcohol and drug problem: a practical approach, *American Journal of Nursing* 14:305, 1990.
27. Sedgwick R: *Family mental health: theory and practice*, St Louis, 1981, Mosby–Year Book.

28. Sedgwick R, Hildebrand S: The adolescent at risk: crisis, the delicate balance. In Howe J, editor: *Nursing care of adolescents,* New York, 1980, McGraw-Hill.
29. Simmons R and others: The impact of cumulative change in early adolescence, *Child Development* 58:1220, 1987.
30. Stelzer J, Elliott C: A continuous-care model of crisis intervention for children and adolescents, *Hospital and Community Psychiatry* 41:562, 1990.
31. Williamson M: The nursing diagnosis of body image disturbance in adolescents dissatisfied with their physical characteristics, *Holistic Nursing Practice* 1:52, 1987.
32. Young M: Parenting during mid-adolescence: a review of developmental theories and parenting behaviors, *Maternal Child Nursing Journal* 17:1, 1988.

ANNOTATED BIBLIOGRAPHY

Cleveland M: Families and adolescent drug abuse: structural analysis of children's roles, *Family Process* 20:295, 1981.

This article provides a structural analysis of sibling roles in families in which adolescents are involved in chemical drug abuse and suggests appropriate clinical interventions.

Hall S, Hall R: Clinical series in the behavioral treatment of obesity, *Health Psychology* 1:359, 1982.

This article compares seven clinical treatment programs for obesity, noting one study (Robin) with college students in which a variety of treatment approaches were used with a high level of success.

Hogarth C: *Adolescent psychiatric nursing,* St Louis, 1991, Mosby–Year Book.

This book provides a theory base and interventions that staff nurses can use in their practice in a variety of settings. It also includes useful information for staff nurses and clinical specialists who train and supervise adolescent psychiatric nurses and faculty members who introduce students to the specialty of psychiatric nursing.

Kizziar J, Hagedon J: *Search for acceptance: the adolescent and self-esteem,* Chicago, 1979, Nelson-Hall Publishers.

The authors address the issue of adolescent self-esteem and discuss ways in which environments can be created that are conducive to the development of healthy self-esteem.

Plant M, Orford J, Grant M: The effects on children and adolescents of parents' excessive drinking: an international review, *Public Health Reports* 104(5):433, 1989.

This article discusses the health risks and long-term consequences on children of parents who drink excessively. Research findings from studies in the United States as well as Western Europe, Latin America, and Japan are reviewed.

After studying this chapter, the student will be able to:

- Discuss the historical developments in treating the young adult
- Discuss various theories of young adult development
- Identify issues of establishing a relationship with a young adult
- Apply the nursing process to the care of the young adult
- Discuss the psychopathology of adjustment disorders as described in the DSM-III-R
- Identify current research findings related to the young adult

Young adult development encompasses maturation and socialization from the ages of 20 to 44 years. Separating from the family of origin, establishing a viable career, developing an intimate adult relationship with a significant other, developing an individual life-style, and establishing and maintaining a social network are all critical tasks of the early adult years.[24] Since the largest component of the US population will be between 25 and 44 years old until the year 2000, health-care providers need to recognize the complex and changing needs of young adults.[23]

Stressors confronting today's young adults are similar to those which confronted their parents as young adults. However, the changes in social values and the various life-styles and family structures compound the decision-making process and may create confusion and anxiety for the young adult. Unemployment, relocation, and retraining affect the life-style of the young adult and shape patterns of marriage, parenting, and relationships with the family of origin.

Young adulthood is a developmental period of rapid change. The young adult faces changes in perception of psychological self and body image, belief systems, values, expectations, and numerous environmental factors. This rapidly changing scenario demands fast assimilation and adaptation, and the young adult's adaptive response is therefore often challenged and confused.

Young adulthood is an active period and requires the individual to make many significant choices with long-term implications. Previously learned behavior that enables good communication, effective interpersonal relationships, and an adequate support system influence how significant choices are made. These same factors are crucial in later coping behaviors in the individual's success as a student, professional, spouse, or parent. The following historical overview outlines the development of research and theories related to the young adult period.

DSM-III-R

A DSM-III-R diagnosis that relates to young adulthood is adjustment disorder. Adjustment disorder may begin at any age. The disorder is a maladaptive reaction to identifiable social stressors. The maladaption is indicated by impairment in occupational or school functioning or usual social activities or relationships with others. There is remission of the disorder after the stressor ceases or when the person develops new coping behavior.

The stressor may be single, such as a divorce, or multiple, such as professional and marital problems. The stressors may be recurrent or continuous, and they may affect a particular person or a group or community. Some stressors

▶ **DIAGNOSES Related to the Young Adult**

MEDICAL DIAGNOSIS	NURSING DIAGNOSES
Adjustment disorder	**NANDA**
	Altered parenting
	Parental role conflict
	Decisional conflict
	PMH
	Altered parenting role
	Altered decision making

DATES	EVENTS
1900	The initial focus on the development of young adults was the problems they experienced. Writings addressed specific areas of the young adult's development, such as marriage and parenthood, instead of a comprehensive approach.
1929	Oakland Growth and Development Study, conducted by the Institute of Human Development of the University of California at Berkeley, began as a longitudinal study that focused on the lives of 171 men and women from birth through age 40.
1938	Harvard University's Grant Study of Adult Development focused on adult men from the classes of 1942 and 1944 who were psychologically healthy.
1939	Valliant, a social psychiatrist from Harvard Medical School, conducted a longitudinal study on developmental issues of 260 male graduates of Harvard from the ages of 20 to 50.
1947	Cox conducted a longitudinal study of 65 young adult men and women who were considered mentally and physically healthy.
1950s	Erikson included the young adult in his writings about psychological development throughout the life cycle.
1960s	Levinson, a Yale psychologist, conducted a 10-year study of the lives of 40 men, identifying two transitional periods and two stable periods. Gould, a psychiatrist at UCLA, conducted a 5-year cross-sectional study of issues and concerns of young adult men and women.
	The establishment of community-based psychiatry and the emphasis on primary prevention and development of crisis intervention theory and technique greatly influenced the nursing management of the young adult in situational or transitional crises.
1970s	Sheehy described the predictable development of the young adult and compared the development of women and men.
1980s	Troll focused on the development of young adults in his writings.
	Baruch, Barnett, and Rivers studied the lives of young adult women; their findings highlighted the importance of the role of a profession in women's lives.
1990s	As the young adult population grows and experiences stress in response to changing societal expectations, nurses are more involved in interventions that prevent the development of chronic problems.
Future	There will be increased emphasis on environmental issues that have an impact on young adults and on changes in demographic patterns and economic factors influencing educational and other resources available to the young adult and new family. In addition, the limited opportunity for upward mobility will be critical.

leading to an adjustment disorder may accompany specific development events, such as getting married, becoming a parent, or going to school.

THEORETICAL APPROACHES

Psychoanalytical

Intrapsychic

Freud[9] identified unconscious conflict in early childhood as crucial to the development and use of defense mechanisms. The period of genital development, from 12 years to early adulthood, sets the stage for the development of sexual maturity and *intimacy* in the adult. Relational problems with members of the opposite sex are thus demon-

strated in subsequent problems, such as impotence, premature ejaculation, divorce, or serial marriages.

Developmental

Erikson[7] identified intimacy as the major developmental task for young adults. Having dealt with issues of identity in adolescence, the individual now begins to develop an interest in an intimate heterosexual relationship. The movement toward commitment includes the development of the ethical strength needed to make sacrifices and compromises to maintain the relationship. Developing a close affiliation with another requires a sense of trust and self-worth. Failure to achieve intimacy results in *isolation*, which can interfere with the development of a meaningful heterosexual relationship. Isolation may delay entry into the stage of generativity.

Interpersonal

The later work of Sullivan[32] focused on the relationships between and among individuals that are primary in development. This inaccurate approach to psychopathology identified stages of personality development as an outgrowth of interpersonal experience. The late adolescent stage of Sullivan's theory of interpersonal growth and development extends from mid-adolescence to the establishment of a deep heterosexual love relationship in early adulthood.

According to Sullivan, the development of productive and effective adult relationships is critical in achieving maturity. Individuals who have not achieved a healthy level of maturity have an inadequate self-system. These individuals use disparagement, or "putting others down," to maintain a feeling of interpersonal security. To Sullivan, mature adults have learned to satisfy important needs, to cooperate and compete with others, to develop and sustain intimate and sexually satisfying relationships, and to function effectively in the society in which they live. The focus of therapy is directed toward understanding and correcting the client's distorted communication process in the context of a client-therapist relationship based on "reciprocal learning situation."[32]

Cognitive

Piaget's theory of development[25] recognizes four major stages in which biological change and maturation usher in new modes of responding. The successful resolution of the formal operations stage, or Piaget's final intellectual developmental stage, culminates in the refinement of the higher-order intellectual functioning of adulthood. The demands of professional education and career development require further refinement and expansion of intellectual operations. Cognitive functioning therefore remains high during early young adulthood.

The decreased *egocentrism* of this period results in a more balanced idealism. However, egocentrism emerges again in senescence as one prepares for death.

Sociocultural

Studies by Gould,[14] Levinson,[21] and Gilligan[12] focus on a sociocultural orientation, which is helpful to the health-care provider in addressing the conflict and ambiguity inherent in those residing in a rapidly changing society. Gould[14] identifies the 29- to 34-year period as critical, when young adults frequently commit to marriage, establish themselves as members of a new family, and assume the responsibility of parenting. This period is also stressful because of increased professional responsibilities.

The 35- to 43-year period is transitional, when values, work, and life-style may be seriously questioned. Gould[14] reported time during this period to be at a premium, the future looming ahead as an unknown. The individual must become goal directed to achieve success personally and professionally. When the individual determines that professional or personal goals are unrealistic in light of previous experience or accomplishments, he must find alternatives to maintain self-esteem. Parents living with an adolescent in the family during this transitional period were identified

in the Gould study as "stressed" when the adolescent family member strives to become his own person and in so doing challenges his parents' values. Additional stress is encountered when the adult parent is confronted with increased responsibilities for an ill or aged parent during this period.

Levinson[21] identified three distinct stages in a male's transition from adolescence to adulthood. They are the Early Adult Transition, or novice period, at 17 to 22 years of age; the Entering the Adult World period at 22 to 28 years of age; and the Age 30 Transition at 28 to 33 years of age. He identified several development tasks essential for the young man entering the first period. These include separating from the family of origin and forming a basis for living in the adult world, establishing more specific goals, making firmer choices, and articulating a clearer self-definition. To master these tasks, the adolescent must learn to separate from family and persons and groups in the world of adolescence. This separation results in loss, grief, and anxiety about the future. Thus internalizing adult behavior and moving into the early adult period may prove stressful to the college student or newly employed worker. The individual begins to articulate more clearly future options and expectations, while continuing to develop personal and professional skills needed for entrance into the adult world.

Entry into the Adult World period requires people to explore self and world, make and evaluate provisional choices, search for alternatives, and construct a more integrated life structure with increased personal and professional commitment. The individual feels a sense of urgency about marrying, establishing a life-long satisfying occupation, and developing a more organized life-style. He may opt for stability in marriage, while continuing to explore career opportunities, or he may focus on a professional career, while continuing to avoid closeness or commitment. This period is fraught with contradiction and inherent problems; mastery of these tasks significantly affects self-worth and adult identity.

Levinson[21] viewed the Age Thirty Transition period as one of opportunity, because the individual now has time for introspection. During this 5-year period the individual feels a sense of urgency. This period provides a second chance to create a more satisfactory life structure. However, this transition period may prove stressful if the individual feels unable to master its developmental tasks and consequently will reactivate unresolved conflicts of adolescence.

Each individual may identify his developmental problems as unique as values are challenged and larger social questions gain considerable attention. However, much remains to be learned about male and female development in this Transition period. (These theoretical approaches are summarized in Table 38-1.)

NURSING PROCESS

Assessment

Physical dimension Physical growth has been essentially completed by young adulthood. Aging and the maintenance of physical integrity are related to individual differences in nutrition, sleep, stress, and genetic variables. Genetic variances need to be explored in this age-group

▼ **TABLE 38-1**   **Summary of Theoretical Approaches**

Theory	Theorist	Dynamics
Psychoanalytical	Freud	Genital development sets the stage for development of sexual maturity in young adulthood.
		Relationship problems with members of the opposite sex are seen in such disorders as impotence and premature ejaculation and such problems as serial marriages and divorce.
	Erikson	The task is intimacy versus isolation. Failure to achieve intimacy interferes with capacity to engage in meaningful heterosexual relationships.
Interpersonal	Sullivan	The development of a productive and effective adult intimate relationship is critical to achieving maturity.
Cognitive	Piaget	Cognitive functioning is refined and remains high during young adulthood.
Sociocultural	Gould	Ages 22 to 28—marriage commitment, creation of a family, parenting, and career advancement.
		Ages 29 to 34—reevaluation of values, work, and life-style.
	Levinson	Ages 17 to 22 (Early Adult Transition)—separation from family, establishment of specific goals, and ability to make firmer choices.
		Ages 22 to 28 (Entering the Adult World)—exploration of self and world, ability to make conditional choices regarding career.
		Age 30 Transition—the period of opportunity to create more satisfactory life.

and have major significance due to child-bearing functions. Physical signs of aging may be evident in the late 20s, with loss of skin elasticity and subsequent wrinkling. Signs of premature graying or balding may also be evident. These and other physical changes may significantly affect the client's self-confidence.

Exploring the client's use of alcohol and drugs is essential in assessing physical status. The young adult client may eat high-calorie foods at home and at fast-food establishments. A rapid weight gain or loss may be a response to caloric intake, a physical response to a high level of stress, or a sign of inadequate coping mechanisms for adaptation. Excessive weight gain or loss may contribute to a poor self-concept.

The nurse's assessment of the client's physical symptoms is an integral part of the health history. Vague somatic complaints may mask underlying mental health problems and delay the client's seeking early intervention for depression or anxiety related to school, work, or interpersonal relationships. Headaches, digestive complaints, and a lack of vigor may signal tension and stress or depression. A thorough assessment of the onset of symptoms, duration, and other related or contributing factors helps the nurse differentiate between physiological stress or psychophysiological manifestations of depression or anxiety. Physical symptoms may be identified as an egocentric response or

a sign of interpersonal conflict as seen in the theories of Piaget and Sullivan.

The young adult may feel increased apprehension about body image and feel unacceptable as a sexual partner. Since Western culture places a high value on youth and beauty, shame about one's own body may greatly inhibit establishing an intimate relationship and thus delay the initiation or achievement of a key developmental task. The nurse needs to assess the client's body image in the initial interview.

The issue of body image and peer acceptance has many implications for the cachectic or obese client. *Cachexia* is a state of malnutrition resulting from excessive dieting. Both malnutrition and overnutrition are often identified as psychogenic. The anorectic client may demonstrate self-starvation after a period of excess weight gain. This client may also eat excessively and exhibit a number of somatic complaints and irrational fears. The anorectic client may also fear the changes of young adulthood and thus demonstrates fear of rejection or of expectations of interpersonal intimacy and increased commitment. The obese client may use ingestion of food to decrease anxiety and stress. This client may be warding off sexuality and subconsciously expressing fear of intimacy. Thus the assessment of weight and nutritional habits are critical in the young adult. The relationship between eating disorders and depression is viewed by Stuart and others[31] as related to

RESEARCH HIGHLIGHT

Early Family Experiences of Women with Bulimia and Depression

• GW Stuart, MT Laraia, JC Ballenger, and RB Lydiard

PURPOSE

This descriptive study investigated both attitudinal measures and behavioral indicators of the bulimia client's early family experiences, including parental rearing practices, family conflict resolution, sexual mistreatment, problematic childhood indicators, and childhood separation experiences.

SAMPLE

A convenience sample of 30 women who had been diagnosed with bulimia nervosa, 15 women diagnosed with a major depressive disorder using DSM-III-R criteria, and 100 women (no psychiatric diagnosis, no psychiatric diagnosis in first-degree relatives, and medically stable) as control group.

METHODOLOGY

Clients and control group members were observed using a full range of sociodemographic variables. Participants completed standardized paper-and-pencil instruments. These included the Childhood Environment Questionnaire and nine-item scale measuring behaviors associated with childhood separatiton anxiety. The Child Environment Questionnaire consisted of the following subsections: EMBU-Memories of Child-Rearing Experiences Scale, Family Violence in Kentucky Questionnaire, Victimization Inventory, and Early Life Events Questionnaire.

FINDINGS

The Memories of Child-Rearing Experiences Scale revealed significant differences between groups in five of the eight subscales. When compared with the control group, bulimics perceived a lack of emotional warmth and rejection; fathers were perceived as more overprotective and rejecting. Patients with depression revealed no overprotection but perceived both mother and father as more rejecting than did the normal controls.

Differences emerge in the way in which family conflict was resolved when data from patient groups were analyzed. The use of threats and coercion to resolve family conflict was evident in families of bulimics, whereas it was not evident in the families of depressives. Significantly less rational family discussion was evident when depressives and bulimics were compared with controls. Neither group differed in use of physical violence when compared with the control population.

This study documents that depressed women perceived their childhood as unhappy, as compared with bulimics who were identified as having twice the number of family problems and three times the number of emotional problems of the control group. Both the bulimic and the depressed populations reported significantly higher levels of childhood separation anxiety than did the control group.

IMPLICATIONS

This study provides descriptive data about the childhood experiences of women with depression or bulimia, which can be useful to those involved in determining a nursing diagnosis and establishing a nursing care plan. Findings can be helpful in identifying target populations at risk. Early intervention programs can be implemented to reduce the incidence of these disorders.

Clinicians working with bulimic and depressed women can benefit from understanding the pattern of perception of childhood rejection and unhappiness that is characteristic of this population and thus focus on the issues of the client's negative cognitions and self-assessment.

Based on data from *Archives of Psychiatric Nursing* 4(1):43, 1990.

early family experiences (see research highlight). See Chapter 31 for additional discussion of eating disorders.

Emotional dimension The ability to function in a stressful environment is critical for the young adult to achieve success in work or school. Stress can serve a useful purpose in motivating the individual to strive for greater achievement. However, an inability to cope effectively with the many stressors of this developmental stage may lead the young adult to seek help in learning new coping behaviors to decrease emotional outbursts. Many emotions may contribute to the client's feeling stressed. Guilt, despair, anger, and loneliness contribute to depression or hopelessness. These feelings result from encounters on the college or university campus, in the workplace, or at home.

To assess the client's perception of emotions experienced, the nurse asks him to identify a current stressful experience and the accompanying feelings or to explore behavior that seems inappropriate or troublesome, underlying feelings, and how these feelings are expressed. It is essential to note that many adjustment disorders have intense emotional components that can be manifested in anxiety or depression.

The nurse assesses the client's perception of how his emotions affect his ability to develop satisfactory relationships or achieve professional goals. These experiences may be used to discuss individual responses to a wide range of economic, social, and intellectual demands. When conflicting demands are placed on the client, the nurse may observe responses ranging from the inability to act and apathy to anger, rage, or destructive behavior.

During the nurse's assessment, the client may become painfully aware of an inability to handle anger effectively. He may find expression of emotions or feelings threatening and thus may resort to using anger to distance others when stressed. The use of anger to ward off feelings of closeness may become an unhealthy defense mechanism. However, in assessing emotional responses in the young adult, the nurse must recognize that depression and guilt may be closely related to anger and manifested in angry outbursts. Anger clearly involves the use of the energy needed for successful resolution of developmental tasks.

Assessment can help both the client and nurse determine how the client uses defense mechanisms, such as repression, to alleviate the expression of anger or to deny feelings of loneliness or depression. Rebellious and immature behavior from adolescence may be evident as the client confronts the demands of college or career. This behavior may have initiated the client's referral to the nurse for assessment and intervention and may continue throughout the nurse-client interaction.

Intellectual dimension Assessing the client's ability to handle cognitive and abstract problems and to appropriately process information provides valuable information that helps the nurse structure interactions. The client may demonstrate an impulsive or irrational decision-making style or markedly vary in style when stressed. He may make decisions soundly by carefully weighing pros and cons or by using a trial-and-error approach.

Limitations identified in intellectual development, such as thinking by intuition or the concrete operations found in earlier stages, may create major adjustment problems for the client. Young adults are required to process large amounts of new information or rapidly develop skills for professional education or succeeding at work. Thus the capacity for a sustained effort and the intellectual ability to manipulate concrete data and comprehend abstract problems are crucial for success. The identification of the capacity to delay gratification and to demonstrate sound decision-making skills is also reflected in the client's ability to establish and maintain interpersonal relationships.

As the young adult is exposed to broader educational or work experiences, the ability to adapt to change becomes evident. Flexibility thus becomes an indicator of identity and self-esteem. Flexibility and risk taking greatly enhance the individual's response to opportunities available for new experiences and result in subsequent mastery in a broader intellectual or interpersonal arena.

Social dimension Assessment of the client's social dimension focuses on interactions or relationships in living, working, or socializing with others. Interaction style has broad implications for success on the job, in an intimate relationship, or in other professional or social situations. Evidence of inadequate communication or failure to develop interpersonal relationships may manifest itself in low self-esteem or alienation. The fear of an intimate adult relationship may inhibit the individual from dating or joining in group activities that involve close interpersonal relationships. Assessment of communication and interpersonal skills are critical in understanding young adult needs.

Changes in technology and increased competition may force the young adult to change employment or expand his educational background to meet employment demands. The young adult may perceive these changes as either a challenge or a threat. Underemployment or unemployment is often a stressor leading to feelings of inferiority, loss of confidence, and fear of economic insecurity. Underemployment often results in disruption or breakdown of social and family relationships. It may be further compounded if the individual has recently married or become a parent, thus appreciably increasing personal and fiscal responsibilities. Developing economic independence, however, goes beyond steady employment and an adequate income; it requires skill in money management.

For professionals, the need to perform in many areas simultaneously and to accept additional responsibility to compete successfully may prove extremely stressful. Support from peers, spouse, and parents is crucial when time and energy are focused on educational or career goals. To deal with conflicting role demands, individuals may quickly find themselves confronted with the need to set priorities to succeed.

Although the capacity for establishing sexual intimacy begins in adolescence, the young adult must develop a personal identity before merging with another in marriage or other long-term intimate relationship. Individuals with similar socioeconomic backgrounds, value systems, role expectations, and interests are most likely to establish a more lasting and secure intimate relationship.

Although fathers' participation in child care has increased in the last two decades,[16] as addressed in Jordon's article "Laboring for Relevance,"[18] the task of early child care is still viewed as primarily the mother's responsibility by both the mother and others (see the research highlight). In light of the ambiguity inherent in the socialization of women, particularly those who are professionals, this responsibility may create role strains not previously anticipated by the new mother.

Assessment of how young women perceive their roles as wage earner (or student), spouse, and parent will give useful clues to sources of stress both on the job and in relationships. The assessment of young men likewise includes a description of how they perceive their role as wage earner (or student), spouse, and parent. Financial pressures or career stressors compound the adjustment of young men and women to marriage and parenthood. Assessment of the importance of the workplace in fulfilling the social needs of young men and women is essential because it identifies areas of ambivalence and stress related to relocation or upward mobility in the organization.

Preparing for marriage is often more emotionally stressful than anticipated. The tasks of the premarital and early marriage period are disengaging from the family of origin and other exceptionally close relationships that may interfere with the spousal relationship and emotionally preparing oneself for the role of spouse and establishing a new life-style that gratifies both partners. Stress and dysfunctional behavior may be encountered in clients who are anticipating marriage or have entered a relationship with unrealistic expectations. Assessment focuses on current experiences from the client's perspective, for example, a loss of parent or inability to accomplish career goals.

Parenting is another major source of stress. Several au-

RESEARCH HIGHLIGHT

Laboring for Relevance: Expectant and New Fatherhood
• PL Jordan

PURPOSE

The purpose of this study was to investigate the experience of being an expectant or new father.

SAMPLE

The study sample consisted of 56 expectant and recent first-time fathers living with their mates. The population was a convenience sample recruited through health-care providers, word of mouth, and media publicity. Of these 56 subjects, 28 volunteered for a longitudinal or cross-sectional group. Ages ranged from 21 to 41 years, with a mean and median age of 30 years. Income ranged from $0 to $90,000/year, and conception ranged from 1 month to 10 years after marriage.

METHODOLOGY

Subjects in the longitudinal sample were interviewed six to seven times over the perinatal period: shortly after conception, after fetal movement felt (20 to 24 weeks of gestation), late pregnancy (36 to 40 weeks of gestation), as soon as possible after birth, and 6 weeks and 6 months postpartum. The fathers in the cross-sectional group were interviewed only one of the above times. The interview was audiotaped and lasted 0.5 to 2.5 hours. Questions asked included broad questions on the experience of being an expectant or new father and specific questions on when and after the baby is born or how individuals acknowledge the subject in his expectant or father role.

Based on data from *Nursing Research* 39(1):11, 1991.

Transcribed interviews were coded and the grounded theory method guided both data collection and analysis.

FINDINGS

Laboring for relevance was identified as a significant component of the expectant and new father experience. He labors to incorporate the paternal role as relevant to his sense of self and repertoire of roles. Three subprocesses were integral to this process: grappling with the reality of the pregnancy and child, struggling for recognition as a parent, and adapting to the role of involved fatherhood. Those individuals interacting with the father were crucial in promoting or impeding evolving fatherhood.

IMPLICATIONS

The nurse providing childbirth or parenting class must be aware of the persistent societal norms related to parental role expectations. Research designed to assist the nurse in understanding the father's experience will lead to reconsideration of nursing therapeutics for the promotion of involved fatherhood. Opportunities for expectant and new fathers to learn basic child care and parenting skills will have an impact on those obstacles impeding role enactment. These changes can positively influence the traditional role of males in today's society.

---

thors have identified potential regression as the predominant risk of parenthood.[3,20] Previous loss of a parent or abandonment increases the new parent's vulnerability. The young adult may be greatly influenced by earlier unresolved losses, thus experiencing a significant deficit in parenting ability. This deficit increases the individual's anxiety and doubt about his ability to succeed as a parent. Even in ideal conditions, parenthood forces the individual to shift the focus from self to the responsibility of caring for another 24 hours a day. The demands of child care may create anxiety and a sense of helplessness, which further compounds the emotional adjustment of the young adult.

The young, married, professional woman with home and family responsibilities may find herself extremely stressed by the parenting role. Assessment of the client's response to the demands of her different roles is helpful in identifying stressors and planning interventions to decrease role conflict. The increased demands on the young father and the changing needs and expectations of his wife may be overwhelming, thus leading to increased anxiety, depression, and strained interpersonal relationships. These tensions may greatly affect the trust and intimacy needed to sustain the marriage relationship and lead to alienation, separation, or divorce.

For single or childless young adults between 20 and 30 years of age, the nurse assesses personal goals and priorities, satisfaction with their quality of life, and their perceived need for increased social contacts or significant changes in life-style. The client may say that overcommitment has been a problem on the job or in social relationships, and failure to meet these commitments has led to feelings of failure or loss of self-esteem. This sense of failure may also considerably affect clients' perception of their ability to marry or assume responsibility for a family.

Individuals with demanding educational or career goals may find little time for social activity and become increasingly isolated from family and peers. Young adults who choose a career over marriage and family or who are too busy professionally to develop a social life or intimate adult relationship may become increasingly aware of a sense of "something missing" as the Age Thirty Transition period approaches. The young adult may choose to make a significant change in life-style at this time to facilitate social contacts, may seek support in reaffirming the value of the current life-style, or may explore other options.

Married couples may reassess decisions to remain childless or to continue to defer childbearing during the Age Thirty Transition period. If the couple fails to satisfactorily resolve conflict over this or other issues at this time, their relationship may become increasingly strained. The young couple is also faced with a growing need to broaden social contacts in this period. They may have been totally involved in careers, education, or the demands of children in the early years of marriage and now have a need to expand beyond the immediate family or work setting. However, this broadening may be perceived by one spouse as a loss of interest in the relationship. This issue needs to be openly addressed to decrease conflict.

The nurse notes the social and emotional implications of separation or divorce when the client has a history of marital discord. The young adult frequently seeks counseling because of depression or feelings of failure from a recent divorce that may be further compounded by feelings of abandonment or rejection. Because divorce demands a major adjustment in life-style for both partners, support may be necessary for both. The stereotype that women have more difficulty coping with divorce may no longer be true. A woman's career can provide not only economic support, but also peer support.

The loss experienced when a significant relationship or traditional marriage breaks up may have an emotional, physical, and financial impact on an individual's sense of well-being. In addition, the stress experienced by being a single parent may greatly decrease the individual's ability to parent successfully.

Spiritual dimension The assessment of the young adult includes determination of current religious practices and value systems. Conflict may be apparent as early values are challenged by the young adult. The young adult may have conflicts related to premarital sexual intercourse, abortion, or living with a person of the opposite sex. Some may resolve these changes in values, however, others may need assistance. Some clients may experience a conflict because of failure to attend religious services as they had as children or adolescents or in making choices in religious affiliation due to changes in value orientation.

As individuals establish themselves in a community and marry, they reflect on ethical and spiritual values. The responsibilities of a family may foster introspection on values and the sharing of philosophical and spiritual orientation with one's children. The focus of the young couple, however, is often primarily on the training of the young children, unless there is a major life crisis, such as divorce, loss of a parent or other family member, a life-threatening accident, or prolonged illness. The nurse may note that the client has begun to search for meaning in life or is actively reassessing spiritual values because of a loss. In today's society, reports of terrorism and destruction, war, and natural disaster confront the individual with many anxiety-producing sights and sounds, thus increasing his vulnerability. Vulnerability also provides an impetus for young adults to assess their value systems and reflect on spirituality.

Students, blue-collar workers, and professionals alike often face moral and ethical situations that demand an assessment in light of individual values. A junior member of a management team or professional group may encounter interpersonal conflict as co-workers engage in business practices that fail to meet the young adult's ethical or moral standards. During the initial assessment, the client may be confused or angry, having become aware of the value con-

ASSESSMENT TOOL: THE YOUNG ADULT

Physical Dimension

Describe your eating habits.
What is your sleep pattern?
What are your thoughts about your body image?
How do you feel about your sexuality?

Emotional Dimension

What do you think and feel when you experience stress?
How does your spouse or significant other respond to you when you experience stress?
What is a stressful experience you are now facing?
How do you handle anger? guilt?
What do you feel hopeful about?
Describe your behavior the last time you were depressed.
What is your response when faced with a conflict?

Intellectual Dimension

What is your response to changes in your life?
How do you make decisions about everyday situations? major situations?
How do you feel about seeking professional assistance?

Social Dimension

How many friends do you have at work?
What type of social events do you participate in with your peers?
How often do you invite friends to your home?
What are your career goals?
What do you think about your performance at your present job?
Describe your marriage.
Describe your parenting behavior.
When faced with several tasks, how do you set priorities?
How do you handle conflicts with your spouse?
Describe the way you manage your finances.
What do you consider your role in the family?
What are your thoughts about assuming this role?

Spiritual Dimension

What are your thoughts about divorce? abortions? infidelity?
How congruent is your value system with your spouse's or significant other's?
How do you behave when faced with a moral or ethical conflict?

---

flicts inherent in entering the adult society. These issues are often stressful to those who have become acutely aware that they cannot continue to compromise their values without loss of integrity. The nurse assists the client in clarifying values and provides an opportunity for the client to explore options and related spiritual and moral values. The accompanying assessment tool contains assessment areas specific to the young adult. It is to be used in conjunction with the assessment tool in Chapter 8, pp. 138-140.

Analysis
Nursing diagnosis

Altered parenting, parental role conflict, and decisional conflict are nursing diagnoses that apply to the young adult. Defining characteristics for these diagnoses are listed in the boxes on p. 777. The following list provides examples of other accepted nursing diagnoses with causative statements for the young adult:

▼ ALTERED PARENTING

DEFINITION

Presence of risk factors during prenatal or childbearing period that may interfere with process of adjustment to parenting.

DEFINING CHARACTERISTICS

- **Physical dimension**

  Perceived threat to own survival

  Evidence of physical or psychosocial abuse

- **Emotional dimension**

  Fear

  Verbalization of perceived or actual inadequacy

- **Intellectual dimension**

  Limited cognitive functioning

  Unreal expectations

- **Social dimension**

  Verbalization of dissatisfaction or disappointment with the infant

  Interruption in bonding process

  Social isolation

  Support system deficit

  Lack of role identity

Modified from Gordon M: *Manual of nursing diagnoses, 1988-1989,* St Louis, 1989, Mosby–Year Book.

1. Powerlessness related to ineffectiveness in parental role
2. Impaired social interaction related to inability to maintain interpersonal relationships
3. Disturbance in self-concept related to obesity
4. Ineffective individual coping related to marital discord
5. Anxiety related to perceived threat to self-concept
6. Social isolation related to depressed mood

The following case example illustrates defining characteristics of altered parenting.

▼ Case Example

Joan's infant son has been seen repeatedly by the nurse, and a diagnosis of failure to thrive has been made. Joan is a single parent and is unable to care for the child because of drug and alcohol abuse. The child lost 2 pounds since the previous clinic visit and also appeared to demonstrate signs of lack of sensory stimulation.

The child is placed in a temporary foster home at Joan's request, and she enters an outpatient rehabilitation program.

The following case example illustrates defining characteristics of parental role conflict.

▼ Case Example

Debbie is a recently divorced single parent of two young children. She has had to resume full-time employment after her divorce and is now expressing many concerns about her parenting skills. She feels she is failing to give her children adequate attention.

▼ PARENTAL ROLE CONFLICT

DEFINITION

Role confusion and conflict in response to crisis experienced by parent or parents.

DEFINING CHARACTERISTICS

- **Emotional dimension**

  Expression of concern or feelings of inadequacy to provide for child's physical and emotional needs during hospitalization or in the home

  Verbalization or demonstration of feelings of guilt, anger, fear, anxiety, and/or frustration about effect of child's illness on family process

- **Intellectual dimension**

  Lack of information related to child development

  Limited understanding regarding parental role

  Expression of concern over perceived loss of control over decisions relating to the child

  Expression of concern about change in family health

- **Social dimension**

  Expression of concerns about change in parental role, family functioning, family communication

  Reluctance to participate in usual caretaking activities, even with encouragement and support

Modified from Gordon M: *Manual of nursing diagnoses, 1988-1989,* St Louis, 1989, Mosby–Year Book.

▼ DECISIONAL CONFLICT

DEFINITION

A state of uncertainty about the course of action to be taken when choice among competing actions involves risks, loss, or challenge to personal values.

DEFINING CHARACTERISTICS

- **Physical dimension**

  Physical signs of distress or tension, such as increased heart rate, increased muscle tension, and restlessness

- **Intellectual dimension**

  Verbalization of undesired consequences of alternative actions being considered

  Verbalization of feeling of distress related to uncertainty about choices

  Vascillation between alternative choices

  Delayed decision making

- **Social dimension**

  Self-focusing

- **Spiritual dimension**

  Questioning of personal values and beliefs while the individual attempts to make a decision

Modified from Kim MJ, McFarland GK, McLane AM: *Pocket guide to nursing diagnoses,* ed 5, St Louis, 1993, Mosby–Year Book.

▼ **TABLE 38-2   NURSING CARE PLAN**

GOALS	OUTCOME CRITERIA	INTERVENTIONS	RATIONALES
NURSING DIAGNOSIS: Anxiety related to perceived threat to self-concept			
LONG TERM			
To develop increased awareness of anxiety	Identifies signs and symptoms of anxiety	Assist client to verbalize perceived threat	Recognize need to begin to identify specific stressors
	Uses constructive strategies in coping with anxiety	Discuss coping strategies	Increasing client coping skills will enhance reduction of anxiety
		Provide opportunity to demonstrate coping ability	To receive feedback and reinforcement
SHORT TERM			
To assist in identifying anxiety as related to perceived threat to self-concept	Increases awareness of factors that threaten self-concept	List anxiety-producing situations related to threat to self-concept	Increased awareness of stress will enhance patient coping skills
To explore individual response to increasing stress	Develops means to monitor increasing anxiety level related to threat to self-concept	Discuss signs of stress and increased anxiety	Stress reduction strategies will increase feelings of competency
To develop skills in coping with perceived threat	Develops adaptive coping skills and uses them in a high-stress situation	Provide opportunity to demonstrate new coping skills	Positive feedback in performance can encourage risk-taking behavior
NURSING DIAGNOSIS: Social isolation related to withdrawn behavior			
LONG TERM			
To reestablish and maintain relationships and a social life	Establishes several significant relationships	Encourage participation in small groups to decrease client apprehension	Participation will enhance risk-taking behavior
	Returns to work and social environment with limited anxiety	Provide opportunity to discuss response to group activity	Response from individuals/group can enhance self-concept
		Assist client to identify individuals/groups that provide support	Skill in interacting with peers will increase social skills
SHORT TERM			
To increase interaction with others and the environment	Identifies behavior that fosters withdrawal	Provide feedback when client withdraws from staff and others	Client may not recognize withdrawn behavior
		Assist in identifying how and when withdrawal is manifested	Recognition of the pattern of withdrawal may help change the behavior
	Initiates interaction with others and environment	Teach client ways to initiate interaction	Lack of skills in social interaction may contribute to withdrawal
		Create situations in which client can practice interacting	Practice can help client feel more secure when he interacts with others
		Encourage client to engage in social activities with others	Provides a frame of reference for evaluating client's social skills

Debbie's family notes that Debbie perceives rather small, insignificant changes in her children's health as directly resulting from her inattention, thus exacerbating her tension and feelings of inadequacy. These feelings have in turn led to periods of depression and anxiety.

The following case example illustrates defining characteristics of decisional conflict.

▼ Case Example

Mark and Betty are experiencing a conflict about when to have their first child. Both want children and before marriage agreed to have the first child during their second year of marriage. Now in the second year of marriage, Mark wants to postpone starting a family for another year when he thinks he will be established in his job as an insurance salesman and financially secure. Betty thinks that because she will continue to work as a computer science technician until shortly before the baby is born, they are financially able to begin the family now. She is pressuring Mark to adhere to the decision they made before marriage.

Planning

Table 38-2 presents a nursing care plan with long-term and short-term goals, outcome criteria, interventions, and rationales. These are examples of the planning stage in the nursing process.

Implementation

Physical dimension Young adults are the healthiest people in the population; thus a major focus for meeting their physical needs is health maintenance. Like other age-groups, young adults need caloric intake based on caloric need to avoid excessive weight gain or loss. Those in non-sedentary occupations and who actively exercise burn more calories than do inactive young adults. Pregnant women require more calories than other young adults. Young adults can decrease their intake of salt and high cholesterol foods that may contribute to the later development of disease.

A young adult who feels worthless and is depressed may think he is not worthy of food and may decrease food intake or avoid meals. This individual may require hospitalization. Careful observation of the client during hospitalization and follow-up to ensure that adequate food intake is maintained may be a short-term goal until the client accepts responsibility for maintaining adequate nutrition.

Young adults who eat and exercise strenuously near bedtime may be unable to sleep restfully. If an infant's needs during the night contribute to interrupted sleep, spouses can take turns getting up so that neither parent loses too much sleep. A young adult with chronic insomnia may need medical or psychiatric assistance.

The nurse ensures that clients understand the hazards of excessive smoking and drinking. Young adulthood is an opportune time for attending a smoking clinic or Alcoholics Anonymous, if necessary. Individuals planning to have a baby must be informed of the potential effects of smoking and drinking on the unborn child.

Genetic counseling is indicated for a couple with family histories of hereditary illness or a condition that is known or suspected to be inherited. Such counseling helps the couple determine their chances of having a normal child.

The nurse or the genetic counselor can discuss with the couple alternative courses of action, such as adoption, artificial insemination, or sterilization. Some couples may benefit from counseling at Planned Parenthood as they decide to start a family.

The nurse informs young adults of the need for an annual physical examination to maintain their health status. Because breast cancer is increasing among women over 35 years of age, young women are taught to examine their breasts monthly, the week after menstruation. The nurse also informs women of the importance of a baseline mammogram between 35 and 40 years of age.

When the stresses of young adulthood cause somatic complaints, such as headaches and stomachaches, the individual needs to have a checkup and have any acute illness treated before the problem becomes chronic. The nurse assists the client to increase his awareness of the relationship between stress and physical symptoms.

Interventions for the person who abuses substances focuses on maintenance of physical well-being. Sleep patterns, nutritional status, and degree of interest in maintaining personal hygiene are monitored. Interventions initially focus on assisting the client to meet his physical needs by providing proper nutrition and encouraging personal cleanliness and grooming. A number of substance abuse programs provide lectures on the physiological effects of drugs, family dynamics in substance or codependent behavior, and other topics. Didactic groups can help to inform clients of the dangers of alcohol or drug ingestion, but these groups clearly focus on specific content and may fail to meet the immediate needs of some clients (see Chapter 18).

Emotional dimension A number of emotional factors are addressed during assessment. It may become apparent that the young adult has failed to manage appropriately the stress of leaving home, establishing successful adult relationships, or achieving professional goals. The client may censor his own feelings, leaving him angry and frustrated. When the client finds that his unexpressed anger results in isolation from his peer group or co-workers, he may seek professional help. Sometimes a client is referred for counseling because of failure at school or work.

The nurse provides the client with the first opportunity to express feelings about the current crisis. How the client identifies the current problem and how he attempts to cope give valuable information. Once the nurse identifies the client's feelings, she and the client together establish and set priorities for short-term and long-term goals. Encouraging the client to identify alternative ways of coping is an effective means of increasing his awareness of the existing problem.

A client's lack of experience in relating to adults may reflect social class differences or feelings of inferiority from previous negative experiences. Role playing, rehearsal, reframing, or other methods assist the young adult in learning new skills. Managing feelings of anger, fear, and conflict is a challenge to the young adult in a rapidly changing, complex society. Increased competence, cultural differences, and changing gender roles today often create frustration for young adults not experienced by previous generations. The nurse provides an opportunity for the client to express feelings and gain confidence.

The client is encouraged to verbalize feelings of failure

or depression resulting from separation or divorce. Support and assistance often aid in resolving feelings of loss and guilt as the client adjusts to the change in life-style. Parents Without Partners and groups for divorcees at churches or community mental health centers allow young adults to express feelings of anger, abandonment, and rejection.

Intellectual dimension Because young adults usually can tolerate high levels of sensory stimulation, coping with multiple stimuli is not generally perceived as a stressor. However, if the client demonstrates low self-esteem or depression, it may be important to assist him in decreasing environmental stimuli until he feels a sense of control. These stimuli can then be increased as the client can tolerate them.

The student who encounters academic stress or failure may need to reassess professional goals and develop a realistic approach to achieve academic success. The nurse and client explore alternatives and establish long-term and short-term goals, which provide the opportunity for academic success and mastery of the developmental tasks of young adulthood. These include intimacy and competency according to Erikson.[7] Involving the client in establishing goals promotes independent decision making and allows the nurse to evaluate the client's decision-making process.

An ongoing evaluation of the client's ability to problem-solve and the client's level of intellectual functioning is essential to help him establish realistic goals that will result in a sense of mastery, thus fostering self-esteem. It is important to recognize that the anxious or depressed client may be unable to perform intellectual functions at a level previously attained and may become angry and frustrated. Continued support from the nurse, family members, and significant others is critical in assisting the client to achieve successfully the level of intellectual functioning he is capable of reaching. Encouraging the client to participate in a therapeutic milieu that necessitates group interaction enhances expressive functions and fosters intellectual responsibility.

Social dimension Interventions for the failure to develop interpersonal relationships using Sullivan's theory focus on increasing self-esteem and improving social interactions. The initial goal is to develop a trusting therapeutic relationship between the client and the nurse. After a relationship has been established, the client is encouraged to talk about the problems he has encountered in his relationships and his feelings about them. The hospitalized client may be assisted to develop intimacy by initially participating in activities such as games and outings with the nurse that are noncompetitive and allow the individual to proceed to additional activities at his own pace. The client is gradually encouraged to interact with peers, first with same-sex peers, then with those of the opposite sex. Then the client may be able to give of self in a relationship that demands intimacy.

The client is encouraged to develop a list of strengths and weaknesses. Positive reinforcement is then given to build on the client's strengths to increase self-esteem. Assertiveness training, role playing, and the modeling of effective communication assist the client in improving interpersonal skills. Group therapy is especially helpful in providing young adults with feedback from peers on their behavior. Group members also provide support and posi-

tive reinforcement as the client makes behavioral changes. Group therapy provides an opportunity to practice interpersonal skills and receive feedback.

When working with young adults having difficulty adapting to the parent role, the nurse must encourage the open expression of feelings. The nurse listens and responds nonjudgmentally as the client verbalizes disappointment and demonstrates lack of parental attachment. The client's expectations of fatherhood or motherhood are explored, and unrealistic expectations discussed. Information about the woman's acceptance of pregnancy and her relationship with her mother often assists her to cope with stress after the delivery.

The nurse assists clients in planning enjoyable activities that they have rarely done since the child's birth. Child care, work schedules, and support from a spouse and other family members can critically affect solution of these problems. The client is also encouraged to seek out other young parents and share experiences and feelings.

Clients can list positive aspects of being a parent, which the nurse emphasizes, the nurse may ask which friend or relative is most admired as a parent. The qualities of this parent are explored. Clients are encouraged to spend time with this admired friend or relative. As clients increase parental attachment, the nurse gives positive reinforcement.

Some women may strive to be "super mom," succeeding both at work and at home, but allocating little time for personal interests or individual needs. Family demands on the young adult may add appreciably to stress on the job, at school, or as a member of the new family. Clients are assisted to realistically examine the basis of their expectations and to adjust their life-styles accordingly. Sometimes family therapy is indicated to help clients adapt to the parenting role.

Interventions for young adults with role conflicts are aimed at reducing stress. The client describes the roles (parent, employee, spouse, boss) that contribute to the conflict. Expectations of self and others are explored, with attention to unrealistic expectations. The client is encouraged to make time for enjoyable activities. The nurse teaches the client relaxation exercises to reduce stress and encourages him to practice them. The nurse also emphasizes the importance of communicating with the person who is the source of stress. Assertiveness training and role playing are useful approaches for intervention in role conflict.

The young adult may be faced with the challenge of relocation for educational or work opportunities. Some may question the value of leaving a close-knit family or community for such purposes. The nurse provides support by carefully listening and helping the client identify advantages and disadvantages of the opportunity and limitations or fears accompanying the proposed change. The opportunity to contact an individual who made a similar move often provides the client with a realistic perception of the adaptation needed to succeed in the new environment.

Young adults may seek treatment or are even hospitalized as a result of marital conflict, separation, or divorce. Intervening with these clients usually requires couple or family therapy or crisis intervention for effective conflict resolution. Conflict resolution includes improved communication, open dialogue, and the establishment of priorities. When these therapies are not possible, the nurse facilitates expression of feelings to increase self-esteem. The client is asked to describe situations or behaviors that precipitate conflict with the spouse. The client is encouraged to accept responsibility for hurtful or destructive behaviors and is asked to try new interaction techniques with the spouse and report the results. Specific measures for intervening in marital conflict are described in Chapter 30.

Spiritual dimension A young couple who experiences a significant loss—for example, loss of a newborn—may seek support and begin to explore their religious values, often for the first time, from an adult perspective. This shared experience either strengthens the relationship or creates tension that inhibits communication and stresses the relationship.

The nurse gains a perspective on the client's response by exploring his value system with him. The client's view of the meaning of life is helpful in assisting with feelings of depression or low self-esteem. The inclusion of the value system and religious orientation in the treatment plan can provide insight into areas of the client's conflict and outside resources or support systems that can be used to change the client's perspective and behavior.

A crisis precipitates a wide range of individual responses. The client with a strong religious orientation may become introspective and respond consistently with the goal of renewal. Thus the successful resolution of a crisis may provide a mechanism for continued growth.

The following case example demonstrates the role of the nurse in assisting the client to resolve an ethical and moral conflict.

▼ Case Example

Mary, a 22-year-old newlywed, contacted the university mental health clinic to see a therapist because of her high level of anxiety was interfering with her success in graduate school. The nurse interviewing Mary provided an opportunity for her to discuss the problem that initiated the contact and sought clues to other issues that may need to be addressed. Mary stated that she had only recently married and that both she and her husband had several more years of education. When questioned about her marriage, she became tearful and said all was going well until she found out she was pregnant a month ago. Her husband had become very angry, said that she was irresponsible, and accused her of tricking him. He refused to talk about the pregnancy and spent a great deal of time away from their apartment in the last month.

The nurse noted that Mary had been feeling a great deal of stress during this period and that her anxiety, sleeplessness, and failure to concentrate were caused by her pregnancy and her husband's reaction to it. Mary expressed a need to talk about options for the pregnancy. The nurse provided information and support as Mary began to deal with her husband's anger and ambivalence about abortion. The nurse also provided an opportunity for Mary and her husband to discuss abortion, adoption, and ways to incorporate a baby into their life-style, as well as information on specific community agencies as requested.

At the next appointment Mary told the nurse that confronting the problem made it possible for her to continue school and that she and her husband had made plans to begin their family. They were looking into child care and other options so that they both could complete their educations without delay. The nurse had assessed the scope of the problem and provided support during a stressful period when the young couple had to address issues of values and morality.

Evaluation

The involvement of the young adult in the evaluation phase of the nursing process is the culmination of the nurse-client relationship. Review of outcome criteria and achievement of short-term and long-term goals are the focus of the evaluation process. During the evaluation process, the level of stress and current methods of coping are also addressed. Because evaluation is an ongoing process, the overall therapeutic plan is reevaluated and updated as the client progresses in treatment and new goals are established.

Positive growth is evident when the client is comfortable in intimate relationships and satisfying work roles and life-styles. This displays that the client has made some choices about his roles as an adult.

BRIEF REVIEW

Young adulthood (ages 20 to 44 years) involves a period of increasing societal expectations. Establishing financial independence from the family of origin, developing an intimate relationship, marrying, and parenting place demands on the individual that produce stress. An individual unable to cope successfully with the demands of this period may experience high levels of stress, demonstrate substance abuse behaviors, or express feelings of unworthiness and depression.

Young adults encounter rapid emotional change. They are also faced with issues about the changing role of women and men in US society. The adaptive response of the young adult is often challenged and confused by an ever-increasing wide range of life-styles from which to choose and which includes single parenting, delayed childbearing, and shared parental responsibilities.

A number of theorists have identified the developmental tasks of this period. The individual's perception of his world greatly influences whether the individual perceives himself as a success or failure. The demands of professional education and career development may prove extremely stressful, although cognitive functioning remains high during this period.

When working with the young adult, the nurse becomes acutely aware of the client's striving to meet the demands of school or work. The client's continued use of coping mechanisms that were successful in earlier developmental stages may interfere with more mature problem-solving activities. Resolution of issues not addressed in earlier developmental periods is a critical task.

REFERENCES AND SUGGESTED READINGS

1. American Psychiatric Association: *Diagnostic and statistical manual of mental disorders, DSM-III-R,* ed 3, Washington, DC, 1987, The Association.
2. Chadrow N: Family structure and feminine personality. In Rosaldo MZ, Lamphere L, editors: *Women, culture and society,* Stanford, Calif, 1974, Stanford University Press.

3. Cohen RS and others: *Parenthood: a psychodynamic perspective,* New York, 1984, The Guilford Press.

4. Colarusso C, Neimiroff RA: *Adult development: a new dimension in psychodynamic theory and practice,* New York, 1981, Plenum Press.

5. Cronenwett LR: Network structure, social support, and psychological outcomes of pregnancy, *Nursing Research* 34(2):93, 1985.

6. Erikson EH: *Childhood and society,* ed 2, New York, 1964, WW Norton.

7. Erikson EH: Generativity and ego integrity. In Neugarten B, editor: *Middle age and aging,* Chicago, 1968, The University of Chicago Press.

8. Fischer KE: Adult children of alcoholics: implications for the nursing professor, *Nursing Forum* 2(4):159, 1987/1988.

9. Freud A: The concept of developmental lines: their diagnostic significance, *Psychoanalytic Study of the Child* 36:129, 1981.

10. Freud S: *Three contributions to the theory of sex,* ed 4, Washington, DC, 1930, Nervous and Mental Disease Publishing Co.

11. Fromm E: *The sane society,* New York, 1955, Holt, Rinehart and Winston.

12. Gilligan C: *In a different voice: psychological theory and women's development,* Cambridge, Mass, 1982, Harvard University Press.

13. Gordon M: *Manual of nursing diagnosis,* St Louis, 1989, Mosby–Year Book.

14. Gould R: *Transformations,* New York, 1978, Simon & Schuster.

15. Haack MR: Collaborative investigation of adult children of alcoholics with anxiety, *Archives of Psychiatric Nursing* 4(1):62, 1990.

16. Hoffman L: Effects of the first child on the women's role. In Miller W, Newman L, editors: *The first child and family formation,* Chapel Hill, NC, 1978, University of North Carolina.

17. Horney K: *The neurotic personality of our time,* New York, 1937, WW Norton.

18. Jordon PL: Laboring for relevance: expectant and new fatherhood, *Nursing Research* 39(1):11, 1990.

19. Keane SM: Challenge within the community: crisis intervention for society's unemployed, *Nurs Forum* 21(3):138, 1984.

20. Lederman RP: *Psychosocial adaptation to pregnancy,* Englewood Cliffs, NJ, 1984, Prentice-Hall.

21. Levinson D and others: *The seasons of a man's life,* New York, 1979, Alfred A. Knopf.

22. Lowenstein SR: Suicidal behavior recognition and intervention, *Hospital Practice* 20:10A, 1985.

23. McFarland G, Wasli E: *Nursing diagnosis and process in psychiatric mental health nursing,* Philadelphia, 1986, JB Lippincott.

24. Owen BD: The young adult. In Hill PM, Humphrey P, editors: *Human growth and development throughout life: a nursing perspective,* New York, 1982, John Wiley & Sons.

25. Piaget J: The stages of intellectual development of the child, *Bulletin of the Menninger Clinic* 26:120, 1962.

26. Ryan RM, Lynch JH: Emotional autonomy versus detachment: revisiting the vicissitudes of adolescence and young adulthood, *Child Development* 60:340, 1989.

27. Selder F: Life transition theory: the resolution of uncertainty, *Nursing and Health Care* 10(8):438, 1989.

28. Sights J, Richards H: Parents of bulimic women, *International Journal of Eating Disorders* 3:3, 1984.

29. Snegroff S: The stressors of non-marital sexual intercourse, *Health Educ* 16(6):21, 1985-1986.

30. *Statistical Abstract of the United States,* 1990, ed 110, Washington, DC, 1990, US Bureau of the Census.

31. Stuart GW and others: Early family experiences of women with bulimia and depression, *Archives of Psychiatric Nursing* 4(1):43, 1990.

32. Sullivan HS: *The interpersonal theory of psychiatry,* New York, 1953, WW Norton.

33. Valliant G: *Adaptation to life,* Boston, 1977, Little, Brown & Co.

34. Walster E, Walster G: *A new look at love,* Reading, Mass, 1978, Addison-Wesley.

35. Watson J: *Nursing, human science and human caring—thing of nursing,* East Norwalk, Conn, 1986, Appleton & Lange.

36. Wolterman MC, Miller M: Caring for parents in crisis, *Nursing Forum* 22(1):34, 1985.

37. Woods NF: *Human sexuality in health and illness,* ed 3, St Louis, 1984, Mosby–Year Book.

ANNOTATED BIBLIOGRAPHY

Goldman HN: *Review of general psychiatry,* ed 2, Norwalk, Conn, 1988, Appleton & Lange.

Excellent review of stress and the mechanisms of defense. Discussion of major developmental landmarks and psychodynamic orientation of Freud, Erikson, Bowly, Piaget, and others provides good overview for understanding of precedents of young adult development.

Schuster CS, Ashburn SS: *The process of human development: a holistic life-span approach,* Boston, Mass, 1986, Little, Brown & Co.

Schuster and Ashburn provide several chapters of interest to those working in the area of young adults. Chapters on changing roles, initiating a family unit, and decision making regarding parenting provide an extensive overview of the issues encountered during the young adult period.

CHAPTER 39

The Middle-Aged Adult

Sophronia R Williams

After studying this chapter, the student will be able to:

- Trace the historical developments related to mental health–psychiatric nursing for the middle-aged adult
- Discuss the psychopathology applicable to the middle-aged adult as described in the DSM-III-R
- Discuss theories related to middle-aged adults
- Apply the nursing process to the care of middle-aged adults
- Identify current research findings related to middle-aged adults

Middle age is one of the fastest growing life spans. The first of the baby boomers, those born between 1946 and 1964, are now entering mid-life. Advances in health science—such as better understanding of the aging body, early recognition and prevention of disease, and more effective treatment of health problems—also contribute to the growth of this age-group. By the year 2000 middle-aged adults will compose 12% of the population. The mental health–psychiatric nurse will play a role in the growth of this age-group by participating in the prevention of mental health problems.

There is no formal discipline that studies the middle years. There is, however, scientific information and systematic theories that contribute to understanding the experiences and needs of individuals in mid-life. This information helps to dispel the myths about middle age.[47] For example, people today are less likely than previously to view middle-aged adults as "over the hill," or the middle-aged woman as floundering in her "empty nest." The stereotype of the middle-aged man who deserts his wife for a woman half his age still exists.

Some view the middle years as the prime of life. It is a time of change, but individuals are usually responsible and in control of their lives. Most middle-aged persons have good physical and emotional health and are financially secure. They have recognized their intellectual abilities, established themselves in the social world, and found ways to meet their spiritual needs. However, they also experience satisfactions and stresses unique to this period of life.

There is no clear agreement on when middle age begins. Chronological age is one means used to determine the beginning of mid-life. It is generally accepted that middle age chronologically begins between 35 and 45 years and ends between 60 and 65 years. Research indicates that the onset of middle age typically occurs at younger chronological ages for the working class and disadvantaged individuals than for the middle class and more advantaged persons.[66]

Levinson and others[58] used a chronological definition of middle adulthood that has five developmental periods:

40 to 45 years: Mid-life transition
45 to 50 years: Entrance into middle adulthood
50 to 55 years: Age 50 transition
55 to 60 years: Culmination of middle adulthood
60 to 65 years: Late adulthood transition

Chronological age may not be the most significant determinant of entrance into the middle years. Culture defines developmental time tables for taking on various roles. The individual internalizes these time tables and then lives up to the predetermined cultural expectations. For example, in western society the age for retirement is predetermined to take place between 65 and 70 years of age. This cultural expectation may force people into retirement, even though some would like to continue working. Social events, such as the last child leaving home or birth of a grandchild, may also signal the beginning of middle age.

▶ DIAGNOSES Related to Middle-Aged Adults

MEDICAL DIAGNOSES	NURSING DIAGNOSIS NANDA
Occupational problem	Impaired adjustment
Other interpersonal problem	Caregiver role strain
Parent-child problem	High risk for caregiver role strain
Other specified family circumstance	

DATES	EVENTS
Pre-1900s	There was no systematic study of the developmental experiences of the middle-aged adult. Philosophers, prophets, and other writers emphasized either characteristic abilities or social and moral responsibilities of the middle-aged adult.
Early 1900s	Popular and professional writers portrayed the middle-aged adult as desolate, gloomy, and more despairing than hopeful. Much information used to describe middle-aged adults came from psychoanalysts' therapy with them. Psychoanalysts viewed the middle years as a series of crises that resulted in pathological behavior. Jung was the first to investigate the middle years while treating his clients.
1920s-1930s	Buhler and others conducted the first formal research on middle-aged adults and recognized them as relatively healthy with strengths. Although their lives were contracting, they could take stock and reassess their lives.
1940s-1950s	Attention was focused on the study of the relatively healthy middle-aged adult.
1960s	The Bethesda Conference on the Middle Years recommended that research be directed toward the potentials of the middle-aged adult instead of their problems. A federal conference on aging recognized that research on the problems of middle age was necessary to solve the problems of the older adult. Professionals became interested in maintaining the health of the middle-aged adult.
1975	The American Journal of Nursing discussed changes in the sexual, physical, and social needs of the middle-aged adult and later compared the middle years with other phases in the life cycle.
1977	The Schweppe Research and Education Fund Conference focused on the interaction between biomedical and social factors in the aging process, with emphasis on the middle-aged adult. Dissemination of information on realities of middle age to middle-aged adults, young adults, health care professionals, educators, and policy makers was emphasized.
	Nursing began demonstrating interest in all aspects of middle age. Stevenson, a nurse, wrote a textbook devoted to issues and crises in the middle years.
1979	Burnside and other nurses comprehensively covered experiences of the middle-aged adult in their text.
1980s	Articles on the middle years are included in journals, and nurses have included a discussion of this age-group in textbooks.
1990s	Interest in this age-group increases as the "baby boomers" now begin their movement through the life span and greater emphasis is given to prevention of mental health problems.
Future	There will be an increase in research of middle-aged adults to determine how different experiences for the "baby boomers" influence their responses to mid-life changes.

Positional cues show middle age as a period between young adulthood and the aged adult period. The position between these two generations increases middle-aged persons' awareness that they are in a different life cycle. For example, the young adult may be having her first child and the aged adult beginning life as a retiree while the middle-aged adult is becoming a grandparent or beginning a second career. Physical and biological changes that are typical for middle age, such as the graying of hair and menopause, occur. The woman without children realizes she will never be a biological mother. Psychological cues, such as valuing the wisdom that comes with mid-life, may be evident. These cues may be used to assess career goals.[66]

The various experiences that make entrance into middle age constitute mid-life transition. *Mid-life transition* begins with the awareness of reproductive and physical changes.

The individual reappraises the meaning of his life—past, present, and future. A goal of this period is to complete three tasks: (1) to terminate the era of early adulthood by reappraising the life goals identified and achieved, (2) to initiate movement into middle adulthood by making necessary changes while trying out new choices, and (3) to deal with conflicts that divide life.[32] The individual's overall goal is to rebuild his life structure. During introspection the middle-aged adult asks himself such questions as, What have I done with my life? What do I really get from and give to my spouse, children, friends, work, community, and self? What are my strengths and liabilities? What have I done with my early dream, and do I want it now? Based on the answers to these questions, the middle-aged adult in transition redefines his own individuality as a mature adult.

The movement into middle adulthood is challenging.

Some people make a smooth transition to this life cycle; others experience a mid-life crisis.

DSM-III-R

The DSM-III-R uses V codes to classify conditions that require treatment or are the focus of attention but are not caused by a mental disorder. Several V codes apply to the middle-aged adult. *Occupational problem* can be applied to the middle-aged adult who seeks assistance because of job dissatisfaction or uncertainty about career choices when laid off or given early retirement. A person in mid-life may seek treatment for a *parent-child problem* that is not due to a mental illness. For example, a typical problem for this age-group may center on the conflict between a mentally healthy adolescent and his middle-aged parents about curfews or choice of friends. Other *specific family circumstances* can apply when the treatment for a mentally healthy middle-aged adult focuses on interpersonal difficulties with a family member other than the person's child or spouse, such as stress related to care of aged parents. *Other interpersonal problems* is a useful classification when a middle-aged adult's reason for seeking treatment is an interpersonal problem with someone other than a family member. For example, the individual may have a problem with a co-worker or romantic partner when neither has a mental disorder.

THEORETICAL APPROACHES

Psychoanalytical

Intrapsychic

Erikson[27] considered the seventh stage of life the middle years. The developmental task is generativity versus stagnation. *Generativity* is a commitment to care for and a willingness to counsel and guide others. Erikson believed that generativity is most meaningful with one's own children. Failure to achieve generativity may cause stagnation. *Stagnation* means excessive concern with oneself. Feelings of stagnation may also be manifested in destructive behavior toward one's children and the community. A person's concern for his own children and for the next generation can help prevent stagnation.

Jung's theories[51] about the middle years, based on a psychological model, addressed aspects of the spiritual dimension. He viewed life as contracting in middle age. Middle-aged people must make a transition to their inner orientation. Such introspection may be threatening. It involves giving up the images of youth and recognizing one's mortality. Middle-aged adults may cling to behavior characteristic of youth. However, in the developmental process of self-individuation, middle-aged adults become more uniquely themselves. This process enables them to balance their psychological functions: thought, feeling, intuition, and sensation.

Buhler's theories[11] about the middle years emphasized goal formulation. Similar to Jung, she viewed life as an expansion and contraction process, with acknowledgment of success or failure as the major task of middle age. Goal achievement depends on (1) satisfaction of needs, (2) ability to expand creatively, (3) adjustment to limitations, and

(4) consistency of inner self. By middle age, a person has either achieved his goals or has failed. Few people achieve all of their life goals. Goals may be identified late in life. The emotional responses to unfulfilled goals are depression, despair, and sometimes suicide.

Peck,[70] expanding Erikson's concepts, described four phases of psychological development for middle age.

1. *Valuing wisdom versus valuing physical powers.* Wisdom is the ability to make the best choices from the available alternatives. Middle age brings a decrease in physical strength, stamina, and beauty. By investing more energy into mental activities, the middle-aged person adjusts. Emotional status and intellectual ability affect task achievement. Persons who define their lives in terms of physical power may become increasingly depressed as that power declines.
2. *Socializing versus sexualizing in human relationships.* The sexual climacteric coincides with the decline in physical powers. This change motivates middle-aged people to redefine men and women in their lives as individuals and companions rather than primarily as sexual objects.
3. *Cathectic flexibility versus cathectic impoverishment.* This task involves shifting emotional investments from one person to another and from one activity to another. Peck believed the task is crucial in middle years. It is generally during middle age when people experience the loss of many relationships. Although middle-aged persons experience losses, they have a wide circle of acquaintances at work and in the community for reinvestment of emotions. People who are unsuccessful in replacing the lost relationships with new ones suffer increasingly impoverished emotional lives through the years.
4. *Mental flexibility versus mental rigidity.* This conflict affects all changes of middle age. Mental flexibility means not being set in one's ways, being open to new ideas, and accepting change in self and society. Flexible adults strive to master life experiences and use them as guides to solving new problems. Rigid middle-aged adults are set in their ways, inflexible in their opinions and actions, and closed-minded to new ideas. Peck believes that mental rigidity is most noticeable during middle age when people have a set of answers to life.

Eclectic

Havighurst[42] defines middle age in terms of specific developmental tasks that the individual needs to achieve between ages 35 to 60 years. He refers to the tasks as "markers of change" along the life span. The tasks are precipitated primarily through biological maturation and changes in social roles. However, he recognizes that the tasks primarily are a combination of biological, psychological, and sociological factors. Each task must be achieved for satisfactory adjustment to middle age and progression to the next developmental stage. The individual needs to master the following tasks:

1. Achieve adult civic and social responsibility
2. Establish and maintain an economic standard of living
3. Help teenaged children become responsible and happy adults

▼ **TABLE 39-1**   **Summary of Theoretical Approach**

Theory	Theorist	Dynamics
Psycho-analytical	Erikson	Achievement of the developmental task generativity versus stagnation is evident in a commitment to care for and a willingness to counsel and guide the next generation. Failure to achieve the task results in excessive concern for oneself.
	Jung	The task for middle age is to make a transition from outer to inner orientation. The transition enables middle-aged people to feel secure about their course in life and to balance their four psychological functions: thought, feeling, intuition, and sensation.
	Buhler	The middle years are characterized by expansion and contraction, during which time the person assesses life goals and acknowledges successes and failures.
	Peck	There are four phases of psychological development for middle age: (1) valuing wisdom versus valuing physical powers, (2) socializing versus generalizing in human relationships, (3) cathectic flexibility versus cathectic impoverishment, and (4) mental flexibility versus mental rigidity.
Eclectic	Havighurst	The developmental tasks of middle age are a combination of biological, psychological, and sociological factors. The tasks are "markers of change" along the life span.

4. Develop adult leisure activities
5. Relate to one's spouse as a person
6. Accept and adjust to the physiological changes of middle age
7. Adjust to aging parents

Table 39-1 presents a summary of the theoretical approaches.

NURSING PROCESS

Assessment

Physical dimension When considering Havighurst's tasks the individual has to accept and adjust to the physiological changes of middle age. The nurse assesses the client's response to these changes that naturally accompany middle age. The most visible changes—such as graying hair, wrinkling skin, and balding—are gradual and genetically determined, with most middle-aged adults manifesting the beginning of these changes by ages 45 to 50.[55] The response to these changes is determined, in part, by the person's contentment with himself in mid-life. Some individuals take the physical changes in stride. People who are insecure may be anxious about these signs of middle age and express their concerns openly or try to conceal the changes. Women are more likely than are men to be bothered by gray hair and may dye or tint the hair. Men may view graying hair as a status symbol, one that helps them to look distinguished.[55]

During the assessment, middle-aged adults are likely to report excess fat in the midsection, regardless of lack of increase in food intake or decrease in exercise. This change is due to redistribution of fat and need not be problematic. However, the change may be a stressor for some individuals.

Some middle-aged adults become obese. Obesity is the physical change that presents the greatest health risk. For people who are 30% or more overweight, the probability of dying in middle age increases by 40%.[83] The causes of obesity are complex. Overeating in response to mid-life changes can result in obesity. Marked obesity in mid-life may follow major emotional stressors such as death in the family, vocational failures, and marital unhappiness. A sedentary life-style may also contribute to excessive weight gain. Individuals who derive feelings of worth from their bodies may be more bothered by physical changes than those who focus on other characteristics to assess their value.[70]

The nurse assesses the functioning of the client's physiological processes (see the box on p. 787). Alterations in these processes affect all body systems, influencing the client's perception of himself and his ability to function and relate to others. Diseases of the cardiovascular system, especially heart disease and stroke, are the main causes of death in middle age. These diseases are stress-related and may also be determined by genetic factors.

The nurse assesses the client's response to *climacteric*. The climacteric is the complex of endocrine, somatic, and psychic changes that occur at the end of the woman's reproductive period. Along with the climacteric, there is a decline in physical strength. Individuals who defined themselves primarily as sexual objects may have difficulty adjusting to changes associated with climacteric.[70]

For women *menopause*, a permanent cessation of menstruation, is a normal physiological response during the climacteric. The age range for menopause is 40 to 60 years, with 50 as the typical age.[40] Menopause results from a loss of ovarian activity and a concomitant decrease in the production of estrogen. With this change comes loss of reproductive function and the ability to bear children. Menopause does not seem to have serious physical symptoms for most women. Typically women experience hot flashes due to the physiological changes. Some have breast pain and dizzy spells. Many women may feel healthier after the menopause and relieved that they no longer need to be concerned about unwanted pregnancy. Other women may experience insomnia, fatigue, headaches, and weight gain.[40]

A side-effect of menopause is osteoporosis, a decrease in bone mass.[7] Some bone loss begins to occur gradually at about age 40 and becomes more pronounced during and after menopausal changes. The physical appearance that results from the bone loss, roundness of the back to the point of being nearly doubled-over, can affect the body image. Of women over the age of 45, 50% are affected with osteoporosis. Of the 25% of Anglo women likely to have

SELECTED PHYSIOLOGICAL CHANGES IN THE MIDDLE-AGED ADULT ACCORDING TO BODY SYSTEMS

Muscular

Mass, structure, and strength slowly decline as a result of decreased muscle use. Changes in collagen fibers result in thicker and less elastic muscles and cause sagging and drooping of breast, facial, and abdominal muscles.

Skeletal

Bone mass begins to decrease, calcium loss and related bone thinning follows menopausal changes, skeletal changes in the thoracic vertebrae lead to height decrease (more pronounced in women than men), and changes occur in the hip joints.

Integumentary

With adequate nutrition and fluid intake, tissues of the integument remain intact and healthy until age 50 to 55. After this age, wrinkles gradually become noticeable; body water content decreases from 60% to 56%, leading to dry skin; and fat content increases from 14% to 30%, leading to sagging folds, such as under the arms and under the eyes. Too rapid weight reduction causes loose folds that do not readily accommodate the loss of fat. Because of loss of water, the skin is more easily bruised and wounds heal more slowly.

Central Nervous

Marked changes usually do not occur until very old age. The high level of intellectual functioning is discussed under assessment of the intellectual dimension. Reflexes begin to slow, and slower response to environmental changes may be observable.

Cardiovascular

Well into middle age, the size of the heart increases to accommodate changes in the arterial system. Functions, rate, and rhythm of the heart are maintained through active work and recreational activities. As sedentary activities increase, the heart begins to lose its tone, and rhythm and rate changes are noticeable.

Respiratory

The respiratory tissues maintain full vital respiratory capacity (maximal breathing capacity) throughout early middle age, barring cigarette smoking and respiratory disease. By age 55 to 60 there is a gradual decrease in breathing capacity caused by thicker, stiffer, and less elastic lung tissues. Cardiopulmonary diseases may accompany the changes in lung tissue.

Renal

With adequate fluid intake, the normal mechanism of kidney functioning is maintained at full capacity throughout middle age.

Gastrointestinal

Normally, secretions from the gastrointestinal tract are maintained at high levels through early middle age. Decreases in the production of digestive enzymes, acids, and juices may be a factor in the increase in incidence of intestinal disorders, cancer, and gastrointestinal complaints of middle-aged clients.

Metabolic

Onset of diabetes mellitus, hypothyroidism, and adrenal tumors is more common after age 45. Proneness to ulcers and vascular lesions increase because of an increased amount of antiinflammatory hormones. This change in hormones may also affect clients' ability to handle stress.

Special Senses

Farsightedness that necessitates correction with glasses or contact lenses develops. Because lenses of eyes gradually become more opaque after age 45, cataract formation becomes a possibility. Blindness may develop as a consequence of diabetes, hypertension, or other cardiovascular conditions.
The sense of hearing, smell, taste, and touch are generally maintained at high levels in early middle age. After age 50, noticeable losses in hearing and smell may occur.

---

one or two fractures by age 65, 70% will be caused by osteoporosis. In addition to menopause, other risk factors for osteoporosis include race (Anglo), a positive family history, small frame, low calcium intake, smoking, and alcohol abuse.[7]

Some of the emotional symptoms that may be a direct result of menopause are anxiety, depression, and irritability. These symptoms are problematic and may be due to the woman's concern about having reached this milestone in her life.

The man's climacteric is referred to as *andropause* because of the decline in the androgen levels during the late 40s and early 50s. Men still produce sperm and are capable of fathering children well into late adulthood.[53] Anxiety and depression may result from a decrease in ability to have an orgasm. This inability may be viewed as sexual inadequacy or imagined loss of sexual power. Some men may have extramarital relationships in an attempt to prove that they can still attract members of the opposite sex.

The nurse assesses for changes in the individual's sleep pattern. The number of hours of sleep that the middle-aged adult needs varies; however, the average person generally requires 6 to 8 hours. As the middle-aged individual approaches his 60s and expends less energy, the need for sleep is approximately 5 to 6 hours a night. More active middle-aged persons may take naps or doze during the day.[55]

Complaints of sleeplessness increase with age. As age increases, middle-aged persons tend to go to bed earlier and awake earlier in the morning and may sleep less well than do older and younger adults.[55] In women there is a sharp increase in sleeplessness around the age of 50.[82]

Emotional dimension Anxiety does not increase appreciably with age for those who have rewarding, nonthreatening life experiences. These people accept and adapt to the visible signs of aging and capitalize on the benefits of middle age. Anxiety may be a positive source that motivates middle-aged persons to reassess themselves and to work further on accomplishing their life goals or identifying new goals.[56] This self-analysis results from a heightened self-awareness when "life is restructured in terms of time-left-to-live rather than time-since-birth.[67]

The nurse is alert for an increased and generalized feeling of anxiety that may arise over irreversible physical and social losses as the person's life begins to contract. Individuals in the high-risk group for osteoporosis may experience anxiety in anticipation of developing the disease. Anxiety may be an emotional response to menopause.

Middle-aged clients who fear growing old may experience a severe level of anxiety. The nurse learns that these individuals are unable to reassess themselves in light of the normal changes of aging. These persons may have a prior history of emotional problems.[70]

Ill health and fear of death cause anxiety for some middle-aged adults. The individual may have numerous presenting physical complaints in response to anxiety about mid-life changes. General malaise; stress-related illnesses, such as peptic ulcers; rheumatoid arthritis; and hypertension are some of the problems the nurse may identify during the assessment.

When using Jung's theory, the nurse assesses the individual's recognition of and response to heightened awareness of his own mortality. As middle-aged adults' parents begin to die and age mates develop life-threatening illnesses such as heart disease and cancer, one's mortality becomes a personal reality.[55] Some middle-aged adults' anxiety and fear about death is evident when they scan the obituary column or write wills in response to the death of age mates, friends, and parents. The threat of sudden death from a heart attack can generate anxiety in men ages 40 to 50. Fear of dying after sustaining a fracture is real, since the occurrence of a hip fracture for individuals with osteoporosis increases the individual's probability of dying within the following year by 5% to 20%.[28]

The nurse assesses for feelings of anger. The work experiences of middle-aged clients may create anger. At work, a middle-aged employee may experience anger when he is at risk for unemployment because of severe economic conditions. This real or imagined threat leads to anger as a defense against the anxiety. Clients may also become angry at work when they perceive others trying to hold them back. For example, a middle-aged employee may not be recommended for promotion because of lack of skills. The individual may believe he was overlooked because of his age.

Anger toward parents and children may occur when the individual's needs are not met. Anger about the role reversal that occurs between middle-aged children and their elderly parents is important to assess. Adult children who perceive themselves as sacrificing their lives for their parents may become frustrated and bitter. The elderly parents may become the objects of rejection and abuse (see Chapter 34).

The nurse may observe pathological guilt during the assessment. Middle-aged adults who have neglected or abused their parents may feel guilty and try to overprotect them.[8] Middle-aged clients may also feel guilt when they think they could have done more to achieve their life goals. On the other hand, some people may feel guilt because they surpassed their parents in achieving career goals. Guilt about how they raised their children may occur, especially when children do not live up to their expectations.

Most persons approaching middle age feel confident of their ability to adjust to mid-life changes and losses. They view mid-life, another milestone in their life, as a challenge and a time for further growth. They are satisfied with their achievements and feel hopeful about the future. These individuals may occasionally have mild depression that is temporary and does not require intervention.

However, there is increased prevalence of major depression in persons over the age of 45.[14,15] Buhler's theory[10] supports assessing for depression in response to unfulfilled goals. The individuals who respond to mid-life with despair and major depression may perceive themselves as failures. They are probably unable to identify new goals without assistance. The persons are unable to accept and adjust to the new mid-life experiences.

Some middle-aged adults experience depression in response to the various losses that are typical of mid-life. The nurse assesses the person's response to losses such as physical decline, job loss, and changes in the family constellation. Lost family ties are traditionally felt more intensely in mid-life. The departure of the last child from home may aggravate an already existing mid-life depression or precipitate the depression.

Job loss is an important consideration when assessing for depression in the middle-aged adult.[36] Depression is most severe for those individuals who attached considerable significance to themselves as workers. The unemployed person may blame himself for the job loss and have low self-esteem and guilt. The person's depression is often intensified if reemployment is prolonged or not a reality because of factors such as age or lack of marketable skills.

Some middle-aged adults use alcohol to cope with the depression related to the loss of a job. When assessing for depression in these persons, the nurse differentiates between depression as a symptom in response to unemployment and as a major psychiatric illness. Depression as a symptom may result from abrupt abstinence of alcohol and may disappear in days or weeks without a need for antidepressant medication. As a psychiatric illness, depression lasts longer and is usually treated with antidepressant medications and sometimes with ECT.[39]

In the past it was believed that hormonal changes associated with menopause played a major role in precipitating depression in middle age. Today many believe that the hormonal changes play no role in the cause of depression in this period. Women who experience severe depression during menopause may be responding to other various losses.[40] Some women interpret menopausal changes as a loss of femininity. The severe depression that occurs is sometimes referred to as *agitated depression.* It is characterized by a moderate to high level of anxiety, bizarre physical complaints, and paranoid ideas. The essential features of depression in the menopausal years do not differ

▼ **TABLE 39-2   Risk Factors for Depression in Middle Age**

Risk Factors	Characteristics
Gender	Female
Age	Declines for women after early 50s; increases for men after late 50s
Social isolation	Absence of intimate, confiding relationships after a change in the nature of the relationship with parents, children, and spouse
Losses	Parental deprivation or loss of a mother before age 14; other losses during midlife, such as a job, career difficulties, marital problems, and physical changes; departure of last child from home; unfulfilled life goals
Family history	History of depression in the family of origin

appreciably from depression in other age-groups. The clinical features of depression in middle-aged men are no different from those at other times of life.[14]

Risk factors that increase the likelihood of depression are summarized in Table 39-2.

The potential for suicide is assessed. Suicide and attempted suicide increase in middle age and are more common among men than women.[16] Suicide is less common between the ages of 40 and 50, after which it increases. Persons who commit suicide are often widowed, separated, or divorced. They may also be socially isolated. Depression and alcoholism in middle age contribute to an increase in the suicide rate. Over 90% of successful suicides in mid-life are by persons who are depressed, alcoholic, or both.[55] See Chapter 14 for additional information on assessment of suicidal behavior.

Intellectual dimension The nurse attends to the senses that are affected in middle age. Most research indicates little change in the ability to taste food up to the age of 60. However, taste buds begin to decrease in men at age 50 to 60 and in women at age 40 to 45. Touch sensitivity remains constant up to about the mid-50s and then gradually decreases. Individual differences affect the ability to smell, although there seems to be an aging effect on the olfactory sense receptors. Visual efficiency declines rapidly after age 40. Bifocals and trifocals are often needed to correct vision.

The client's ability to retain information is assessed. Short-term memory is believed to decline in middle age. However, the situations in which clients are tested need to be considered when assessing individual memory differences. For example, individuals generally retain information acquired visually longer than that which they hear.

Middle-aged adults who actively use their intellectual functions have little if any loss of mental ability, whereas those who do not engage in productive mental activities may experience a decline in intellectual performance. In middle age, people may have a wealth of previous experiences that they use to improve their present functioning. This ability is termed *wisdom.*[70] Wisdom is the ability to

make the best choices from the available alternatives.[70] The middle-aged adult who ages successfully gives higher priority to wisdom than physical power.[70]

For some middle-aged adults, vocabulary and verbal skills continue to improve. There also may be improvement in the middle-aged adult's ability to organize and process incoming information and handle larger vocabularies.

When using Peck's theory,[70] the nurse assesses the individual's mental functioning for flexibility or rigidity. Some middle-aged adults are flexible in their thinking and open to new ideas and changes in behavior. They accept and adapt to new experiences and continue to grow. Others are set in their ways. These individuals are inflexible and resist new experiences. They display an unwillingness to accept the need for normal mid-life changes, viewing them instead as change for change's sake.[21] Generally women are more flexible than are men in their capacity for change and growth in middle age.[29]

The nurse is alert for the type of defense mechanisms the client uses to deal with anxiety. Some individuals engage in pathological use of the defense mechanisms of denial and rationalization. Use of dissociation, repression, and sublimation may also increase in mid-life. Some individuals may become paranoid, blaming others for their failure to achieve their life goals. They may be bitter and envious of those who succeed. Buhler[10] describes these individuals as lacking the insight into their own limitations that lead to a lack of success.

When doing an assessment the nurse may observe signs and symptoms of Alzheimer's disease and Pick's disease, organic mental disorders that prevent the individual from achieving many of the tasks of mid-life. These diseases are discussed in Chapter 33.

Social dimension Abuse of alcohol is a major problem in middle age. The nurse encounters middle-aged clients who have abused alcohol since young adulthood and in some cases since adolescence; these clients may increase consumption of alcohol in middle age in response to changes in their lives. Sometimes clients who have secretly abused alcohol may do so openly when the children leave home. Other clients may lead stable lives before reaching middle age and begin abusing alcohol in their early 40s.[74] These clients seem to resort to alcohol abuse in an effort to cope with various mid-life changes.

Sometimes one spouse becomes less tolerant of the other's consumption of alcohol after the children leave. Separation or divorce may be the result. The threat of loss of the spouse motivates some alcoholic partners to seek treatment. Middle-aged individuals with alcoholism may also seek treatment because of problems on the job, with family, or with physical health.

The nurse assesses for changes in the nature of the person's roles and social relationships. Many middle-aged adults are caring for their dependent children. Children of middle-aged parents typically range from late adolescent to their late 20s. Because some parents are having children later in life, the children may be in their mid-teens or younger. For others the children may be married with young children of their own. Caring for the adolescent tends to be a challenge for some parents since mid-life stress occurs simultaneously with adolescent stress. Using Erikson's theory,[27] the nurse inquires about the parents' ability to give the adolescent guidance and support as he becomes a responsible adult. The parents' willingness to devote time and energy to caring for the adolescent enables them to achieve Erikson's task, generativity.[40] Some conflict is natural as adolescents struggle to find themselves. Parents who foster the adolescents' independence and responsibility, allowing them to develop their own identity, are likely to have less conflict with them.[48] When the parents use pressure to guide the adolescent and disallow the individual to be autonomous, intense conflict, resentment, and hostility are likely to be the result. Generally, parents who were successful in their parenting role with young children are likely to have few problems with adolescents.[83]

When middle-aged parents have children younger than adolescents, they may feel out of sync with their peers. These parents have child-rearing responsibilities that require more time and direct involvement than do their age mates. During assessment, the nurse may observe parents of young children who take their responsibilities in stride. Other parents may become hostile and have marital conflicts.[83]

The nurse needs to assess the individual's adjustment to stepparenting as a new role. After a divorce some middle-aged adults remarry and become stepparents. The role of stepparent may be the most difficult in mid-life.[57] The greatest area of conflict is discipline and handling the children. Stepparents may contribute to problems in the relationship when they feel insecure and so afraid of failure that they try to establish the relationship too quickly. Such behavior does not allow sufficient time for the child to resolve feelings about the previous marriage.

A stepparent may have problems when he tries to replace the biological parent. The child compares the stepparent with the biological parent and may expect the same treatment. When the treatment is not forthcoming the child is likely to express hostility. Children may also be resentful and angry when they think that the stepparents favor their biological children.[57] Some stepparents are successful in meeting the needs of stepchildren. These individuals create a positive experience for the children and guide and support them as they recover from the divorce of their parents. These stepparents achieve the task of generativity.

Attention is given to the parents' response to the departure of the last child from home. Many middle-aged parents respond positively to the last child's leaving home, seeing it as an opportunity for freedom from child-rearing responsibilities.[35] The parents who best adapt to the "empty nest" are those who have encouraged their children's independence. The departure of the last child from the home is experienced as a negative stressor by parents who have focused most or all of their attention and time on children.[55] These parents often become depressed, feeling that they have nothing to live for. These parents have difficulty "letting go."

Many of today's middle-aged adults are caring for their dependent children and their aging parents at the same time. These middle-aged adults are referred to as the sandwich generation, caught between competing obligations to their children and to their parents.[78]

The nurse assesses the individual's adjustment to aging parents. Generally a daughter is the caregiver for aging parents. The changing relationship between the middle-aged adult child and aging parents involves *role reversal.* Many adults want to care for aging parents and do so willingly. These individuals view the responsibility as reciprocating for the care the parents gave them in the past. The middle-aged caregiver may also see the activity as role modeling for their own children who will one day need to care for them.[8] Care of aging parents can contribute to the middle-aged adults' achievement of Havighurst's task, adjustment to the reality of the aging parent.[42]

The role reversal involved in caring for aging parents may be a source of strain. Meeting the needs of parents who have any form of dependency—cognitive, physical, or financial—entails a great burden for the middle-aged adult.[78] The responsibility for parents prevents or delays the middle-aged adult child's achievement of Erikson's task, generativity.[27] The time needed for the aging parent may lead to marital discord. Middle-aged adult caregivers sometimes experience restrictions on their time and freedom, as well as their social and recreational activities.[49]

Caring for the aging parent reminds the client of his own aging and eventual death. When the client is unprepared to deal with this reality, his experiences with his aging parents may motivate him to come to grips with his own aging and eventual death. If the client's parents are dead, the past relationship needs to be explored.

The decision to institutionalize an aging parent is one of the most difficult and engenders strong feelings of ambivalence, guilt, and shame. The adult child may be reluctant to make a decision for nursing home placement, especially if the parent does not want to go to a nursing home. (See research highlight.)

The combination of caring for aging parents; rearing adolescents, stepchildren, or young children; and possibly bearing the financial pressures of putting one or more children through college can be a heavy burden for middle-aged parents. These experiences and departure of children from the home may force individuals to take stock of their marriage. The nurse inquires about the result of the individuals' examination of their marital relationship. The partners' reassessment of their marriage either leads to a strengthening of the relationship or reveals problems. One or both marital partners may become dissatisfied and seek an extramarital relationship. Some partners turn to a younger person in actuality or fantasy in a desire to maintain youth. Men are more likely than women to have extramarital affairs with younger partners. Although society disapproves of an older man in an extramarital affair with a younger woman,[31] it is commonly more accepted than a woman having a young partner. However, acceptance of the latter is increasing.

Strong marriages survive the reassessment of middle age and may improve as the marital partners spend more time together. Maladaptive marriages tend to survive the midlife crisis because most people in such marriages are so insecure that they do not question the nature of the marital relationship.[31] These people maintain the marriage because they are neurotically dependent on their spouse, are fearful of being alone, feel guilty, or are financially dependent on the spouse.

Divorce is a possible outcome when reassessment of the marital relationship in middle age reveals serious problems. Partners who divorce after 20 years have usually been in-

RESEARCH HIGHLIGHT

Nursing Home Placement: The Daughter's Perspective

• MA Johnson

PURPOSE

The purpose of this study was to explore the experiences of adult daughters resulting from the admission of a parent to a nursing home.

SAMPLE

The convenience sample consisted of 16 daughters who had admitted a parent to a skilled care nursing facility with anticipation of long-term or permanent residence during the 7 days preceding the study. The daughters ranged in age from 33 to 67 years. Of the respondents, 50% were working outside the home; 72% were married, and the remaining were equally distributed between divorce and widow status.

METHODOLOGY

An unstructured format that allowed for in-depth probes was used for most of the interviews. Eight specific open-ended questions were used when the daughters did not spontaneously offer information. The investigator interviewed the subjects in a location designated by the daughter. Of the interviews, 62% were conducted in the daughter's home and 11% were conducted by telephone. The other interviews were held at the daughter's place of business, the investigator's office, or a restaurant. The first interview was face-to-face. Three interviews were scheduled, with each respondent covering the first 2 months after admission. Seven of the parents were not in the nursing home at the final interview time. Two were discharged before Time 2, two died before Time 2, and three died before Time 3. Each daughter was interviewed at least two times for a total of 45 taped interviews: 7 to 10 days after admission, 30 to 35 days after admission, and 60 to 70 days after admission.

Based on data from *Journal of Gerontological Nursing* 16(11):6, 1990.

FINDINGS

The data compiled from the interviews were categorized into four groupings related to the decision for nursing home placement: lack of control over the decision, rationale suggested for the decision, dilemmas encountered, and revisiting the decision. The daughters described a lack of control of the decision because another person made or the situation dictated the decision—physician, parent, nursing home as only option. Most daughters expressed ambivalence about following through with the decision. They reported ethical dilemmas (1) when having to make a choice between the needs of their parents and the rest of their family, (2) in relation to depriving the parent of autonomy and usual life-style, and (3) when questioning the choice of nursing home. Guilt and concern about hurting the other parent and other family members was a theme. By the end of the study, six of the daughters reported that they had been able to reconcile their feelings about the placement; seven were still distressed about the need for placement.

IMPLICATIONS

The findings indicate the need for nursing intervention before the parent is actually placed in a nursing home. Nurses can discuss the possibility of nursing home care with the family before admission. Nurses can facilitate the decision-making process by encouraging discussion about appropriateness of nursing home placement. They can provide an opportunity for the family to examine thoughts and feelings about placement of a parent in a nursing home.

---

compatible throughout their marriage. Divorce during the postparental years may result when a marriage was maintained for the sake of the children. The external restraints that traditionally bound couples together have been removed for some people. For example, the woman who works outside the home is not financially dependent on the husband and thus is more likely to divorce if the marriage is not strong. However, divorce in mid-life occurs less frequently than continuing in an unhappy, incompatible marriage. The couple may then cope by attempting to ignore the difficulties with emotional and physical withdrawal, extramarital relationships, spending extra time at work, or abuse of alcohol.

The nurse assesses the client's response to the death of a spouse, one of the most stressful experiences of middle age. Women's tendencies to marry older men and the increasing death rate among middle-aged men, especially from cardiovascular disease, increase the potential for widowhood in middle age. Some women begin preparing for widowhood in middle age by becoming involved in managing the financial activities related to the household. Others begin or resume a career to become financially secure.

Bereavement often leads to the death of widowed persons within 5 years of the spouse's death.[81] Men and women tend to react differently to the loss of a spouse. Men are likely to feel that they have lost a part of themselves, whereas women may feel deserted and abandoned. Men find it more difficult to express grief than do women. However, men tend to recover from the loss more quickly than do women and remarry sooner after the death. Women are likely to feel alone once the support of friends and family is no longer available. The majority of widowed persons in their late 40s and early 50s remarry because they want companionship, to avoid loneliness, and to have a partner for social activities. Few women in their middle to late 50s remarry.[38]

Grandparenthood is a major life event that needs to be

explored. Some middle-aged parents eagerly await the day they will become grandparents and may directly or indirectly pressure their children to begin a family. If the children will not accommodate the parent, a conflict may emerge. Transition into the role of grandparent involves a change in the parent-child relationship: for the first time, parents share their parental role with an adult child.

The grandchild establishes a bond of common interest between the parent and the grandparent. A comprehensive study by Neugarten and Weinstein[67] indicated that most grandparents derive pleasure and satisfaction from their role. The grandparents in their study had negative experiences when differences arose between the adult child and the parents over child discipline and when grandparents were exploited for baby-sitting services.

Information on the meaning of the role of grandparent is valuable for the assessment. Neugarten and Weinstein[67] have ascribed five meanings to the role of grandparent:

1. Grandparenthood is a source of biological renewal or continuity with the future. In this instance the grandparents view the grandchildren as an extension of themselves, through whom they vicariously experience renewed life.

2. Grandparenthood provides emotional self-fulfillment by giving the grandparents an opportunity to perform the emotional role of grandparent better than they did the role of parent.

3. For a few persons grandparenthood means being a resource person. The grandparents can gain satisfaction by financial or experiential contributions to the grandchild's welfare.

4. A few persons view the grandchild as an extension of the self who will accomplish what neither they nor their children could. Thus the grandchild provides an opportunity for grandparents to aggrandize their ego.

5. Some persons have relatively remote feelings or psychological distance. In Neugarten and Weinstein's study, some of the grandmothers attributed their remoteness to busy work and social schedules. The reasons given seem to have been rationalizations.

Although middle-aged adults are often the givers rather than the receivers of social support, they need supportive relationships. Social support mobilizes the personal resources necessary for coping with stress. Social support comes through interaction with family, friends, and acquaintances in informal and formal situations. An assessment of the number and quality of the relationships and the frequency of the interactions provides valuable information on middle-aged clients' support systems.

Because middle-aged adults are often between the older and younger generations in the family, opportunities for them to receive social support may be greatly decreased. Once the children leave the home, depending on the status of the marital relationship, the spouses may or may not be able to provide mutual social support. When social support is not forthcoming within the marital relationship, the partners may seek support from friends or children, if they are parents.

The nurse determines the extent to which the individual has achieved stability in social competence. Many middle-aged persons have attained social competence. They have established patterns of socializing that are compatible with their skills and income. This social competence is used to maintain relationships with friends.

Friendships are important to middle-aged persons' well-being. They may serve both as sources of emotional support and as means for integrating the individual with the larger society. However, middle-aged adults may have few friends. Fewer friends in middle age is attributed to a decrease in energy available for investment in relationships rather than a loss of popularity. The relationships with friends that married couples maintain are close and generally develop when children are at home.

Single middle-aged women and men may have been working on friendships since early adulthood. Although some of their friends may be married, most are unmarried. The friendship patterns of unmarried persons vary little in middle age. The single woman generally has a strong, stable support system in a group of female friends with whom she has traveled, socialized, and turned to for support. There seems to be no clear pattern of social behavior and friendship patterns for men. The single middle-aged man is likely to have fewer friends than acquaintances. Thus acquaintances may compose the single man's support system.[46]

The friendship circle diminishes considerably if divorced middle-aged persons do not remarry. The change in marital status decreases the opportunity for support from friends at a time when the need is great.[46] Relatives may become the divorced person's closest friends and support system. Divorced, middle-aged parents who have children at home have limited time for friendships and socializing.

The newly widowed person may at first be flooded with invitations. Later the bereaved person is invited to social functions as an "extra." Gradually this person builds friendships in a small group of other unattached middle-aged individuals.

The nurse encounters middle-aged adults who avoid meaningful interaction with their peers. These persons may not have developed social skills. During the parenting years these individuals often failed to maintain their social relationships with peers. Sometimes persons who are ill at ease in situations with their peers will establish a "pal" relationship with their adolescent children. This "pal" relationship may have begun when the parent attended social activities with their young children. These parents encounter problems when their children broaden their social horizons beyond them.

Havighurst's theory[42] supports assessment of middle-aged adults' use of leisure time and involvement in civic organizations. Middle-aged adults may be more involved in formal organizations than are young adults. The increased participation in various types of voluntary associations reaches its peak at about age 50 and plateaus at the end of middle age.[81]

It is important for the nurse to determine the client's response to the changing sense of self resulting from all of the issues that characterize middle age, such as a changing physical appearance, being a parent of adolescent children, caring for aging parents, and work. A number of studies indicate that a positive increase in self-concept usually occurs with advancing age.[44] Neugarten[64] described the self-concept of middle-aged clients in terms of their perception of changes in their careers, families, and status and how they deal with both inner and outer worlds. Women tend to shift their self-image from relationships with others to their own abilities and feelings. Men tend to be more occupationally minded in self-image and have more difficulty as they age.[2] The client who has adjusted well to the changes of middle age will have a positive self-concept. Clients who are insecure and lack self-confidence have a negative self-concept.

Middle-aged adults experience a balance between dependence and independence. Healthy dependence may be expressed in any of their life situations. At the same time, middle-aged adults have a healthy degree of self-reliance. Men in this age-group tend to be passive and dependent, which increases with age, whereas women are likely to become more assertive. As a result of middle-aged adults' development of self, they appreciate the significance of interdependence. For example, parents need their children as vehicles for generativity and spouses rely on each other. Manifestations of an unhealthy imbalance between dependence and independence can be seen in the middle-aged businessman who has cardiac disease yet strives for independence as a defense against dependence.

Middle-aged clients are more likely than younger workers to be laid off when economic losses are severe.[36] When these clients lose a job, unemployment is often prolonged. Some employers are prejudiced against older job seekers. Employers may perceive a middle-aged job seeker as someone who will become ill or disabled or who will be costly in such fringe benefits as insurance and pension. The experiences of job hunting may lead to emotional distress. After middle-aged clients find work, many of them may continue to be subjected to displacement through less attractive occupational assignments, lower earnings, and perhaps some damage to their physical and mental well-being.[36]

Implications of the person's preparation for retirement are assessed. The meaning of work to middle-aged adults affects their plans for retirement. For some clients, their work gives meaning and structure to their lives. Without preparation for retirement, these clients may become physically or mentally ill. Some retiring persons are concerned about finding interests in common with their partner. These persons often think of retirement as a joint endeavor. If only the husband is employed, he may anticipate retirement with pleasure, whereas the wife worries that his presence in the home all day will interfere with her routine. Some single, divorced, or widowed persons avoid thinking about retirement if they view it as a loss of a position of value in society. Managing with a fixed income is also a realistic concern for many of these individuals.

Spiritual dimension In an effort to cope with some of the changes in mid-life, many people turn to religion. Generally, church membership and attendance rise sharply for those in their 40s and 50s, but both decline after age 60. The middle-aged adult may think he will find a reason for being that gives meaning to life in organized religion. If his involvement does not achieve this purpose, he may feel hopeless and in despair.

HOLISTIC ASSESSMENT TOOL: THE MIDDLE-AGED ADULT

Physical Dimension

What is your reaction to changes in your physical appearance?

What changes have you noted in your sleep pattern?

What are your thoughts about your current weight?

What changes have occurred in your eating habits, for example, the amount of food you eat?

What is your response to menopausal changes? (for women) andropause? (for men)

Since becoming middle aged, how would you rate your sexual experiences on a scale of 1 to 10, with 10 being high?

What measures are you taking to decrease the risk of osteoporosis?

What changes have you noticed in your vision?

Emotional Dimension

What are your feelings about the changes in your life?

In what ways do you express your emotional responses to changes in your life?

What changes have you observed in situations or experiences that you would normally respond to with feelings of anger? guilt? depression?

What are your feelings about your responsibility for your aging parents? your children?

Intellectual Dimension

How well do you recall recent events? remote events?

Describe how you have coped with mid-life changes.

As you enter middle age, what changes have you noticed in your ability to express yourself? in your vocabulary?

What method of presenting information allows you to best retain it—visual? verbal?

Social Dimension

What do you consider the major role change you have experienced since entering mid-life?

Describe your relationship with your spouse now that you are middle-aged.

What effect did the last child leaving home have on your marriage? on your life in general?

Describe your adjustment to the death of your spouse. (if a spouse has died)

How is your relationship with your parents different since you entered mid-life?

Describe your relationship with your grandchildren. (if a grandparent)

How many friends do you have?

How often do you get together with friends?

Who are the people who constitute your support system?

In what ways have your life goals changed?

What changes have you made in the amount of alcohol you consume?

What preparation are you making for retirement?

Spiritual Dimension

In what ways have your beliefs, thoughts, and feelings about death and dying changed since you reached middle age?

What changes have occurred in your church attendance?

What changes have you made in your purpose in life?

The specific content of the individual's religious beliefs and the cultural norms associated with a particular religion need to be considered in the assessment. For example, a woman from a Catholic background facing divorce may find her distress increased by the church's position against divorce. A man from a Protestant background who has grown up with a strong commitment to the work ethic may find facing unemployment especially hard to take.

Using Jung's theory,[51] the nurse assesses the extent to which persons have accepted the inevitability of their own death. Events that precipitate a struggle with the meaning of life can be stressful for the middle-aged adult. For example, loss of meaningful relationships and the illness and death of significant others can lead to issues related to one's own mortality. The perception of death as a reality leads to taking stock of one's marriage, career, personal relationships, values, and other commitments made earlier in life.

The assessment tool on p. 793 contains assessment areas specific to the middle-aged adult. It is to be used in conjunction with the assessment tool in Chapter 8 (p. 139).

Analysis
Nursing diagnosis

Impaired adjustment, caregiver role strain and high risk for caregiver role strain, are NANDA-accepted nursing diagnoses related to mid-life. The defining characteristics of impaired adjustment and caregiver role strain are listed in the accompanying boxes.

The following case example illustrates a client's impaired adjustment to an impending divorce.

▼ Case Example

Mary Jo, a 45-year-old mother of two adolescent sons, became severely depressed when the divorce she initiated was in process.

▼ IMPAIRED ADJUSTMENT

DEFINITION

The state in which an individual is unable to modify his life-style/behavior in a manner consistent with a change in health status.

DEFINING CHARACTERISTICS

- **Emotional dimension**

  Extended period of shock and disbelief or anger regarding health status change

- **Intellectual dimension**

  Verbalization of nonacceptance of health status change
  Nonexistent or unsuccessful ability to be involved in problem solving or goal setting

- **Social dimension**

  Lack of movement toward independence

- **Spiritual dimension**

  Lack of future-oriented thinking

Modified from Kim MA, McFarland GK, McLane AM, editors: *Pocket guide to nursing diagnoses,* ed 5, St Louis, 1993, Mosby—Year Book.

She cried constantly, could not sleep, and was unable to make plans to move out of her apartment. Although she gave a long list of reasons for the divorce, she felt ambivalent about leaving the relationship after 20 years of marriage. She expressed anger at herself for having difficulty adjusting to ending the marriage, which she believed was a mistake from the beginning. She was concerned that her husband would not provide financial support for the boys. She believed she could not manage financially with her salary as a receptionist. Mary Jo sought professional assistance with the depression associated with ending the marriage.

The following case example illustrates the characteristics of caregiver role strain.

▼ Case Example

Charlotte, a 50-year-old homemaker and mother of two teenagers, has been caring for her 75-year-old mother since she had a heart attack 1 year ago. The mother fractured her hip 2 years ago, and it never healed properly; however, she was able to manage with minimal assistance from her daughter until her husband's death and the heart attack a year ago. The mother lives alone in her own house. Charlotte goes to her mother's house at least three times a day and assists her in getting in and out of bed in the morning, for a midday nap, and at night. In addition, Charlotte does the housecleaning, meal preparation, laundry, and handles her mother's financial matters. Charlotte is aware that caring for her mother along with the responsibility for her own family is severe pressure, but her mother will not let anyone else help. Charlotte feels an obligation to respect her mother's wishes. She is also concerned that an outside caregiver may not be patient

---

▼ CAREGIVER ROLE STRAIN

DEFINITION

A caregiver's felt difficulty in performing the family caregiver role.

DEFINING CHARACTERISTICS

- **Emotional dimension**

  Worry about the care receiver's health and emotional state
  Worry about having to put the care receiver in an institution
  Worry about who will care for the care receiver if something should happen to the caregiver
  Feel that caregiving interferes with other important roles in their lives
  Feel loss because the care receiver is like a different person compared to before caregiving began
  Feel stress or nervousness in their relationship with the care receiver
  Feel depressed

- **Intellectual dimension**

  Family conflict around issues of providing care

- **Social dimension**

  Have insufficient resources to provide the care needed
  Find it hard to do specific caregiving activities

Modified from North American Nursing Diagnosis Association Classification of Nursing Diagnosis: Proceedings of the tenth conference, 1992 (in press).

with her mother who has become very angry and demanding as her health declines. Charlotte reported that her life has completely changed since she has become the caregiver for her mother. The time she spends caring for her mother has put a strain on her marriage, the family no longer goes out for dinner, and they have not had a vacation since Charlotte assumed caregiver role. While Charlotte's husband wants his wife to help her mother, he thinks she should hire an outside helper. Charlotte is aware that her mother's health is declining and that other arrangements will soon have to be made. She is dreading the day when it becomes necessary to place her mother in a nursing home.

The following list provides examples of other NANDA-accepted nursing diagnoses with causative statements related to the middle-aged adult:

1. Disturbance in self-concept related to obesity
2. Sleep pattern disturbance related to anxiety secondary to menopausal changes
3. Anxiety related to changes in body image
4. Grieving related to departure of children from home
5. Impaired social interaction related to divorce
6. Disturbance in self-concept related to lack of updated job skills
7. Powerlessness related to lack of assertiveness

8. Spiritual distress related to inability to accept own mortality

Planning

Long-term and short-term goals, outcome criteria, interventions, and rationales appropriate for the middle-aged adult are shown in the nursing care plan in Table 39-3.

Implementation

Physical dimension The nurse provides information about the physical changes that naturally accompany middle age. She reinforces the client's healthy responses to these changes by verbalizing her observation of these responses. Depending on the client's needs, the nurse shares information about the importance of avoiding excess sun to slow down the drying of skin. If the client lacks knowledge, the nurse mentions creams and lotions that may help decrease the drying of skin and help conceal wrinkles. Some clients may be sufficiently concerned about physical changes to inquire about cosmetic surgery. The nurse supports the client's decision.

▼   **TABLE 39-3   NURSING CARE PLAN**

GOALS	OUTCOME CRITERIA	INTERVENTIONS	RATIONALES
NURSING DIAGNOSIS: Ineffective Individual Coping related to role reversal with aging parent			
LONG TERM			
To develop adaptive coping responses	Uses existing coping abilities	Assist client to identify coping abilities	Knowledge of abilities will decrease threat
		Have client role play use of coping abilities	Increases confidence in abilities
	Uses effective problem-solving abilities	Determine existing problem-solving abilities	To establish baseline for developing plans
		Teach problem-solving approach	An ability to problem solve will improve coping responses
SHORT TERM			
To discuss thoughts and feelings about role reversal	Verbalizes thoughts and feelings	Provide a private setting that promotes expression of thoughts and feelings	Increases chances that client will share thoughts and feelings
	Discusses reasons for thoughts and feelings	Assist client to explore reasons for thoughts and feelings	Knowledge of reasons may decrease uncertainty
To adapt life-style to accommodate responsibility for parents	Makes statements about parents' and own need for dependence and independence	Determine client's knowledge of the needs of each for dependence and independence	Recognizing that each has a need for dependence and independence may increase acceptance of role change
	Makes statements indicating knowledge of need for change in relationship	Provide factual information about the developmental changes for the aged	Increase in knowledge helps client adjust to role change
		Give positive reinforcement which conveys recognition of the need for role reversal	Positive reinforcement will encourage the continuation of the behavior

An adjustment to increased periods of wakefulness and less deep sleep may be achieved as the nurse helps the client understand changing biological rhythms. Restful sleep provides added energy. The client may know how to relieve insomnia by bedtime rituals, such as a warm bath. Relaxation and exercise may also induce sleep. Medications such as estrogen may be prescribed to reduce sleeplessness.

The importance of sound nutrition and exercise in maintaining health can be taught. Exercise in middle age helps restore strength to muscles not used regularly. The nurse encourages jogging, swimming, and biking to improve cardiovascular strength and blood circulation. These activities may also decrease the risk of osteoporosis.[84] Neugarten[64] uses the term *body monitoring* for activities in which clients engage to keep the body in shape. A good balance of rest and exercise in middle age contributes to slowing the aging process. The nurse encourages middle-aged clients to relax and participate in active and passive leisure activities.[24] Today a wide range of methods such as relaxation exercises, meditation, and self-hypnosis are used to help clients learn to relax.

Intervention in obesity contributes to decreased morbidity and mortality in middle age. Heart disease, hypertension, and diabetes may be prevented if middle-aged clients keep their weight within the limits established for their height and frame (see Chapter 31).

There are two essential features of a weight maintenance program. They are (1) controlling caloric intake and (2) expending sufficient energy to burn the calories consumed because of the changes in eating habits and exercise. The nurse helps the client develop a successful plan for losing and maintaining weight. If the client's program involves major weight loss, he is referred to his physician for a complete physical and a nutritionist for assessment before beginning a diet.

When recommending a caloric intake, the nurse should follow the rule of thumb of 15 calories per day per pound. Specific information on diets can be found in many books. The hazards of fad diets, crash dieting, and fasting are discussed in Chapter 31.

Regular exercise is an essential aspect of a weight maintenance program. Before clients begin a strenuous exercise program, the nurse encourages them to consult their physician or exercise physiologist. Less rigorous exercises are listed in Table 39-4. Aerobics are beneficial for middle-aged clients. The nurse recommends a comprehensive book on aerobics that presents a scientifically sound exercise program and activities for middle-aged women and men. The nurse informs the client that adhering to a weight control program may be difficult but not impossible.

Middle-aged clients need information on the relationship between stress and physical disorders. This knowledge helps to decrease the potential for developing stress-related illnesses. A general focus for education is the relationship between emotional and physical health. Stress reduction methods and measures used to reduce anxiety (see Chapter 10) are useful. The nurse discusses risk factors that contribute to coronary problems, such as smoking, diet, intake of alcohol and coffee, and a sedentary life-style.

The nurse discusses with the client the pros and cons of estrogen replacement to eliminate the physiological symptoms of menopause. She listens to concerns the client

TABLE 39-4   **Nature and Examples of Activities and Calories Burned**

Nature of Activities	Examples of Activities	Calories Burned per Hour
Sedentary activities	Writing, reading, and watching television	About 100
Light activities	Slow walking, household activities such as dusting and washing dishes, and average office work	About 150
Moderate activities	Walking at brisk pace, scrubbing, playing golf, bowling, and gardening	About 200
Vigorous activities	Athletic activities usually done away from home such as tennis, walking rapidly, and jogging	300 to 1000

expresses about the increased risk of cancer with estrogen therapy. The individual is referred to her physician for additional information.

Sometimes climacteric changes lead to sexual difficulties. The nurse teaches postmenopausal women about vaginal dryness and recommends lubricants. Sexual counseling by nurses with specialized preparation is helpful. The nurse encourages clients to identify and examine several areas that may contribute to sexual problems such as physiological and role changes, communications, and changing attitudes about sexuality.

In preparation for the gradual changes in mid-life sexuality, the nurse provides information about expected changes and their effects on sexual performance. Such interventions often prevent unnecessary anger, resentment, fears, withdrawal, or blaming the partner. Information on sexuality in mid-life may also decrease the need for the spouse to have extramarital affairs.

Emotional dimension   Expressing anger rather than internalizing it prevents physical disorders, such as coronary problems and ulcers. Today's middle-aged clients are likely to feel guilty about expressing anger and fear loss of control. The nurse can use role playing to provide an opportunity for the client to express anger in a safe situation.

The nurse assists the widowed person to examine feelings of guilt to see whether they are realistic. For example, the nurse assists a widow to dispel her belief that she could have prevented her husband's death by examining how her headstrong husband disregarded her suggestions that he stop smoking. Widows who have a fear of living alone will benefit from information about security measures, such as outdoor lights, a timer for indoor lights, and deadbolt locks. The nurse also suggests that the middle-aged person maintain a relationship with a neighbor who knows her whereabouts.

The nurse assists the grieving widowed, middle-aged person. The individual's anxiety is generally reduced by learning that certain thoughts and feelings are normal for the grieving person. Middle-aged clients who do not work through the grieving process are likely to feel sustained anger and despair that adversely affect their functioning. The anger and despair may be manifested as chronic depression. The nurse provides these people with an opportunity to complete the grieving process (see Chapter 13).

Individuals who have lost a spouse through death can be supportive to one another. The nurse recommends mutual self-help groups for widowed persons. These mutual support groups provide an opportunity for widowed persons to talk about the experiences related to their loss with a peer group that understands the pain.[77] The nurse directs or assists the individual to find a mutual support group by looking in the yellow pages of the telephone directory under Mental Health, calling the community mental health center, or asking a pastor or religious leader. If no such group is available in the client's community, the nurse assists the individual to organize such a group. The nurse can serve as a resource for the group.

Suicide and suicide potential are problems that require immediate intervention (see Chapter 14). Specific interventions for anxiety, anger, guilt, and despair are discussed in Chapters 10, 11, 12, and 14, respectively.

Intellectual dimension The nurse capitalizes on the intellectual strengths of middle-aged clients. She encourages them to maintain and enhance intellectual functioning by being actively involved in new tasks that are challenging and require flexibility.[47] She encourages them, for example, to enroll in refresher courses, continuing education courses, workshops, or courses for college credit. These educational experiences are beneficial for using leisure time, developing a second career, or planning for retirement. Middle-aged clients can also be encouraged to renew past interests in creative activities.

Assisting clients to be flexible and to accept new experiences requires patience and tolerance. If the inflexibility existed before middle age, the client may need to be referred for psychotherapy for help in changing the lifelong pattern of coping. A matter-of-fact presentation of information about normal mid-life changes may decrease the client's resistance to change. The nurse and the client together identify the mid-life changes that are most bothersome to the client and explore alternative behavior to meet the client's needs. The nurse encourages the client to participate in self-help groups composed of middle-aged adults with problems with flexibility. These groups help clients become aware of the maladaptive nature of the problems and work on changing the behavior.

The nurse guides clients to examine how they cope with mid-life changes and stresses. For example, a person who is unemployed may be coping with systematic job hunting or by joining a support group composed of others with the same problems. The nurse helps the person recognize the positive aspects of such coping behavior.

Clients who develop physical illnesses to cope with problems of mid-life are referred for psychotherapy. Some nursing measures for intervention in these problems are discussed in Chapter 19. The nurse provides information to families about behavior that indicates the beginning of Alzheimer's and Pick's disease (see Chapter 33). Since the disease results in gradual deterioration of intellectual functioning, it is essential for the nurse to include family members in the teaching.

Social dimension The nurse assists middle-aged couples in adjusting to the postparental marriage. They need to know that their marital relationship in middle age is a new one, one which requires revitalization. The partners explore revitalization of the marriage based on commitment, communication, and compromise.[24] Commitment entails a willingness to understand each other and to renegotiate the terms of the present marital relationship, instead of focusing on what has been or may have been. Commitment may be based on the survival of the marriage to middle age. This survival suggests a solid foundation on which to build a postparental marital relationship. The nurse guides each partner to recognize the other's uniqueness and the right of each to grow in flexible roles, one of Havighurst's tasks for mid-life.[42]

Communication is perhaps the most important component in the new middle-aged marital relationship.[24] Some couples have to learn to risk sharing their feelings and needs. The steps for sharing feelings are (1) to try to get in touch with one's own emotions, (2) to ask the partner when he would be receptive to an expression of feelings and needs and then share these to the best of one's ability, and (3) to learn to listen to all levels of the partner's communication. A simple exercise for beginning to learn to listen is (1) for one spouse to state how he or she feels as clearly as possible and (2) for the other spouse to try to rephrase what was expressed in his own words to make sure he has understood.

Compromise involves negotiations in which neither person wins nor loses. The partners choose a mutually agreed time and place for discussion of differences. The nurse emphasizes the need to keep the focus of the discussion on the issues at hand. Open communication of thoughts and feelings, listening, and understanding are essential for resolution of conflict.[24]

The middle-aged couple may have problems revitalizing their relationship. Divorce does not usually come easily to clients who have endured a relationship into mid-life. In this case, the couple may seek professional guidance. The nurse can suggest marriage counseling. First, she can share self-help methods such as those previously described with the couple. If the couple's efforts are unsuccessful, the nurse provides marital counseling or refers them to another professional who specializes in marriage counseling. If the marriage is in serious trouble, even counseling may not help. Counseling prevents divorce in only about 10% to 15% of cases and changes unhappy marriages into happy ones in less than 5% of cases.[24]

If a marriage ends in divorce, each spouse needs assistance to adjust to the changed roles. The nurse informs the clients that even though the marriage was unhappy, they will respond as they would to any loss. Each needs to complete the grieving process. Clients are encouraged to explore approaches to reorganizing their lives as single middle-aged persons and perhaps as single parents of adolescents. Clients who become single parents can be referred to Parents Without Partners, the most widely known peer group. Divorced Anonymous is another organization that may be of value. These organizations help the divorced client to develop a new social life.

The nurse often helps middle-aged adult children who have responsibility for aging parents. The nurse shares information on resources and professional services for aged parents. The nurse provides a list of the services that are available at agencies for the aged. Adult children may benefit from anticipatory guidance in what to expect as the parents age and what they can do to help meet the parents' needs before a crisis develops (see Chapter 40).

Group interventions provide guidance for adults caring for aging parents. When feasible, the adult child and parent attend community-based educational groups.[54] At these meetings, adult children and aging parents learn about the aging process and changes resulting from illness. The needs of the parents and the availability of resources may also be presented. Adult children and their parents learn what to expect. In groups such as these, middle-aged caregivers and their parents can discuss their problems from a personal perspective.

Support groups for middle-aged caregiving adults provide them with an opportunity to discuss their concerns in the absence of their parents. The caregivers discuss concerns such as adjustments to the role reversal, decisions about living arrangements for aging parents, and strategies for coping with their parents' aging. They can also express feelings such as despair, anger, guilt, and conflict. Kaplan[54] reports that some group members maintain contact after the group is terminated and function as a valuable support system.

The nurse may recommend an intergenerational family group, which allows all of the children of aging parents to explore feelings and concerns. For example, anger or conflict over who will assist the parents can be expressed. Drawing up a will and making preplanned burial arrangements can also be discussed.

Clients may seek mental health services as they adjust to unemployment or the role of unemployed job seeker. Interventions for unemployment problems include allowing the client to express his thoughts and feelings about the experiences. The client may be referred to appropriate community agencies for job counseling. Some special programs are available to prepare middle-aged women for entrance into or return to the work force.

Retirement planning is essential. During early middle age, retirement seems remote. But as individuals near retirement, they are encouraged to plan for retirement. An important factor that influences retirement planning is the person's financial status. Will the client's income be sufficient for him to live on? Clients need to include inflation in their assessment of finances. Anticipatory guidance in retirement issues helps potential retirees make a smooth transition into retirement.

Spiritual dimension Middle-aged clients may need help reassessing their meaning of spirituality and the purpose it serves in the current transition to mid-life. The nurse needs to be aware of this and not impose her own spiritual values. Middle-aged clients' increased focus on religious practices is reinforced when important to their value system. When not, other activities are suggested such as community services and volunteering to enrich their lives.

The nurse provides an opportunity for the client to express his concerns about death. She supports his involvement in religious activities as one means for handling the prospect of his own death. The nurse assists the individual to find some meaning in life. She guides the client in an examination of what he has accomplished and provides support as the client identifies new goals that are attainable.

Evaluation

Middle-aged clients may participate in the ongoing evaluation of their responses to the nursing intevention. When evaluating the extent to which goals have been achieved, the nurse bases her evaluations on change that is realistic for the client. Middle-aged clients may overemphasize change and want change for the sake of change. They may end up with a chaotic life. During evaluation the nurse emphasizes the continuing potential for growth and fulfillment after therapy is terminated.

BRIEF REVIEW

The middle-aged adult population is currently the fastest growing group in the United States. Although study of this stage of the life cycle is not yet a distinct discipline, nurses and other professionals have begun scientific exploration of the mental health care needs of middle-aged people and interventions to meet these needs.

A person begins transition into the middle years at age 40 and works toward completing the tasks of this stage until age 65. Chronological age may not be the best indicator of movement into mid-life, because social, positional, physical, and biological cues also indicate the beginning of change.

Havighurst, Erikson, Jung, and Peck have made lasting contributions to the theoretical explanation of the experiences of middle age. Havighurst identifies seven tasks related to assuming a position of social responsibility and guidance of others. The task of developing generativity versus stagnation is Erikson's approach to describing the need for middle-aged adults to counsel and direct others. If the client is excessively concerned about himself, he stagnates. Jung and Buhler have similar views that middle-aged people become inner oriented as they engage in a critical assessment of themselves. Peck believes individuals in mid-life need to invest their energy in various people and activities. This action fills the void left by the loss of many significant relationships. His four tasks for middle-aged adults are (1) valuing wisdom versus physical powers, (2) cathectic flexibility versus impoverishment, (3) mental flexibility versus rigidity, and (4) socializing versus sexualizing in human relationships.

Some of the major stressors of middle age result from losses and role changes. Physical changes such as obesity, departure of the last child from the home, renegotiating the marital relationship, and role reversal with aging parents are some of the major events confronting the middle-aged adult. Most middle-aged adults cope effectively with these stressors. If they do not, they may become depressed and abuse alcohol, which may necessitate professional assistance.

REFERENCES AND SUGGESTED READINGS

1. Ainlay SC, Smith DR: Aging and religious participation, *Journal of Gerontology* 39(3):357, 1984.
2. Back KW: Transition to aging and the self-image, *Aging and Human Development* 2:4, 1971.
3. Barbee EL, Baur JA: Aging and life experiences of low-income, middle-aged African-American and caucasian women, *Canadian Journal of Nursing Research* 20(4):5, 1988.
4. Benedek T: Parenthood during the life cycle. In Anthony E, Benedek T, editors: *Parenthood: its psychology and psychopathology,* Boston, 1970, Little, Brown & Co.
5. Birren JE, Schaie KW, editors: *Handbook of the psychology of aging,* ed 3, San Diego, 1990, Academic Press.
6. Blazer D and others: Major depression with melancholia: a comparison of middle-aged and elderly adults, *Journal of American Geriatric Society* 31(10):927, 1987.
7. Bourguet CC, Hamrick GA, Gilchrist VJ: The prevalence of osteoporosis risk factors and physician intervention, *The Journal of Family Practice* 32(37):265, 1991.
8. Brody E: *Women in the middle: their parent-care years,* New York, 1990, Springer Publishing Co.
9. Buck MM, Gottlieb LN: The meaning of time: Mohawk women at midlife, *Health Care of Women International* 12(1):41, 1991.
10. Buhler C: The general structure of the human life. In Buhler C, Massarik F, editors: *The course of human life: a study of goals in the humanistic perspective,* New York, 1968, Springer Publishing Co.
11. Buhler C: The course of human life as a psychological problem. In Looft WR, editor: *Development psychology: a book of readings,* New York, 1972, Holt, Rinehart & Winston.
12. Burrows GD, Dennerstein L: Depression and suicide in middle age. In Howells JD, editor: *Modern perspectives in the psychiatry of middle age,* New York, 1981, Brunner/Mazel.
13. Butler RN: Psychiatry and psychology of the middle-aged. In Freedman AM, Kaplan HI, Sadock BJ, editors: *Comprehensive textbook of psychiatry,* ed 4, Baltimore, 1985, Williams & Wilkins.
14. Chapman AH: *Textbook of clinical psychiatry: an interpersonal approach,* ed 2, Philadelphia, 1976, JB Lippincott.
15. Chiriboga DA: Stresses and loss in middle age. In Kalish RA, editor: *Midlife loss: coping strategies,* Newbury Park, Calif, 1989, Sage Publications.
16. Ciernia JR: Myths about male mid-life crises, *Psychological Reports* 56:3, 1985.
17. Coe RN and others: Correlates of a measure of coping in older veterans: a preliminary report, *Journal of Community Health* 15(5):287, 1990.
18. Colarusso CA, Nemiroff RA: *Adult development: a new dimension in psychodynamic theory and practice,* New York, 1981, Plenum Press.
19. Cooke DJ: Social support and stressful life events during midlife, *Maturitas* 7(4):303, 1985.
20. DeLucci MF and others: The men's adult life experiences inventory: an instrument for assessing developmental concerns of middle age, *Psychological Reports* 64(2):479, 1989.
21. Desmond TC: America's unknown middle-agers. In Vedder CB, editor: *Problems of the middle-aged,* Springfield, Ill, 1965, Charles C Thomas.
22. *Diagnostic and statistical manual of mental disorders,* ed 3 revised, Washington, DC, 1987, American Psychiatric Association.
23. Diekelmann N and others: The middle years: a special supplement, *American Journal of Nursing* 75:993, 1975.
24. Donohugh DL: *The middle years,* Philadelphia, 1981, WB Saunders.
25. Ecklein JL: Obstacles to understanding the changing role of women in socialist countries, *Insurgent Sociologist* 12(1-2):7, 1984.
26. Edinberg MA: *Talking with your aging parents,* Boston, 1987, Shambhala.
27. Erikson EH: *Childhood and society,* ed 2, New York, 1964, WW Norton.
28. European Foundation for Osteoporosis and Bone Disease: Concensus development conference: prophylaxis and treatment of osteoporosis, *British Medical Journal* 295:914, 1987.
29. Fiske M: *Middle age: the prime of life?* New York, 1979, Harper & Row.
30. Foxall MJ, Ekberg JY, Griffith N: Adjustment pattern of chronically ill middle-aged persons and spouse, *Western Journal of Nursing Research* 7(4):443, 1985.
31. Friedman HJ: The divorced in middle age. In Howells JG, editor: *Modern perspectives in the psychiatry of middle age,* New York, 1981, Brunner/Mazel.
32. Frieberg KL: *Human development: a life span approach,* ed 3, Boston, 1987, Jones & Bartlett.
33. Gallo JJ: The effect of social support on depression in caregivers of the elderly, *The Journal of Family Practice* 30(4):430, 1990.
34. Ganong LH, Coleman M: Remarriage and health, *Research in Nursing and Health* 14:205, 1991.
35. George LK: *Role transition in late life,* Monterey, Calif, 1980, Brooks/Cole.
36. George LK, Gold DT: Job loss in middle age. In Kalish RA, editor: *Midlife loss: coping strategies,* Newbury Park, Calif, 1989, Sage Publications.
37. Golan N: *Passing through transitions: a guide for practitioners,* New York, 1981, The Free Press.
38. Golan N: *The perilous bride: helping clients through midlife transitions,* New York, 1986, Free Press.
39. Gordon VC: Growth-support intervention for the treatment of depression in women of middle years. *Western Journal of Nursing Research* 8(3):281, 1986.
40. Grambs JD: *Women over forty: visions and realities,* New York, 1989, Springer.
41. Hanks RS: The impact of early retirement incentives on retirees and their families, *Journal of Family Issues* 11(4):424, 1990.
42. Havighurst RJ: *Developmental tasks and education,* New York, 1972, David McKay.
43. Hayward MD, Hardy MA: Early retirement processes among older men: occupational differences, *Research on Aging* 7(4):491, 1985.
44. Hess AL, Bradshaw HL: Positiveness of self-concept and ideal self as a function of age, *Journal of Genetic Psychology* 117:57, 1970.
45. Holliday SG, Chandler MJ: *Wisdom: explorations in adult competence,* Basel, New York, 1986, Kruger.
46. Howells JG, editor: *Modern perspectives in the psychiatry of middle age,* New York, 1981, Brunner/Mazel.
47. Hunter S, Sundel M, editors: *Midlife myths: issues, findings and practice implications,* Newbury Park, Calif, 1989, Sage.
48. Huyck MH: Midlife parental imperatives. In Kalish RA, editor: *Midlife loss: coping strategies,* Newbury Park, Calif, 1989, Sage.
49. Jarvik LS, Small G: *Parentcare: a common sense guide for adult children,* New York, 1988, Crown.
50. Johnson MA: Nursing home placement: the daughter's perspective, *J Gerontol Nurs* 16(11):6, 1990.
51. Jung CG: *Modern man in search of a soul,* New York, 1933, Harcourt Brace & Co.
52. Jung CG: Collected works, vol 17, *The development of personality,* New York. 1954, Pantheon Books.
53. Kalish RA, editor: *Midlife loss: coping strategies,* Newbury Park, Calif, 1989, Sage.
54. Kaplan BH: An overview of interventions to meet the needs of aging parents and their families. In Ragan PK, editor: *Aging*

parents, University Park, Calif, 1979, Ethel Percy Andrus Gerontology Center, University of Southern California.

55. Katchadourian H: *Fifty: midlife in perspective,* New York, 1987, WH Freeman & Co.

56. Kuhlen RG: Developmental changes in motivation during adult years. In Birrin JE, editor: *Relation of development and aging,* Springfield, Ill, 1964, Charles C Thomas.

57. LeMaster EE, DeFrain J: *Parents in contemporary America: a sympathetic view,* Homewood, Ill, 1983, The Dorsey Press.

58. Levinson D and others: *The seasons of a man's life,* New York, 1978, Alfred A Knopf.

59. Masserman JH: *Psychiatry and health,* Port Washington, New York, 1986, Human Science Press.

60. Mattila VJ: Paranoid-hallucinatory functional psychoses in later middle age, *Psychiatric Fennica* 16:19, 1985.

61. Meek D, Thorne P, Luker A: Support groups for older women, *Nursing Times* 85(46):15, 1989.

62. Miller B, Montgomery A: Family care-givers and limitations in social activities, *Research on Aging* 12(1):72, 1990.

63. Mirkin PM, Meyer RE: Alcoholism in middle age. In Howells JG, editor: *Modern perspectives in the psychiatry of middle age,* New York, 1981, Brunner/Mazel.

64. Neugarten BL, editor: *Personality in middle and later life: empirical studies,* New York, 1964, Atherton Press.

65. Neugarten BL: Adult personality: toward a psychology of the life cycle. In Neugarten BL, editor: *Middle age and aging,* Chicago, 1968, The University of Chicago Press.

66. Neugarten BL: The awareness of middle age. In Neugarten BL, editor: *Middle age and aging,* Chicago, 1968, The University of Chicago Press.

67. Neugarten BL, Weinstein KK: The changing American grandparent. In Neugarten BL, editor: *Middle age and aging,* Chicago, 1968, The University of Chicago Press.

68. Neugarten BL and others: Women's attitudes toward menopause. In Neugarten BL, editor: *Middle age and aging,* Chicago, 1968, The University of Chicago Press.

69. Patsdaughter CA, Killien M: Developmental transitions in adulthood: mother-daughter relationships, *Holistic Nursing Practice* 4(3):37, 1990.

70. Peck RC: Psychological development in the second half of life. In Neugarten BL, editor: *Middle age and aging,* Chicago, 1968, The University of Chicago Press.

71. Pett MA and others: Intergenerational conflict: middle-aged women caring for demented older relatives, *American Journal of Orthopsychiatry* 58(31):405, 1988.

72. Platzer H: Aging in men and the crisis of age, *Nursing* (Lond), 3(26):963, 1988.

73. Rife JC, First RJ: Discouraged older workers: an exploratory study, *International Journal of Aging and Human Development* 29(3):195, 1989.

74. Rosin AJ, Glatt MM: Alcohol excess in the elderly, *Quarterly Journal of Studies on Alcohol* 32:53, 1971.

75. Schlossberg NK: *Counseling adults in transition: linking practice with theory,* New York, 1984, Springer.

76. Schuster CS, Ashburn SS: *The process of human development: a holistic life-span approach,* Boston, 1986, Little, Brown & Co.

77. Silverman PR: *Widow-to-widow,* New York, 1986, Springer.

78. Sommers T, Shields L: *Women take care: the consequences of caregiving in today's society,* Gainesville, Fla, 1987, Triad.

79. Stephens MAP and others: Stressful situations in caregiving: relations between caregiver coping and well-being, *Psychology and Aging* 3(2):208, 1988.

80. Thomson J, Oswald L: Effect of estrogen on sleep, mood and anxiety of menopausal women, *British Medical Journal* 2:1317, 1977.

81. Troll LE: *Early and middle adulthood: the best is yet to be—maybe,* Monterey, Calif, 1975, Brooks/Cole.

82. Tune GS: The influence of age and temperament on the adult human sleep-wakefulness pattern, *British Journal of Psychology* 60:431, 1969.

83. Turner JS, Heims DB: *Contemporary adulthood,* ed 2, New York, 1982, Holt, Rinehart & Winston.

84. US Public Health Service: *Healthy people 2000: health promotion and disease prevention objectives,* US Dept of Health and Human Services, Washington, DC, 1989, Government Printing Office.

85. Waring J: *The middle years: a multidisciplinary view—a summary of the Second Annual Conference on Major Transitions in the Human Life Course,* New York, 1978, Academy for Educational Development.

86. Willits FK, Crider DM: Health rating and life satisfaction in the later middle years, *Journal of Gerontology* 43(5):517, 1988.

ANNOTATED BIBLIOGRAPHY

Brody EM: *Women in the middle: their parentcare years,* New York, 1990, Springer.

The content in this book was obtained from middle-aged parent-caring women. The book presents a description of the feelings, experiences, and problems of these women and the effects of these experiences on the women's mental and physical well-being, life-styles, and family relationships.

Golan N: *The perilous bridge: helping clients through midlife transitions,* New York, 1986, The Free Press.

This text presents theoretical perspectives on the late mid-life period and uses case situations of actual clients to highlight common emotional reactions to the stressors in this period. The author includes the range of treatments that were offered to these clients, as well as additional interventions she considers effective for assisting middle-aged adults through the transitional period of mid-life.

Grambs JD: *Women over forty: visions and realities,* New York, 1989, Springer.

This text presents some of the realities, stereotypes, myths, and social practices and policies that influence the experiences of women over the age of 40. Attention is given to dispelling some of the myths by presenting the normal experiences in the development of women over age 40 and the unique rewards and problems that arise that the person can solve. Generalizations, conclusions, and speculations are based on scholarly research and analysis. The book includes a chapter on older women who are of ethnic minority groups and a cross-cultural perspective of older women.

Hunter S, Sundel M: *Midlife myths: issues, findings, and practice implications,* Newbury Park, Calif, 1989, Sage.

The intent of this book is to dispel some of the myths surrounding mid-life by providing knowledge about physical, cognitive, and social aspects of middle-aged personality development, mental health, and personal development. A chapter addresses application of research findings and their implications for practice.

Kalish RA: *Midlife loss: coping strategies,* Newbury Park, Calif, 1989, Sage.

The intent of this book is to contribute to any reader's understanding of the middle-aged adult. This book clearly presents a variety of topics that address losses and rewards experienced by middle-aged adults and the impact of these losses on the person's life and some coping strategies.

Katchadourian H: *Fifty: midlife in perspective,* New York, 1987, WH Freeman.

This easy-to-read book presents factual information about various aspects of mid-life. The author describes the common physical, social, and psychological changes of middle adulthood.

Christine Gorman Walton
Cornelia Kelly Beck

After studying this chapter, the student will be able to:

- Discuss historical developments related to mental health–student psychiatric nursing for the aged adult
- Describe theoretical explanations of the aging process
- Apply the nursing process to the mental health care of aged individuals

- Describe specific forms of treatment frequently used for the mental health care of the aged
- Identify current research findings relevant to the aged adult

The age of 65 is the socially accepted time for designating a person as aged. However, experience with the aged has shown that chronological and psychological aging differ. Each person ages at a unique rate because of physical, emotional, intellectual, social, and spiritual factors.

The current trend is to separate older ages into phases: the young-old are 65 to 75 years, the old-old are 75 to 90 years, and the elite old are older than 90 years. With the recent change in the mandatory retirement age in some industries, 70 may become the norm for designating someone as aged. However, in this chapter, persons who are older than 65 years are considered to be in their later years, and the terms "elders," "the aged," "the old," and "the elderly" are used interchangeably.

Although older people generally function well, a significant number of them need mental health care to function at an optimal level. About 1% of the elderly are in mental hospitals, and 15% to 25% in the community have significant mental health problems; also, the National Nursing Home Survey[63] found that 30% of nursing home clients had a "diagnosable psychiatric disorder" and 61% had one or more mental impairments or conditions.

Older people are more likely than younger people to have multiple chronic disorders and to have encountered major object losses. They are also less likely to have supportive people and services available. Despite these difficulties, older people for the most part adapt to their circumstances. In fact most older people go through life with success, equanimity, and good humor.[34]

THEORETICAL APPROACHES

Psychoanalytical

Erikson[25] saw the final stage of life, ego integrity versus despair, as a time when individuals evaluate their accomplishments and failures and search for meaning in their lives. If older persons can find some meaning in their lives and accept the course that their lives have taken, they can look back with a sense of integrity. Older persons who evaluate their lives as a waste of time fall prey to a sense of loss, contempt for others, and despair.

Peck[48] discussed the following three developmental tasks of the older adult:

TASK	EXAMPLE
Body transcendence versus body preoccupation	Establish satisfying relationships and engage in creative activities to transcend self-centeredness and illness
Ego differentiation versus work role preoccupation	Redefine self in terms of roles other than those in the work situation
Ego transcendence versus ego preoccupation	Have one's life extend into the future through children, friendships, and contributions to society

Cognitive

Beck[3] contends that persons' cognitive appraisal of themselves and their situation predominates in establishing equi-

HISTORICAL OVERVIEW

DATES	EVENTS
1900s	Freud advised that psychoanalysis and other forms of psychotherapy were not useful with people over 50 years because of the inelasticity of their mental processes and their ineducability
1919	Although he agreed with Freud, Abraham was one of the first clinicians to show optimism concerning treatment of the elderly; he found that the weakening of their ego defenses facilitated change in the therapeutic process.
1950	The first nursing textbook on care of the elderly, *Geriatric Nursing,* by Norton[46] was published.
1958	Hanna Segal published the first clinical material describing analytic sessions with an elderly client.
1962	The first gerontological nursing research was published in Britain by Norton and colleagues.
	A small group of geriatric nurses appealed to the American Nurses' Association (ANA) for recognition of geriatric nursing as a specialty and held its first national meeting.
1963	Melanie Klein published theoretical formulations on the normal adaptation of the elderly as it affects children and family members.
	Of the aged mentally ill 40% were in psychiatric institutions, whereas 53% were in nursing homes.
1964	The first American study in gerontological nursing, *The Elderly Ambulatory Patient,* addressed patient health care knowledge, medication errors, food patterns, ambulation, and travel profiles.
	Levin described the impact of loss and change in the therapeutic process with the elderly.
1966	The ANA established the Division on Geriatric Nursing.
1969	The first nursing research was conducted with aged clients in a psychiatric facility.
	Of the mentally ill aged 75% were in nursing homes, making them the successor to state mental hospitals as the community treatment component of the deinstitutionalization of older mentally ill persons.
1970s	The elderly banded together socially and politically, using "senior power" against being cast as second-class citizens.
1973	Congress established a network of state and area agencies on aging to develop a coordinated system of comprehensive services to meet the needs of older Americans.
	The ANA's division on geriatric nursing published the "Standards for Geriatric Nursing Practice."
1974	The National Institute on Aging was established within the National Institutes of Health to support and conduct biomedical, social, and behavioral research and training related to the aging process.
1977	The term "geropsychiatric nursing" first appeared in the Cumulative Index to Nursing and Allied Health Literature.
1981	At the Third White House Conference on Aging, the American Psychiatric Association and the Committee on Long-Term Care recommended that mental health be an integral part of a comprehensive health and social service delivery system.
	The ANA's division on gerontological nursing prepared a statement that included a definition and philosophy of gerontological nursing practice and presented this statement to the participants in the White House Conference on Aging.
1984	The Middle Atlantic Geropsychiatric Nurses' Association was formed; the group comprises clinical nurse specialists with an interest in the mental health needs of the older adult.
1990s	Of the voting population 35% is 60 years or above and strongly support legislation for comprehensive mental health services.
	Economic issues and a growing shortage of long-term care beds dictate a major rise in the number of aged clients cared for in their own homes.
Future	Standards of practice and ANA certification in geropsychiatric nursing will be added to the existing age-specific specialty groups.
	There will be scarce resources because of the large number of "baby boomers" who will greatly influence how money is spent for health care.
	The aged may again become second-class citizens.

librium during the process of adjusting to losses. He proposes that when a negative view of the future, environment, and self is the basis for evaluating a loss, the impact of this negative view is greater than the loss. This cognitive triad is frequently characteristic of older people, and thus their personal cognitive distortions may increase their emotional reactions to loss. For example, they frequently believe that nothing is left in which they can invest their energies. The lack of meaningful roles ascribed to older people by our culture reinforces these appraisals.

Sociocultural

The theory of disengagement developed by Cummings and Henry[14] is one of the earliest and most controversial sociological theories on aging. According to the theory, the aging individual realizes his mortality and begins to reduce involvement with others. At the same time, society is disengaging itself from the individual. Individuals can use this freedom from restrictions to enjoy old age.

An opposing view is the activity theory. Havighurst[30] proposes that activity promotes well-being and satisfaction in aging. Older adults who remain active, engage in social activities, and establish new roles, relationships, hobbies, and interests will age with a sense of satisfaction.

The continuity theory proposed by Neugarten[45] suggests that individuals' personalities do not change as they age and that their behavior becomes more predictable. They maintain continuity in their habits, commitments, preferences, and particularly the way they adapt to social situations. Thus their pattern of aging can be predicted from knowledge of these factors.

The interactionist theory proposed by Spence[59] views age-related changes as resulting from the interaction of the individual characteristics of the person, circumstances in society, and the history of social interaction patterns of the person. Interactionist theory focuses on roles that the individual fills during a lifetime. People try to plan and balance their roles, move from one role to another, and assume a complex pattern of roles. However, with aging, people's major roles end and they choose new roles.

Biological

Physiological changes have been explored to explain the emotional changes that accompany aging. Researchers suggest that manic-depressive illness and recurrent depressive disorders in older individuals are caused primarily by lack of physiological energy and that lithium is effective in treating these disorders because it normalizes the physiological system and prevents wide swings of physiological energy.[64] They also propose that the aging of the hypothalamus and the hormonal system reduces the ability to withstand depression.[28] The synthesis of catecholamines decreases and the production of monoamine oxidase (MAO) increases to compensate. Increased levels of MAO are especially common in women because of the inverse relationship between levels of estrogen and MAO.[30]

There are normal neurological changes that can interfere with the older person's ability to communicate with others.[33] These neurological changes occur in three general areas: (1) receiving of messages from the sensory organs, (2) integrating messages, and (3) sending messages to the sensory affector neurons.

Reception of messages in the brain is decreased by the losses of hearing and vision. Hearing decreases because of losses of fibers of the auditory nerve and losses of neurons throughout the auditory pathways. Also, the tympanic membrane becomes more rigid and occasionally thickens. Vision is affected by many changes. The visual field is decreased by a loss of receptors, recession of the eye due to a loss of retroorbital fat, and loss of elastic tissue in the upper and lower lids. By the age of 60 the pupil becomes fixed at only one third the size it was at age 20, resulting in a decline in accommodation for near vision. In addition, corneal edema, hazing, and opacities of the lense are common.

Though cerebral oxygen consumption and glucose utilization is maintained, cerebral blood flow providing these nutrients is decreased. There is also a loss of neurons throughout life, which decreases the rate of conduction between two or more neurons. Both of these changes in the brain can result in problems with integrating or interpreting messages.

The ability to send messages to the sensory affector neurons and organs is decreased because of nerve cell loss. The motor function of the older cerebral cortex may continue to respond after stimulation, resulting in shaking, head nodding, and tremors that interfere with new messages.

Data on the association between genetic factors and mental functioning are limited. However, genetic factors have been found to be involved in the preservation of mental functioning into old age. Chromosome loss has been found to correlate with loss of certain cognitive functions, such as memory.[39] Table 40-1 summarizes theories of aging.

NURSING PROCESS

Assessment

Physical dimension The presence of physical illness increases with age, resulting in 80% of individuals over age 70 suffering from significant physical illness and 50% of the elderly having an illness that interferes with independence.[40] Also, physical illness can precede or follow an emotional problem, especially depression. Physical illness and events surrounding the onset of physical complaints are assessed.

Since the older person's physiological tolerance for sleep deprivation is lower than that of the younger person, insomnia is important to note. The older adult may have certain changes in sleep patterns (see the research highlight on p. 805). The first alteration relates to the time it takes a person to fall asleep, known as the latency period. A latency period of about 10 minutes is typical until 60 years of age. At 70 to 79 years the latency period reaches a mean of 23 minutes.[27]

The second alteration is the frequency and length of periods of wakefulness during the night. Awakenings are often caused by the need to urinate or by anxiety and depression about declining health and death.[38] These awakenings may interrupt rapid eye movement (REM) sleep. REM sleep is particularly important to the older person's central nervous system. The elderly person's amount of stage 4 non-REM sleep is cut in half. Mental agility declines

▼ **TABLE 40-1   Summary of Theories of Aging**

Theory	Theorist	Dynamics
Psychoanalytical	Erikson	Acceptance of one's life experiences leads to integrity; viewing one's life as a waste of time results in despair.
	Peck	Achievement of body transcendence, ego differentiation, and ego transcendence leads to successful aging.
Cognitive	Beck	Older persons' negative view of the future, the environment, and themselves increases their negative emotional reactions to loss.
Sociocultural		
Disengagement	Cummings and Henry	The individual voluntarily reduces involvement with society as society disengages itself from the individual.
Activity	Havighurst	The individual who remains active ages with a sense of satisfaction.
Continuity	Neugarten	Individuals maintain a consistent level of activity as they age.
Interactionist	Spence	Individuals move from one role to another depending on their characteristics and circumstances.
Biological	Wolpert; Frolkis	The lack of physiological energy results in reduced ability to cope with stress.

as stage 4 sleep declines, and the person finds it more difficult to learn psychomotor skills. Also, older people who go to bed early in the evening may awaken early in the morning and complain of insomnia because they are unable to return to sleep.[26] Frequent daytime napping because of boredom can also lead to difficulties in sleeping at night.

The time of day during which the older person naps is important. REM sleep predominates during morning naps and is a continuation of nighttime sleep. The client awakens refreshed because it is a light stage of sleep. In addition, REM sleep helps to organize recent memory data, and morning naps enable the client to think more clearly. Afternoon naps, on the other hand, predominate in stage 4 sleep, the deepest level of sleep. On awakening the client is likely to feel groggy and exhausted. The more stage 4 sleep in the afternoon, the longer the latency—or falling-asleep—stage will be that evening.[27]

Because of the way appearances change with aging and the value that American society places on a youthful appearance, elderly persons may have problems with their body image and self-esteem. The nurse assesses and records any comments made by the older person regarding his body, such as aging skin, thinning hair, or the loss of teeth. A summary of the physical changes in aging is presented in Table 40-2.

Emotional dimension Researchers generally agree that physical decline and the need to conserve energy may cause the older person to express emotion more subtly than at an earlier age. Also, when older people were growing up, they were encouraged not to show their feelings. For these reasons, the overt clues for assessing the older person's emotional dimension may be fewer, and sensitivity is needed to detect subtler clues.

According to Erikson, individuals evaluate their accomplishments and failures during the final stage of life. The older person who views life as primarily consisting of failures is more likely to develop emotional problems. Thus the older person's cognitive appraisal of himself and his situation is important. If the older person's appraisal of his situation is negative, emotional problems such as anxiety and depression can result.

Anxiety is common in old age and is frequently caused by the losses experienced by the aged, particularly the loss of self-esteem and the ability to adapt. Severe anxiety is not as common in elderly persons, because they have developed strategies to handle stress. The common manifestations of anxiety in the aged person are similar to those in other age-groups (see Chapter 10). However, because of changes in the larynx with normal aging, voice changes—which may be a sign of anxiety—are not as easy to detect in the older person as they are in the younger person. Anxiety can also result in insomnia. Drastic changes in the semantic content of conversation may signal mounting anxiety. Individuals may manifest their anxiety by turning their heads away, watching television, closing their eyes, or looking out the door or window to avoid eye contact.

Older people have a tendency to reminisce. Although this process can serve a function, as discussed later in this chapter, it can also result in reality-based or imagined guilt feelings. Because most older people grew up in an environment that promoted a strict conscience, they may have strict rules for themselves. When they do not live up to these standard, they may feel guilty and have a tendency to ruminate over past failures. The presence of guilt can worsen depression and anxiety.

Older persons may hide their feelings about themselves and the way they are treated. This often means that their anger is repressed and is manifested by depression. They may be unable to accept that they even feel anger because they have learned to suppress it. Aphasia, brain damage, or various other physical, emotional, and social factors may also block the expression of anger. Often older persons talk about their anger only indirectly. For example, they may complain about the hospital food and staff, relatives, or world events instead of talking about feelings of anger.

On the other hand, some people may be more apt to express anger in their later years. These people may become less inhibited with age, or their defenses may be less effective in helping them control their anger. Aggressive reactions by disturbed older persons often arise out of a need to gain attention, a need to feel in control, or violations of lifelong dietary preferences and privacy needs.[2] The re-

RESEARCH HIGHLIGHT

A Comparative Study of the Bedtime Routines and Sleep of Older Adults
• JE Johnson

PURPOSE

The purpose of the study was to identify and describe the self-reported nocturnal sleep patterns and bedtime routines of older men and women living in their own home. The relationship between these routines and patterns according to gender were also investigated.

SAMPLE

The sample consisted of 45 men and 42 women who were randomly selected from a list of clients of three family practice and three internal medicine physicians. The subjects ranged in age from 65 to 97 years, with a mean age of 82.2 years. Clients with illnesses and medications that interfered with sleep were excluded from the study.

METHODOLOGY

Data were collected with the Bedtime Routine Questionnaire (BRQ) and the Sleep Pattern Questionnaire (SPQ). The BRQ consisted of six questions designed to obtain information about the activities involved in the bedtime routine. Each subject was observed for 2 nights to see whether activities performed corresponded with the reported routine. The SPQ contained a set of questions completed just before retiring and questions to be answered immediately on arising in the morning. Data were analyzed using descriptive statistics, correlation procedures, and Analysis of Variance (ANOVA).

Based on data from *Community Health Nursing* 8(3):129, 1991.

FINDINGS

All subjects perceived some disturbance in their sleep pattern, with older women perceiving their patterns to be more disturbed than did older men. Subjects with a bedtime routine had fewer sleep complaints than those without a routine. Older men who followed a routine had the least disturbed sleep. Older women without a routine reported the most disrupted sleep patterns.

IMPLICATIONS

When planning care for the noninstitutionalized older client, it is important for the nurse to take into consideration that sleep patterns change with age and that older men and women are likely to express concerns about unsatisfactory sleep. Because insufficient sleep can interfere with daytime alertness and functioning, the nurse needs to caution older clients about engaging in activities that require alertness and attention to safety. The nurse needs to encourage bedtime routines as one means for improving sleep patterns of older adults.

---

sponses interfere with proper care, cause distress to the individual and others, may induce serious emotional problems, and often aggravate physical disorders.

Depression is the most common psychiatric disorder in older adults and is often related to age-related losses.[19,58] Exposure to losses can decrease the older adult's perception of control and can result in anxiety, loneliness, hopelessness, and even suicide.[58] As many as 40% of the cases of depression are severe and require hospitalization.[43] Severely depressed older adults may be unable to verbalize their problems or even talk intelligibly. They often have neglected themselves by not eating or bathing. Symptoms of depression in general can be similar to anxiety and include guilty ruminations, withdrawal, avoidance, or lack of eye contact. However, depressed persons will have less energy than do anxious persons, resulting in slowness of movement and fatigue.

Older people who have a progressive loss of intellectual faculties often become depressed. It is important for the nurse to distinguish depression from dementia. In fact, depression as an early feature of dementia has been observed so frequently that depression was believed at one time to progress to dementia. However, when dementia becomes severe, the loss of psychological capacity is so great that the individual has little or no ability to react with depression. The symptoms of depression are overshadowed by the forgetfulness, poor judgment, and confusion of organic disorders.

Because the verbal response patterns and overt behaviors of depressed persons and those of persons with organic mental disorders are similar, the depressed older person may be misdiagnosed as cognitively impaired. However, a number of signs distinguish between depression, delirium, and dementia (Table 40-3).

In some older persons, nocturia unaccompanied by daytime urinary frequency is a symptom of depression. Thus if the explanation of nocturia is inadequate, depression needs to be considered as a possible cause. The psychomotor agitation sometimes present in depression tends to disappear as the person ages, except when the depression is severe.[53] This is probably due to the weakened emotional tone that accompanies aging.

Related to depression is hopelessness. The losses inherent in aging that can precipitate depression can also result in a decreased perception of control. Persons who view loses as irrevocable and cannot conceptualize that any effect on their part can improve the situation are suffering from hopelessness.[4] When older people view the future as hopeless, they are at great risk for suicide and subintentional suicidal behavior.[50] The nurse assesses older clients' losses and their ways of coping with these losses.

Suicide is the leading cause of death in the elderly. Al-

▼ **TABLE 40-2   Physical Assessment Findings in the Elderly**

Characteristics	Findings
CARDIOVASCULAR CHANGES	
Cardiac output	Heart loses elasticity; therefore decreased heart contractility in response to increased demands
Arterial circulation	Decreased vessel compliance with increased peripheral resistance to blood flow resulting from general or localized arteriosclerosis
Venous circulation	Does not exhibit change with aging in the absence of disease
Blood pressure	Significant increase in the systolic, slight increase in the diastolic, increase in peripheral resistance and pulse pressure
Heart	Dislocation of the apex because of kyphoscoliosis; therefore diagnostic significance of location is lost
	Increased premature beats, rarely clinically important
Murmurs	Diastolic murmurs in over half the aged; the most common heard at the base of the heart because of sclerotic changes on the aortic valves
Peripheral pulses	Easily palpated because of increased arterial wall narrowing and loss of connective tissue; feeling of tortuous and rigid vessels
	Possibility that pedal pulses may be weaker as a result of arteriosclerotic changes; colder lower extremities, especially at night; possibility of cold feet and hands with mottled color
Heart rate	No changes with age at normal rest
RESPIRATORY CHANGES	
Pulmonary blood flow and diffusion	Decreased blood flow to the pulmonary circulation; decreased diffusion
Anatomic structure	Increased anterior-posterior diameter
Respiratory accessory muscles	Degeneration and decreased strength; increased rigidity of chest wall
	Muscle atrophy of pharynx and larynx
Internal pulmonic structure	Decreased pulmonary elasticity creates senile emphysema
	Shorter breaths taken with decreased maximum breathing capacity, vital capacity, residual volume, and function capacity
	Airway resistance increases; less ventilation at the bases of the lung and more at the apex
INTEGUMENTARY CHANGES	
Texture	Skin loses elasticity; wrinkles, folding, sagging, dryness
Color	Spotty pigmentation in areas exposed to sun; face paler, even in the absence of anemia
Temperature	Extremities cooler; decreased perspiration
Fat distribution	Less on extremities; more on trunk
Hair color	Dull gray, white, yellow, or yellow-green
Hair distribution	Thins on scalp, axilla, pubic area, upper and lower extremities; decreased facial hair in men; women may develop chin and upper lip hair
Nails	Decreased growth rate
GENITOURINARY AND REPRODUCTIVE CHANGES	
Renal blood flow	Because of decreased cardiac output, reduced filtration rate and renal efficiency; possibility of subsequent loss of protein from kidneys
Micturition	In men, possibility of increased frequency as a result of prostatic enlargement
	In women, decreased perineal muscle tone; therefore urgency and stress incontinence
	Increased nocturia for both men and women
	Possibility that polyuria may be diabetes related
	Decreased volume of urine may relate to decrease in intake but evaluation needed
Incontinence	Increased occurrence with age, specifically in those with dementia
Male reproduction	
Testosterone production	Decreases; phases of intercourse slower, lengthened refractory time
Frequency of intercourse	No changes in libido and sexual satisfaction; decreased frequency to one or two times weekly
Testes	Decreased size; decreased sperm count; diminished viscosity of seminal fluid
Female reproduction	
Estrogen	Decreased production with menopause
Breasts	Diminished breast tissue
Uterus	Decreased size; mucous secretions cease; possibility that uterine prolapse may occur as a result of muscle weakness
Vagina	Epithelial lining atrophies; narrow and shortened canal
Vaginal secretions	Become more alkaline as glycogen content increases and acidity declines

▼ **TABLE 40-2** **Physical Assessment Findings in the Elderly—cont'd**

Characteristics	Findings
GASTROINTESTINAL CHANGES	
Mastication	Impaired because of partial or total loss of teeth, malocclusive bite, and ill-fitting dentures
Swallowing and carbohydrate digestion	Swallowing more difficult as salivary secretions diminish
	Reduced ptyalin production; therefore impaired starch digestion
Esophagus	Decreased esophageal peristalsis
	Increased incidence of hiatus hernia with accompanying gaseous distention
Digestive enzymes	Decreased production of hydrochloric acid, pepsin, and pancreatic enzymes
Fat absorption	Delayed, affecting the rate of fat-soluble vitamins A, D, E, and K absorption
Intestinal peristalsis	Reduced gastrointestinal motility
	Constipation because of decreased motility and roughage
MUSCULOSKELETAL CHANGES	
Muscle strength and function	Decrease with loss of muscle mass; bony prominences normal in aged, since muscle mass decreased
Bone structure	Normal demineralization, more porous
	Shortening of the trunk as a result of intervertebral space narrowing
Joints	Become less mobile; tightening and fixation occur
	Activity may maintain function longer
	Normal posture changes; some kyphosis
	Range of motion limited
Anatomic size and height	Total decrease in size as loss of body protein and body water occur in proportion to decrease in basal metabolic rate
	Increased body fat; diminished in arms and legs, increased in trunk
	Decreased height from 2.5 to 10 cm from young adulthood
NERVOUS SYSTEM CHANGES	
Response to stimuli	All voluntary or automatic reflexes slower
	Decreased ability to respond to multiple stimuli
Sleep patterns	Stage 4 sleep reduced in comparison to younger adulthood; increased frequency of spontaneous awakening
	Stay in bed longer but get less sleep; insomnia a problem
Reflexes	Deep tendon reflexes responsive in the healthy aged
Ambulation	Kinesthetic sense less efficient; may demonstrate an extrapyramidal Parkinson-like gait
Voice	Decreased range, duration, and intensity of voice; may become higher pitched and monotonous
SENSORY CHANGES	
Vision	
Peripheral vision	Decreases
Lense accommodation	Decreases, requires corrective lenses
Ciliary body	Atrophy in accommodation of lens focus
Iris	Development of arcus senilis
Choroid	Atrophy around disk
Lense	May develop opacity, cataract formation; more light necessary to see
Color	Fades or disappears
Macula	Degenerates
Conjunctiva	Thins and looks yellow
Tearing	Decreases; increased irritation and infection
Pupil	May be different in size
Cornea	Presence of arcus senilis
Retina	Observable vascular changes
Stimuli threshold	Increased threshold for light touch and pain
	Ischemic paresthesias common in the extremities
Hearing	Less perceptible high-frequency tones; hence greatly impaired language understanding; promotes confusion and seems to create increased rigidity in thought processes
Gustatory	Decreased acuity as taste buds atrophy; may increase the amount of seasoning on food

From Ebersole P, Hess P: *Toward healthy aging: human needs and the nursing process,* ed 3; Data from Malasanos L and others: *Health assessment,* ed 3, Mosby–Year Book; Blake D: *Physiology and Aging Seminar for Nurses,* Napa, Calif., May; and Wardell S, editor: *Acute interventions: nursing process throughout the life span,* Reston, Va, 1979, Reston Publishing Co.

▼ **TABLE 40-3**   **Distinguishing Depression, Delirium, and Dementia**

Features	Depression	Delirium	Dementia
Confusion	Client may complain of problems with remembering; concern with these problems; impairment probably mild	Client is likely to deny problems exist, selective impairment, major disruption in daily living	Confusion is noticed by others, staff, family; major memory disturbance
Hallucinations and delusions	Absent (usually)	Vivid hallucinations and well-developed delusional systems	Sometimes paranoid accusations present; illusions, personality changes possible
Onset	Can be abrupt or gradual; look for a precipitant: life changes, losses, change in health	Abrupt and rapid	Slow and insidious
Progress	Not progressive	Symptoms become severe in a few days	Gradual or step-wise progression
Fluctuations	Client may feel worse in the morning	Large fluctuations, even hour to hour	Some change in severity possible, but not large (clients with multiinfarct dementia exhibit greater fluctuations in mental status and behavior than do clients with Alzheimer's disease)
Duration	From 2 weeks to 6 months; may last years	A few days or weeks	Months or years
Mental status exam	Usually no errors, or no more than one	Connotative errors likely	Two or more errors (number or errors correlates to severity of disease)
Neurological	Normal aging pattern; performance on tests requiring speed	Selective impairment, especially attention	Global deficit that becomes worse as the disease progresses

Modified from Goss A, King K: Based on data from Zarit S, Orr N, Zarit J: *The hidden victims of Alzheimer's disease: families under stress,* New York, 1985, New York University Press.

though the elderly make up about 11% of the population, they account for roughly 25% of reported suicides. In 80% of older persons' suicide attempts, depression is present; 12% of elderly persons who attempt suicide try again within 2 years, usually in a setting identical to that of the first attempt.[44] The risk of suicide is highest among elderly Anglo men than any other group. For women the rate of suicide peaks in middle age with a male/female suicide ratio overall of 3:1. By age 85 this male/female ratio rises to 12:1.[50]

Older persons may choose suicide so that they can die while they are still physically and mentally able to make decisions; this is especially true if they are facing a debilitating terminal illness and are alone. They may attempt suicide as a way of controlling or beating death. They may consider suicide as a way to rejoin deceased loved ones and commonly attempt suicide on the anniversary date of an important loss. Even when they have been taught that suicide is wrong, their guilt feelings may be overcome by a strong belief that they have a right to choose when and how to die.

Older people are more likely to succeed in their suicide attempts because they generally choose more lethal methods. The ratio of attempts to completed suicides is 10:1 among all ages and 1:1 for those over the age of 65.[50] Thus the elderly person who states a wish to die is considered at high risk. This is especially true if plans include a violent method and a suicide note is left.

Although elderly persons' active suicide attempts are more violent, they are not nearly as common as the indirect self-destruction called benign suicide or subintentional suicide. This self-destructive behavior is frequently seen in the older person who finds it impossible to deal with widowhood and dies shortly after the spouse's death. It also occurs frequently among the aged who reside in nursing homes. Examples of subtle self-destructive behavior are refusing to eat, refusing medication, and not taking care of one's physical needs. These behaviors often are not viewed as suicide attempts by those caring for the elderly, and the intent behind such suicidal behavior is often ignored. Thus if clients refuse medications or refuse to eat, their behavior may be interpreted as being stubborn, cantankerous, or confused; their neglect of their physical needs could be viewed as forgetfulness or carelessness. However, any behavior that may harm the individual needs to be explored for self-destructive intent.

N **Intellectual dimension** According to the biological theory, there are many normal physical changes that can result in both communication and psychological problems. Sensory changes can affect aged persons' perceptions of their world. For example, the decline in peripheral vision in the elderly may result in viewing others as intruding on their personal space without warning. The nurse assesses the older client for sensory changes such as decreased hearing and vision problems. It is important to assess the older client's ability to integrate messages and the time needed by the individual to respond to others. It is futile to begin asking clients questions if they cannot hear you. Also, if clients have vision problems, touch may be needed to let them know you are present. Awareness of the older client's special needs for communication decreases frustration for the client and the nurse when establishing a therapeutic relationship.

Although long-term memory for past events usually remains intact in the older person, short-term memory for recent events is frequently impaired. The loss of neurons in the brain that accompanies aging decreases the older person's ability to store short-term memories.[13] Also, the preservation in memory of past events may be the result of the greater importance of these events or the frequent mental rehearsal of them by the older person.

Data on an older person's orientation and memory indicate the reliability of the information given by that person. Also, having data on the person's level of understanding assists the nurse in asking questions and giving the client information at an appropriate level. Because the older person is frequently distracted by irrelevant stimuli, questions must contain only one thought and be clear and concise. Older persons' increased response time requires that questions be paced to their speed in answering. For the confused older client whose attention span is short, the nurse provides a rest period between data collection sessions.

Sensory deprivation is a common problem among the elderly, particularly those in institutions. It may result from body changes, such as hearing loss, that alter the reception or perception of sensations; a decrease in life space, such as with a loss of mobility; or a decrease in the amount or variety of environmental stimuli. Thus stimulation in the older person's environment is particularly important as his life space decreases. Sources of stimulation to each of the five senses, contacts with other people, and the meaningfulness of the stimuli to clients are important areas for assessment.

If the older person's activities are limited to a particular community, building, or room, sensory deprivation is more likely. For example, the older person who is transferred from home to a high-rise apartment building may stay primarily in the apartment where there is inadequate sensory stimulation. Such sensory deprivation is believed to exacerbate the loss of functional cells in the central nervous system and thereby speed up normal degeneration. In general, isolation leads to sensory deprivation, loss of mental function, and personality disintegration in the elderly.[2]

Many older adults think of physical problems as more acceptable than psychological problems. The aged tend to use physical complaints to express emotional problems, especially depression, even when they are well. Of geriatric outpatients, 60% have significant somatic preoccupations.[40]

Many of the physical complaints resulting from depression are wrongly considered by nurses to be a part of normal aging, and therefore depressive states often are not diagnosed. For example, an older person with the classical depressive picture of perpetual fatigue and the gastrointestinal symptoms of anorexia, epigastric distress, and constipation can easily be viewed as experiencing the normal processes of aging rather than as being depressed.

An intense, almost morbid preoccupation with health, called *hypochondriacal preoccupation,* may be present. Frequently, this preoccupation is concerned with the gastrointestinal and cardiovascular systems. These complaints may have a bizarre quality and may be the beginning of somatic delusions. This preoccupation with one's body may provide elderly persons with an acceptable "sick role" and allow them to deny their loss of independence, success, and prestige.

Older persons' degree of defensiveness about their aging is assessed as an indicator of their adaptation. Patterns of denial may interfere with their acceptance of aging and their recognition of physical limitations. An example is elderly people who are secretive about their age, overuse hair dyes and cosmetics to appear young, exaggerate their physical prowess, and ignore physical impairments. This denial impedes healthy adaptation to the reality of aging. The older person who refuses to plan may be failing to face the decline of aging and may awaken one day with the realization that "I am old."

The older client, especially when confused, may engage in compulsive or repetitive behaviors. An example of these behaviors is wandering. *Wandering* is a tendency to move about either in a seemingly disoriented fashion or in pursuit of an unobtainable goal. The client who wanders is particularly troublesome to families and institutions who have a moral and legal obligation for the client's safety.

Wandering most often is an avoidance behavior in response to stress. In comparison to clients who do not wander, wanderers move about more, spend more time screaming or calling out, spend less time in social behavior, and are more disoriented.

In assessing wandering, the following questions are considered[17,35]:

1. What is the person's pattern of wandering?
2. Is it searching behavior, combined with calling out or looking for an unobtainable person or goal—for example, a dead spouse?
3. Is it searching behavior directed toward an obtainable but lost object—for example, dentures?
4. Is it apparently non–goal-directed, characterized by multiple goals and aimlessness or a poor attention span?
5. Is it the result of a lifelong pattern of coping with stress, as in walking or running away from stress?
6. Is it related to previous work roles, such as mail carrier?
7. Is the individual searching for security in the face of fear or anxiety?
8. What is the individual's usual route?
9. What is the timing of the wandering; is it seasonal or at a particular time of day?
10. What is the individual's usual affect and behavior during wandering?

Expressive functions may also be affected by aging or by the disease processes that frequently accompany aging.

Incoherent or repetitious speech, sometimes called *sounding,* can also result from nonorganic causes. It often occurs when meaningful communication has been interrupted and is frequently seen as meaningless babble. However, sounding can serve several purposes for older people, including (1) reaffirming their presence, (2) testing how people respond to their needs, (3) discharging pent-up tension, (4) providing self-stimulation, and (5) establishing their personal space or territorial boundaries.[20]

Social dimension According to Peck's developmental theory,[48] older adults must accomplish tasks that result in satisfying relationships and activities, that redefine self in terms other than the work role, and that exemplify their contributions to society and younger generations as extending past their own lives. Accomplishing these tasks prevents a preoccupation with the work role, body functions, and death. Also, the activity theory proposes that continued activity during old age promotes well-being and satisfaction, and interactionalist theory focuses on the need to choose new roles as major roles end during old age.

One of the developmental tasks of older persons is adjusting to changes in their relationships with significant others, including spouses, siblings, friends, children, and grandchildren. Retirement, decreased mobility, illness, and the death of significant relatives or friends often increases the significance of people who remain. The significance of remaining relationships is assessed by the nurse. For example, children's returning home for special occasions may become extremely important to the aged parent.

Accomplishing these developmental tasks can be made more difficult by the prevailing attitude of society that glamorizes youth and disparages old age. This frequently results in low self-esteem that can lead to depression. Low self-esteem is usually expressed in subtle statements such as "I'm useless now" or "You don't need to waste your time on me." Some depressed older persons believe that they are of no value; they think of themselves as ugly, lonely, hopeless, and undeserving. They are unable to see that their thoughts are unrealistic; they do not understand that these beliefs do not represent them.

Older persons' relationship with their spouse is an important assessment area. Generally, the pattern of satisfaction with marital relationships continues into old age. Frequently older people believe that since their children have grown and they are more free to do as they please, they will be drawn closer together by mutual leisure interests. However, many potential marital stressors may emerge, including retirement, financial concerns, disagreements about moving, and health problems. As in any other life stage, these stressors may draw the couple together or separate them.

Role reversal may occur in the marriages of older persons. Older men who have been actively involved with the world may become more introverted and submissive. Women who have been passive earlier in life may become more outgoing and sometimes domineering and aggressive. The degree to which roles are reversed depends on the characteristics of the couple and their past patterns of decision making. It may range from the woman's simply sharing more in decision making to her assuming the role of family authority and primary decision maker.

The older person's social interaction and social support need to be assessed. These include the loss of relationships because of the deaths of friends and family, relocations, and retirement. Elderly persons often have some definite expectations of their children, such as believing that they should visit or write often. Aged parents need to begin viewing their children as adults.

The nurse assesses changes in the older person's relationships and expectations of relationships. When the older person's expectations for relationships are not met, loneliness may develop. Loneliness is the emotional response to the discrepancy between desired and available relationships.[49] The older person is especially vulnerable to loneliness because of the many changes they encounter in their relationships. Loneliness is painful and undesirable. The accompanying research highlight shows that the presence of hopelessness worsens feelings of loneliness, whereas the presence of spiritual well-being or transcendence decreases the possibility of loneliness.

According to disengagement theory, retirement is a significant event in which society and the individual are disengaging. Most retired persons are able to adapt over time and use this freedom to enjoy old age. However, important areas of data collection are the following:

1. The meaning that work held for the older person
2. How the older person views his retirement
3. Whether the retirement was mandatory or voluntary
4. How prepared the person is for retirement
5. How the spouse reacts to retirement
6. Whether the older person is involved in non-work activities or hobbies or interests

Some older people may view retirement as a privilege, welcome the relief from a rigid schedule, and look forward to leisure years. Others may view retirement as a threat and vigorously oppose it, especially if their self-worth is based primarily on work. If work played a central and significant role in the person's life, the loss of work may be felt severely. When retirement is compulsory, older people may think that they are being discriminated against or that their dignity has been affronted. Thus they may enter retirement resentful toward society. The feelings of loss may hinder the person from finding substitutes for work. In these cases the aged individual is likely to become depressed. What appears to be a problem with retirement may actually be a reaction to aging, or vice versa, and this also is considered in the assessment. Persons who are able to make their own decisions about retirement are generally happier in their retired years. Voluntary retirees have significantly greater satisfaction, feelings of usefulness, emotional stability, self-confidence, and motivation.

Some wives of retirees look forward to their husbands' retirement, and others have grave reservations. Unemployed wives may find that having their husbands home all day interferes with their routines and necessitates major adjustments. When the wife is still employed and the husband retires, the wife may experience stress, especially if she retains responsibility for most household chores.

The older person's participation in leisure activities is assessed. Persons who become more active after retirement usually experience greater satisfaction than those whose participation decreases or remains unchanged.

Although financial needs may decrease after retirement,

RESEARCH HIGHLIGHT

Psychological Correlates of Loneliness in the Older Adult
• CG Walton, C Shultz, C Beck, and R Walls

PURPOSE

To establish a better understanding of loneliness in older adults. This was accomplished by exploring the relationship between loneliness with the presence of age-related losses, hopelessness, self-transcendence, and spiritual well-being.

SAMPLE

The sample was composed of 107 subjects who were attending classes offered by universities throughout the spring and summer of 1989. The mean age of subjects was 71.24 years (sd = 6.05), with 57.7% being female and 42.5% being male.

METHODOLOGY

Subjects completed a demographic questionnaire and five likert scales on loneliness, age-related losses, hopelessness, self-transcendence, and spiritual well-being.

Based on data from the *Archives of Psychiatric Nursing* 5(3):165, 1991.

FINDINGS

The data were analyzed using a regressive decision tree. Higher loneliness scores were associated with higher scores for age-related losses and higher scores for hopelessness. Lower loneliness scores were associated with higher scores for self-transcendence and higher scores for spiritual well-being.

IMPLICATIONS

This research enhances the understanding of loneliness in older adults. Older adults who encounter age-related losses and/or hopelessness may be at greater risk for loneliness. Additional research is needed to identify and test interventions that could decrease loneliness by increasing self-transcendence and/or spiritual well-being or decreasing hopelessness.

---

financial matters are a concern of retirees and account for many of the problems in adjusting to retirement. Economic problems often necessitate adjustments in older persons' life-styles. For example, they may be unable to join or maintain memberships in organizations, to give gifts to family or friends, or to retain their homes. Most older people who have had adequate incomes are able to adjust their life-styles and find adequate financial resources. However, the onset of health problems commonly causes a financial crisis.

Housing can have a decisive impact on the well-being of older persons. Because most older people prefer to live independently in their own homes, the loss of this meaningful possession can be a major stressor; living with children or other relatives causes more stress.

Many people move to the Sunbelt after retirement. The function of such relocations in achieving life satisfaction is inconclusive. Some of these "transplanted" people become lonely for the family and friends they left behind and find it difficult to cope with an unfamiliar environment and to adapt to one-season weather. For others a new environment leads to renewed vitality.

Maintaining trust in oneself and the world is a challenge for the person facing the multiple losses of aging and living in an environment in which he fears physical harm. Older people who manifest trust have usually been able to achieve the developmental tasks discussed earlier in this chapter. Those who have not developed trust and are under stress are likely to exhibit symptoms ranging from suspiciousness to paranoia.

The dulling of the senses, especially loss of hearing, has been associated with suspiciousness. Failing memories may also lead to suspiciousness in aged persons who choose to project their problems onto others rather than accept a decrease in memory. Major environmental changes, such as moving to a nursing home, may lead to suspiciousness.

Environmental changes involve the stress of adjusting to an unfamiliar environment and new relationships. Social isolation is also highly correlated with the development of paranoia.

Older adults may make vague complaints that external forces—such as landlords, nurses, or relatives—are controlling their lives. These may be generalized feelings of desertion or of being abused by the younger generation, the government, or outside forces. This suspiciousness may be a lifelong style that becomes exaggerated as a result of the situational changes accompanying aging. Individuals who have consistently used the defense mechanism of projection may be predisposed to heightened suspiciousness in their later years when multiple losses occur.

The older person's suspiciousness is not to be dismissed without ruling out a justifiable cause. The older person's view may be accurate; the bank officer may indeed be reluctant to give the older person a loan, the store clerk may avoid answering questions, or someone may be planning to steal his Social Security check.

While true paranoid disorders sometimes start in old age, most of the paranoid symptoms seen in elderly persons reflect social isolation and misinterpretations of environmental events rather than delusions. When multiple losses challenge people's sense of control over the world, they may search for some explanation for the losses. If they are unable to find an explanation, they may attempt to reduce the ambiguity of the unknown by resorting to mystical or primitive interpretations of their world. This is especially true in individuals whose personality predisposes them toward suspiciousness.

Important areas of assessment include the older person's level of independence, his ideas about dependence-independence, and his reaction to the loss of independence. Independence is also related to many other factors including health, income, mobility, housing, and life-style. These factors need to be assessed to determine the older person's ability to remain independent.

Most individuals between 65 and 75 years of age continue with normal activities and by 85 years are usually showing the effects of age and may need assistance with normal activities. Older people usually dislike dependence. Adjusting to dependence then becomes a major task of old age.

Most older people highly value independence and often become unhappy when placed in a dependent situation.[64] The desire to remain independent in one's later years can be adaptive or maladaptive, depending on the reason for and the degree of this desire. In a society that values independence highly, making decisions and doing things for themselves give older persons pride. They may also want to remain independent to avoid being a burden on others.

In addition, mistrust may be a motive for remaining independent. The older person may fear being used or manipulated. Older people may isolate themselves from others because they are afraid of losing their independence. This isolation helps them avoid any negative reactions from others to their disabilities. These last two motives are maladaptive because they can lead to withdrawal and isolation. Therefore the motives that the aged person has for maintaining independence are important in the assessment.

In contrast, some older people may enjoy dependence, particularly those for whom it has been a lifelong pattern. They may use helplessness to attract and hold the love of family, friends, or caregivers. This can put a strain on relationships and may lead to abuse of the older person (see Chapter 34). Dependence may be culturally influenced; for example, some elderly southern women were socialized to depend on their husbands. An older person may have a need for dependence that originated early in life but lies dormant until many of the resources are lost; these losses affect the individual's sense of mastery and may activate feelings of helplessness.

The majority of older men and women with intact relationships continue to enjoy themselves sexually and consider sensual pleasure a rewarding part of being an older person. More time is needed to reach orgasm and the period of orgasm decreases, but the overall pattern of sexual activity of a couple remains intact.

Older people often distinguish between intercourse and intimacy. Some research suggests that the nonintercourse aspects of love peak in the later years, since more and more persons are likely to have experienced the full range of human loving. However, the expression of sexuality may be hampered by lack of privacy, unavailability of partners, or negative caregiver attitudes.[35]

In the assessment, nurses are concerned with the status of past as well as present loving relationships and the degree to which the client was or is satisfied with these relationships. Even if a person is no longer sexually active, asking questions about sexuality shows recognition of the individual's past and present. The nurse inquires about the older person's current sexual outlets, the importance of sexual activity in his life, and any problems regarding sex.

Spiritual dimension The final stage of life often provides time to think about spiritual matters. Mortality and immortality, love relationships, and transcendence take a new meaning as death approaches; these are important areas of assessment for the nurse. The spiritual dimension can be broken down into two subcategories: existential well-being and religious well-being. Existential well-being consists of a set of beliefs that life is purposeful, meaningful, and positive.[47] Religious well-being means that the person relates those beliefs to God or the church. Spirituality can provide the means for the older adult to obtain integrity as described by Erikson.[25] Also, spiritual well-being and self-transcendence can assist older people to believe that their lives have meaning and their contributions to others will extend past their own lives as described in Peck's developmental theory.[48]

Spirituality has been found to correlate with feelings of happiness, usefulness, greater socialization, and personal adjustment in older people, especially in men and those older than 70 years.[7,8,36,37] When the older people of today were being reared, religion and church- or temple-related activities were emphasized and church activities were often the main social events. Most studies indicate that older people who have grown up with these values continue these activities if possible. Those who have not been active church or temple members during their young and middle adult years often reestablish ties as they become older. Membership in a church or synagogue is often retained longer than membership in any other voluntary organization. Religious activities may decrease only when the older person becomes ill or cannot find transportation. When religious activities outside the home decrease, those within the home—such as listening to religious services on the radio or television—may increase. The nurse assesses whether the older person is currently involved in religious activities or has participated in religious activities in the past.

Also important in the assessment is the older person's ability to transcend. *Self-transcendence* is the ability to look beyond or overcome self-concerns in order to remain actively involved in relationships, activities, and life in general. The many losses experienced by older adults increase the likelihood of dwelling on self-concerns. Two primary components of self-transcendence, body transcendence and ego transcendence, are found in Peck's theory.[48] The nurse assesses *body transcendence* by determining the client's ability to accept the physical signs of aging and to transcend pain or discomfort to maintain satisfying human relations and creative activities. *Ego transcendence* is the ability to accept inevitable mortality and maintain the belief that one's actions and contributions will endure after death. The nurse assesses the older person's relationships with others, involvement in creative activities, and whether bodily concerns and thoughts of death interfere with relationships or activities.

The finiteness of life takes on added significance in later years; at this time persons may achieve their last developmental task, the acceptance of death. Their readiness for death and their fears about dying are important factors in the assessment of the spiritual dimension. Having put their affairs in order and having achieved their major goals, many older persons are ready for death while continuing to live their lives to the fullest. For many of these people, estab-

HOLISTIC ASSESSMENT TOOL: THE AGED ADULT

Physical Dimension
Genetic history

At what age did members of your family die?
Is there any history of Alzheimer's disease or multi-infarct dementia in your family?

Activities of daily living
DIET AND ELIMINATION
Describe any problems you have with incontinence.
EXERCISE AND ACTIVITY
Describe physical limitations you have that prohibit adequate exercise.
SLEEP AND REST
Describe any fears you have that keep you from falling asleep at night or keep you awake during the night.
Do you take naps and at what time of the day?
What is your consumption of tobacco, alcohol, and drugs?

General appearances
BODY IMAGE
In what ways has the aging process altered your body image?

Sexuality
Describe any vaginal pain or irritation.
Describe any difficulty you have with sexual functioning.

Emotional Dimension
How have you responded to your own aging?
What losses have occurred as an older adult? What have these losses meant to you? In what ways have you coped with the losses of aging?
Describe your feelings about your aging and your present circumstances.
Does anything about your physical health concern you?
In what ways are you satisfied with your accomplishments?
Describe any major regrets you have about your life.

Intellectual Dimension
What changes have occurred in your vision, hearing, taste, smell, and feeling? In what ways have you compensated for these sensory changes?
Describe any difficulty you have with your memory. What strategies have you used to help with your memory?
In what ways have you been able to adapt to the changes taking place in your world?

Social Dimension
Self-concept
In what ways has your self-concept been altered by the aging process?

Interpersonal relations
In what ways has your relationship with your spouse and children changed during your older adulthood.
What kinds of social interactions do you engage in? Describe your satisfaction with your level of social interaction.

Environmental factors
Are you retired? If so, was it a mandatory or voluntary retirement? Was retirement forced because of illness?
Describe any preretirement preparation.
Describe any difficulty in adjusting to retirement.

Trust-Mistrust
Do you feel safe going out during the day or night?
Describe your satisfaction with your level of control of your life.

Dependence-Independence
In what areas have you been required to become more dependent because of the aging process? How have you adjusted to this change in dependence?

Spiritual Dimension
How has your philosophy of life changed during your later years?
What meaning does your life have?
Describe your sense of purpose and usefulness.
What do you fear about your own dying?
Describe how you have achieved the major goals in your life.

---

lishing a legacy is important. Clients who are discussing the meaning of life may despair. They may think that God is punishing them for their sins and turn away from God. A few older people feel cheated by life. These people may approach death with despair.

Many older people do not fear death, and older people with strong religious beliefs are generally less anxious about death than those who are not religious. Those who are anxious usually have fears about the process of dying rather than about death itself. They fear losing control as death approaches, being unable to get help when they need it, and being abandoned.

The holistic assessment tool above contains assessment information specific to the aged adult. It is to be used in conjunction with the assessment tool in Chapter 8.

Measurement tools

Table 40-4 lists measurement tools that are useful in assessing the older adult.

Analysis
Nursing diagnosis

Relocation stress syndrome is a nursing diagnosis approved by NANDA that applies to the aged adult. The defining characteristics of this nursing diagnosis are listed in the box on p. 814.

The following case example illustrates the characteristics of the nursing diagnosis, relocation stress syndrome.

▼ Case Example

Mr. Brown, an 87-year-old father of one daughter and two sons, was moved from the home of his daughter to a nursing home after his condition became such that he needed 24-hour care. Mr. Brown reluctantly agreed with his children that relocating him to a nursing home was the best solution, but he still felt that he was being abandoned by his children. Following the move, Mr. Brown showed significant depressive behavior such as crying, difficulty sleeping, loss of appetite, and social withdrawal. There also was a

▼ **TABLE 40-4   Measurement Tools**

Instrument	Description
Home Assessment Checklist	A 50-item questionnaire that evaluates environmental and safety conditions of the older person's general household, kitchen, bathroom, and bedroom
Older Americans' Resources and Services Instrument (OARS)	A multidimensional functional assessment tool that covers social and economic resources, mental health, and activities of daily living
Short Portable Mental Status Questionnaire (SPMSQ)	A 10-item questionnaire that assesses the presence and degree of cognitive deficit in regard to orientation, long-term and short-term memory, and information necessary for activities of daily living

degree of disorientation to place; he sometimes thought he was still at his daughter's home. Mr. Brown became more dependent on the nursing home staff, requiring assistance with some daily routines that he did for himself at his daughter's home. He ex-

▼ **RELOCATION STRESS SYNDROME**

DEFINITION

Physiological and/or psychosocial disturbance as a result of transfer from one environment to another.

DEFINING CHARACTERISTICS

• **Physical dimension**

Sleep disturbance
Change in eating habits
Gastrointestinal disturbance
Weight change

• **Emotional dimension**

Anxiety
Apprehension
Depression
Insecurity
Sad affect
Restlessness
Vigilance

• **Intellectual dimension**

Increased confusion
Verbalization of unwillingness to relocate
Increased verbalization of needs
Unfavorable comparison of posttransfer with pre-transfer staff
Verbalization of being concerned or upset about transfer

• **Social dimension**

Loneliness
Dependency
Lack of trust
Withdrawal
Change in environment or location

Modified from North American Nursing Diagnosis Association Classification of Nursing Diagnosis: proceedings of the tenth conference 1992 (in press).

pressed concern that the staff would not care for him as well as his daughter. He complained of too few visits from his children, who visited him at least once and sometimes twice a day.

The following list provides examples of NANDA-accepted diagnoses with causative statements:

1. Disturbed self-concept related to the aging process
2. Potential for violence self-directed related to loss of spouse
3. Social isolation related to relocation to nursing home
4. Powerlessness related to recent retirement

Planning

Table 40-5 provides a nursing care plan with long- and short-term goals, outcome criteria, interventions, and rationales for diagnoses related to the aged adult. These serve as examples of the planning stage of the nursing process.

Implementation

Physical dimension Older persons' rest and sleep can be promoted by helping them become aware of their biorhythms and synchronize their activities and rest with their body functions. They also need information about the normal changes in the sleep patterns of people in this age-group.

Plans should be made for a balance between activity and rest during the day. Older people can take up to three times as long to get to sleep in the evening if they take afternoon naps. Therefore it is helpful to schedule social and recreational activities in the afternoon and to allow ample time for a nap before lunch. Scheduling purposeful activities in the afternoon also helps prevent boredom and provides exercise conducive to evening sleep. Short intermittent rest periods during the day—such as sleeping, reading, watching television, or listening to the radio—help increase the efficiency of activities that follow. Rest periods of about 20 minutes in a reclining position are particularly helpful after the noon and evening meals. Before the person rests, the nurse or client loosens clothing around the neck, wrists, ankles, and pelvic girdle to allow for proper circulation.

▼ **TABLE 40-5   NURSING CARE PLAN**

GOALS	OUTCOME CRITERIA	INTERVENTIONS	RATIONALES
NURSING DIAGNOSIS: Feelings of powerlessness related to admission to a nursing home			
LONG TERM			
To develop a feeling of hope about existence	Makes future-oriented statements	Encourage client to make likes and dislikes known to caregivers	Fosters hope by encouraging the client to make choices and exert control over daily activities
To maintain control over existence	Is assertive in asking for needs to be met	Encourage openness and expression of feelings related to loss of independence	Assists the client in maintaining control over his life by actively planning daily schedule
		Encourage family and friends to visit and to allow the client some choices as to the time and day of visits	Allows client to have some control in relationship with significant others
SHORT TERM			
To exercise self-determination	States that his actions have an influence on the outcome of events or experiences	Encourage client to make preadmission daily schedule known to caregivers	Fosters self-determination by encouraging and assisting the client to make decisions about daily living
To make decisions about important aspects of daily living	Assumes responsibility for as much self-care as possible	Assist client in setting up a daily schedule of activities (ADL, meals, social interactions) similar to his preadmission schedule	Fosters self-determination by encouraging and assisting the client to make decisions about daily living
	States preferences about activities such as bedtime and frequency and timing of baths	Encourage and assist client to individualize his room by decorating and/or placing familiar objects where he can view them	To increase familiarity and feeling of security
NURSING DIAGNOSIS: Social isolation related to the recent loss of a spouse			
LONG TERM			
To develop needed or desired intimate relationships and roles	Describes present relationships and roles that are meaningful	Encourage the use of skills by teaching others or participating in volunteer programs, such as a foster grandparent program	Increases socialization with peers and younger people and stimulates interest in living
	Expresses feelings of belonging and being needed	Encourage participation in church activities and groups	To improve self-image and promote attainment of self-transcendence and spiritual well-being through acceptance in a group
SHORT TERM			
To complete grieving process accompanying loss of sources of intimacy	Decreases frequency of feelings of sadness over loss	Provide time for the person to talk about the deceased spouse	Provides human contact and intimacy for grieving
To decrease frequency of feelings of loneliness	Prepares for contacts with people for high-risk periods such as evenings, meals, holidays, and anniversaries	Schedule regular contacts with children and other family members who may also be grieving	Provides support while completing grieving process
	Seeks out surrogates for human intimacy, such as pets	Explore resources for buying a pet or the loan-a-pet program	Provides a nonthreatening source of intimacy

Clients are encouraged to nap in their beds because when they nap in a chair, the neck is often hyperflexed or hyperextended. This may compress the arteries in the neck; changes in cerebral blood flow and decreased vascular resistance may lead to mental confusion or hypotension.

If older persons are institutionalized, arrangements are made to follow their usual bedtime rituals, including allowing time for these rituals before retiring. Since older clients sometimes fear that other people will enter their room or home during the night, their safety and the safety of their personal belongings are ensured. A call or telephone system that is answered promptly may provide the sense of security needed for rest. Foods rich in protein and milk products before bedtime help promote sleep and provide alternatives to sleep medications.

By their acceptance and positive regard for older persons, nurses can promote a positive body image. Encouraging older persons to take pride in their appearance is also important and may include discussing hairstyles or the use of cosmetics to cover blemishes. In an institution, nurses can help prevent any unsightly appearance that may be caused by stained dentures, soiled clothing, and unkempt hair, fingernails, and beards. Older people sometimes fail to maintain their appearance because their hands are crippled with arthritis or they lack awareness, energy, or incentive; the strategic placement of mirrors can improve their awareness.

If changes in body image have produced negative self-evaluations, older people need reassurance and positive reinforcement for the aspects of themselves that transcend physical appearance. For example, because of a client's problems with hearing and vision, the nurse sits in a chair in full view of the client, eliminates extraneous noise, and ensures that rooms are well lit. Female nurses should consider wearing dark lipstick, which can assist older people who read lips. Use of visuals that have limited detail and are composed of the primary colors can activate senses.

Emotional dimension It is often effective to combine several techniques when dealing with anxiety in elderly clients. Attentive listening or touch can alleviate anxiety. Anxiety can also be treated by using deep muscle relaxation after systematic desensitization. Then, positive reinforcement can be used to condition alternate or competing responses. A combination of self-efficacy training, modeling, operant shaping of alternate responses, and supportive counseling is especially effective if feelings of helplessness underlie the anxiety.[16]

Exercise is an excellent intervention for anxiety. In older adults, exercise has been shown to decrease anxiety, depression, and health worries and improve self-image, sleep quality and quantity, and short-term memory and concentration. For exercise to be effective, it must be long-term.[25,41,60] Psychological benefits occur after 4 to 6 weeks of exercise and diminish if exercise is discontinued.[41] The older person should exercise three times a week for at least 20 minutes. The intensity of the exercise is not as important as the length of time. Research has shown that older persons taking yoga classes can reap similar psychological benefits as older persons participating in high-intensity aerobic exercise.[60] It is important to assist the older adult in choosing an exercise that is convenient. Older persons are more likely to continue exercising if they exercise with a friend

or within a group. When older adults exercise in groups, they may have the added benefit of decreased loneliness and improved social life.[25] A popular form of individual or group exercise for older adults is mall walking.

Older people need encouragement to express their anger. Letting them know their anger is sensed and accepted is important. Because older people frequently hold in angry feelings, outbursts may be strong when they are given a chance to express them. They need to be encouraged to explore the causes for their feelings and to receive direction in getting back to the initial cause or loss. After finally exposing their anger, they may need assistance in reestablishing relationships with loved ones. Initially, constructive physical activities may also provide for some release of anger. Examples of such activities are hammering, digging in a garden, painting, and squeezing clay.

Older persons often do not understand the relationship between their physical complaints and their depression. It is helpful to first establish rapport by listening to clients' complaints fully and intently; then assistance can be given in helping them be as comfortable as possible. This conveys understanding and hope. The nurse explains that some of the physical symptoms may be manifestations of depression and that in dealing with the depression some of their physical symptoms may be relieved.

Since repetitious talking about symptoms does not help the client, behavior modification may be useful. For example, expressions of feelings and interest in activities, people, and living can be reinforced with positive responses. Preoccupation with self and physical symptoms is given no response or minimal matter-of-fact attention. "How are you?" is not an appropriate opening remark because it may encourage statements about physical complaints. Instead, conversation can be directed to the person's emotional state, to important past experiences, or to present interests.

Preoccupations or actual problems with defecation, particularly constipation, frequently accompany depression in the older person. However, because of their habit-forming effect, laxatives and enemas are used only when necessary. When an enema is used, its meaning to the depressed older person needs to be considered, since it can be viewed as an invasion, a well-deserved punishment, or a means of control. Natural laxatives, such as raw or bulk food, are preferable. Fluid intake and exercise are also encouraged.

Electroconvulsive therapy (ECT) is commonly used for severe depression, especially in the older person who may not be able to tolerate psychopharmological interventions (see Chapter 14). In elderly persons, ECT is frequently the treatment of choice instead of antidepressants. Older people are more likely to have concurrent medical problems in which antidepressants, due to their cardiotonic and hypotensive (anticholinergic) effects, are contraindicated.[6] Also, if depression is accompanied by suicidal tendencies, which is common in elderly persons, a drug trial of 4 to 6 weeks may place the client at undue risk.

Complications that can interfere with ECT include cardiorespiratory problems, severe confusion, and falls.[66] These complications do not usually present a serious problem. In the majority of cases, a treatment course can be resumed and carried to completion.

Of those older persons who receive ECT, 80% respond favorably.[67] However, controlled trials in younger clients have shown short-term response rates to ECT are much more successful than are long-term responses.[6] Therefore, even if the client no longer appears depressed after treatment, the use of ECT must be followed by some form of psychotherapy to increase the probability of a positive long-term response.

Cognitive psychotherapy is helpful in treating depression in older persons. Cognitive restructuring is a way for them to cope with situations that cannot be changed in reality but can be changed in the way they are perceived.

The nurse refrains from being overly optimistic in dealing with depression in older people. The depressed older person with a severe physical illness may not be helped substantially by psychotherapy. The physical illness decreases the person's vitality that is already reduced by aging and depression.

Intellectual dimension According to the biological theory, there are many normal physical changes associated with old age that can result in problems with cognition and communication and in psychological problems. Some older adults have short-term memory problems. For these persons, orientation to time, place, and person may help to improve memory. Reminders, such as brief notes or instruction cards that are concise and well organized help the individual cope with excessive stimuli and function more independently. Giving the older person a choice of responses or offering alternative solutions when asking questions is also helpful, since recognizing information is usually easier than recalling information.

When short-term memory problems are present, it is best to present information that is congruent with the person's present knowledge base. This can be done by adapting information to the individual's past experiences. Memory can improve when the older person demonstrates what has been taught. Also, summarizing information and providing time for questions and answers can reinforce information. Older people require more time to receive and react to messages. When teaching older clients, it is best to allow them control over the pace of learning. Speech patterns should be paced at 140 words per minute. It is important to convey that the interaction may be paced slower and that the nurse has time for the slower pace.

Memory training can also be used for older adults to assist with short-term memory problems. Generally this training consists of *mnemonic techniques* such as visual imagery associations. For example, the older person learns a series of logical steps for reconstructing a person's name or presentation of the face, as follows[65]:

1. Identify a prominent facial feature (such as a large nose).
2. Derive a concrete, high-imagery transformation of the person's name ("Beck" becomes "Beak").
3. Form a visual image associating the prominent facial feature with the name transformation.

Combining relaxation with training helps the elderly persons to benefit from memory programs.[66]

A series of games called Eldergames has also been used to work with the memory problems of older clients. They concentrate, for example, on evoking earlier memories when short-term memory, but not long-term memory, has begun to erode.[51]

Sensory deprivation is a problem for many older adults, especially those in nursing homes. Activities that activate all five senses provide excellent interventions. Arts and crafts that use colorful materials and different textures can activate senses. For example, older adults who work with different colors of yarn to create a hook rug experience different textures and colors. Older adults who work with clay experience different smells, textures, and subtle colors. Pointing out these different sensations can enhance the older adult's experience.

Nature can provide many long-forgotten sensory experiences for older adults. Morganett[12] suggests nature hikes to provide stimulation to all five senses. If older adults are too frail for nature hikes, the nurse can conduct nature demonstrations using available plants and animals. During nature hikes or demonstrations, vision is stimulated by seeing the differences in colors or examining differences in animals and plants. Hearing is stimulated by listening to different sounds of birds, frogs, or insects. Touch is stimulated by feeling different textures of nonpoisonous plant leaves. Smell can be stimulated by smelling flowers, or the nurse can crush a plant leaf for the group to smell. Taste can be stimulated by bringing berries or jams to have as a snack after the hike or demonstration. These types of activities not only stimulate all the senses but also can facilitate discussion of the experiences and sharing of childhood memories.

In teaching-learning situations with the elderly, the nurse assures older persons that they will be given ample time and that their efforts will be accepted without ridicule. A task that seems overwhelming to the older person can be divided into smaller, more manageable parts, increasing the chance of success. Other suggestions for teaching older adults are presented in Table 40-6.

Social prejudice has fueled the belief that older persons are too old to learn. However, for the retired person who is free from many of the responsibilities and obligations of younger adults, learning can be very important. Learning opportunities provide for personal enrichment, creativity, socialization, and pleasure. Classes that combine older and younger people can improve attitudes about the other as people as they share and discover common concerns.[52] Retired professors and professionals can provide valuable resources as teachers.[56] The research highlight on p. 819 reviews the positive psychological outcomes of older people who experienced late-life learning through taking computer classes.

Cognitive functioning in older persons may be stimulated by physical exercise and music and may be improved by adequate sleep. Those who participated in exercise therapy for a 12-week period were found to have a significant improvement in cognitive functioning. Music therapy also improves the older person's memory and cognitive functioning.[9] Since lack of sleep interferes with cognitive functioning, any of the activities discussed earlier for promoting sleep are also helpful in improving cognitive functioning.

The most common approach to the management of wandering behavior is the use of medications, door locks, gerichairs, and other restraints. However, these actions may produce or exacerbate wandering behavior. Restraints may increase hostility, as well as decrease security, orientation, and stimulation.

The interventions for wandering are tailored to the

▼ **TABLE 40-6   Strategies for Teaching Aged Adults**

Instructional Variable	Strategies
Rate of presentation of information	Present new information at a fairly slow rate
	Let adult learner proceed at his own rate whenever feasible
	Provide adult learner with ample time to respond to questions
	Present a limited amount of material in any single presentation to prevent swamping effects
Organization of information	Present new information in a highly organized fashion
	Use section headings, handouts, summaries, and so on, so that adult learner can get a "handle" on material
	If memory processes are taxed in a learning project, encourage adult learner to use retrieval plans
	Avoid introduction of irrelevant information to prevent confusion
	If visual displays are used, employ simple stimulus configurations
Mode of presenting information	Use auditory mode of presentation when presenting discrete bits of information to be used immediately
	Use visual mode when presenting textual materials to capitalize on opportunity for review during reading
	Utilize models to facilitate strategy development
Covert strategies	Encourage adult learner to generate his own mediators
	Supply adult learner with mediators when necessary
	With concrete material, imagery mediators are superior to verbal mediators and interacting images better than conjunctive images
	Whenever feasible, train adult learner in use of mnemonic devices
	Encourage adult learner to generate covert monitoring verbalizations and provide training when necessary
Meaningfulness of material	Present information that is meaningful to adult learner
	Assess cognitive structure of adult learner to ensure that material is introduced at appropriate level
	Use examples, illustrations, and so on, which are concrete
Degree of learning	Provide ample opportunity for adult learner to over-learn material before moving on to new material
	Remove time constraints from instructional and evaluation process
Introduction of new material	As initial step in learning, identify and eliminate inappropriate responses that may "compete" with appropriate response
	Organize instructional units so that potentially interfering materials are spaced far away from each other
	Stress differences between concepts before similarities
	Make instructional sequence parallel hierarchy of knowledge in any given area
	Instructional procedures should be premised on knowledge of conditions required for a type of learning based on task analysis
	Introduce a variety of techniques for solving problems
Transfer effects	Take advantage of experience the adult learner possesses
	Relate new information to what adult learner already knows
	Develop learning sets that maximize opportunity for positive transfer effects
Feedback effects	Provide verbal feedback concerning correctness of responses after each component of task is completed
	Do not assume that initially poor performance on a novel, complex task is indicative of low aptitude
Climate	Establish a supportive climate
	Engage adult learner in information-oriented, collaborative evaluation
	Encourage adult learner to take educated guesses

Modified from Burnside IM: One-to-one relationship therapy. In Burnside IM: *Nursing and the aged,* ed 2, New York, 1981, McGraw-Hill; based on data from Okun MA: *Adult Education* 27(3):139, 1977.

mood of the wanderer. The placid wanderer who may be bored or repeating a real or imagined activity needs to be approached casually and perhaps channeled into a less disturbing behavior. Agitated wanderers—who may be releasing frustration and tension through motor activity—need to be listened to, kept at a fair distance, and given outlets for their aggression. "Happy wanderers," who may

be exploring, need to be left alone but watched or taken on "guided tours." In general, wandering decreases if a regimen of exercise, walking, or getting outside is established.[34]

Social dimension According to Erikson[25] the final stage of life occurs when individuals evaluate their accomplishments and failures. Self-esteem is promoted by reinforcing positive past and present achievements. One ap-

RESEARCH HIGHLIGHT

Older Adults and Computer Education: "Not to Have the World a Closed Door"

• ML Eilers

PURPOSE

To describe the characteristics of older people who participate in computer classes.

SAMPLE

Sixty-two older adults aged 61 to 70 participated in the computer courses and were surveyed about their experiences.

METHODOLOGY

The computer courses were written by a 73-year-old man and taught by older adults. Qualitative data were collected by questioning older participants about their experiences with learning to use the computer.

FINDINGS

Increased self-esteem was reported by 49% of participants, and 17.5% reported that attitudes of others toward

Based on data from *International Journal of Technology and Aging* 2(1):56, 1989.

them were much better. Participants also reported self-perceived improvement in cognitive function, enjoyment of the mental challenge, and feelings of accomplishment and control over the environment. Several participants were excited about their increased ability to communicate with younger people in new, mutually rewarding ways. Overall, the computer classes enhanced supportive social interaction and provided the opportunity for new friendships based on shared interests. Many participants reported future plans for using their computer knowledge, including writing simple income tax programs, computerizing business records, and becoming computer consultants.

IMPLICATIONS

These findings help dispel the persistent belief that recipients of microprocessor technology are exclusively young scholars and professionals. Also, older adults can learn new and challenging information.

---

proach is asking the client to list his attributes and then to assess them as positive, negative, or neutral. Another technique is to use a prepared self-concept scale on which the client is asked to characterize his usual functioning. The nurse then interjects traits the client may not have included and helps the client set up goals for improving the negative qualities. Usually, the number of positive traits suggested by clients outweighs the number of negative traits. This in itself is helpful, because it suggests to clients that they are not totally negative.[34]

Elderly persons tend to attribute their negative physical symptoms to aging. Therefore another approach to improving self-esteem involves redirecting the negative attributes that the client associates with aging to environmental factors. For example, when the client attributes his tiredness to "being old," he can be reminded that he was awakened at 5:30 AM. Explanations for feelings and behavior are thus refocused on factors that can be changed. This type of intervention improves self-esteem in the older person by changing negative, defeatist attitudes into hopeful, problem-solving approaches.[51]

The recognition by elderly persons and by society of the continuing need for social interaction is promoted through mass media, pamphlets, posters, and discussion groups. On an individual basis, the nurse uses skillful interviewing to help the elderly person become aware of social interaction needs, validate the person as important, and accept the need for interactions as normal. Clients are then assisted in identifying realistic and acceptable solutions and, if possible, in making their own choices. The nurse may need to introduce older persons to neighbors or others in the community, help them form new relationships by identifying common interests and experiences,

help them revive old relationships, or involve them in group activities. The choices that the older person makes to meet social interaction needs are supported; the nurse also assists in evaluating the choice.

According to Peck's developmental theory[48] older adults must engage in satisfying relationships and activities, redefine self in terms other than the work role, and view their contributions to society and younger generations as extending past their own lives. The nurse may form small discussion groups with elderly clients to provide opportunities for social interaction, to teach social skills, or to offer a continuing support system. The use of alcoholic beverages during social events has also helped increase the socialization of elderly persons. Friendly visitor services and telephone reassurance programs are examples of community-based services that have been successful in providing social support to the elderly.

Elderly widowed persons' needs for assistance vary, depending on their ability to adjust to the loss of a spouse. When the older person needs support from others who understand or assistance in becoming involved in old or new activities, the nurse helps by providing the client with information about support groups.

According to disengagement theory, retirement is a significant event in which society disengages itself from the individual. Preretirement counseling is a way to prevent some of the problems that elderly persons encounter during retirement. A postretirement program is also needed to help retirees review their accomplishments, cope with the realities of retirement, adjust to the new role, and identify ways they can continue to contribute to society. For example, some firms offer retired workers part-time employment in a special workshop; volunteer groups may provide workshops and craft centers for the elderly; and elderly business people may advise businesses. Several programs for retired persons have been sponsored by the US government. The Retired Senior Volunteer Program (RSVP) helps aged persons meet the expenses incurred doing volunteer work; in the Foster Grandparent Program elderly people are paid a small fee for providing emotional support to children in institutions, families at high risk for child abuse, and young juvenile offenders. A sense of comradeship and community is fostered by such participation, which also diminishes feelings of hopelessness and social rejection.

Although nurses cannot usually directly affect the income of the elderly, they can be advocates for them in supporting governmental and other efforts to ensure an adequate income in retirement. Nurses can also help elderly clients get information on budgeting, tax benefits, insurance, wills, estates, investments, and reduced rates offered to senior citizens.

The nurse counsels older people on their decision to move or with their selection of housing. The present residence must be evaluated and other residences thoroughly investigated before the client makes the decision to relocate. If the client decides to relocate, a trial move may be suggested. For the older person with brain dysfunction, any relocation—even within the same facility—is disruptive. Therefore the nurse provides a thorough orientation to the new environment.

If the client has paranoid behavior related to isolation, as may be present in the client who recently moved, the nurse intervenes in the process that created the isolation. Restoring social communication is essential; relocating the older individual may be necessary. Because the individual's paranoia may cause people to stay away from him and thus worsen the condition, "shuttle diplomacy" may be necessary.[21] This involves contacting individuals living in close proximity to the client who are aware of the client's condition and may have been targets of the client's accusations. The client's condition is explained to these people, and they are informed that the client is being treated and that the prognosis is good. This prevents further isolation. Planned visits to the client by members of an outreach team help resocialization.

Giving the older person control and participation in decision making may help to prevent suspicion. Older persons may also benefit from help in organizing their possessions or from techniques that will help their memory, such as those described earlier. Aged persons need to have control over the basic decisions affecting their lives, rather than to have the decisions of others imposed on them. For example, they can participate in decisions about relocation, rather than having their children decide for them that their home is no longer an appropriate place for them to live. Aged persons also need to know that others will accept their decisions. Just as clients are given the chance to take part in planning their care, they need the opportunity to make choices as the plan is put into effect.

Interventions for helping the older person maintain as much independence as possible for as long as possible involve social policy issues, such as providing adequate supplementary income, and expanding community services, such as homemaker services, visiting nurses, Meals on Wheels, and adequate public transportation. Nurses can be advocates for elderly persons in securing such services.

Negative reactions to dependence can be reduced by respecting older people's desire for independence and by giving them as many choices as possible. For example, individuals in an institution can be allowed to choose meals, recreational activities, or the timing of their baths.

Excessive disability or dependence is discouraged by not hurrying or assisting a client who is capable of self-care. This approach also discourages helplessness, which fosters further dependence. Examples include eliminating a wheelchair when a client can walk or establishing a bladder-restraining program rather than using catheterization.[38]

Spiritual dimension Spirituality provides the means for the older adult to obtain integrity as described by Erikson.[25] Also, spiritual well-being and self-transcendence can assist older people to believe their lives have meaning and their contributions to others will extend past their own lives as described in Peck's developmental theory.[48]

Some of the interventions that assist with spirituality—such as being a foster grandparent, engaging in late-life learning, and reminiscing—have been discussed within the framework of the other dimensions. Intervening in religious well-being frequently involves collaboration with clergy. Nurses should recognize the support that religious institutions offer to elderly persons. Nurses can also become involved in encouraging churches to develop services and opportunities for aged persons. They may provide opportunities for the older and younger generations to interact and for older people to interact with each other through sharing resources, crisis assistance, or programs such as Adopt-a-Grandparent.

Self-transcendence assists people in attaining spiritual well-being. The nurse fosters self-transcendence through the use of visualization and meditation to increase the meaning of existence for the client. Connecting a present need with a memory can ease the former. For example, aged persons recently relocated to a nursing home may long for the familiar environment of their home. Directing them to visualize their past familiar environment in as much detail as possible helps reconstruct these perceptions, eases the need for the familiar, and provides comfort. Nurses may also teach clients to meditate and encourage them to keep a dream diary, practice yoga, recite poetry, or play a musical instrument.

Another mode of self-transcendence for the older person is the mentor relationship. This mode is infrequently used but can add meaning to older people's lives, and others may benefit from their wisdom. The nurse can encourage the aged person to advise younger persons. For example, an aged person with business experience can assist a younger person in business.

The nurse can help older people meet their needs for transcendence by encouraging them to share their experiences in an oral or written record, to teach skills to others, to share assets, or to donate organs. Establishing a legacy may become a major concern before a person's death. Legacies can extend one's meaning to others by handing down something from the past. Sharing experiences allows older persons to see how their lives have had an impact and prepares them to leave the world with a sense of meaning. It can also give a feeling that one's life will continue, will be tied with survivors, and will provide younger generations with a sense of continuity.[20]

Often older people have particular objects that represent important memories and express the person's transcendence of self. For example, one woman who had owned many cats and had also collected figurines of cats kept the figurines near her bed at the nursing home. These objects represented important memories and were her most cherished possession. She guarded them with great care and needed to make decisions concerning when and to whom these objects would be given. Insensitive distribution of these objects by staff or family members conveys a negative message to the older person, such as "Your death is imminent." When older people approach death, they may want to give away their important possessions or plan for this distribution as a way of expressing their transcendence; nurses help and support the client in this process, as well as help family members graciously accept these gifts.

To help older people establish legacies, the nurse may ask clients what has been the most meaningful contribution in their lives, what impact their generation has had on the world, or what they would like to leave to the younger generation. After the person's interests are determined, a method is established for recording the legacy, identifying the recipients, and distributing the legacy. The older person also needs feedback on how the legacy is received.[20]

If older persons are unable to gain satisfaction by recalling their individual accomplishments, another approach is to tap into their past. Questions about the accomplishments of their generation may be asked. Mentioning important historical events, eliciting their reactions to these events, and asking questions such as "What happened during your lifetime that changed the world?" may give the person a feeling of collective accomplishment.

Other people, particularly if they are angry or are denying their mortality, may not be concerned with a legacy and need not be pushed to do so. These persons need assurance of God's or a supreme being's love and need help to find hope. The assistance of clergy may be needed.

Evaluation

Nursing interventions are evaluated by the extent to which they build on the older client's strengths and do not encourage disability. Care is appropriate if the unique characteristics and needs of the elderly person are taken into consideration. The effectiveness of nursing interventions is related to the extent to which needed changes are incorporated into the older person's long-established life patterns. Finally, the issue of efficiency in caring for elderly persons needs to address the increased time required for nursing care of those in this age-group.

By this stage in their lives, older people often have the self-awareness to assess changes in their sense of well-being. Therefore their reports can be an important aspect of the evaluation.

SPECIFIC TREATMENT MODALITIES

Each of the treatment modalities discussed in Part III of this text can be used with the aged client. Reality orientation, validation therapy, resocialization, reminiscent therapy, and pet therapy are discussed in this chapter because these are used most often with older persons.

Reality Orientation

Reality orientation (RO) was one of the first psychological therapies used with institutionalized elderly persons. Though this therapy may be very effective in some cases, it can be very frustrating and ineffective for those with dementia.[31] It is a behavioral approach that attempts to increase an individual's awareness to time, place, and person. Two basic approaches are used in RO: 24-hour RO and classroom RO. Twenty-four-hour RO involves everyone who comes in contact with confused elderly clients. All present the client with basic information about time, place, and person. For example, when bringing supper to the elderly client, the nurse says "Hello, Mr. Darrell. I am Ms. Kelly. It is 6 o'clock in the evening. Here is some meat loaf and black-eyed peas for your supper." This is a team approach in which every contact with the person helps reorient him. It is often an early phase of rehabilitation used in conjunction with more traditional techniques such as activity therapy, physical and occupational therapy, and remotivation. As a supplement to 24-hour RO, many institutions provide RO classes. These may be scheduled on a daily to a weekly basis. Classes are divided into basic and advanced courses. The therapist works best with only three or four moderately to severely confused clients, but six or eight are usually involved in the advanced class for those who are less confused.

Since the goal of RO is to reduce confusion, its effectiveness as a treatment is evaluated by progress in the individual's ability to accurately state time, place, and date. Changes in other behavioral indicators of confusion also need to be monitored.

Validation Therapy

It is possible that disoriented behavior is not meaningless and that continually correcting a client's disoriented responses (language or behavioral) systematically neglects the true meaning of the confused behavior.[67] Such neglect not only is perceived by the client, but also increases his anxiety and isolation. For example, cooperative nursing home residents who believe that they are still at home may become upset when an RO program is aimed at removing this belief. If an individual is happier in a confused state than in an oriented one, the wisdom of using RO with this person is addressed.

This concern about RO led to the development of *validation therapy*[22] for use with the confused client. This therapy involves searching for the meaning and emotion in the client's words and validating these with the client. For example, if a nursing home client tells the nurse that she has to leave because she has to see her mother (who has been dead for many years), the nurse would respond as follows:

Client: I have to go. I have to see my mother.
Nurse: What does she look like? You must have loved her very much. Do you still miss her?

This dialogue leads to a warm discussion of the client's

relationship with her mother. If the same client had been forced to face the reality that her mother is dead, the client would likely have become uncooperative.

Resocialization

Studies designed to explore the relative effectiveness of reality orientation and *resocialization* have generally found that resocialization is more effective.[10,18,55] Each study reported increased responsiveness, increased socialization with staff and with each other, increased participation in self-care, and less disruptive behavior. Some techniques reported to facilitate socialization and group interaction include the following:

1. Creation of unity and a sense of belonging through touching and joined hands to both initiate and terminate a session
2. Planning of group time so that it is least likely to be changed or disrupted by other activities
3. Minimizing of outside distractions by holding the group session in a convenient but quiet room; establish the norm with other staff that clients are not to be disturbed during group time
4. Structure the group session as follows:
   a. Announce a topic that is familiar
   b. Stimulate memories through associated foods, objects, and pictures
   c. Incorporate activities that are likely to evoke relevant memories and encourage active participation of all members (for example, cutting cake, stirring lemonade, singing a familiar theme-related song)
5. Keeping friends together and sitting next to a member who seems particularly anxious or confused
6. Being careful to design activities to meet the needs of the group members. Activities that evolve from the needs of the leader or staff are likely to be too abstract or complicated

Reminiscent Therapy

Reminiscent therapy involves reminiscing to assign new meanings to past experiences. Whether it is used as an individual or group process, *reminiscent therapy* is a summation of one's life in which the client integrates experiences into his self-concept by mentally reliving them. Repressed and painful material is reviewed, and some of the sting is taken out of the past by altering the perception of it. Early memories may be reconstructed in such a way that they serve the individual's needs, and interests and alleviate fears. Or reminiscence may be used to reduce the dissonance between older people's expectations of themselves from the past and their present situation and behavior.

As in other group work with aged persons, the number of group members is kept at about eight or nine. Persons who have been isolated and who have not had much chance to explore and resolve long-held conflicts are at psychological risk in a reminiscent group; feelings of guilt and remorse, which often emerge during the life review process, may develop into obsessive rumination and even suicidal panic.[11,17] Older people who are confused or suffering from brain damage can also participate in reminiscent therapy. However, caution is needed to prevent the heightened

anxiety, called catastrophic reaction, that occurs when they cannot answer or perform.

Reminiscing groups can be conducted by professionals from a variety of disciplines, including nurses; art, occupational, or music therapists, and social workers. The life review process is more likely to succeed if the person is able to experience it in a cohesive, supportive group in which trust and security are available. Since the group is a support rather than a therapy group, skills in listening and communication are adequate preparation for leading it.

The life review is a crucial process in the aged person's adaptation and, if successful, assists in the following[15]:

1. Personal reintegration
2. Serenity
3. Acceptance of life as meaningfully resolved
4. Greater understanding of life's ambiguities
5. Transfer of culture and value to others
6. Examination of intrapsychic conflicts
7. Reconciliation of family relationships
8. Richer sharing of present experiences
9. Acceptance of death

Unstructured reminiscing groups may be spontaneously stimulated by a special occasion at which people begin remembering the past. More structured groups may be short-term (about 10 weeks) or may go on indefinitely with a periodic evaluation of the goals.

Pet Therapy

The use of pets in therapy with the elderly has many beneficial effects. In some institutions, dogs, cats, birds, and rabbits have been given permanent residence. In other situations, animals are brought in daily or weekly. Since animals show affection without restraint, they often help effect positive mental and physical changes. All clients, especially those who have poor eyesight or are hard of hearing, can benefit from the tactile stimulation that pets provide. Pet therapy is not a replacement for human contact, but it is an alternative that is especially useful for reaching the frail or withdrawn older client.[34]

Humor

The use of humor as an intervention can be effective in stressful situations to diffuse anger and frustration. Humor stimulates endorphins, enhances feelings of well-being, decreases anxiety, increases cardiac and respiratory rates, and enhances metabolism and muscle tone.[61] These positive physiological changes can last up to 45 minutes. In group or interpersonal situations, humor can be used to alter the client's perception of the situation, assist the client to cope more effectively, and encourage bonding. Humor decreases defensiveness while increasing trust and openness to communication.

Humor must be used with caution because of the possibility of clients' viewing the humor as making light of their situation. Humor should never be at the expense of another. Humor involves a high level of cognition and is not used with clients who are confused, paranoid, or severely depressed.

Simon[57] suggests several structured activities that nurses can use to incorporate humor into group therapy for elders.

The nurse can show videotapes of comedies such as Keystone cops, Marx brothers, or modern comedies. Local colleges usually have theater departments from which clowns or comedians can be accessed. Recordings of old radio programs such as George Burns and Gracie Allen can be used. The nurse schedules discussion groups after structured activities to encourage the awareness of humor and humorous situations in daily life and to promote reminiscing and interaction among participants.

BRIEF REVIEW

As the number of aged persons has grown, attention to their mental health care has increased. Nursing has had a primary role in the care of this age-group, and the geropsychiatric nurse has a prominent role in caring for their mental health.

Although a variety of theories have been proposed to explain the changes in the aged, this remains a fertile field for new understanding. Erikson describes the major developmental task of this age-group as ego integrity versus despair. Peck describes their tasks as (1) ego differentiation versus work role preoccupation, (2) body transcendence versus body preoccupation, and (3) ego transcendence versus ego preoccupation. Other relevant theories are cognitive, sociocultural, and biological.

The nurse's attitude toward aged persons is an important consideration in establishing a therapeutic relationship with an elderly client. Older people, because of their years of experience, are often uniquely qualified to participate in planning their care.

The nurse is frequently involved in designing interventions to prevent and treat the loneliness, depression, and paranoid behavior common to those in this age-group. The issues of retirement, relocation, dependence, and death are also paramount concerns for elderly persons. The behavioral manifestations and dynamics of these conditions have some distinctive features that are important to consider when assessing the older person and deciding which aspects of intervention are most crucial.

A number of specific individual and group treatment approaches have been used successfully with the older client. These include reality orientation, validation therapy, resocialization, reminiscent therapy, pet therapy, and humor.

REFERENCES AND SUGGESTED READINGS

1. American Nurses' Association: *Standards of gerontological practice*, Kansas City, 1976, The Association.
2. Aronson MK, Bennett R, Gurland BJ, editors: *The acting-out elderly*, New York, 1983, Haworth Press.
3. Beck AT: The development of depression: a cognitive model. In Friedman RN, Katz MM, editors: *The psychology of depression: contemporary theory and research*, Silver Springs, Md, 1974, VH Winston & Sons.
4. Beck AT: *Cognitive therapy and emotional disorders*, New York, 1976, International Universities Press.
5. Beck AT and others: The relationship between hopelessness and ultimate suicide: a replication with psychiatric outpatients, *American Journal of Psychiatry* 147:2, 1990.
6. Benbow SM: The role of electroconvulsive therapy in the treatment of depressive illness in old age, *British Journal of Psychiatry* 155:147, 1989.
7. Bilrine GLG: Old age: its liabilities and its assets. A psychobiologic discourse. In Lowenstein R, editor: *Psychoanalysis:*

8. *a general psychology*, New York, 1980, International Universities Press.
8. Blazer D, Palmore E: Religion and aging in a longitudinal panel, *Gerontologist* 16:82, 1976.
9. Burnside IM: *Nursing and the aged*, ed 3, New York, 1988, Mosby–Year Book.
10. Burnside IM: *Working with the elderly: group process and techniques*, ed 2, Monterey, Calif, 1987, Wadsworth.
11. Butler RN, Lewis MI: *Aging and mental health*, ed 3, St Louis, 1982, Mosby–Year Book.
12. Clunn, P: *Psychiatric–mental health nursing*, New York, 1985, Medical Examination Publishing, 1986.
13. Copstead LE: *Normal neurological changes of aging* (videotape), Philadelphia, 1988, JB Lippincott.
14. Cummings E, Henry WE: *Growing old*, New York, 1961, Basic Books.
15. Davis AJ, Kalkman ME: *New dimensions in mental health–psychiatric nursing*, ed 5, New York, 1980, McGraw-Hill.
16. Davison GC, Neale JM: *Abnormal psychology: an experimental clinical approach*, New York, 1982, John Wiley & Sons.
17. Dawson P, Reid DW: Behavioral dimensions of patients at risk for wandering, *Gerontologist* 27(1):104, 1987.
18. Donahue E: Reality orientation: a review of the literature. In Burnside I, editor: *Working with the elderly*, Monterey, Calif, 1984, Wadsworth.
19. Draper B: The effectiveness of services and treatment in psychgeriatrics, *Australian and New Zealand Journal of Psychiatry* 24:2, 1990.
20. Duke University Center for the Study of Aging and Human Development: Duke University Medical Center, Durham, NC, 1975.
21. Ebersole R, Hess R: *Toward healthy aging: human needs and nursing response*, ed 3, St Louis, 1990, Mosby–Year Book.
22. Eisdorfer C: Conceptual models of aging: the challenge of a new frontier, *American Psychologist* 38:197, 1983.
23. Eilers ML: Older adults and computer education: "not to have the world a closed door," *International Journal of Technology and Aging* 2(1):56, 1989.
24. Emery CF, Blumenthal JA: Perceived change among participants in an exercise program for older adults, *Gerontologist* 30:4, 1990.
25. Erikson EH: *Childhood and society*, ed 2, New York, 1964, WW Norton & Co.
26. Feil N: *Validation: the Feil method*, Cleveland, Ohio, 1982, Edward Feil Productions.
27. Feinberg I: Functional implications of changes in sleep physiology with age. In Terry RD, Gershon S, editors: *Neurobiology of aging*, New York, 1976, Raven Press.
28. Frolkis VV: Physiological aspects of aging. In von Hahn HP, editor: *Practical geriatrics*, Basel, Switzerland, 1975, S Karger, AG.
29. Hagebak JE, Hagebak BR: Serving the mental health needs of the elderly: the case for removing barriers and improving service integration, *Community Mental Health Journal* 16:4, 1980.
30. Havighurst RJ: Successful aging. In Williams RH, Tibbits C, Donahue W, editors: *Processes of aging*, vol 1, New York, 1963, Atherton Press.
31. Heacock P and others: Caring for cognitively impaired older people: reconceptualizing disability and rehabilitation, *Journal of Gerontological Nursing* 17:3, 1991.
32. Kales JD: Aging and sleep. In Goldman R, Rockstein K, editors: *The physiology and pathology of human aging*, New York, 1977, Academic Press.
33. Kenny RA: *Physiology of aging: a synopsis*, ed 2, St Louis, 1989, Mosby–Year Book.
34. Kermis MD: *Mental health in late life*, Boston, 1986, Jones & Bartlett Publishers.

35. Kermis MD: *The psychology of human aging: theory, research and practices,* Newton, Mass, 1984, Allyn & Bacon.

36. Koenig HG, George LK, Siegler IS: The use of religion and emotion-regulating coping strategies among older adults, *Gerontologist* 28:3, 1988.

37. Koenig HG, Kvale JN, Ferrel C: Religion and well-being in later life, *Gerontologist* 28:1, 1988.

38. Lewis C: Facilitating a better reality: a treatment approach for the confused and disoriented. In Horton AM, editor: *Mental health interventions for the aged,* New York, 1982, Praeger Publishers.

39. Matsuyama SS, Jarvik LR: Genetics and mental functioning in senescence. In Birren JE, Sloane RB, editors: *Handbook of mental health and aging,* Englewood Cliffs, NJ, 1980, Prentice-Hall.

40. Meyers BS, Alexopoulos GS: Geriatric depression, *Medical Clinics of North America* 72:4, 1988.

41. Morgan WP: Affective beneficence of vigorous activity, *Medicine and Science in Sports and Excercise* 17(1):94, 1985.

42. Morganett BA: Nature hikes for nursing home residents, *Geriatric Nursing (Lond)* 8:4, 1987.

43. Murphy E: The prognosis of depression in old age, *British Journal of Psychiatry* 142:111, 1983.

44. Murray R, Huelskoetter M, O'Driscoll D: *The nursing process in later maturity,* Englewood Cliffs, NJ, 1980, Prentice-Hall.

45. Neugarten BL: *Personality in middle and late life,* New York, 1964, Atherton Press.

46. Norton K: *Geriatric nursing,* St Louis, 1950, Mosby–Year Book.

47. Paloutzian RF, Ellison CW: Loneliness, spiritual well-being and the quality of life. In Peplau LA, Perlman D, editors: *Loneliness: a sourcebook of current theory, research and therapy,* New York, 1982, John Wiley & Sons.

48. Peck R: Psychological developments in the second half of life. In Neugarten B, editor: *Middle age and aging,* Chicago, 1968, The University of Chicago Press.

49. Peplau LA, Micelli M, Morasch B: Loneliness and self-evaluation. In Peplau LA, Perlman D, editors: *Loneliness: a sourcebook of current theory, research and therapy,* New York, 1982, John Wiley & Sons.

50. Richardson R, Lowenstein S, Weissberg M: Coping with the suicidal elderly: a physician's guide, *Geriatrics* 44(9):43, 1989.

51. Rodin J, Langer E: Aging labels: the decline of control and the fall of self-esteem, *Journal of Social Issues* 36(2):12, 1980.

52. Rose JB: Age barriers fall: a high school creative writing class for two kinds of seniors, *Aging* 352:10, 1986.

53. Roybal ER: Federal involvement in mental health care for the aged, *American Psychologist* 39:163, 1984.

54. Schelsbusch L, Wessels W: Hopelessness and low-intent in parasuicide, *General Hospital Psychiatry* 10:209, 1988.

55. Schuster CS, Ashburn SS, editors: *The process of human development,* Boston, 1986, Little, Brown & Co.

56. Sheppard S: Learning as a life long high, *Aging* 352:20, 1986.

57. Simon JM: The therapeutic value of humor in aging adults, *Journal of Gerontological Nursing* 14:8, 1988.

58. Slimmer LW and others: Perceptions of learned helplessness, *Journal of Gerontological Nursing* 13:5, 1988.

59. Spence DL: The meaning of engagement, *International Journal of Aging and Human Development* 6:193, 1975.

60. Stevenson JS, Topp R: Effects of moderate and low intensity long-term exercise by older adults, *Research Nursing and Health* 13:4, 1990.

61. Sullivan JL, Deane DM: Humor and health, *Journal of Gerontological Nursing* 14:1, 1988.

62. Thomasma DC: Freedom, dependency and the care of the very old, *Journal of the American Geriatrics Society* 32:906, 1984.

63. U.S. National Center for Health Statistics: The national nursing home survey—1977 Summary for the United States, Hyattsville, Md, U.S. Department of Health, Education, and Welfare, PHS, 1979.

64. Wolpert EA: Manic-depressive illness as an actual neurosis. In Anthony EJ, Benedek T, editors: *Depression and human existence,* Boston, 1975, Little, Brown & Co.

65. Woodruff DS, Birren JE, editors: *Aging: scientific perspective and social issues,* Monterey, Calif, 1983, Brooks/Cole.

66. Yesavage JA: Imagery pretraining and memory training in the elderly, *Gerontology* 29:271, 1983.

67. Zorumski CF, Rubin EH, Burke WJ: Electroconvulsive therapy for the elderly: a review, *Hospital and Community Psychiatry* 39:6, 1988.

68. Zung W: A self-rating depression scale, *Archives of General Psychiatry* 12:63, 1965.

ANNOTATED BIBLIOGRAPHY

Burbank PM: Psychosocial theories of aging: a critical evaluation, *Advances in Nursing Science* 9:73, 1986.

This article presents a summary and evaluation of the three major theories of aging: activity theory, disengagement theory, and continuity theory. Some important problems are identified with each theory.

Burnside IM, editor: *Working with the elderly: group process and techniques,* North Scituate, Mass, 1987, Duxbury Press.

A useful guide for learning to work with groups of elderly persons. The text presents a brief history of group work with the elderly and an overview of a variety of types and levels of the group process. Theoretical concepts are adapted for group work with the elderly, and many practical suggestions are given. The book includes a discussion of curriculum changes needed to prepare professionals for group work with the elderly.

Busse EW, Blazer DS, editors: *Geriatric psychiatry,* Washington, DC, 1989, American Psychiatric Press.

This text presents valuable information about the scientific base of aging and geriatrics. It addresses the knowledge and skills that are necessary for the professional to care effectively for clients with the disorders of late life.

Ebersole P: *Caring for the psychogeriatric client,* New York, 1989, Springer.

This textbook emphasizes management strategies that are effective with aged persons with a variety of emotional and behavioral problems. The book includes most of the common issues that must be understood to provide humanistic and holistic care to the aged. The major focus is long-term care. One chapter is devoted to geropsychiatric disorders requiring short-term hospitalization.

PART V

Issues and Trends

The practice of mental health–psychiatric nursing, while having its foundation in the one-to-one therapeutic relationship, occurs within the context of a social structure in which legal, ethical, and professional issues exert a significant influence on the care provided. Informed deliberation on these issues is a dynamic, ongoing process essential to the accountable, caring practice of mental health–psychiatric nursing.

The nurse is continually faced with situations in which value judgments are made, thus necessitating the clarification, reaffirmation, or reexamination of values. Chapter 41 presents major ethical orientations and discusses ethical issues in mental health–psychiatric nursing over the life cycle.

In Chapter 42 an overview of the legal system is presented as a background for understanding the federal and state laws of concern to mental health–psychiatric nursing practice. Malpractice, assault and battery, false imprisonment, confidentiality, commitment, and consent are explicated, and the nurse's role in influencing changes in the law is discussed. Content on patient classification systems is presented.

As the body of knowledge that provides a basis for the professional practice of mental health–psychiatric nursing is expanded through research, the quality of client care is enhanced. In Chapter 43 the development of research in mental health–psychiatric nursing is discussed and major research studies are highlighted. The measurement of behavior is described, and particular measurement, ethical, and legal considerations in mental health–psychiatric nursing research are examined.

Society has a right to expect a reasonable degree of excellence in the provision of mental health–psychiatric nursing care. Chapter 44 presents the approaches that have been developed for ensuring a standard of care. Protocols, peer review, and auditing are discussed as mechanisms for implementing the ANA's Standards of Nursing Care in Psychiatric–Mental Health Nursing. Professional development, credentialing, and third-party payments are examined within the context of mental health–psychiatric nursing practice.

Finally, psychiatric consultation liaison nursing is discussed in Chapter 45. Types of consultation-liaison are explained, and qualifications for the role of psychiatric consultation-liaison nurses are presented. A conceptual model that describes the processes of consultation and liaison and an integration of the two processes is examined. Practice issues related to psychiatric consultation liaison nursing are addressed.

Elsie L Bandman
Bertram Bandman

After studying this chapter, the student will be able to:

- Discuss the origin and development of moral issues in the treatment of the mentally ill
- Examine ethical issues in mental health–psychiatric nursing from a historical perspective
- Analyze each of the ethical views presented in relation to client problems encountered in mental health–psychiatric nursing

- Identify the major ethical issues in mental health–psychiatric nursing of the infant, the child, the adolescent, and the adult
- Analyze the ethical principles relevant to individual, group, and family therapy
- Apply logical principles to the examination of ethically justifiable norms in mental health–psychiatric nursing

The value placed on the care of the mentally disabled is a measure of the ethical sensitivity of a society. The worth placed on the mentally ill as human beings by religious, educational, social, and health care institutions of society determines whether they are to be treated as persons in need of help, punished as objects possessed, or simply rejected and ignored.

Current psychiatric nursing emphasizes the role of the nurse as a therapeutic agent. Such responsibility inevitably raises moral questions. Psychiatric nurses are faced with choices regarding the continuation of medication or electroconvulsive therapy when the client refuses. Conversely, some clients demand medications or treatment that nurses regard as unnecessary. Nurses are confronted by involuntarily admitted clients who refuse recommended individual, group, or family therapy. Such situations raise dilemmas regarding the client's right to respect and to receive and to refuse treatment versus the client's best interests.

The moral issues that affect mental health–psychiatric nursing often conflict. This makes ethics seem complicated and multifaceted, appearing as a science, sometimes as an art, sometimes as a religion, and at other times as a game or business. Whatever ethical orientations the nurse chooses as the "right" ones and no matter how hard the struggle to avoid imposition of the nurse's values on clients, the selection of therapeutic interventions is laden with moral choices. The selection of one intervention over another supports or opposes a particular moral framework that emphasizes rights, justice, duty, goals, love, power, or

self-interest. Thus the nurse is inescapably a moral agent in relation to clients, her own good, and the good of society.

VALUE CLARIFICATION

To act ethically, people must identify their notions of right and wrong. Value clarification is a three-stage process for making a person's preferences and priorities explicit. It begins with a choice of a value from among alternatives, then moves to a prizing of that value, and finally to a decision to act on that value.[19] In the first stage, one sifts through one's preferences and ranks them; in the second stage, one reflects on which of the chosen values are worthwhile; and in the third stage, one maps a strategy of action to achieve the values one has chosen and prized on reflection (Figure 41-1).

Expression of an individual's preferences does not imply that these preferences are justifiable or should be preferred. No matter how much a person reflects on his choice of values, the value that he prizes may not be morally justifiable to other persons and groups. Value clarification is an initial stage in value deliberation and must be followed by moral justification. This further development involves the study of ethics.

ETHICAL ORIENTATIONS

Ethical issues arise whenever there is a possibility of good or harm. Almost anything one does in the practice of

DATES	EVENTS
500 BC	The Greeks and Romans subjected mentally ill persons to cruel and inhumane treatment. A few ancient societies, however, treated mentally ill persons as prophets who possessed insight and vision.
500 AD	For Europeans, treatments such as hydrotherapy, music, gymnastics, rocking, and massage were available mainly for the rich with acute disorders. Chronically ill patients were thought to be incurable.
1200s	Care of the sick was considered a religious duty.
1200s-1500s	There was a vigorous rebirth of interest in human personality, values, and affairs. Books on depression, mother-child relationships, and the mentally retarded were published.
1500s	At the time of the Reformation and the Inquisition, mentally ill persons were persecuted as witches and allies of the devil.
1600s	Moral treatment of mentally ill persons included respect, individualized care, privacy, confidentiality, and forms of occupational therapy, drama, and psychotherapy based on commitment to a rational, scientific approach and rejection of supernatural causation.
1700s-1800s	Benjamin Rush introduced moral treatment and scientific investigation of mentally disabled individuals in the United States in 1783. Dorothea Dix reformed the brutal care and neglect of mentally ill persons and created or expanded hospital facilities in America, Canada, and Europe.
1884	The American Psychiatric Association advocated humanization of treatment of mentally ill individuals through specialized care for alcoholic, acute, and chronic patients; family care; and legislative reform.
1908	The National Committee for Mental Health was organized to make issues of mental health and care of mentally ill persons a matter of national concern.
1980s-1990s	The role of the psychiatric nurse as client advocate is developed.
Future	The mental health–psychiatric nurse will become increasingly involved in ethical issues affecting clients.

nursing may cause good or harm. The difficult aspect of ethics concerns how one defines good or harm. What is the good? How can one be sure that it is really the best choice? Another difficulty lies in deciding whose good or which good is given priority. Good for whom? And what about the other people affected by the decision? Several major ethical orientations are presented in the following discussion along with several major moral positions. These positions provide reasoned answers without definitive conclusions to major ethical controversies in mental health–psychiatric nursing.

Paternalism Versus Libertarianism

A major ethical orientation that affects the treatment of psychiatric clients is paternalism versus libertarianism. Paternalism holds that the state, or, literally, "one's father," knows best and that each individual is subordinate and duty bound to comply with the authority figure, be it a parent, physician, nurse, or hospital, who is said to know best. The antithesis of paternalism is libertarianism, which holds that the individual is sovereign and may choose without interference as long as the individual does not harm others. For example, a 24-year-old psychiatric client is seriously disturbed and suspicious but is no danger to others. She can

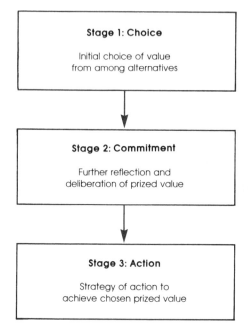

FIGURE 41-1 Value clarification process. *(Modified from Steele SM, Harmon VM: Values clarification in nursing, New York, 1979, Appleton-Century-Crofts.)*

improve if given drug "X," which has a side effect of undesirable automatic movements, but she values her appearance more than improving her mental state. If the client refuses drug "X," but the nurse knows that this drug will restore the client's rationality by reducing paranoid thoughts, the nurse is justified in giving the drug to the client on paternalist grounds of doing what is in the client's best interest. On libertarian grounds, however, the client has the right to refuse to take drug "X" based on a fully informed choice.

Egoism Versus Altruism

A second moral orientation that affects mental health–psychiatric nursing is that of egoism versus altruism. Egoism holds that one thinks and acts in one's own interest.

A difficulty with egoism is its denial of the fact that people generally live together, work together, and need one another. Therefore they need to control one another's behavior by avoiding harm and giving help. For every person to act without considering others is inappropriate when the sensitivities and welfare of others are involved.

Some difficulties with egoism and paternalism lead to another moral-based view, sometimes identified as altruism, or love-based ethics. Most notable in this regard is the ethics or Christianity, which holds that one should love God and love one's neighbor as oneself. Love-based ethics also means teaching disturbed clients the importance of developing love, care, affection, and consideration for the needs of others.

One difficulty with a love-based view of ethics is that "love" is ambiguous. It may refer to child-parent relationships, romantic or sexual relationships, or an ideal, such as "brotherhood" or "sisterhood" between people. Second, people sometimes discriminate unfairly, singling out some to be loved while rejecting or ignoring others. A third difficulty of a love-based ethics is that it is difficult for any one to show or to give love to more than a small number of persons on a continuing basis. Despite these difficulties, love is an antidote to selfishness.

Majority Rule Versus Absolute Principles

Mill, chief advocate of the greatest happiness for the greatest number principle, or majority rule (also known as *utilitarianism*), held that "actions are right in proportion as they tend to promote happiness, wrong as they tend to produce the reverse of happiness."[14]

In contrast, Kant,[11] a major proponent of principled morality, believed that an act is good if everyone ought, in similar circumstances, to do the same act without exception. This is known as the *universalizability principle*. In practice, the universalizability principle means that no one may commit suicide and that everyone must tell the truth, help others, keep every promise, and develop his or her own talents.

A close philosophical cousin to Mill's utilitarianism is the *doctrine of double effect*. This doctrine holds that a lesser good or even harm is morally permissible if done to achieve a greater good, provided that certain conditions are fulfilled. One condition is that the harmful side effect is not intended directly. Violating the psychiatric client's confidentiality by warning the police of the client's intent to kill a particular person is a lesser wrong if it prevents the greater wrong of murder. Critics of double effect, however, say that the harm done has nothing to do with the intended good. In different terms, the end does not justify the means.

Acts of utilitarianism and double effect are sometimes viewed as unprincipled expediency and a mockery of morality. Defenders of utilitarianism and double effect counter that ethics, being practical, is contaminated by the conditions in the real world. For example, if a drug stabilizes a seriously disturbed person but has side effects, administering the drug is justified on double effect grounds because of the good it does for the client.

A strength of Kantian ethics is that it reminds persons of ideals and principles that should govern human conduct. Telling the truth, for example, is a vital obligation in treating psychiatric clients. By comparison, a strength of utilitarian ethics is that it often minimizes disaster and harm and maximizes benefits to the majority, such as giving behavior-controlling drugs to disturbed clients. A difficulty of utilitarian ethics, however, is that appeal to the majority may overload minorities, such as mentally afflicted persons in need of long-term help. The needs of mentally afflicted persons may require taxes that the majority opposes. In psychiatric client care, the scarcity of personnel, facilities, or resources allocated to their care may be used to rationalize custodial or inadequate treatment of clients.

Omissions Versus Commissions

A fourth moral orientation is whether omissions are equivalent to commissions. In psychiatric nursing terms, the issue is whether failing to treat a client, such as a homeless mentally ill person, is morally equivalent to providing merely custodial care.

The philosophical justification for rating omissions with commissions comes from existentialism. This ethical model holds that one exists by taking responsibility for all decisions in all aspects of one's life in which one has a conscious, reflective process at work. For example, a person who recognizes the plight of a psychiatric client is responsible for correcting that client's plight insofar as possible. To fail to correct an evil is to show "bad faith" and is as bad as doing evil. Watching another person being abused without intervening is as bad as being the abuser. To evade decisions is to make decisions that support the existing situation.

A strength of existentialism is its emphasis on honest and responsible human relationships. A difficulty of existentialism is the practical impossibility of being responsible for all the world's difficulties.

Absolute Rights Versus Prima Facie Rights

A fifth moral orientation concerns the view that rights based on justice are absolute versus the view that rights can be overridden, since they are rights on the surface or face, that is, *prima facie* rights.

Three conditions accompany any right. To have a right is to be free to exercise it or not as one chooses. Second, to have rights implies that others have corresponding duties to comply with the terms and provisions of one's rights.

Third, to have rights means that one's rights are consistent with rationally defensible principles of justice. Rights then imply freedom, duties or responsibilities, and justice. In the absolute view of rights the contention is that individual rights to property or to refuse treatment can never be overridden by any other moral considerations. In contrast, treating rights as prima facie means that rights may be overridden by stronger conflicting rights or by other values. For example, a psychiatric client's right to the freedom of the nursing unit may be overridden by seclusion or restraints if the client physically abuses others.

A strength of the prima facie view is that an individual's absolute right may be overridden in favor of the rights of others or the person's own best interests. In the prima facie view the rights of a larger number of persons morally outweigh the rights of a small number when the rights of the two groups conflict. Another strength of the prima facie view is its practical advantage in coping with conflicts of rights and in suggesting priorities among rights, to avoid arbitrariness, for example. A difficulty, however, is that prima facie rights may be treated as weaker than rights need to be; rights are then too easily overturned by every pressure that comes along. Rights without built-in constraints against their erosion are not worth the respect accorded them as rights. On the other hand, rights written in stone, without possibility of change, are too brittle to withstand the rigors of practical moral life. The ideal is to have rights that are well entrenched, sturdy, and well respected, but open to reasoned modifications. At any rate, the differences between these two views of rights are a matter of degree, but both views hold that rights are important to moral discourse.

Human rights are generally regarded as the union of self-determination and subsistence rights, or the right to be helped when one is in need. The limits and extent of such rights are frequently debated. One issue is that some subsistence rights impose intolerable burdens on those expected to provide for such rights. For example, giving all psychiatric clients optimal psychiatric care, including prolonged psychoanalysis, is regarded by opponents of subsistence rights as too expensive. In relation to other urgent social goals, such as education or care of elderly persons, this means of reducing mental illness consumes an inordinate amount of available resources.

A summary of the models of ethics, their characteristics, leading figures, advantages, and drawbacks is presented in Table 41-1.

A Trilogy of Clients' Moral Rights

Despite the controversies over the meaning, limits, and significance of rights, three important moral rights of psychiatric clients emerge: (1) the right to respect, (2) the right to receive treatment, and (3) the right to refuse treatment. Each of these rights has an impact on nurse-client relations and issues of care.

The right to respect includes the right to dignity and regard for a psychiatric client as a potentially rational person. The client is not seen as a means or instrument of someone else's will. The right to respect also implies the right to privacy, confidentiality, and informed consent.

The right to receive treatment includes the client's right to know the diagnosis, proposed treatment, procedures and processes, and expected results.

The remaining right in this trilogy of health care rights is the client's right to terminate or refuse treatment at any time. If after a true and adequate explanation, including a statement of consequences, the client believes that the proposed treatment is either too risky, burdensome, or painful to bear, or, if the competent client simply wishes to discontinue treatment, he has the right to do so.

Macklin[12] cites three reasons clients give for refusing treatment: (1) the client perceives inhumane conditions; (2) drugs or treatments have undesirable side effects; and (3) the client's consenting organ, the mind, is affected. A ground for overriding a psychiatric client's right to refuse treatment is that treatment would increase the client's rational powers and autonomy. In Macklin's view, only for the third reason may a client's right to refuse be overridden.

There are several views on whether to override a mental client's right to refuse treatment. Table 41-2 summarizes the views held by a libertarian, a paternalist, a utilitarian, and a rational paternalist.

Competence and the Rights of Psychiatric Clients

The judgment that a person is competent gives reason to trust that the person will avoid doing harm. This judgment is a basis for awarding or denying a person's right to decide. The concept of competence is ambiguous. The scenes presented in Table 41-3 help clarify the concept.[7]

These scenes and moral-philosophical positions show that no position seems appropriate for all cases. Libertarian values are what psychiatric clients' rights are largely about. But to restore clients' rationality, paternalism or rational paternalism requiring treatment may be appropriate. In other cases, utilitarian values of the greatest good to the greatest number are required.

ETHICAL ISSUES THROUGHOUT THE LIFE CYCLE
Infancy and Childhood

The mental health–psychiatric nurse who counsels prospective parents must consider several moral issues. Couples with a family history of mental illness fear the genetic transmission of schizophrenia or major affective disorders. The nurse is able to inform these couples that the nature versus nurture controversy is unresolved. Only a few genetic defects out of a vast number of possibilities can be identified. The nurse counselor can clearly recommend genetic screening to identify such diseases as Tay-Sachs, sickle cell anemia, and hemophilia. The nurse can also recommend amniocentesis as a test for Down syndrome with the choice of aborting the pregnancy. However, only as the scientific evidence regarding genetic vulnerability to mental illness develops can the nurse definitively answer questions about the inheritance of mental illness. Until then, nurses must clearly identify their moral positions regarding sterilization, contraceptives, or abortion for a mentally disabled person. The mentally ill or defective person greatly needs information, education, counseling, and concrete help in avoiding an unwanted pregnancy. If pregnant, the client needs prenatal care, delivery support, and help for

▼ **TABLE 41-1   Models of Ethics**

Model	Characteristics	Leading Figures	Advantages	Drawbacks
Paternalism	"Father knows best"; emphasis on single authority figure as sole decision maker; in nursing and health care, "captain of the ship" doctrine	Plato Hobbes Lord Patrick Devlin	One authority figure, unity; line and staff authority; appropriate if one person knows better than others what to do, for example, some physicians and psychiatrists	Denies pluralism, variety, democracy, shared decision making, and distribution of rights, responsibilities, and powers; inappropriate if person in charge is less competent than subordinate co-workers
Libertarianism	Premium placed on individual liberty; unjustified interference is morally impermissible; taxation is used solely to minimize "force and fraud"; other forms of taxation for social and economic causes constitute "forced labor"	JS Mill R Nozick R Sade M Friedman	Liberty is a cherished value and is related to individual initiative, achievement of merit (sometimes identified as meritocracy), and individual independence, principle of informed consent respects individual liberty	Undue attention to good aspects of individual liberty and not enough regard paid to social and communal responsibilities such as public education, hospitals, and sanitation
Utilitarianism	Greatest happiness for greatest number, emphasis on consequences of acts aimed at maximizing pleasure and minimizing pain; provides basis for calculation of cost/benefit/risk ratio	JS Mill J Bentham	Pleasure and desire for happiness come easily to people; one can appeal to people to seek happiness; concerned with acts and consequences, leading to prudence and care to achieve one's desired results (for example, avoidance of sexually transmitted diseases); also based on cost/benefit/risk ratio; considers majority interests	Ignores minorities; fails to give attention to nonnegotiable values such as justice, truth telling, doing good for its own sake, and avoiding evil for the same reason, if necessary (for example, not torturing or killing even though these may pay off)
Kantian ethics	Emphasis on moral character, good will, intentions, obligations rather than inclination, interests, or desires; emphasis on principled action no matter what the personal consequences; acts are moral only if universal, result of free will, rational, impartial, and exceptionless	I Kant J Rawls	Values such as promising, helping the needy, truth telling, and being just are uncompromising (for example, slavery is absolutely wrong and is never made right by consequences); torture, murder, lying, and injustice are always wrong	Fails to consider aspirations, interests, drives, motivations, consequences, and contexts that call for adaptation of principles; inflexible
Existentialism	Conscious human beings have a free will and are therefore responsible for their acts; human acts include commissions and omissions (This issue arises if one considers whether not doing is morally equivalent to doing; for example, is failure to treat tantamount to murder?); according to theory, one is as responsible for not acting as for acting; according to Descartes, a forerunner of existentialism, one is responsible for what one is con-	S Kierkegaard J-P Sartre	Increases responsibility for omissions, negligence, unconcern (for example, Kitty Genovese murdered in a New York apartment with 37 neighbors looking on and doing nothing; the 37 onlookers are regarded as being as evil as the murderer)	To identify omissions with commissions places undue burden of responsibility on people's shoulders; we cannot, as a practical matter, be held responsible for all the starvation and suffering in the world

TABLE 41-1 Models of Ethics—cont'd

Model	Characteristics	Leading Figures	Advantages	Drawbacks
Existential-ism—cont'd	scious about; to know, for example, that a client needs help and to do nothing is as serious as harming that client (that is, passive euthanasia is the same as active euthanasia)			
Absolute rights versus prima facie rights	Absolute rights stress exceptionless rights and their application to all contexts; prima facie rights refer to rights that are assumed until further notice, and these may be overridden if more morally compelling interests arise	J Feinberg J Rawls R Dworkin RB Brandt	Absolute rights: the people of a society know that some values in the form of rights have priority over all other values; prima facie rights: flexible, practical	Absolute rights too stringent; prima facie rights treated as interests that may be overridden by more powerful interests; rights are not steadfast or assured values

planning what to do with the baby. The nurse uses the nursing process and the moral principles of striving to do good and to do no harm.

Other examples of ethical problems threatening the mental health of the family are the birth of a baby with Down syndrome or serious deformities. Technology can save many infants, and the decision to treat or not to treat is not always considered. Parents need time to evaluate the facts and advice to make their own decision. The decision is not the pediatrician's, neonatologist's or the obstetrician's. It is an ethical decision with which the couple lives for the rest of their lives; they must give serious consideration to their own resources and to the rights of the infant.

Moral questions arise about how far a family must go in subordinating its energies, goals, and resources to the care of the abnormal child. Choices are between the sanctity of

TABLE 41-2 Ethical Positions Toward a Psychiatric Client's Right to Refuse Treatment

Position	Attitude
Libertarian	The client may refuse any treatment if he does not harm others.
Paternalist	The mental health–psychiatric nurse (acting on behalf of the state) may override a client's rights for the good of the client.
Utilitarian	The mental health–psychiatric nurse (acting on behalf of the state) may override the client's rights if doing so serves the greatest happiness of the greatest number.
Rational paternalist	The client's right may be overridden if the client would later, retrospectively, regard such an action as being in his rational interest, in contributing to his autonomy as a person.

life and the rights of the parents and siblings to a full life without the lifelong expense and anguish of caring for the handicapped child. In all cases any contemplated treatment must be carefully explained in nontechnical language so that the parents understand exactly the prognosis, risks, and alternatives, especially when impairment and dependence will be lifelong. The nurse who is aware of the ethical orientations previously discussed can assist the parents by explaining the moral basis of the choices.

Adolescence

Increasingly, adolescents seek health care such as counseling, contraceptives, or abortion on a confidential basis without parental knowledge. The age of 18 is now the age of majority in all states, but adolescents who are minors may be provided health care without parental consent in the following situations: in emergencies; when abortion services are required (in litigation in some states); when parental abuse or neglect threatens the adolescent; when treatment of venereal disease is needed; when detection of pregnancy is requested; when the adolescent is married, a parent, divorced, or self-supporting and living away from her parents (emancipated minors); and when the adolescent is age 16 and older and requesting admission to a psychiatric hospital for treatment.[21] Persons who fall into these categories have not only the right to respect and the right to receive treatment but also the right to refuse treatment. This means that adolescents' rights to self-determination entitle them to receive a full explanation of the risks and benefits of the proposed treatment, the diagnosis, prognosis, and the alternatives as the basis for informed consent, as does any adult. However, there are limits to the rights of even emancipated adolescents, such as the right to be sterilized, to donate an organ, and to receive electroconvulsive therapy. Parental consent, a court order, or both are required for these procedures. When parents disagree over health services provided or refuse lifesaving treatment for their dependent adolescent, the health care facility usu-

▼ **TABLE 41-3   Five Scenes Showing How "Competence" Gives a Reason for Overriding a Psychiatric Client's Right to Receive or Refuse Treatment**

Scene	Conflict	Conclusion
Dr. Doe: "I cannot prescribe drug "X" for you because it will do you physical harm." **Mr. Roe:** "But you are mistaken. It will not cause me physical harm."	Dr. Doe and Mr. Roe disagree factually about drug "X."	Mr. Roe is factually incompetent (the layperson is presumed wrong when disagreeing with a physician).
Dr. Doe: "I cannot prescribe drug "X" to you because it will cause you physical harm." **Mr. Roe:** "That's just what I want. I want to harm myself."	Dr. Doe and Mr. Roe disagree whether drug "X," which harms Mr. Roe, is good.	Mr. Roe is incompetent (it is presumed that Mr. Roe's values in wanting to harm himself are irrational).
Dr. Doe: "I cannot prescribe drug "X" to you because it is likely to do you physical harm." **Mr. Roe:** "I don't care if it causes me physical harm. I'll get a lot of pleasure first, so much pleasure, in fact, that it is well worth running the risk of physical harm. If I must pay a price for my pleasure, I am willing to do so."	Dr. Doe and Mr. Roe disagree that drug "X," which harms Mr. Roe, causes enough pleasure to justify drug "X" despite its harm.	Mr. Roe is competent (moral stalemate between Dr. Doe and Mr. Roe).
Dr. Doe: "You need a blood transfusion to stay alive." **Mr. Roe:** "A blood transfusion is against my religious principles as a Jehovah's Witness. I'd rather die first."	Dr. Doe and Mr. Roe disagree that a blood transfusion will serve Mr. Roe's ultimate good.	Mr. Roe is competent (moral, religious conflict values between Dr. Doe and Mr. Roe).
Dr. Doe: "I cannot release you because of your continuing insistence that you are the historical Napoleon and the savior of France." **Mr. Roe:** "I refuse to stay in your institution precisely because I am the historical Napoleon, and I am urgently needed in the immediate liberation of France."	Dr. Doe and Mr. Roe disagree on Mr. Roe's identity, with Mr. Roe believing himself to be the historical Napoleon.	Mr. Roe is incompetent (no stalemate exists, since there is a factual basis for going against Mr. Roe's claim).

ally seeks a court order appointing a guardian to protect the best interests of the minor or adolescent.

The adolescent's right to psychiatric treatment has not received the same degree of support from the courts, from family, and from public opinion as has the adolescent's right to medical care for physical illness. Parents may deny an adolescent's right to psychiatric treatment on the grounds of shame, guilt, or threat to their status as "good parents." Where public community mental health facilities are available, the adolescent's right to treatment and to moral self-determination is respected. In recent years no psychiatrist, physician, or surgeon has been found liable by the courts for the proper treatment of minors 15 years of age and older without parental consent.[10] Most states now permit minors to consent to medical treatment without specifying psychotherapy. Seemingly, this immunity from parental interference includes standard forms of psychotherapy given by recognized professionals. However, the right of the adolescent to receive nontraditional or bizarre forms of treatment, such as those emphasizing sexual expression, presents moral dilemmas to even those parents most supportive of adolescents' rights to self-determination. The parents' right to care for their children in ways they consider beneficial may in this case conflict with the adolescent's right to receive treatment. Parents sometimes resolve this di-

lemma by appeal to the adolescent on grounds of love or utilitarian ethics, since resorting to paternalism usually harms the relationship between parent and child. The ultimate parental appeal is based on their overriding concern for the adolescent's best interests. A lawsuit by the parents charging that the nontraditional treatment contributes to the delinquency of a minor may be the last resort and may irreparably damage the parent-child relationship.

The adolescent's right to refuse treatment is complicated by the adolescent's struggle toward individual values. If these are radically different from those of the parents, the parents may require psychiatric care for what they consider abnormal behavior. The adolescent's refusal of psychiatric treatment undertaken on grounds of parental objection to long hair, sexual activity, use of marijuana, and failure to attend church, for example, is justified by the adolescent's right to his own values. The parents can impose curfews, or limit allowances and use of the family car to curb behavior, but forcing an adolescent to participate in treatment is difficult and antitherapeutic. Such force violates the individual's right to self-determination.

It is difficult to support the adolescent's unqualified right to refuse treatment when confronted with an adolescent's suicidal or homicidal tendencies. Yet, as the commitment of "normally" rebellious minors to mental hospitals by parents demonstrates, parents do not always have the best interests of the child at heart. The adolescent so treated has the right to refuse treatment and to receive available help and protection in exercising due process rights. The same rigorous standards for commitment that apply to adults—danger to self and others—apply to adolescents. An adolescent's rights and an adult's rights differ in degree, however. An adolescent's autonomy cannot be as extensive as an adult's because of the general dependence, inexperience, and needs of an adolescent.

Instances in which adolescents leave home and family to join religious groups that control all aspects of the young person's life cause genuine dilemmas. In such groups, the adolescent is conditioned into total obedience to the community and is regarded as communal property. Desperate parents have abducted adolescents from such groups and placed them in psychiatric care involuntarily. Some adolescents in this situation have refused psychiatric intervention and returned to the religious community. Others were relieved at the actions of their parents and participated in therapy. The moral dilemma is whether the adolescent is able to make a rational decision to refuse treatment or is responding in terms of the behavior control by the group.

In most cases involving adolescents, the dilemma is between the adolescent's right of self-determination and parental duty to respect the young life by preserving it in whatever ways are possible and necessary. Clearly, the facts and ethical issues of the situation require careful evaluation by parents, mental health–psychiatric nurses, and others involved in providing care. In this way, a decision is the result of careful assessment and deliberation justified on the moral principles deemed most appropriate to save the young life. Appeals to love, principles, or utilitarian ethics may be included in the decision by parents, nurses, and other health professionals who respond to the adolescent's difficulties.

Adulthood

Not all adults can achieve developmental tasks of independence and ego-enhancing interdependence. Persons with psychiatric problems sometimes behave and dress in ways that are odd, distasteful, disgusting, or unacceptable to the public. A fundamental ethical issue for the community becomes the extent to which it tolerates deviant behavior. One example is whether harmless "bagladies" carrying their belongings in shopping bags, dressed in layers of long-worn, shabby clothing, and sometimes smelling of urine should be allowed to roam the subways, train stations, and streets of cities. One view is that such persons are to be regarded as mentally ill and placed in public institutions involuntarily. Another view is that they are vagrants and deserve prison. Still another view is that they be placed as mandatory residents in community facilities. Vagrants, beggars, alcoholics, and delusional and hallucinating persons in the streets are individuals whose behavior poses a problem mainly to themselves. The issue concerns individual liberties versus the offense given to the general public. One libertarian argument is that, since the offensive behavior falls short of actually harming anyone else, interference is unjustified. The counter-argument by legal paternalists is that these persons set a negative example by demeaning

themselves and disrespecting others. To allow them to continue is to sanction their behavior.

Ethical dilemmas arise concerning the right to end one's life. The value that all life is sacred conflicts with the value of self-determination and freedom. The moral principle of autonomy is pitted against the rights of individuals in families and in society to preserve life. One view holds that all suicidal clients be locked up "for their own good" until their ideas change. This may take years or may never occur. One concern is with the hospitalized client who, despite therapy and drugs, makes repeated attempts to end his life. The paternalistic person, who believes that all life is sacred, cares for the mentally ill and prevents all suicide on the assumption that such persons are unable to care for themselves. The counter-argument is that the chronically ill, institutionalized client discharged into an indifferent community suffers isolation, loneliness, and alienation. These conditions may be enough to make the person wish to end his life. In this view, an individual has a fundamental right to control his life. However, a dilemma concerns the individual's right to end his life when the impaired organ is the organ of judgment. This argument for autonomy is supported in the case of clients who decide to end their lives at lucid intervals. The issue of valuing the freedom of an individual versus interfering in people's lives by protecting them against their own wishes is virtually unsolvable. Critics of paternalism view the increasing use of behavior control techniques of all kinds as threatening the freedom of choice over one's own body.

▼ ....
THE AMERICAN NURSES' ASSOCIATION CODE FOR NURSES WITH INTERPRETATIVE STATEMENTS

1. The nurse provides services with respect for human dignity and the uniqueness of the client unrestricted by considerations of social or economic status, personal attributes, or the nature of health problems.
2. The nurse safeguards the client's right to privacy by judiciously protecting information of a confidential nature.
3. The nurse acts to safeguard the client and the public when health care and safety are affected by the incompetent, unethical, or illegal practice of any person.
4. The nurse assumes responsibility and accountability for individual nursing judgments and actions.
5. The nurse maintains competence in nursing.
6. The nurse exercises informed judgment and uses individual competence and qualifications as criteria in seeking consultation, accepting responsibilities, and delegating nursing activities to others.
7. The nurse participates in activities that contribute to the ongoing development of the profession's body of knowledge.
8. The nurse participates in the profession's efforts to implement and improve standards of nursing.
9. The nurse participates in the profession's efforts to establish and maintain conditions of employment conducive to high quality nursing care.
10. The nurse participates in the profession's effort to protect the public from misinformation and misrepresentation and to maintain the integrity of nursing.
11. The nurse collaborates with members of the health professions and other citizens in promoting community and national efforts to meet the health needs of the public.

From American Nurses' Association: *Code for nurses with interpretative statements,* Kansas City, Mo, 1976, The Association.

The principle of fully informed consent, contained in the *Code for Nurses* (see the box on p. 833) and other codes, is a necessary condition for all forms of therapy. It is especially significant in the relationship of nurse to client if trust is to grow into a therapeutic alliance in which nurse and client work together. An ethically justifiable relationship is based on clearly stated presumptions of the client's autonomy to enter into treatment, have a say in the direction of the treatment, seek consultation freely, and end treatment at will, after analysis of the reasons for ending therapy. Clients have these rights and can expect that they will be supported by the nurse. The client with clearly expressed problems has the right to expect that therapy will be directed toward problems, rather than toward satisfaction of the nurse's need. In a therapeutic relationship, the nurse respects the client in every way possible, including the client's nondestructive values, even if different from social norms. Respect for clients means that they are not used for the nurse's ego aggrandizement or sexual satisfaction. Respect includes the client's right to privacy and confidentiality. Clients are not discussed in any way with another client, family member, health professional, or agency without the client's knowledge and consent. A patient's Bill of Rights is shown in the accompanying box.

All persons seeking psychiatric help may be asked basic questions of value, such as whether the client, family, or group want to change behavior; to what extent; and for what purpose. In some therapeutic relationships the client's values are in harmony with those of the nurse and with societal norms. But the nurse's values may oppose the client's in other cases.

The central ethical issue in family therapy may be the balance among the rights of an individual and the rights of other individuals in the family and society. For example, if a father continues incestuous sexual relations while in family therapy, the nurse must decide to refuse to continue therapy because of the father's use of the child as a means to satisfy his sexual drives, to report the practice to the police, or to continue therapy aimed at ending incest. The nurse may use this issue as the focus of family therapy to help clarify the rights and duties of parents and children to each other. Another issue is whether the nurse has the

▼
THE AMERICAN HOSPITAL ASSOCIATION STATEMENT: A PATIENT'S BILL OF RIGHTS

The American Hospital Association presents a Patient's Bill of Rights with the expectation that observance of these rights will contribute to more effective patient care and greater satisfaction for the patient, his physician, and the hospital organization. Further, the Association presents these rights in the expectation that they will be supported by the hospital on behalf of its patients, as an integral part of the healing process. It is recognized that a personal relationship between the physician and the patient is essential for the provision of proper medical care. The traditional physician-patient relationship takes on a new dimension when care is rendered within an organizational structure. Legal precedent has established that the institution itself also has a responsibility to the patient. It is in recognition of these factors that these rights are affirmed.

1. The patient has the right to considerate and respectful care.
2. The patient has the right to obtain from his physician complete current information concerning his diagnosis, treatment, and prognosis in terms the patient can be reasonably expected to understand. When it is not medically advisable to give such information to the patient, the information should be made available to an appropriate person in his behalf. He has the right to know, by name, the physician responsible for coordinating his care.
3. The patient has the right to receive from his physician information necessary to give informed consent prior to the start of any procedure and/or treatment. Except in emergencies, such information for informed consent should include but not necessarily be limited to the specific procedure and/or treatment, the medically significant risks involved, and the probable duration of incapacitation. Where medically significant alternatives for care or treatment exist, or when the patient requests information concerning medical alternatives, the patient has the right to such information. The patient also has the right to know the name of the person responsible for the procedures and/or treatment.
4. The patient has the right to refuse treatment to the extent permitted by law and to be informed of the medical consequences of his action.
5. The patient has the right to every consideration of his privacy concerning his own medical care program. Case discussion, consultation, examination, and treatment are confidential and should be conducted discreetly. Those not directly involved in his care must have the permission of the patient to be present.

6. The patient has the right tot expect that all communications and records pertaining to his care should be treated as confidential.
7. The patient has the right to expect that within its capacity a hospital must make reasonable response to the request of a patient for services. The hospital must provide evaluation, service, and/or referral as indicated by the urgency of the case. When medically permissible, a patient may be transferred to another facility only after he has received complete information and explanation concerning the needs for and alternatives to such a transfer. The institution to which the patient is to be transferred must first have accepted the patient for transfer.
8. The patient has the right to obtain information as to any relationship of his hospital to other health care and educational institutions insofar as his care is concerned. The patient has the right to obtain information as to the existence of any professional relationships among individuals, by name, who are treating him.
9. The patient has the right to be advised if the hospital proposes to engage in or perform human experimentation affecting his care or treatment. The patient has the right to refuse to participate in such research projects.
10. The patient has the right to expect reasonable continuity of care. He has the right to know in advance what appointment times and physicians are available and where. The patient has the right to expect that the hospital will provide a mechanism whereby he is informed by his physician or a delegate of the physician of the patient's continuing health care requirements following discharge.
11. The patient has the right to examine and receive an explanation of his bill regardless of source of payment.
12. The patient has the right to know what hospital rules and regulations apply to his conduct as a patient.

No catalog of rights can guarantee for the patient the kind of treatment he has a right to expect. A hospital has many functions to perform, including the prevention and treatment of disease, the education of both health professionals and patients, and the conduct of clinical research. All these activities must be conducted with an overriding concern for the patient, and, above all, the recognition of his dignity as a human being. Success in achieving this recognition assures success in the defense of the rights of the patient.

From the American Hospital Association, 1975, Chicago, AHA.

right or duty to remain morally neutral while the family works through its choices, as in the case of drug-abusing parents, adversely influencing their child.

Another ethical issue concerns the role of the nurse in family therapy in relation to the family's values. The nurse may see her role as that of a referee who takes a neutral stance, helping the family to develop its own norms, or, in contrast, she may communicate her ethical views to the family in problematic situations. Moral problems arise concerning whether the nurse can deny her own values in evaluating behavior.

Whatever ethical orientation nurses choose and no matter how hard nurses try not to impose their values on families, the very process of selecting interventions is loaded with value judgments. Selected interventions are for or against a particular framework of ethics. For example, if a nurse asks family members deadlocked in a conflict of rights what they think about a situation in terms of greatest individual need and the least advantaged person in the family, the nurse is using a framework based on justice. If, on the other hand, the nurse asks the same family what would make the most people happy in this situation, the nurse is intervening from a utilitarian orientation. If the nurse asks what would be right for everyone with no exception, the nurse is intervening on the basis of an absolute principle orientation.

The nurse cannot remain neutral when values oppose a common morality as in cases of violence or incest. Yet nurses may not express their ethical orientations in all situations. It may be unnecessary when the family has well-defined moral principles and a common morality for guiding conduct. In most cases, however, nurses can help families explore their moral choices on the basis of mutual respect. Such principles as autonomy, beneficence, and justice are continually refined through dialogue and applied toward strengthening human relationships.

ETHICAL APPROACHES TO RESOLUTION OF VALUE CONFLICTS

Ethical principles apply to nursing practice and health care throughout life. A wide range of choices is available in most situations of health and illness. Moreover, one cannot not decide in matters of health and illness, since to do nothing is to decide in favor of the situation as it is. The availability of options has important implications for the client, since every choice carries a different degree of intrusiveness. Generally, clients expect to maintain control and to make decisions based on their values and goals, an application of the principle of self-determination. On the other hand, the nurse possesses expertise because of her education and experience. Serving the client's well-being by improving health is the justification for the existence of all health care disciplines. The justification of nursing is to look after the well-being of clients by applying the principles of beneficence (to do good, to be just, and to give equal consideration) and nonmaleficence (to prevent harm). The union of these principles with autonomy is essential to shared decision making. Shared decision making provides consideration of the family's goals, values, and well-being. The principle of equity (treating like cases alike) is also considered in shared decision making. Appli-

> ▼
> ### STEPS IN ETHICAL DECISION MAKING
>
> 1. Define the problem through nursing assessment
> 2. Clarify the client's problem in relation to life-style, values, goals, resources, and relationships
> 3. Assess the client's competence, communication, and understanding as the basis of consent or refusal
> 4. Separate ethical issues from administrative, medical, or legal considerations
> 5. Identify major ethical issues in relation to desires and competing or conflicting options
> 6. Justify the moral choice through ethical principles
> 7. Evaluate the moral choice and justification in relation to professional codes, the law and the institutional mission
> 8. Carry out the moral decision based on fully informed, freely given rational choice
> 9. Appeal an irrational or coerced decision not supportive of the client's well-being through legitimate channels of authority.

cation of this principle suggests that nursing resources are fairly distributed and that nurses treat all clients with equal respect as individuals.

Conflict between principles is at times unavoidable. In psychiatric nursing practice, an acutely psychotic, violent, and assaultive client must be restrained to prevent harm to self or others. This is an example of the use of the principle of beneficence (to do good and prevent harm) to override the principle of the client's self-determination. Clearly, the safety of the client and others overrides the client's need to physically express his rage and frustration against himself or others. The principle of equity (treating like cases alike) is applied to the client by the use of restraints and explanations exactly as they would be applied to similarly violent and assaultive clients.

Shared decision making helps clients assume responsibility for decisions relating to their lives and health. See the accompanying box for suggested steps in ethical decision making.

The ethical principles and guidelines discussed are illustrated in the following case example.

▼ Case Example

Betty, a beautiful 19-year-old college student with schizophrenia, is urged to take medication "X," which is known to benefit clients with similar symptoms by making their behavior less irrational. Possible side effects include uncontrollable muscular and facial movements that do not always respond to medication. Betty refuses to take drug "X."

The question in this case is whether paternalism, libertarianism, or utilitarianism is the best philosophy to use. The nurse can choose from several moral orientations. For example, a nurse, Ms. N., may be a libertarian and supports Betty's right to refuse medication. Another health team member with a utilitarian orientation may ask Ms. N. in a moral dialogue, "Have you considered what effects Betty's refusal will have on her as well as on her family? Betty may never function in a responsible position without drug "X." Or a paternalist-oriented nurse may ask Ms. N., "Are you thinking of Betty's long-term good? Her chances of a hospital discharge and return to college will be helped by taking drug "X" and hindered by not taking it."

By referring to the suggested steps in decision making, Betty's problem can be summarized as follows:

1. The problem is Betty's refusal to take drug "X" because of its side effects.
2. Possible side effects affecting her appearance can interfere with her single life-style, intimate relationships, and hopes for a successful career and marriage.
3. The client can understand the options.
4. Administrative and legal considerations emphasize her well-being.
5. The major ethical issues are the client's right to refuse treatment versus the paternalistic position of forcing drug administration in support of her best interests.
6. The client's right to free choice can be justified by the principle of liberty rights to her own body. The paternalist position of requiring the drug can be supported by principles of beneficence (do good), nonmaleficence (do no harm), equal consideration, and utility (the greatest good for the greatest number).
7. Nursing and medical professional codes of ethics support principles of doing good and avoiding harm. The client may be seriously harmed by failure to take the drug for control of her symptoms.
8. The nurse as client advocate implements the decision by educating the client about the significant aspects of this drug in relation to her life-style, her career and marriage goals, and the control of side effects by the selective use of additional drugs and drug moratoriums. As a result of the nurses's relationship and educational activities, Betty agrees to take the drug for control of her symptoms with monitoring and systematic follow-up visits.

There are two difficulties with ethical decision making. The first is that ethical values are part of the very process of identifying and selecting data and considering who should decide. The second is that after the nurse considers the alternatives, she still has to make a justifiable decision as to what to do. There is no verification that shows that libertarianism, paternalism, utilitarianism, love, or any other position has the conclusive and justifiably right answer.

Each moral or ethical view sets out its catalog of virtues or priorities. The mental health–psychiatric nurse, knowing alternative views not as closed systems but as overlapping, dynamic priorities, has to decide in particular cases. The decisions and each part of the process are laden with value judgments. Some moral decisions seem right, others wrong. Approximately a dozen ethical views merit consideration without providing the absolutely right answer. Yet some ethical principles provide a relatively stable core of moral strength, shared by neighboring moral views. Some behaviors and conditions are justifiably regarded as bad, such as slavery, segregation, abuse, torture, rape, and murder. By implication, their opposites, freedom, desegregation, kindness, and consideration are regarded as good.

However, the nurse can apply principles of evaluation to supplement ethical decision making in mental health–psychiatric nursing. She observes logical *do's* and *dont's*, such as not having more in the conclusion than there is in the premises or not concluding more than the evidence warrants. Knowing what is unwarranted may sometimes be as valuable as knowing what is warranted.

Ethical alternatives may be considered in a nondogmatic way. A general rule is to begin with the libertarian presumption of respect for the personhood of the client and seriously consider the client's word but to override the client if compelling reasons justify doing so. Knowing the strengths of paternalism and utilitarianism helps when the libertarian view is too frail to help the client. For example, restoring a depressed, suicidal client to rationality and autonomy may justify coercing the client into taking medications.

One philosophical move is to take the principles that apparently conflict and categorize some of these as "ends" principles and others as "means" principles. One then works toward harmonizing ethical ends and means. For example, autonomy may be regarded as a goal of mental health–psychiatric nursing. The means for achieving a client's autonomy or liberty may then be temporary control of a client's behavior. But such control is only a means toward achieving the goal (end) of the client's autonomy.

Another philosophical move is to convert apparently conflicting ends into harmonious ends and means as an identifiable goal, such as a client's autonomy (a Platonic-Kantian value) with other ends such as self-realization and happiness (Aristotelian and utilitarian values). An example is the psychiatric nurse who strengthens the client's autonomy and helps him to be productive and satisfied. In this way, both the nurse and the client achieve greater self-realization, and moral principles are maximized. The closer the ties between means and ends, the closer moral dilemmas come to satisfactory resolution. Stalemates and tragedies exist where minimal moral principles operate. To fail to recognize stalemates is to ignore the human predicament, which is that not everything in this world is tidy and clear as some persons would like. However, one can still work to improve the human relations that can be improved. That is what the ethics of mental health–psychiatric nursing is largely about.

BRIEF REVIEW

Ethical issues in the treatment of mental health–psychiatric clients include paternalism versus libertarianism, egoism versus altruism; majority rule, or utilitarian ethics, versus absolute principles; omissions versus commissions; absolute versus prima facie rights; and negative versus positive rights. The moral "-isms" also present ways of looking at issues. No absolute standard of right and wrong can be applied to mental health–psychiatric nursing. However, some values and principles, such as respect for rights and the golden rule morality implied by utilitarianism, have good reasons behind them.

Three client rights—the right to respect, the right to treatment, and the right to refuse treatment—have major roles in moral values. But dilemmas easily arise in dealing with the rights of mentally disturbed persons. A case in point is the psychiatric client's right to refuse the kind of treatment that the client needs to become more rational. Further dilemmas surrounding the right to respect, to receive treatment, and to refuse treatment arise in individual, group, and family therapy. The emphasis is on a rights-based view, one that shows respect for clients as ends rather than as means.

REFERENCES AND SUGGESTED READINGS

1. Annas GJ: *The rights of doctors, nurses, and allied health professionals,* New York, 1983, Avon Books.
2. Annas GJ: *The rights of patients,* ed 2, Carbondale, Ill, 1989, Southern Illinois University Press.
3. Bandman EL, Bandman B: *Critical thinking in nursing,* Norwalk, Conn, 1988, Appleton & Lange.
4. Bandman EL, Bandman B: *Nursing ethics through the life span,* ed 2, Norwalk, Conn, 1990, Appleton & Lange.
5. Bloch DA: The family of the psychiatric patient. In Arieti S, editor: *American handbook of psychiatry,* vol 1, ed 2, New York, 1974, Basic Books.
6. Davidhizar R: Beliefs and values of the client with chronic mental illness regarding treatment, *Issues in Mental Health Nursing* 6:261, 1984.
7. Feinbers J: *Social philosophy,* Englewood Cliffs, NJ, 1973, Prentice Hall.
8. Flanagan L: Psychiatry: a question of ethics, *Nursing Times* 82(35):39, 1986.
9. Hobbes T: *The leviathan,* Oxford, England, 1861, Blackwell Press.
10. Holder AR: *Legal issues in pediatrics and adolescent medicine,* ed 2, New York, 1985, John Wiley & Sons.
11. Kant I: *Fundamental principles of the metaphysics of morals,* Indianapolis, 1948, Bobbs-Merrill (originally published in 1785).
12. Macklin R: *Man, mind, and morality: the ethics of behavior control,* Englewood Cliffs, NJ, 1982, Prentice Hall.
13. Mill JS: *Utilitarianism, liberty and representative government,* London, 1910, JM Dent & Sons (originally published in 1859).
14. Mill JS: *Utilitarianism,* Indianapolis, 1957, Bobbs-Merrill (originally published in 1859).
15. Peplau HE: Some reflections on earlier days in psychiatric nursing, *Journal of Psychosocial Nursing and Mental Health Services* 20(8):17, 1982.
16. Plato: *The republic,* Indianapolis, 1974, Hackett (translated by GMA Grube).
17. Sandelowsi M: The politics of parenthood . . . competing maternal-fetal, parent-child, and individual-family claims, *Maternal-Child Nursing* 11(4):235, 1986.
18. Sharfstein SS, Beigel A, editors: *The new economics and psychiatric care,* Washington, DC, 1985, American Psychiatric Press.
19. Steele SM, Harmon VM: *Values clarification in nursing,* New York, 1979, Appleton-Century-Crofts.
20. Trotter CMF: I never promised you a rose garden but I must remember to tell you about the thorns: the ethics involved in psychotherapy, *Journal of Psychosocial Nursing and Mental Health Services* 23(4):6, 1985.
21. Wieczorek RR, Natapoff JN: A conceptual approach to the nursing of children, Philadelphia, 1981, JB Lippincott.

ANNOTATED BIBLIOGRAPHY

Bandman EL, Bandman B: *Nursing ethics through the life span,* ed 2, Norwalk, Conn, 1990, Appleton & Lange.
This book addresses the moral issues and problems of everyday nursing practice throughout the life span of clients, beginning with the procreative family and ending with the dying client. Models of nurse-client-physician relationships are analyzed. Professional codes of ethics are evaluated. Approaches to making ethically justifiable decisions based on nursing strategies, guidelines, and canons of critical reasoning are presented separately and in conjunction with developmental stages. Example cases with analysis are used throughout the text.

Virginia Trotter Betts

After studying this chapter, the student will be able to:

- Identify sources of mental health law
- Describe common potential civil liability interactions
- Explain the role of a nurse witness in client consent and legal proceedings
- Identify how guaranteed rights may be applied to mental health settings
- Describe the civil and procedural rights of clients with mental health problems

- Distinguish between voluntary and involuntary commitment of adults and minors
- Identify issues in the commitment of mentally ill criminal clients
- Identify the main issues in client consent to and refusal of treatment
- Describe ways in which a nurse can influence legislation

Laws are an important aspect of U.S. society, and there are significant relationships between the legal and health care systems. Because of some of the special characteristics of mental health–psychiatric care, there needs to be recognition by the professional nurse of the laws that impact client care and the mental health system. Nurses not only must function effectively within the boundaries of current law but also must be able to analyze the need for legal change and participate in the political processes required to bring about successful change.

OVERVIEW OF THE LEGAL SYSTEM

When analyzing the legal trends throughout the United States on matters of mental health, it is necessary to know the relevant Supreme Court decisions and federal statutes. Because laws may differ between levels of government as well as from state to state, particular state mental health codes and subsequent interpretations by both the state courts and the federal appeals court need to be determined. State statutes can then be compared with national precedents.

Civil Law

Civil law involves relationships and disputes between citizens and resolves such disputes in various ways, usually with a law suit that seeks monetary settlement. The most common civil actions brought against nurses working in

mental health settings include malpractice, assault and battery, false imprisonment, and breach of confidentiality.

Malpractice

Malpractice is a civil action that may be brought against a professional when failure to meet a professional standard of care causes injury to the client. The nurse's professional standard of care is to do what a reasonably prudent nurse would do for the client. To assess and keep up to date on what a reasonably prudent nurse would do, the nurse:

1. Practices within national standards of practice
2. Follows the policies and procedures of an agency
3. Reads and discusses current articles and texts written for mental health–psychiatric nursing
4. Attends professional continuing education courses

If the nurse does not act as the prudent nurse would have done in a similar situation and the act or failure to act injures the client, the client, through a lawsuit or settlement, may receive monetary compensation for damages. Typically the injury of the client must be actual physical harm. However, some courts are beginning to recognize severe emotional distress and economic deterioration as compensable injuries.

In 1980 a Connecticut hospital was successfully sued for $3.6 million for the malpractice of its nurses. Ms. Pisel had been placed in a seclusion room as her orientation deteriorated. According to the chart, no one checked her for 4 hours, after which time she was found semicomatose,

	DATES	EVENTS
HISTORICAL OVERVIEW	1700-1800s	The mentally ill lost many of their rights with institutionalization: the right to vote, to make wills or contracts, and to keep their professional licenses.
	Early 1900s	The state legislature created an alternative to state involuntary commitment proceedings by providing care and permitting voluntary hospital admissions.
	1951	Almost every state permitted the mentally ill to avoid involuntary commitment by volunteering themselves for confinement.
	Late 1960s	The rights of the mentally ill experienced renewed attention as a spin-off of the civil rights movement.
	1970s	There was legal recognition that confinement in a mental hospital involves a massive curtailment of liberty; the courts and lawmakers began to examine the question of who can be institutionalized and how this institutionalization is to be accomplished.
	1980s	Increasing policies of deinstitutionalization caused societal strain to redirect mental health care in the community.
	1990s	Health care costs and efforts to manage such costs are increasing use of managed care and case management options for mental health clients.
	Future	National research on Effectiveness and Quality of Care will significantly affect psychiatric care and will evaluate cost and benefit of numerous regimens.

having wedged her head between the mattress and rail of a metal bed. In this case there were multiple instances of failing to meet nursing standards of care, including failure to promptly monitor a secluded client and failure to notify the physician of a change in the client's condition. A nurse also revealed that, a few days after the injury, the nursing director told the staff to rewrite the nursing notes, which they did, raising a legal and ethical issue in addition to malpractice (*Pisel v. Stamford Hospital*, 1980).

Most psychiatric malpractice cases arise from care received in inpatient settings. Sexual abuse, physical harm, poor observation or supervision, and premature release are frequently litigated incidents.[31]

The most common malpractice cases against psychiatric nurses are those dealing with inadequate observation or judgment.[4] An example is failure to prevent a suicide by not synthesizing data that indicate that the client needs closer supervision and/or not initiating precautions to ensure the client's safety. A client who is despondent, has threatened suicide, and has some means for self-injury needs to be closely observed.

Assault and Battery

The legal definition of *assault* is a threat of touching without consent. *Battery* is the actual unconsented touch. An assault and battery suit can be brought both as a civil suit by a person and as a criminal suit by the state. A person can sue civilly for assault and battery without an injury. In the health care setting (except in an emergency), any treatment of a client is a battery if the treatment is given without proper consent. If the client is incompetent, a guardian must give consent before treatment.

False Imprisonment

False imprisonment is the wrongful confinement of a person in such a way that he or she cannot escape. A potential for false imprisonment arises when the client is locked on a ward or placed in seclusion or restraint or when a voluntarily hospitalized client wishes to leave but is not released. To avoid suits for false imprisonment, a hospital needs to have a policy defining when a client may be confined. Confinement is permitted when the client is dangerous to himself or others. Documentation of the events justifying such restraint is critical. Continued observation and adherence to policy on releasing the client are also important.[3]

Confidentiality of Communications

Under the American Nurses' Association's (ANA's) *Code of Ethics* and certain state statutes, the nurse has the responsibility to keep information about a client confidential. This means that information received from clients or their records should be released only by an appropriate release of information protocol.

In law, there is a concept called *privileged communication*. Privileged communication means that, even in court proceedings, selected persons do not have to reveal a client's communication to them. When called to court to tell what the client said about any feelings, thoughts, or actions, the nurse needs to assess the applicability of privileged communication to the professional nurse. Only a few states provide "privilege" for nurses. In the other states, the nurse is required to reveal client communication if instructed to do so by the judge during a court proceeding. Thus a dilemma of professional ethics and legal responsibility can arise if the nurse is called as a witness. If the nurse in a state without privilege refuses to speak, her behavior may be considered criminal contempt of court.

Whether the nurse is called as a witness for or against the client affects the status of the communication. In court the general rule is that the client may at any time permit the professional to release information. It is the client's privilege, not the professional's. Therefore if the client asks the professional to testify, the professional must truthfully give all information, including any communication of the client. Only when the nurse is a witness against the client and the privileged communication statute covers nurses must the nurse keep the information confidential.

The issue of confidentiality may arise in a commitment hearing. If the nurse is asked by the client or the client's attorney to testify, the nurse has no choice. However, if the nurse is asked by the state to testify in order to commit the client, the nurse should refuse to speak about client communications unless she is instructed by the judge and the law does not recognize communication to the nurse as privileged.

In a malpractice suit, privileged communication is not an issue. When a client is suing a nurse for the care given, the client has already put the issue of nursing care before the court and therefore waived his privilege of confidentiality. Thus the nurse is free to reveal all communications with the client.

The nurse may also be asked to appear at court as an expert witness on the standard of care for nursing. As an expert witness, the nurse's testimony is based on experience and education as a nurse, so there is no problem with client confidentiality. Before giving a deposition or appearing in court, the nurse examines the records of the case and is asked to give an opinion as to the appropriateness of the nursing care.

In an evolving legal trend, professionals are being required to disclose confidential information outside court proceedings. Some states have now imposed a duty on professionals to disclose confidential information when a known potential victim is at serious risk of harm. This duty was first recognized in the case of *Tarasoff v. Board of Regents of the University of California* (1976). In this case the client confided to his psychotherapist that he intended to kill Tatiana Tarasoff. Although the therapist did contact legal authorities, he did not warn the intended victim or her parents of the threat. When the client later killed the woman, her parents won a lawsuit based on the therapist's failure to warn. This case clearly set new legal precedent commonly called the *duty to warn.*

The evolving case and statutory law has not gone so far as to say a therapist must warn of every threat. A therapist must warn about threats that pose a serious danger to an identifiable victim.[5] This study has been imposed by courts on psychiatrists, psychotherapists, and other mental health workers.

The argument against further expansion of this duty to warn victims is that the effectiveness of therapy will be reduced if therapists must breach their clients' confidences to warn potential victims. If a client's trust is diminished, the client may cease to admit anger, and successful treatment may be impossible. The duty to warn has placed mental health workers in a double bind.[19] If they break a client's confidence, they may be sued for breach of confidentiality. If they fail to break the confidence and a potential victim is injured, the mental health professional may be sued for negligence in a failure to warn.

CURRENT AND EVOLVING MENTAL HEALTH LAW

The U.S. Constitution, its interpretations by the U.S. Supreme Court, and selected federal and state laws need to be examined with application to mental health. These discussions focus on civil rights, commitment proceedings, and consent issues.

Federal Law

In the 200 years since the passage of the Bill of Rights, several constitutional amendments have had significant application to mental health law (Table 42-1).

The First Amendment states: "Congress shall make no law respecting an establishment of religion, or prohibiting the free exercise thereof; or abridging the freedom of speech." Freedom of speech as guaranteed by the First Amendment has been interpreted in one court to include a person's mental processes and the communication of ideas (*Kaimowitz v. Department of Mental Health,* 1973). This means that persons have the right to their own thoughts, even if the thoughts are bizarre. However, this interpretation is not accepted by most states.

Freedom of religion has been held to mean the right to practice one's religion even when institutionalized. This includes the right to refuse medication or treatment on the grounds that it conflicts with religious beliefs (*Winters v. Miller,* 1971). Although a client does have a right to practice a religion, the courts have not recognized an absolute right to refuse treatment on religious grounds.

▼ **TABLE 42-1   Amendments to the U.S. Constitution as Related to Mental Health Care**

Amendment	Possible Interpretations
First: Freedom of speech	Right to generate abnormal thought
	Right to express abnormal thought
First: Freedom of religion	Right to practice religion
	Right to refuse treatment if it conflicts with religious beliefs
Fifth: Federal right to due process of law	Procedural rights
Eighth: Freedom from cruel and unusual punishment	Freedom from treatment used as punishment
	Freedom from poor institutional conditions
	Freedom from excessive medication
Fourteenth: State right to due process of law and equal protection	Procedural rights
	Privacy
	Equal treatment

The Eighth Amendment to the Constitution says that "Excessive bail shall not be required, nor excessive fines imposed, nor cruel and unusual punishment inflicted." It is still unclear in the law whether freedom from cruel and unusual punishment applies only to criminals or can be applied to noncriminal hospitalized mentally ill clients. It does apply to the mentally ill when treatments such as medications, restraints, seclusion, aversive stimuli, electroconvulsive therapy, and psychosurgery are used as punishment rather than therapy. Other violations of the Eighth Amendment have been considered to be institutional conditions such as unsanitary living conditions, inadequate exercise or nutrition, and insufficient staffing (*Lessard v. Schmidt,* 1974). It has also been argued that an excess of medication and forced medication are cruel and unusual punishment (*Lessard v. Schmidt,* 1974).

The Fifth Amendment to the Constitution states: "No person . . . shall be compelled in any criminal case to be a witness against himself, nor be deprived of life, liberty, or property, without due process of law." The Fourteenth Amendment, Section 1, states: "Nor shall any State deprive any person of life, liberty, or property, without due process of law; nor deny to any person within its jurisdiction the equal protection of the laws." These provisions require that citizens be guaranteed due process of law. Due process means that certain procedural safeguards, such as the right to notice, counsel, a hearing, access to documents, client's own professional examination, client's presence at the hearing, and client's cross-examination of witnesses, must be provided before the state can place such clients in hospitals against their will. The Fifth Amendment applies due process to the federal government, and the Fourteenth Amendment applies the due process principle to all states. Because the Supreme Court has recognized that involuntary commitment to a mental hospital involves a grave deprivation of liberty, any law that commits a person to a mental hospital must meet due process requirements (*Humphrey v. Cady,* 1972). State statutes, state courts, and lower federal courts have defined due process procedures. These procedures are further discussed in the section later in this chapter on civil commitment.

Besides creating a fundamental right to be free from incarceration and requiring due process before commitment, the Fifth and Fourteenth Amendments guarantee a fundamental right to privacy. Privacy has thus far been used by courts to protect family and physical privacy. The most familiar privacy case is *Roe v. Wade* (1973) in which the Supreme Court case granted a woman the right to a first-trimester abortion. The right to privacy may also apply to a mental health client's right to refuse treatment. The concept of privacy is still being defined by the courts and new mental health precedents may be set. Limitations of *Roe v. Wade* as set out in *Webster v. Reproductive Health Services* (1989) have yet to be applied to mental health care.

Equal protection under the law, which is also mandated by the Fourteenth Amendment, means that neither the federal nor the state government can treat one group of people differently than another unless there is a rational reason to do so. If the government has an appropriate reason for unequal treatment, it can proceed differently. For example, if a mentally ill criminal is committed to a mental hospital, under the guarantee of equal protection, the criminal should have the same procedural safeguards and the same rights as those of a noncriminal client committed to a mental institution. However, the state has a rational reason (to protect the community from the criminal) for treating the criminal and noncriminal unequally.

Civil Rights

Constitutional rights apply to all citizens as well as to clients in all settings: inpatient, outpatient, and community. However, these rights are broad and difficult to apply.

Besides the rights that courts find in U.S. and state constitutions, other sources of clients' rights exist. In 1980 Congress passed the Mental Health Systems Act [PL 99-319], creating a recommended bill of rights for mentally ill clients.[23] The rights found in the Act are only a model from the Congress to the states; they are not law. However, this act reflects federal lawmakers' agreement on what rights states should adopt. The rights that a state adopts as actual legal rights in its mental health code have the force of law for that state's residents. Following are the rights most frequently listed in state statutes for residential clients.[30]

1. Right to completeness and confidentiality of records
2. Right to access to records
3. Right to access to personal belongings
4. Right to freedom from restraints and isolation
5. Right to treatment, including individual medical plan, least restrictive alternatives, and periodic review of examinations
6. Right to daily exercise
7. Right to access to visitors
8. Right to use of writing materials and uncensored mail
9. Right to use of telephone
10. Right to access to courts and attorneys
11. Right to employment compensation
12. Right to be informed of rights

The Mental Patient's Bill of Rights should be compared with the state's mental health code, federal and state statutes, federal and state constitutions, and hospital or ward policies.

All rights, whether constitutional or statutory, are merely theoretical unless the client knows them and can use them. The nurse acts as the client's advocate by informing the client of his legal rights and then supporting his decision on how or whether a right is pursued. Some state statutes provide a grievance procedure for clients who believe their rights are being violated, but other states have no grievance procedure. In the latter case, clients may secure their rights through lawsuits. A violation of a right guaranteed by the U.S. Constitution may be brought before federal or state court, and clients may sue an individual state or federal government official if that official violated their constitutional right by ignoring the law or acting maliciously (*Wood v. Strickland,* 1975).

Rights may be withdrawn under certain circumstances. If state law is unclear on when such rights can be curtailed, a written agency policy should define the criteria for denial of rights. For example, despite the right to freedom from physical isolation, a client who has attacked another client may be placed in isolation. When the right to freedom is denied, documentation in the client record should state the events. Agency policy for activities that may abridge rights should be carefully written and followed. For example, the policy might state, "Isolation must take place within 15 minutes of an incident; there must be a written order; the order is valid for a maximum of 3 hours; the client shall have access to toilet facilities every hour and exercise every 3 hours while in isolation." Nursing notes should indicate that the client's behavior was assessed before isolation, and that all agency criteria for isolation procedures were followed.[38]

State Law
Commitment

The commitment of a client to a mental institution is the exercise of a strong power of state government. The state is able to commit a person under its police power to protect others or under its *parens patriae* power to "care for" the person. A person may be committed to a mental hospital through the civil court of the criminal court system. The civil court system requires that the person meet commitment criteria set up in the state mental health code. The criminal system requires that the person is being prosecuted for a crime but is either incompetent to stand trial or is citing a claim of being not guilty of the crime because of insanity. Civil commitment may be initiated by the client, a physician, the policy, a state attorney, a family member, or others listed in state statute. There are two types of civil commitments: voluntary and involuntary.

Civil commitment

Voluntary entry into the hospital is by consent of the client or someone acting for the client. Almost every state permits voluntary admission[7] for mental health treatment, although public hospital bed space is increasingly limited, and admission to public facilities requires acute symptoms.

When admission is voluntary, the client has a statutory right to be released. However, some time lag to go through hospital exit procedures (about 48 hours) is reasonable and gives the mental health team time to initiate involuntary commitment proceedings if necessary.

Voluntary clients are considered competent unless a court finds otherwise, and therefore they have the right to refuse treatment, including psychotropic medications, unless they are dangerous to themselves or others, as in a violent episode on the treatment unit (*Rennie v. Klein,* 1981). This right to refuse medications is one important difference between the care of voluntary clients and that of involuntary clients. Nurses must be able to clearly identify the admission status of their clients at all times.

State codes have two types of involuntary commitment: *emergency* and *indefinite.* The indefinite involuntary commitment usually has subdivisions of *initial* and *extended* commitments.

When a person's conduct poses an immediate danger of serious harm to himself or others, the client may be held temporarily for initial treatment through the emergency involuntary commitment statutes in most states. Unfortunately, it may be a police officer who first encounters the client, and the client may be held at a jail until transfer to a health facility is possible. In a health facility an examination is performed to determine that an emergency exists.

The person required to perform the admitting examination varies from state to state and can be the psychiatrist, physician, or, in some states, the psychiatric nurse.

Statutes specify when the examination must be done and how long emergency detention can last. The suggested statute on civil commitment of the American Bar Association (ABA) recommends no longer than 72 hours for an emergency.[37] Because no hearing is required, emergency treatment can be started, although no review or diagnosis takes place. It is in everyone's best interest to keep the detention period for an emergency commitment short and to hold a hearing quickly.

If the initial screening does not validate the existence of an emergency, the client must be released. The client must also be released when the emergency ceases or at the expiration of the state statutory emergency detention time if no petition for involuntary commitment has been filed.

Due process

The exact procedures for involuntary commitment that meet due process are created by each state's legislature in its mental health code. The state mental health code defines what a mental disorder is, the conditions that must be met to commit someone involuntarily, the procedure for the hearing, the length of an initial and extended commitment, and the rights of the client. If the state legislature does not create a constitutionally acceptable code, the courts will. In 1975, the U.S. Supreme Court in *O'Connor v. Donaldson* said that the presence of mental illness alone was not enough to justify involuntary institutionalization. In this case, Mr. Donaldson was 50 years old with delusional ideation when his father successfully had the state of Florida commit him to a state mental hospital. Mr. Donaldson was diagnosed as paranoid schizophrenic, but he had never committed a dangerous act. He was institutionalized for 15 years despite his repeated requests for release. For this 15 years he received little treatment and at times he was kept in a room with 60 other clients. The Supreme Court decided that "a state cannot constitutionally confine without more [sic] a nondangerous individual who is capable of surviving safely in freedom by himself or with the help if willing and responsible family members or friends" (*O'Connor v. Donaldson,* 1975, p. 578). "Without more" means the client must at least receive more than milieu therapy. The court, however, did not specify what treatment would be enough to justify confinement of a nondangerous person. Future court cases will be necessary to define the minimal treatment.

It is clear that a state may commit a person for mental illness plus dangerousness. By 1979, 46 states adopted the criteria of mental illness and danger to self or others as the grounds for involuntary commitment. About 30 states also declared that nondangerous mentally ill persons can be committed if they are "gravely disabled" or "in need of care or treatment." Gravely disabled or in need of care or treatment typically means that because of a mental condition the client is unable to care for his basic needs of nutrition, clothing, shelter, safety, and medical care.[36] An example of a gravely disabled client is one who does not eat because of disorientation.

Almost every state permits indefinite involuntary commitment on the grounds of danger to self or others. It is important to know what this means. Danger to self may include a range of behavior from attempted suicide to neglecting basic needs. Danger to others may include behavior ranging from threats of violence to actual attacks. In all these situations, exact statutory language is important. When language is specific, the client's actual conduct must reflect the statutory language. For example, if the state commitment statute requires substantial threat of imminent harm and the statement "I feel so bad I would like to die" is the client's only action, there may not be sufficient evidence to commit the client. However, if the client's statement were accompanied by the act of holding a loaded gun to the temple, the conduct would then become specific to the statute.

Using dangerousness as the criterion for state commitment has been criticized. Research shows that no one, including psychiatrists and judges, can accurately predict who will be dangerous.[11] Research also shows that mentally ill clients are no more apt to be dangerous than people in the general population.[11] Thus to place mentally ill persons in hospitals when they have committed no dangerous act is to place them there merely for their mental illness.

The ABA recommends in its model act the following criteria for involuntary commitment[37]:

1. Severe mental disorder
2. Likelihood of inflicting serious physical harm on self or others as manifested by an overt act
3. Incompetency to make own treatment decisions
4. Treatability (including availability of treatment resources as well as improvements in condition)

The model act does not recommend involuntary commitment of the gravely disabled but suggests a legal incompetency hearing and appointment of a guardian.

In any civil commitment proceedings, the state will have to prove by clear and convincing evidence (a higher standard of proof than in most civil litigation) that the client meets the state's criteria for commitment (*Addington v. Texas,* 1979). What constitutes clear and convincing evidence depends on the facts of the case. An example of clear and convincing evidence of dangerousness is found in *In the Matter of N.B.* (1980). The client in this case was hostile and aggressive to the hospital staff and tried to choke an-

other client. The court determined that he was dangerous and therefore an appropriate candidate for involuntary commitment. However, public opinion conflicts frequently over the dangerousness standard, for example, *Boggs v. New York City Health and Hospitals* (1988).

Besides meeting the state criteria for commitment, nonemergency involuntary commitment of an adult must also be procedurally fair to meet the constitutional right of due process of law. This means that certain procedures have been recognized as giving the client a fair chance at presenting his version of the situation. The typical procedural rights for short- or long-term commitment are found in the accompanying box. The commitment hearing is conducted with all rights that the state constitution recognizes. Then the judge finds either clear and convincing evidence for commitment or insufficient evidence, in which case the client is not hospitalized.

The ABA recommends that the initial involuntary commitment be no more than 90 days. If during that 90 days the client exhibits new threats or acts of harm, another 90-day commitment is sought.[37] Most states, however, permit initial commitments of 6 months to 1 year.

Commitment of minors

Commitment of minors differs from commitment of adults because minors, who are persons under 18 years of age, are considered legally incompetent to perform adult activities. Therefore parents make decisions for their children, traditionally deciding when they need to receive counseling or medication and if they need to be placed in a mental hospital. The unique situation with minors is that their parents voluntarily commit them, although in fact the child may strongly protest. The question is whether this situation is actually voluntary or involuntary commitment. If it is a type of involuntary commitment, the minor needs to be allowed some constitutional procedural safeguards because his liberty is being taken away.

Cases dealing with children represent a clash between two legal concepts: the right of the family to be free from state intrusion and the *parens patriae* responsibility of the state to protect citizens with a disability, in this case, minors. In the past most states did not intervene when parents

STATE COMMITMENT PROCEDURAL RIGHTS

1. Right to remain silent—client does not have to say anything that can be used to determine if commitment criteria are met, for example, talking about acts of violence during examination or hearing. Not in majority of states.
2. Right to notice*—client must be given information about time, date, place of hearing, witnesses who will speak for commitment, and what they will speak about.
3. Right to counsel*—client has a right to an attorney who will represent the client's interest, including private talks with his attorney, uncensored communication, and absolute right to call. In a few states, counsel has the right to be present at mental examination.
4. Right to hearing*—client has a right to a meeting with a judge, including presentation of evidence and witnesses on client's behalf before nonemergency detention can continue. May be held at hospital.

5. Right to jury—client has a right to a jury hearing if long-term commitment is being sought (long term means 90 days or more). No U.S. constitutional right in civil commitment hearings and not a right in majority of states.
6. Right to review documents*—the chart, Kardex, medication sheets, as well as the psychiatrist's examination report must be made available to client's counsel.
7. Right to own professional examiner*—client can choose psychiatrist to do an independent examination and testify in the hearing.
8. Right to be present at hearing*—client can hear full testimony about his mental illness and dangerousness unless the judge finds client disruptive in the proceedings. It can be argued that the client who is excessively medicated is not present.
9. Right to cross-examine witnesses*—client or attorney can ask questions of any witnesses, including health professionals.

*Most frequently found in state statute.

voluntarily committed their children to mental institutions.[12]

However, over time, states have changed their statutes to include more procedural safeguards before the institutionalization of children.[13] Typically, these rights include a right to counsel for the child and a right to a hearing.

The issue of whether states could permit voluntary commitment of minors to mental institutions without substantially increased procedural safeguards was finally decided by the U.S. Supreme Court in 1979. The case, *Parham v. J.L.* (1979), challenged the Georgia statute permitting voluntary commitment without an adversarial hearing. The Supreme Court held that, although the child has a right to be free of unnecessary physical restraint and not to be labeled erroneously, parents could place their children in institutions without a hearing. The court said that the child's rights are adequately safeguarded by a physician's examination and review of the child's history. The court considers the physician to be a neutral fact finder who determines whether a child meets the state's statutory requirements for commitment. If, in the physician's judgment, the child does not, the parent may not admit the child to the hospital. Instead of a formal hearing, the physician's examination can counteract potential parental force. Although this is the current law, state statutes that do require a hearing are valid, since a state can always have more stringent safeguards than the U.S. Constitution requires; however, a state may not have fewer safeguards. In the Supreme Court decision in the *Parham* case, three justices dissented, saying that children need even more procedural safeguards than adults because they are confined longer, are more vulnerable, and bear an emotional scar for life if erroneously labeled. The *Parham* decision has been criticized in both the legal and the psychiatric fields, and it is possible that, as a result of this dissent, the Supreme Court will recognize more procedural safeguards for minors in the future. Clearly more safeguards are available for the involuntary commitment of the child (*Johnson v. Solomon,* 1979). The mental health nurse must pay careful attention to the protection of the rights of the minor client, especially when treatment approaches "for the good of the child" are perceived differently by the parents and the child.[33]

Criminal commitment

Persons may also be placed in mental institutions through criminal proceedings. When citizens are accused of a crime, they may plead that they should not be found guilty because they were insane. Criminal law defines insanity differently from the health care perspective, which is concerned with descriptive symptoms and prognosis, not merely a time-specific state of mind. Currently, state courts recognize three different definitions of criminal insanity.[8]

1. The M'Naghten Rule—at the time of committing the act, the person under defect of reason did not know the nature and quality of the act or did not know it was wrong.
2. The Irresistible Impulse Test—at the time of the act the person was of such mental condition that even if he knew the act to be wrong, his actions were beyond control.
3. The American Law Institute, Model Penal Code Section 4.01(1)—at the time of the conduct, as a result

of mental disease or defect, the person lacked substantial capacity either to appreciate the wrongfulness of his conduct or to conform his conduct to the requirements of law.

Whichever definition a state uses for an insanity defense, if the accused is found by a jury to meet the criteria, the accused is found not guilty of the crime. The client is then committed to a mental hospital for evaluation and treatment. The client is treated as long as he meets commitment criteria. When no longer mentally ill by state criteria, the client is released.

Controversy continues over the appropriateness of this approach to the criminal treatment problem, including statutes that call for a plea of "guilty but insane" and giving criminals a time sentence in a mental institution if mental illness is present.[21] This standard allows treatment of the mental illness if resources are available while still holding the client responsible and punishable for the crime.

Sometimes criminals are found mentally ill after they are already in jail. They have a right to be treated for their illness; however, they are not automatically transferred to a mental institution just because a psychiatrist now finds them mentally ill. They have a right to counsel and a hearing before a change in their commitment from a jail to a mental hospital (*Vitek v. Jones*, 1980).

The criminal system also funnels clients into mental institutions because of questions of competence to stand trial. *Competence to stand trial* refers to a criminal defendant's ability to (1) confer with an attorney about his defense, (2) understand the charges against him, and (3) understand courtroom procedure. If a criminal defendant cannot because of mental disorder meet these criteria, the client is placed (without a commitment hearing) in a mental hospital for evaluation or treatment. Periods of observation and treatment can be long, and if the standard for competence is never regained, the client has in fact received a lengthy sentence.[20] To remedy this problem, the Supreme Court held in *Jackson v. Indiana* that a 27-year-old client who was incompetent to stand trial for a theft of $9 worth of property could not be "held more than a reasonable time necessary to determine whether there is substantial probability that he will attain capacity in the foreseeable future" (*Jackson v. Indiana*, 1972, p. 728). If regaining competence is not foreseeable, a civil commitment proceeding may be initiated if state criteria are met; otherwise, the client is released. Minors who are charged with crimes but who are also mentally ill typically have their criminal charges dropped or are placed on probation if they spend a specified time in a mental institution or receive outpatient treatment.

Right to treatment and least restrictive alternative

Two emerging concepts affect the commitment process: the right to treatment and the least restrictive alternative principle. The theory behind a right to treatment comes from the concept of due process in that a state should not institutionalize a person unless it can provide active treatment. If a person is gravely disabled and there is no treatment, it would be more appropriate to appoint a guardian than to institutionalize the person without treatment. A right to treatment was first articulated in a criminal case *(Rouse v. Cameron)* in 1966, when Mr. Rouse applied for release from a mental hospital on the grounds that he had received no treatment. He had avoided a criminal charge of carrying a dangerous weapon when he was found to be insane and then had spent 4 years involuntarily committed to a mental hospital without treatment. However, the maximum sentence for carrying a dangerous weapon was only 1 year. Interpreting the Washington, D.C. statute that said mental patients are entitled to treatment, the judge ruled that a criminal had a right to treatment if he were insane or a right to be released if he were no longer insane.

By 1979, following the rule in *Wyatt v. Stickney* (1974), 27 states had some form of right to treatment through statutory or case law.[30] Some states have explicit rules about what treatment entails, including a treatment plan with objectives, activities, and evaluation criteria. Others are not specific, stating only that a right to treatment exists. Laws are vague about whether a right to treatment entails an obligation to treat or is merely a right to be released from a hospital when treatment is not available.

The *least restrictive alternative (LRA) principle* means that the least restrictive treatment and placement possible should be ordered for a client. The principle can be applied to any mentally disabled client, from mentally ill to developmentally delayed. LRA ensures that when a state has the right to intervene, the state will do so with minimal intrusion into the client's life. The LRA principle has been applied to the commitment process by some federal courts and by at least 10 states.[36] The following are some examples of the application of the LRA principle:

1. Placing a client in the care facility closest to his home rather than in a state hospital far from his home.
2. Placing a client who can maintain daily employment in a weekend and night care facility rather than a 24-hour hospital.
3. Providing home care services instead of full-time hospitalization to a gravely disabled client.

Unfortunately, one of the difficult problems with the LRA principle is the continuing limited availability of outpatient and community services that serve the mentally ill.

The LRA principle has sometimes been applied to conditions within the institution after commitment.[42] This means that other medications are to be tried before psychotropic medications, psychotherapy must be tried before medication, and closer observations before seclusion (*Wyatt v. Stickney*, 1974; *Rennie v. Klein*, 1981).

Consent to treatment

In legal terminology *consent* has three elements: capacity, voluntariness, and information.[29] All three must be present for consent to be valid.

Capacity means the ability to understand, although total comprehension is not necessary. The law says certain classes of people do not have capacity: minors (usually persons under 18 years of age), persons declared incompetent by the court, and criminals who have successfully proved incompetency. Individuals may have varying degrees of capacity. For instance, a mentally disabled client may have the capacity to know that he does not want electroconvulsive therapy but may be unable to understand a complex contract or manage financial matters.

For persons who are recognized as lacking capacity under the law, a guardian may be appointed to give consent.

Parents of a minor are automatically the guardians. In the case of an adult, a court proceeding must first take place to determine if the adult is competent. Competency hearings usually take place when a client refuses hospitalization or treatment; when parental rights over children are at issue; or when the validity of a will is in question. Unfortunately, there is no single national definition of legal incompetency. Incompetency is the legal conclusion that, because of an impairment, the person is no longer able to make responsible decisions for himself, his dependents, or his property.

If a court determines that an adult is incompetent, it appoints a guardian. Typically the court appoints a family member as the guardian. If no family member is available, a friend, a staff member, or other interested person can be appointed. The guardian the court appoints may have power of consent for the person; the power to use his property as necessary; or power over both the person and his property. Most courts have held that the guardian must represent the judgment the client would make, not what the guardian believes is best for the client.[29] For example, a mentally ill client is declared incompetent and the guardian is asked to consent to electroconvulsive therapy. Although the guardian may believe strongly that the client would benefit from the treatment, the guardian's beliefs should not be controlling. If the client had previously said that electroconvulsive therapy was not personally desirable, or if the client had experienced electroconvulsive therapy and indicated that it would be unacceptable in the future, the guardian should present these views.

Secondly, valid consent must also be *voluntary*, not forced, threatened, or given under fraud or distress. Some abuses in this area have arisen in forced or uninformed experimental projects (for example, treatment for syphilis with placebos) or in requiring the client to be part of an experiment in order to gain admittance to a particular unit or residential center (for instance, admittance only if consent is given for a hepatitis study).

Several gray areas may constitute duress. The client who is voluntary but who is threatened with discharge or involuntary commitment if he does not consent to medications, treatment, or continued hospitalization may be a victim of coercion. It has also been suggested that because of the inherent inequality of the physician-client relationship, it is impossible for the client to escape coercion totally (*Kaimowitz v. Department of Mental Health*, 1973).

The third party of valid consent is that it must be *informed*, that is, the person must have sufficient information to make a choice about the treatment (*Cobbs v. Grant*, 1972). Typically the following information must be given a client about the treatment, experiment, or surgery (*Salgo v. Leland Stanford Jr. University Board of Trustees*, 1957):

1. Procedure to be performed
2. Purposes of the procedure
3. Expected result
4. Risks involved
5. Medical alternatives

How much information needs to be given to the client is determined by what other professionals would do in similar circumstances. Legally, most states require that the practitioner tell the client what other practitioners would tell him, although some courts hold that at a minimum the client needs to be told of any risk of death, permanent injury, or delayed recuperation (*Cobbs v. Grant*, 1972). The medical alternatives include only these recognized by medicine. They do not include information on nontraditional treatments, such as those of Indian medicine men. It is also necessary to inform the client of the probable results of refusing the treatment or medications (*Young v. Group Health Cooperative of Puget Sound*, 1976). In *Canterbury v. Spence*, clients were said to be truly informed only if all things "the patient would find significant" in making a decision were shared.[9]

The person who is to perform the procedure is legally responsible for explaining the procedure. Informed consent is the result of one or more conversations between client and physician and is usually evidenced by a written document between the parties. An oral consent is as valid as a written consent but more difficult to prove.

Typically, the more intrusive the procedure, the more likely that a written consent will be obtained because the written document can be used as proof that consent was given. A written consent, however, does not always mean the consent is valid. If any of the three elements of consent is missing, the consent is not valid. A lack of valid, informed consent makes health professionals vulnerable to suits for battery (see earlier discussion). In such a lawsuit, if the treatment and its results have had a serious negative consequence on the client, the court will likely examine the prior presence of each element of consent.

It is advisable for the nurse to be present during the physician's explanation of the procedure so information can be used to teach and care for the client. The nurse may also witness the client's signature to the consent. When nurses act as consent witnesses, they are acknowledging that the client was the one who signed the form. The remainder of the nurse's role as a consent witness is unclear in the courts. The nurse may be responsible for observing indications of disorientation or noting that the information was understood. If the client is very disoriented or indicates misunderstanding, the nurse does not have the client sign the form but notes the disorientation and informs the physician. The major issue in informed consent in the mental health arena is the client's capacity to be *truly* informed. Therefore documentation and assessment by the nurse as to capacity and knowledge are significant.

In certain circumstances treatment may be given even though consent was not obtained or a full explanation was not given to the client. Treatment may be begun if there is an emergency and the client is unable to consent. An emergency is defined differently under each state's law but usually refers to the possible loss of life, an extremity or an eye, or other potentially serious, irreversible physical harm. The client may be unable to consent to treatment because he is semiconscious as a result of a medication overdose. An emergency may also exist if a client is about to injure another person. In an emergency, an attempt to obtain consent from a relative, court, or hospital administrator may be required by state statute. However, if serious consequences may result from such a delay, treatment may be begun without consent.

Consent of minors

The ABA recommends that children be given some independent right to consent to specific forms of treatment.[40]

- Children over 14 years old can consent for themselves to psychotherapy, whereas children under 14 years must have parental consent.
- Parental consent is required for all minors' medication, but a child over the age of 14 years has an independent right to refuse medication. The refusal by the child may be overturned by a court.

Right to refuse treatment

Another evolving issue in mental health law is the right to refuse treatment or to withhold consent. Usually every person has a right to accept or refuse medication or other treatment for any reason, even whim. There is, however, a tension between the client's right to his body and what the physician or society may decide is best for that person.

The mentally ill client's right to refuse medical treatment is not absolute. Clients can usually refuse treatment because it is against their religious beliefs. This was established for mental health clients in *Winters v. Miller* in 1971. Ms. Winters, a 59-year-old client with no dependents, had been involuntarily placed in a New York hospital. Although a practicing Christian Scientist, she was continually medicated despite her objections on religious grounds. She had never been declared by a court to be mentally incompetent. A federal district court found that if a person is competent, the person may refuse treatment. Many states have now included in their statutes a right to refuse treatment because of religious beliefs.[29]

Even when refusal is not on religious grounds, a right to refuse treatment is generally recognized. However, unique problems arise with mental health clients. First, competent clients always have the right to refuse treatment. The problem is determining whether a mentally ill client is in fact competent. Most states, in statute or through case law, hold that, until a separate hearing determines legal incompetency, the client who acts incompetently has all the rights of a competent person, including refusing treatment. Once a person is legally incompetent, the guardian has the power of consent. A guardian does not rely on his own beliefs but should decide as the client would if the client were competent using the client's previous decisions and religious beliefs; the complications of the treatment; and the prognosis in determining whether to consent to or refuse treatment (*Superintendent of Belchertown State School v. Saikewicz*, 1977; *In the Matter of Guardianship of Richard Roe III*, 1981).

In 1979 the voluntary and involuntary clients at the Massachusetts state mental health facilities asked for a clear delineation of when clients could be forcibly medicated. The federal appeals court said that medication could be forced only after legal determination of incompetency, unless there was an emergency. However, the court said that even before a declaration of incompetency, an emergency could be defined as including not only physical harm but also mental deterioration. Because state laws are clear in stating that an emergency treatment can begin without the client's consent, this broad interpretation of emergency situations has far-reaching consequences (*Mills v. Rogers*, 1982). To protect the client's rights, the court did say that in an emergency, psychotropic medications can be forced on the client only after other alternatives had been ruled out. In other words, forced medication in a psychiatric emergency is subject to the LRA principle.

Some states have determined that the right to refuse treatment is based not on a client's competency but on whether the client has a voluntary or an involuntary admission. Such states conclude that voluntary clients have a right to refuse treatment but involuntary clients do not.[1] The Mental Health Systems Act of 1980 (Section 9501) recommends that all states adopt a right to refuse treatment for voluntary clients but does not mention this right for involuntary clients. The issue of whether a competent involuntarily committed client can refuse medication when there is no emergency was introduced in the case of *Rennie v. Klein* (1981). Mr. Rennie, 38 years old, was involuntarily committed to a New Jersey psychiatric hospital in 1976. He had a history of suicidal, homicidal, and delusional episodes and eleven prior hospitalizations. He was not declared incompetent. When Mr. Rennie refused medication, the lower federal court found that involuntarily committed clients have a partial right to refuse treatment. But because the state also has a right to protect other hospitalized clients, there may be some instances in which medication can be forced on involuntarily committed competent clients. To protect the involuntary client's right to refuse treatment, the appeals court said that state regulations which provide review of medication refusal by a treatment team must meet the constitutional due process requirement.

The rights of involuntarily committed clients to refuse medication remain less clearly defined, necessary to be addressed by professionals, and open to further litigation. Institutional policies should be congruent with case law and acknowledge that as treatments become more risky, invasive, or have questionable prognosis, the client's right to refuse is strengthened.

NURSES' INFLUENCE ON CHANGES IN THE LAW

Nurses should be sure their informed opinions are heard and their special advocacy for clients work to influence changes in the law. Expert witnesses, especially on the nursing standard of care, will change case law by increasingly demanding a national standard of nursing practice using generic and psychiatric–mental health standards promulgated by the American Nurses' Association.

When state and federal legislators introduce bills, they collect input from their constituents. Nurses should respond in depth to better develop rights and obligations for mental health care.

The first step in ensuring that legislation reflects nurses' input is to elect legislators who have the views the nursing profession supports. A nurse can do this by being informed about candidates' positions, campaigning for a sympathetic candidate, and voting. There is an American Nurses' Association Political Action Committee (ANA-PAC) with state branches. ANA-PAC and its state political action committees are organized to support candidates who are proponents of health care resources and alternative providers.

After electing a candidate who listens to nurses, the next step is to know what bills are being presented to the state or federal legislatures. To affect the bill, nurses must lobby. This can be done individually or through group efforts, usually the state nurses' association. Individually, nurses can attend committee hearings on the bill and at times testify.

Nurses can also express viewpoints to representatives or senators by telephone, telegram, or letter. A nurse who has helped with a legislator's campaign or is a voter in the legislator's district may get a better reception. A viewpoint should be objective and based on factual data that are presented to validate a position.

Although it is not easy to affect legislation, it is very possible. In one state a nurse who attended a state subcommittee meeting on the mental health code was able to influence the bill so that it reflected a nursing concern. The proposed bill stated that institutionalized clients were required to have a complete physical examination every 2 years. The nurse knew this was too infrequent and reported this to the committee. The committee then adopted the nurse's suggestion that a physical examination be done every 6 months. In another state, psychiatric nurses worked persistently for months to achieve passage of third-party reimbursement for nurse therapists, which would increase access to mental health care in their state.

Belonging to professional associations and lobbying through them is essential. Each state nurses' association has a legislative committee and usually a paid lobbyist who is aware of state legislation affecting nursing and who knows how to influence that legislation. Often state associations have workshops during legislative sessions to teach nurses about the legislative process. The workshops are worthwhile and enable a nurse to watch a representative in action and become familiar with the lobbying process. Special interest groups in the area of mental health, such as the state mental health associations and the ANA Council on Psychiatric Mental Health Nursing also are aware of pending mental health legislation, both federal and state.

BRIEF REVIEW

Legally, the mental health client has many rights, and the nurse has concurrent obligations. Laws that influence mental health care are made by state legislators, Congress, and state and federal courts. To know the law for the state in which the nurse practices, it is necessary to know both state and federal statutes as well as recent cases decided by the state courts, the federal circuit courts and courts of appeals, and the Supreme Court.

The nurse is vulnerable to a malpractice suit when the nursing standard of care is breached and a client is injured. The nurse may also be sued for assault and battery, false imprisonment, or breach of confidentiality. Quality care and accurate documentation are essential protections for the nurse. The nurse may reveal a client communication if the client consents; if the client brings a malpractice action against the nurse; or if there is a duty to warn a known potential victim of a client's threat of serious harm. The nurse must reveal client confidences in a court proceeding unless a state's privileged communication statute applies to nurses.

The U.S. Constitution and state laws have given the mentally ill client many rights. Constitutional amendments have been interpreted in courts as permitting mental health clients to be free from punishment, to be given due process of law, and to have the right to have or refuse treatment. Congress has suggested that states adopt certain civil rights for mentally ill clients, and many states have guaranteed rights.

Mentally ill clients may be institutionalized either by their own consent or through the power of the state. A client may not be involuntarily committed by the state merely for being mentally ill, but most states permit commitment when a client is dangerous to himself or others or when he is gravely disabled. Proving that the client meets the state criteria for commitment involves numerous procedural safeguards concerning the hearing, counsel, and length of commitment. If clear and convincing evidence of the client's dangerousness or grave disability is presented and due process is followed, the state may involuntarily commit the client. A right to treatment and the LRA principle are two emerging trends influencing the commitment process. Minor children may also be committed to mental hospitals, but the law typically does not guarantee them the full due process rights guaranteed to adults. Criminal clients enter mental hospitals if they are found not guilty by reason of insanity or are found imcompetent to stand trial.

In dealing with the mental health system the client has the right to consent to treatment if the client has the mental capacity, has voluntarily given consent, and is informed. The client who is competent has a right to refuse treatment, but the courts have still not fully decided if involuntarily committed clients can refuse treatment. If a client is not competent, a legal guardian may consent to what the client would permit if the client had the capacity to consent.

Mental health laws will change with new statutes and court decisions. The nurse must be aware of the most recent legislation to know the client's rights and the nurse's obligations. The nurse may also influence the law by testifying about the nursing standard of care as an expert witness and by active participation in the political process.

REFERENCES AND SUGGESTED READINGS

1. AA Law: *Psychiatry and mortality essays and analysis,* Washington, DC, 1984, American Psychiatric Press.
2. *Addington v Texas,* 441 U.S. 418, 1979.
3. Amicus brief in *Okin v Rogers, Mental Disability Law Reporter* 2:43, 1977.
4. Andrade P, Andrade J: Malpractice of psychiatric nurse, *Proof of Facts* 2d 26:363, 1981.
5. Beck JC: *The potentially violent patient and the Tarasoff decision in psychiatric practice,* Washington, DC, 1987, American Psychiatric Press.
6. *Boggs v N.Y. City Health and Hospitals,* 523 NY S271; 525 NY S2796, 1988.
7. Brakel SJ, Rock RS, editors: *The mentally disabled and the law,* Chicago, 1971, The University of Chicago Press.
8. Brooks AD: *Law, psychiatry, and the mental health system,* Boston, 1974, Little Brown & Co.
9. *Canterbury v Spence,* 464 F2 772, 1977.
10. *Cobbs v Grant,* 8 Cal. 3d 229, 104 Cal. Rptr. 505, 502 P.2d 1, 1972.
11. Diamond BL: The psychiatric prediction of dangerousness, *University of Pennsylvania Law Review* 123:439, 1974.
12. Ellis J: Volunteering children: parental commitment of minors to mental institutions, *California Law Review* 62:840, 1974.
13. Ellis J: Commitment proceedings for mentally ill and mentally retarded children. In Schetky DH, Benedek EP, editors: *Child psychiatry and the law,* New York, 1980, Brunner/Mazel.
14. *Humphrey v Cady,* 405 U.S. 504, 1972.
15. *In the Matter of Guardianship of Richard Roe III,* 421 N.E. 2d 40 (Mass. 1981).
16. *Jackson v Indiana,* 406 U.S. 715, 1972.
17. *Johnson v Solomon,* 484 F.Suppl. 278, 1979.
18. *Kaimowitz v Department of Mental Health,* 2 Prison L. Rptr. 433 (Cir. Ct. Mich. 1973).
19. Kjervik DK: The psychiatric nurse's duty to warn potential victims of homicidal psychotherapy outpatients, *Law, Medicine and Health Care* 9(6):11, 1981.
20. Laben JK, McLean CP: *Legal issues and guidelines for nurses who care for the mentally ill,* ed 2, Owings Mills, Md, 1984, National Health Publishing.
21. Legal issues in state mental health care: proposals for change—civil commitment, *Mental Disability Law Reporter* 2:75, 1977.
22. *Lessard v Schmidt,* 349 F.Suppl. 1078 (E.D. Wis. 1972) remanded 414 U.S. 473 (1974), on remand 379 F.Suppl. 1379 (1974), remanded 421 U.S. 957 (1975).
23. Mental Health Systems Act, PF 96-398. U.S. Congress, 96th Congress, 1980.
24. *Mills v Rogers,* 102 S.Ct. 2442, 1982.
25. *O'Connor v Donaldson,* 442 U.S. 584, 1979.
26. *Parham v J.L.,* 442 U.S. 584, 1979.
27. *Pisel v Stamford Hospital,* 180 Conn. 314, 430 A2d I, 1980.
28. *Rennie v Klein,* 476 F.Suppl. 1294 (D.N.J, 1979), modified and remanded 653 F.2d 836 (3rd Cir. 1981), cert. denied 49 U.S.I.W. 3911 (U.S. 1981).
29. Right to refuse treatment under state statutes, *Mental Disability Law Reporter* 3:350, 1979.
30. Rights of disabled persons in residential facilities, Mental Disability *Law Reporter* 3:350, 1979.
31. Rinas J, Clyne-Jackson S: *Professional conduct and legal concerns in mental health practice,* San Mateo, Calif, Appleton and Lange, 1988.
32. *Roe v Wade,* 410 U.S. 113 (1973).
33. Ross AM, Betts VT: Legal issues pertinent to the specialty of child and adolescent mental health nursing. In West P, and Evans C, editors: *Child and adolescent mental health nursing,* Rockville, Md, Aspen Publishers, 1992.
34. *Rouse v Cameron* 373 F (D.C. Circuit) 2451 1966.
35. *Salgo v Leland Stanford, Jr., University Board of Trustees,* 154 Cal 2 560, 317 P.170 (1st District, 1957).
36. State laws governing civil commitment, *Mental Disability Law Reporter* 3:206, 1979.
37. Suggested statute on civil commitment, *Mental Disability Law Reporter* 2:127, 1977.
38. Suggested statute on mental health standards and human rights, *Mental Disability Law Reporter* 2:305, 1977.
39. Suggested statute on mental health treatment for minors, *Mental Disability Law Reporter* 2:305, 1977.
40. *Superintendent of Belchertown State School v Saikewicz,* 370 N.E.2d 417 (Mass. 1977).
41. *Tarasoff v Board of Regents of the University of California,* 131 Cal Reptr 14, 551 P 2d 334, 1976.
42. Turnbull HR, editor: *The least restrictive alternative: principles and practices,* Washington, DC, 1981, American Association on Mental Deficiency.
43. *Vitek v Jones,* 445 U.S. 480, 1980.
44. *Webster v Reproductive Health Services,* 109 S.C. 3040 (1989).
45. *Winters v Miller,* 446 F.2d 65 (2nd Cir. 1971), cert. denied, 404 U.S. 985, 1971.
46. *Wood v Strickland,* 420 U.S. 308, 1975.
47. *Wyatt v Stickney,* now *Wyatt v Aderholt,* 325 F.Suppl. 781 (M.D. Ala. 1971), 344 F.Suppl. 373 (M.D. Ala. 1972), 344 F.Suppl. 387 (M.D. Ala. 1972), aff'd 503 F.2d 1305 (5th Cir. 1974).
48. *Young v Group Health Cooperative of Puget Sound,* 535 F.Suppl. 776 (D. Ark. 1976).

ANNOTATED BIBLIOGRAPHY

American Bar Association: *Mental Disability Law Reporter,* Washington, DC.

This bimonthly magazine focuses on the disabled, including the mentally ill. It presents current cases and laws that affect this population. Although it is written mainly for lawyers, it is the most comprehensive summary of current law on the disabled.

Cavadina M: *Mental health law in context,* Brookfield, Vt, 1989, Dartmouth Publishing Co.

In depth view of mental health law. Law for the lawyer and advocate.

Ennis BJ, Emergy RD: *The rights of mental patients,* New York, 1978, Avon Books.

This is an American Civil Liberties Union handbook for mental patients. It presents current law in lay terms on involuntary hospitalization, civil and criminal commitment, and rights in or out of the hospital. It also has fact sections on the problem of defining mental illness and an appendix on drug descriptions, side effects, and dosages.

Klein JI, MacBeth JE, Onek JN: *Legal issues in the private practice of psychiatry,* Washington, DC, 1984, American Psychiatric Press.

Excellent review of private practice psychiatry issues and concerns.

Nursing malpractice: the nurses's duty to follow orders, 90 W.Va. L. Review 1291, 1988.

Legal review of the nursing legal responsibilities in client care.

Parry J, editor: *Mental disability law: a primer,* ed 3, Washington, DC, 1988, American Bar Association.

Brief current look at mental health legal concepts.

Perlin M: *Mental disability law,* Charlottesville, Va, 1989, Michie Company.

Legal treatise that addresses in-depth concepts first touched on in this chapter.

Simon RI: *Clinical psychiatry and the law,* Washington, DC, 1986, American Psychiatric Press, Inc.

An up-to-date review and instructive commentary on legal concerns in the psychiatric practice.

Turnbull HR, editor: *The least restrictive alternative: principles and practices,* Washington, DC, 1981, American Association on Mental Deficiency.

This is a guide to understanding the meaning of the legal term "least restrictive alternative." Its descriptions of various alternatives are useful for client referrals.

CHAPTER

43 Research

Lenora Richardson
Lynne Goodykoontz

After studying this chapter, the student will be able to:

- Describe historical events significant of mental health–psychiatric nursing research
- Explain research approaches in mental health–psychiatric nursing
- Identify studies related to five dimensions of the person

- Discuss challenges of measuring human behavior
- Outline major sources of researchable questions in mental health–psychiatric nursing
- Discuss legal, ethical, and future considerations

Psychiatric–mental health nursing research provides the basis for developing theory and testing clinical approaches that improve the nurse's ability to work therapeutically with clients in a variety of settings.[39] The interpersonal nature of psychiatric nursing lends itself to a combination of subjective and objective data. However, designing research studies of human behavior is difficult. Variables used are often abstract and hard to precisely define. Measurements of human behavior are mostly indirect. Smoyak[68] reports that mental health–psychiatric nurses have trouble applying research findings to practice. Therefore research from other disciplines involving human responses is often used in nursing interventions.

However, there is an increase in research conducted by psychiatric nurses to guide their practice. The Western Interstate Commission for Higher Education compiled the last published summary of the number and topics of studies in mental health–psychiatric nursing; the period covered was 1954 through 1980.[76] These data show a significant increase in nurse-directed research. Most of the studies concerned the nurses themselves, although investigation of clinical issues was evident.

In psychiatric nursing's growth as a specialty, nurses have contributed significantly to the development of clinical research. In a review of research in mental health journals between 1979 and 1991, the authors noted a continued growth in the frequency of mental health–psychiatric nursing research, particularly clinical research. With the recent shift in emphasis from a psychological to a biological view of mental illness (see Chapter 4), psychiatric–mental health nurses are broadening their scope to meet the overall

research needs in the field, including making contributions to neuroscience research.

The most recent statement of the need for psychiatric–mental health nursing research was put forth by the National Institute of Mental Health (NIMH) Task Force on Nursing. The Task Force defined psychiatric nursing research as focusing on the following three areas[51]:

1. Fostering mental health, preventing mental illness, and improving the understanding, treatment, and rehabilitation of the mentally ill
2. Facilitating care of persons who are acutely and chronically mentally ill
3. Improving the delivery of mental health nursing services

Involvement in research is a growing expectation of nurses in all settings. Research is included in the American Nurses' Association's (ANA) Standards of Psychiatric and Mental Health Nursing Practice (see the box on p. 852). Mental health–psychiatric nurses should be familiar with the structure, process, and outcome criteria outlined in Standard XI.[3]

APPROACHES TO RESEARCH

A detailed discussion of the various research approaches, including conditions under which each is most appropriately applicable, may be found in Campbell and Stanley,[13] Kerlinger,[41] Fox,[31] Polit and Hungler,[56] and Seaman and Verhonick.[65] However, several research approaches deemed particularly relevant for mental health–psychiatric nursing will be briefly discussed, with examples of their use.

DATES	EVENTS
1915	Tucker conducted one of the earliest surveys in mental health–psychiatric nursing service that demonstrated the conditions under which mental health–psychiatric nurses functioned.
1928	Taylor did a study on educational qualifications of mental health–psychiatric nurses.
1946	The training grants provided by the National Mental Health Act of 1946 had a significant impact on psychiatric nursing research.[16]
1949	The establishment of the National Institute of Mental Health (NIMH) and psychiatric nursing as a clinical specialty provided funds for psychiatric nursing education and enabled psychiatric nurses to develop research expertise.
1950s	Early studies on nursing care of neuropsychiatric patients exceeded research in all other clinical fields in volume and quality.[61] Nurses participated in and co-authored broad studies of psychiatric care with other professionals.
1956	At the First Midwest Conference on Psychiatric Nursing, Marian Kalkman emphasized the pressing need for nursing research in state hospitals.
1960s	After the community mental health movement, psychiatric nursing research began to deal with the nurse-client relationship.
1983	*Monograph* reported that the number of studies on psychiatric nursing care increased from 28 between 1954 and 1959 to 825 from 1975 to 1980.[76]
1987	Creation of a Task Force on Nursing to examine ways of increasing the participation of nurses in the NIMH.[48]
1990s	Psychiatric nurses are conducting more research on biological aspects of mental illness in collaboration with other professionals.
Future	With increasing emphasis on short-term hospitalization and prevention of illness, nurses will conduct research to promote mental health.

Experimental

One basic distinction in research is that between experimental and nonexperimental. In experimental research the investigator manipulates some condition or phenomenon to assess the effects on some other condition or phenomenon. Therefore the effect of various approaches can be determined. An example of experimental research is seen in the research highlight on p. 853.

Quasi-experimental

Because of the nature of clinical situations in which psychiatric nurses collect data, studies may be conducted under less than controlled situations. When researchers cannot select subjects or assign treatments, a quasi-experimental design may be used. They are similar to experimental studies but are less rigorously controlled. Investigators are challenged with recognizing limitations of their work.[51]

An example of a quasi-experimental design is a study by Courtright and others[18] in which the use of music during mealtime was assessed for effects on acting out behaviors of a group of 109 mentally ill clients. Music was the variable manipulated. Client behaviors were tallied during the din-

ing period. Music was played during two of the 4-week periods and absent during two of the 4-week periods. The results suggested that the use of background music in the dining environment was effective in reducing disruptive behaviors in chronic psychiatric clients.[18]

Nonexperimental

In nonexperimental research the investigator centers on the description of existing conditions or phenomena without manipulation of variables. An example of nonexperimental research follows.

Burgess and others[12] conducted a study in which fifteen juveniles who had committed murders produced five drawings to assist in recalling memory and replicating images of themselves and the murders. Assessment was made of the phases of murder and motivational dynamics. Information was provided to understand what triggered the violent act and underlying beliefs of the offender.

Causal Comparative Research

Causal comparative research is an extension of correlational research in that the researcher attempts not only to discover relationships among variables of interest but also to identify the possible cause after the effects have occurred. With this approach, as with other descriptive approaches, the researcher cannot manipulate the variables. The investigator selects groups that differ on some phenomenon and tries to find variables that might explain the differences.

For example, a researcher who is interested in depression in the elderly may wish to identify factors that are related to depression in this group. The researcher may begin by selecting a sample of elderly persons who were either clinically diagnosed as depressed or scored in the depressed range on an instrument designed to identify depressed persons, such as the Depression Inventory.[5,6] The researcher may then select a sample of elderly persons who are identified either clinically or by the instrument to be within the normal range. The researcher then gathers data on a variety of factors that are determined to be related to depression.

The researcher must recognize that causal comparative research is descriptive; that is, factors that are identified are not interpreted as causative of the condition being investigated. Because the variables are uncontrolled and the subjects are not randomly selected as assigned to groups, any relationships identified may be interpreted only as possible causes. A more rigorous approach is needed to establish a causal relationship.

Qualitative Comparative Analysis

Another method or approach to research is that of qualitative comparative analysis, or grounded theory, described by Glaser and Strauss.[34] This approach is important for theory development, especially in an area in which theoretical bases for explaining phenomena are lacking. Using the qualitative comparative analysis approach, the researcher enters the situation without having formulated specific hypotheses or questions, armed only with the general area of interest. Observations are made in great detail and with great breadth. The researcher then leaves the situation and attempts to discover, from the qualitative data gathered, the variables in the situation. Gradually, as variables and relationships are identified through entries into the situation followed by study of the data, the researcher constructs the theory. The theory is grounded in the phenomena in question through this process. The theory then must be tested using formal research to validate it.

Recognized methods of qualitative research include phenomenological and ethnographical. In phenomenological research, data are structured by subjects' description of experiences and the investigators' interpretation of the descriptions. Data are obtained by interview and written descriptions by subjects. The researcher analyzes and describes the participants' descriptions of the phenomenon. In ethnonursing research, data are structured by the lived experience of the group and the researcher's interpretation of the experience. Data are collected by interview and observations of participants as they normally function in real life. The researcher observes, clarifies, and verifies with the group living the experience of the phenomenon.[56]

The phenomenological research method was used by Hamel-Bissell[37] in generating propositions to explain nurses' reactions to actively suicidal clients. Tape recordings were obtained of 36 female psychiatric nurses who were asked to recall their reactions to actively suicidal clients. The nurses were asked to describe their predominate mood states during experiences with actively suicidal clients. Consistent with the qualitative method of research, the researcher obtained the tape recorded interactions and analyzed them for major themes. The results of the study revealed that nurses have similar feeling states in response to suicidal clients and these feeling states follow a specific pattern. The investigator identified four distinct phases that the nurse goes through when dealing with suicidal clients: naivete, recognition, responsibility, and individual choice. The validity of the model may be further tested using a formal research approach and a larger sample.

Case Study

The case study is a descriptive survey that focuses on one or a limited number of units. The unit of study may be an individual, a group, or an institution. The method involves an attempt to discover, in depth, multiple attributes of the unit. Typically, the case study involves intense study of changes that occur over time. Data may not be subject to statistical interpretation but may require qualitative analyses.

Case studies are often conducted to aid in understanding phenomena or to fully understand a problematic situation in which intervention is needed. The study may provide a

RESEARCH HIGHLIGHT

Leisure: How to Promote Inpatient Motivation After Discharge
• SW Johnson, M McSweeney, and RE Webster

PURPOSE

The purpose of this study was to examine interventions that psychiatric nurses could use to motivate psychiatric clients to be involved in leisure activities after discharge from the hospital.

SAMPLE

Ninety matched volunteer subjects were placed in one of three groups. The diagnosis of 90% of the subjects was depression. The psychiatric inpatients were given classes on participation in leisure activities after discharge. Two additional approaches were used with one group involved in written contracts and the other group involved in written contracts and musical entertainment.

METHODOLOGY

King's Goal Attainment Theory was the basis for examining the transaction of communication between the nurse and client. Three treatment approaches were used. The control group received only leisure planning classes.

In addition to the classes, one of the experimental groups

completed written contracts concerning clients' leisure activity plans after discharge and the other experimental group received the same written contracts and musical entertainment as a reward. All participants completed assessment forms to determine their leisure participation activities before and after hospitalization.

FINDINGS

Both experimental groups were significantly more involved in leisure activities following hospital discharge than the control group that received the classes only intervention. Also, the group receiving the class and contract had more positive changes in leisure activities than the group with the class, contract, and music.

IMPLICATIONS

The educational approach alone does not seem to motivate clients to participate in leisure activities. The addition of the contract appears to have a major influence on clients' behavior. A written contract may facilitate a nurse-client transaction.

Based on data from *Journal of Psychosocial Nursing* 27:9, 1989.

---

baseline from which to proceed. The researcher is able to employ a dynamic process, moving in the most appropriate direction, as information unfolds and interpretations are made. Many researchers in mental health–psychiatric nursing have used the case study method. For example, Prim[57] used the case study method to determine the effectiveness of specific theory based interventions in decreasing the amount of fluids ingested by clients with the syndrome of self-induced water intoxication and psychosis (SIWIP). The unit of study was a 47-year-old male, chronic schizophrenic client with symptoms compatible with idiopathic polydipsia with water intoxication. The researcher used nursing theory to conduct a comprehensive analysis of factors contributing to the polydipsia. Interventions were developed and implemented based on the analysis.

Because case studies focus on an in-depth analysis of a limited number of subjects, they are helpful as a means of identifying areas requiring further study. They may also serve as a means of obtaining information to plan and conduct formal research. A weakness of the case study research method, however, is vulnerability to subjective biases because of the narrow focus and the degree of involvement by the researcher throughout the study.[75]

FIVE DIMENSIONS OF THE PERSON

Research in psychiatric–mental health nursing reflects the five dimensions of the client. Because clients who are diagnosed as mentally ill frequently present with problems in each of these dimensions, research in each is essential to facilitate nurses' understanding of these aspects and to

provide them with a basis for intervening. Examples of research in each of these dimensions will be discussed.

Physical dimension Brown and Tanner[10] conducted a study to determine the reliability and validity of a measure of Type A behavior when used with a preschool group. The sample consisted of 155 preschool children, 2½ years of age to 6½ years of age. The Mathews Youth Test of Health (MYTH) was completed on each of the children to test for the presence of Type A behavior, including hostility, competitiveness, impatience, and leadership subscales. In addition, measures of cardiovascular reactivity (systolic and diastolic blood pressures and pulse), locus of control, and self-esteem were included in the study. Using a standard procedure, the child's blood pressure and pulse were taken in a relaxed state and repeated while the child actively participated in the memory games. Other measures included in the study were obtained 2 weeks after completion of the MYTH. Results of the study indicated that those preschoolers who scored in the Type A range of the MYTH responded with significantly greater systolic blood pressures (SBP) when participating in assigned activities than those preschoolers who scored in the Type B range of the MYTH. The Competitiveness subscale on the MYTH was the most predictive of SBP rsponse to the game involvement, followed by the Hostility and Inpatient subscales. Reliability values of the MYTH were acceptable, indicating that the instrument is a reliable measure of Type A behavior in preschool children. The link of the MYTH to cardiovascular reactivity provides a strong statement for construct validity of the instrument when used with preschoolers. The researchers concluded that the

MYTH is an adequate measure of Type A behavior in preschoolers.

Emotional dimension Kovarsky[42] compared the grief reactions of two types of sudden untimely deaths: the loss of a child (ages 15 to 29 years) by accidental death or by suicidal death. The sample consisted of 31 parents who lost a child to suicide and 21 parents who lost a child to other types of death. Participants in the study completed the Texas Revised Inventory of Grief, the Revised UCLA Loneliness Scale, and the Personal Inventory Sheet. Results of the study indicated that both sets of parents experienced a high degree of disturbed grief and loneliness. However, the grief and loneliness of parents who lost a child by accident abated over time, while the grief and loneliness of parents who lost a child by suicide tended to remain constant or increase over time. The study also indicated that suicide survivors and their families blame themselves and their physicians more often than accident survivors and their families.

Social dimension Stuart and others[69] described the early family experiences of adult women with bulimia and those with depression and contrasted their experiences with those of a nonpsychiatric population of women. The sample consisted of 30 women with bulimia, 15 women diagnosed with a major depressive illness, and a normal control group of 100 women. Participants completed the Memories of Child-Rearing Experiences Questionnaire, Family Violence in Kentucky Questionnaire, Victimization Inventory, and the Early Life Events Questionnaire. Results of the study revealed that the three groups were different with regard to their descriptions of early family experiences. Women with bulimia described a family characterized by problems, tension, threats, and physical coercion. They perceived themselves as being rejected by both parents, with their mother as lacking in warmth and caring and their father as overly controlling. Women with depression identified both parents as rejecting and perceived less warmth from their fathers. Depressed women in the sample also experienced more deaths and chronic physical illnesses than women who were not depressed or bulimic. The researchers concluded that the study allows one to identify children at risk for these disorders by examining childhood perceptions of family experiences.

Intellectual dimension Buckwalter and others[11] examined the behavioral effects of communication interventions on speech-impaired clients. The sample consisted of 23 aphasic and/or dysarthric clients. Clients were exposed to individualized brief speech tasks 10 minutes per shift, one-to-one interactions on any topic 10 minutes per shift, and a control period in which there was no therapy. Results of the study indicated that while clients performed significantly better during the period when they received the speech tasks, they were more satisfied with the intervention of regular staff-client interactions. Further, the benefits of the individualized speech tasks were not maintained throughout the study, except for a few specific areas of dysfunction. The authors concluded that brief daily therapeutic interactions can positively influence the socialization level of communication-impaired clients and interrupt the adverse process of withdrawal.

Spiritual dimension Carson and others[14] examined the relationship between hope and spiritual, religious, and existential well-being. Sixty-five adult male clients known to have HIV antibodies participated in the study. Clients were being treated at an outpatient setting. The study group was divided into those persons with a reported diagnosis of HIV positive, persons diagnosed with AIDS, and persons diagnosed with ARC. Participants completed the Hopelessness and the Spiritual Well-Being Scales. Results of the study indicated that those subjects who were higher in spiritual, existential, and religious well-being tended also to be higher in hope. The results of the study also indicated that the group of participants were both hopeful and spiritually well. Study participants received treatment in a large, well-known, and prestigious research center and persons in another setting may have different levels of hope and spiritual well-being.

MEASUREMENT OF BEHAVIOR

Research in mental health–psychiatric nursing often involves the measuring of behavior. The measurements can be indirect or direct. Most direct measures are physiological, such as laboratory tests and blood pressure, pulse, and respiration measurements. Accurate measurement of psychological characteristics such as anxiety, dependency, and hope are more technical and therefore difficult to achieve. In mental health–psychiatric nursing, instruments such as questionnaires are used most often in research. These instruments may be constructed by investigators or borrowed from other researchers. Instruments may be found in journals or books. A number of authors have prepared collections of instruments for the mental health–psychiatric nursing researcher.[15,17,54,58,60]

The researcher tries to identify instruments that measure the variables of the study as accurately and precisely as possible, which generally is not easy in psychiatric—mental health nursing. Without an accurate measure of the variables of interest, the research conducted is useless.

The many difficulties with instrumentation have been addressed by nurse researchers; an entire issue of Nursing Research (September-October 1981) was devoted to this problem. Reliability and validity of instruments especially are areas of concern in the study of human behavior. Reliability refers to the ability of the instrument to consistently measure the same trait upon repeated measurements. The two most common types of reliability are stability and internal consistency. Stability, as measured by the test-retest method, is expressed as the correlation between the scores from two administrations of the same test to the same subjects. Internal consistency refers to the consistency of performance of a group of individuals on the items of a single test.[38] It is difficult to establish reliability in behavioral research, in part because many of the traits of interest change over time, independently of the stability of the measure. In addition, clients may actually change as a result of the first administration. Poorly standardized instruction, errors resulting from subjectivity, and fluctuations in the individual are examples of influences that lower the reliability of psychological measurements. The nurse can improve reliability by (1) writing clear items for the measuring instrument, (2) adding more items of equal kind and quality, and (3) writing clear and standard instructions.[41]

More doubt is expressed by professionals concerning

the validity rather than reliability of psychological measurement. Validity refers to the extent to which an instrument measures what it intends to measure. A precondition for validity is reliability. An instrument cannot be useful for the purposes for which it is intended if it does not measure consistently. Instruments often work well on physical qualities and relatively simple characteristics. They work less well on the measurement of complex behavior. The nurse can attempt to validate the measurement instrument by (1) content validation—determining the adequacy of the instrument in measuring the content of the particular situation under consideration, (2) criterion validation—a comparison of the study instrument with other measurements known or believed to measure the same traits or characteristics, and (3) construct validation—determining the extent to which certain components of the phenomenon being studied account for performance on the instrument. Construct validity examines the theory that explains the differences in the behavior measured.

Foreman[30] conducted a study to assess and compare reliability and validity of three mental status questionnaires using a group of 66 elderly hospitalized clients. Instruments were the Short Portable Mental Status Questionnaire (SPMSQ), Mini-Mental State Examination (MMSE), and the Cognitive Capacity Screening Examination (CCSE). Internal consistency reliability as well as content, criterion-related, and construct validity were assessed. Internal consistency reliability was determined by conducting the statistical procedure Kuder-Richardson 20 to determine if all of the items on the questionnaire were measuring just one attribute or phenomenon. Construct validity was determined by conducting a factor analysis statistical procedure to determine if within each of the mental status exams, various components of cognitive functioning were effectively identified. Criterion related validity was determined by correlating each of the mental status questionnaires with the client's clinical diagnosis of global cognitive impairment as determined by physicians and nurses. Content validity was determined by reviewing and summarizing the research and clinical literature about the three mental status questionnaires. The results of the study indicated that only the CCSE consistently exceeded minimally acceptable standards of reliability and validity. Therefore the validity and reliability of the CCSE was supported for the sample in the study.

Dingeman and others[21] conducted a study to determine the reliability and factor structure of the Nurses' Observation Scale for Inpatient Evaluation (NOSIE) using a group of 247 short-stay psychiatric clients. Items were grouped into seven factors: social competence, social interest, personal neatness, irritability, manifest psychosis, retardation, and depression. The clients were rated on each item of the NOSIE by two psychiatric nurses independently. The results were very similar among American, English, and Dutch clients (except for the social competence and personal neatness subscales in the Dutch). Therefore the instrument's reliability and validity were supported.

The competence of clients to complete the instrument as expected is also a concern. Medication and particular symptoms, such as psychosis, may affect clients' ability to respond validly. Differences in the measurement settings and investigators may affect the results of the study. Therefore researchers must be thoroughly familiar with the research instruments, setting, and protocol, that is the manner in which the research is to be conducted.

SOURCES OF RESEARCHABLE QUESTIONS

Researchable questions or problems in mental health–psychiatric nursing may stem from a variety of sources, including theory, the literature, and nurses' own experiences. The practitioner in mental health–psychiatric nursing collaborates with the nurse researcher to develop questions and problems for study directly relevant to clinical practice. Questions arise in daily practice that, when placed in an appropriate framework and properly developed, can be researched. Questions about the clinical area are frequently initiated this way. A study may flow from a specific problem or a more general need. In either case research questions may involve the client, nurse, client-nurse interactions, interventions, or anything of curiosity. The research conducted by Nokes and Kendrew[52] on experiences of loneliness among HIV infected veterans and its relationship to the development of infections is an example of research on clinical problems.

Dawkins and others[20] demonstrate research on the nurse. They examined factors that contributed to the job stress of 43 psychiatric nurses. Many questions about the interaction between the client and the nurse can be posed. An example is an investigation of the effect of the nurse's leadership style on client behavior in group therapy. Questions about the setting may include a comparison of the effects of rape victim counseling in the hospital emergencyroom with counseling in the victim's home. Many studies have been done to evaluate interventions. A 1989 study by Johnson and others[40] evaluated the effectiveness of three different interventions to motivate psychiatric inpatients to become involved in leisure activities after discharge.

A number of questions have come from researcher curiosity:

1. What are the characteristics of elderly persons who choose to attend a program on human sexuality?
2. What are differences among various cultural groups in coping styles?
3. What changes occur in relationships with significant others in younger compared with older bereaved individuals in the first year after death?

To establish priorities in mental health–psychiatric research, a study was conducted using the Delphi technique. The Delphi technique is a methodological tool used for problem-solving, planning, and forecasting. It consists of several rounds of questionnaires completed by experts on a specific topic of interest. The goal is to obtain group consensus of opinions without face to face meetings.

Opinions of 367 Veterans Administration (VA) nurses were gathered to identify areas in which nurses needed to conduct research.[74] As seen in Table 43-1, a top priority was to identify factors that contributed to repeated admissions and effective assessment and interventions. Client teaching, care planning, and methods to assist staff with motivation were also seen as high priorities.

The ANA standards of nursing practice provide ideas for research that focus on testing relationships between nursing interventions and client outcome (Table 43-2). An example is a study designed to determine interventions ef-

▼ **TABLE 43-1**   The Highest Fifteen Priorities of Mental Health–Psychiatric Nurses in Veterans Administration Institutions

Rank	Item
1	After identifying factors that contribute to repeated hospital admissions, determine and evaluate interventions that reduce readmission among VA clients with chronic problems.
2	Explore the factors that relate to continuity of care after hospitalization, with emphasis on the nurse's role.
3	After developing criteria to assess the client's compliance, explore those interventions that enhance the client's response to the health maintenance program.
4	After examining contributing factors to staff burnout, determine various ways to deal with this phenomenon in the VA system.
5	Identify factors that influence and increase psychiatric symptomatology in hospitalized VA clients.
6	Identify assessment criteria to predict potentially suicidal clients and preventive nursing interventions for self-destructive behavior.
7	Evaluate the effectiveness of various approaches to care planning on client care and nursing staff satisfactions.
8	Develop reliable and valid criteria to assess the client's readiness to learn, and evaluate the effects of teaching clients.
9	Explore and evaluate supportive measures to enhance the care of terminally ill clients and their families (for example, hospice, Brompton's solution, and family counseling).
10	Explore the effects of treatment approaches such as milieu therapy, chemotherapy, and specific nursing interventions for clients with psychiatric problems.
11	After exploring the role of the VA in providing health maintenance and prevention programs, identify and evaluate effective methods for accomplishing this.
12	Determine effective approaches to motivate staff to provide quality care for veterans.
13	Define quality nursing care and develop valid and reliable criteria to measure it.
14	Identify factors that contribute to successful implementation of primary nursing in VA health care settings.
15	Explore nursing comfort measures to help clients manage and tolerate pain.

Modified from Ventura MR, Waligora-Serafin B: Study priorities identified by nurses in mental health settings, *International Journal of Nursing Studies* 18:41, 1981.

▼ **TABLE 43-2**   Ideas for Research from ANA Standards

Nursing Intervention	Client Outcome
Psychotherapeutic	Regains or improves previous coping ability.
Health teaching	Prevents further disability. Demonstrates acquisition of knowledge.
Activities of daily living	Attains level of ability in self-care in acute and rehabilitation phases.
Somatic therapies	Incorporates knowledge of somatic and drug therapies into self-care activities.
Therapeutic environment	Is oriented to schedule and rules for milieu. Knows reasons for and condition of release from restraint or seclusion. Demonstrates awareness of environmental effects on health.
Psychotherapy (individual, group, or family)	Articulates elements of therapeutic contract. Demonstrates responsibility for therapeutic work. Shows movement toward goals of therapy.

From Western Interstate Commission for Higher Education: *A sourcebook: research in psychiatric nursing,* Boulder, Colo, 1983, Western Interstate Commission for Higher Education.

or methods may suggest a project. Often a study may be replicated with another sample, another setting, or some variation that can increase knowledge about the problem being investigated.

Theory may serve as a source of researchable problems. According to Stevens,[70] theory describes or explains, whereas research is designed to test the description or explanation. Research is necessary to determine the accuracy of theory.

Researchable questions may develop as the nurse interacts with professionals from related disciplines. The nurse researcher may wish to compare aspects of her practice with those of others. For example, how do nursing interventions compare with interventions used by social workers or clinical psychologists. Because nursing is a practice discipline, theories of many other disciplines have stimulated ideas for nursing research and are likely to continue to do so in the future. Theories on stress, families, change, and adaptation are only a few that are relevant to mental health–psychiatric nursing. Behavioral theories are particularly significant.

fective in reducing a client's level of anxiety. Anxiety levels may be reduced through teaching techniques that benefit both clients and staff.[61]

Research questions may also arise from the literature. Studies published in *Nursing Research* and other journals often conclude with suggestions for related research. Juxtaposition of several studies may create an idea for another.

Descriptions of particular interventions, an instrument,

HUMAN AND LEGAL CONSIDERATIONS

The ANA's Human Rights Guidelines[2] for Nurses in Clinical and Other Research provide a framework for involving clients in investigation. They identify human rights—the right to freedom from intrinsic risk or injury and the right of privacy and dignity. Informed consent means that a person knowingly, voluntarily, intelligently, and in a clear and manifest way gives consent to participate in experimental procedures.[22]

The issue of informed consent for psychiatric clients presents special challenges. A psychiatric client's ability to understand information relevant to participating in the study may vary from time to time, depending on psychiatric symptoms, for example, inability to concentrate or mood fluctuations.[19] These same characteristics compromise the client's ability to respond accurately to research instruments, leading to an inaccurate portrayal of the phenomenon being studied. Therefore researchers in mental health–psychiatric nursing need to assess that clients are competent to give informed consent and accurately respond to research instruments.

Several principles in the ANA's Code for Nurses[1] emphasize the nurse's obligation to safeguard confidential information about a client obtained from any source. The researcher explicitly ensures confidentiality by the consent form given to each prospective subject asked to participate in research.

FUTURE RESEARCH

The question of what lies ahead for nursing was the subject of an issue of The American Nurse.[1] The future of nursing will likely be focused on prevention, the aging population, and distributive care. Research emphasis will continue to move from basic to applied areas of excesses, such as smoking and obesity.

Sill's[66] work of 14 years ago still has implications for psychiatric nursing today and will continue to have implications in the future. Sill[66] proposed that mental health–psychiatric nursing research focus on determination of boundaries of health care, which include the boundaries of nursing care. Sills also recommended research on healthy individuals and quality of life rather than illness.

McBride[49] urged that research be done to understand the illness experience of clients and to evaluate the cost effectiveness of nursing services provided. McBride also urged nursing research that focuses more on nursing care than doing therapy. More recently McBride[48] has suggested that research in nursing should combine recent gains made in knowledge about brain function with the psychological, social, and cultural factors that also influence human behavior. Such research would involve psychiatric nurses in managing side effects of medications, to monitoring mood states and circadian rhythms, to understanding environmental effects, such as parental discord, on the brain chemistry and functioning in children. Fleming[29] urged that research be done in areas of preventive health, nursing care, and conditions likely to persist in the future.

In the 1984 and 1985 forum to discuss issues in psychiatric nursing, the Council of Directors of Graduate Programs identified the need for research studies to examine the relationship between clinical research and public policy. The Council also stated that research must examine the concept of reversibility in organic disorders and that research must demonstrate what nurses offer as clinicians. Research also needs to examine the effects of rapid societal changes.

A Task Force on Nursing appointed by the National Institute of Mental Health emerged because of a growing need for research efforts to decrease a rapidly expanding population at risk for the development of major mental disorders and to develop strategies to reduce disability associated with psychiatric disorders.[48] These problems continue to be research priorities for researchers in psychiatric–mental health nursing.

Smoyak[68] wrote that research on interactions between therapists and clients is needed. Generally, she identified a need for research that documents which interventions work and when they work with families. Specifically, she gave direction to an area of study by investigating the contract between therapist and client. Smoyak raises the question, "Is the contract one that the therapist wants or the client wants?"

The uses of psychotherapy and family therapy are instances of the nurse's expanded role that need to be explored. Interpersonal systems theories and crisis and rhythm theory have a bearing on the expanded role.[27]

Classifying psychiatric clients according to their needs for nursing care also requires research. The problems of identifying behaviors and the less defined procedural emphasis make classification difficult largely because of the interpersonal nature of mental health–psychiatric nursing. Confidence in a given system depends on being certain of its validity and reliability. Some systems sufficiently classify clients according to nursing care needs, whereas other systems have not been adequate. Psychiatric client classification systems need to incorporate indentifiable behaviors specific to this population and have less emphasis on procedural aspects. Loomis[46] has gone far in developing a classification system for psychiatric–mental health nursing (see Chapter 8). Studies like that of Schroder and others[64] need to be done to determine the validity and reliability of this and other client classification systems in psychiatry.

The future direction of research in this field is toward health and wellness. Attention will be given to incorporating a more holistic approach to client care.

BRIEF REVIEW

Psychiatric–mental health nursing research provides the basis for developing theory and testing clinical approaches to improve nursing pratice. Psychiatric nurses continue to make contributions to nursing research, especially clinical research. With the recent change in emphasis from a psychological to a biological view of causes of mental illness, psychiatric nurses have begun making contributions to neuroscience research. The NIMH Task Force on Nursing's definition of psychiatric nursing research also provides some direction for the focus of psychiatric–mental health nursing research.

Methodological approaches relevant to mental health–psychiatric nurse researchers include experimental, quasi-experimental, and nonexperimental approaches, such as casual comparative research. Phenomenological and ethnographical are two types of qualitative research used by psychiatric nurses. Many researchers in mental health–psychiatric nursing have used the case study.

Recent research in psychiatric–mental health nursing

has focused on one or more of the five dimensions of the client. Research that focuses on the five dimensions facilitates the nurse's understanding of the client's behavior and provides a basis for intervention.

Measurement of behavior is problematic because of the individual's complexity. An important prerequisite to reliable and valid research is the selection of instruments that appropriately measure the variable in question. Traditional standardized tests and other instruments can be found in publications on nursing or psychological variables and not in published and unpublished studies. Uniformity in administration is essential for valid research.

Research questions may be generated within nursing practice or a related area. Other sources of researchable questions include theory and published literature. The nurse's curiosity is a source for research questions.

Informed consent for psychiatric clients presents a challenge. The client's ability to understand information relevant to participating in the research may vary. The client may not be able to appropriately respond to the instrument.

Future research in mental health—psychiatric nursing is likely to be applied as opposed to basic, focusing on healthy individuals, prevention health issues, and problems that are likely to persist. Also, theory testing and classification systems will be investigated.

REFERENCES AND SUGGESTED READINGS

1. American Nurses' Association: *Code for nurses with interpretive statements,* Kansas City, Mo, 1976, American Nurses' Association.
2. American Nurses' Association: *Human rights guidelines for nurses in clinical and other research,* Kansas City, 1975, The Association.
3. American Nurses' Association: *Standards of psychiatric and mental health nursing practice,* Kansas City, 1982, The Association.
4. Baker B, Lynn M: Psychiatric nursing consultation: the use of an inservice model to assist nurses in the grief process, *Journal of Psychiatric Nursing and Mental Health Services* 17(7):43, 1979.
5. Beck AT: *Depression,* Philadelphia, 1967, University of Pennsylvania Press.
6. Beck AT and others: An inventory for measuring depression, *Archives of General Psychiatry* 4:561, 1961.
7. Brandt P, Weinert C: The PRQ: a social support measure, *Nursing Research* 30:277, 1981.
8. Brower H, Tanner L: A study of older adults attending a program on human sexuality: a pilot study, *Nursing Research* 28:36, 1979.
9. Brown E: *Newer dimensions of patient care. II. Improving staff motivation and competence in the general hospital,* New York, 1962, Russell Sage Foundation.
10. Brown MS, Tanner C: Measurement of Type A behavior in pre-schoolers, *Nursing Research* 39(4):207, 1990.
11. Buckwalter KC and others: The behavioral consequences of a communication intervention on institutionalized residents with aphasia and dysarthia, *Archives of Psychiatric Nursing* 2(5):289, 1988.
12. Burgess A and others: Juvenile murderers: assessing memory through crime scene drawings, *Journal of Psychosocial Nursing* 29(1):26, 1990.
13. Campbell D, Stanley J: Experimental and quasiexperimental designs for research, Skokie, Ill, 1963, Rand McNally & Co.
14. Carson V and others: Hope and spiritual well-being: essen-
tials for living with AIDS, *Perspectives in Psychiatric Care* 26(2):28, 1990.
15. Cattell J, Warburton F: Objective personality and motivation tests, Chicago, 1967, University of Illinois Press.
16. Chamberlain J: The role of the federal government in developing of psychiatric nursing, *Journal of Psychosocial Nursing and Mental Health Services* 21(4):11, 1983.
17. Churn K, Cobb S, French J Jr: *Measures for psychological assessment,* Ann Arbor, Mich, 1975, Survey Research Center.
18. Courtright P and others: Dinner music: does it affect the behavior of psychiatric inpatients? *Journal of Psychosocial Nursing* 28(3):37, 1990.
19. Davis A, Underwood P: The competency quagmire: clarification of the nursing perspective concerning the issues of competence and informed consent, *International Journal of Nursing Studies* 26(3):271, 1989.
20. Dawkins JE, Depp FC, Selzer NE: Stress and the psychiatric nurse, *Journal of Psychosocial Nursing* 23(11):9, 1985.
21. Dingeman PM and others: A cross-cultural study of the reliability and factorial dimensions of the nurses' observation scale for inpatient evaluation (NOSIE), *Journal of Clinical Psychology* 40(1):169, 1984.
22. Downey M: A bill to regulate Defense Department experimental procedures in human subjects (HR 13457), U.S. Senate, 94th Congress, second session, April 29, 1976. In Arniger B Sr: Ethics in nursing research, *Nursing Research* 26:334, 1977.
23. Downs FS: *A sourcebook of nursing research,* ed 3, Philadelphia, 1984, FA Davis.
24. Downs F: The relationship of findings of clinical research and development of criteria: a researcher's perspective, *Nursing Research* 29:94, 1980.
25. Dracup K, Meleis A: Compliance: an interactionist approach, *Nursing Research* 31:31, 1982.
26. Fawcett J: A declaration of nursing independence: the relationship of theory and research to practice, *Journal of Nursing Administration* 10(6):36, 1980.
27. Fitzpatrick JJ and others: *Nursing models and their psychiatric mental health applications,* Bowie, Md, 1982, Robert J. Brady Co.
28. Flaskerud J: Perceptions of problematic behavior by Appalachians, mental health professionals, and lay non-Appalachians, *Nursing Research* 29:140, 1980.
29. Fleming J: The future of nursing research. In Downs F, Fleming J, editors: *Issues in nursing research,* New York, 1979, Appleton-Century-Crofts.
30. Foreman M: Reliability and validity of mental status questionnaires in elderly hospitalized patients, *Nursing Research* 36(4):216, 1987.
31. Fox D: *Fundamentals of research in nursing,* ed 4, New York, 1982, Appleton-Century-Crofts.
32. Fox D, Leeser I: *Readings on the research process in nursing,* New York, 1981, Appleton-Century-Crofts.
33. Friedeman J: Development of a sexual knowledge inventory for elderly persons, *Nursing Research* 28:372, 1979.
34. Glaser B, Strauss A: *The discovery of grounded theory: strategies for qualitative research,* Chicago, 1967, Aldine Publishing Co.
35. Gortner S: Nursing research: out of the past and into the future, *Nursing Research* 29:204, 1980.
36. Haller K, Reynolds M, Horsley J: Developing research based innovation protocols: process, criteria, and issues, *Research in Nursing and Health* 2:45, 1979.
37. Hamel-Bissell B: Suicidal casework, assessing nurses' reactions, *Journal of Psychosocial Nursing* 23(10):20, 1985.
38. Huck SW and others: *Reading statistics and research,* New York, 1974, Harper & Row.
39. Hoeffer B, Beeson L, Gowdy V: Mental health nursing. In Tan-

ner C, Lindeman CA, editors: *Using nursing research*, New York, 1989, National League for Nursing.

40. Johnson S and others: Leisure: how to promote inpatient motivation after discharge, *Journal of Psychosocial Nursing* 27(9):29, 1989.

41. Kerlinger R: *Foundations of behavioral research*, New York, 1964, Holt, Rinehart and Winston.

42. Kovarsky RS: Loneliness and disturbed grief: a comparison of parents who lost a child to suicide or accidental death, *Archives of Psychiatric Nursing* 3(2):86, 1989.

43. Krampitz S, Pavlovich N, editors: *Readings for nursing research*, St Louis, 1981, Mosby—Year Book.

44. Larson E and others: Comparison of two schema for classifying nursing research, *Image: Journal of Nursing Scholarship* 23(3):161, 1991.

45. Liaschenko J: Changing paradigms within psychiatry: implications for nursing research, *Archives of Psychiatric Nursing* 3(3):153, 1989.

46. Loomis M: Discussion: psychosocial nursing diagnosis, *Archives of Psychiatric Nursing* 2(6):357, 1988.

47. Marram G: Barriers to research in psychiatric—mental health nursing: implications for preparing the nurse researcher, *Journal of Psychiatric and Mental Health Services* 14(4):7, 1976.

48. McBride AB: Psychiatric nursing in the 1990's, *Archives of Psychiatric Nursing* 4(1):21, 1990.

49. McBride A: Present issues and future perspectives of psychosocial nursing, *Journal of Psychosocial Nursing* 24(9):27, 1986.

50. Miller T: Life events scaling: clinical methodological issues, *Nursing Research* 30:316, 1981.

51. National Institute of Mental Health: Report of the task force on nursing, Rockville, Md, 1987, National Institute of Mental Health.

52. Nokes K, Kendrew J: Loneliness in veterans with AIDS and its relationship to the development of infections, *Archives of Psychiatric Nursing* 4(4):271, 1990.

53. Norman J and others: Psychiatric patients view of their life before and after moving to a hostel: a qualitative study, *Journal of Advanced Nursing* 15(9):1036, 1990.

54. Pfeiffer J, Heslin R: *Instrumentation in human relations training*, Iowa City, 1973, University Associates.

55. Pincus HA, Pardes H: Clinical research careers in psychiatry, Washington, DC, 1986, JB Lippincott.

56. Polit D, Hungler B: Nursing research: principles and methods, ed 2, Philadelphia, 1987, JB Lippincott.

57. Prim R: Water intoxication and psychosis syndrome, *Journal of Psychosocial Nursing* 26(11):16, 1988.

58. Robinson J, Shaver P: Measures of social psychological attitudes, Ann Arbor, Mich, 1973, Institute for Social Relations, University of Michigan.

59. Rose LE: Ethical considerations of patient involvement in clinical psychiatric research, *Canadian Mental Health* 34(2):8, 1986.

60. Rugh J, Schwitzgebel R: Instrumentation for behavioral assessment. In Ciminero A, Calhoun K, Adams H, editors: *Handbook of behavioral assessment*, New York, 1977, John Wiley & Sons.

61. Sadow D, Syder M: Anxiety reduction lessons that benefit students and patients, *Journal of Psychosocial Nursing* 28(9):29, 1990.

62. Schanding D and others: A small study of how the staff of an inpatient psychiatric unit spends its time, *Perspectives in Psychiatric Care* 10(2):91, 1982.

63. Schmidt S: Withdrawal behavior of schizophrenics: application of Roy's model, *Journal of Psychosocial Nursing and Mental Health Services* 19(11):26, 1981.

64. Schroder PJ and others: Testing validity and reliability in a psychiatric patient classification system, *Nursing Management* 17(1):49, 1986.

65. Seaman C, Verhonick P: *Research methods*, ed 2, New York, 1982, Appleton-Century-Crofts.

66. Sills G: Research in the field of psychiatric nursing: 1952-1977, *Nursing Research* 26:201, 1977.

67. Slavinsky A, Kerauss J: Two approaches to the management of long-term psychiatric outpatients in the community, *Nursing Research* 31:285, 1982.

68. Smoyak S: Clinical practice: institute or based on research, *Journal of Psychosocial Nursing and Mental Health Services* 29(4):9, 1982.

69. Stuart GW and others: Early family experiences of women with bulimia and depression, *Archives of Psychiatric Nursing* 4(1):43, 1990.

70. Stevens B: *Nursing theory: analysis, application, evaluation*, Boston, 1979, Little, Brown & Co.

71. Stricklin ML: The mental health patient assessment record: interobserver reliability, *Nursing Research* 28:11, 1979.

72. Topf M, Dambacher B: Predominant source of interpersonal influence in relationships between psychiatric patients and nursing staff, *Research in Nursing and Health* 2(1):35, 1979.

73. Ventura M, Hinshaw A, Atwood J: Intrumentation: the next step, *Nursing Research* 30:257, 1981.

74. Ventura MR, Waligora-Serafin B: Study priorities identified by nurses in mental health settings, *International Journal of Nursing Studies* 18:41, 1981.

75. Waltz C, Bausell R: *Nursing research: design, statistics and computer analysis*, Philadelphia, 1983, FA Davis.

76. Western Interstate Commission for Higher Education: *A sourcebook: research in psychiatric mental health nursing*, Boulder, Colo, 1983, Western Interstate Commission for Higher Education.

77. Williams M and others: Nursing activities and acute confusional states, *Nursing Research* 28:25, 1979.

78. Wilson H: *Deinstitutionalized residential care for the mentally disordered: the Soteria House approach*, New York, 1982, Grune & Stratton.

79. Wilson HS, Hutchinson SA: *Applying nursing research*, Reading, Mass, 1986, Addison-Wesley.

80. Youssef FA: Adherence to therapy in psychiatric patients: an empirical investigation, *International Journal of Nursing Studies* 21(1):51, 1984.

ANNOTATED BIBLIOGRAPHY

Brooking J, editor: *Psychiatric nursing research*, New York, 1986, John Wiley & Sons.

This book presents a collection of research studies that give the reader an overview of relevant research in the field of psychiatric nursing in the mid 1980s. The studies still are beneficial in posing questions about methodology and presenting hypotheses for future research. The book is useful for nursing students, nurse educators, nurse researchers, and nurse managers.

Fitzpatrick JJ, Wykle ML, Morris DL: Collaboration in care and research, *Archives of Psychiatric Nursing* 4(1):53, 1990.

The authors present a model of research in geriatric—mental health nursing to exemplify psychiatric—mental health nursing care and research in collaboration with other health professionals. The article addresses the NIMH Task Force on Nursing's definition of psychiatric mental health nursing research. Strategies to enhance collaboration for improved client health are presented.

Liasachenko J: Changing paradigms within psychiatry: implications for nursing research, *Archives of Psychiatric Nursing* 3(3):153, 1989.

This article addresses the change in focus from a psychological paradigm to a biological one for determining the causes of mental illness. The author explores the implications of this change for psychiatric nursing research. The article includes useful application of Sills' 1977 views on research in psychiatric nursing.

McBride AG: Psychiatric nursing in the 1990s, *Archives of Psychiatric Nursing* 4(1):21, 1990.

This article reviews the accomplishments of psychiatric nursing and addresses some of the limitations in the field. The author describes some of the challenges for the 1990s, with attention to the need to integrate the biological sciences and behavioral sciences in the practice of psychiatric nursing. The article includes useful content on setting a research practice agenda for the future.

Western Interstate Commission for Higher Education: *A sourcebook: research in psychiatric mental health nursing,* Boulder, Colo, 1983, Western Interstate Commission for Higher Education.

This monograph discusses issues in psychiatric–mental health nursing. A summary of topics of master theses and literature and a listing of studies in psychiatric–mental health nursing are presented.

Quality Assurance/Quality Improvement

Elizabeth B Brophy
Diane M Hedler

After studying this chapter, the student will be able to:

- Define quality assurance and quality improvement
- Recognize the evolving character of quality assurance and improvement
- Critique the American Nurses' Association standards of care in mental health–psychiatric nursing

- Give examples of protocols and a quality assurance program for nurses
- Analyze modes of professional development in terms of their effects on client care
- Differentiate between licensure and certification
- Show how quality assurance and improvement can be applied to nursing models

The rules are changing in health care. Quality assurance (QA) is currently evolving into *quality improvement* (QI), or *continuous quality improvement* (CQI), building on the positive characteristics of it's predecessor. How do the two differ? How have they developed?

Quality assurance is a process by which excellence in health care is sought. For nurses, as for other health care professionals, it involves professional standards of care, ways to measure the effectiveness of interventions, and, if necessary, corrective action to improve client care. *Quality improvement* is also a process based on the philosophy that quality care is the responsibility of each individual within the system and that all health-related tasks must fit together to meet client expectations and institutional goals.

Quality assurance/quality improvement is an important aspect of mental health–psychiatric nursing for several reasons. First, quality assurance programs help nurses monitor their practice in a systematic way. Mental health–psychiatric nurses want to ensure that their care contributes to the mental health of the person, the family, and the community. By developing and using procedures that improve the quality of care, nurses can maintain the standards they have developed.

Second, federal funds, particularly those provided through Medicare, Medicaid, and maternal and child health programs, are available only after standards of care have been met. State agencies have similar requirements and accrediting groups such as the Joint Commission on Accreditation of Healthcare Organizations (JCAHO) require formal assessment programs.

Finally, quality assurance/quality improvement is important to public confidence in health care professionals.

The increased involvement of insurance companies and other private and public organizations in the evaluation of health care systems suggests that confidence in the quality of health has eroded. Quality assurance/quality improvement programs are one way for nurses to regulate their profession, maintain a high level of performance, and retain the confidence of the public.

THE EVOLUTION OF QUALITY ASSURANCE

In 1986 the JCAHO recognized that the Quality Assurance guidelines were not providing an adequate evaluation of hospital performance. An Agenda for Change, that is, a plan of action, was developed. The focus of the Agenda for Change is to challenge health care providers to consistently improve every aspect of the institutions' functions. One idea about how to proceed came from industry.

After World War II, W. Edwards Deming worked with Japanese manufacturers to introduce quality control and emphasize improvement in productivity. The Deming method became known as the total quality management (TQM), or the continuous quality improvement (CQI) approach.[21] In a review of related literature, Masters and Schmele[36] pointed out that "opportunities to improve quality care were mainly related to problems of process or structure and generally were not related to employee behaviors" (p. 8). Deming thought that a lack of quality is seldom a consequence of a lack of motivation in the individual, but rather of the procedures used within the system.

During the mid-1980s, the Deming method was applied to health care institutions. In 1989 Batalden and Buchanan[12] described the process as it was utilized by the Hospital

HISTORICAL OVERVIEW

DATES	EVENTS
1858	Florence Nightingale documented her attempts to raise the standards of health care during the Crimean War.
1912	E.A. Codman introduced the first system of medical audit.
1913	The American College of Surgeons introduced accreditation for medical education and performance.
1923	The Goldmark Report recommended closing substandard nursing schools, instituting 48-hour workweek, and encouraging staff nurses rather than student nurses to assume responsibility in hospitals.
1948	The Brown Report, funded by the Carnegie Foundation, recommended national accreditation for nursing schools and affiliation of hospital schools with universities.
1955	*Hospital Progress* made reference to evaluation by means of nurses' notes. American Nurses' Foundation was formed to conduct, sponsor, and stimulate research.
1956	The Commission on Professional and Hospital Activities, Inc. was formed.
1957	Thayer Hospital, Waterville, Maine, developed the nursing audit plan.
1960	Sr. M. Deeken developed a guide for the nursing service audit.
1965	The American Nurses' Association (ANA) wrote its position paper on entry into practice. National League for Nursing (NLN) provided a self-evaluation guide to assess nurses' functions and skills.
1967	Yura and Walsh defined evaluation as one of the four functions of the nursing process. D. Slater developed a rating scale with six dimensions of nursing behavior. Amendments were made to Medicare and Medicaid legislation. Utilization review committees were created.
1970	Wandelt and Agar developed the Quality Patient Care Scale (Qual-PaCS), based on observation and rating. The JCAH shifted focus from provision of minimal to optimal care by means of retrospective medical care audits.
1971	The ANA Commission on Economic and General Welfare and Congress for Nursing Practice recommended work on peer review, joint practice, and audits.
1972	Carter and others developed the nursing process criteria. Phaneuf published *The nursing audit: profile for excellence.* Amendments to the Social Security Act created the PSROs in an effort to overcome the deficiencies of the utilization review committees; this shifted the responsibility for assessing care from hospitals to local groups of physicians. American Hospital Association's Patient Bill of Rights, Social Security amendments (PL92-603), and patient evaluation procedure (PEP) for health professionals were introduced.
1973-1974	The ANA published generic and division standards based on the nursing process.
1974	Medicus/Nursing Care Systems recommended development of process and outcome criteria and use of retrospective and concurrent monitoring. The JCAH developed discharge outcome criteria and critical management elements for disease-oriented diagnostic categories.
1975	The federal government reviewed regulations regarding institutional review requirements consistent with Professional Standards Review Organizations (PSRO) system.
1976	The ANA formed the interdivisional Council on Certification. The ANA set forth a model for implementing standards of care and published the *Quality Assurance Workbook.* A section on the quality of professional services was added to JCAH *Accreditation Manual for Hospitals.*

▶ DATES	EVENTS
1979	The credentialing study was reported in Madison, Wisconsin.
	Revision of mental health–psychiatric standards of practice was initiated.
	JCAH accreditation manual for hospitals was totally revised, with problem-focused approach to quality assurance activities.
1982	Revised standards of psychiatric–mental health nursing practice were published.
1983	Passage of H.R. 1900 (PL98-21), the Social Security Amendment of 1983, established prospective payment system based on 467 diagnostic-related group (DRG) categories for pretreatment diagnosis billing.
1984	Psychiatric, rehabilitation, and substance abuse hospitals of units were exempted from DRGs.
1989	The federal government established the Agency for Health Care Policy and Research (AHCPR) that investigates and defines outcome measures of quality health care.
1990s	Revolutionization of quality in health care.
	The development of client classification systems and nursing diagnoses for psychiatric clients contributes to effective utilization of mental health–psychiatric nurses and more precise interventions.
	Quality assurance programs are recognized as essential to the health of clients.
	A shift occurred from emphasis on the process of care to addressing the outcomes of care.
	A shift occurred from a quality assurance philosophy to a quality improvement philosophy with emphasis on continuous quality improvement.
	The Joint Commission has begun the development of outcome indicator sets that will eventually require data collection.
Future	Nurses will be challenged to develop nurse-sensitive indicators of quality.
	Research findings will be used to guide nurses to more accurately diagnose and treat clients with psychiatric problems.
	Nursing care will be based on scientific data in order to achieve the most efficient and least costly care.

Corporation of America. Because of intense physician interest, the JCAHO initiated the progression from QA to CQI, noting that CQI builds on the strengths of the prior QA program.

The 1991 quality assurance standards emphasized monitoring and evaluation. It included a 10-step process, focused on such activities as the identification of important aspects of care, indicators for monitoring care, and the collection and organization of data for the identification of problems which, when resolved, would provide improved client care. The tendency was for each unit or discipline to apply the 10-step process internally, thereby fragmenting the delivery of health care. The 1992 Quality Assessment and Improvement guidelines are based on the principles that health care services are frequently carried out jointly by several groups and that these processes must be integrated and efforts coordinated throughout the entire organization. Emphasis is on all key activities of the agency, with the expectation that every single member of the group, beginning with administrators, will work every minute of every day to provide the most intelligent care that is possible. Full implementation of continuous quality improve-

ment will probably take several years to accomplish. A comparison of some aspects of QA and CQI may be seen in Table 44-1.

Difficulty in identifying and measuring "quality" care remains in spite of efforts to introduce a new, positive approach to evaluation programs. In the next few years, nurses will be challenged to develop nurse-sensitive indicators of quality.

The JCAHO was founded by physicians. The American Hospital Association has representation on the governing board of JCAHO, but there is no representation from professional nursing groups.[33] However, in December 1989, a new public health care service agency called the Agency for Health Care Policy and Research (AHCPR) was established.[34] Recognizing the need for interdisciplinary approaches to the drafting of practice guidelines, seven panels were established, of which three are chaired or cochaired by nurses.[26] It seems that the JCAHO recognizes that nurses have an important role to play in quality assurance/quality improvement and that the skills of nurse clinicians and nurse researchers will be critical factors in the development of new evaluation programs focused on client care.

▼ **TABLE 44-1   A Comparison of QA and CQI**

Quality Assurance	Continuous Quality Improvement
• Emphasis on monitoring, evaluation	• Broad emphasis on process
• Problem identification and corrective action	• Problem prevention by improving process
• Focus on the individual, department, and/or discipline	• Focus on the complex series of activities involved in any key functions
• Clinical aspects of care	• Interrelated governance, managerial, support, and clinical processes
• Negative perceptions of personnel; meeting external accreditation standards	• Cooperative effort, sense of involvement or ownership
• No significant participation of staff in resolution of cost and quality problems	• Involvement of all personnel, including administrators and managers

KEY COMPONENTS IN QUALITY ASSURANCE/ QUALITY IMPROVEMENT

Quality assurance programs involve several key components. *Standards of care* in mental health–psychiatric nursing practice, *indicators,* or measures, used to evaluate key functions of practice, and *protocols* for nursing interventions provide the basis for developing a review of care procedures of institutions, departments, or units. *Reviews* may be conducted in an *individual* or *peer-review* format and may also address the *levels of practice.*

Professional development may be reviewed as a part of a quality assurance program within a hospital or agency. This may be implemented through a continuing education program in the institution being reviewed or through participation in a formal graduate educational program. Nurses may enroll in master's or doctoral programs in clinical practice, research, education, administration, or a combination of these. Professional development is an important factor in the maintenance and upgrading of care.

Allied concepts, for example, *credentialing,* are related to quality assurance. Credentials provide evidence of clinical competency. Two types of credentials are commonly considered in an evaluation of client care. *Licensure* involves the legal right of nurses to provide nursing services for pay. *Certification* is a nongovernmental recognition of the achievement of standards in a specialized area of nursing.

The quality assurance and improvement process may vary, depending on the practice model being used. Mental health–psychiatric nurses work in institutional and noninstitutional settings, with a variety of age groups and illnesses. Quality assurance and improvement programs explore the aspects of care that are pertinent to a specific setting.

Many nurses today believe that access to and quality of care is linked to *third-party reimbursement* for their services.[29] To get such reimbursement, nursing care must be differentiated from care provided by allied health professionals. Finally, participation in professional activities is a mark of the professional individual and is linked with quality assurance and improvement.

Quality assurance and improvement programs look for evidence of effectiveness, efficiency, and accountability. The information may be used to request funding, report costs, gain community support, provide immediate feedback to nurses, and improve care. Overall, the major effects of quality assurance and improvement are an increased awareness and upgrading of mental health–psychiatric nursing care. For truly professional nurses, this systematic kind of evaluation, both positive and negative, is desirable.

Standards of Care

In mental health–psychiatric nursing standards are drawn from knowledge about human behavior, the norms of the groups who care for the mentally ill, and the values of those who call themselves mental health–psychiatric nurses. Such norms and values include the right of clients to be safe in the settings where they receive care, to feel a sense of acceptance, and to be provided with appropriate therapy. Standards of care derived from such bases suggest professional behaviors through which the desired quality of care can be achieved. The ANA *Standards of Psychiatric and Mental Health Nursing Practice*[8] constitute just such a firm and carefully developed basis for nursing interventions.

For a number of reasons the implementation of the ANA standards in everyday practice is difficult. First, the complexity of each client—his situation, personal dynamics, and responses—must not be underestimated and must be considered. At the same time, the role of the nurse may vary according to the setting. For example, the clinic nurse may assume primary responsibility for individual therapy, while the hospital nurse may be expected to implement written orders. Consequently, nursing care should be applied in a manner that is consistent with the needs of the client and the characteristics of the setting.

Second, nurses are frequently involved in dependent functions (such as implementing physicians' orders) and independent functions (such as assessment of nursing care) at the same time. The psychiatrist and the nurse basically share responsibility for planning treatment. Realistically, however, not all physicians accept this position. Therefore nurses strive to implement standards of care based on the expectations of the nursing profession and of the institution. The standards may or may not be accepted by other health professionals with whom nurses work. To add to the complexity of the situation, each nurse has unique knowledge and skill. When procedures are designed to assess whether the standards of care have been implemented, it becomes difficult to identify which aspects of client outcome are directly attributable to nursing intervention. When psychiatrists and nurses collaborate in therapy, four factors regarding standards of care are in operation: (1) the ANA standards representing the expectations of the nursing profession, (2) the nurse's personal values, (3) the American Medical Association (AMA) standards representing the expectations of the medical profession, and (4) the psychiatrist's personal values.

Nurses owe primary loyalty to the client rather than to the institution, the profession, or the physician. However, institutional regulations often impinge on care. Nurses functioning as client advocates may find themselves in conflict with the institution, a psychiatrist, or both. The physician and the nurse together may not agree with the institution. For example, a psychiatrist and a nurse may believe that a female client can benefit from visits by her 15-year-old son, who is her only child. However, the institution has a strict rule that does not allow minors to visit in the psychiatric unit. Obviously, important factors have been introduced, including the nurse's relationship and responsibility to the employer as well as to the client. Nurses are not able to use the ANA standards of care or any other set of standards in isolation but need to generalize the intent while using their own judgment to determine effective behaviors in the setting in which they are working.

Standards of nursing care have many sources; however, the question "Who really sets standards of nursing care?" may legitimately be asked. In many cases specific nursing standards and nursing protocols have been developed in response to the requirements set by the JCAHO. Nurses, particularly those in middle management, tend to seek guidelines from professional nursing organizations. Consequently, publicatons such as the ANA's *Standards of Psychiatric and Mental Health Nursing Practice*[10] significantly influence nurses in setting standards. Concepts presented in ANA and NLN publications are reviewed by nurses in clinical practice and evaluated in light of clinical realities. In addition, input is available and often mandated by government agenices, state boards of nursing, state nursing organizations, and state health departments. The result is a unique combination of ideas flowing from experience, situational realities, professional ideals, and individual personalities.

Some common points in nursing standards may be identified from hospital to hospital and agency to agency. At the same time, features peculiar to one situation may be found and are often related to the availability of technological facilities or to different cultural viewpoints. This is desirable because the institutions in which nurses practice are indeed different, and the standards of nursing care must be appropriate to the setting. For example, the behavior of a female nurse who places her hand on a male client's shoulder in a moment of client panic may be perfectly acceptable to an Irish-American client but not to a client of Japanese descent.

The way standards for mental health–psychiatric nursing practice are developed in a particular hospital often involves committees and statements of standards to the nurses in that setting. Nurses who are most influential in the development of standards are those who have achieved a significant level of expertise in an area, who have completed graduate education, and who have been recognized by their peers as being outstanding in the professional nursing role.

Indicators

Indicators are aspects of the health care process, usually related to appropriate nursing interventions, developed by health care professionals against which the health care practices in a given setting are compared.[58] Until recently indicators were commonly called criteria. Indicators are defined differently by different authors.[45] In this chapter, *indicators* are considered tools used to gather information for the evaluation of the quality of care[40] in order to maintain professional standards. Indicators must be objective, clearly defined and measureable.[52] Three types of indicators are generally used: structure, process, and outcome indicators. During the last 10 years, the focus in nursing has been on process indicators, however with the changes implied in quality improvement, the emphasis is currently on process and outcome indicators. At the same time, nurses involved in quality assurance/quality improvement, as Schroeder clearly indicates, cannot "look at outcomes totally in isolation from the structure and process of care."[48] Unit based nursing indicators are those formulated by the nurses who are responsible for direct client care in a particular unit or service. This allows for a great deal of specificity in identifying the goals of nursing care and for an appropriate nursing response to changing factors in a given unit, for example, the use of new technological devices or procedures. However, in the context of quality improvement, all client-focused services are evaluated in an integrated fashion so that client care is enhanced.

Structure indicators focus on the aims of the institution, the client, or the nurse. In structure indicators, statements may be made about the philosophy and objectives of the institution, the physical facilities, the administrative organization, financial management, government and accreditation standards, and the policies and procedures of the institution. Examples of structure indicators in mental health–psychiatric nursing practices are (1) the expectation that staff nurses have completed a course in group therapy and (2) the requirement that each client in the unit be assigned a primary and associate nurse. Accreditation manuals provide additional structure indicators. Accreditation agencies require that administrators record the specific processes by which structure indicators are used during a quality assurance review. When structure indicators are used, it is necessary to verify that adequate resources are available to provide necessary services. In other words, nurses need adequate knowledge, equipment, support personnel, and facilities to provide quality care.

Process indicators are used to evaluate actions and the sequence of events in client care. During a concurrent review the activities of professional and nonprofessional personnel during the assessment and management phases of client care are evaluated at the same time. Examples of a process review in mental health–psychiatric nursing include (1) documentation of the nurse-client relationship and the client's movement toward identified goals, (2) evidence that clients for whom medication has been ordered receive instruction about the medication, and (3) data to indicate whether the nursing care plan was developed with input from the client and the primary nurse within 72 hours of administration.

The use of process indicators is an opportunity to take immediate action to improve the final outcome of care.

These indicators also enable the nursing department to evaluate (1) the extent to which nursing activites are completed, (2) the implementation of policy and procedures, and (3) the activities of the coordinator of each component of care.

Outcome indicators are developed to evaluate the results of care, that is, a change in the health of the client after he receives medical and nursing care. Only when outcome factors are compared to pertinent indicators can the nurse know that the goals of care have been achieved.[4] Examples of outcome criteria are the previously confused client's orientation to time, place, and person and his responsibility for activities of daily living when discharged.

One problem with outcome indicators is the fact that only the effects of intervention are reviewed. If the outcomes are evaluated as not reaching the level stated in the predetermined criteria, it is difficult to determine whether some aspects of the nursing process were poorly implemented or whether the client was poorly motivated or uncooperative. For example, a withdrawn client may be discharged without having responded verbally, except with close family members. If the client's communication patterns were apparently unchanged, it would help to analyze the steps of the nursing process as they were implemented and the client characteristics and behaviors observed by the caregivers. In such a situation a process review becomes desirable.

Once the indicators are chosen, quality assurance administrators may need to consider whether the unit review is to apply only to a certain discipline. Nurses may choose to audit only a particular aspect of nursing care within their clinical specialty, such as the administration of medications. A structure indicator could be: Are the correct medications available? A process indicator could be: Was the correct dose given? An outcome indicator could be: Was the client's anxiety relieved? In terms of quality improvement, other indicators could be developed that would involve not only the nurses' functions but the interaction between the nurses and the physicians who ordered the medication.

Protocols

A *protocol* is "an instrument that guides a practitioner in the collection of data and recommends specific action based on that data.[15] Protocols are used primarily by nurses in primary care facilities and in rural areas. Usually, a protocol is a written statement of signs and symptoms, with a list of necessary or desirable laboratory or other diagnostic procedures, and of specific indications of therapeutic interventions that may be followed by a care provider who is not a physician. Another type of protocol is composed of guidelines to be used by health care providers in overseeing the progression of a chronic illness. Interventions may be limited, and, during acute phases, referrals to physicians will be made.

In hospital quality assurance and improvement programs, protocols may be defined as statements of discrete steps used by nurses in the clinical role. Nurses assist the client to attain long- and short-term goals. By stating nursing behaviors precisely and in sequence, nurses are able to recognize whether specific stages in client care have been accomplished well or poorly.

In mental health–psychiatric nursing, particularly in community mental health nursing, protocols involving medications may become common. For example, the physician frequently approves the use of mild sedatives in certain types of hyperactive clients. The acceptability of protocols is influenced by such factors as the number and availability of psychiatrists, the difficulty in evaluating symptoms, the frequency with which specified conditions are encountered, and the expected severity of the client's responses.

Protocols for mental health–psychiatric nurses are usually developed by a multidisciplinary committee of professional health care providers who work in the setting where the protocols will be used. Members of the committee are most often physicians because they are recognized as health team leaders and have the right to prescribe medications. It is acceptable for such a committee to review published protocols for adaptation and use in a given setting.

Such committees may use literature on biochemistry, psychiatric disorders, and appropriate treatments as a basis for setting up the role expectations and functions. Pathological conditions that may be seen commonly need to be identified and diagnostic tests specified. For example, the protocol used for a client who comes into a community mental health clinic complaining of being depressed and unable to cope with life may include such biological assessments as a complete physical examination, urinalysis, SMA-18, chest x-ray exam, and perhaps the rapid dexamethasone suppression test or the thyrotropin stimulation test. Psychological tests may include the Minnesota Multiphasic Personality Inventory, the Beck Depression Scale, and the standardized National Institute of Mental Health Diagnostic Interview. Finally, guidelines related to intervention should be stated clearly and concisely.

While protocols are being developed, arrangements are made for emergency referrals to appropriate consultants or, at a later time, to the psychiatrist responsible for the unit or agency. Nurses using protocols also need to seek a periodic review of client records to validate the effectiveness of the treatment methods.

The most critical problem with protocols is legal constraints on nursing practice. Many states limit the definition of nursing functions. Only physicians are licensed to sign prescriptions for medications and order x-ray and laboratory studies. In using protocols nurses seek to perform functions within their area of expertise, making certain procedures available to clients when a physician is not present and furnishing the physician with data about complex conditions that require medical review, diagnosis, and treatment. The standardized procedures found in protocols may also be viewed as limiting nursing interventions. The degree of restriction in what a nurse is allowed to do is governed by legal factors and the availability of physicians.

Protocols may be written to reduce the legal vulnerability of the health care provider or the agency. For example, the required number of diagnostic procedures may be excessive. The freedom to order basic diagnostic tests as recommended in the protocol without being forced to order unnecessary tests is critical if nurses are to be able to use protocols effectively.

In summary, protocols may be used in several ways: (1) to direct nursing interventions, (2) to intervene in client care when physicians are not available, and (3) to serve as specific statements of nursing behaviors that can be incorporated into quality assurance activities.

Nursing Case Management

Case management is focused on the planning, coordination, and sequencing of client care during a specific hospitalization or period of treatment. Zander[53] states that "it is often preferable to have an interdisciplinary team participate in the planning and delivery of care" (p. 201). She suggests that physicians and nurses "need to agree on process and outcome standards, as well as to design monitoring and documentation tools" (p. 201). This approach seems to be consistent with the "new" concept of CQI, emphasizing the interdisciplinary character of client care. Zander also speaks of a *critical pathway* as a case management tool to be used in the implementation of the case management plan. Vantassel[50] defined a critical pathway as a written plan and timetable for client care that identifies routine treatments, activities, medications, diet, and expected length of stay. Each day is clearly identified and the expected activities for each day specified. Interactions among members of the health team are focused on achieving client goals on a daily basis. Discharge planning assumes a new importance and the probability of cooperative planning is enhanced. Case management would facilitate the goal of QI within the institutional structure. It could possibly shorten the length of the hospital stay and reduce hospital costs.

Patient Classification Systems

To the professional nurse today, patient classifications and nursing diagnoses are important and related. Both can help to identify the knowledge and behaviors that are specific to mental health–psychiatric nurses.

The term *patient classification system* refers to the "identification and classification of patients into care groups or categories, and to the quantification of these categories as a measure of the nursing effort required."[24] Classification systems may be used to estimate staffing patterns for nurses by describing what nurses do. A major problem in the care of mentally ill clients is the difficulty in establishing broad categories and/or methods of quantification—for example, when the focus of care is on an adolescent who is "acting out."

In an attempt to use the nursing diagnoses developed by NANDA in the care of mentally ill clients, many mental health–psychiatric nurses have tended toward the DSM-III-R classification system because it includes behavioral terms and is used by allied health professionals, such as psychiatrists and psychologists. However, in 1984, because of a lack of relevant psychiatric nursing diagnoses, a task force was set up by the Executive Committee of the ANA Division of Psychiatric and Mental Health Nursing Practice to identify and classify nursing diagnoses that can be used by mental health–psychiatric nurses. The task force developed a system organized into three response classes: individual, interpersonal/family, and community/environment. The committee concentrated its initial work in developing 12 response patterns within the individual response class.[35] See the appendix for the classification system.

Patient classification systems and nursing diagnoses may foster effective use of nurses and precise interventions; however efficiency does not guarantee quality care.[24]

Reviews

Nursing care reviews, formerly called "audits," are written verifications that the nursing care is appropriate and in accord with the standards in a particular clinical area. The JCAHO has expanded the term to mean client care review and evaluation. This expanded term implies not only that many indicators of the quality of care should be examined but also that the review process must continue as the framework for assessment of care.

JCAHO standards require that professionally qualified nurses direct nursing care, that an organizational working plan and written procedures related to nursing care be maintained, that evidence of safe therapeutic care be presented, and that ongoing plans to update nurses' knowledge and skills be developed. Federal and state governments also require quality assurance and improvement activities on client care involved in federal- or state-funded health care programs.

Publications such as the *Statement on Psychiatric and Mental Health Nursing Practice*[5] and *A Plan for Implementation of the Standards of Nursing Practice*[3] provide guidelines for client care and nurses' actions. The ANA Congress of Nursing Practice also publishes a *Quality Assurance Update* to address issues in the quality assurance process. Administrators may choose to develop standards and review procedures specific to their own setting or to adapt standardized review plans that are commercially available. Another important source of information is the *Journal of Nursing Quality Assurance.* The name of this journal was changed in October, 1991, to the *Journal of Nursing Care Quality.*

Review programs developed by individual hospitals or agencies have the advantage of being specific to the setting and therefore probably have a high degree of validity. However, such plans may suffer from some unclear, untested, and unreliable statements. On the other hand, carefully developed standardized audit programs or instruments contain clear, tested statements with indexes of reliability and validity.

One such standardized review program is Medicus, which was developed jointly by the Rush-Presbyterian–St. Luke's Medical Center in Chicago, the Baptist Medical Center in Birmingham, and the Medicus Systems Corporation. The Medicus Nursing Quality Assurance Monitoring System may be used in a mental health–psychiatric nursing unit.[39]

Six major objectives and 32 subjectives are used in the Medicus Nursing Monitoring System. The major objectives are[19]:

1. Formulation of a nursing care plan
2. Attention to the client's physical needs
3. Attention to the client's emotional, mental, and social needs
4. Evaluation of nursing care objectives
5. Attention to unit procedures for the protection of all clients
6. Collaboration in the delivery of nursing care by administrators and managerial personnel

This monitoring system is implemented by applying client-specific criteria at the various levels of care.

Other instruments that may be used as part of an ongoing audit are also available. The Slater Nursing Competencies Rating Scale includes 84 items related to observable or measurable nursing behaviors that represent the critical elements of the nursing process. The following items, focused on actions directed toward meeting the psychosocial needs of individual clients, are taken from the Slater Nursing Competency Rating Scale.[51]

1. The nurse gives full attention to the client.
2. The nurse is a receptive listener.
3. The nurse approaches the client in a kind, gentle, and friendly manner.
4. The nurse responds in a therapeutic manner to the client's behavior.
5. The nurse recognizes anxiety in the client and takes appropriate action.

As implied in its title, this scale requires a nurse observer and allows for ratings from "best nurse" to "poorest nurse."[51] The Quality Patient Care Scale (Qual-PaCS) is a 68-item instrument derived from the Slater Scale. The Slater Scale is focused on the nurse's performance and involves observation of nursing interventions, whereas Qual-PaCS is focused on the client. Both scales permit comparison of the quality of care received from different care-providing groups in a variety of settings. The greatest challenge to persons using such standardized programs or instruments is to adjust them to the specific needs and characteristics of the setting.

Review programs are a way to assess and verify the quality of client care. By referring to JCAHO, PSRO, ANA, and government requirements for health care agencies, nurses can develop or adapt quality assurance and improvement activities that are specific to their area of practice and can become part of client care review and evaluation.

There are three types of review: concurrent, retrospective, and prospective. These types of review are discussed within the context of nursing care, although the concept may be applied to care provided by any group of health professionals, such as physicians and pharmacologists, as well as care provided by members of several groups of health care professionals working collaboratively.

A *concurrent review* is a method of evaluating ongoing activities (Table 44-2). In mental health–psychiatric nursing, concurrent reviews involve an assessment of one particular aspect of care provided to clients who are in treatment. For example, in a psychiatric unit the evaluators may want to find out whether side rails are up on the beds of confused, elderly clients. Client charts, care plans, staff and client interviews, and observations of nursing care are components of a concurrent review. This type of review allows corrective action to be taken immediately, thereby quickly improving the quality of care being rendered in the area. Immediate feedback also gives the nurse an opportunity to develop clinical capabilities.

In a *retrospective review* the nursing process as it was applied during treatment is evaluated after services have been rendered (Table 44-2). In this type of review direct observation of nursing care is impossible; the completed medical record, nursing care plans, nurses' charts, interviews with staff members and former clients, staff conferences, and questionnaires are used to form a picture of events. This kind of evaluation is the means by which actions that would improve the quality of care in similar cases in the future may be identified. One potentially serious problem in the retrospective review is that people are often forgetful. The length of time since treatment and the impact of the experience on the client or nurse influence the degree of retention of some of the facts that are essential for the evaluation. This emphasizes the importance of accurate recording.

A *prospective review* resembles a descriptive study. Criteria are set, and a review of a defined number of clients with a specific diagnosis is made. For example, the care given to the next 20 clients diagnosed as being depressed may be studied. After a prospective review, it is possible to develop criteria based on the observation of the care provided to the selected client sample.

In the future nurses will be more involved in *multidisciplinary reviews* than they are at the present time. In this approach a particular client problem or diagnosis is selected. A multidisciplinary group establishes specific indicators as appropriate to this problem or diagnosis. The multidisciplinary review involves an evaluation of the performance of the various health professionals, such as the psychiatrist, psychologist, psychiatric nurse, and psychiatric social worker. Reviewers may elect to review the specific assessment procedures of the team in working with suicidal clients. In multidisciplinary reviews the total treatment will be evaluated in order to improve the care provided by the team.

Operation of a Quality Assurance Program

In large institutions it is common for quality assurance committees to oversee all nursing review activities. The nursing quality assurance committee usually sets standards

▼ **TABLE 44-2** **Types of Reviews: Differentiating Factors**

Factors	Concurrent	Retrospective	Prospective
Time of care	Ongoing	Past	Future
Data	Observation	Records	Predetermine criteria and
	Records	Interviews	plan of care
	Interviews		
Significant consideration	Provides immediate feedback	Danger of forgotten or nonrecorded data	Focus on a specific diagnostic group

of care and may suggest specific criteria to be used in evaluation. This group generally organizes the mechanical details of the program, setting up review deadlines and frequently arranging for analysis of data.

When the review takes place, it is important to isolate the factors that negatively affect client care. Such factors can be identified from external and internal unit or area sources.[18] External sources include government reports of care in similar situations, client complaints, suggestions from other units, professional literature, and agency or department lists of nursing goals and objectives. Internal sources include the unit's medical records, incident reports, surveys of clients and staff members, research and evaluation by staff members, previous audit results, and staff members' suggestions.

When possible improvements in the quality of care have been identified, the type of indicator is chosen by the unit quality assurance committee members, unit administrator, and unit staff nurses. Decisions on the number and type of clients to be surveyed are then made. Indicators include statements of what is measured (for example, assessment of emotional needs), what source of data is used (for example, client interviews, medical records, and nursing care plans), and at what level the criteria need to be met (for example, 100% or 85%). Any exceptions to the indicators are stated (for example, disoriented clients will not be interviewed).

The topic, rationale, and criteria are then submitted to the quality assurance committee for evaluation before the study can be undertaken. Final approval for the study occurs on the unit level but only after the recommendations of the nursing quality assurance committee have been taken into account.

When the study plan is ready for implementation, data may be collected by the nursing quality assurance committee, unit staff members, or a person designated by the committee. After the data are obtained, it is advisable for the unit staff nurses and supervisors to review the study process and make comments. The data are then analyzed either by institutional personnel or by computer. Computers are used more commonly because of the volume and complexity of the data collected and the time required for analysis.

When the data analysis is complete the unit staff nurses are informed of the results of the review. Problems and probable causes are identified, criteria are reviewed with the nursing staff, actions for improving the quality of care are recommended, and a follow-up plan is formulated. A summary report of the review is then submitted to the quality assurance committee.

Peer Review

Peer review is a process by which the quality of nursing care rendered by an individual nurse is evaluated by other mental health–psychiatric nurses actively involved in clinical nursing practice. The ANA[8] has identified peer review as a vital component of a quality assurance and improvement program, and it is now required for eligibility for third-party reimbursement by Civilian Health and Medical Program of Uniformed Services (CHAMPUS). Evaluation of individual nurse performance in quality assurance and im-

provement programs is different from the general evaluation of performance often initiated by employers. The goal of quality assurance and improvement programs is primarily to improve overall client care.

Standards of care now constitute the foundation of the evaluation in quality assurance and improvement programs. Protocols provide step-by-step guidelines for nursing interventions, reviews verify the appropriateness and outcomes of client care, and peer review allows the contributions of individual nurses to be appraised.

At present a staff nurse's performance is frequently assessed by self-evaluation, peer evaluation, and supervisor evaluation. Peer review procedures promote individual accountability and are often the primary way of recognizing clinical expertise. Peer review documents nursing care and establishes the degree to which practice is based on identified standards.

Record keeping by nurses must be carefully incorporated into the peer review process. The use of Diagnostic Related Groups (DRGs) in the care of hospitalized Medicare clients has influenced the nursing role. Because the allocation of federal funds is based on categories of treatment, the documentation of effective interventions has become essential for reimbursement. Nurses have always been expected to chart care. Currently, however, nurses are asked to document nursing interventions and specific outcomes of these interventions. They are expected to review the charting of client services in auxiliary departments and to note the completeness of medical reports and diagnoses.

A number of variables are included in peer review. Client care includes the nursing processes of assessment, analysis, planning, implementation, and evaluation, as well as collaboration with other health professionals. Professional development may include self-direction, consistently high standards of care, and attendance at educational activities. Client teaching may be considered to be one aspect of nursing care or a separate nursing function. Leadership and management skills may be considered another part of the role, including delegation of responsibility, planning and implementation of in-service programs, and consultation. Research has long been recognized as a function of the nursing role, but it is only now being considered in performance appraisal activities.

Levels of Practice

The concept of *levels of practice* may be defined as a ranking of performance based on knowledge and skill. Specific nursing behaviors that reflect comparable levels of practice are identified.

Client care may be evaluated using accepted standards of care, recognizing that all staff nurses are capable of the basic nursing tasks. However, care can be enhanced if attention is systematically given to the "fit" between the client's needs and the nurse's expertise. The inclusion of the levels of practice concept in a quality assurance program provides a more precise description of the unit being evaluated and the level of care being rendered.

In mental health–psychiatric settings it is necessary to know the beginning levels of theoretical knowledge and clinical skill that can be expected of staff nurses. The activities in this clinical area differ from those in other clinical

▼ **TABLE 44-3   Indicators Related to Levels of Practice in Mental Health–Psychiatric Nursing**

Function	Level of Practice	Indicators
Communication	I	Uses communication skills of listening and problem-solving goals in the stages of the nurse-client relationship.
		Participates in regular supervision of own nursing interventions.
	II	Uses communication skills of confrontation and reflection to intervene in the expression of feelings and provide for attainment of therapeutic goals.
		Participates in regular supervision of own nursing interventions.
	III	Uses a therapeutic framework (for example, psychoanalytical, interpersonal, gestalt): interventions reflect appropriate communication responses and insight into nursing therapy.
		Participates in regular supervision of own nursing interventions.
	IV	Uses appropriate communication responses in the implementation of interventions; nursing therapy reflects a theoretical framework and definition of therapy issues and goals.
		Participates in regular supervision of own nursing interventions.
Education	I	Identifies need for personal and professional growth; attends all required unit and hospital in-service programs.
		Attends formal education programs or earns a minimum of 8 to 12 continuing education units each year.
	II	Initiates topics for in-service programs.
		Identifies in-service needs for self and unit to continuing education committee member and unit nursing managers.
	III	Conducts a minimum of one in-service program each year.
		Provides orientation session for new graduate nurses.
	IV	Plans, implements, and evaluates a continuing education or client education program.
		Plans, implements, and evaluates an educational program relating to a mental health issue on or off the unit at least once a year.

specialties and need to be clearly defined. Levels of practice must be related to reasonable skill development; for example, the new baccalaureate graduate can be expected to participate in group therapy but not to assume full responsibility for a weekly therapy group of clients. Specific examples of indicators related to levels of practice are represented in Table 44-3.

Levels of practice are based on the institutional philosophy and objectives, the nursing department's philosophy and objectives, and the ANA standards of practice. The ANA standards for mental health–psychiatric nursing are used when mental health–psychiatric nurses are involved.

Initially, a levels of practice committee is organized. This committee is composed of representatives of the different groups of nurses, such as administrators, clinical specialists, and staff nurses. After fundamental nursing criteria are complete and approved by the nursing department, the mental health–psychiatric nursing group develops specific additional criteria.

When specific nursing behaviors are correlated with levels of practice, staff nurses have a system in which (1) increased knowledge and skills can be used efficiently, and (2) professional development can be recognized. Until the concept of levels of practice was used, staff nurses who sought promotion usually had to seek status in administration or education. Nurses who remained at the bedside may have received salary increments based on length of service, but the staff nurse role remained static, placing the new graduate and veteran nurse on the same level in the or-

ganization. A recognition of levels of practice provides a way to acknowledge the experienced nurse as well as to differentiate skills among nurses with similar preparation and experience.

The need for precision in the use of nursing resources and for documentation of nursing care has been reemphasized with the advent of DRGs and similar cost-containment measures. Medicare funding for client care depends on the achievement of specific client goals, accurately reflected in written records that are clearly understood by the hospital community and funding agencies. With time such groups as the major insurance companies may not only review the skill level of the professional nurse who provided a particular aspect of client care but even require that specific functions be done only by those who can provide evidence of advanced skill.

Integration of Key Components in Quality Assurance/Quality Improvement

When standards of care, protocols, review procedures, peer review, and levels of practice are discussed, it is important to be able to translate the ideas into practices that are observable and related to client care. Behavioral interpretations of three standards of care are presented in Table 44-4. These standards are among the ANA standards for mental health–psychiatric nursing.[10]

It is also important to recognize that evaluation, when considered as part of an institutional review, involves all

▼ **TABLE 44-4**   **Application of Three ANA Standards of Mental Health–Psychiatric Nursing Practice to Three Quality Assurance Components**

Protocol	Review	Peer Review
STANDARD V-A—PSYCHOTHERAPEUTIC INTERVENTIONS: THE NURSE USES PSYCHOTHERAPEUTIC INTERVENTIONS TO ASSIST CLIENTS IN REGAINING OR IMPROVING THEIR PREVIOUS COPING ABILITIES AND TO PREVENT FURTHER DISABILITY		
Involvement of primary nurse in one-to-one therapeutic care	Review nursing care plan and progress notes to assess nursing interventions with alternate behavior patterns, limit setting, and interpersonal relationships Informally discuss progress and direction of therapy Interview client about nurse's attention to client's time and needs Interview other health professionals who are collaborating in client care about apparent changes in client problems identified in nursing care plan	Interview unit nurses about primary nurse's attention to client conferences, awareness of client problems, and so on Report progress of therapy, with expectation of peer feedback; provide evidence of appropriate consultation Provide written process recordings, audiotapes, and videotapes of individual sessions
Clarification of communication as part of coordination of client care, with professional personnel such as physicians, other nurses, and administrators and with nonprofessional personnel such as aides and nursing assistants	Ascertain effectiveness of communication among health professionals at unit staff conferences Review written progress notes Monitor end-of-shift report about understanding and implementation of care plan Interview nonprofessional personnel about their knowledge of care plan and awareness of pertinent intervention in a given situation based on information received from the primary nurse	Observe input provided by primary nurse at the multidisciplinary conferences Evaluate, over an extended period, the effectiveness of the end-of-shift report Review written progress notes Expect peers to substitute for primary nurse, using her care plans
STANDARD VIII—CONTINUING EDUCATION: THE NURSE ASSUMES RESPONSIBILITY FOR CONTINUING EDUCATION AND PROFESSIONAL DEVELOPMENT AND CONTRIBUTES TO THE PROFESSIONAL GROWTH OF OTHERS		
Determine quality of informal educational methods of professional development for individual nurse by means of discussions with peers and supervisors, consultations with other professional personnel, and use of institutional information resources on unit	Interview nurse Interview supervisory personnel Review number and types of professional books and periodicals checked out of library by nursing staff Note verbal or nonverbal indications of new awareness of therapeutic concepts, theories, or strategies	Evaluate informal discussions Note introduction of new ideas or concepts in unit meetings or reporting sessions Note any tendency to share new insights or strategies that can improve client care in unit
Determine extent of organized informational experience planned to improve knowledge and skills in areas of clinical expertise that have not been well developed in nurse	Review all continuing education activities at least annually Review budget in terms of amount of money made available for continuing education on a given unit Provide evidence of attendance at meetings, courses, and the like Confer with nurses involved in continuing education program to determine if they disseminate information obtained at workshops, courses, and the like Interview nurses on regular basis to review learning needs and achievements	Document whether or not new knowledge has been incorporated in provision of client care Invite persons to present in-service program based on workshops attended Interview peers in terms of improvement of care provided
Determine if any contributions were made to client care in units in which student nurses are placed	Observe staff nurses' responses when student nurses are functioning in area Interveiw clients about collaboration between staff nurses and student nurses in therapeutic matters Use interview or questionnaire to determine staff nurses' perceptions regarding student nurses on unit	Interview peers about perceptions of individual staff nurses regarding presence of student nurses on unit Interview student nurses in terms of their acceptance and learning experiences in psychiatric area

Continued

▼ **TABLE 44-4** **Application of Three ANA Standards of Mental Health–Psychiatric Nursing Practice to Three Quality Assurance Components—cont'd**

Protocol	Review	Peer Review
STANDARD XI—RESEARCH: THE NURSE CONTRIBUTES TO NURSING IN THE MENTAL HEALTH FIELD THROUGH INNOVATIONS IN THEORY AND PRACTICE AND PARTICIPATION IN RESEARCH		
Encourage an awareness of need for and appreciation of nursing research	Interview nurses about attempts to incorporate research findings in nursing practice and willingness to participate in research projects Review unit research activities on an annual basis Review budget in terms of funds requested or allocated for research purposes	Determine if staff members incorporate research factors in case presentations Interview staff nurses regarding their attitudes toward nursing research by identifying degree of support and assistance provided for individual research projects planned and implemented by individual nurses

From The American Nurses' Association: *Standards of psychiatric and mental health nursing practice,* Kansas City, Mo, 1982, The Association.

professional nurses who function in a particular area of the institution. Although the data for quality assurance and improvement programs are obtained from individuals, final reports are made in terms of the group. If the findings indicate a need for change, this is considered in terms of the group, not the individual.

It is critical to coordinate standards of care, protocols, review procedures, and peer review in such a way as to complete the quality assurance activities with a sense of accomplishment. These activities improve care. However, to attain the level of nursing care desired, it is important to critique nursing interventions in a constructive manner to avoid dampening the enthusiasm of those involved. For example, criticisms can be made by describing a specific behavior instead of assuming that one knows the nurse's rationale for her actions. If, while making an emphatic statement, the nurse has the habit of shaking her finger at the person with whom she is speaking, this can be pointed out as an observed behavior. The pointing out of a specific action may allow the criticism to be accepted and remedied.

PROFESSIONAL DEVELOPMENT

The JCAHO staff requires staff development in health care institutions. This requirement is based on the assumption that such programs provide a way to correct negative findings in personnel and outcome audits. The objective of this attempt to remove deficits and to encourage participation in specialized roles and functions is better client care.

The ANA[2] says that professional nurses have the serious responsibility to become involved in a continuous learning process that builds knowledge and skill. The evaluation procedures of a quality assurance program provide a way to improve skills and the quality of care. Professional development and quality assurance programs are closely allied, and the relationship benefits the facility, clients, and nurses.

The term *professionalism* implies certain levels of competence and education, reflecting a breadth of knowledge, skills, and maturity. Nurses most commonly become involved in continuing education or graduate education.

Continuing Education

Continuing education includes short-term planned programs or courses provided by staff educators or academicians. Learning is designed to enhance knowledge and skill. Situational needs in each hospital or agency influence the content in continuing education programs. When planning in-service programs, staff directors may refer to several ANA publications, such as the *Standards for Nursing Services*[1] and the *Standards for Continuing Education in Nursing.*[6]

If continuing education programs are to be successful, nurse administrators must approve of them and facilitate their implementation. To do this, nurse administrators need to be in a position of authority, with the ability to channel the funds and personnel required for well-organized programs.

Interinstitutional cooperation is one way to contain the cost of continuing education. Audiovisual hardware, library materials, and personnel of one health agency may be used in programs in another agency.

College based programs, sometimes called *degree-completion* or *educational mobility programs,* are a form of continuing education. This enterprise is characterized by an effort on the part of nurse educators to differentiate between content considered essential to a generic baccalaureate nursing program and content that may be lacking for registered nurses working for a bachelor's degree in nursing. One solution is to require nurses to complete challenge examinations. This approach seems reasonable if the evaluators have a clear idea of what content is essential.

Graduate Education

Graduate education includes organized programs of study under professional educators in a college or university. The primary function of graduate education in nursing is to prepare nurse specialists, providing the specialized knowledge and skills needed to exercise independent judgments in a particular specialty area. The graduate of the basic baccalaureate program is considered a generalist; the graduate of the clinical master's program is considered a specialist. In other words, the professional nurse, the generalist, is expected to understand the basic principles of nursing as it is applied in multiple clinical areas, such as medical-surgical and psychiatric nursing. On the master's level the nurse studies a specific clinical area in depth, becoming a specialist in that area of practice.

Nursing programs that lead to a clinical master's degree usually focus on a common core of knowledge, expertise in a specialty area of nursing, and a research orientation designed to foster inquiry in that clinical specialty. In graduate mental health–psychiatric nursing programs, emphasis is usually on assessment, awareness of the most frequently encountered emotional problems, and pathological conditions, appropriate nursing interventions, modes of evaluation, and research in that clinical area. Nursing skills usually include practice in individual therapy, group therapy, and marital or family therapy. Students work in a variety of settings and collaborate with other health professionals. Graduates are also expected to understand issues relevant to mental health–psychiatric nursing and the promotion of mental health.

The doctorate is a critical degree for the advancement of the nursing profession. Members of any discipline who are prepared at this level are expected to preserve, expand, and transmit the knowledge that is critical to the discipline. Nurses with doctorates are needed to teach in graduate programs, to work in clinical and administrative positions, and to conduct research in every aspect of nursing. Each year more doctoral programs in nursing are made available. As a result, the degrees of Doctor of Nursing Science (DNSc), Doctor of Nursing Education (DNEd), Doctor of Philosophy in Nursing (PhD), Doctor of Public Health (DPh), and others are awarded in much larger numbers than in the past.

In summary, professional development, whether through continuing education or graduate education, is important in order to retain quality assurance and quality nursing care. Nurses returning to the clinical area with master's or doctoral degrees contribute not only specialized knowledge but also broadened perspectives on their own capabilities and on the health care system itself.

Use of structure, process, and outcome indicators for review of educational programs as well as for clinical practice helps identify and maintain the levels of excellence essential to quality of care.

CREDENTIALS

A *credential* attests to the institution's or person's qualifications in a particular area of expertise. To acquire a credential, an institution or individual is identified by a recognized authority as having met a set of standards at a given time. The purpose of credentials is to ensure quality care and to protect the public. This purpose is inherent in any quality assurance program, with possession of the credentials constituting a part of the audit process.

Any discussion of credentials is incomplete without reference to *The Study of Credentialing in Nursing*[7] conducted in Milwaukee in 1978 and 1979. The report identified four fundamental features of the process of acquiring credentials: quality, identity, protection, and control. These features will be referred to in the following comments. In clinical nursing, critical credentials include licensure and certification.

Licensure

Licensure is the process by which a state gives a person the legal right to practice nursing. It is the oldest, most familiar mechanism used in the United States to regulate the quality of services. In most states, once a license is issued, the person is required to pay only the annual fee and seek renewal of the license. Therefore licensure is used to identify the practitioner. In addition, it protects the recipient of care because practices that do not reach minimal standards leave the practitioner open to legal action.

Programs involving licensure of nurses are developed in state legislatures. Various states define the scope of practice differently and allow varying degrees of diagnosis and intervention by registered nurses. Furthermore, as the nursing profession has expanded, the states have granted the same licensure to graduates of diploma, associate degree, and baccalaureate degree programs.

In the 1978 ANA statement of resolutions, the profession identified two categories of nursing practice: the professional and the technical. Similar resolutions were upheld at the 1986 ANA Convention. The underlying premise is that the minimal preparation for entry into professional nursing practice needs to be the baccalaureate degree. In 1982 the NLN agreed with the underlying premise that the minimal preparation for entry into professional nursing practice needs to be the baccalaureate degree and reaffirmed this agreement at the 1983 NLN National Convention[42] and again in 1986.[41]

Under the present system a board of nurse examiners or a similar group is part of the state structure involving the licensing of nurses. This gives nurses some power in the implementation of the law. Currently, in some states, consideration is being given to a type of institutional licensure. This approach places the power to grant or withhold licenses in the hands of hospital and agency administrators.

On the one hand, advocates of institutional licensure imply that state nursing licensure boards are self-serving. Proponents of institutional licensure suggest that this practice will cut costs and promote efficiency by (1) providing opportunities for evaluation of individual on-site performance, (2) allowing for innovative continuing education programs in hospitals, and (3) facilitating career mobility. On the other hand, nurses focus on individual accountability for the quality of nursing care. If institutional administrators were to develop job descriptions for all health workers, nurses would probably no longer determine the scope of their own practice, job mobility might be hindered, formal nursing educational programs could be considered inappropriate, and nurses could be hired because of a salary category rather than on the basis of level of expertise.[26] Several basic questions deserve to be posed. Would institutional licensure improve the quality of health care? Would the current standards of nursing practice, as published by the ANA, be influenced by institutional licensure? Would the cost of an institutional licensing program be passed on to the consumer?

Certification

Certification is the process by which a nongovernmental agency provides a reliable endorsement that a person has met predetermined standards in a specialized area of nursing. Certification procedures in nursing have been developed to protect the consumer and to recognize clinical expertise. This type of credentialing is voluntary and nurses who elect to forego this process can still practice. Professional organizations are primarily involved in certification procedures, although states and institutions have started programs to recognize clinical competency, particularly in areas of clinical specialization.

Specialty organizations, for example, the Association of Operating Room Nurses, provide certification for members of their group. Mental health–psychiatric nurses are among those who have chosen to use the ANA certification program. Two levels of certification are available for mental health–psychiatric nurses. Registered nurses may apply for certification as mental health–psychiatric nurses after having practiced direct client care for at least 4 hours weekly, with 2 years of mental health–psychiatric nursing experience within the last 4 years, with access to supervision during that period. Certification as a clinical specialist may be obtained in adult or child and adolescent care. Requirements include a master's degree in nursing or a higher degree, with a specialty in mental health–psychiatric nursing, access to supervision, and experience in clinical practice in at least two kinds of treatment modes. Applicants on both levels must complete a comprehensive examination.

In 1987 the ANA reported that 8214 mental health–psychiatric nurses had been certified at the generalist level, 2756 at the clinical specialist level in adult psychiatric nursing, and 317 at the clinical specialist level in child psychiatric nursing.[2]

The major problem in any consideration of certification is the lack of a standardized system that can be recognized by the profession and by the public. A major advantage to an acknowledged professional system of certification is the recognition of competency as a basis for treatment and third-party payments.

PARTICIPATION IN PROFESSIONAL ACTIVITIES

Acquiring professional credentials involves evaluation of both individuals and institutions. By belonging to professional organizations either as an individual or as a member of a group, the professional nurse contributes to the quality of care. Following is a list of nursing organizations to which the mental health–psychiatric nurse may belong:

- American Association of Colleges of Nursing
- American Nurses Association
    - Cabinet on Nursing Education
    - Cabinet on Nursing Practice
    - Cabinet on Nursing Research
    - Cabinet on Human Rights
    - Council on Psychiatric–Mental Health Nursing
- American Academy of Nursing
- American Hospital Association
    - Assembly of Hospital Schools of Nursing
    - Staff Specialists in Nursing Education
- International Council on Nursing

- National League for Nursing
    - Council of Baccalaureate and Higher Degree Programs
    - Council of Home Health Agencies and Community Health Services

Many mental health–psychiatric nurses also belong to non-nursing groups, which include the following:

- American Association of Suicidology
- American Orthopsychiatric Association
- American Personnel and Guidance Association
- American Psychological Association
- American Red Cross
- American Society of Allied Health Professionals
- Association for Specialists in Group Work
- Health Standards and Quality Bureau (formally the Bureau of Quality Assurance)
- International Academy of Professional Counseling and Psychotherapy
- National Alliance for Mental Illness
- Women and Health Care

Although these lists are not exhaustive it is apparent that many nursing groups emphasize a particular clinical area or minority interest. This diversification of interest may reflect fragmentation among professional nurses, however, participation in professional organizations is a critical aspect of professional development.

Ineffective communication among the various interest groups may tend to foster parochialism among professional nurses. *Networking* is a system of sharing information that creates links among people. This system focuses on reciprocal relationships. For example, a mental health–psychiatric nurse, working as a team member in an alcohol abuse program, contacts a nurse educator, requests and receives help in locating a research instrument, and, at the same time, is invited to be a guest speaker in a class focused on the care of alcoholic clients. Networking helps participants satisfy their professional needs and expand their professional interests. It allows for collaborative planning and the development of effective techniques for identifying, storing, retrieving, and linking resources.

THIRD-PARTY PAYMENT

A third-party payment is a reimbursement by a person or group who is neither the provider nor the receiver of services, for example, payment by an insurance company. For years nurses have sought a change in reimbursement policies. Nurses believe that they can provide health maintenance programs and community-based care, especially in long-term illnesses, that would reduce the need for hospitalization and the overall cost of health care. Much of this is impossible because reimbursement policies, for the most part, are focused on the delivery of medical care. This approach emphasizes pathology and reinforces the practice of hospitalization.[30]

Although third-party payment to nurses is not common, one event that may prove to be significant to a general acceptance of third-party reimbursement is the approval in 1982 of CHAMPUS, a provision in the Defense Appropriations Act. CHAMPUS is a federally supported medical program designed specifically for active and retired military personnel and their spouses and children. Certified psychiatric nurses and nurse practitioners are eligible for direct reimbursement for their services under CHAMPUS.

State insurance laws must be considered in any discussion of third-party payments. Many health care providers and consumers recognize that the law in each state defines the limits of nursing practice, but not everyone realizes that the state insurance laws allow or disallow reimbursement to specific health professionals. In many states registered nurses may not be reimbursed by third parties. For example, in August 1984, a bill providing third-party reimbursement for nursing services was vetoed by Governor Mario Cuomo of New York. In his veto message Governor Cuomo recognized this approach as a cost-effective alternative for health care but found the bill "unacceptable" because it would lead to "fragmentation of payment."[11]

Mental health–psychiatric nurses in Michigan, Washington, New Jersey, and West Virginia may be reimbursed for health care services, but under varying conditions. Consequently, professional nurses seeking third-party reimbursement must examine not only the definition of nursing in each state but also the insurance laws of the state. In practice many mental health–psychiatric nurses work as therapists in community clinics or outpatient departments where third-party payments are made to the agency. In this way mental health–psychiatric nurses fill a therapeutic role but are not paid directly.

In late 1990 new legislation was passed in the Congress that would allow direct reimbursement to nurse practitioners, certified nurse midwives, and clinical nurse specialists under the Federal Employees Health Benefits Program. The new law allows federal employees and their dependents to choose a nurse as a health care provider. These nurses can then be reimbursed "if the federal employee's insurance plan reimburses for the service that the nurse provides."[48] A large number of insurance plans are available, and federal employees may, with time, choose plans that allow for this reimbursement. The consequences of this legislation for clients and for nurses will become more apparent as health care services provided by nurses are utilized by the public.

It is obvious then that changes are needed. Jennings[30] pointed out, however, that whereas technological advances in the health care industry have occurred rapidly, changes in the economics of health care have tended to lag. Professional nurses must work to be recognized by physicians and by the public as essential health care providers. Policymakers on the state and national levels may not allow third-party payment for professional nurses until the evidence is available to show that quality health care rendered by nurses is cost-effective.

PRACTICE MODELS

Practice models are various patterns in the delivery of nursing services by which health care is made available to diverse groups in different settings. The most obvious distinction in practice models can be made when comparing nursing practice in institutional and noninstitutional settings. In the institutional settings the administrators delegate the responsibility for client care to the health professionals they employ. In noninstitutional situations the individual health professional is held directly responsible for care. It is especially important that nurses in noninstitu-

tional facilities review procedures regularly because individual nurses have a degree of responsibility that is shared by several people in a hospital setting.

In the psychiatric hospital or the psychiatric unit of a general hospital, the staff nurse is usually responsible for a specific number of clients. The nurse is expected to confer with the psychiatrist, be sure the client receives the medications ordered, and assess the client in terms of nursing interventions that may include individual or group therapy. There is a certain sense of security in this practice site because the client is safeguarded during the entire period of hospitalization.

Joint practice represents another institutional practice model. Shortly after The National Joint Practice Commission was established in 1971, a study funded by the Kellogg Foundation allowed professional personnel in four American hospitals to work together to explore nurse-physician relationships. The five elements found to be essential in joint practice were (1) a joint practice committee, (2) primary nursing, (3) individual decision making by nurses, (4) an integrated client record, and (5) a joint client care record review. The final evaluation of the project indicated that the quality of care improved with joint practice.

The role of the clinical nurse specialist in either the hospital or the agency setting involves direct care responsibilities. In addition, the clinical specialist serves as a consultant for staff nurses and other nursing personnel, organizes and presents in-service educational programs, and identifies research findings that may be pertinent to clinical interventions. Whether the clinical specialist functions in a staff or line position depends on the organizational structure of the agency or institution and on the conditions of employment set when the clinical specialist becomes a member of the clinical staff.

In the outpatient department of a hospital or in a community mental health center, the nurse is assigned a caseload and arranges appointments for individual, group, marital, or family therapy. In this setting the nurse has more autonomy than in the hospital units because clients are exposed to multiple stimuli outside the health center. Frequent intraagency conferences involving health professionals provide opportunity for consultation.

The mental health–psychiatric nurse who works in a school, industrial plant, or military agency is also a member of an institutional group. Although the nurse in the school or the factory may work alone or as one of a small group of nurses, the nursing activities in the role are usually clearly described and may be limited.

The clinical nurse specialist in a noninstitutional setting is involved with clients in a way that is considerably different from that seen in hospital settings. The nurse in private practice is the most obvious example. A mental health–psychiatric nurse in private practice works on a fee-for-service basis, not unlike that used by the private duty nurses of the 1950s. The major difference, however, is that the private duty nurse only assumes responsibility for carrying out the physician's orders. In contrast, the nurse practitioner in private practice is responsible for data collection, problem identification, and intervention. This professional collaborates with a medical doctor or a group of health professionals.

In a 1985 issue of *Pacesetter*,[9] the newsletter of the

Council on Psychiatric and Mental Health Nursing, guidelines for mental health–psychiatric nurses in private practice were provided. Some of these guidelines are presented here. Clinical nurse specialists in psychiatric and mental health nursing should do the following:

- Identify themselves to clients as members of the nursing profession and display or have credentials to show if they are requested
- Be certified, eligible for, or in the process of becoming certified by the ANA or a state nurses' association or both
- Carry malpractice and premises liability insurance
- Conform the ANA *Standards of Psychiatric and Mental Health Nursing Practice*
- Respect client's rights to confidentiality; maintain and safeguard appropriate records; when such data are to be shared (with other professionals on referral, with courts or lawyers in case of lawsuits), inform the client in advance; when such data are used for professional publications, reframe data to prevent recognition of the client.
- Avoid engaging in social, sexual, or business contacts with the client or those close to the client; may engage in professional contacts with the client or those close to the client.
- Be available to the client outside regular business hours in emergencies; when unavailable for such reasons as illness or vacations, provide a qualified substitute who will respond to emergency calls.
- Recognize limits of statutory accountability in relation to client needs and use referrals to other professionals for necessary services, such as medications or hospitalization; collaborate with these professionals when appropriate and authorized by the client.

Finally, mental health–psychiatric nurses are also active as nursing consultants in medical-surgical settings, hospices, convalescent homes, and other agencies and programs. Consultation is discussed in Chapter 45.

BRIEF REVIEW

Quality assurance and improvement programs are now a formal part of hospital and agency care. Standards of nursing care developed with the professional organization are the bases for quality assurance and improvement activities. The most difficult aspect of quality assurance is developing realistic indicators and designing monitoring procedures in constantly changing conditions.

The concepts of levels of practice and the use of protocols provide an opportunity for mental health–psychiatric nurses to expand the nursing role based on the development of clinical competencies. Peer review and professional development through continuing education or graduate education are ways for professional nurses to enhance their knowledge and skill. Credentials protect the consumer by providing identification of nurses' qualifications in particular clinical areas.

It is important to note that systematic evaluation of nursing care is a priority for professional nurses, not only in terms of their responsibility to the public but also in their commitment to themselves and to the profession.

REFERENCES AND SUGGESTED READINGS

1. Aidroos N: Use and effectiveness of psychiatric nursing care plans, *Journal of Advanced Nursing* 16(2):177, 1991.
2. American Nurses' Association: *Certification catalog,* Kansas City, Mo, 1988, The Association.
3. American Nurses' Association: *A plan for implementation of the standards of nursing practice,* Kansas City, Mo, 1975, The Association.
4. American Nurses' Association: *Quality assurance workbook,* Kansas City, Mo, 1976, The Association.
5. American Nurses' Association: *Statement on psychiatric and mental health nursing practice,* Kansas City, Mo, 1976, The Association.
6. American Nurses' Association: *Standards for continuing education in nursing,* vol 1, Kansas City, Mo, 1979, The Association.
7. American Nurses' Association: *The study of credentialing in nursing: a new approach,* Kansas City, Mo, 1979, The Association.
8. American Nurses' Association: *Pacesetter,* Kansas City, Mo, 1981, The Association.
9. American Nurses' Association: Guidelines for private practice, *Pacesetter* 12:3, Spring 1985.
10. American Nurses' Association: *Standards of psychiatric and mental health practice,* Kansas City, Mo, 1982, The Association.
11. American Nurses' Association: Legislature passes reimbursement bill, Governor vetoes it, *The American Nurse* 16(9):19, 1984.
12. Batalden P, Buchanan D: In Goldfield N, Nash DB, editors: *Providing quality care: the challenge to clinicians,* Philadelphia, Pa, 1989, American College of Physicians.
13. Bentley J, Boojawon D: Measuring quality in a psychiatric hospital: quality of psychiatric care, *Nursing Times,* 86(42):46, 1990.
14. Bulechek GM, Maas ML: Nursing certification: a matter for the professional organization. In McCloskey JC, Grace HK, editors: *Current issues in nursing,* ed 3, St Louis, 1990, Mosby–Year Book.
15. Bullough B: *The law and expanding nursing role,* NY, 1980, Appleton-Century-Crofts.
16. Calder K: Quality improvement: a new approach to quality assurance, *AARN Newsletter* 47(5):109, 1991.
17. Clark AP and others: Legal implications of standards of care, *DCCN* 10(2):96, 1991.
18. Cooke RA, Rousseau DM: Behavioral norms and expectations: a quantitative approach to the assessment of organizational cultures, *Group and Organizational Studies* 13:245, 1988.
19. *Coordinators manual: nursing quality monitoring methodology,* May 1983, Medicus Systems Corp.
20. Day G: Evaluating a nursing quality assurance program, *Journal of Quality Assurance* 12(3):22, 1990.
21. Deming WE: *Out of the crisis,* Cambridge, Mass, 1986, Massachusetts Institute of Technology, Center for Advanced Engineering Study.
22. Filos MS and others: Quality assurance through use of self evaluation tool: methods of a pilot study, *Journal of AAOHN* 39(1):20, 1991.
23. Fralic MF, Kowalski PM, Llewellyn FA: The staff nurse as quality monitor, *American Journal of Nursing* 91(4):40, 1991.
24. Giovannetti P: Understanding patient classification systems, *Journal of Nursing Administration* 9(2):4, 1979.
25. Goldstein LS: Linking utilization management with quality improvement, *Psychiatric Clinics of North America* 13(1):157, 1990.
26. Grippando GM: *Nursing perspectives and issues,* Albany, NY, 1977, Delmar Publishers.

27. Hegyvary ST: Issues in outcome research, *Journal of Quality Assurance* 5(2):1, 1991.

28. Hurley ML: What do the new JCAHO Standards mean for you? *RN* 54(6):42, 1991.

29. Jacob A: Forward, *Journal of Nursing Quality Assurance* 5:x, 1991.

30. Jennings CM: Nursing's case for third party reimbursement, *American Journal of Nursing* 79:111, 1979.

31. Joint Commission on Accreditation of Hospitals: *The quality assurance guide: a resource for quality assurance,* Chicago, 1980, The Joint Commission.

32. Joint Commission on Accreditation of Health Care Organization: *Accreditation manual for hospitals,* Chicago, 1991, The Joint Commission.

33. Kerfoot K: Standards of regulatory agencies. In McCloskey JC, Grace HK: *Current issues in nursing,* St Louis, 1985, Mosby—Year Book.

34. Lang NM, Marek KD: The policy and politics of patient outcomes, *Journal of Nursing Quality Assurance* 5(2):7, 1991.

35. Loomis ME and others: Development of a classification system for psychiatric—mental health nursing: individual response class, *Archives of Psychiatric Nursing* 1(1):16, 1987.

36. Masters F, Schmele JA: Total quality management: an idea whose time has come, *Journal of Nursing Quality Assurance* 5(4):7, 1991.

37. McCormick KA: Future data needs for quality of care monitoring, DRG considerations, reimbursement and outcome measurements, *Image: A Journal of Nursing Scholarship* 23(1):29, 1991.

38. Meisenheimer CG, editor: *Quality assurance,* Rockville, Md, 1985, Aspen Systems Corp.

39. Miller MC, Knapp RG: *Evaluating quality of care,* Germantown, Md, 1979, Aspen Systems Corp.

40. Nadzam DM: The agenda for change: update on indicator development and possible implications for the nursing profession, *Journal of Nursing Quality Assurance* 5:18, 1991.

41. National League for Nursing: *Interpretive statement on NLN position in support of two levels of nursing practice,* Publication No 11-2158, NY, 1986, National League for Nursing.

42. News: NLN reaffirms its BSN stance despite "technological nursing" rift, *American Journal of Nursing* 83:985, 1983.

43. O'Leary D: President's column, CQI-a step beyond QA, *Joint Commission Perspectives* 10:2, 1990.

44. O'Toole A, Loomis M: Revision of the phenomena of concern for psychiatric—mental health nursing, *Archives of Psychiatric Nursing* 3:288, 1989.

45. Podgorny KL: Developing nursing-focused quality indicators: a professional challenge, *Journal of Nursing Care Quality* 6:1, 1991.

46. Redfern SJ, Norman IJ: Measuring the quality of care: a consideration of a different approach, *Journal of Advanced Nursing* 15(11):126, 1990.

47. Sandella D: Cost versus quality: in the balance, *Nursing Administration Quarterly* 14:31, 1990.

48. Schroeder PS: From the editor, *Journal of Nursing Quality Assurance* 5:2, 1990.

49. U.S. Department of Health and Human Services, Public Health Service, nursing advisory panel for guideline development: summary, Rockville, Md, 1990, Agency for Health Care Policy and Research.

50. Vantassel M: Effective application of critical pathways... written plan for efficient and precise delivery of health care, *Michigan Nurse* 63(5):5, 1990.

51. Wandelt M, Stewart D: *The Slater Nursing Competency Rating Scale,* NY, 1975, Appleton-Century-Crofts.

52. Williams AD: Development and application of clinical indicators for nursing, *Journal of Nursing Care Quality* 6:1, 1991.

53. Zander K: Case management: a golden opportunity for whom? In McCloskey JC, Grace HK: *Current issues in nursing,* St Louis, 1985, Mosby—Year Book.

ANNOTATED BIBLIOGRAPHY

Albiez-Gibbons A: Mental health acuity system: the measure of nursing practice, *Journal of Psychosocial Nursing and Mental Health Services* 24(7):16, 1986.

This article presents the development of an acuity system in a mental health—psychiatric setting that reflects the variable intensity of client care on each shift. By nursing staff developing standards of care for clients in behavioral crises, the quality of care is addressed without increasing documentation during crisis periods. The use of a mental health acuity system in projecting staffing needs is also discussed.

Finkelman A: *Quality assurance for psychiatric nursing,* Gaithersburg, Md, 1991, Aspen Publishers.

This text presents an overview of the quality assurance process. The content includes strategies for implementing or refining a quality assurance program on a psychiatric unit. The book serves as a practical and detailed guide to applying quality assurance principles.

Kaplan KO, Hopkins JM, Longabaugh R: *Quality assurance guide for psychiatric and substance abuse facilities,* Chicago, 1981, Joint Commission on Accreditation of Hospitals.

This book provides a comprehensive, problem-focused approach to quality assurance from the point of view of the Joint Commission. It includes goals and objectives, identification and resolution of problems, priority setting, sample programs, critiques of quality assurance plans, and examples of assessment methods.

Shroeder P, editor: *Issues and strategies for nursing care quality,* Gaithersburg, Md, 1991, Aspen Publishers.

This text presents a broad look at quality issues and programs in health care. It describes an application of quality concepts to quality assurance activities found within clinical areas. The book addresses issues that will play a role in quality assurance in the nineties and into the 21st century. The content is written by experts in the field of nursing care quality.

Joyce Levy

Anita Lewis

After studying this chapter, the student will be able to:

- Define psychiatric consultation liaison nursing
- Identify the historical facts that have influenced the development of psychiatric consultation liaison nursing
- Identify the steps in the psychiatric consultation liaison process
- Identify the overall goals of psychiatric consultation liaison nursing

- Describe models of practice within psychiatric consultation liaison nursing
- Identify techniques and strategies for building a consultee-consultant alliance
- Identify the sources of power, benefits, and challenges of consultation liaison work
- Describe the educational preparation, professional experience, and clinical supervision of the psychiatric consultation liaison nurse

Mental health consultation is "the provision of clinical expertise regarding the delivery of psychological care in response to a request from a health care provider."[28] *Liaison* is "the facilitation of the relationship that exists between the patient, the illness, the consultees, and the hospital/ward milieu."[28]

The goals of liaison practice are consistent with the goals of consultation, and a dynamic, complementary relationship exists between consultation and liaison work. Consultation is the rendering of an expert opinion. Liaison work activates, expands, and brings to life that expert opinion. Consultation practice precedes liaison practice. Slowly, they become mutually dependent. The following example illustrates this relationship. A consultation was requested to determine why a client was refusing to complete a course of intravenous antibiotic treatment. He gave no reason for his refusal. The assessment by the psychiatric consultation liaison nurse revealed that the major reason for the client's refusal was not related to his feelings or any misunderstanding regarding the treatment but rather to his loss of confidence in his primary nurse. The consultation developed into a need for liaison practice.

A *consultation alliance* is a relationship between consultant and consultee, characterized by an understanding that clinical problems will be approached together. A *liaison alliance* is a relationship between the consultant and the consultee that indicates some clinical dilemmas can be resolved by reflecting on the interactions among care providers and clients. In the previous example, a liaison alliance is essential before the client's loss of confidence in his primary nurse can be addressed. The primary nurse needs to feel comfortable and safe with the liaison nurse to be able to openly discuss her relationship with the client.

The essence of consultation is personal and professional respect. Consultants are "invited in." Regardless of the type of consultation being provided, the consultee is ultimately responsible for the client. A second invitation to consult is rarely issued when the consultee feels devalued. If the consultant behaves or is viewed as a supervisor, an arrogant expert, or a judge, the effectiveness of clinical practice is impaired. The terms *consultation liaison nurse, consultants,* and *liaison nurse* will be used interchangeably in the chapter. The types of mental health consultation are listed below[7]:

1. Client centered
2. Consultee centered
3. Program centered administrative
4. Consultee centered administrative

Client-centered and consultee-centered consultation are discussed in this chapter.

CHARACTERISTICS OF THE PSYCHIATRIC CONSULTATION LIAISON NURSE

Qualifications

The psychiatric consultation liaison nurse is a registered nurse with a master's degree, clinical experience in general nursing, advanced clinical skills in psychiatric nursing, and administrative or supervisory experience. The psychiatric

	DATES	EVENTS
HISTORICAL OVERVIEW	1934	Rockefeller Foundation provided funds for five psychiatric liaison departments in general hospitals.
	1940s	Psychiatric nursing consultation was provided in general hospitals.
	1950s	Mental health consultation and psychiatric units in general hospitals were further expanded.
	1960s	Nursing departments in many general hospitals recognized the need for the role of consultation liaison nurses.
		Discussion of the concept of nursing consultation appeared in the literature.
	1970s	Gerald Caplan published research and development data relating to mental health consultation.
		Formal graduate education programs in consultation liaison nursing were developed at the University of Maryland and Yale University.
	1974	*Liaison nursing: a psychological approach to patient care* was the first textbook published on psychiatric consultation liaison nursing.
	1982	*Psychiatric liaison nursing: the theory and clinical practice* by Anita Lewis and Joyce Levy was published. This book established a theoretical base for practice.
	1987	First National Psychiatric Liaison Nursing Conference was held.
	1989	American Nurses' Association published Standards for Psychiatric Consultation Liaison Practice.
	1990s	With increased awareness of and interest in the psychosocial needs of clients in the general hospital, the skills of the psychiatric consultation liaison nurse are in greater demand.
	Future	With short-term hospitalization, there will be increased requests for the expertise of the psychiatric consultation liaison to assist in preparing the client and family for discharge to home-based care.

consultation liaison nurse should be clinically competent, proficient in assessing complicated nursing care situations, and insightful and knowledgeable about transference and countertransference.

The hallmarks of psychiatric consultation liaison nursing are objectivity, flexibility, and personal and professional maturity. The ability to take reasonable risks and to tolerate the intolerable is important because the liaison nurse often deals with the most painful clinical situations. Expert skills in the art of listening for process, themes and agendas are required. Problems presented for consultation are frequently complex and filled with hidden agendas. Identifying the essence of the problems, expanding consultation to include liaison principles, and formulating and implementing the interventions form the core of practice. The ability to practice autonomously is essential. Autonomy has advantages, but it also can create a feeling of isolation. A liaison nurse may not have a peer group within the hospital.

Roles

The major focuses of the liaison nurse are enhancement of the delivery of psychological nursing care and the effective management of care. She also serves as a catalyst in negotiations with staff and clients and promotes a profes-

sionally supportive, nonevaluative, collaborative relationship with the consultee. The liaison nurse practices predominantly in the general hospital, although the role has been successfully implemented in community settings.[19]

Development and implementation of the role are a continuous process. This process is altered, tested, and influenced by the liaison nurse, the health care system, and external forces. When she enters a health care system to provide psychiatric consultation liaison nursing, the liaison nurse carefully assesses the hospital or organization. Appraisal of reporting relationships, formal and informal power, job descriptions, history of the system, and identification of subsystems are important. High visibility, availability, flexibility, and credibility in response to requests are essential, while the liaison nurse strives to achieve clinical goals. The pressure to gain acceptance may tempt the newly hired liaison nurse to act in inappropriate situations. For example, a consultee may be warm, friendly, and welcoming to the liaison nurse and attempt to involve her in a struggle with the administration.

The role can be implemented in many ways beyond the established structure of the nursing department through inservice and orientation programs and committee participation. The liaison nurse can be helpful to nurses and clients dealing with the ramifications of devastating conditions such as AIDS, organ transplantation, cancer, chronic illness, trauma, and addiction. Liaison nurses may also implement the role by participation in educational programs.

Goals

The clinical responsibilities of liaison nurses are based on the goals of practice. Clear goals are the foundation of practice and continue to serve as guidelines as the role develops. The goals are:

1. To teach the concepts of effective psychological care and its implementation
2. To support nursing staff in providing psychological nursing care
3. To aid in maintaining alliances, respect, and esteem with the consultee
4. To encourage acceptance and tolerance of insolvable care issues

The goals may be implemented by formal or informal teaching, direct or indirect client intervention, client care conferences, support groups for consultees, multidisciplinary conferences and role modeling.

CONCEPTUAL MODEL

Although consultation and liaison practice are a part of every encounter with a client or a consultee, for purposes of clarity, they are discussed separately.

The Consultation Process

The consultation process involves the four steps listed below. These steps are carefully thought through and expanded in building an alliance with the consultee.[28]

1. Invitation
2. Evaluation of appropriateness
3. Problem identification
4. Direct or indirect care

The first step, the *invitation to consult*, is accompanied by assessment of several issues. First is identification of the consultee. Who is requesting consultation—nurse, doctor, social worker, family member, or client? The psychiatric consultation liaison nurse then reviews prior experience with the consultee making the request. It is also important to consider when consultation is sought in the course of hospitalization and illness and to identify whether there is any significance to the "timing" of the request. For example, has the client been admitted the day of the request, and has this somehow created sufficient anxiety among the consultees to warrant immediate consultation? Has the client been in the hospital for weeks, being managed by the consultee and now consultation is indicated? What has changed to warrant this request?

The second step involves *evaluation of the appropriateness of the consultation request*. All requests for consultation are, at the very least, opportunities to illustrate and clarify the role of the liaison nurse and explore issues relative to the psychological care of clients. Each consultation request is a potential opportunity to be a role model for, to teach, or to learn more about the consultee, the unit, and the system. Some common consultation requests are shown in the accompanying box. Every request is a poten-

▼ ....
COMMON CONSULTATION REQUESTS

A consultation is frequently requested for the client who:
Is depressed
Is manipulative
Is frequently asking for pain medication
Wants staff to do everything for him
Is refusing treatment
Is threatening to leave AMA
Is an addict or abuses drugs and alcohol
Has a psychiatric history
Has a terminal illness
Refuses surgery
Needs support
Is verbally abusive
Is physically abusive
Is seductive

tial springboard for enhancing consultation alliances, since each request is a call for help.

Problem identification is the third step of the consultation process. Clarifying the nature of the request and the focus of the problem is important if the consultation is to be useful and the goals of practice achieved.

Consultation requests are both overt and covert. The former usually reflects a legitimate difficulty (for example, a client who is noncompliant with medical treatment). The latter typically reflects the consultee's wish for or fear of the client or an emotional reaction to the situation that may be unacceptable. Often the covert question reflects unconscious reactions. In the noncompliant client, the covert level of the request may be "This client is infuriating. Tell us that we've tried long enough and can be angry and abandon him." Noting the descriptive language used in expressing the problem is helpful.

The problem necessitating consultation is initially defined by the consultee. Indications for requesting consultation are illustrated in the box on p. 881. Just as the client may accurately or inaccurately identify his problems, so may the consultee. Perhaps the language is misleading. Perhaps the consultee's diagnosis of the problem is incorrect. While maintaining a client care focus, the liaison nurse tries to "diagnose the total consultation." This process involves comprehensively assessing aspects of the consultation that are beyond the consultant-client interaction.[28] (See the box on p. 881.) Reviewing issues pertinent to the client's family, other health care providers, the doctor, the ward, the medical illness and reviewing the client's chart, aid the consultant in clarifying the consultation problem before determining the intervention. Consultees may have unrealistic or unconscious expectations of the liaison nurse and her ability to solve the problem, and such expectations become apparent as the total consultation is diagnosed.

The final step of the consultation process involves a *decision about a direct or an indirect model of care*. This determination is based primarily on the nature (seriousness, intensity, or impact) and the focus (client, consultee, family, or other) of the consultation request. In direct con-

▼ **INDICATIONS FOR REQUESTING PSYCHIATRIC NURSING CONSULTATION**

Assessment—unable to assess the problem and/or formulate a nursing diagnosis

Containment—problem has been managed but not solved

Escalation—problem out of control

Painful—problem well known but always difficult to manage

Danger—potential or actual to client and/or others

Implementation—problem acknowledged but unable to make effective interventions

Need—problem requires expert psychiatric intervention

▼ **ELEMENTS OF DIAGNOSING THE TOTAL CONSULTATION**

1. Consultation request
2. Consultee
3. Doctor and other members of thte health care team
4. Unit
5. Family
6. Medical illness
7. Chart
8. Client (direct consultation model)

From Lewis A, Levy J: *Psychiatric liaison nursing: the theory and clinical practice*, Reston, Va, 1982, Reston Publishing Co.

sultation, the liaison nurse interviews the client and/or family and then provides psychological intervention. In indirect consultation, a consultee-centered/case-centered conference is held, and intervention is planned. Follow-up, reassessment, and evaluation are ongoing and essential to both models. These activities are best shared by consultant and consultee as their alliance strengthens. Documentation in the client's record is the consultee's responsibility with the indirect model. The liaison nurse is responsible for documentation with the direct model.

The following guidelines may help determine a direct or an indirect approach.

Direct care is indicated when:

1. The problem presented remains unclear or complex
2. The consultant's role is new or not well understood; clinical involvement may help her enter the system
3. The required intervention is beyond the level of the consultee's expertise
4. Consultee anxiety is high and inhibits problem resolution
5. Consultee resistance is rigidly fixed
6. The same or similar problem(s) have been previously presented by the same consultee, at which time an indirect model was unsuccessful
7. Alliances would be enhanced
8. The problem is of special interest to the consultant and a direct model will not hamper alliances

Indirect care is indicated when:

1. The problem is clear and easily formulated
2. The consultee has formulated an appropriate intervention plan and is merely asking for support and validation from the consultant
3. Consultee anxiety is sufficiently low and her clinical skill is sophisticated enough to implement the required intervention
4. The consultee is appropriately motivated to carry out the intervention
5. Resistance to carrying out the intervention is low and chances are high that the plan can be successfully implemented
6. The problem can be resolved fairly easily by the consultee, who has become too dependent on the consultant
7. The problem is not client focused but rather consultee focused
8. A direct model would weaken alliances and may be in-

terpreted as a lack of confidence in the consultee on the part of the consultant

The Liaison Process

Liaison is a method by which to detect, prevent, and manage psychiatric problems and to resolve difficulties between clients and consultees. Liaison is part of the supportive, educative, clinical partnership between the consultant and consultee. Liaison also denotes an abstract process that the consultee may regard as manipulative, interpretive, or intrusive.

The following elements comprise the liaison process:

1. Education and socialization
2. Developmental level of the system and the consultee(s) within the system
3. The value and necessity of an alliance
4. Language
5. Developing the "ear" of the client and the "ear" of the consultee
6. Speaking the unspeakable
7. Confirmation of reality

Each element emerges from the one that precedes it. All of the elements are of equal importance for understanding liaison work and enacting the process.

Education and socialization

As nurses are educated and then socialized into their profession, they often assume three basic beliefs:

1. What they "can do"
2. What they "should do"
3. What they "can't do"

When nurses begin professional practice, they often believe that they "can do" everything for clients. With additional experience, they believe that they "should do" everything. This "should do" belief frequently results in nurses experiencing frustration and discouragement in their efforts to intervene with clients. The final result is that nurses may feel they "can't do" anything. Each clinical situation may emphasize one of these beliefs or blend all three of them. The unsophisticated liaison nurse may hold these same beliefs.

A brief example illustrates. When the inexperienced consultee encounters her first help-rejecting client, she discovers that sympathy, time, energy, alternative teaching methods, or threats of future illness are ineffective ("can do"). She may then feel responsible, believing that she "should" be able to intervene. Through increased experience with help-rejecting clients, the consultee may feel defeated at the onset ("can't do"). With additional clinical experience, consultee and liaison nurse learn to set priorities and become more skillful in predicting client care outcomes. The liaison nurse notes where the consultee is in regard to her beliefs.

Other factors that influence the attitudes and interventions of the consultee include the milieu of the ward, nursing leadership, the impact of continuing education programs, performance expectations, client/family responses, the illness and identification, and transference.

Developmental level of the system and the consultee(s) within the system

The developmental level of the system refers to the level of nursing practice, leadership, relationships among health care providers, and the psychological sophistication within a health care system. As some consultees remain and others move on and as leaders develop, a dynamic, ever changing system is created. The developmental stage of each consultee is reflected in her level of education and/or socialization, her relationships with other health care providers, and the quality of care she provides. For example, when the consultee adheres to the "can do" position, believing she can always meet the client's needs, a therapeutic intervention may be difficult.

▼ Case Example

Mrs. Rose, a 59-year-old woman, was hospitalized on a general surgical unit in a small community hospital, having a radical mastectomy for breast cancer 3 days earlier. She was attempting to conceal her grief by constantly requesting "little things" of her nurse, and the nurse attempted to meet her requests. Although these unending requests enabled her to have frequent contact with her nurse, they also prevented the client and nurse from discussing Mrs. Rose's psychological reaction to her mastectomy.

With education and experience, nurses increase their knowledge about the meaning of a client's behavior. There are nurses who tend to hold on to the "should do" position, sometimes demonstrated in the belief that all clients should be as independent as possible and that the nurse should consistently encourage their independence. For example, to Mrs. Thomas, a 42-year-old woman, status post subarachnoid hemorrhage, dependency meant renewed closeness with her estranged husband. This was evidenced by his attentiveness, including feeding her. Although she was able to feed herself, Mrs. Thomas found this very supportive. The nurse's attempt to intervene in this dependency would have proven nontherapeutic. There are situations in which independence is not the most desirable goal for the client.

The value and necessity of an alliance

The potential power of consultation and liaison alliances is reflected in the honest valuing of the consultee's work, views, and expertise. It is important to tactfully recognize gaps in knowledge and not question the consultee unnecessarily. The consultant communicates to the consultee her belief that the request was appropriate, that she tried in some way to deal with the problem, that anxiety can be detrimental to problem solving.

Anxiety can influence the consultee's approach to the psychiatric consultation liaison nurse in other ways, as shown in the case example below.

▼ Case Example

A highly competent staff nurse with years of clinical experience, angrily approached the liaison nurse. The staff nurse demanded that the liaison nurse help her stop a 51-year-old business executive, who had had abdominal surgery 5 days earlier, from regressing. "He's refusing to do anything for himself. He's on the light constantly and always pointing out my inefficiencies," she said. The consultee's affect was hostile and demanding. It was apparent that she had not approached the client about her concerns. This behavior was uncharacteristic of her. The consultee was affectively doing to the consultant what the client was doing to her. In addition to solving the stated problem, it would be appropriate for the liaison nurse to diagnose the total consultation with special attention to the hidden problem—the esteem needs of the consultee.

Language

The language used by the consultee to describe the problem in nursing care is significant. The quality, intensity, potential symbolic meaning, and concurrent affect expressed in the language are noted by the liaison nurse in diagnosing the total consultation. It is important to ask the consultee whether the client describes the problem in the same way as the consultee. A consultee may label a client "manipulative and seductive," whereas the client describes himself as "angry and frightened." For example, Mr. Michael, a 46-year-old, married father of four, 2 days after femoral-popliteal bypass graft, is described by the nurse as "doing well, but very withdrawn for no apparent reason." However, Mr. Michael describes himself as not doing well because he is still in the intensive care unit, his family has not visited, and he is experiencing mild confusion with poor memory and is trying to conceal it.

Developing the "ear" of the client and the "ear" of the consultee

This element of the liaison process involves perfecting the clinical skill of hearing issues from the perspective of the client as well as the consultee. This results in the development of a "larger" ear. If the client is described as "appropriately depressed," questions the consultant may raise are: How are his behavior and responses to illness being heard and felt? By whose standards are the client's psychological responses being judged? Understanding the affects coloring the experience, the possible perceptions and feelings of all involved, and the quality of their communication are crucial in developing the larger ear. This understanding is primarily for the use of the liaison nurse. Depending on the intensity of the problem and the strength of the alliance, such understanding may or may not be shared directly with consultees or clients.

The liaison nurse remains sensitive to everyone's opinion. By gathering views, the consultant illustrates that although consensus may not be possible, an intervention that takes each view into consideration may be developed. This is the value of developing the larger clinical ear.

Speaking the unspeakable

There are times when offering an interpretation—putting into words what others are unaware of and therefore unable to say—can be useful. The value of speaking the unspeakable is often illustrated in the clarification of transference and identification issues for a consultee who may be suffering in the course of her attempts to care for a client.

▼ **Case Example**

Mr. Fine, a 28-year-old law student, diagnosed with acute renal failure necessitating dialysis, was described as tearful, compliant and withdrawn. The client was overwhelmed with the loss of a normal body function.[1] The nursing staff knew he was depressed but could not move beyond their own sadness and identification. The liaison nurse intervened by speaking the unspeakable, which involved addressing the consultee's fear, vulnerability, and helplessness.

Assessing alliances is crucial when speaking the unspeakable. Will speaking out help or hinder? Will interpretation open the door for additional understanding and intervention? Caution is necessary. If the consultee is feeling vulnerable, suspicious, or her image of herself has been injured, an interpretation may pointlessly add unwelcome insight to injury.

Confirmation of reality

This final element of the liaison process involves describing and examining a situation as it actually is. This perspective is useful in labeling intolerable situations, some of which must be endured. It involves saying what others are painfully aware of, but too frightened or inhibited to say. There are situations in which confirming reality provides clarity and helps to solve problems.

▼ **Case Example**

When a 31-year-old client with AIDS began to throw his urine and feces at the nurses, prompt intervention was in order. The liaison nurse stated that in reality the client needed his health care team more than they needed him, and the nurses do not have to tolerate such behavior. This resulted in an increased willingness to understand what may have motivated the client's actions. Empathic limits were developed.

In chaotic, provoking, clinical situations, a sense of reality may become elusive. Confirming reality can dramatically reduce the tension experienced by consultees. It can lead not only to a solution to the problem, but also to the enhancement of alliances.

Assessment of Consultations

A holistic approach consisting of five dimensions for assessing consultations serves as an additional tool in psychiatric consultation liaison practice. The significance of each dimension varies with the problem, the client, and the consultee.

Physical dimension The liaison nurse assesses the physiological impact of the illness. All physical illness is a psychological event; it is rarely possible to experience an illness exclusively in the body or the mind. Data are compiled concerning biological causes of the illness, natural history, treatment, symptoms, present and projected degree of debilitation, absence or presence of pain and prognosis. The typical experience of a particular illness and whether this is an unusual or expected presentation are key in formulating useful interventions. How have normal body processes been effected by the illness? Is the illness visible, and has this influenced body image? Visible signs and symptoms of illness are not a prerequisite for distortion of body image. When a young woman with a long-standing diabetes was asked to describe how she felt about her body, she tearfully responded, "That's easy, I feel terrible; my body is dirty and marked."

The client's physical status, health history, and usual health care practices before becoming ill are noteworthy. The possibility of an underlying organic cause for the psychological presentation of a physical illness is considered. For example, pancreatic cancer can often be first expressed as a clinical depression. In addition, medications, treatments, and metabolic imbalances can alter cognitive status and influence physical presentation. It is imperative to note that the relationship between the physical and psychological causes and presentations of illness are fluid.

Emotional dimension The client's psychological and emotional responses to illness and hospitalization are best evaluated in the context of his premorbid status. Significant psychological history, personality style, defensive structure, mode of adaptation, affect, mood, and present level of psychological functioning are relevant. Four psychological behaviors are necessary to work through an illness. These include "egocentricity, constriction of interests, emotional dependency, and hypochondriasis."[28] These behaviors are expected stages in the client's response to illness. They also may not occur or may vary in intensity. The behaviors are individualized. The client who is having difficulty sharing his nurse with other clients may be described as egocentric. The client intensely focused on his intravenous line is demonstrating constriction of interests. The client who is unable to make even the smallest decision on his own is exhibiting emotional dependency. Hypochondriasis is evident in the client who becomes focused on minor body aches and pains and is unable to give them up. The client may move from one stage to another as well as return to a previously experienced stage.

The experience of giving and receiving care is filled with emotion, mutual expectations and assumptions, identifications and transference responses among clients and health care providers. Sorting out these issues is crucial. The psychological developmental levels of client and consultee are also significant. Illness often holds special meaning for the client and consultee. Depending on the nature of the illness, its symptoms, its treatment course, the nursing care required, the part of the body affected and previous knowledge or experience, meanings of illness may vary. The following eight categories have been identified in the psychological meanings of illness: a challenge, an enemy, a punishment, a weakness, a relief, a strategy, irreparable loss or damage, a value.[31]

The degree of emotional conflict the client feels may be a result of the meaning illness has and/or the life disruption it precipitates. These facets of the emotional dimension may be difficult to assess directly.

Intellectual dimension This dimension includes a mental status examination of the client. The neurological and metabolic ramifications of the illness; potential side effects of medication and treatments; and symptoms of pseudodementia, dementia, and delirium are noted.

The liaison nurse evaluates whether a formal mental status examination is appropriate. The evaluation is based on the overall psychological presentation of the client, degree of physical illness and discomfort, and the nature of the problem. The client's education, intellectual capacity, memory, and ability to apply knowledge are factors.

Identifying the consultee's understanding of the problem and her ability to understand and carry out a psychologically based nursing care intervention are also useful.

Social dimension This dimension can be especially powerful. When social norms and family dynamics and the values of the client and consultee are at odds, the conflict may precipitate the request for consultation. These situations are often very tense.

Clinical problems symptomatic of conflicts in the social dimension, often present as interpersonal problems among clients and consultees or between consultees. These kinds of clinical situations represent complex challenges to intervention.

Important areas for consideration include the atmosphere of the ward; leadership or management style; the degree, nature, and sources of professional esteem and cohesion among consultees; and relationships among care providers. Environmental factors also necessitate review, for example, the location and social significance of the hospital to the client; the consultee; the community; whether the client is in a private room, a semiprivate room, or a ward; and whether room change occurs and why. The degree of life disruption that illness and hospitalization create for the client and his family is significant. Culture and ethnicity mold the relationship between client and consultee. They may also color the client's and the consultee's beliefs concerning the liaison nurse and the use of consultation.

Spiritual dimension Assessment of religious and philosophical beliefs concerning general life values, ethical standards, views of illness, death, hope, and the purpose of life provide the liaison nurse with an even richer understanding of the client, the consultee, and their responses to each other. Recognizing the importance of religious teachings in the life of client and consultee is central. For example, the refusal to have an abortion or to receive blood products reflects not only a religious viewpoint but also a potential area of conflict between client and consultee. Clients, consultees, and liaison nurses may find their values in conflict when faced with defining comfort measures for the terminally ill client. Clients who have strong, supportive religious beliefs may be better equipped to face the stresses of a long and complex illness.

PRACTICE ISSUES

The issues of identification, transference, countertransference, and resistance are the most difficult to assess, understand, and intervene in. Assessment requires an understanding of these issues, which can influence the consultee, the client, and the liaison nurse.[14] It is often these issues that are roadblocks to the liaison nurse's implementation of her recommendations.

The experience of illness and hospitalization and the regression that accompanies the experience are among the precipitants for identification, transference, and countertransference.

Identification, a conscious process, raises issues that are usually recognized and more easily understood than transference or countertransference. Identification may develop around similarities between client and consultee (age, sex, type of illness, appearance, or occupation). A staff nurse may overidentify with a client who is also a nurse, the same age, and suffering from a dreaded disease such as cancer of the reproductive system. On an unconscious level, the client may evoke in the nurse previous feelings such as rivalry, rage, or depression. These powerful feelings cloud the path to intervention. At these times postponing action while observing and listening is advisable.

Identification issues can also evoke the unconscious process of transference or countertransference and complicate the consultee-client relationship. There are behavioral clues to transference and countertransference (see the accompanying box). Transference and countertransference can be positive or negative and can benefit or interfere with the client-nurse relationship. *Transference* includes unconscious feelings and expectations related to relationships and events in the past. An important aspect of understanding clients who are physically ill is speculating on possible unconscious motives for their present adaptation. Why is the client overcompliant? What does it mean when a young man cannot bear to be separated from his wife before surgery? Why does an elderly woman become hostile when her CAT scan is postponed? Is it simply fear or is there a reawakening of feelings from the past or could this just be an expression of her compulsiveness?

Clients may revive unresolved conflicts in the health care provider.[59] These conflicts may interfere with the care of the client. *Countertransference* can either lead to defensive maneuvers that destroy the alliance with the client, as with Mr. Josh in the following case example, or lead to positive steps that help the client overcome isolation and suffering, as exemplified by Ms. Patrick in the second case example on p. 885.

▼ ·····

BEHAVIORAL AND EMOTIONAL CLUES TO TRANSFERENCE AND COUNTERTRANSFERENCE

Increased or decreased interest in the client
Depression
Affectionate feelings
Inability to set limits
Arguing with the client
Desire to impress the client
Sadistic, hostile feelings
Disapproving and angry feelings
Special need to be reassuring
Provoking acting-out behavior
Thinking or dreaming about the client
Desire to assist client in special ways
Strong desire to provide care for client
Deriving unusual satisfaction or gratification from the care of the client

▼ Case Example

Mr. Josh, a 32-year-old lawyer with an 8-year history of drug abuse was demanding, disruptive, and threatening to sign out against medical advice. Mr. Josh had been admitted with an infected leg. A multidisciplinary case conference was organized to address his nursing needs and to formulate a management plan. The primary nurse described Mr. Josh's behavior as obnoxious and divulged without embarrassment the hostile techniques she used to maintain control. She further revealed how she used these techniques with her children. What effect did Mr. Josh's issues have on the nurse and on his care? It is possible that he raised conflictual issues that had not been resolved for the nurse.

▼ Case Example

Ms. Patrick, in contrast to the other nurses, approached an elderly woman client in a warm, caring, solicitous manner that was out of proportion to the client's nursing care needs. Ms. Patrick was constantly doing things for the client. The extra attention clearly helped. The client had demonstrated increasingly demanding behavior after her CAT scan was rescheduled. It is important for the liaison nurse to recognize that Ms. Patrick's behavior may be a positive countertransference response that has led to a positive adaptation for the client.

The consultant refrains from discussing the consultees' countertransference issues when diagnosing the total consultation. The nurse is responsible for her own behavior. However, if the nurse's personal struggles or conflicts interfere with safe care, if there is potential for harm to the client, or if the nurse asks for help, tactful intervention, including a recommendation for psychotherapy, may be indicated.

As attention is concentrated on both positive and negative effects of transference and countertransference, the impact on the consultee and the client becomes more obvious. The more a consultee seeks direct personal satisfaction from caring for the client, the more likely that emotionally charged issues will be avoided or acted out by either party instead of being felt or discussed in a helpful manner. It is also possible that the nurse can use client care as a defense against the emotions evoked by the client. What does it mean for the client who, after expressing fear and sadness about pending renal transplant surgery, is provided prompt attention to his physical needs and then is left to rest—alone with his worries? If the nurse's wish is to have her sense of competence and self worth mirrored by the client's appreciation and recovery, the client's affect may be intolerable. She may provide him with competent care in one dimension while also abandoning him in another.

Liaison nurses are not immune to identification, transference, and countertransference. The role as consultant does allow some distancing from the clinical situation. However, psychiatric education and clinical supervision assist the consultant in remaining vigilant about these issues in clinical situations and in professional interactions. What does it mean when the staff nurse compliments the nurse consultant by saying, "We knew you would figure something out" or "I'm so glad to see you. We don't know what to do—we've tried everything." Does the consultee want the consultant to magically fix it? Does the consultant wish to be viewed as superior?

When a clinical case is presented for consultation, a parallel process may occur among the consultee, client, and liaison nurse. *Parallel process* refers to the reenactment of the relationship between client and consultee within the relationship between consultee and consultant. For example, the client may express hopelessness to his nurse (consultee). The consultee may then tell the consultant that the client's clinical situation is hopeless. The liaison nurse must be attuned to feelings of helplessness, depression, anger, or hopelessness in herself and recognize the presence of parallel process. It is possible that the consultee unwittingly is communicating and reenacting the clients feelings to the consultant. After a careful assessment and analysis, if a consultation remains unclear, the diagnosis may be parallel process.

▼ Case Example

The liaison nurse was asked to see Mr. Alexander, a 41-year-old married father of three, who was in the intensive care unit (ICU) after suffering from angina. Mr. Alexander was accepting of his care, the experience of being in the ICU, and his diagnosis.[44] The ICU nurses described him as a "real nice guy" without any problems, but they thought he would need some support when he left their unit. Since it was stressful in the ICU with many admissions and transfers, the liaison nurse intervened directly. The liaison nurse had the same impression of Mr. Alexander as the consultee but began to wonder why the consultation was requested. More importantly, she found herself visiting the client more often than his psychological discomfort warranted. When Mr. Alexander casually mentioned his hope for the television he had requested 2 days ago, the liaison nurse, quite out of character, bypassed the usual procedure for obtaining TV sets and personally issued the second request. The next day when Mr. Alexander still had not received his TV, the liaison nurse tracked down the TV hostess and insisted that he get his set immediately.

The client's passivity was probably the reason for the consultation, and the active role of the liaison nurse mirrored the active role the ICU nurses assumed in requesting consultation. Perhaps Mr. Alexander evoked identification, transference, or countertransference.

An ongoing challenge for the liaison nurse is determining how to deal with these issues. Acknowledgment of personal conflicts with a consultee may best be addressed by a general statement such as "It seems that this client is really getting to you." It is important to recognize that sometimes conflicts with clients are based on inexperience rather than on unconscious wishes or fantasies. The inexperienced nurse who becomes too involved with the depressed client may want to be therapeutic and may not be experiencing countertransference. As the liaison nurse continues to observe and study behavior and relationships, more questions arise about the relationships among consultee, client, and the liaison nurse.

Resistance is another issue that influences the practice of psychiatric consultation liaison nursing. Resistance is an overt or covert force that is opposing in nature. Resistance may emanate from conscious and unconscious feelings and may often not be understood. It is not simply rejection. As the liaison nurse continues to develop alliances and become more credible in the system, resistance takes on a variety of forms. Some examples of resistance, as demonstrated by the consultee, are:

• Reluctance or refusal to carry out interventions

- Asking for help but failing to allocate time to discuss the problem
- Failure to communicate major changes in a client's condition
- Consistently stating that there are no physiological care problems

The risk for the liaison nurse rests with personalizing the resistance, becoming hurt, angry, or withdrawn. The liaison nurse listens to what the consultees are saying, recognizes verbal as well as nonverbal communications, and hears the urgency in their requests and their discomfort, fear, or terror. These observations are combined with the consultant's own feelings as a mirror to the parallel process that may be occurring. The goal of psychiatric consultation liaison nursing is always to guide intervention. However, if the observation or recognition of resistance is not included, diagnosing the total consultation may never be achieved. The liaison nurse needs to be cautious and not view all questioning of psychiatric consultation as resistance. There may be realistic reasons for this questioning; perhaps the consultee feels that the client's unstable medical condition would make an intervention impossible or inadvisable.

The liaison nurse can be more effective when she considers all of the possibilities regarding resistance rather than limiting herself to one interpretation. A skilled liaison nurse considers that resistance may be present but recognizes that it is not the only force opposing successful interventions. Clinical supervision by an experienced psychiatric consultation liaison nurse helps to identify resistance and its effect on practice. For example, a liaison nurse who was new to her role was troubled by the consultees' lack of interest in intervening directly with their clients. The consultees insisted that the consultant see every client. Her supervisor suggested that perhaps the consultees felt inadequate, were overworked, or were showing resistance by requesting the liaison nurse to do what they were clinically capable of doing. Their resistance may have been a wish that the liaison nurse "work" and not just talk to them. Perhaps the consultation alliance was not strong enough. The goals of psychiatric consultation liaison nursing practice are not attainable without understanding resistance.

Other practice issues that warrant attention are the benefits and hazards of practicing psychiatric consultation liaison nursing in one system over time. Benefits occur when the liaison nurse remains in a system enduring resistance while maintaining alliances. These benefits include the following:

1. The system is likely to reward the demonstrated competence of the consultant with power.
2. Explanation of roles and goals decreases.
3. The quality of consultations increases.
4. Increased competence of the consultee results in a trend away from crisis intervention and toward preventative management.
5. There is an increase in the quantity of consultations.

Hazards that may result when the liaison nurse remains in a system are:

1. Increased clinical competence and acceptance can lead to entitlement, elitism, false safety, and boredom.
2. Consultees may want to continue to ascribe magical attributes to the liaison nurse. The consultant may no longer try to dispel the myth. The following is an example of the hazard of deemphasizing this mystical conception. Dr. Adam requested Ms. Gottlieb, the liaison nurse, to assess Mr. Philip's depression following his pneumonia. He told the nurse manager that no one was as efficient or thoughtful as Ms. Gottlieb. The hazard for Ms. Gottlieb is feeling flattered, complimented, honored, or superior rather than assessing the meaning of this statement in terms of the total consultation.
3. Sharing secrets and becoming more involved with the group that was initially taboo is tempting.

This is the time to identify new and productive professional paths and to avoid the pitfalls of staying in the system.

The consultation liaison process is illustrated through application to a clinical case.

▼ Case Example

Consultation request

"I need your help with Mr. Slaten. He's screaming, being impossible, and refusing care!"

Assessing the consultation request

Who: Request for consultation is initiated by the client's primary nurse, Ms. Brown.

What: The request is for help in dealing with Mr. Slaten, a 53-year-old divorced father of one 19-year-old daughter. The client has a 15-year history of diabetes mellitus. Two years ago he had a mild, right-sided cerebrovascular accident. He is legally blind, has chronic congestive heart failure, and presently suffers from a severely infected leg. Approximately 6 months before admission, he developed a chronic deep vein thrombosis of the left leg. After delaying hospitalization and trying to "follow doctor's orders at home," Mr. Slaten felt he no longer had a choice but to be admitted to the hospital. Severe vascular insufficiency to his lower left leg and foot were diagnosed. A below-knee amputation is recommended. Despite intense pain, Mr. Slaten is refusing the procedure.

When: Consultation is requested on day 6 of hospitalization.

How: The request is expressed by telephone to the consultant. Ms. Brown is talking rapidly. She sounds frightened and upset and asks if the consultant can be available today.

Why: Mr. Slaten's behavior and responses to his illness, hospitalization, and prescribed treatment are interfering with the delivery of comprehensive care. The consultee is clearly worried, frustrated, and distraught about Mr. Slaten's physical and emotional status.

Consultation questions

Overt consultation question: "Why is Mr. Slaten, who is familiar with this hospital and staff, being so disruptive and refusing care? Please evaluate his behavior and possible depression."

Covert consultation question: A strong, implied wish on the part of the consultee that the consultant "get Mr. Slaten to stop being crazy and sign the surgical permit—how can he treat us like this?"

Analysis: Problem identification

The type of consultation being requested is client centered.

The consultee—The liaison nurse has worked with the consultee before. Ms. Brown has been a registered nurse for 2 years and is frequently in charge of the ward on the night shift. Ms. Brown is bright, insightful, and highly motivated, encourages client participation in care planning and delivery, individualizes care plans, and sets realistic care goals. Ms. Brown is convinced that the consultant will know what to do. Of note is that Ms. Brown has a tendency to respond personally to clinical nursing failures.

The doctor—Dr. Martin has been caring for Mr. Slaten for many years. He is clearly quite angry with Mr. Slaten, and tells the liaison nurse that Mr. Slaten "should have come in sooner, does as he pleases, and is merely taking up our time. If he doesn't want the amputation, he doesn't have to have it." It is apparent from the ensuing discussion that Dr. Martin has made an enormous effort with Mr. Slaten. Dr. Martin is worried and upset with him and convinced that the client's decision to refuse surgery is not in his best interest. The liaison nurse has never worked with Dr. Martin, who has a reputation for rarely seeking psychiatric consultation, preferring to manage things himself. Dr. Martin is friendly and polite, but obviously skeptical of what may be accomplished.

The unit—The unit is a busy 35-bed medical-surgical unit. It is well staffed, and primary nursing is practiced. The nurse manager has been in her position for many years and is supportive to staff but only occasionally calls the consultant. However, the nurse manager does support and encourage her staff in their requests for consultation.

The family—Mr. Slaten has one child, Amy. She had been living with him, but recently moved in with her fiancé and is very involved in planning her wedding. There has been no contact with Mrs. Slaten for many years. Amy visits her father daily, sometimes accompanied by her fiancé. Reportedly, the client is in better spirits when his daughter is present. There is no other family. Mr. Slaten was working and living independently until he developed the thrombosis. This, coupled with his chronic illnesses, forced him to retire from a 20-year career as an art critic. Mr. Slaten gave up his apartment and moved to a low-cost housing development.

The medical illness—Mr. Slaten is an insulin-dependent diabetic. His present medical regimen includes neutral protamine hagedorn (NPH)-insulin, methyldopa (Aldomet), furosemide (Lasix), a low-salt, 1200 calorie diet, and mild fluid restriction warranted by congestive heart failure. Mr. Slaten suffers from bilateral vascular insufficiency and peripheral neuropathy. His left leg is the most seriously effected, with many deep, infected skin lesions and probable osteomyelitis. The leg is quite swollen, extremely painful, and is not responding to routine wound care, intravenous Keflex, and elevation. Meperidine (Demerol) and hydroxyzinepamoate (Vistaril) are not successful in controlling pain, and the client is refusing to try other analgesic, stating that they make him feel "sick" and "cloud" his head. Dressing changes are painful and Mr. Slaten sobs and swears—when he allows them to be done. He is on strict bed rest, is sleeping poorly with minimal appetite, constipation, low-grade fevers, and headaches. He has never been as ill as he is now.

The chart—Mr. Slaten's chart reflects a long association with the hospital. He has always complied with prescribed medical regimen. He has been hospitalized over the years for pneumonia, pulmonary edema, a foot ulcer, and most recently the CVA. Mr. Slaten was well known and loved by the staff and was previously described as "quiet, cooperative, appreciative, and a fighter." Notes in the present chart suggest that the client's present behavior is uncharacteristic of him—"hostile, demanding, uncooperative, and verbally abusive to staff." The chart is now filled with notations concerning the progressive, deterioration of Mr. Slaten's leg and his equally deteriorating emotional state. At times, he refuses to bathe and eat and is further described as "depressed, irritable, and mildly confused." The chart indicates that Mr. Slaten is in metabolic balance, and his neurological evaluation is normal.

Determination of model of care

Direct consultation—Ms. Brown's efforts to solve the problem herself by client education, support, and empathic limit setting have failed. Ms. Brown feels she has failed because she is unable to change Mr. Slaten's behavior. Ms. Brown's anxiety is quite high.

The problem is complex. Identification and or transference may be involved (consultee is similar in age to client's daughter). Direct service may provide an opportunity to intervene regarding Mr. Slaten and also to further assess, understand, and perhaps intervene with Ms. Brown's concerns. Also, Dr. Martin is resistant and doubtful regarding the usefulness of psychiatric consultation. Direct service may clarify the clinical work of the psychiatric consultation liaison nurse. Additional factors include the busy pace of the unit and Mr. Slaten's limited social supports.

In further diagnosing the total consultation, each dimension necessitates careful assessment, either by direct examination or indirectly by observation and listening.

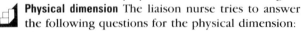 **Physical dimension** The liaison nurse tries to answer the following questions for the physical dimension:

- What would have been Mr. Slaten's overall psychological state if he were a healthy 53-year-old man?
- Was his behavior a direct result of persistent, unremitting physical deterioration?
- Is his behavior a typical presentation? (With recognition of the effects of diabetes on the body, consideration is given to factors such as sexual potency, energy level, and neuropathy.)
- What is it like to experience the worst complications of diabetes?
- How did Mr. Slaten deal with the deterioration of sight?
- What is the illness experience with a severely infected leg?
- Is there much pain?

Emotional dimension The liaison nurse tries to answer the following questions for the emotional dimension:

- If Mr. Slaten was described as a fighter, what happened to that spirit?
- What is the experience of viewing oneself as a competent fighter and now as hopeless, incompetent, and useless?
- What does it mean when a passive, self-contained gentleman is shouting obscenities at nurses and doctors?
- What has been the general psychological meaning of illness for Mr. Slaten? Has this meaning changed?
- If Mr. Slaten no longer views illness as a challenge, is he struggling with whether he can continue to fight?
- Do the visible signs of deterioration have a special emotional impact on Mr. Slaten?

Intellectual dimension The liaison nurse tries to answer the following questions for the intellectual dimension:

- Is it possible that Mr. Slaten has mental status changes?
- What is his performance on the mental status examination?
- Is he experiencing organic changes that are altering his behavior?
- Has his loss of short-term memory been induced by depression?
- Is his behavior an example of externalization as a defense against anxiety, emotional dependence, and/or ambivalence regarding the recommended amputation?
- Has his previous pride in his intellectual abilities contributed to his response to illness?

Social dimension The liaison nurse tries to answer the following questions for the social dimension:

- Will Mr. Slaten be able to maintain his present living situation?

- What has the impact of his daughter's recent separation from him and her future marriage had on his response to the illness?
- Would it be helpful for Mr. Slaten to explore the issues regarding his daughter with Ms. Brown?
- To what degree has Mr. Slaten become isolated because of the progressive illness?

 Spiritual dimension The liaison nurse tries to answer the following questions for the spiritual dimension:

- What part has hope and faith served in Mr. Slaten being a fighter?
- Does he want to die now?
- What was involved in his earlier trusting belief in God?
- Does he now feel betrayed by God?
- Does he believe that he has been given more than he can bear?

The practice issues raised for Dr. Martin and Ms. Brown are different. These issues were influenced by the course of Mr. Slaten's illness, and these two consultees' previous personal and caregiving experiences. Some of the caregiving issues are:

- Was Dr. Martin experiencing sympathy, depression, and sadness?
- Was Ms. Brown feeling manipulated and angry?
- What accounts for Ms. Brown's tendency to personalize her caregiving failures?
- Does Mr. Slaten hold some special significance for Ms. Brown?
- What did Ms. Brown's upset and concern mean to Mr. Slaten?
- What unconscious issues were raised for Dr. Martin and Ms. Brown by Mr. Slaten's affect and behavior?
- How was Mr. Slaten's psychological conflict experienced by Dr. Martin and Ms. Brown?
- What meaning does Mr. Slaten's illness and his struggle with whether he can continue to fight hold for Dr. Martin and Ms. Brown?
- How are these issues experienced by the psychiatric consultation liaison nurse?

NURSING DIAGNOSES

The following list provides examples of NANDA approved nursing diagnoses with causative statements to be considered in the case:

1. Ineffective individual coping related to being overwhelmed by complex medical illness
2. High risk for self-directed violence related to abandonment and depression
3. High risk for dysfunctional grieving related to an alteration in support system
4. Powerlessness related to complications of illness
5. Noncompliance with nursing and medical care measures related to ineffective coping
6. Disturbance in self-concept related to alterations in body image
7. Dysfunctional grieving related to retirement, major life changes, and separation from daughter
8. Social isolation and lack of diversional activity related to the ramifications of medical illness

Liaison Elements

In further assessing the consultation and determining intervention, the liaison nurse endeavors to answer the following questions: Does Ms. Brown believe that she "should" or "can," with consultation, provide Mr. Slaten with successful interventions? Does Dr. Martin believe that he "should" intervene but knows that he "can't"? How did the previous relationship between Ms. Brown and the consultant influence this case? How can the developing alliance with the nurse manager and Dr. Martin be addressed? Did Mr. Slaten's language communicate criticism, despair, or helplessness? Was it heard as manipulation or devaluation? Did Mr. Slaten hear things differently? Was the unspeakable issue the wish for the client to leave or to die?

Intervention

The following are the interventions planned for Mr. Slaten:

1. Direct assessment of Mr. Slaten and ongoing grief work by the liaison nurse.
2. Consultation with a psychiatrist for psychotropic and pain medication and evaluation of competency and suicidality.
3. Social service consultation with daughter and fiancé for evaluation of needs.
4. Team meeting—liaison focus, includes the nurse manager. Mr. Slaten's internal conflict is explained, his psychological status and affect are described, and a plan of care is developed.
5. Care plan
   a. Therapeutic limit setting
      (1) Meals and snacks are provided as usual; if Mr. Slaten refuses these, he is not offered special foods.
      (2) Verbal abuse is to be ignored, but when Mr. Slaten becomes physically abusive, he is to be restrained.
      (3) Struggles over bathing and dressing changes are to be avoided; offer several different times for care and assistance while making Mr. Slaten responsible for refusing care.
   b. The consultees are encouraged to recognize the real stresses in Mr. Slaten's life and that his behavior is a mirror of his internal conflict. (Ms. Brown and Dr. Martin are not responsible for Mr. Slaten's responses, reactions, or care choices.)
   c. The liaison nurse is consistently visible and available.
   d. Regular team meetings are held.

BRIEF REVIEW

Historically, psychiatric consultation liaison nursing emerged as a subspecialty of psychiatric nursing and developed in response to recognition of the mind-body relationship in physical illness and recovery, additional clinical responsibilities of nursing staff, and technological advances in medicine.

Mental health consultation is "the provision of clinical expertise regarding the delivery of psychological care in response to a request from a health care provider."[28] Liaison is "the facilitation of the relationship that exists between the patient, the illness, the consultees and the hospital/

ward milieu."[28] The goals of psychiatric consultation liaison practice are (1) to teach the concepts and implementation of psychological care, (2) to support nursing staff in providing psychological care, (3) to aid in maintaining alliances, respect, and esteem with the consultee, and (4) to encourage acceptance and tolerance of insolvable care issues. Consultation and liaison alliances are crucial and develop as the work progresses. The liaison nurse remains available, visible, objective, nonevaluative, and collaborative with consultees. Consultation and liaison alliances are strengthened as the psychiatric consultation liaison nurse implements the steps of the consultation process—assessment of the invitation to consult, evaluation of the appropriateness of the request, problem identification, and the determination and implementation of a direct or indirect intervention. The total consultation is diagnosed to further understand the needs of the client and the consultee.

Consultation practice is complementary to liaison practice. The elements of the liaison process are (1) education and socialization, (2) developmental level of the system and the consultee(s), (3) value and necessity of an alliance, (4) language, (5) developing the "ear" of the client and the "ear" of the consultee, (6) speaking the unspeakable, and (7) confirmation of reality. Liaison symbolizes the clinical partnership between the consultant and consultee.

Practical issues that affect the consultation liaison process are identification, transference or countertransference, parallel processing, or resistance involved in the consultation liaison relationship.

Psychiatric consultation liaison nursing practice can become quite powerful in the creation of a respectful, competent, clinical partnership with consultees. Utilizing the skills and knowledge of a nurse, a psychiatric clinician, and a consultant, the many pieces of the consultation liaison process are identified and implemented to enhance client care.

REFERENCES AND SUGGESTED READINGS

1. Backman ME: *The psychology of the physically ill patient: a clinicians guide*, New York, 1989, Plenum.
2. Badger T: Mental health consultation with a surgical unit nursing staff, *Clinical Nurse Specialist* 2:3, 1988.
3. Barbiasz J and others: Establishing the psychiatric liaison nursing role: collaboration with the nurse administrator, *Journal of Nursing Administration* 14:8, 1982.
4. Barry P: *Psychosocial nursing assessment and intervention*, Philadelphia, 1989, JB Lippincott.
5. Blumenfield M and others: Survey of nurses working with AIDS patients, *General Hospital Psychiatry* 9:58, 1987.
6. Boyd JN and others: The merit and significance of clinical nurses specialists, *Journal of Nursing Administration* 21:9, September 1991.
7. Caplan G: *The theory and practice of mental health consultation*, New York, 1970, Basic Books.
8. Chisholm NM: The psychiatric consultation-liaison nurse and the challenge of AIDS: caring for nurses, *Clinical Nurse Specialist* 5(2):123, 1991.
9. Chitty K, Maynard C: Managing manipulation, *Journal of Psychosocial Nursing* 24:6, 1986.
10. Davitz LI, Davitz JR: *Nurses' responses to patients' suffering*, New York, 1980, Springer.
11. Fife B, Lemler S: The psychiatric nurse specialist: a valuable asset in the general hospital, *Journal of Nursing Administration* 13:14, 1983.
12. Fife B: Establishing the mental health clinical specialist role in the medical setting, *Issues in Mental Health Nursing* 8(1):15, 1986.
13. Fishel AH: Psychiatric consultation: improving the work environment, *Journal of Psychosocial Nursing and Mental Health Services* 29(11):31, 1991.
14. Groves J: Taking care of the hateful patient, *New England Journal of Medicine* 296(16):883, 1978.
15. Hamric A, Spross J: *The clinical nurse specialist in theory and practice*, New York, 1983, Grune & Stratton.
16. Hart CA: The role of psychiatric consultation liaison nurses in ethical decisions to remove life-sustaining treatments, *Archives of Psychiatric Nursing* 4(6):370, 1990.
17. Hendler N, Wise T, Lucas MJ: The expanded role of the psychiatric liaison nurse, *Psychiatric Quarterly* 51:135, 1979.
18. Holstein S, Schwab J: A coordinated consultation program for nurses and psychiatrists, *Journal of the American Medical Association* 194:5, 1965.
19. Jackson H: The psychiatric nurse as a mental health consultant in a general hospital, *Nursing Clinics of North America* 4:327, 1969.
20. Jenike MA: *Geriatric psychiatry and psychopharmacology: a clinical approach*, Chicago, 1989, Mosby–Year Book.
21. Jurchuk M: Competence and the nurse-patient relationship, *Critical Care Clinics of North America* 2:3, 1990.
22. Kahana R, Bibring G: Personality types in medical management. In Zinberg NE, editor: *Psychiatry and medical practice in a general hospital*, New York, 1964, International Universities Press.
23. Kohnke MF: *The case for consultation in nursing designs for professional practice*, New York, 1977, John Wiley & Sons.
24. Kucharski A, Groves J: The so-called "inappropriate" psychiatric consultation request in a medical or surgical ward, *International Journal of Psychiatry in Medicine* 7:209, 1976-1977.
25. Kuntz S, Stehle J, Marshall R: The psychiatric clinical specialist: the progression of a specialty, *Perspectives in Psychiatric Care* 18:2, 1980.
26. Kurlowicz LH: Psychiatric-liaison nursing intervention with nurses of hospitalized AIDS patients, *Clinical Nurse Specialist* 5(2):124, 1991.
27. Langman-Dorwart N: A model for mental health consultation to the general hospital, *Journal of Psychiatric Nursing and Mental Health Services* 17(3):29, 1979.
28. Lewis A, Levy J: *Psychiatric liaison nursing: the theory and clinical practice*, Reston, Va, 1982, Reston Publishing.
29. Lipowski ZJ: Consultation liaison psychiatry: an overview, *American Journal of Psychiatry* 131:623, 1974.
30. Lipowski ZJ: Liaison psychiatry, liaison nursing and behavioral medicine, *Comprehensive Psychiatry* 22:6, 1981.
31. Lipowski ZJ: Physical illness: the individual and the coping process, *International Journal of Psychiatry in Medicine* 1(2):98, 1970.
32. McKegney FP, Beckhardt R: Evaluative research in consultation liaison psychiatry: review of the literature 1970-1981, *General Hospital Psychiatry* 4:197, 1982.
33. Meyer E, Mendelson M: Psychiatric consultations with patients on medical and surgical wards: patterns and processes, *Psychiatry* 24:199, 1961.
34. Minarik P: The psychiatric liaison nurse's role with families in acute care, *Symposium on Family Nursing in Acute Care* 19:1, 1984.
35. Moos RH: *Coping with physical illness*, New York, 1977, Plenum Medical Book Co.
36. Murray MG, Synder JC: When staff are assaulted: a nursing consultation support service, *Journal of Psychosocial Nursing and Mental Health Services* 29(7):24, 1991.

37. Nelson J and Schilke D: The evolution of psychiatric liaison nursing, *Perspectives in Psychiatric Care* 14(9)61, 1976.
38. Newton L, Wilson KG: Consultee satisfaction with a psychiatric consultation-liaison nursing service, *Archives of Psychiatric Nursing* 4(4):264, 1990.
39. Parsons WA, Myrick RD, Gunnoe J: The case of Mr. W: mental health consultation, *Journal of Gerontological Nursing* 14(8):14, 1988.
40. Pasanau RO: *Consultation-liaison psychiatry*, New York, 1976, Grune & Stratton.
41. Pati B: Nursing consultation: a collaborative process, *Journal of Nursing Administration* 10(11):33, 1980.
42. Poteet J: A closer look at the concept of support, *General Hospital Psychiatry* 4(1):19, 1982.
43. Rankin E, editor: Psychiatric/mental health nursing, *Nursing Clinics of North America* 21:3, 1986.
44. Riegel B, Ehrenreich D: *Psychological aspects of critical care nursing,* Rockville, Md, 1989, Aspen Publishers.
45. Roberts S: *Behavioral concepts and the critically ill patient,* Norwalk, Conn, 1986, Appleton-Century-Crofts.
46. Robinson L: *Liaison nursing: psychological approach to patient care,* Philadelphia, 1974, FA Davis.
47. Robinson L: Psychiatric liaison nursing 1962-1982: a review and update of the literature, *General Hospital Psychiatry,* 4:189, 1982.
48. Robinson L: Psychiatric consultation liaison nursing and psychiatric consultation liaison doctoring: similarities and differences, *Archives of Psychiatric Nursing* 4(1):73, 1987.
49. Rutherford DE: Consultation: a review and analysis of the literature, *Journal of Professional Nursing* 4(5):339, 1988.
50. Samter J, Scherer M, Shulman D: Interface of psychiatric clinical specialists in a community hospital setting, *Journal of Psychiatric Nursing and Mental Health Services* 19(1):20, 1981.
51. Schwab JJ: The psychiatric consultation, *Journal of Continuing Education in Psychiatry* 40(2):17, 1979.
52. Simmons MK: Psychiatric consultation and liaison. In Critchey D, Mourin J, editors: *The clinic specialist in psychiatric mental health nursing,* New York, 1985, John Wiley & Sons.
53. Simons RC, Pardes H, editors: *Understanding human behavior in health and illness,* Baltimore, 1977, Williams & Wilkins.
54. Skiba K, VanSteinberg P: Use of a psychiatric consultation team on medical surgical units. Innovations, AONE Council, *American Hospital Association* 2:12, December 1991.
55. Sneed NV: Power: its use and potential misuse by nurse consultants, *Clinical Nurse Specialist* 5(1):58, 1991.
56. Sparacino P, Cooper D, Minarik P: *The clinical nurse specialist implementation and impact,* Conn, 1990, Appleton & Lange.
57. Stein H: *In the psychodynamics of medical practice: unconscious factors in patient care,* Berkeley, 1985, University of California Press.
58. Stickney S, Moir G, Gardner E: Psychiatric nurse consultation: who calls and why, *Journal of Psychiatric Nursing and Mental Health Services* 19(10):22, 1981.
59. Strain J, Grossman S: *Psychological care of the medically ill,* New York, 1975, Appleton-Century-Crofts.
60. Tally S and others: Effect of psychiatric liaison nurse specialist consultation on the care of medical-surgical patients with sitters, *Archives of Psychiatric Nursing,* 44(2):114, 1990.
61. Termini M, Ciechoski M: The consultation process, *Issues in Mental Health Nursing* 3(1):77, 1981.
62. Yoest M: The clinical nurse specialist on the psychiatric team, *Journal of Psychosocial Nursing* 27:3, 1989.

ANNOTATED BIBLIOGRAPHY

Barry P: *Psychosocial nursing assessment and intervention.* Philadelphia, 1989, JB Lippincott.

General psychiatric concepts are used to develop a psychosocial assessment and intervention model for nonpsychiatric settings. The emphasis is on the functioning of nonpsychiatric clients who are having psychological responses to physical illness. The first part of the book presents a theoretical base, including the implications of psychosocial issues and stress in physical illness, organic brain syndromes, use of defense mechanisms, and major personality styles. The second part includes nursing interventions with the emotionally complex client, psychosocial aspects of specific physical conditions, and the coping challenge of chronic illness. This book is a helpful guide for the psychiatric consultation liaison nurse.

Yoest MA: The clinical nurse specialist on the psychiatric team, *Journal of Psychosocial Nursing and Mental Health Services* 27(3):27, 1989.

This article describes the establishment of the role of the psychiatric liaison nurse within a multidisciplinary team of a medical hospital. Problems and issues encountered as a member of the team are presented. Various theoretical approaches that serve as a philosophical foundation for the psychiatric liaison nurse's role as a member of the team are discussed. Case studies are used to illustrate the interactive role of the psychiatric liaison nurse as a team member.

DSM-III-R Classification: Axes I-V Categories and Codes

All official DSM-III-R codes are included in ICD-9-CM. Codes followed by an asterisk (*) are used for more than one DSM-III-R diagnosis or subtype in order to maintain compatibility with ICD-9-CM.

A long dash following a diagnostic term indicates the need for a fifth digit subtype or other qualifying term.

The term *specify* following the name of some diagnostic categories indicates qualifying terms that clinicians may wish to add in parentheses after the name of the disorder.

NOS means *not otherwise specified.*

The current severity of a disorder may be specified after the diagnosis as:

Mild   Currently
Moderate   meets
Severe   diagnostic
         criteria
    In partial remission (or residual state)
    In complete remission

DISRUPTIVE BEHAVIOR DISORDERS

314.01	Attention-deficit hyperactivity disorder
	Conduct disorder
312.20	group type
312.00	solitary aggressive type
312.90	undifferentiated type
313.81	Oppositional defiant disorder

ANXIETY DISORDERS OF CHILDHOOD OR ADOLESCENCE

309.21	Separation anxiety disorder
313.21	Avoidant disorder of childhood or adolescence
313.00	Overanxious disorder

EATING DISORDERS

307.10	Anorexia nervosa
307.51	Bulimia nervosa
307.52	Pica
307.53	Rumination disorder of infancy
307.50	Eating disorder NOS

GENDER IDENTITY DISORDERS

302.60	Gender identity disorder of childhood
302.50	Transsexualism
	Specify sexual history: asexual, homosexual, heterosexual, unspecified
302.85*	Gender identity disorder of adolescence or adulthood, nontranssexual type
	Specify sexual history: asexual, homosexual, heterosexual, unspecified
302.85*	Gender identity disorder NOS

TIC DISORDERS

307.23	Tourette's disorder
307.22	Chronic motor or vocal tic disorder
307.21	Transient tic disorder
	Specify: single episode or recurrent
307.20	Tic disorder NOS

ELIMINATION DISORDERS

307.70	Functional encopresis
	Specify: primary or secondary type
307.60	Functional enuresis
	Specify: primary or secondary type
	Specify: nocturnal only, diurnal only, nocturnal and diurnal

SPEECH DISORDERS NOT ELSEWHERE CLASSIFIED

307.00*	Cluttering
307.00*	Stuttering

DISORDERS USUALLY FIRST EVIDENT IN INFANCY, CHILDHOOD, OR ADOLESCENCE

Developmental Disorders
NOTE: These are coded on Axis II

Mental Retardation

317.00	Mild mental retardation
318.00	Moderate mental retardation
318.10	Severe mental retardation
318.20	Profound mental retardation
319.00	Unspecified mental retardation

Pervasive Developmental Disorders

299.00	Autistic disorder
	Specify if childhood onset
299.80	Pervasive developmental disorder NOS

Specific Developmental Disorders

	Academic skills disorders
315.10	Developmental arithmetic disorder
315.80	Developmental expressive writing disorder
315.00	Developmental reading disorder
	Language and speech disorders
315.39	Developmental articulation disorder
315.31*	Developmental expressive language disorder
315.31*	Developmental receptive language disorder
	Motor skills disorder
315.40	Developmental coordination disorder
315.90*	Specific developmental disorder NOS

Other Developmental Disorders

315.90*	Developmental disorder NOS

OTHER DISORDERS OF INFANCY, CHILDHOOD, OR ADOLESCENCE

313.23	Elective mutism
313.82	Identity disorder
313.89	Reactive attachment disorder of infancy or early childhood
307.30	Stereotype/habit disorder
314.00	Undifferentiated attention-deficit disorder

ORGANIC MENTAL DISORDERS

Dementias Arising in the Senium and Presenium

Primary degenerative dementia of the Alzheimer type, senile onset

290.30	with delirium
290.20	with delusions
290.21	with depression
290.00*	uncomplicated

(Note: code 331.00 Alzheimer's disease on Axis III)

Code in fifth digit:
1 = with delirium, 2 = with delusions, 3 = with depression, 0* = uncomplicated

290.1x	Primary degenerative dementia of the Alzheimer type presenile onset, _____
	(Note: code 331.00 Alzheimer's disease on Axis III)
290.4x	Multiinfarct dementia, _____
290.00*	Senile dementia NOS
	Specify etiology on Axis III if known
290.10*	Presenile dementia NOS
	Specify etiology on Axis III if known (e.g., Pick's disease, Jakob-Creutzfeldt disease)

Psychoactive Substance-Induced Organic Mental Disorders

Alcohol

303.00	intoxication
291.40	idiosyncratic intoxication
291.80	Uncomplicated alcohol withdrawal
291.00	withdrawal delirium
291.30	hallucinosis
291.10	amnestic disorder
291.20	Dementia associated with alcoholism

Amphetamine or similarly acting sympathomimetic

305.70*	intoxication
292.00*	withdrawal
292.81*	delirium
292.11*	delusional disorder

Caffeine

305.90*	intoxication

Cannabis

305.20*	intoxication
292.11*	delusional disorder

Cocaine

305.60*	intoxication
292.00*	withdrawal
292.81*	dilirium
292.11*	delusional disorder

Hallucinogen

305.30*	hallucinosis
292.11*	delusional disorder
292.84*	mood disorder
292.89*	Posthallucinogen perception disorder

Inhalant

305.90*	intoxication

Nicotine

292.00*	withdrawal

Opioid

305.50*	intoxication
292.00*	withdrawal

Phencyclidine (PCP) or similarly acting arylcyclohexylamine

305.90*	intoxication
292.81*	delirium
292.11*	delusional disorder
292.84*	mood disorder
292.90*	organic mental disorder NOS

Sedative, hypnotic, or anxiolytic

305.40*	intoxication
292.00*	Uncomplicated sedative, hypnotic, or anxiolytic withdrawal
292.00*	withdrawal delirium
292.83*	amnestic disorder

Other or unspecified psychoactive substance

305.90*	intoxication
292.00*	withdrawal
292.81*	delirium
292.82*	dementia
292.83*	amnestic disorder
292.11*	delusional disorder
292.12	hallucinosis
292.84*	mood disorder
292.89*	anxiety disorder
292.89*	personality disorder
292.90*	organic mental disorder NOS

Organic Mental Disorders Associated with Axis III Physical Disorders or Conditions, or Whose Etiology is Unknown

293.00	Delirium
294.10	Dementia
294.00	Amnestic disorder
293.81	Organic delusional disorder
293.82	Organic hallucinosis
293.83	Organic mood disorder
	Specify: manic, depressed, mixed
294.80*	Organic anxiety disorder
310.10	Organic personality disorder
	Specify if explosive type
294.80*	Organic mental disorder NOS

PSYCHOACTIVE SUBSTANCE USE DISORDERS

Alcohol

303.90	dependence
305.00	abuse

Amphetamine or similarly acting sympathomimetic

304.40	dependence
305.70*	abuse

Cannabis

304.30	dependence
305.20*	abuse

Cocaine

304.20	dependence
305.60*	abuse

Hallucinogen

304.50*	dependence
305.30*	abuse

Inhalant

304.60	dependence
305.90*	abuse

Nicotine

305.10	dependence

Opioid

304.00	dependence
305.50*	abuse

Phencyclidine (PCP) or similarly acting arylcyclohexylamine

304.50*	dependence
305.90*	abuse

Sedative, hypnotic, or anxiolytic
304.10   dependence
305.40*   abuse
304.90*   Polysubstance dependence
304.90*   Psychoactive substance dependence NOS
305.90*   Psychoactive substance abuse NOS

SCHIZOPHRENIA

Code in fifth digit:
1 = subchronic, 2 = chronic, 3 = subchronic with acute exacerbation, 4 = chronic with acute exacerbation, 5 = in remission, 0 = unspecified.

Schizophrenia
295.2x   catatonic, _____
295.1x   disorganized, _____
295.3x   paranoid, _____
          Specify if stable type
295.9x   undifferentiated, _____
295.6x   residual, _____
          Specify if late onset

DELUSIONAL (PARANOID) DISORDER

297.10   Delusional (Paranoid) disorder
          Specify: erotomanic, grandiose, jealous, persecutory, somatic, unspecified

PSYCHOTIC DISORDERS NOT ELSEWHERE CLASSIFIED

298.80   Brief reactive psychosis
295.40   Schizophreniform disorder
          Specify: without good prognostic features or with good prognostic features
295.70   Schizoaffective disorder
          Specify: bipolar type or depressive type
297.30   Induced psychotic disorder
298.90   Psychotic disorder NOS (Atypical psychosis)

MOOD DISORDERS

Code current state of Major Depression and Bipolar Disorder in fifth digit:
1 = mild, 2 = moderate, 3 = severe, without psychotic features, 4 = with psychotic features (*specify* mood-congruent or mood incongruent), 5 = in partial remission, 6 = in full remission, 0 = unspecified
For major depressive episodes, *specify* if chronic and *specify* if melancholic type.
For Bipolar Disorder, Bipolar Disorder NOS, Recurrent Major Depression, and Depressive Disorder NOS, *specify* if seasonal pattern.

Bipolar Disorders

Bipolar disorder
296.6x   mixed, _____
296.4x   manic, _____
296.5x   depressed, _____
301.13   Cyclothymia
296.70   Bipolar disorder NOS

Depressive Disorders

Major Depression
296.2x   single episode, _____
296.3x   recurrent, _____
300.40   Dysthymia (or Depressive neurosis)
          Specify: primary or secondary type
          Specify: early or late onset
311.00   Depressive disorder NOS

ANXIETY DISORDERS (or Anxiety and Phobic Neuroses)

300.21   Panic disorder
          with agoraphobia
          Specify current severity of agoraphobic avoidance
              Specify current severity of panic attacks
300.01   without agoraphobia
              Specify current severity of panic attacks
300.22   Agoraphobia without history of panic disorder
          Specify with or without limited symptom attacks
300.23   Social phobia
          Specify if generalized type
300.29   Simple phobia
300.30   Obsessive compulsive disorder (or Obsessive compulsive neurosis)
309.89   Post-traumatic stress disorder
          Specify if delayed onset
300.02   Generalized anxiety disorder
300.00   Anxiety disorder NOS

SOMATOFORM DISORDERS

300.70*   Body dysmorphic disorder
300.11   Conversion disorder (or Hysterical neurosis, conversion type)
          Specify: single episode or recurrent
300.70*   Hypochondriasis (or Hypochondriacal neurosis)
300.81   Somatization disorder
307.80   Somatoform pain disorder
300.70*   Undifferentiated somatoform disorder
300.70*   Somatoform disorder NOS

DISSOCIATIVE DISORDERS (or Hysterical Neuroses, Dissociative Type)

300.14   Multiple personality disorder
300.13   Psychogenic fugue
300.12   Psychogenic amnesia
300.60   Depersonalization disorder (or Depersonalization neurosis)
300.15   Dissociative disorder NOS

SEXUAL DISORDERS

Paraphilias

302.40   Exhibitionism
302.81   Fetishism
302.89   Frotteurism
302.20   Pedophilia
          Specify: same sex, opposite sex, same and opposite sex
          Specify if limited to incest
          Specify: exclusive type or nonexclusive type
302.83   Sexual masochism
302.84   Sexual sadism
302.30   Transvestic fetishism
302.82   Voyeurism
302.90*   Paraphilia NOS

Sexual Dysfunctions

Specify: psychogenic only, or psychogenic and biogenic (Note: If biogenic only, code on Axis III)
Specify: lifelong or acquired
Specify: generalized or situational
Sexual desire disorders
302.71   Hypoactive sexual desire disorder
302.79   Sexual aversion disorder
Sexual arousal disorders
302.72*   Female sexual arousal disorder
302.72*   Male erectile disorder

Orgasm disorders
302.73   Inhibited female orgasm
302.74   Inhibited male orgasm
302.75   Premature ejaculation
Sexual pain disorders
302.76   Dyspareunia
306.51   Vaginismus
302.70   Sexual dysfunction NOS

Other Sexual Disorders

302.90*   Sexual disorder NOS

SLEEP DISORDERS
Dyssomnias

Insomnia disorder
307.42*   related to another mental disorder (nonorganic)
780.50*   related to known organic factor
307.42*   Primary insomnia
Hypersomnia disorder
307.44   related to another mental disorder (nonorganic)
780.50*   related to a known organic factor
780.54   Primary hypersomnia
307.45   Sleep-wake schedule disorder
Specify: advanced or delayed phase type, disorganized type, frequently changing type
Other dyssomnias
307.40*   Dyssomnia NOS

Parasomnias

307.47   Dream anxiety disorder (Nightmare disorder)
307.46*   Sleep terror disorder
307.46*   Sleepwalking disorder
307.40*   Parasomnia NOS

FACTITIOUS DISORDERS

Factitious disorder
301.51   with physical symptoms
300.16   with psychological symptoms
300.19   Factitious disorder NOS

IMPULSE CONTROL DISORDERS NOT ELSEWHERE CLASSIFIED

312.34   Intermittent explosive disorder
312.32   Kleptomania
312.31   Pathological gambling
312.33   Pyromania
312.39*   Trichotillomania
312.39*   Impulse control disorder NOS

ADJUSTMENT DISORDER

Adjustment disorder
309.24   with anxious mood
309.00   with depressed mood
309.30   with disturbance of conduct
309.40   with mixed disturbance of emotions and conduct
309.28   with mixed emotional features
309.82   with physical complaints
309.83   with withdrawal
309.23   with work (or academic) inhibition
309.90   Adjustment disorder NOS

PSYCHOLOGICAL FACTORS AFFECTING PHYSICAL CONDITION

316.00   Psychological factors affecting physical condition
Specify physical condition on Axis III

Personality Disorders
NOTE: These are coded on Axis II

Cluster A
301.00   Paranoid
301.20   Schizoid
301.22   Schizotypal

Cluster B
301.70   Antisocial
301.83   Borderline
301.50   Histrionic
301.81   Narcissistic

Cluster C
301.82   Avoidant
301.60   Dependent
301.40   Obsessive compulsive
301.84   Passive aggressive
301.90   Personality disorder NOS

V CODES FOR CONDITIONS NOT ATTRIBUTABLE TO A MENTAL DISORDER THAT ARE A FOCUS OF ATTENTION OR TREATMENT

V62.30   Academic problem
V71.01   Adult antisocial behavior
V71.02   Childhood or adolescent antisocial behavior
V65.20   Malingering
V61.10   Marital problem
V15.81   Noncompliance with medical treatment
V62.20   Occupational problem
V61.20   Parent-child problem
V62.81   Other interpersonal problem
V61.80   Other specified family circumstances
V62.89   Phase of life problem or other life circumstance problem
V62.82   Uncomplicated bereavement

V40.00   Borderline intellectual functioning (Note: This is coded on Axis II)

ADDITIONAL CODES

300.90   Unspecified mental disorder (nonpsychotic)
V71.09*   No diagnosis or condition on Axis I
799.90*   Diagnosis or condition deferred on Axis I

V71.09*   No diagnosis or condition on Axis II
799.90*   Diagnosis or condition deferred on Axis II

MULTIAXIAL SYSTEM

Axis I   Clinical Syndromes
            V Codes
Axis II   Developmental Disorders
            Personality Disorders
Axis III   Physical Disorders and Conditions
Axis IV   Severity of Psychosocial Stressors
Axis V   Global Assessment of Functioning

SEVERITY OF PSYCHOSOCIAL STRESSORS SCALE: ADULTS

Examples of Stressors

Code	Term	Acute events	Enduring circumstances
1	None	No acute events that may be relevant to the disorder	No enduring circumstances that may be relevant to the disorder
2	Mild	Broke up with boyfriend or girlfriend; started or graduated from school; child left home	Family arguments; job dissatisfaction; residence in high-crime neighborhood
3	Moderate	Marriage; marital separation; loss of job; retirement; miscarriage	Marital discord; serious financial problems; trouble with boss; being a single parent
4	Severe	Divorce; birth of first child	Unemployment; poverty
5	Extreme	Death of spouse; serious physical illness diagnosed; victim of rape	Serious chronic illness in self or child; ongoing physical or sexual abuse
6	Catastrophic	Death of child; suicide of spouse; devastating natural disaster	Capitivity as hostage; concentration camp experience
0	Inadequate information, or no change in condition		

SEVERITY OF PSYCHOSOCIAL STRESSORS SCALE: CHILDREN AND ADOLESCENTS

Examples of Stressors

Code	Term	Acute events	Enduring circumstances
1	None	No acute events that may be relevant to the disorder	No enduring circumstances that may be relevant to the disorder
2	Mild	Broke up with boyfriend or girlfriend; change of school	Overcrowded living quarters; family arguments
3	Moderate	Expelled from school; birth of sibling	Chronic disabling illness in parent; chronic parental discord
4	Severe	Divorce of parents; unwanted pregnancy; arrest	Harsh or rejecting parents; chronic life-threatening illness in parent; multiple foster home placements
5	Extreme	Sexual or physical abuse; death of a parent	Recurrent sexual or physical abuse
6	Catastrophic	Death of both parents	Chronic life-threatening illness
0	Inadequate information, or no change in condition		

GLOBAL ASSESSMENT OF FUNCTIONING SCALE (GAF Scale)

Consider psychological, social, and occupational functioning on a hypothetical continuum of mental health-illness. Do not include impairment in functioning caused by physical (or environmental) limitations.

NOTE: Use intermediate codes when appropriate, for example, 45, 68, 72.

Code

90

81
Absent or minimal symptoms (e.g., mild anxiety before an exam), **good functioning in all areas, interested and involved in a wide range of activities, socially effective, generally satisfied with life, no more than everyday problems or concerns** (e.g., an occasional argument with family members).

80

71
If symptoms are present, they are transient and expectable reactions to psychosocial stressors (e.g., difficulty concentrating after family argument); **no more than slight impairment in social, occupational, or school functioning** (e.g., temporarily falling behind in school work).

70

61
Some mild symptoms (e.g., depressed mood and mild insomnia) **OR some difficulty in social, occupational, or school functioning** (e.g., occasional truancy, or theft within the household), **but generally functioning pretty well, has some meaningful interpersonal relationships.**

60

51
Moderate symptoms (e.g., flat affect and circumstantial speech, occasional panic attacks) **OR moderate difficulty in social, occupational, or school functioning** (e.g., few friends, conflicts with co-workers).

50

41
Serious symptoms (e.g., suicidal ideation, severe obsessional rituals, frequent shoplifting) **OR any serious impairment in social, occupational, or school functioning** (e.g., no friends, unable to keep a job).

40

31
Some impairment in reality testing or communication (e.g., speech is at times illogical, obscure, or irrelevant) **OR major impairment in several areas, such as work or school, family relations, judgment, thinking, or mood** (e.g., depressed man avoids friends, neglects family, and is unable to work; child frequently beats up younger children, is defiant at home, and is failing at school).

30

21
Behavior is considerably influenced by delusions or hallucinations OR serious impairment in communication or judgment (e.g., sometimes incoherent, acts grossly inappropriately, suicidal preoccupation) **OR inability to function in almost all areas** (e.g., stays in bed all day; no job, home, or friends).

20

11
Some danger of hurting self or others (e.g., suicide attempts without clear expectation of death, frequently violent, manic excitement) **OR occasionally fails to maintain minimal personal hygiene** (e.g., smears feces) **OR gross impairment in communication** (e.g., largely incoherent or mute).

10

1
Persistent danger of severely hurting self or others (e.g., recurrent violence) **OR persistent inability to maintain minimal personal hygiene OR serious suicidal act with clear expectation of death.**

ANA Standards of Psychiatric and Mental Health Nursing Practice

STANDARD I—THEORY

The nurse applies appropriate theory that is scientifically sound as a basis for decisions regarding nursing practice.

STANDARD II—DATA COLLECTION

The nurse continuously collects data that are comprehensive, accurate, and systematic.

STANDARD III—DIAGNOSIS

The nurse utilizes nursing diagnoses and standard classification of mental disorders to express conclusions supported by recorded assessment data and current scientific premises.

STANDARD IV—PLANNING

The nurse develops a nursing care plan with specific goals and interventions delineating nursing actions unique to each client's needs.

STANDARD V—INTERVENTION

The nurse intervenes as guided by the nursing care plan to implement nursing actions that promote, maintain, or restore physical and mental health, prevent illness, and effect rehabilitation.

STANDARD V-A—PSYCHOTHERAPEUTIC INTERVENTIONS

The nurse (generalist) uses psychotherapeutic interventions to assist clients to regain or improve their previous coping abilities and to prevent further disability.

STANDARD V-B—HEALTH TEACHING

The nurse assists clients, families, and groups to achieve satisfying and productive patterns of living through health teaching.

STANDARD V-C—SELF-CARE ACTIVITIES

The nurse uses the activities of daily living in a goal-directed way to foster adequate self-care and physical and mental well-being of clients.

STANDARD V-D—SOMATIC THERAPIES

The nurse uses knowledge of somatic therapies and applies related clinical skills in working with clients.

STANDARD V-E—THERAPEUTIC ENVIRONMENT

The nurse provides, structures, and maintains a therapeutic environment in collaboration with the client and other health care providers.

STANDARD V-F—PSYCHOTHERAPY

The nurse (specialist) utilizes advanced clinical expertise in individual, group, and family psychotherapy, child psychotherapy, and other treatment modalities to function as a psychotherapist and recognizes professional accountability for nursing practice.

STANDARD VI—EVALUATION

The nurse evaluates client responses to nursing actions in order to revise the data base, nursing diagnoses, and nursing care plan.

STANDARD VII—PEER REVIEW

The nurse participates in peer review and other means of evaluation to assure quality of nursing care provided for clients.

STANDARD VIII—CONTINUING EDUCATION

The nurse assumes responsibility for continuing education and professional development and contributes to the professional growth of others.

STANDARD IX—INTERDISCIPLINARY COLLABORATION

The nurse collaborates with interdisciplinary teams in assessing, planning, implementing, and evaluating programs and other mental health activities.

STANDARD X—UTILIZATION OF COMMUNITY HEALTH SYSTEMS

The nurse (specialist) participates with other members of the community in assessing, planning, implementing, and evaluating mental health services and community systems that include the promotion of the broad continuum of primary, secondary, and tertiary prevention of mental illness.

STANDARD XI—RESEARCH

The nurse contributes to nursing and the mental health field through innovations in theory and practice and participation in research.

Reprinted with permission of the American Nurses' Association: *Standards of psychiatric and mental health nursing practice,* Kansas City, Mo, 1982, Pergamon Press.

Glossary

abreaction Process whereby repressed material is brought back to consciousness and reexperienced affectively.

absolute rights Veto powers that moral agents have against majorities or rulers.

abstract thinking Stage in the development of cognitive thought processes. Thoughts are characterized by adaptability, flexibility, and the use of abstractions and generalizations.

abuse Excessive use of a substance that differs from accepted social practice.

accommodation Process of change that enables the individual to manage situations that were previously beyond his abilities.

acquaintance rape A rape committed by a man known to the victim.

acrophobia Fear of high places.

acting out Indirect expression of feelings through behavior, usually nonverbal, that attracts the attention of others.

active listening Alert hearing, with an attitude of wanting to hear what the client has to say.

active-passive Concept that characterizes persons as either actively involved in shaping events or passively reacting to events.

actualized religions Religions that stress trust in one's own nature and encourage self-direction and growth.

activity theory Theory in which Havighurst proposes that activity promotes well-being and satisfaction in aging.

acute or functional grief The process of acknowledging and expressing feelings associated with loss.

acute pain A subjective sensation of hurt, caused by a harmful stimulus, that warns of current or impending damage to tissue.

adaptation Striving to find equilibrium between oneself and one's environment.

adaptive dependence Behavior in which a person is dependent when the external and internal environments preclude autonomous functioning.

adaptive independence Behavior that occurs when the individual is able to act according to his own judgment.

adaptive maneuvering Manipulative responses of newborns.

addiction Physical dependence on a substance.

addictive behavior Unrestrained seeking for gratification.

adjunctive groups Groups with specific activities and focuses, such as socialization, perceptual stimulation, sensory stimulation, and orientation to reality.

administrative consultee-centered consultation Expert advice to caregivers in conflict.

administrative program-centered consultation Expert advice regarding a program or a policy of an organization.

Adult ego state Part of the self that computes and solves problems, using information received from the Parent and Child ego states.

affect Outward manifestation of a person's feelings and emotions.

affection Feeling or emotion expressed toward another; a loving attachment; fondness.

affiliation Closeness or connection with another (as achieved by affiliative behavior).

agape Greek for the highest form of love.

agapeism Practice of love-based ethics.

aggression Forceful, self-assertive action or attitude that is expressed physically, verbally, or symbolically. It may arise from innate drives or occur as a defensive mechanism and is mani-

fested by either constructive or destructive acts directed toward oneself or against others.

aggressive maneuvering Type of destructive manipulative behavior that is characterized by multiple demands, threats, requests for special consideration, and playing members of the health care team against each other.

aggressive-radical therapy Therapy that proposes that clients should be radicalized through the therapeutic process. Making all values explicit results in the client's viewing the solution of emotional conflict and the raising of political consciousness as one and the same.

agnosia Total or partial loss of the ability to recognize familiar objects or persons through sensory stimuli as a result of organic brain damage.

agoraphobia Anxiety disorder characterized by a fear of being in an open, crowded, or public place, where escape may be difficult or help not available in case of sudden incapacitation.

agraphia Impairment in intellectual functioning characterized by the loss of the ability to write.

aim Characteristic of an instinct directed toward removing a body need.

akathisia Side effect of antipsychotic medication that is manifested by a feeling of restlessness and frequently accompanied by complaint of a twitching or crawling sensation in the muscles.

akinesia Impaired motor function.

Al-Anon Self-help group in which family members and friends of alcoholics are taught how to understand and give healthy support to the drinker.

alarm reaction (AR) Initial response to stress characterized by a generalized expression of the body's defense system; first stage of the general adaptation syndrome.

Alateen Self-help group for teenagers that teaches them how to understand and give healthy support to the drinking family member.

alcohol dementia A general state of intellectual deterioration and personality change that occurs late in severe alcoholism.

Alcoholics Anonymous (AA) Organization of recovering alcoholics whose purpose is to help alcoholics stop drinking and maintain sobriety through group support, shared experiences, and faith in a power greater than themselves.

alcoholism Condition in which a person's drinking behavior constitutes a social and health problem, characterized by psychosocial and biochemical causes, physiological effects, including brain damage, and public and personal consequences.

alexia Impairment in intellectual functioning characterized by the inability to comprehend written words.

all-channel pattern of communication Messages may originate at any point, and all members may interact.

altruism Love-based ethics that involve loving and doing for others what one does for oneself.

ambivalence Simultaneous conflicting feelings or attitudes toward a person or object.

amnesia Loss of memory of a specific time or event or a loss of all past memories.

anaclitic depression Syndrome occurring in infants usually after sudden separation from the mothering person and characterized by severe impairments in the infant's physical, emotional, intellectual, and social development.

analysis Categorization of data, identification of gaps in data, and determination of patterns from pieces of data. Used to interpret and give meaning to collected data.

andropause Change of life in men when a reordering of their life takes place, for example, career change and divorce.

anger Strong feeling of annoyance or displeasure.

anhedonia Inability to feel pleasure or happiness for experiences that are ordinarily pleasurable.

anilingus Oral stimulation of the anal area.

anima Female archetype in the male.

animus Masculine archetype in the female.

anorexia General loss of appetite resulting from physical and psychosocial causes, contributing to a state of malnutrition and related mental health problems.

anorexia nervosa Extreme form of anorexia, usually seen in adolescent girls, characterized by distorted body image and prolonged inability to eat, with marked weight loss, amenorrhea, and other symptoms resulting from emotional conflict. Creates life-threatening condition and retarded growth.

anticholinergic Pertains to the blockade of acetylcholine receptors resulting in inhibition of transmission of parasympathetic nerve impulses.

anticipatory adaptation Act of adapting in advance of a potentially distressing situation, such as when a person tries to relax before calling to receive the results of a laboratory test.

anticipatory grief Feelings experienced in anticipation of a loss that has not yet occurred.

anticipatory guidance Helping persons anticipate vivid details of an expected challenge and consider the accompanying unpleasant emotions and fantasies.

antisocial behavior Lack of socialization with behavior patterns that bring a person repeatedly into conflict with society.

antisocial personality disorder Disorder characterized by repetitive failure to abide by social and legal norms and to accept responsibility for own behavior.

anxiety State of feeling of apprehension, uneasiness, agitation, uncertainty, and fear resulting from anticipation of a threat or danger, usually of intrapsychic origin, whose source is generally unknown or unrecognized.

anxiety disorders Emotional illness characterized by the feeling of fear and by symptoms associated with the autonomic nervous system, such as palpitations, tachycardia, dizziness, and tremor.

anxiety hierarchy Hierarchical relationships among anxiety-producing stimuli.

anxiolytic An antianxiety medication.

aphasia Abnormal neurological condition in which language function is defective or absent because of an injury to certain areas of the cerebral cortex.

apnea absence of spontaneous respirations.

approach-approach conflict Conflict resulting from the simultaneous presence of two or more incompatible impulses, desires, or goals, each of which is desirable.

approach-avoidance conflict Conflict resulting from the presence of a single goal or desire that is both desirable and undesirable.

apraxia Impairment in the ability to engage in purposeful activities, even though muscle strength and coordination are present.

arbitrary inference Type of cognitive distortion in which a negative conclusion is drawn from insufficient evidence.

archetypes Symbols that are derived from the collective experiences of the race.

Arica therapy Alternative therapy founded by Oscar Ichazo that focuses on consciousness and provides tools to systematize and describe the human psyche. The goal of therapy is to increase the powers of the mind.

art therapy Type of therapy that focuses on expressing oneself and portraying one's feelings by use of various forms of artwork.

asceticism Defense mechanism commonly used in adolescence that involves repudiation of all instinctual impulses.

assault Threat of touching without the client's consent.

assertiveness Behavior that is directed toward claiming one's rights without denying the rights of others.

assessment First phase of the nursing process, which involves the collection of data about the health status of the client.

assimilation Process by which the child develops the ability to handle new situations and problems with his existing mechanisms.

assurance Process that includes the identification of values and standards, specification of criteria, measurement of observable aspects of care, and remedial action if indicated.

asterixis Hand-flapping tremor often accompanying metabolic disorders.

atman Innermost spirit and highest controlling power of a person.

atypical somatoform disorder Physical symptoms and complaints that appear to be a preoccupation with some imagined defect in physical appearance or ability.

audit Review and evaluation of nursing care procedures.

authenticity Quality of being trustworthy and genuine; emotional and behavioral openness in a relationship.

authoritarian personality Constellation of traits indicative of one who advocates obedience and strict adherence to rules.

autism Preoccupation with the self and with inner experiences.

autistic thought Ideation that has a private meaning to the individual.

autoerotic Sensual, self-gratifying.

automatic thoughts Type of habitual shorthand conclusion about a situation that is not subjected to critical evaluation.

aversion therapy Application of the behavioral model of psychiatric care. A painful stimulus is given to create an aversion to another stimulus, which leads to a behavior that the individual wishes to change.

avoidance responding Performing a behavior before a conditioned stimulus appears.

avoidance-avoidance conflict Conflict resulting from the confrontation of two or more alternative goals or desires that are equally aversive and undesirable.

avoidant personality disorder Condition characterized by hypersensitivity to rejection, a need for uncritical acceptance, and low self-esteem.

awareness context of death What each individual involved with a dying client knows of the client's defined status or condition and the client's recognition of others' awareness.

balancing factors Events that contribute to the production and outcome of a crisis.

basic anxiety Profound insecurity and vague apprehensiveness.

battered wife Any woman who is beaten by her mate, regardless of the legality of the marital relationship.

battery Touching the client without his consent.

battle fatigue Physically and psychologically disabling condition caused from participation in a war.

behavior Any observable, recordable, and measurable act, movement, or response of an individual.

behavior modification Type of therapy that attempts to modify observable, maladaptive patterns of behavior by the substitution of a new response or set of responses to a given stimulus.

behavioral treatment Modality of treatment that helps the individual modify behavior by changing learned behavior responses.

benign suicide Indirect self-destructive behavior; also called subintentional suicide.

benzodiazepines Group of chemically related antianxiety drugs.

bereavement Process used to work through the response to a loss

bibliotherapy Type of group therapy in which articles, books, poems, and newspapers are read in the group to help stimulate thinking about events in the real world and secondarily to foster relating to each other.

biofeedback Process providing a person with visual or auditory information about the autonomic physiological functions of his body, as blood pressure, muscle tension, and brain wave activity, usually through the use of instrumentation.

biorhythms Any cyclic biological event or phenomenon, such as the sleep cycle, the menstrual cycle, or the respiratory cycle.

bipolar disorder Subgroup of the affective disorders that is characterized by the occurrence of at least one episode of manic behavior, with or without a history of episodes of depression.

bisexuality Ability to achieve orgasm with a partner of either sex.

blocked communication Incongruent verbal and nonverbal messages; also, discrepancies and inconsistencies in messages.

blocking Spontaneous loss of thought.

blunting Decreased intensity of emotional expression from that which one would normally expect.

body image Person's subjective concept of his physical appearance.

body language Transmission of a message by body position or movement.

body monitoring Activities in which individuals engage to keep the body in shape.

borderline personality disorder Condition characterized by instability in many areas, with no single feature present. Some characteristics are unstable interpersonal relationships, impulsive behavior, and wide mood swings.

boundary Index of family health in which the generations are clearly marked and issues are dealt with by the appropriate generation; the limit set between the family and the larger society.

bruxism Grinding of the teeth.

bulimia nervosa Form of anorexia nervosa in which the victim alternates periods of anorexia and fasting with periods of gorging and then purging with induced vomiting. Victims may rapidly consume up to 50,000 calories of food in a few hours and then induce vomiting, sometimes repeating the behavior as often as three or four times in one day.

butyrophenones Group of chemically related antipsychotic drugs.

cachectic State of malnutrition resulting from excessive dieting.

caffeinism Condition of nervous stimulation resulting from excessive use of caffeine-containing beverages or drugs. Characterized by typical drug withdrawal symptoms when caffeine intake is restricted or removed.

cao gio Folk practice that consists of applying oil to the back and chest of a child with cotton swabs, massaging the skin until warm, and then rubbing it with the edge of a copper coin until marks appear.

capacity Ability to understand or comprehend. Total comprehension is not necessary.

caring Refers to a phenomena related to assisting, supporting, or enabling another person with evident or anticipated needs to ameliorate or improve a human condition.

case management The planning, coordination, and sequencing of client care during a specific hospitalization or period of treatment. Also, an approach to providing treatment for the chronically mentally ill in the community.

case study Descriptive survey that focuses on one or a limited number of units; a unit may be an individual, a group, or an institution.

catastrophic reaction Heightened anxiety that occurs in confused persons when they are not able to answer or perform.

catatonic State of psychologically induced immobilization, at times interrupted by episodes of extreme agitation.

catatonic excitement State of extreme agitation that occurs when a person is unable to maintain catatonic immobility.

catatonic stupor Apparently unresponsive state that is related to a fear of loss of impulse control.

catharsis Release that occurs when the client is encouraged to talk about things that bother him. Thoughts and feelings are brought out in the open and discussed.

causal comparative research Extension of correlational research in which, in addition to discovering relationships among variables of interest, the researcher also identifies the possible cause after the effects have already occurred.

causal connecting statements Process by which the nurse helps the client relate the cause and effect between two events that are the outcome of the client's specific feelings, behavior, or responses.

certification Process by which a nongovernmental agency provides a reliable endorsement that a person has met predetermined standards in a specialized area of nursing.

chain pattern of communication Messages are initiated at one point and are passed from one receiver to the next until the message reaches the end of the chain.

chakras In Hindu belief, centers of swirling pranaic energy that act as centers of consciousness.

chemical dependence Extreme pathological dependence on a chemical substance.

ch'i In Chinese philosophy, fundamental life energy that flows in orderly ways through the body along meridians.

child abuse or neglect Physical or mental injury, sexual abuse, negligent treatment, or maltreatment of a child under eighteen years of age.

Child ego state Part of self that includes feelings, wishes, and memories; part of this ego state is the natural use of feelings as they arise, and part is learned behavior as one responds to others by adapting to their wishes or by rebelling.

child psychiatry Subspecialty area of psychiatry that focuses on the study and treatment of emotionally disturbed children.

chlorpromazine equivalent Approximation of the quantity of drug necessary to equal 100 mg of chlorpromazine's antipsychotic efficacy.

chromosome Any of the threadlike structures in the nucleus of a cell that function in the transmission of genetic information.

chronic care Modality of care, usually clinic based, requiring monitoring of a chronic, long-standing clinical health problem.

chronic mental distress Set of behaviors representing a role created by society as a result of observations of individuals exhibiting behaviors troublesome to society and labeled mentally deviant.

chronic pain Subjective sensation of hurt, with or without pathological findings and of longer duration.

chronicity The continuation of a health disruption until it has a possibly permanent impact on the overall identify and life style of the client.

chronopsychophysiology Science that studies the physiological cyclic processes in the body.

circadian rhythm Pattern based on a 24-hour cycle, especially the repetition of certain physiological phenomena, such as sleeping and eating.

circumstantial speech Type of speech in which there is the inclusion of many unnecessary and trivial details before the person reaches his goal.

civil suit Dispute between two persons that is resolved by a variety of remedies, most often monetary.

clang associations Combining of words that rhyme.

clarification Intervention technique designed to guide the client to focus on and recognize gaps and inconsistencies in his statements.

claustrophobia Fear of closed places.

client-centered consultation Expert advice regarding care of person needing service.

climacteric Menopausal period in women; sometimes used to refer to the corresponding period in men.

clinical psychologist Psychologist who specializes in the selection, administration, and interpretation of psychological tests.

closed awareness context of death Attempts are made to prevent the client from knowing of his possible death.

closed groups Groups in which all members are admitted at the same time and vacancies occurring in membership are not filled.

coaching Method of engaging spouses in dialogue about alternative actions while leaving the choice to clients.

coalitions Family members uniting with one parent against the other.

codependency Stress induced preoccupation with the addicted person's life leading to extreme dependence and excessive concern with the dysfunctionally addicted person.

cognition Process of logical thought.

cognitive Referring to the mental process of comprehension, judgment, memory, and reasoning, as contrasted with emotional and volitional processes.

cognitive appraisal Process that probably takes place in the cerebral cortex and intervenes between the environmental stimulus and the reaction.

cognitive restoration Intervention technique designed to restore cognitive functioning.

cognitive structuring The therapist reviews with the client the changes that have occurred in a client's thinking in order to give the client a sense of change and a sense of playing an active role in producing the change.

cohabitate To live together in a sexual relationship when not legally married.

coitus Sexual intercourse with a partner of the opposite sex.

collective bargaining Use of collective action in negotiating client care and economic issues with one's employer, including wages, hours, and work conditions.

collective unconscious Inherited, racial foundation of the personality structure.

collusion Active process by which each mate unconsciously chooses a partner based on his unmet infantile needs with the expectation that the partner chosen will meet the need.

community mental health–psychiatric nursing The application of specialized knowledge to populations and communities to provide and maintain mental health and to rehabilitate populations at risk that continue to have residual effects of mental illness.

communication Totality of human behavior, including both how people behave and how they exchange meanings about their behavior.

companion animals Animals that serve as substitutes for people.

compensation Defense mechanism by which the individual attempts to make up for real or fancied deficiencies.

competence to stand trial Mental condition necessary for a criminal defendant so that he may confer with an attorney about his defense, understand the nature of charges against him and understand courtroom procedure.

complementary transactions Transactions that can go on indefinitely as the persons keep relating from the same ego states.

compulsion Insistent, repetitive, intrusive, and unwanted urge to perform an act that is contrary to one's usual wishes or standards.

compulsive personality disorder Disorder characterized by limited ability to express tender emotion, the need for perfection, and irrational adherence to order; rules and rituals interfere with functioning.

concreteness Difficulty with abstract thinking manifested by the literal interpretation of messages.

concrete thinking Stage in the development of the cognitive thought processes in which thoughts are logical and coherent.

The individual is able to sort, classify, order, and organize facts but is incapable of generalizing or dealing in abstractions.

concurrent audit Method of evaluating ongoing activities.

confabulation Fabrication of experiences or situations, often recounted in a detailed and plausible way to fill in and cover up gaps in memory.

confession Act of seeking expiation through another from guilt for an actual or imagined transgression.

confidentiality Disclosure of certain information only to another specifically authorized person.

confinement deprivation Disorder that occurs when individuals are separated from familiar surroundings or denied contact with familiar persons or objects, as when one is confined to a single hospital room or one-room apartment.

conflict Opposition between two drives that are experienced simultaneously in response to the same situation.

confrontation Communication that invites another to examine some aspects of his behavior that exhibit a discrepancy between what he says and what he does.

congruent communication Communication pattern in which the sender is communicating the same message on both verbal and nonverbal levels.

conjoint family therapy Therapy in which a single nuclear family is seen and the issues and problems raised by the family are addressed by the therapist.

conscience Prohibiting aspect of the ego that relates to that which is morally wrong.

conscious Experiences within awareness at the moment.

consensually validated symbols Symbols that are accepted by enough people that they have an agreed upon meaning.

consensus Device individuals use to establish unanimous social meaning.

consent Voluntary agreement by the person who has the capacity to do so, given the appropriate information.

consort abuse Battering of an emancipated minor or female 18 years of age or older, involving an intentional act or acts of physical violence that occur during the course of an intimate, interpersonal relationship with a spouse or male partner.

constructive manipulation Using one's strengths and abilities in interpersonal situations to promote successful relationships.

consultation alliance Relationship between the consultant and the consultee characterized by an understanding that clinical dilemmas will and can be approached together.

consultee-centered consultation Expert advice to the consultee to clarify the details of the client's situation to increase the consultee's cognitive understanding and awareness of her feelings involved in caring for the client.

continuity theory Theory about aging which suggests that people's personalities do not change as they age and that their behavior becomes more predictable.

contract Agreement within the one-to-one relationship involving setting goals and a plan of action for carrying out the goals to achieve behavior change.

conversion disorder Somatoform disorder characterized by a loss of, or alteration in, physical functioning that is an expression of psychological conflict.

coping Active process of using personal, social, and environmental resources to manage stress.

coping mechanisms Balancing factors that affect individuals' ability to restore equilibrium following a stressful event.

corrective emotional experience Process by which the client gives up old patterns of behavior and learns and relearns new patterns through reexperiencing early unresolved feelings and needs.

counterconditioning Process used by the behavioral therapist in which a learned response is replaced with an alternative response that is less disruptive for the person.

countertransference Conscious or unconscious emotional response of a psychotherapist to a client.

couples therapy Therapy in which couples, married or unmarried and living together, are seen in therapy.

craving Persistent psychological or physiological hunger or need for a substance.

credential Global term referring to a recognition that a person or institution has attained a predetermined set of standards at a given point in time. In this text, licensure, certification, and accreditation are discussed as types of credentials.

crisis Event experienced when a person faces an obstacle to important life goals that is, for a time, insurmountable through the use of usual problem-solving methods.

crisis intervention Active entering into the life situation of an individual, family, or group experiencing a crisis to decrease the impact of the crisis event and to assist the client or clients to mobilize personal resources and regain equilibrium.

crisis-prone person Individual who has no available support system, or, if social supports are available, is unable to use them in his efforts to cope with everyday stress.

crisis resolution Development of effective adaptive and coping devices to resolve a crisis.

criteria Specific rules or principles against which health care practice may be compared. In this text, structure, process, and outcome criteria are discussed.

critical pathway A written plan and timetable for client care that identifies routine treatments, activities, medications, and expected length of stay in the hospital.

cross dependence A condition in which one substance can prevent withdrawal symptoms caused by a different substance in the same pharmacological class.

cross tolerance A condition in which tolerance to one substance results in reduced response to another, resulting in tolerance to both substances.

cue Stimulus that determines the nature of the person's response.

cultural group Class of people who share some common characteristics but do not necessarily share a culture.

culturally relativistic perspective Understanding the behavior of transcultural clients within the context of their culture.

cultural relativity Fitting within the context of a particular culture.

culture Learned patterns of values, beliefs, customs, and behaviors that are shared by a group of interacting individuals.

cunnilingus Oral stimulation of the female genitals.

curandero Type of folk healer used by Hispanics.

cyclothymia A chronic mood disturbance involving numerous hypomanic episodes and numerous periods of depressed mood. It is severe enough to be diagnosed as major depression or a manic episode

dance therapy Type of therapy that involves expression of feelings through the rhythmic body movements of dance.

daydreams Future states during which the child withdraws from the real world to a world of fantasy and wish fulfillment.

death instincts Instincts aimed at destruction.

defense mechanism Unconscious intrapsychic reaction that offers protection to the self from a stressful situation. Also called "ego defense."

deinstitutionalization At the individual client level, this means the transfer to a community setting of a client who has been hospitalized for an extended period of time, generally many years; at the mental health care system level, this means a shift in the focus of mental health care from the large, long-term institution to the community-based care. This is accomplished by discharging long-term clients and avoiding unnecessary admissions.

deja vu Sensation that what one is experiencing has been experienced before.

delayed, or dysfunctional, grief Syndrome that results when there is failure to experience or express grief at the time of loss.

delirium Acute organic mental disorder characterized by confusion, disorientation, restlessness, clouding of the consciousness, incoherence, fear, anxiety, excitement, and often illusions, hallucinations, and delusions.

delirium tremens Mental diagnostical term that has been replaced with the diagnosis "alcohol withdrawal delirium."

delusion Fixed false belief contrary to evidence. It may be persecutory, grandiose, nihilistic, or somatic in nature.

delusion of grandeur False belief that one has great money, power, and prestige. It is frequently manifested in the belief that the individual is a famous person.

delusion of persecution False belief that one has been singled out for harassment.

delusion of poverty False belief that one is impoverished.

dementia Chronic organic mental disorder characterized by personality disintegration, confusion, disorientation, stupor, deterioration of intellectual capacity and function, and impairment of control of memory, judgment, and impulses.

denial Defense mechanism used to resolve emotional conflict and allay anxiety by disavowing thoughts, feelings, wishes, needs, or external reality factors that are consciously intolerable.

density Concentration of people in a given location.

dependence on a substance Compulsion to take a substance either on a continuous or periodic basis in order to experience its effects and to avoid the discomfort of its absence.

dependent personality disorder Mental disorder characterized by an inability to function independently and lack of self-confidence.

depersonalization disorder Emotional disorder characterized by a feeling of self-estrangement in which a dream-like atmosphere pervades.

depression Mood disturbance characterized by feelings of sadness, despair, and discouragement resulting from some loss or disappointment.

depression position Normal stage of development during which the child learns to modify ambivalence and sustain loss of the "good mother."

dereistic thought Type of mental activity in which fantasy is not tempered by the laws of logic, experience, and reality.

destructive manipulation Using or "playing" others for one's own purposes.

detoxification Process of withdrawal from alcohol in a controlled environment.

detriangle Process by which one avoids participating in a triangular interpersonal situation.

developmental crisis Stress that occurs when a person is unable to complete the tasks of a psychosocial stage of development and is thus unable to move on to the next stage.

developmental lines Concept developed by Anna Freud that considers the child's chronological age and expectations for ego maturation at each stage of development.

deviant behavior Everyday transactions that exceed the usual accepted behavior and involve failure to comply with a social norm.

dietician Health professional who is concerned with the nutritional needs of the client.

differentiation Degree to which the emotional and intellectual systems of a person are integrated. High differentiation results in goal-directed, mature behavior. Also called *individuation.*

direct practice roles Roles in which the nurse meets the mental health needs of the community through various treatment modalities.

discounts Actions that devalue by not recognizing a person, a problem or a problem's importance and solvability, or the person's ability to solve the problem.

disengagement Term describing the rigid, fixed boundaries that can exist between subsystems in a family. These rigid boundaries lead to distance and discourage communication.

disjunctive Relationship in contextual therapy characterized by distancing.

disorientation Inability to correctly identify the self in relation to time, place, or person.

disparaging maneuvering Type of destructive manipulative behavior exemplified by reprimands and self-pity.

displacement Shift of an emotion from the person or object toward which it was originally directed to another, usually neutral or less dangerous, person or object.

dissociation System of processes for minimizing or avoiding anxiety by which parts of the individual's experience called "not me" are kept out of consciousness.

dissociative disorders Conditions characterized by a sudden, temporary alteration in the integrative functions of consciousness, identity, or motor behavior.

distancing Movement away from another.

distracting maneuvering Type of destructive manipulative behavior exemplified by changes of subject, flattery, expressions of helplessness, tearfulness, dawdling, and last-minute stalling.

disturbed communication Communication that is not clear and is impeded by various factors.

diurnal mood variation Changes in mood that are related to the time of day.

doctrine of double effect Doctrine that a lesser good or an evil is morally permissible if done to achieve a greater good, provided that certain conditions are fulfilled.

dominance Fact or state of controlling or prevailing over others.

double approach-avoidance conflict Conflict resulting from the presence of two goals, both of which are desirable and undesirable.

double blind Two conflicting messages from someone who is crucial to one's survival. One message is usually verbal, one nonverbal. See also *incongruent communication*.

dream analysis Primary method of gaining access to uncensored material from the unconscious.

drive Stimulus that has sufficient strength to impel the person into activity.

dual diagnosis Alcohol and/or drug dependence simultaneously with mental illness.

dysarthria Impaired, difficult speech, usually a result of organic disorders of the nervous system or speech organs.

dysfunctional thought record Record on which a client is instructed to recod his thoughts whenever a strong emotion is experienced; this record is explored by the therapist and the client to examine the evidence that supports or refutes the automatic thoughts and to explore alternative interpretations.

dysfunctional stereotype Stereotyping in which the dysfunctional aspects of a culture are emphasized.

dyskinesia Impairment of the ability to execute voluntary movements.

dysmnesia Impairment in the ability to retain and recall information.

dyspareunia Pain during sexual intercourse.

dystonia Side effect of antipsychotic medication that is characterized by muscle spasms, particularly of the head, neck, and tongue.

dysthymia A chronic mood disturbance involving depressed mood for a period of at least 2 years.

echolalia Repeating exactly what is heard.

echopraxia Imitation of the body position of another.

eclectic approach Use of a combination of theories from more than one framework.

ecology Study of organisms in their home; the study of people as they influence and are influenced by one another and their environment.

ectomorph Person whose physique is characterized by slenderness and fragility. See also *endomorph; mesomorph*.

egalitarian group leadership Groups led by coleaders of equal status; a collegial relationship.

ego Executive of the personality that maintains harmony among the id, the superego, and the external world.

ego boundaries Individual's perception of the boundary between himself and the external environment.

ego dystonic Elements of a person's behavior, thoughts, impulses, drives, and attitudes at variance with the standards of the ego and inconsistent with the total personality. Also called "ego alien."

ego state Consistent pattern of feelings accompanied by a related set of consistent behavior patterns.

ego syntonic Aspects of a person's behavior, thoughts, and attitudes viewed as acceptable and consistent with the total personality.

egoism Ethical position that one does and should think and act in one's interest exclusively.

elderly abuse Any willful or negligent act that results from negligence, malnutrition, physical assault or battery, or physical or psychological injury inflicted against an elderly person by other than accidental means.

electroconvulsive therapy (ECT) Electric shock delivered to the brain through electrodes placed on the temple(s) to artificially produce a grand mal seizure.

emancipated minor An individual under the legal age of majority who is married, a parent, divorced, or self-supporting and living away from his or her parents.

embarrassment State of feeling self-conscious or ill at ease.

emic Defining of normal and abnormal behavior by members within a cultural group.

emotion An affective state; a feeling.

emotional abuse Use of implicit or explicit threats, verbal assault, or acts of degradation that are injurious or damaging to an individual's sense of self-worth.

emotional cutoff Breaking away from an emotional attachment to family to differentiate oneself.

emotional object constancy Ability to hold a mental symbolic picture of the loved object when the object is absent.

emotional neglect Lack of maintaining an interpersonal atmosphere conducive for psychosocial growth and development of a sense of personal worth and well-being.

emotional system Emotional chain reactions that occur among family members and tie the emotional functioning of one family member integrally to that of another.

emotionally disturbed child Child whose personality development is arrested or interfered with so that he shows impairment in reasonable and accurate perceptions of the world, impulse control, learning, and social relations with others.

empathy Ability to recognize and, to some extent, share the emotions and states of mind of another and to understand the meaning and significance of that person's behavior.

enabling behavior Behavior that results from codependency and that helps to maintain addiction.

encopresis Fecal incontinence.

encounter group Group that focuses more on emotional experiencing; especially valued are emotional honesty, self-exposure, confrontation, and obtaining an intense positive emotional experience.

enculturation Process by which culture is transmitted from one generation to the next.

endomorph Person whose body build is characterized by a soft, round physique with a large trunk and thighs, tapering extremities, an accumulation of fat throughout the body. See also *ectomorph; mesomorph*.

enmeshment Excessive tightness at the expense of individual independence; occurs in families in which sharing is intense and engulfing.

entitlement Underlying assumption of people which holds that the world owes them something.

enuresis Incontinence or involuntary urination; particularly problematic for children. Also called "bed-wetting."

environmental modification Intervention that focuses on making changes in the client's environment that decreases stress and the potential for another crisis.

equilibrium Balance among the parts of a system.

erogenous zones Areas of the body (mouth, anus, and genitals) in which tension becomes concentrated and can be relieved by manipulation of the region.

eros Lust or sexual drive; a type of physical love.

ethic Standard of valued behavior or beliefs adhered to by an individual or group; a goal to which one aspires.

ethical dilemma Issue for which moral claims conflict with one another: (1) a difficult problem that seems to have no satisfactory solution or (2) a choice between equally unsatisfactory alternatives.

ethnocentricity Attitude that one's own cultural group is superior.

ethnocentric perspective One's judgment of the behaviors of persons of a different culture by the standards of one's own culture.

etic Defining of normal and abnormal behavior by persons outside a cultural group.

evaluation Category of the nursing process in which a determination is made and recorded regarding the extent to which the established goals of care have been met.

excess disability The loss of function that is associated with the perceptions of the client or nurse but is not a true disability.

exhibitionism Achievement of sexual pleasure by exposing one's sexual organs to another, usually a stranger.

existential School of philosophical thought that focuses on the importance of experience in the present and the belief that people find meaning in life through their experiences.

experimental research Research in which the investigator deliberately manipulates some condition or phenomenon to assess the effects of intervention on some other condition or phenomenon.

expiatory behavior Repentant, atoning, or some kind of reparative behavior resulting from a guilty conscious.

exploitative character Term used by Fromm to describe a person who takes what he wants by exploiting or using everyone, enhancing his stance of interpersonal power in the process.

expressive aphasia Inability to express ideas in words.

expressive functions Observable behaviors from which mental activity is inferred, including speaking, writing, drawing, physical gestures, facial expressions, and movements.

expressive groups Groups that focus on feelings. In groups for the elderly, these are contrasted with the more concrete and structured groups commonly used, such as remotivation, reminiscence, and life review groups.

external locus of control Belief that an outcome is determined by fate, chance, or powerful others and is thus beyond personal control.

extinction Decrease in the occurrence of a behavior when the behavior is not reinforced.

extrapyramidal effects Side effects of an antipsychotic medication that resemble the symptoms of parkinsonism, including tremor, drooling, and altered gait.

extrasensory perception (ESP) Awareness or knowledge acquired without using the physical senses.

factitious disorders Symptoms of illness that are caused by the deliberate effort of the person, usually to gain attention. Attempts to gain attention by this means are often repeated even when the individual is aware of the hazards involved.

false personification Security operation that involves stereotyping, such as labeling or prejudging others.

false transactions Transactions in which communication is stopped or crossed up by one individual relating from a different ego state than the other person expected.

family myths Series of fairly well-integrated beliefs shared by all family members concerning each other and their mutual position in the family life.

family projection process Primary mechanism by which the multigenerational transmission process operates; the family members attribute their thoughts and impulses to other family members.

family therapy Therapy modality that focuses treatment on the process between family members that supports and perpetuates symptoms; a way of conceptualizing human relationship problems that focuses on the context in which an emotional problem is generated.

fan pattern of communication Messages originate at one source and are directed downward to several receivers who do not interact with each other.

fear Emotion that results from tension and pessimism arising from the danger of actual physical harm to one's existence.

feedback Response to the sender of a message.

fellatio Oral stimulation of the male genitals.

female sexual dysfunction Medical term for psychosomatic and pathological conditions that interfere with normal female sexual activity.

fetal alcohol syndrome A type of intellectual impairment of the fetus that results from the mother's abuse of alcohol during pregnancy.

fetishist Person who obtains sexual pleasure from an inanimate object, such as a shoe or leather garment.

first-order change Change within a system that itself remains unchanged.

fixation Arrest at a particular stage of psychosexual development, such as anal fixation.

fixed feature space Internal and external design of a building and its relationship to other buildings and environmental factors.

flat affect Affect of a client who does not communicate feelings in verbal or nonverbal responses to events.

flexibility Ability to adapt or to respond to changing conditions; the state of mind that permits consideration of new ideas and information.

flight of ideas Alteration in thought processes resulting in a sudden rapid shift from one idea to another before the preceding one has been concluded with some relatedness of the train of thought.

flight to health Resistance process occurring when the client chooses to abruptly terminate therapy, seeing himself as "cured," rather than experiencing a reactivation of painful feelings.

flight to illness Client's effort to demonstrate to the therapist that he is too ill to terminate therapy and continued support is needed.

flooding Form of desensitization that uses real or imaginary situations to evoke strong feelings of anxiety.

focused activity Technique that serves the purpose of actively focusing the client toward his adaptive coping abilities and away from maladaptive ones.

folk illnesses Illnesses that are attributed to nonscientific causes; two major categories are naturalistic and personalistic illnesses.

formative evaluation Judgments made about the effectiveness of nursing interventions as they are implemented.

free association Spontaneous verbalization of thoughts and emotions entering the consciousness during psychoanalysis.

free-floating anxiety Type of neurotic anxiety that is characterized by general apprehensiveness and pessimism.

Freudian character Term used by Fromm to describe a miserly person who holds on to what he has.

frigidity Inability of the female to achieve orgasm.

frustration Feeling resulting from an interference with one's ability to attain a desired goal, satisfaction, or security.

function of communication That which communication accomplishes for the person or persons involved (as distinguishable from the structure of communication).

functional analysis Discovery of the sequence of events involved in producing and maintaining undesirable behavior.

functional disorder Mental or emotional impairment that is believed to be psychosocial in origin.

fusion Tendency of two people experiencing an intense emotional attraction to unite.

fusion-exclusion Compensatory mechanism by which two people can stay in close contact with each other and avoid fusion-generated anxiety either by excluding a third person from their relationship or by focusing their energies on a third person.

galactosemia Genetic condition in which one is unable to metabolize galactose.

Gamblers Anonymous Self-help group that helps gamblers and uses a modified version of the Alcoholics Anonymous program as its approach.

game Series of learned, unconscious maneuvers that lead to a well-defined payoff; an ulterior transaction that leaves the players with bad feelings.

gender identity Inner sense of maleness or femaleness that identifies the person as being male or female.

gender role Image a person presents to others and to himself that declares him to be male or female.

general adaptation syndrome (GAS) Process by which the body's nonspecific responses to stress or noxious agents evolve through stages of adaptation.

general anxiety disorder Anxiety state characterized by persistent anxiety of at least a month's duration, excluding symptoms associated with a phobic, panic, or obsessive-compulsive disorder.

general female sexual dysfunction Condition in which the female feels no sexual pleasure from sexual stimulation and is unable to have erotic feelings and responses.

generic approach A treatment approach to crisis based on the premise that certain identifiable patterns of behavior are characteristic of each type of crisis and that psychological tasks specific to the type of crisis are required if the crisis is to be successfully resolved.

genetic insight Deepest level of self-understanding.

genetics Branch of biology dealing with the phenomena of heredity and the laws governing it.

genogram Multigenerational diagram of a family.

genuineness Quality characterized by openness, honesty, and sincerity. The nurse possesses genuineness when she is self-congruent and authentic and relates to the client without a defensive facade.

geropsychiatric nursing Mental health–psychiatric nursing care of the older adult.

gestalt Whole picture.

globus hystericus Feeling of a lump in the throat that interferes with swallowing.

grandiosity Overappraisal of one's worth and ability.

grandstanding Form of manipulation of others to satisfy one's needs.

gravely disabled Because of a mental condition, the client is unable to care for his basic needs of nutrition, clothing, shelter, safety, and medical care.

grief Emotional response that follows loss or separation.

group content Work of a group; specific tasks and problems; goals to be accomplished.

group dynamics All that takes place within a group from the time of its inception until termination.

group norms Acceptable group behaviors. These will vary from one group to another. In one group it is acceptable to be open with feelings, but this is not acceptable in another group that is primarily concerned with accomplishing a concrete task.

group process Interaction continually taking place between members of a group.

group therapy Modality of therapy in which common problems are confronted in a group setting by individuals experiencing similar difficulties.

guilt Remorseful awareness of having done something wrong.

guilty fear Emotional response that occurs when a person is in the process of doing something that is immoral, disapproved of, or illegal. The fear is of getting what is deserved.

habeas corpus Right retained by all psychiatric clients that provides for the release of an individual who claims he is being deprived of his liberty and detained illegally. The hearing for this determination takes place in a court of law in which the client's sanity is at issue.

habit Link or association between a stimulus and a response.

half-life Time it takes for half of a medication to be eliminated, destroyed, or decayed in the body.

hallucinations Sensory perception that does not result from an external stimulus. It can occur from any of the senses and is classified auditory, gustatory, olfactory, tactile, or visual.

hatha yoga Step-by-step system of physical training that involves use of the entire body, stretching exercises, and holding postures.

helplessness Belief that no one can do anything to aid one; an inability to make autonomous decisions.

hepatic encephalopathy Brain damage caused by liver disease and consequent ammonia intoxication and by deficiency of thiamin and other nutrients. Usually seen as a consequence of alcoholism and its attendant malnutrition.

heterogeneous groups Groups composed of members of both sexes, with a variety of ages, backgrounds, behaviors, and needs.

histrionic personality disorder Mental disorder characterized by dramatic and exaggerated behavior that draws attention to oneself.

holism Philosophy in which all entities are viewed more in terms of relationships and processes than as separate parts that can be adequately analyzed in isolation.

homeostasis Maintenance of a normal steady state in the body.

homogeneous groups Groups composed of members of the same sex and similar ages, backgrounds, behaviors, and needs.

homosexuality Sexual orientation toward someone of the same sex.

homunculism Notion that children are miniature adults.

hope Mental state characterized by the desire to gain an end or accomplish a goal combined with some expectation that what is desired is attainable.

hopelessness Belief that no help can be obtained.

hospice System of family-centered care provided outside the hospital designed to assist the dying client to maintain a satisfactory life-style through the terminal phases of dying.

hostile aggressiveness Pattern of behavior ranging from threatening physical violence to voicing challenging, demeaning, and criticizing remarks.

hostility Feeling of anger and resentment characterized by destructive behavior.

hot flash Common symptom of menopause in which the body becomes warm with an excessive period of perspiration followed by chills; may involve only the face and neck or may extend over the entire body.

human ecology Study of people in their multiple environments.

human potential movement Social transition of values from a child-centered focus to an adult-centered focus on development potential.

humanism Philosophy in which people, as well as their interests, developments, fulfillment, and creativity, are made central and dominant.

hydrotherapy   Various forms of therapy entailing the use of water to bring about a therapeutic and tranquilizing effect.

hyperkinesis   Unusual or excessive activity in children with resulting behavioral problems and learning difficulties. Theories of the cause vary and include allergies and sensitivities to food additives.

hypertensive crisis   Syndrome characterized by rapidly changing neurological abnormalities. Occurs after eating certain foods containing a high concentration of tyramine in reaction to the ingestion of MAO inhibitors.

hypervigilance   Increased state of watchfulness.

hypnosis   An altered state of consciousness whereby distraction is minimized and concentration is heightened to reduce pain.

hypnotic   A trancelike state.

hypochondriacal pain   Pain described by persons who have a constant preoccupation with their bodies, fear disease or body dysfunction, and experience pain.

hypochondriacal preoccupation   An intense, almost morbid, preoccupation with health.

hypochondriasis   Somatoform disorder characterized by an exaggerated concern for one's health, an unrealistic interpretation of signs or sensations as abnormal, and preoccupation with the fear of having a serious disease.

hypomania   Clinical syndrome that is similar to, but less severe than, that described by the term *mania* or "manic episode."

hypothesis   A level of interpretation based on theoretical formulations that can be validated but are tentative and can be changed as new data are collected.

hysteria   Disorder in which symptoms of physical illness appear without any underlying organic pathological condition. Also known as *conversion reaction.*

hysterical pain   A type of conversion disorder brought on by a specific, highly charged emotional event related to earlier unconscious emotional conflicts.

id   Basic system of the personality structure that consists of all psychological processes that are present at birth.

ideas of reference   Obsessive delusion that the statements or activities of others refer to oneself, usually taken to be deprecatory.

identification   Unconscious defense mechanism by which a person patterns his personality on that of another person, assuming the person's qualities, characteristics, and actions.

identity   Organizing principle of the personality system that account for the unity, continuity, uniqueness, and consistency of the personality. It is the awareness of the process of "being oneself" that is derived from self-observation and judgment and is the synthesis of all self-representations into an organized whole.

identity confusion   Lack of clarity and consistency in one's perception of the self, resulting in a high degree of anxiety.

idiosyncratic behavior   Variation from the dominant cultural pattern encountered in one person.

illusions   False interpretation of an external, usually visual or auditory, sensory stimulus.

imagery   Formation of mental concepts, figures, and ideas.

immediate memory   Type of memory that involves the fixation of information that is selected for retention during the registration process.

immobility deprivation   Inability to respond to physical stimulation resulting from decreased physical activity, such as that caused by traction, casts, or paralysis.

impetus   Stength or force of an instinct.

implementation   Phase of the nursing process in which nursing actions are carried out that assist the client to maximize his health capabilities and provide for client participation in health promotion, maintenance, and restoration.

implosive therapy   Form of desensitization therapy in which there is repeated exposure to a highly feared object.

impotence   Inability by the male to obtain or maintain an erection of sufficient strength to allow performance of the act of intercourse.

incest   Sexual activity performed on a child by a member of the child's family group, not limited to sexual intercourse but including any action performed to sexually stimulate the child or use of the child to stimulate other persons.

incompetency   Legal status that must be proved in a special court hearing. As a result of the hearing the person can be deprived of many of his civil rights. Incompetency can be reversed only in another court hearing that declares the person competent.

incongruent communication   Communication pattern in which the sender is communicating a different message on the verbal and nonverbal levels and the listener does not know to which level he should respond. See also *double bind.*

indirect practice roles   Roles in which the nurse participates in care by providing clinical expertise and knowledge to other health care providers who use that knowledge to meet the mental health needs of the community.

individual approach   A treatment approach to crisis that emphasizes assessment of the intrapsychic and interpersonal processes of the person in crisis by a mental health professional.

individual family therapy   Therapy in which each family member has a single therapist and the family may meet together occasionally with one or two of the therapists to see how the members are relating to one another and work out specific issues that have been defined by individual members.

individualization   Caring for each client as an individual and unique being with a singular outlook on the world and life situations.

individuation   Gradual development of psychological autonomy—self that is separated from the mother; sense of separate identity but simultaneously a deep attachment to the family. Also called *differentiation;* interrelated with *separation.*

indoklon therapy   Treatment with indoklon, a colorless, volatile liquid given with oxygen inhalation to induce convulsions, used for emotional disturbances.

informal space   Personal distances maintained in interpersonal encounters.

informed consent   Disclosure of a certain amount of information to the client about the proposed treatment and the attainment of the client's consent, which must be competent, understanding, and voluntary.

infradian rhythms   Encompassing cycles that are longer than 24 hours, such as the menstrual cycle.

injunctions   Covert script messages given from the Child ego state of the father and mother.

insight   Self-understanding; extent of one's understanding of the origin, nature, and mechanisms of behavior.

instincts   Inborn psychological representation of a need.

insulin coma therapy (insulin shock therapy)   Insulin given in progressive amounts to a fasting client to produce hypoglycemia and coma for the treatment of psychiatric disorders.

integration   Stage, as described in Moreno's theory of emotional release, that the individual feels restored with self and others following the release of anger; also, the tendency for all aspects of a culture to function as an interrelated whole.

intellectualization   Defense mechanism in which reasoning is used as a means of blocking a confrontation with an unconscious conflict and the emotional stress associated with it.

intentionality   General goal of self-mastery in psychotherapy; seen as self-actualization by Maslow and congruence by Rogers.

interactional synchrony   Nonverbal body positioning and adjustments very young children make to adult verbalizations that enhance learning the relationships of verbalizations and gestures.

interactionist theory   Theory about aging that views age-related changes as resulting from the interaction between the individual characteristics of the person, the circumstances in society, and the history of social interaction patterns of the person.

internal locus of control   Belief that an outcome is a consequence of the individual's actions and is thus under his personal control.

interpersonal communication   Communication between two or more persons, characterized by expressive action, the conscious or unconscious perception of that action by another or others, and the perception that the expressive action was perceived by others.

interpersonal perceptions   Concept of norms, social responsibility, and justice growing from role taking and understanding of the meaning of situations to other people.

interpretation   Assigning an underlying cause or meaning to a behavior.

intervention   Any act by the nurse that implements the nursing care plan or any specific objective of the plan.

intimacy   Capacity to commit; reciprocal involvement with othes personally, sexually, occupationally, and socially.

intimate zone   The area within 18 inches of the body; the space in which physical activity occurs.

introjection   Intense type of identification in which the person incorporates qualities or values of another person or group into his own ego structure.

introspection   Act of examining one's own thoughts and emotions by concentrating on the inner self.

isolation   Defense mechanism in which an unacceptable idea, impulse, or act is separated from its original memory source, thereby removing the emotional charge associated with the original memory.

Johari's window   A two-way matrix that provides an analysis of the known and unknown aspects of self as they relate to self-awareness and awareness of others.

kinesic behaviors   Nonverbal cues of communication that function to achieve and maintain bonds or attachments between people.

kinesiology   Scientific study of muscular activity and of the anatomy, physiology, and mechanics of the movement of body parts.

Korsakoff's syndrome   Form of amnesia often seen in chronic alcoholism, characterized by a loss of short-term memory and an inability to learn new skills.

kwashiorkor   Form of protein malnutrition, seen in weaned infants, characterized by physical and mental growth intervention and fluid-electrolyte imbalances.

lability   Frequent or unpredictable mood changes.

language   Collection of signs or symbols of which two or more communicators or interpreters understand the significance.

language acquisition device (LAD)   Innate, schematic central nervous system neuromotor structure that is species specific and matures as the child develops, providing the mechanisms for speech.

latency   Stage of development occurring between the ages of 6 and 12 years in which the major task is the achievement of a sense of competence.

learned helplessness   Behavioral state and personality trait of a person who believes that he is ineffectual, that his responses are futile, and that he has lost control over the reinforcers in his environment.

learning disorder   Condition affecting children and characterized by difficulties in reading, writing, and numerical calculation.

leftover guilt   Type of guilt resulting from early conditioning and shaped by patterns of thinking, feeling, reacting, and behavior within the family.

lesbian   Woman whose sexual orientation is toward another woman.

lethality   Estimation of the probability that a person who is threatening suicide will succeed based on the method de-

scribed, the specificity of the plan, and the availability of the means.

levels of practice   Identified nursing behaviors related to degrees of knowledge and skill development.

leverage   Therapeutic influence developed by the helping person as a result of the helping person's efforts on the client's behalf.

liaison   The facilitation of the relationship that exists between the client, the illness, the consultees, and the hospital/ward milieu.

liaison alliance   A relationship between the consultant and the consultee that signifies some clinical dilemmas can be understood and resolved by reflecting on the interactions among care providers and clients.

libertarianism   Ethical orientation that the person is sovereign and may choose without interference as long as he does not harm others.

libido   See *psychic energy.*

licensure   Process by which the legal right to practice nursing is accorded a person in a given state and based on evidence of minimal standards of competence.

life change units   Term assigned to the kinds of social changes an individual experiences and the amount of stress that the changes cause.

life instincts   Instincts directed toward survival and propagation of the species.

life review   Reminiscence usually occurring in old age as a consequence of the realization of the inevitability of death.

limit setting   Act of making a person aware of his rights and responsibilities while communicating the expectation that he will respect the rules; also, the application of appropriate sanctions if the person does not obey the rules.

locus of control   Person's perception of the power he has over events that affect his life.

logotherapy   Approach to psychotherapy based on the existential model and developed by Viktor Frankl. The focus is on the search for meaning in present experiences.

long-term memory   Type of memory that is also referred to as learning and involves a person's ability to store information.

loneliness   The absence of expected relationships.

loose associations   A communication pattern characterized by lack of clarity or connection between one thought and the next.

loss   An actual or potential state in which a valued object, person, or body part that was formerly present is lost or changed and can no longer be seen, felt, heard, known, or experienced.

love   Strong affection for another arising out of personal relations.

lunacy   Archaic term referring to the belief that the moon affects behavior, especially psychopathological behavior.

machismo   Hispanic concept of the man, which includes their culturally desirable traits of courage and fearlessness and the dysfunctional behaviors of heavy drinking, seduction of women, and domineering and abusive spouse behaviors.

magical thinking   Belief that merely thinking about an event in the external world can cause it to occur; result of regression to an early phase of development.

magnification   Cognitive distortion in which the effects of one's behavior are magnified.

maladaptive behavior   Behavior that does not adjust to the environment or situation and interferes with mental health.

maladaptive independence   Behavior that interferes with an individual's ability to attain a high level of health.

male sexual dysfunction   Medical term for psychosomatic and pathological conditions that interfere with normal male sexual activity.

malingering   Willful and deliberate feigning of the symptoms of a disease or injury to gain some consciously desired end.

mal ojo   The practice of casting the "evil eye."

mandala   Universal religious symbol spontaneously drawn by most children.

mania Condition characterized by a mood that is elevated, expansive, or irritable.

manipulation Process of influencing another to meet one's own needs and desires, regardless of the needs and desires of another.

manipulative religions Religions that emphasize the inability of individuals to trust their own nature and encourage helplessness.

mapping Process of handing down a set of patterns from one generation to another.

marasmus Form of protein and calorie malnutrition in infants and young children, often associated with maternal and other deprivation with life-threatening physical and mental consequences.

marathon group Form of group originated by George Bach that meets for an extended time, for example, several days in a row or a whole weekend. The intensity of the group and its extended time frame are believed helpful in the breaking down of defenses built to protect one from knowing and understanding one's inner self.

marketing character Term used by Fromm to describe a person who takes in whatever the authority of others provides.

marriage contract (couple contract) Situation in which two people join in a committed relationship, each with a separate understanding of expectations within the relationship.

Maslow's hierarchy of needs Pyramid of human needs (physiological, safety, security, love and belonging, self-esteem, and self-actualization) theorized by Abraham Maslow.

masochism Pleasure derived from physical or psychological pain inflicted either by oneself or by others.

masochist One who gains feeling of satisfaction by allowing another to inflict pain.

massage Technique of some alternative therapies that involves rubbing or kneading of the body, usually with the hands, to stimulate circulation.

matter-of-factness Avoidance of emotional responses and reassurance; treatment of requests, pleas, or manipulative maneuvers with casualness.

material abuse The theft or misuse of an individual's property or money.

matiasma The beliefs and practices surrounding the healing practice of the "evil eye."

maturational crisis Transitional or developmental periods within a person's life when his psychological equilibrium is upset.

mechanical restraints Any of several means of restricting a client's freedom of movement. Includes camisoles, wrist and ankle restraints, sheet restraints, and sheet packs.

meditation Technique of tension reduction in which the person closes his eyes, relaxes the major muscle groups, and repeats a cue word silently to himself each time he exhales.

megavitamin therapy Treatment that includes giving the psychiatric client large doses of special vitamins and minerals.

melancholy Feeling of deep sadness or depression.

menopause Termination of menstruation, usually between the ages of 48 and 50.

mental health A state of well-being whereby a person functions comfortably in society and is generally satisfied with oneself and one's achievements.

mental health consultation The provision of clinical expertise regarding the delivery of psychological care in response to a request from a health care provider.

mental health–psychiatric nurse A nurse who specializes in the care of clients with mental health problems.

mental health–psychiatric nursing Interpersonal process that strives to promote and maintain behavior that contributes to integrated functioning. It employs the theories of human behavior as its science and purposeful use of self as its art. It is directed toward both preventing and treating mental disorders and promoting optimal mental health for society, the community, and the individuals who live within it.

mental illness A substantial disturbance of thoughts or mood that significantly impairs judgment, behavior, and capacity to recognize reality or to cope with the ordinary demands of life.

mentor One who guides; a teacher.

mesomorph Person whose physique is characterized by a predominance of muscle, bone, and connective tissue. See also *ectomorph; endomorph.*

metacommunication Communication that refers to how a given message is to be understood.

mid-life transition Bridge between early adulthood and middle adulthood that lasts from 40 to 45 years of age.

milieu Environment or setting.

milieu therapy Use of the total environment of a setting for treatment purposes.

minimization Cognitive distortion in which the effects of one's behavior are minimized.

misuse of substances Use of a substance for purposes other than those for which it was intended or used incorrectly as prescribed.

mnemonic techniques Techniques for improving memory such as visual imagery associations or categorization.

modal operators Term within neurolinguistic programming that refers to grammatical structures which imply contingencies, possibilities, and necessities.

momentary adaptation Ability to be effective at the moment a distressing situation actually occurs.

monoamine oxidase (MAO) inhibitors Group of chemically related antidepressant medications.

mood A prolonged feeling.

moral anxiety Type of anxiety that is experienced in response to fear of the ego.

morbid grief reaction Delayed or distorted reaction to the loss of a significant person.

morphogenic families Families characterized by flexible rules and communication that are appropriate to the developmental level of family members.

mourning All psychological processes set in motion within the individual by a loss. The process of mourning is resolved only when the lost object is internalized, bonds of attachment are loosened, and new object relationships are established.

multidisciplinary audit An audit done by a group of health care professionals.

multigenerational transmission process Emotional process by which unresolved family problems are carried from one generation to another.

multiinfarct dementia Condition in which a succession of strokes has destroyed enough brain tissue to cause dementia.

multiple family therapy Therapy in which four or five families meet weekly to confront and deal with problems or issues they have in common.

multiple impact therapy Therapy in which families come together for intensive work, usually over a 3-day weekend or week-long encounter.

multiple personality disorder Condition characterized by the existence of two or more complete personality systems that are usually very different from one another.

Munchausen's syndrome Term applied to persons who repeatedly come to acute care setting with convincing but false symptoms of illness or injury, and with falsified documents to support evidence of the disease.

muteness Disorder characterized by a complete loss of speech.

mutual collaboration Concept that emphasizes the nurse and client working together to identify client problems and plan desired outcomes.

mutual pretense context of death The client and others know that he is dying but pretend otherwise.

myoclonus   Spasm of a muscle or a group of muscles.

narcissism   Abnormal interest in oneself, especially in one's own body and sexual characteristics; self-love.

narcissistic personality disorder   Condition characterized by an exaggerated sense of self-importance.

narcotherapy   Intravenous administration of barbiturates or stimulants to produce a physiological effect conducive to therapeutic change.

Naroctics Anonymous   Organization similar to Alcoholics Anonymous for drug-dependent individuals.

National Alliance for the Mentally Ill (NAMI)   National organization for family members of psychotic persons.

naturalistic illnesses   Illnesses caused by impersonal factors, that is, entities without regard for the persons.

nature versus nurture controversy   Long-standing debate as to a child's personality potential, with "nature" proponents emphasizing instincts, genetics, and biological factors and "nurture" proponents emphasizing environment and socialization.

negative reinforcers   Events or conditions that reward a desired behavior.

neglect   Condition that occurs when a caregiver is unable to or fails to provide minimal emotional and physical care to a person entrusted to his care.

neologisms   Words that are invented by the person and understood only by him.

networking   Informal communication system by means of which resources and information are pooled or shared.

network therapy   Therapy conducted in people's homes in which all persons interested or invested in a problem or crisis that a particular person or persons in a family are experiencing take part.

neuroleptic   Medication that produces an altered state of consciousness, characterized by quiescence, reduced motor activity, and reduced anxiety.

neurotic anxiety   Type of anxiety that arises when perception of danger is from the instincts of the id.

Neurotics Anonymous   Self-help group for persons with emotional problems that uses the format of the Alcoholics Anonymous program.

neurotic behavior   Behavioral dysfunction that is characterized by anxiety but in which reality is not distorted.

neurotransmitter   Chemical compounds serving as transmitters of neuromuscular impulses. A number of these substances have nutrient precursors and hence may be affected by diet.

night terrors   Nightmares after which the child has difficulty reorienting to reality.

nightmare   Frightening dream accompanied by feelings of helplessness and suffocation.

nihilistic delusion   False belief that the self, part of the self, or another object has ceased to exist.

nodal events   Occurrences that may cause anxiety, such as birth, death, divorce, marriage, or a child leaving home.

noncompliance   Failure of the individual to carry out the self-care activities prescribed in a health care plan.

nonexperimental research   Research in which the investigator centers on description of existing conditions or phenomena.

nonpossessive warmth   Nurse's warm acceptance of the client's experience as being part of that person with no conditions on acceptance.

nonverbal communication   Messages that do not involve the spoken or written word and are conveyed by behavior.

normal grief reaction   Syndrome manifested by bereaved people that consists of somatic distress, preoccupation with the image of the deceased, guilt, hostile reactions, and generally increased anxiety.

norms   Ideal cultural patterns that represent what most members of the society believe persons ought to do in a particular situation.

nuclear family emotional system   How a single generation deals with their level of differentiation.

nuclear problem   Underlying reason for an individual's reaction to a precipitating event.

numinous   Spiritually elevating.

nursing audit   Type of clinical evaluation of nursing care that may focus on a nursing activity (process audit) or on the behavior of a client in response to the nursing care that has been provided (outcome audit).

nursing care reviews   Written verifications that the nursing care is appropriate and in accord with the standards in a particular clinical area (formerly called audits).

nursing diagnosis   Statement of a health problem or a potential problem in the client's health status that a nurse is licensed and competent to treat. A number of nursing diagnoses have been identified and accepted by the National Group on the Classification of Nursing Diagnosis (Fifth National Conference).

nursing process   Process that serves as an organizing framework for the practice of nursing. It encompasses all of the steps taken by the nurse in caring for a client: assessment, analysis, planning, implementation, and evaluation. The rationale for each step is founded in theory.

obesity   Condition in which the individual weighs at least 20% more than his ideal weight.

object   Means by which the aim of an instinct is achieved.

object permanence   Capacity to perceive that things exist even when not seen.

object relations   Emotional bonds between one person and another, as contrasted with interest in and love for the self; usually described in terms of capacity for loving and reacting appropriately to others.

obsession   Intrusive, repetitive thought, image, or impulse that the person finds distressing and unwanted because of its repulsive or inane nature. Content may be of aggressive, sexual, blasphemous, or obscene quality.

obsessive-compulsive   Characterized by or relating to the tendency to perform repetitive acts or rituals, usually as a means of releasing tension or relieving anxiety.

occupational therapist   Health professional who assists the client in activities of daily living, the development of work tolerance, the development of muscle strength and skills, and resocialization.

oculogyric crisis   Side effect of antipsychotic medication that is characterized by the uncontrollable rolling upward of the eyes.

one-to-one relationship   Mutually defined, collaborative goal-directed client-therapist relationship for purpose of psychotherapy.

open awareness context of death   The client and others know that he is dying and relate to each other openly.

open groups   Groups that admit new members whenever vacancies occur in membership.

operant behavior   Behavior whose strength is controlled by the stimulus events that precede and follow it.

operant conditioning   Process by which the results of a person's behavior determine whether the behavior is more or less likely to occur in the future.

operationalization of behavior   Stating the client's complaints or problems in specific, observable behavioral terms.

organic brain syndrome (OBS)   Any psychological or behavioral abnormality associated with transient or permanent brain dysfunction caused by a disturbance of the physiological functioning of brain tissue.

organic mental disorders   Psychological or behavioral abnormalities associated with brain dysfunction caused by a disturbance of the physiological functioning of brain tissue with a known etiology.

orgasmic dysfunction   Inability of the female to achieve orgasm in sexual activity.

orientation   Ability to correctly relate the self to time, place, and person.

orientation phase   Phase of the therapeutic relationship in which the nature and purpose of the relationship is explained.

orthostatic hypotension   Drop in blood pressure related to change in position. A common side effect of psychotropic medications.

outcome criteria   Criteria developed to evaluate the end result of the care and services provided to the client.

overgeneralization   Cognitive distortion in which that which is true for one event is assumed to be true for all others.

overloading   Talking too much and too fast; a common way for the elderly to handle anxiety.

overreaction   Term applied to responses that are appropriate to a situation but go beyond what one would normally expect from the situation.

pain prone person   Person who expresses pain predominantly in response to loss, anger, hostility, rejection, and guilt.

panic   Attack of extreme anxiety that involves the disorganization of the personality. Distorted perceptions, loss of rational thought, and an inability to communicate and function are evident.

panic disorder   Anxiety state characterized by recurrent panic (anxiety) attacks that occur at times unpredictably, although certain situations may become associated with a panic attack.

panic state   Type of neurotic anxiety that is accompanied by acute and extreme anxiety, intense physiological arousal, and disorganization of personality and functional abilities.

paradoxical interventions   Approach to treatment of dysfunctional communication that address difficulties in problem formulation and resolution.

parallel process   Reenactment of the relationship between client and consultee within the relationship between consultee and consultant.

paranoid delusion   False belief that one is being persecuted.

paranoid disorders   Mental disorders with persistent delusions or persecution or jealousy.

paranoid ideation   Exaggerated belief or suspicion, not of a delusional nature, that one is being harrassed, persecuted, or treated unfairly.

paranoid personality disorder   Mental disorder characterized by extreme suspiciousness and mistrust of others, a fear of losing independence, and a desire to be dominant.

parapsychology   Study of experiential phenomena that occur outside of the usual limits of sensory awareness, including extrasensory perception and precognition.

parataxic distortion   Use of a parataxic mode of thinking by an adult.

parataxic mode of experience   Type of thinking in which the person thinks there is a causal relationship between events that occur at the same time but are not logically related.

parens patriae   Power of the state to commit a person to protect others from harm.

Parent ego state   Part of self with messages (tapes) that sound like one's parents; the tapes contain advice and value messages with many *oughts* and *dont's*.

Parents Anonymous   Self-help group for abusive parents.

Parents Without Partners (PWP)   Self-help group for single parents, whether widowed, separated, or divorced.

passive   Behavior that subordinates the individual's own rights to the demands of others.

passive-aggressive personality disorder   Disorder characterized by an indirect resistance to social and occupational demands, procrastination, and inefficient functioning.

paternalism   Ethical orientation that the state knows best and that each person is subordinate and duty bound to comply with the authority figure who is said to know best.

pathological or morbid grief   Excessive grief response resulting in health problems.

patient classification system   Identification and classification of clients into care groups or categories and the quantification of these categories as a measure of the nursing effort required.

patterned operations   Patterns of behavior that are observable and manifested either verbally or nonverbally.

pedophile   Person whose sexual preference is for a child.

peer review   Process by which the quality of nursing care rendered by one nurse is evaluated by other nurses actively involved in clinical nursing practice.

perception   Process by which a person interprets stimuli.

perceptual deprivation   Inability to recognize stimuli from the environment often because of medications that alter the level of consciousness, cerebral dysfunction, or thought disorders.

performationism   Theory that all human life has some form and function and that the embryo is a tiny, fully formed adult that has to grow in size and stature only.

perseveration   Involuntary and pathological persistence of an idea or response.

persona   Social mask that a person wears in social situations.

personalistic illness   Illness resulting from punishment or aggression, directed specifically toward the individual.

personal set   Sensory apparatus, beliefs, and patterned operations that the nurse brings to the relationship with a client.

personal unconscious   The aspect of the mind that consists of experiences that were once conscious but that have been transformed by repression, suppression, or other mechanisms.

personal zone   Similar to a protective zone, the boundaries of which expand and contract according to contextual characteristics; from 18 inches to approximately 4 feet.

personalistic illnesses   Illnesses that result from punishment or aggression that are specifically directed toward a person.

personification   Image that individuals have of themselves and others.

pet therapy   Use of pets to bring about positive changes in the client's physical and mental status.

phenomenological groups   Groups that focus on the experiencing of persons: getting to know and understand them as "real people."

phenomenology   Study of phenomena.

phenothiazines   Group of chemically related antipsychotic medications.

phenylketonuria (PKU)   Genetic disease caused by lack of the cell enzyme that controls metabolism of the essential amino acid phenylalanine. Accumulated abnormal metabolites cause severe mental retardation in unscreened and untreated infants. Therapy is nutritional: low phenylalanine diet with special formula and foods.

philosophy   Search for understanding about the basic truths and principles of the universe, life, and morals by logical reasoning.

phobic reaction   Persistent fear of some object or situation that presents no actual danger to the person or in which the danger is magnified out of proportion to its actual seriousness.

photophobia   Intolerance or fear of light.

photosensitivity   Excessive response to sunlight.

physical abuse   Intentional injury, harmful deed, or destructive act inflicted by a parent, guardian, mature child, or caregiver on another person with whom an interpersonal or advocacy relationship is shared.

physical dependence   Characteristic of drug addiction that is present when withdrawal of the drug results in physiological disruptions.

physical neglect   Volitional deprivation of essential care necessary to sustain life, growth, and development.

physiological conversions   Physiological changes that accompany anxiety and serve no constructive purpose. However, they can form the basis for pathological changes in function that may progress to structural changes and irreversible organic changes.

placebo Any medical or nursing measure that is effective because of its implicit or explicit therapeutic intent rather than its specific chemical or physical properties.

planning Act of determining what can be done to assist the client in restoring, maintaining, or promoting health. This phase involves judging priorities, establishing goals, developing objectives, and identifying strategies for implementation.

pleasure-pain Concept that characterizes persons as drawn to events that are positively reinforcing versus repelled from those that are negatively reinforcing.

pleasure principle Seeking immediate gratification of needs in order to experience pleasure and avoid pain.

point behaviors Refers to how body parts move within space and how they orient themselves in some direction.

polyaddiction Dependence on several substances, not necessarily similar in effect, such as alcohol, cocaine, and cigarettes.

polypharmacy The use of many different medications prescribed by more than one physician and dispensed by more than one pharmacy.

positive regard State of conveying attitudes of warmth, caring, liking, interest, and respect to another.

positive reinforcement Reward for a response.

positive thinking Coping strategy that serves as a defense against environmental obstacles and encourages a pursuit of happiness.

possession trance Belief that the body has been taken over in its function by a spiritual entity.

postcrisis period Period characterized by a return to the steady state, with the person resuming his precrisis level of functioning or perhaps a higher or lower state of functioning, depending on the effectiveness of the crisis resolution.

posttraumatic stress disorder Anxiety state precipitated by a traumatic even that involves reexperiencing the traumatic event.

posturing Voluntary assumption of inappropriate or bizarre posture.

poverty of speech State in which one's vocabulary is increasingly diminished.

practical nurse Nurse who works under the supervision of a registered nurse.

pragmatic Belief that ideas are valuable only in terms of their consequences.

prana Life energy that unites the physical body into a whole and organizes the life processes.

precognition Having foreknowledge of events.

preconscious Perceptions and memories that are outside awareness but are immediately available to consciousness when the need arises.

precrisis period Period during which the person maintains his equilibrium through the use of his usual coping mechanisms.

precursor therapy Type of treatment relating chemical compounds that are influenced by diet to neurological clinical conditions.

predisposing factors Conditioning factors that influence both the type and amount of resources that the individual can elicit to cope with stress. They may be biological, psychological, and sociocultural in nature.

preformationism Dominant theory before the seventeenth century that viewed all human life with the same form and function (for example, children are small adults).

preinteraction phase First phase of the nurse/client relationship whereby the nurse becomes aware of her thoughts and feelings about the interaction.

premature ejaculation Lack of voluntary control over the reflex of ejaculation by the male before the female has achieved orgasm in the act of sexual intercourse.

premonition Sense of an impending event without prior knowledge of it.

premorbid personality Characteristics of one's personality occurring before the development of disease.

preparatory grief Preparation of oneself for separation and impending losses; occurs in stage IV of the process of dying.

prepubescent period Period of development before puberty; period of accelerated growth preceding gonadal maturity.

pressured speech A rapid type of speech in which the person appears driven to continue.

preventive psychiatry Use of theoretical knowledge and skills to plan and implement programs designed to achieve primary, secondary, and tertiary prevention.

prima facie rights Rights on the surface or face that may be overriden by stronger conflicting rights or by other values.

primary anxiety First stage of anxiety related to the developmental process and that evolves out of the birth process.

primary care Phase of health care that is considered to be the initial entry into the health care system, usually community-based care.

primary drives Drives that are innate and in close contact with physiological processes.

primary gain Decrease in anxiety resulting from the individual's efforts to cope with stress.

primary process thought Primitive thought processes that are normally kept unconsciously by use of the coping mechanism of repression; impulsive infantile ideation that involves the use of an image of an object to relieve tension.

primitive anxiety Fearlike state induced by the anxiousness of the mothering one.

privileged communication legal term that applies only in court-related proceedings and means that the right to reveal information belongs to the person who spoke and the listener cannot disclose the information unless the speaker gives permission. It exists between a client and health professional only if a law specifically establishes it.

process criteria Criteria used in the evaluation of actions, sequence of behaviors, and events during the provision of client care.

process of communication Manner in which something is said or done, as in asking a direct question; content of communication; literal meaning of words and symbols.

procrastination Putting off doing something until some future time.

professional development Enhancement of the theoretical knowledge and level of skill in the nurse in order to remain effective in the nursing role.

projection Attributing one's own thoughts or impulses to another person. Through this process the individual can attribute his own intolerable wishes, emotional feelings, or motivations to another person.

projective character Term used by Fromm to describe a person who is unable to use his powers and to realize the potentiality inherent in him.

prospective audit Audit that reviews a defined number of clients with a specific set of criteria.

protocol Guideline or statement of behaviors identified as discrete steps to be taken by nurses in the clinical role.

prototaxic mode of experience Type of primitive experience characterized by sensations, feelings, and fragmented images of short duration andwhich are not logically connected.

proxemics Study of the interaction of spatial features of an environment.

pseudocyesis Condition in which a person has nearly all the usual signs and symptoms for pregnancy such as enlargement of breasts, weight gain, cessation of menses, and morning sickness but is not pregnant.

pseudodementia Delirium that masquerades as dementia.

pseudodenial Client's denial of his illness to another person or failure to tell another person about his illness to protect that person.

pseudohomosexuality Occurring during adolescence when there is a preference for members of the same sex and inordinate amounts of time are spent with members of the same sex.

pseudohostility Term used to describe families that quarrel excessively to cover up their real need and affection for each other.

pseudomutuality An extreme family defense against individualization.

pseudoparkinsonism Having Parkinson's disease-like symptoms which include tremors and muscle rigidity.

pseudoplacidity Characteristic of individuals who use a limited range of human emotions because of their rigidity and excessive control of their emotions.

pseudoposition Compensatory mechanism in which spouses assume "pretend" polarized positions with one another.

pseudoself That part of the self that fluctuates with the emotionality of the moment.

psychiatric nursing See *mental health–psychiatric nursing.*

psychiatric social workers Social workers who deal with the social and psychological problems of clients.

psychiatric technician Technician who assists the nurse in performing client care activities.

psychiatrist Physician who specializes in the treatment of mental disorders.

psychic energy (libido) Body energy used for psychological tasks such as thinking, perceiving, and remembering.

psychoanalysis Branch of psychiatry founded by Sigmund Freud devoted to the study of the psychology of human development and behavior; a system of psychotherapy based on the concept of a dynamic unconscious and the use of techniques such as free association, dream interpretation, and analysis of defense mechanisms.

psychoanalytical treatment Process of therapy in which the irrational belief systems from the unconscious realm are eradicated through gaining of insights and correcting the system so that normal functioning can be assumed by the individual.

psychodrama Therapeutic use of dramatic techniques developed by Moreno, enabling group members to act out and receive feedback about stressful life experiences.

psychodynamics Explanation of the forces that motivate behavior; emphasizes the influence of past experiences on present behavior and the influence of mental forces on development and behavior.

psychodynamic insight Behavioral change resulting from uncovering the roots of origin of one's behavior.

psychogenic Originating within the mind.

psychogenic amnesia Condition characterized by either a partial or total inability to recall the past.

psychogenic fugue Condition characterized by amnesia and physical flight from an intolerable situation.

psychogenic pain Pain in the absence of adequate physiological explanations when psychological explanations may clarify the cause.

psychogenic pain disorder Somatoform disorder characterized by the complaint of pain in the absence of physical findings and evidence of an etiological role for psychological factors.

psychological dependence Characteristic of drug addiction that is manifested in a craving for the abused substance and a fear that it will not be available in the future.

psychological testing Diagnostic tool used by the psychologist to aid in assessment of the client; includes administration of a battery of cognitive and projective tests.

psychology Study of the mind.

psychomotor retardation Slowing of motor activity related to a state of severe depression.

psychosexual development Series of developmental phases throughout the life cycle that promotes growth of the individual in the areas of psychological and sexual development.

psychosomatic Relating to, characterized by, or resulting from the interaction of the mind, or psyche, and the body; the expression of emotional conflict through physical symptoms.

psychosurgery Surgical interruption of selected neural pathways that involve the transmission of emotional impulses in the brain.

psychosynthesis Alternative therapy developed by Robert Assagioli that focuses on three levels of the unconscious: lower, middle, and higher conscious, or superconscious. The goal of the treatment is the recreation or integration of the personality.

psychotherapy Any of a great number of related methods of treating mental or emotional disorders by psychological techniques rather than by physical means.

psychotic behavior Severely dysfunctional behavior characterized by a panic level of anxiety, personality disintegration, and regression behavior. The person experiences a reduced level of awareness and has great difficulty functioning adequately.

psychotic disorders Category of health problems distinguished by the following characteristics: severe mood disorder, regressive behavior, personality disintegration, reduced level of awareness, great difficulty in functioning adequately, and gross impairment in reality testing.

puberty Developmental period during which the secondary sexual characteristics begin to appear and sexual reproduction capability is present.

pubescence Stage of maturation in which the individual becomes physiologically capable of reproduction.

public space Space that extends outward from approximately 12 feet, with the individual in the center.

qualitative comparative analysis Research approach used to generate theory from a combination of inductive and deductive reasoning; also referred to as "grounded theory."

quality assurance Process by which (1) appropriate criteria related to client care are identified and (2) mechanisms to ensure the measurement and achievement of specified criteria are developed.

quality improvement A process based on the philosophy that quality care is the responsibility of each individual within the health care system and that all health-related tasks must fit together to meet client expectations and institutional goals.

radical therapy Alternative therapy that is really more an attitude about the therapeutic process than a specific type of treatment. The focus is on the social and political value systems of the therapist, client, and society. The goal is for the client to be better able to cope with society and to become active politically for change.

rage Violent, intense, and short-lived anger.

rape Legally defined as the forcible perpetration of the act of sexual intercourse on a woman. A more contemporary definition would include acts of oral and anal sodomy and allow for its occurrence within marriage as well.

rapport Sense of mutuality and understanding; harmony, accord, confidence, and respect underlying a relationship between two persons; an essential bond between a therapist and a client in psychotherapy.

rational responses Alternative interpretations that support or refute automatic thoughts.

rationalization Defense mechanism in which the individual attempts to justify or make consciously tolerable, by plausible means, feelings, behavior, and motives that otherwise would be intolerable.

rational suicide A type of suicide in which a person carries out his death in a planned manner using his method of choice and with the cooperation and participation of family and/or friends at a time selected by the individual.

reaction formation Defense mechanism in which a person avoids anxiety through overt behavior and attitudes that are opposite of his repressed impulses and drives and that serve to conceal those unacceptable feelings.

reality anxiety   Type of anxiety that is equated with fear and is based on the perception of danger in the external world.

reality principle   Postponement of immediate gratification of needs until a more appropriate object for satisfaction of needs is available.

reality testing   Process of evaluating one's environment so as to differentiate between external reality and one's inner imaginative world.

recent memory   Type of memory that involves retention of information for an hour or so to 1 to 2 days.

reception deprivation   Inability to receive stimuli properly because of damage in tissue receptors, resulting in partial or total loss of sensation.

receptive aphasia   Inability to recognize or manipulate words as symbols of ideas.

receptive character   Term used by Fromm to describe a person who takes in whatever the authority of others provide.

receptive functions   Functions that involve one's ability to acquire, process, classify, and integrate information.

reciprocal inhibition   Response inhibitory to anxiety that occurs in the presence of the anxiety-evoking stimuli, thus weakening the connection between the stimuli and the anxiety response.

Recovery   Self-help group that provides support for persons discharged from inpatient psychiatric hospitals.

referential index deletions   Term in neurolinguistic programming that refers to the omission of the specific person being discussed.

reflecting   Communication technique in which the nurse picks up the feeling tone of the client's message and repeats it back to the client. Reflection encourages the client to continue with clarifying comments.

reframing   Finding alternative ways for viewing behavior.

regression   Return to an earlier, more primitive form of behavior.

reinforcement   Any event, contingent on the response of the organism, that alters the future likelihood of that response.

rejunctive   Relationship in contextual therapy characterized by moves toward trustworthy relatedness.

relapse   Reestablishment of addiction after a period of abstinence.

relaxation therapy   Type of therapy that focuses on learning and practicing relaxation techniques in a group using such modalities as deep breathing exercises, muscle relaxation, fantasies of being in one's favorite place, fantasizing with music, and guided imagery.

religiosity   Excessive concern with spiritual and religious matters.

reminiscent therapy   Therapy that aims at integrating the client's life experiences into their self-concept by mentally reliving them.

remotivation group   Type of group that uses a give-step format developed for regressed or withdrawn persons.

repetition compulsion   Concept central to the psychoanalytical explanation of play, which states that when a child is exposed to experiences unable to be understood he will set up the experience in play and reexperience the situation again and again until the overload is reduced.

repression   Involuntary exclusion of a painful or conflictual thought, impulse, or memory from awareness. It is the primary ego defense, and other mechanisms tend to reinforce it.

repressive-inspirational approach   Approach used in some groups that discourages the breaking down of defense mechanisms. Members are encouraged to focus on positive feelings and group strengths. This approach is commonly used in groups of chronically mentally ill clients.

resentment   Indignation or ill will resulting from a real or imagined offense.

resistance   Attempt of the client to remain unaware of anxiety-producing aspects within himself. Ambivalent attitudes toward self-exploration in which the client both appreciates and avoids anxiety-producing experiences are a normal part of the therapeutic process.

resocialization   Use of the techniques to facilitate socialization and group interaction, usually among cognitively impaired persons.

restating   Reflecting back that which has been said, using the client's choice of words.

retarded ejaculation   Condition in which the male fails to complete an orgasm with the act of ejaculating semen.

retrospective audit   Audit that evaluates services after they have been rendered.

rigidity   Inability to acquire new responses to changing conditions. The state of mind that rejects information and remains unyielding and opinionated.

ring pattern of communication   Messages that are initiated at one point and are passed from one receiver to another with the last receiver reporting to the sender.

risk factors   Situations in the environment that are potentially hazardous to the child's mental health.

role ambiguity   Form of role stress that occurs when one or more roles are not clearly articulated in terms of behavior or levels of expected performance.

role behaviors   Behaviors used repeatedly by individuals; specific behaviors recognized as part of one's usual way of relating.

role change   Occurs in situations in which status is retained but role expectations remain the same.

role conflict   Role stress that occurs when a person is required to enact roles that are in conflict with his value system or to play two or more roles that conflict with one another.

role incompetence   Role stress that results from a person's inability to fulfill role obligations.

role incongruence   Role stress that occurs when an individual undergoes role transitions, requiring a significant modifcation in attitudes and values.

role induction interview   Therapeutic technique that provides information to the client in advance of ways the client is expected to behave.

role overload   Type of role stress that occurs when excessive demands are made of a person in a particular role and insufficient time is available to fulfill obligations.

role overqualification   Type of role stress that occurs when a role position does not require full use of a person's resources.

role playing   Psychotherapeutic technique in which a person acts out a real or simulated situation as a means of understanding intrapsychic conflicts.

role reversal   Act of assuming the role of another person in order to appreciate how the person feels, perceives, and behaves in relation to himself and the other.

role stress   Situation that occurs when the demands for a person's position in the social structure are difficult, conflicting, or impossible.

roles   Patterns of behavior expected of persons.

romanticism   Social and esthetic movement in art, literature, and music characterized by a revolt against society and social institutions.

rumination   Persistent thinking about and discussion of a particular subject.

sadist   Individual who gains a feeling of power by inflicting pain on others.

sadomasochism   Pleasure derived from pain and suffering inflicted on self by self or others and the inflicting of physical or psychological pain or suffering on others.

samadhi   State of total enlightment in which the body, mind, and spirit function as a harmonious whole.

Santero   A type of folk healer used by Hispanics.

scapegoat   Person who bears the blame for others.

schema   Innate knowledge structure that allows the child to organize in his mind ways to behave in his environment.

schizoid personality disorder   Disorder characterized by aloofness, lack of warmth, indifference to the feelings of others, and a serious defect in interpersonal relationships

schizophrenia   Manifestation of anxiety of psychotic proportions, primarily characterized by inability to trust other people and disordered thought processes, resulting in disrupted interpersonal relationships.

schizotypal personality disorder   Emotional illness characterized by unusual speech, behavior, and thought content. There are also problems in interpersonal relationships.

school phobia   Child's state of anxiety related to separating him from his parents by his attending school. It is a form of separation anxiety; the child is not afraid of school per se.

script   Transactional analysis term that refers to a person's life plan that was adopted during childhood.

seclusion   Form of physical restraint in which the individual is placed in a single room, which may be locked, to decrease stimuli and allow the agitated client to gain control of his behavior.

secondary drives   Drives that evolve during the process of growth and incite and direct behavior.

secondary gain   Indirect benefits, usually obtained through an illness or disability.

secondary intervention   Early diagnosis and prompt and effective treatment to reduce the duration of a significant number of psychiatric disorders that occur.

secondary process thought   Conscious thought processes that are under the control of the ego and are characterized by logic.

secondary reinforcers   Events or conditions that are associated with or supplemental to positive reinforcers.

second-order change   Change that changes the system itself.

security operations   Term related to the interpersonal model of psychiatric care that refers to mental mechanisms which are developed to deal with anxiety-provoking experiences.

sedative   Substance that has a calming effect.

selective abstraction   Type of cognitive distortion in which focus on one aspect of an event negates all other aspects.

selective inattention   Security operation occurring when the person avoids anxiety by not attending to what is said or what is happening.

self-actualization   Tendency toward maximal realization and fulfillment of one's human potential.

self-care model   Framework for nursing care directed toward self-care by the client to the greatest degree possible. The model requires an assessment of the client's capability for self-care and need for care.

self-concept   Composite of ideas, feelings, and attitudes that a person has about his own identity, worth, capabilities, and limitations. Such factors as the values and opinions of others, especially in the formative years of early childhood, play an important part in the development of self-concept.

self-destructive behavior   Any behavior, direct, or indirect, that if uninterrupted, will ultimately lead to the death of the individual.

self-disclosure   The process of voluntarily revealing information about one's self, ideas, values, feelings, and attitudes.

self-esteem   Judgment or evaluation of one's worth in relationship to one's ideal self and to the performance of others.

self-help groups   Therapeutic groups without health professional leadership. Some have been started jointly by health professionals and lay persons, but group members take on the leadership responsibility.

self-ideal   Perception of how one should behave based on certain personal standards. The standard may be either a carefully constructed image of the kind of person one would like to be

or merely a number of aspirations, goals, or values that one would like to achieve.

self-imposed guilt   Restrictive type of guilt that the individual is aware of and from which he is unable to free himself.

self-management approach   Treatment approach in which the client assumes responsibility for his behavior, for changing his environment, and for planning his future.

self-other   Concept that characterizes persons believing that sources of power are within the self as opposed to those who believe the source of power is in others.

self-responsibility   One of the concepts of holism by which individuals assume responsibility for their own health.

self-system   Significant aspect of personality that develops in response to anxiety.

semifixed feature space   Objects in the environment that have some degree of mobility, for example, furniture.

sensitivity training group   Group developed for the purpose of increasing self-awareness, increasing understanding of group process, or increasing awareness of the effects of one's behavior in groups.

sensory deprivation   Involuntary loss of physical awareness caused by detachment from external sensory stimuli; often results in psychological disorders such as panic, mental confusion, depression, and hallucinations.

sensory overload   Bombardment by multiple sensory stimuli as in an intensive care unit.

sensory-based language   Nonverbal behavior.

separation   At the end of infancy, psychological disengagement from the mother, who is now perceived as distinct and apart from oneself, interrelated with *individuation*.

separation anxiety   Anxiety that becomes manifest at separation from a significant person, especially and beginning with the mother. This is normal behavior toward the end of the first year.

set   Predisposition to behave in a certain way.

sexual abuse   Engagement of dependent children or developmentally immature individuals in forms of exploitive or physically intimate sexual activity.

sexual dysfunction   Psychosomatic disorder experienced as a difficulty for individuals to have/or enjoy sexual encounters.

sexuality   Totality of sensations, attitudes, thoughts, feelings, and actions related to one's maleness or femaleness.

sexual masochism   Sexual pleasure and gratification derived by experiencing physical or mental pain and humiliation.

sexual sadism   Sexual pleasure and erotic gratification obtained from inflicting physical or psychological pain on another person.

sexual therapy   Modality of counseling that aids in the resolution of pathological conditions so that a healthy sexuality can be maintained to allow life and relationships to be enjoyed.

shadow   Archetype that represents the unacceptable aspects and components of behavior.

shame   Painful emotion caused by a strong sense of guilt, embarrassment, or disgrace.

sibling position   Birth order of the person in relation to his siblings.

Simple deletions   Term in neurolinguistic programming that refers to the omission of detailed information.

simple phobia   Irrational fear of a specific object or situation, such as fear of snakes or elevators. The fear seldom persists beyond adolescence.

situational crisis   Crisis that occurs when a specific external event upsets an individual's psychological equilibrium.

situational loneliness   Loneliness precipitated by a specific life event.

situational supports   Persons who are available in the environment and who can be depended on to help the individual solve problems.

skills training   Teaching of specific verbal and nonverbal behaviors and the practicing of these by the client.

sleep apnea Absence of spontaneous respirations occurring during sleep.

sleep deprivation Inability to receive adequate rest resulting in fatigue, heaviness of eyelids, tremors, apathy, and visual distortions.

social anxiety Discomfort in the presence of others.

social character Set of characteristics common to most people in a cultural group or society.

social ideal Society's conception of the ideal behavior pattern.

social interaction Action mutually affecting two or more persons.

social interaction pattern Milieu treatment pattern wherein the physician, client, and staff are viewed as team members, all of whom have information valuable to the client's care.

social learning theory Theory that explains the development of aggressive behavior as part of the socialization process.

social phobia Irrational fear of being observed or scrutinized, such as fear of speaking or performing in public.

social radical therapy Intent to bring about change by merging into the larger radical political movement.

social relationship Continuing pattern of social interaction.

social roles Patterns of attitudes, values, goals, and behaviors that are expected of individuals by virtue of their position.

social skills training Type of training that focuses on assisting the person to function more effectively in everyday social interaction.

social space Area about 4 to 12 feet from the person; in this zone no touching is possible.

social support systems Members of one's social environment who are perceived by the individual as "significant others" and who provide some degree of emotional support, task-oriented help, feedback and evaluation, social relatedness and integration, and access to new information.

socialization Basic process by which the human organism becomes a person, acquires norms and values, and becomes a functioning member of society.

societal regression How society deals with the anxiety generated by dwindling food and material sources and increasing threats of atomic annihilation.

sociogram Diagram or picture portraying people relating to each other. Usually people are indicated by circles. Lines drawn between circles represent people relating to each other.

solid self That part of the self that is thought out and not influenced by attempts at emotional negotiation.

somatic Pertaining to the body.

somatic delusion False belief that all or a part of the body is impaired in some way.

somatic therapies Specific medical intervention techniques used to treat an emotional disorder.

somatization disorder Somatoform disorder characterized by repeated and multiple physical complaints of several years' duration for which no physical cause can be identified, although medical attention has been sought.

somatoform disorders Group of disorders characterized by recurrent and multiple physical symptoms for which there are no demonstrable organic findings or identifiable physiological bases.

somnambulism Dissociative manifestation of sleepwalking.

somniloquy Dissociative manifestations of talking while sleeping.

sounding incoherent or repetitive speech resulting from non-organic causes.

source Body needs related to instincts.

specificity Component of psychotherapy that facilitates the clear, explicit expression of thoughts and feelings.

spiritualism Any philosophy, doctrine, or belief emphasizing the spiritual rather than the material.

spirituality Core of an individual's existence, integrating and transcending the physical, emotional, intellectual, and social dimensions.

spontaneity An energy force that propels an individual toward a creative state of being.

stage of exhaustion (SE) Third stage of the general adaptation syndrome that results from prolonged experiences with stress.

stage of resistance (SR) Second stage of the general adapatation syndrome characterized by resistance to change in body organs that leads to homeostasis and survival.

standards of care Comprehensive statements indicating the level of nusing care expected of the practitioner.

status Position in society.

status epilepticus Medical emergency characterized by continual attacks of convulsive seizures occurring without intervals of consciousness.

statutory rape Legal term for the act of sexual intercourse with a female under the age of consent determined by state law.

stereotype Opinion held by a group that is represented by a lack of critical judgment.

stigma Attribute that is deeply discrediting.

stimulus hierarchy List of arousing aspects of a phobic object in increasing order of the level of fear produced.

stranger anxiety Anxiety at the appearance of unfamiliar persons, normal and expected at 6 to 9 months of age. This is a sign of development of the awareness of the existence of a special, loved person.

stress Body's arousal response to any demand, change, or perceived threat.

stress inoculation Procedure useful in helping clients control anxiety by substituting positive coping statements for statements that bring about anxiety.

stress management Methods of controlling factors that require a response of change within the person by identifying the stressors, eliminating negative stressors, and developing effective coping mechanisms to constuctively counteract the response.

stressors Stimuli that the individual perceives as harmful or threatening and produce a state of tension.

strokes Transactional analysis term that refers to unit of recognition that one person can give another or that a person can give to himself.

structural analysis Segregation and analysis of ego states.

structural modification Technique of structured family therapy in which the therapist changes the structure of the boundaries between generations.

structure criteria Criteria that indicate the aims and purposes of the institution, agency, or program.

subculture Group of individuals within a society who share values, beliefs, and behaviors that differ from those of the dominant society.

sublimation Unconscious process of substituting socially more acceptable activity patterns that partially satisfy a need for an activity that would give rise to anxiety.

submission Type of kinetic reciprocal activity in which one person resigns themselves to another.

subsequent anxiety Second stage of anxiety that is experienced with maturation of the ego and superego.

substance abuse Use of any mind-altering agent to such an extent that it interferes with the individual's functioning.

substance dependence Physiological dependence on drugs characterized by the development of tolerance for drugs or withdrawal symptoms when drugs are not taken.

succorance Act of client seeking help following loss of parent or friend by asking the nurse to take the part of a significant other.

succession The state of every system being in a constant state of change.

suicide Self-inflicted death.

suicide attempt Any action deliberately undertaken by the individual that, if carried to completion, will result in his death.

suicide gesture Suicide attempt that is planned to be discovered in an attempt to influence the behavior of others.

suicide threat Direct, indirect, verbal, or nonverbal warning that the individual plans to attempt suicide.

summative evaluation Judgments about the effectiveness of nursing care when it is terminated.

superego Aspect of the personality concerned with prohibitions of parental figures.

supervision Process by which a nurse of lesser experience is assisted by a nurse clinician of greater experience to develop self-awareness and therapeutic skills.

supportive psychotherapy Therapy designed to assist the client to modify interpersonal relationships, change perceptions and cognitions, and reward behavior contingencies.

suppression Process that is the conscious analogy of repression. It is the intentional exclusion of material from consciousness.

surface structure Term within neurolinguistic programming that refers to the meaning expressed in the sentence as spoken, which is usually not well formed or complete.

suspicion awareness context of death When client becomes suspicious, usually because of personal physical clues, that information about his condition is being withheld.

symbiosis Mutually reinforcing relationship between two persons who are dependent on each other.

Synanon Residential center that uses a therapeutic community approach to provide rehabilitation for drug abusers.

syntaxic mode of experience Type of thinking that is logically interrelated with experience and involves the use of consensually validated symbols.

synesthesia Perceptual distortion that involves the tasting of color.

system Set of parts meshing with each other within a boundary.

systematic desensitization Technique of behavior therapy that involves the pairing of deep muscle relaxation with imagined scenes depicting situations that cause the client to feel anxious. The assumption is that if the person is taught relaxation rather than anxiety while imagining such scenes, the real-life situation that the scene depicted will cause much less anxiety.

system recomposition Technique of structured family therapy in which the therapist intentionally changes the composition of roles so that all members have an opportunity to interact within their designated role.

symptom focusing Technique of structured family therapy in which the therapist takes control of the symptom by prescribing that the client intensify the symptom.

tabula rasa Description of the receptive "blank stare" condition of the child's mind at birth.

tangential speech Loss of goal direction in communication; failure to address the original point of discussion.

tardive dyskinesia Serious side effect of antipsychotic medication characterized by the buccolinguomasticatory movement of the extremities, and tonic contractions of the back and neck muscles.

telegraphic speech Type of language disturbance commonly experienced by persons with OBS and characterized by irrelevant replies to questions.

telepathy Communication of thought from one person to another by means other than the physical senses.

temper tantrums Unpredictable, violent outbreaks of anger during which the person is out of control, screaming, kicking, and striking at others.

termination phase Conclusion of the nurse-client relationship in which both participants evaluate outcomes achieved and project future changes.

thanatology Study of dying and death.

theme interference Type of transference reaction often identified during consultation.

theme interference reduction Method of consultation that reduces the potential displacing of conflict on future clients.

themes Underlying issues or problems experienced by the client that emerge repeatedly during the course of the nurse-client relationship.

therapeutic alliance Joining of the client's rational adult ego with the therapist in a collaborative effort to study the client's conflicts.

Therapeutic communication Communication in which there is an intent of one or more of the participants to bring about a change in the communication pattern of the system.

therapeutic community Use of a treatment setting as a community with the immediate aim of full participation of all clients and the eventual goal of preparing clients for life outside the treatment setting.

therapeutic impasse Roadblock in the progress of the nurse-client relationship that arises for a variety of reasons and may take different forms.

therapeutic milieu General setting where treatment occurs, regardless of the philosophy of treatment.

therapeutic nurse-client relationship Mutual learning experience and a corrective emotional experience for the client in which the nurse uses herself and specified clinical techniques in working with the client to bring about behavioral change.

therapeutic reminiscing Sharing events about the past in a way that makes one feel good about the past.

therapeutic touch Specialized kind of touching in which there is an intent to heal.

therapist Person in charge of directing the change of another person who skews communication in such a way that the client is exposed to situations and message exchanges that eventually bring about more gratifying social relations.

theraplay Form of treatment that uses active physical contact and control of the child.

third-party payment Reimbursement for nursing services provided by a person or group, neither of which is the provider or recipient of the services.

thought retardation Disturbance of thought characterized by extremely slow thought formation.

thought stopping Type of behavior modification that helps the client to limit negative thoughts about himself.

tolerance Characteristic of drug addiction that refers to the progressive need for more of the abused substance to achieve the desired effect.

tort Civil wrong for which the injured party is entitled to compensation.

total institution Institution that provides complete facilities for personnel who choose to use them.

trance Generally interpreted as soul absence of some kind and frequently linked to hallucinations or visions.

transaction Stimulus from an ego state of one person and the corresponding response from the ego state of another person.

transactional analysis (TA) Therapeutic modality based on the communications model of psychiatric care and developed by Eric Berne. Therapy takes place through the identification and interpretation of communication units (transactions) leading to understanding of interpersonal games that underlie behavioral disturbances. The goal is to develop the ability to communicate directly without using games.

transcendent Pertaining to the ability to go beyond one's ordinary everyday limits and to experience more than one's usual existence.

transcutaneous electrical nerve stimulators Use of an electrical current at or near the pain site to control pain.

transference Unconscious mechanism by which feelings and attitudes originally associated with important people and events in one's early life are attributed to others in current interpersonal relationships.

transformation rules Reordering of words into sentences to convey meaning in the process of learning language.

transient loneliness Loneliness that lasts only a few minutes or hours and is relieved by the client.

transitional crisis Crisis period related to the movement from one stage of development to another.

transsexual Person who is genetically an anatomical male or female but expresses, with strong conviction, that he or she has the mind of the opposite sex, lives as a member of the opposite sex either part or full time, and seeks to change his or her original sex legally, through hormonal and surgical sex assignment.

transvestite Person who cross-dresses, or puts on the garments of the opposite sex, by choice.

triadic childbearing Parental constellation in which the father and mother are equally significant to the child's personality, maturation and development.

triangle Emotional process that deflects the conflict in a dyad by focusing on a third person, issue, or thing.

tricyclics Group of chemically related antidepressant medications.

tyramine Amino acid; restricted in diet for persons on monoamine oxidase (MAO) inhibitor drugs used as antidepressants because of the nutrient-drug interaction, which may bring on a hypertensive crisis.

ulterior transactions Transactions that are bilevel. The first level is usually of relevant statement; the second level is usually nonverbal and has hidden psychological meaning.

ultradian rhythms Pattern based on a cycle of less than 24 hours such as stomach contractions and brain wave rhythms.

unconscious Level of awareness that characterizes memories, thoughts, and feelings that have undergone repression.

underlying assumption Set of rules one holds about oneself, others, and the world; these rules are regarded as unquestionably true.

undifferientiated family ego mass Emotional fusion in families in which all members are similar in emotional expression.

undoing Defense mechanism in which something unacceptable and already done is symbolically acted out in reverse, usually repetitiously, in the hope of relieving anxiety.

universal qualifiers Term within neurolinguistic programming that refers to general impressions of limitations; all, common, every, only, and never are examples of universal qualifiers.

universalizability principle Principle that an act is good if everyone should, in similar circumstances, do the same act without exception.

unspecified verbs Term within neurolinguistic programming that refers to verbs that are more or less specific to observable actions.

vaginismus Condition in the female in which normal genitalia are present, but the vaginal muscle tightly closes when penal penetration is attempted.

validation Agreement of the nurse with certain elements of the client's communication.

validation therapy Therapy that involves searching for the meaning and emotion in the client's words and validating these with the client.

value clarification Method whereby a person can discover his own values by assessing, exploring, and determining what his personal values are and what they hold in personal decision making.

values Concepts that a person holds worthy in his personal life.

They are formed as a result of one's experiences with family, friends, culture, education, work, and relaxation.

vector Direction of forces related to change in behavior.

venting Technique that allows the client to freely express his thoughts and feelings about a crisis situation.

verbal communication Written and spoken messages exchanged in the form of words as the elements of language.

violation of rights Form of elderly abuse that occurs when an individual is forced from his home or coerced into a nursing home unnecessarily.

violence Acting out of destructive aggression by assaulting people or objects in the environment.

visualization Intervention aimed at guiding the client in a relaxed state to visualize positive experiences and promote more effective use of one's imagination.

voluntary consent Consent that is not forced, threatened, or given under fraud or distress.

voyeurism Achievement of sexual pleasure by observing the nudity or sexual activity of others.

wandering Tendency to move about either in a seemingly aimless or disoriented fashion or in pursuit of an indefinable or unobtainable goal.

we-group Group that provides the chronically mentally ill client with safe opportunities to socialize with others who are familiar with the problem of chronic mental illness.

Wernicke's syndrome Syndrome associated with thiamine and sometimes niacine deficiency that consists of memory loss, confabulation, progressive dementia, ataxia, clouding of consciousness, and maybe coma. The disorder mainly affects alcoholics.

wheel pattern of communication Messages originate at a central position; interaction may occur between the message sender and any one of the receivers as well as between the receivers positioned next to each other.

wisdom The ability to make the best choices from the alternatives that are available.

withdrawal Attempt to avoid interaction with others and thus avoid relatedness; also, the occurrence of specific physical symptoms when substance intake is reduced or discontinued.

withdrawal syndrome Occurrence of specific symptoms when a person who is physically addicted to a chemical substance discontinues its use.

word salad Communication pattern characterized by a jumble of disconnected words.

work of worrying Coping strategy by which inner preparation through worrying increases the level of tolerance for subsequent threats.

working phase Phase of the nurse-client relationship in which dysfunctional patterns of behavior are identified and new ways of coping with stress are explored and tested.

working through Process by which repressed feelings are released and reintegrated into the personality.

worry Concern at the present time about a future situation or event.

yang Polarized aspect of *ch'i* that is active or positive energy.

yin Polarized aspect of *ch'i* that is passive or negative energy.

yoga (hatha) Alternative therapy of ancient lineage that focuses on the body's musculature, posture, breathing mechanism, and consciousness. The goal of this ancient practice is attainment of physical and mental well-being through mastery of the body, achieved by exercising, holding postures and proper breathing, and "one-pointedness" meditation.

zoophile Person whose sexual preference is for an animal.

Index

Nursing process—cont'd
  guiding principles in, 136
  helping factors and, 135-137
  historical overview of, 135
  implementation phase of, 156-157; *see also* Implementation
  levels of, 134
  nursing standards and, 136-137
  planning phase of; *see* Planning
  recording in, 162-163
  theoretical perspectives in, 136
Nursing research on mental illness, 13-14
Nursing systems in Orem's self-care model, 74-75
Nursing theory, 71-86
  historical overview of, 72
  Johnson's, 78-80
  King's, 76-78
  Orem's, 74-76
  Peplau's, 71-74
  philosophical foundations and assumptions of, 83t
  Roger's, 80-81
  Roy's, 81-83
  studies based on, 84t
Nutrition; *see also* Diet; Food(s)
  altered, 615
    case example of, 620
    definition and characteristics of, 620, 627
    in dementia, 660
  historical overview of, 616
  loneliness and, 437
  during middle age, 796
Nutritional status, 19-20
Nyctophobia, 184t
NYU Loneliness Scale, 441t

O

Oakland Growth and Development Study, 770
Obayuwana scale, 264t
Obesity, 615-623
  assessment of
    emotional dimension, 617-618
    intellectual dimension, 618
    physical dimension, 617
    social dimension, 618, 620
    spiritual dimension, 620
  causes of, 786
  defined, 615-623, 620
  DSM-III-R diagnoses related to, 615
  genetics and, 616
  implementation related to, 620-623
    emotional dimension, 620
    intellectual dimension, 621
    physical dimension, 620
    social dimension, 621-623
    spiritual dimension, 623
  in middle age, 786
  nursing care plan related to, 621t
  nursing process and, 617-623
  physical activity and, 616
  planning related to, 620
  support groups and, 622

Obesity—cont'd
  theoretical approaches to, 615-617, 617t
    biological, 615-616
    cognitive, 616
    learning, 617
    psychoanalytical, 616
    sociocultural, 617
Object permanence, development of, 701
Object relations theory, assumptions of, 601
Object relations therapy in couples therapy, 601
Obsessional personality, psychoanalytic definition of, 288t
Obsessional Scales, 295t
Obsessions
  behavioral continuum of, *288*
  characteristics of, 288
  defined, 288
  physical illnesses associated with, 292
  psychoanalytic definition of, 288t
  somatic, 297
Obsessive-compulsive disorders
  characteristics of, 287
  cortisol levels in, 289
  cultural factors in, 294
  family of client with, 300
  interaction with client with, 301-302
  intervention in, evaluation of, 302
  prevalence of, 286
  psychiatric disorders in relatives of children with, 290
  psychoanalytic definition of, 288t
  sexuality and, 294
  treatment of, 298-299
    definitions and examples of, 298t
Obsessive-Compulsive Group, purpose or goal of, 567t
Obsessive-compulsive personality disorder
  characteristics of, 287
  psychoanalytic definition of, 288t
Occupation, DSM-III-R diagnoses related to, 785
Occupational therapist, functions of, 513
Occupational therapy for depression, 272
OCD; *see* Obsessive-compulsive disorders
O'Connor v. Donaldson, 842
OCPD; *see* Obsessive-compulsive personality disorder
Odor, sensory impact of, 512
Older Americans' Resources and Services Instrument, 814t
Omnibus Budget Reconciliation Act of 1989, 525, 526t
Omnipotence in rigid personality, 289
Omniscience in rigid personality, 289
Operant conditioning, 61, 157
Ophidiophobia, 184t
Opiates, drug detection period for, 376t
Opinion about Mental Illness, 521t
Opium
  anxiety and, 190
  uses and effects, 374t-375t
Oppositional defiant disorder, 208, 749
  characteristics of, 751

Oral contraceptives
  interaction with diazepam, 497
  sexual function affected by, 606
  vitamin B6 deficiency and, 266
Oral stage of development, fixation at, 308
Orcutt, J., on boredom, 454
Orcutt's Scale, 459t
Orem, Dorothea
  nursing theory of
    basic assumptions of, 83t
    strengths and weaknesses of, 85t
    studies based on, 84t
  self-care model of, 74-76
    clinical application of, 75-76
    concepts of, 74-75
    holistic perspective in, 75
Organic anxiety disorders, characteristics of, 651
Organic brain syndromes, 143
Organic delusional disorders, characteristics of, 651
Organic hallucinosis, characteristics of, 651
Organic mental disorders
  associated with DSM-III-R axis III, 651
  codes in, 892
  psychoactive drug-induced, 650
Organic mood disorders, characteristics of, 651
Organic personality disorders, characteristics of, 651
Orgasm
  disorders of, 600
  inhibited female, defined, 600t
  inhibited male, defined, 600t
Orientation
  assessment of, 143
  disorders of, in schizophrenia, 341
Orlando, I.J., and therapeutic relationship, 109
Orthostatic hypotension
  from antidepressants, 493
  from antipsychotic medications, 486-487
  from psychotropic medications, nursing interventions for, 499t
Osteoporosis
  during middle age, 796
  risk factors for, 786-787
Outcome indicators, 866
Outcome statements
  client culture and, 154-155
  components of, 152-153
  feasibility of, 155
  realistic, 154
  short-term versus long-term, 153-154
Outpatient care, 12
Overcompliance in schizophrenia, 338t
Overeaters Anonymous, 29, 622
Overgeneralization, 62
Overweight, defined, 620
Oxazepam
  absorption of, 496
  for alcoholic client, 368
  for anxiety, daily dose range, 202t
  dosages and half-lives, 496t
  nursing considerations, 369

Peptic ulcer, physical, emotional, and environmental components of, 394t
Perception, 23
  alterations in, definition and characteristics of, 344
  defined, 76
  difficulties in, in schizophrenia, 340-341
  disorders of, 143, 143t
Perceptual isolation, 454
Perceptual reversals, 724
Perfection, assumptions about, 63
Perfectionism
  assessment of, 313
  guilt and, 230
Peridol; *see* Haloperidol
Perlman, D., loneliness theory of, 433, 435t
Perls, Frederick (Fritz), 64-65
  key concepts of, 67t
  theory applied to group therapy, 565t
Perpetrator
  characteristics of, 673-674
  in cycle of violence, 673
  in nursing process, 675
  of sexual abuse, 680
Perphenazine
  daily dosage range, 348t
  diluents for, 488t
  equipotent dosages and side effects, 483t
Perrigault, J., theory of flexibility-rigidity, 291t
Persecution
  delusions of, 339t
  ideas of, defined, 144
Perserveration, defined, 144
Persistence, assessment of, in children, 729t
Persona, Jungian concept of, 56
Personal Inventory Sheet, 854
Personal space, cultural attitudes toward, 176
Personality
  authoritarian, 286
  Beck's theory of, 62
  behavioral theories of, 61
  body build and, 19
  cognitive theory of, 61-63
  crisis-prone, 546
  Ellis's theory of, 62
  Freudian theory of, 53-55
  general systems theory of, 63-64
  Jungian theory of, 55-57
  obsessional, psychoanalytic definition of, 288t
  Piaget's theory of, 61-62, 62t
  self-actualizing, 65
  sociocultural theory of, 63
  in somatization disorders, 405-406
  Sullivan's theory of, 58
  type A
    characteristics of, 389
    research on, 853-854
Personality disorders, 328, 330
  borderline; *see* Borderline personality disorder
  characteristics of, 307

Personality disorders—cont'd
  codes in, 894
  DSM-III-R definition of, 452
  organic, characteristics of, 651
Personality Inventory for Children, 727t
Personality tests for children, 727t
Personality traits
  addictive behavior and, 359-360
  characteristics of, 307
  DSM-III-R definition of, 452
  in somatization disorders, 399
Personifications
  false, 289
  Sullivan's concept of, 58
Perspiration, emotional arousal and, 22t
Pertofrane; *see* Desipramine
PET; *see* Positron emission tomography
Pet therapy
  for elderly, 822
  for lonely client, 445-446
Peyote, uses and effects, 374t-375t
Pfeiffer Short Portable Mental Status Questionnaire, 446
Phencyclidine
  drug detection period for, 376t
  uses and effects, 374t-375t
Phenelzine
  daily dose range, 268t
  dose, sedation, and anticholinergic symptoms, 492t
Phenmetrazine, uses and effects, 374t-375t
Phenobarbital, drug detection period for, 376t
Phenothiazines, equipotent dosages and side effects, 483t
Phenylbutazone, interaction with lithium, 494
Philosophy(ies), 40-52
  ancient Greek, 44, 47t
  asceticism, 44-45, 47t
  Chinese, 43, 47t
  East Indian, 43-44, 47t
  existentialism, 46, 47t
  health care and, 41
  holistic, 46-48, 47t
    health care and, 46-48
  and human nature, 40-41
  humanism, 45-46, 47t
  influence on views of human nature, health care, and nursing, 47t
  mental health-psychiatric nursing and, 41-42
  overview of, 42-46
  personal, 40
    effect on nursing care, 41-42
    evolution of, 40
  pragmatism, 45, 47t
  preliterate, 42-43, 47t
  romanticism, 45, 47t
  significance of, 40-42
Phobia(s), 182
  common types of, 288
  examples of, 184t
  fear and, 285
  function of, 288

Phobia(s)—cont'd
  incidence of, 286
  psychoanalytical definition of, 288t
  psychoanalytical theory of, 185
  simple, 183
    characteristics of, 183
  social, 184
Photosensitivity from antipsychotic medications, 487
Physical abuse; *see also* Abuse
  assessment for, 312
  characteristics of, 534
  chronic pain and, 416
  defined, 671
  in dependent client, 323
Physical examination, 138
Physical fitness, emotional aspects of, 20
Physical neglect, defined, 671
Physical restraints for angry client, 216-217
Physical therapy, 158
Piaget, Jean
  on adolescence, 751
  cognitive theory of, 61-62, 62t, 722
  developmental theory of, 720, 722t
  infant development theory of, 700-701, 701t
  intellectual development stage of, 771, 772t
  key concepts of, 67t
  mistrust theory of, 331t
  on moral judgment, 228
  rigid response theory of, 291
  theory of flexibility-rigidity, 291t
  trust development theory of, 333-334
Pick's disease during middle age, 789, 797
Pilomotor response, emotional arousal and, 22t
Pinel, Philippe, 505, 522
Piperazine, equipotent dosages and side effects, 483t
Piperidine
  absorption and distribution of, 484
  equipotent dosages and side effects, 483t
Pisel v. Stamford Hospital, 839
Placebos for pain, 425
Plan for Implementation of the Standards of Nursing Practice, A, 867
Planning, 151-156
  in ANA Standards of Psychiatric and Mental Health Nursing Practice, 151
  discharge, 155-156
  outcome statements in, 152-153
  purposes of, 151-152
  in SOAP format, 162
Plato, 44
Play
  child's communication through, 737
  growth and development fostered by, 732, 737
  by type and age groups, 738t-740t
Play therapy, 745
Pleasure principle, 53
Polyaddiction, defined, 359
Polypharmacy in elderly, 360
POR; *see* Problem-oriented record

DSM-III-R MEDICAL DIAGNOSES AND NANDA NURSING DIAGNOSES

DSM-III-R	NANDA Diagnoses
Chapter 10, Anxiety	
Agoraphobia	Anxiety
Depersonalization	Sleep Pattern Disturbance
Simple Phobia	Post-Trauma Response
Social Phobia	
Post-Traumatic Stress Disorder	
Sleep Disorders	
Psychophysiological Disorders	
Chapter 11, Anger	
Intermittent Explosive Disorder	High Risk for Violence
Passive Aggressive Personality Disorder	
Chapter 12, Guilt	
	Spiritual Distress
Chapter 13, Loss	
Uncomplicated Bereavement	Anticipatory Grieving
	Dysfunctional Grieving
	High Risk for Dysfunctional Grieving
Chapter 14, Hope-Hopelessness	
Bipolar Disorder	Body Image Disturbance
Major Depression	Personal Identity Disturbance
Seasonal Affective Disorder	Self-Esteem Disturbance
	Chronic Low Self-Esteem
	Situational Low Self-Esteem
	High Risk for Violence: Self-Directed
	Self-Care Deficit
	Hopelessness
Chapter 15, Flexibility-Rigidity	
Pathological or Compulsive Gambling	Fear
Kleptomania	
Obsessive-Compulsive Disorders	
Obsessive-Compulsive Personality Disorder	
Pyromania	

DSM-III-R	NANDA Diagnoses
Chapter 16, Dependence-Independence	
Avoidant Personality Disorder	Powerlessness
Dependent Personality Disorder	
Histrionic Personality Disorder	
Chapter 17, Trust-Mistrust	
Delusional Disorders	Sensory/Perceptual Alterations
Paranoid Personality Disorder	Altered Thought Processes
Schizoid Personality Disorder	Impaired Verbal Communication
Schizophrenia	
Schizotypal Personality Disorder	High Risk for Self-Mutilation
Chapter 18, Addictive Behavior	
Psychoactive Substance Dependence	Defensive Coping
Psychoactive Substance Abuse	Ineffective Denial
Chapter 19, Somatization	
Somatoform Disorders	Ineffective Individual Coping
Conversion Disorder	
Somatization Disorder	
Hypochondriasis	
Chapter 20, Pain	
Somatoform Pain Disorder	Pain
Factitious Disorders	Chronic Pain
Conversion Disorder	
Hypochondriasis	
Chapter 21, Loneliness	
	Impaired Social Interaction
	Social Isolation
Chapter 22, Boredom	
Borderline Personality Disorder	Diversional Activity Deficit
Narcissistic Personality Disorder	
Chapter 23, Manipulation	
Antisocial Personality Disorder	
Adult Antisocial Disorder	
Malingering	